Coronavirus Disease 2019 (COVID-19): A Clinical Guide

Coronavirus Disease 2019 (COVID-19): A Clinical Guide

Edited by

Ali Gholamrezanezhad, MD
Keck School of Medicine, University of Southern California (USC)
Los Angeles, California, USA

Michael P. Dube, MD
Keck School of Medicine, University of Southern California (USC)
Los Angeles, California, USA

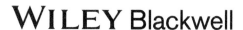

Registered Offices
John Wiley & Sons, Inc., 111 River Street, Hoboken, NJ 07030, USA
John Wiley & Sons Ltd, The Atrium, Southern Gate, Chichester, West Sussex, PO19 8SQ, UK

For details of our global editorial offices, customer services, and more information about Wiley products visit us at www.wiley.com.

Wiley also publishes its books in a variety of electronic formats and by print-on-demand. Some content that appears in standard print versions of this book may not be available in other formats.

Library of Congress Cataloging-in-Publication Data applied for
ISBN: 9781119789680 (hardback)

Cover Design: Wiley
Cover Image: © koto_feja/Getty Brandon K.K. Fields, Natalie L. Demirjian, Ali Gholamrezanezhad

Set in 9.5/12.5pt STIXTwoText by Straive, Pondicherry, India

SKY10039240_120122

This book is dedicated to healthcare workers around the world and those who support them. We especially wish to recognize Frances Marie Canchola, RN, a beloved HIV research nurse at the University of Southern California. Frances fell ill in November 2020 and ultimately lost her life to complications of COVID-19 in January 2021—a month after the first SARS-CoV-2 vaccines received Emergency Use Authorization in the United States. There are countless people who now will no longer need to be hospitalized or die as a result of this disease once they choose to be vaccinated.

—*Michael P. Dube and Ali Gholamrezanezhad*

To my mother, Fatemeh
For her endless support and devotion to making my life most fulfilling . . .

my wife
for her unconditional love and patience . . .

my brother
for his support in silence!

and to the "hand of god,"
a person whose company has been the greatest honor of my life, saved me in a critical time, and succored and shaped me into the person I am proud of!

—*Ali Gholamrezanezhad*

Contents

List of Contributors

Behnoosh Afghani, MD
Department of Pediatrics, University of California
Irvine School of Medicine, Irvine, CA, USA
Hospitalist, CHOC Children's, Orange, CA, USA
Pediatric Infectious Diseases, University of California
Irvine School of Medicine, Irvine, CA, USA

Hashem Al-Marzouki, MD
Department of Ophthalmology, College of Medicine,
King Saud bin Abdulaziz University for Health
Sciences, King Abdulaziz Medical Center, Jeddah,
Saudi Arabia

Kiarash Aramesh, MD, PhD
The James F. Drane Bioethics Institute, Edinboro
University of Pennsylvania, Edinboro, PA, USA

Shadi Asadollahi, MD
Department of Radiology, Keck School of
Medicine, University of Southern California, Los
Angeles, CA, USA
Russell H. Morgan Department of Radiology and
Radiological Science, Johns Hopkins University
School of Medicine, Baltimore, MD, USA

Isaac Asante, MS, PhD
Clinical Pharmacy Department, School of
Pharmacy, University of Southern California, Los
Angeles, CA, USA
Roski Eye Institute, Keck School of Medicine,
University of Southern California, Los
Angeles, CA, USA

Mobin Azami
Student Research Committee, Kurdistan University
of Medical Sciences, Sanandaj, Iran

Arnold S. Baas, MD
Division of Cardiology, Department of Medicine,
UCLA Health, Los Angeles, CA, USA

Glenn Baumann
Keck School of Medicine, University of Southern
California, Los Angeles, CA, USA

Alexis Bennett
Laboratory of Neuro Imaging, USC Stevens
Neuroimaging and Informatics Institute, Keck School
of Medicine, University of Southern California, Los
Angeles, CA, USA

Amy Bellinghausen, MD
Division of Pulmonary, Critical Care, and Sleep
Medicine, Department of Medicine, University of
California San Diego, La Jolla, CA, USA

Alexander A. Bruckhaus
Laboratory of Neuro Imaging, USC Stevens
Neuroimaging and Informatics Institute, Keck School
of Medicine, University of Southern California, Los
Angeles, CA, USA

Mauricio Bueno, MD
Department of Family Medicine, Adventist Health
White Memorial, Los Angeles, CA, USA

Angela N. Buffenn, MD, MPH
The Vision Center, Children's Hospital Los
Angeles, Roski Eye Institute, Keck School of
Medicine, University of Southern California,
Los Angeles, CA, USA

Amanda M. Burkhardt, PhD
Clinical Pharmacy Department, School of
Pharmacy, University of Southern California,
Los Angeles, CA, USA

Aidan Burrell
Australian and New Zealand Intensive Care Research
Centre, School of Public Health and Preventative
Medicine, Monash University, Melbourne, VIC,
Australia
Intensive Care Unit, The Alfred Hospital,
Melbourne, VIC, Australia

Andrew T. Catanzaro, MD
Adventist Healthcare, Gaithersburg, MD, USA

Ching-Fei Chang, MD
Division of Pulmonary and Critical Care, Department
of Medicine, Keck School of Medicine, University of
Southern California, Los Angeles, CA, USA

Lee-anne S. Chapple, PhD
Adelaide Medicine School, University of Adelaide,
Adelaide, SA, Australia
Intensive Care Unit, Royal Adelaide Hospital,
Adelaide, SA, Australia
Centre for Research Excellence in Nutritional
Physiology, Adelaide, SA, Australia

Vijay K. Chaudhary, PhD
Centre for Innovation in Infectious Disease Research,
Education and Training, University of Delhi South
Campus, New Delhi, India

Subhana Chaudhri, MD
Greater Manchester Mental Health NHS Foundation
Trust, Manchester, United Kingdom

Peter Chen, MD
Department of Medicine, Division of Pulmonary
and Critical Care Medicine, Cedars-Sinai Medical
Center, Los Angeles, CA, USA

Sarah Cherukury
USC Master of Public Health Program,
University of Southern California,
Los Angeles, CA, USA

Desmond Chin, MD
Department of Radiology, Keck School of
Medicine, University of Southern California,
Los Angeles, CA, USA

Meshe Chonde, MD
Division of Cardiology, Department of Medicine,
UCLA Health, Los Angeles, CA, USA

Erin Chung
Department of Pediatrics, University of
Washington, Seattle Children's Hospital,
Seattle, WA, USA

Dalia Copti, MSN, FNP-C, AGACNP-BC
Department of Nursing, Suzanne Dworak-Peck
School of Social Work, University of Southern
California, Los Angeles, CA, USA

Daniel Crouch, MD
Division of Pulmonary, Critical Care, and Sleep
Medicine, Department of Medicine, University of
California San Diego, La Jolla, CA, USA

Jacek Czubak, MD
Department and Clinic of Otolaryngology, Head
and Neck Surgery, Wroclaw Medical University,
Wrocław, Poland

Kalpana Dave
USC Master of Public Health Program,
University of Southern California, Los
Angeles, CA, USA

Michael DiVita, MD
Division of Cardiology, Department of Medicine,
UCLA Health, Los Angeles, CA, USA

Michael P. Dube, MD
Department of Medicine, Division of
Infectious Diseases, Keck School of Medicine,
University of Southern California, Los
Angeles, CA, USA

Dominique Duncan, PhD
Laboratory of Neuro Imaging, USC Stevens
Neuroimaging and Informatics Institute, Keck
School of Medicine of USC, University of Southern
California, Los Angeles, CA, USA

Liesl S. Eibschutz, MS
Department of Radiology, Keck School of
Medicine, University of Southern California, Los
Angeles, CA, USA

Masoomeh Faghankhani, MD
Tehran University of Medical Sciences,
Tehran, Iran

Jeremy Falk, MD
Department of Medicine, Division of Pulmonary and
Critical Care Medicine, Cedars-Sinai Medical Center,
Los Angeles, CA, USA

Ashley M. Fan, PharmD
Department of Pharmaceutical Services, UCLA
Health, Los Angeles, CA, USA

Fabrizio Fantini, MD
Department of Dermatology, ASST Lecco,
Alessandro Manzoni Hospital, Lecco, Italy

Kate Fetterplace
Allied Health Department (Clinical Nutrition),
Royal Melbourne Hospital, Melbourne, VIC,
Australia
Department of Critical Care, Melbourne Medical
School, The University of Melbourne, Melbourne,
VIC, Australia

Wojciech Flieger
School of Medicine, Medical University of Lublin,
Lublin, Poland

Hector Flores, MD
Department of Family Medicine, Adventist Health
White Memorial, Los Angeles, CA, USA

Lucia Flors, MD, PhD
Department of Radiology, Keck School of
Medicine, University of Southern California, Los
Angeles, CA, USA

Marcin Frączek, MD, PhD
Department and Clinic of Otolaryngology, Head
and Neck Surgery, Wroclaw Medical University,
Wrocław, Poland

Amy Freeman-Sanderson, PhD
Graduate School of Health, University of
Technology Sydney, Sydney, NSW, Australia
Speech Pathology Department & Intensive Care Unit,
Royal Prince Alfred Hospital, Sydney, NSW,
Australia
Critical Care Division, The George Institute for
Global Health, Sydney, NSW, Australia

Tianyuan Fu, MD
Department of Radiology, University Hospitals
Cleveland Medical Center, Cleveland, OH, USA

Rachael Garner
Laboratory of Neuro Imaging, USC Stevens
Neuroimaging and Informatics Institute, Keck
School of Medicine of USC, University of Southern
California, Los Angeles, CA, USA

Mehdi Ghasemi, MD
Department of Neurology, University of
Massachusetts Medical School, Worcester,
MA, USA

Ali Gholamrezanezhad, MD
Department of Radiology, Keck School of
Medicine, University of Southern California, Los
Angeles, CA, USA

Amit Gupta, MD
Department of Radiology, University Hospital
Cleveland Medical Center, Cleveland, OH, USA

Sanjay Gupta, PhD
Independent Scholar (former Head, Centre for
Emerging Diseases, Department of Biotechnology),
Jaypee Institute of Information Technology,
Noida, India

Vandana Gupta, PhD
Department of Microbiology, Ram Lal
Anand College, University of Delhi, New Delhi,
India

Benjamin P. Hammond, MD
Flaum Eye Institute, University of Rochester
Medical Center, Rochester, NY, USA

Diana L. Hanna, MD
Division of Medical Oncology, Norris Comprehensive
Cancer Center, University of Southern California,
Los Angeles, CA, USA
Hoag Cancer Center, Newport Beach, CA, USA

Elham Hatami, MD
Department of Pathology, University of
California San Diego Medical Center, San
Diego, CA, USA

Kaidi He, MD
Department of Pediatrics, Children's Hospital of
Los Angeles, Los Angeles, CA, USA

Janett A. Hildebrand, PhD, FNP-BC, CDE
Department of Nursing, Suzanne Dworak-Peck
School of Social Work, University of Southern
California, Los Angeles, CA, USA

Jeffrey J. Hsu, MD, PhD
Division of Cardiology, Department of Medicine,
UCLA Health, Los Angeles, CA, USA
Division of Cardiology, Department of Medicine,
Veterans Affairs Greater Los Angeles Healthcare
System, Los Angeles, CA, USA

Wendy W. Huang, MD
Phoenix Children's Hospital, Ophthalmology,
Phoenix, AZ, USA

Jennifer H. Johnston, MD
Department of Radiology, McGovern School of
Medicine, UT Houston, Houston, TX, USA

Sean K. Johnston, MD
Department of Radiology, Keck School of
Medicine, University of Southern California, Los
Angeles, CA, USA

Narges Jokar, MD
Department of Molecular Imaging and Radionuclide
Therapy, The Persian Gulf Nuclear Medicine
Research Center, Bushehr Medical University
Hospital, Bushehr, Iran

Arturas Kalniunas, MD
West London NHS Trust, London, United Kingdom

Megan Kamath, MD
Division of Cardiology, Department of Medicine,
UCLA Health, Los Angeles, CA, USA

Sanaz Katal, MD, MPH
St Vincent's Hospital Medical Imaging Department,
Melbourne, Victoria, Australia

Simran P. Kaur, BSc
Department of Microbiology, Ram Lal Anand
College, University of Delhi, New Delhi, India

Kiandokht Keyhanian, MD
Department of Neurology, University of
Massachusetts Medical School, Worcester, MA, USA

Akhilesh Kumar, MSc
Ochsner Clinical School, University of Queensland,
New Orleans, LA, USA

Heinz-Josef Lenz, MD
Division of Medical Oncology, Norris Comprehensive
Cancer Center, University of Southern California, Los
Angeles, CA, USA

Grace Y. Lin, MD, PhD
Department of Pathology, University of California
San Diego Medical Center, San Diego, CA, USA

Angelena Lopez, MD
Department of Medicine, Division of Pulmonary and
Critical Care Medicine, Cedars-Sinai Medical Center,
Los Angeles, CA, USA

Stan Louie, PharmD
Clinical Pharmacy and Ophthalmology
Clinical Experimental Therapeutics Program,
Ginsburg Institute of Biomedical Technology,
USC School of Pharmacy,
USC Keck School of Medicine, University of
Southern California, Los Angeles, CA, USA

Angela Lu, MS
Department of Pharmacology and Pharmaceutical Sciences, School of Pharmacy, University of Southern California, Los Angeles, CA, USA

Andrea P. Marshall, PhD
Gold Coast Health, Southport, QLD, Australia
School of Nursing and Midwifery, Griffith University, Southport, QLD, Australia

Yuri Matusov, MD
Department of Medicine, Division of Pulmonary and Critical Care Medicine, Cedars-Sinai Medical Center, Los Angeles, CA, USA

Cameron McGuire, MD
Division of Pulmonary, Critical Care, and Sleep Medicine, Department of Medicine, University of California San Diego, La Jolla, CA, USA

Brooke McNeilly, DO
Department of Neurology, University of Massachusetts Medical School, Worcester, MA, USA

David E. Michalik, DO
Department of Pediatrics, University of California Irvine School of Medicine, Irvine, CA, USA
Division of Pediatric Infectious Diseases, Miller Children's and Women's Hospital, Long Beach, CA, USA

Babak Mohit, DrPH
Sleep Disorders Center, Division of Pulmonary and Critical Care Medicine, Department of Medicine, University of Maryland School of Medicine, Baltimore, MD, USA

Shabnam Mortazavi, MD, MPH
Assistant Professor of Radiology, David Geffen School of Medicine at UCLA, Los Angeles, CA, USA

Wakana Murakami, MD
Visiting Researcher of Radiological Sciences, David Geffen School of Medicine at UCLA, Los Angeles, CA, USA
Department of Radiology, Showa University Graduate School of Medicine, Tokyo, Japan

Sabha Mushtaq, MD
Department of Dermatology, Venereology and Leprology, Government Medical College and associated hospitals, University of Jammu, Jammu, India

Lee Myers, MD
Keck School of Medicine, University of Southern California, Los Angeles, CA, USA

Niyousha Naderi, MD
Keck School of Medicine, University of Southern California, Los Angeles, CA, USA

Saeideh Najafi
Department of Radiology, Keck School of Medicine, University of Southern California, Los Angeles, CA, USA

Ary Serpa Neto, MD, MSc, PhD
Australian and New Zealand Intensive Care Research Centre, School of Public Health and Preventative Medicine, Monash University, Melbourne, VIC, Australia

Binh T. Ngo, MD
Department of Dermatology, Keck School of Medicine, University of Southern California, Los Angeles, CA, USA

Delma Nieves, MD
Department of Pediatrics, University of California Irvine School of Medicine, Irvine, CA, USA
Division of Pediatric Infectious Diseases, CHOC Children's, Orange, CA, USA

Mazen Odish, MD
Division of Pulmonary, Critical Care, and Sleep Medicine, Department of Medicine, University of California San Diego, La Jolla, CA, USA

Sharon O'Neill, DNP, FNP-BC, PPCNP-BC, PMHNP-BC
New York University Rory Meyers College of Nursing, New York, NY, USA

Anna Orzeł
School of Medicine, Medical University of Lublin, Lublin, Poland

Sofia Pappa, MD, PhD
West London NHS Trust, London, United Kingdom
Faculty of Medicine, Department of Brain Sciences, Imperial College London, London, United Kingdom

Isabel Pedraza, MD
Department of Medicine, Division of Pulmonary and Critical Care Medicine, Cedars-Sinai Medical Center, Los Angeles, CA, USA

Caroline I. Piatek, MD
Jane Anne Nohl Division of Hematology, Keck School of Medicine, University of Southern California, Los Angeles, CA, USA

Raffaella Pizzolato Umeton, MD
Department of Neurology, University of Massachusetts Medical School, Worcester, MA, USA
Department of Neurology, Massachusetts General Hospital, Harvard Medical School, Boston, MA, USA

Brian P. Pogatchnik, MD
Clinical Instructor in Radiology, Stanford University School of Medicine, Stanford, CA, USA

Phillip Quiroz, MPH
Keck School of Medicine at the University of Southern California, Los Angeles, California, USA

Sebastiano Recalcati
Department of Dermatology, ASST Lecco, Alessandro Manzoni Hospital, Lecco, Italy

Michael Jovan Repajic
Department of Radiology, Keck School of Medicine, University of Southern California, Los Angeles, CA, USA

Katarzyna Resler
Department and Clinic of Otolaryngology, Head and Neck Surgery, Wroclaw Medical University, Wrocław, Poland

Emma J. Ridley, PhD
Australian and New Zealand Intensive Care Research Centre, School of Public Health and Preventative Medicine, Monash University, Melbourne, VIC, Australia
Nutrition Department, The Alfred Hospital, Melbourne, VIC, Australia

Alexandra Rose, MD
Division of Pulmonary, Critical Care, and Sleep Medicine, Department of Medicine, University of California San Diego, La Jolla, CA, USA

Hana Russo, MD, PhD
Department of Pathology, University of California San Diego Medical Center, San Diego, CA, USA

George W. Rutherford, MD
Department of Epidemiology and Biostatistics, School of Medicine, and Institute for Global Health Sciences, University of California San Francisco, San Francisco, CA, USA

Charlotte Sackett
USC Master of Public Health Program, University of Southern California, Los Angeles, CA, USA

Nikoo Saeedi, MS
Medical School of Islamic Azad University of Mashhad, Mashhad, Iran

Elpitha Sakka, MRes
School of Pharmacy and Biomolecular Sciences, University of Brighton, Brighton, United Kingdom

Vorada Sakulsaengprapha, MS
Johns Hopkins University School of Medicine, Baltimore, MD, USA

Wala Salman, MD
West London NHS Trust, London, United Kingdom

Cynthia Sanchez, DNP, FNP-C
Department of Nursing, Suzanne Dworak-Peck School of Social Work, University of Southern California, Los Angeles, CA, USA

Mohd Fardeen Husain Shahanshah, BSc
Department of Microbiology, Ram Lal Anand
College, University of Delhi, New Delhi, India

Bhawna Sharma, BSc
Department of Microbiology, Ram Lal Anand
College, University of Delhi, New Delhi, India

Anurag Singh, BSc
Department of Microbiology, Ram Lal Anand
College, University of Delhi, New Delhi, India

Calvin M. Smith, MD
Department of Internal Medicine, Nashville
General Hospital at Meharry, Nashville, TN, USA

Juliana Sobczyk, MD
Department of Pathology, Memorial Satilla
Hospital, HCA Healthcare, Waycross, GA, USA
Laboratory Director, St. Augustine Foot & Ankle, Inc.,
St. Augustine, FL, USA

Karolina Stolarczyk
Department and Clinic of Otolaryngology, Head
and Neck Surgery, Wroclaw Medical University,
Wrocław, Poland

Victor Tapson, MD
Department of Medicine, Division of Pulmonary and
Critical Care Medicine, Cedars-Sinai Medical Center,
Los Angeles, CA, USA

Salar Tofighi, MD
Department of Radiology, Keck School of
Medicine, University of Southern California, Los
Angeles, CA, USA

Erlinda R. Ulloa, MD
Department of Pediatrics, University of California
Irvine School of Medicine, Irvine, CA, USA
Division of Pediatric Infectious Diseases, CHOC
Children's, Orange, CA, USA

Victoria Uram, MPH
Department of Clinical Research, University
Hospitals, Cleveland, OH, USA

Christian Vega
Keck School of Medicine, University of Southern
California, Los Angeles, CA, USA

Yasaswi V. Vengalasetti, MS
Department of Epidemiology and Population
Health, Stanford University School of Medicine,
Stanford, CA, USA

Elzbieta Vitkauskaite
West London NHS Trust, London, United Kingdom

Darko Vucicevic, MD
Division of Cardiology, Department of Medicine,
UCLA Health, Los Angeles, CA, USA

Jenny Yang
Division of Pulmonary, Critical Care, and Sleep
Medicine, Department of Medicine, University
of California San Diego, La Jolla, CA, USA

Boniface Yarabe
Department of Radiology, Keck School of
Medicine, University of Southern California,
Los Angeles, CA, USA

Michelle Zappas, DNP, FNP-BC
Department of Nursing, Suzanne Dworak-Peck
School of Social Work, University of Southern
California, Los Angeles, CA, USA

Tomasz Zatoński, MD
Department and Clinic of Otolaryngology, Head
and Neck Surgery, Wroclaw Medical University,
Wrocław, Poland

Yujia Zhang
Laboratory of Neuro Imaging, USC Stevens
Neuroimaging and Informatics Institute, Keck
School of Medicine of USC, University of
Southern California, Los Angeles, CA, USA

Preface

The astounding speed and global impact of the coronavirus disease 2019 (COVID-19) pandemic was unforeseen when the first cases of this illness were reported in December 2019 from Wuhan, China. By the end of January 2020, nearly 8000 cases had been reported globally from 19 countries, and the World Health Organization declared a Public Health Emergency of International Concern. It soon became apparent this was not going to be a focal or controllable outbreak. In the more than two years that have followed, the world has truly been turned upside down with countless severe disruptions to life and economies worldwide.

The challenges to the healthcare systems in high-, middle-, and low-income countries alike have been enormous. The strain on individuals and institutions has been dealt with by interventions of varying success. The mental and physical health of workers have been a prime focus in the global response to the pandemic.

The scientific community has responded rapidly, if imperfectly at times, to the death and disability imposed by severe acute respiratory syndrome coronavirus 2 (SARS-CoV-2). Important and dramatic advances in the care of critically ill inpatients have been made, primarily using potent anti-inflammatory interventions such as glucocorticoids and tocilizumab. Multiple effective vaccines have been developed with record speed using multiple different vaccine platforms and have been disseminated globally. Much work still needs to be done in combatting vaccine hesitancy worldwide and providing vaccines in the developing world.

Outpatient management and prevention of hospitalization and disease progression have made slow but steady progress, with the availability in some settings of anti-SARS-CoV-2 monoclonal antibodies. Subsequently, studies of promising oral antiviral agents have reported beneficial effects of preventing hospitalization with a more generally applicable form of treatment.

Sadly, the pandemic has further exposed health disparities around the globe. Minority and lower-income people have disproportionally borne the brunt of COVID-19 illness and mortality, the result of environmental and structural disadvantages and greater noninfectious medical comorbidity. Viral mutation has led to emerging SARS-CoV-2 variants that have properties of increased infectivity and reduced responses to vaccines and monoclonal antibodies. The Delta variant exploded worldwide in the summer of 2021, challenging but not fully overcoming current therapies. The world will continue to monitor for variants of concern, more recently with the Omicron variants, and science will adapt with new vaccines and therapeutics as necessary.

In spite of terrible loss of life, disabling post-COVID syndromes, and damage to global economies, there is reason for optimism. The first-generation messenger RNA and viral vector vaccines appear to be maintaining protection against severe disease, and vaccines promising better protection from variants are emerging. As the world sorts out how to make vaccines more generally available in lower-income countries, there is an expectation that infection with SARS-CoV-2 will eventually become a more manageable virus along the lines of other respiratory viruses such as influenza.

1

COVID-19: Epidemiology

Phillip Quiroz[1], George W. Rutherford[2], and Michael P. Dube[3]

[1] Keck School of Medicine at the University of Southern California, Los Angeles, California, USA
[2] Department of Epidemiology and Biostatistics, School of Medicine, and Institute for Global Health Sciences, University of California San Francisco, San Francisco, CA, USA
[3] Department of Medicine, Division of Infectious Diseases, Keck School of Medicine, University of Southern California, Los Angeles, California, USA

Abbreviations

ACE2	angiotensin-converting enzyme 2
CDC	US Centers for Disease Control and Prevention
CFR	case fatality rate
MERS	Middle East respiratory syndrome
MERS-CoV	Middle East respiratory syndrome coronavirus
mRNA	messenger RNA
SARS	severe acute respiratory syndrome
SARS-CoV-2	severe acute respiratory syndrome coronavirus 2
WHO	World Health Organization

On 1 December 2019, the first report of a pneumonia of unknown etiology was recognized in Wuhan, China, presenting with fever, malaise, dry cough, and dyspnea [1]. Based on clinical criteria, diagnostic tests, and imaging, this respiratory disease was determined most likely to be that of viral origin. Although its presentation resembled that of other well-known viral pneumonias in the region (i.e. influenza, severe acute respiratory syndrome [SARS], Middle East respiratory syndrome [MERS]), it was clear this was a novel disease. The World Health Organization (WHO) announced an epidemic cluster of outbreaks of this disease in Wuhan, Hubei Province by 31 December 2019 [2]. This aggressive increase in cases understandably caught the attention of epidemiologists in the region, who conducted origin-related field studies in the community and nearby health facilities. Nose and throat specimens were collected for viral genomic sequencing and analysis. On 12 January 2020, the Chinese government publicly shared the genetic sequence of the causative agent, a novel coronavirus that the International Committee on Taxonomy of Viruses later would christen severe acute respiratory distress syndrome coronavirus 2 (SARS-CoV-2).

SARS-CoV-2 is a novel coronavirus that belongs to the viral family Coronaviridae. A relatively large classification, these viruses are enveloped, positive-sense, single-stranded RNA viruses. Typically, these cause mild to moderate upper respiratory tract illnesses, but they can cause enteric, hepatic, and neurologic diseases as well [3]. Four of the seven known coronaviruses cause only mild to moderate disease. However, three new coronaviruses have emerged from animal reservoirs over the past two decades that cause widespread serious illness and death. The first of these is SARS coronavirus (SARS-CoV), which emerged in November 2002 and causes SARS. The second is known as the MERS coronavirus (MERS-CoV), which causes MERS. MERS was first identified in September 2012 and continues to cause sporadic and localized outbreaks largely in Saudi Arabia and South Korea [4]. The third and most recent novel coronavirus to emerge in this century is SARS-CoV-2; it is the seventh member of the coronavirus family known to infect humans.

The first death from the novel SARS coronavirus was announced by Chinese health officials on 11 January 2020 [2]. The WHO named this illness coronavirus disease 2019 (COVID-19) according to its nomenclature on 11 February 2020 and would eventually declare the outbreak a pandemic on 11 March 2020 [5]. At the time of this writing in August 2021, the SARS-CoV-2 pandemic has left entire countries crippled and in desperate recovery. Worldwide spread has left more than 4 million people dead, ranking it among the top 10 most deadly pandemic illnesses in human history.

Origin

In the early stages of the pandemic, most cases were associated with individuals who had previously visited the Huanan wholesale seafood market in the city of Wuhan. It is important to note that in this market, along with seafood, large collections of various wild animals were also available for purchase and consumption during this time. SARS-CoV-2 was isolated from environmental samples of the market by Chinese Center for Disease Control and Prevention. Suspicions arose that this may have originated from the same animal host, masked palm civets (*Paguma larvata*), as SARS-CoV. Early viral sequencing showed that SARS-CoV-2 shares only 79.6% sequence identity with SARS-CoV based on full-length genomic comparisons. However, at the whole-genome level, it is highly identical (96.2%) to bat-CoV RaTG13, which was previously

detected in the horseshoe bat *Rhinolophus affinis* from Yunnan Province, more than 1500 km from Wuhan [6]. In addition, similar strains of SARS-CoV-2 were found earlier in other regions of China. Bats are likely reservoir hosts for SARS-CoV-2; however, whether bat-CoV RaTG13 directly jumped to humans or transmitted to intermediate hosts to facilitate animal-to-human transmission remains inconclusive, and epidemiologic investigations are still being conducted.

Animal Host

In China, SARS-like viruses (SARS and MERS) have largely made bats their natural hosts. However, bat SARS, like other coronaviruses, will not normally directly infect humans unless mutation or recombination occurs in intermediate animal hosts. There are hundreds of different coronaviruses, most of which circulate among such animals as pigs, camels, and bats. Generally, bat habitats are far from human activity, so this recombination event rarely results in disease. However, further human encroachment into animal habitats has increased interaction between humans and animal hosts. Although this is still being studied, the first hypothesized mechanism by which this virus obtained virulence in humans is thought to be what is termed a zoonotic "spillover event," in which a virus reaches a certain mutagenic threshold and gains the ability to transmit from one species to another, which, in the case of humans, can lead to disease (Figure 1.1) [7].

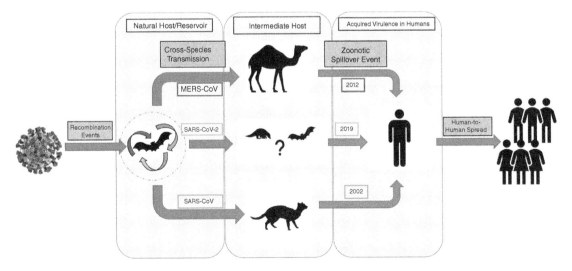

Figure 1.1   Diagram depicting historical examples, along with the proposed mechanism for SARS-CoV-2, of other Coronaviridae theorized recombination events leading to circulation in animals and zoonotic spillover into humans.

These events, although rare, are thought to have led to similar outbreak-type events several times in human history. Intermediate animal hosts of SARS-CoV and MERS-CoV were determined to be the masked palm civets (*P. larvata*) and the dromedary (*Camelus dromedarius*), respectively, before transmission to humans occurred [8, 9]. With respect to COVID-19, genomic evidence has pointed to the Sunda pangolin (*Manis javanica*) as a suspected intermediate host of SARS-CoV-2. Sequence identity between pangolin-origin coronavirus and SARS-CoV-2 is 99%, indicating that SARS-CoV-2 may have been passed on to humans as a result of exposure with these mammals [10]. In addition, SARS-CoV-2 and other coronaviruses from pangolins use receptors (angiotensin-converting enzyme 2 [ACE2] receptor) with similar molecular structures to infect cells, bolstering the argument for the virus being enzootic in these animals. However, others have questioned the relationship between pangolin and human infection, and this hypothesis is still being studied [11].

Infectivity and Incubation

The precise interval that an individual with SARS-CoV-2 infection can transmit infection to others is uncertain. However, it is estimated that infected individuals are likely to be the most contagious in the earlier stages of illness when viral RNA levels from upper respiratory specimens are the highest. Modeling studies have estimated that infectivity begins two days before symptom onset, peaks, and then lasts for approximately seven days. Infectivity rapidly declines after 8–10 days after presentation of illness [12, 13]. Nucleic acid detection studies (reverse transcriptase-polymerase chain reaction) support this infectious period by demonstrating SARS-CoV-2 RNA detection in people one to three days before their symptom onset, with the highest viral loads observed around the day of symptom onset and a gradual decline over time [12]. The duration of nasopharyngeal reverse transcriptase-polymerase chain reaction positivity generally appears to be one to two weeks for asymptomatic persons, up to three weeks or more for patients with mild to moderate disease, and even longer for patients with severe COVID-19 disease and/or immunocompromise [12]. It is important to note that prolonged viral RNA detection does not indicate prolonged

infectiousness, and that the duration of viral RNA shedding is variable and may increase with age and illness severity [14]. Furthermore, the short-term risk for reinfection (e.g. within the first several months after initial infection) is low, because prior infection has been shown to reduce the risk for infection in the subsequent six to seven months by 80–85% [15].

Modes of Transmission

Overview

The US Centers for Disease Control and Prevention (CDC) confirmed person-to-person transmission on 30 January 2020. Many transmission routes have been considered, such as surface-to-surface contact, fecal-oral, bloodborne, and sexual contact, but evidence points to droplet spread via the respiratory pathway to be the most likely principal mode of transmission [16, 17].

Respiratory Droplets

Inhalation of droplets allows the transmitted virus's spike (S) protein to bind to the host ACE2 receptor on respiratory epithelial tissue, a critical step for cell entry and infection [18]. Entry then allows for replication and, as the viral load increases, an increased risk for transmission when an infected individual coughs, sneezes, sings, or talks in the proximity of an uninfected individual. Viral load is highest in the upper respiratory tract (nasopharynx and oropharynx) early in disease and increases in the lower respiratory tract over time. This further suggests that the upper respiratory tract is the initial site of viral replication, with subsequent descending infection [17].

Aerosolization

Although transmission most likely occurs through prolonged close-range contact (i.e. within approximately 6 ft or 2 m) and involves large respiratory droplets, transmission also can occur more distantly via smaller respiratory droplets that can remain in suspension or be recirculated through ventilation systems. In addition, it is likely that during aerosol-generating procedures (e.g. fiberoptic bronchoscopy) the virus may be transmitted at a greater distance [17, 19]. Although SARS-CoV-2 also can be potentially transmitted over such longer distances via an airborne route, in a nonprocedural setting this would primarily occur in specific scenarios where proximity and viral load are optimized (i.e. sneezing and/or coughing in close contact). The precise extent to which aerosol transmission has contributed to the overall pandemic is uncertain and is not thought to be the major contributor to overall pandemic transmission [17, 20]. Regardless, there are numerous examples suggesting aerosol transmission in some settings and evidence supporting proximity as a key determinant of risk, along with duration of contact, indoor settings (i.e. households, healthcare settings, college dormitories, homeless shelters, detention facilities, superspreader events), and poor ventilation [17, 19, 21].

Direct Surface Contact and Fomites

Early reports of clustered infections from China raised concern of possible surface contact transmission of SARS-CoV-2. Although it is plausible that touching a contaminated surface and subsequently contacting a mucosal surface (the eyes, nose, or mouth) could lead to infection, there is currently no conclusive evidence for fomite or direct contact transmission in humans. Early concerns of events suggesting fomite transmission were circumstantial [22, 23]. In these early reports, individuals using shared facilities (such as elevators and restrooms) proposed either fomite or respiratory transmission in those settings. In a detailed investigation of a large nosocomial outbreak linked to 119 confirmed cases at a hospital in South Africa, fomite transmission was proposed given the separated distribution of cases in multiple wards [22]. However, the hospital did not have a universal mask policy, lacked adequate ventilation, and had a substantial burden of infection among health care workers. As a result, respiratory transmission from infected staff could not be excluded [24]. Among healthcare workers, poor hand hygiene has been shown to be associated with increased risk for infection with SARS-CoV-2. Although this might suggest increased risk for contamination via direct contact or fomite spread, it is difficult to separate this from other hygienic practices. As will be discussed in subsequent sections, hand hygiene precautions have been shown to be highly associated with practices that decrease risk overall (mask wearing, ventilation, adequate distancing, etc.) [17]. In addition, providers should always practice good surface hygiene, with the precautions that evidence may provide different conclusions in the future. In short, collective data suggest that live virus persists transiently on surfaces, and although it is beneficial to practice good sanitary hygiene overall, fomites are not thought to be a major route of transmission [17].

Fecal-Oral

SARS-Cov-2 has been detected in nonrespiratory specimens, including stool, blood, ocular secretions, and semen, but their role in infection also appears to be minimal. Fecal-oral transmission was theorized early in the outbreak because of the known high concentration of ACE2 receptors in the small bowel [25]. Although viral RNA is commonly detected in stool, live virus has only rarely been isolated. Currently, no evidence supports fecal-oral transmission in humans, and studies with intragastric inoculation of SARS-CoV-2 in macaques did not result in infection [17]. This is supported by an official joint report released by the WHO and China in February 2020 stating transmission through the fecal-oral route did not appear to be a significant contributing factor for viral spread [26].

Bloodborne

Bloodborne transmission was also hypothesized early on, but the proportion of persons with viral RNA detectable in blood is currently unknown and likely very small. An early study found viral RNA in only 3 of 307 blood specimens. However, no replication-competent virus has been isolated from blood samples to this date, and there have been no documented cases of bloodborne transmission [27]. Moreover, there have been documented reports of recipients of platelets or red blood cell transfusions from donors diagnosed with SARS-CoV-2 in which the transfused individuals did not experience COVID-19-related symptoms, nor did they test positive for SARS-CoV-2 [26, 28].

Semen and Vaginal Secretions

Sexual transmission of SARS-CoV-2 was also an initial concern. However, no current evidence supports sexual transmission of SARS-CoV-2 in semen or vaginal fluids. Although viral RNA has been found in semen, infectious virus has not been isolated [29]. In addition, vaginal fluid studies have been negative except for a small number of case reports showing RNA with low viral levels [30].

Asymptomatic Transmission

People who express symptoms convey the highest risk for transmission. However, one of the more insidious aspects of this virus is its ability to spread among individuals who are minimally symptomatic or asymptomatic. Multiple studies have demonstrated that asymptomatic or presymptomatic persons have the ability to spread infection, and this has been well documented throughout the pandemic [31–33]. Some models estimate the proportion of spread attributable to asymptomatic and presymptomatic transmission at greater than 50% [34]. However, it is important to note that the risk for transmission from an individual who is asymptomatic appears to be less than from a presymptomatic individual, who also carries lesser risk than that from one who is symptomatic [33]. The impact of asymptomatic spread on the pandemic is undoubtedly considerable and has led to difficulties in quantitatively tracking exposure in populations. Nevertheless, the concern for undetected spread has shaped policy and national decisions across the globe, forcing implementation of multiple unprecedented global infection prevention measures that will be briefly discussed in later sections.

Virulence and Mortality

Case Fatality Rate

Case fatality rate (CFR) is the total number of deaths from disease divided by the total number of confirmed cases. As of June 2021, there have been 178 180 208 confirmed cases and 3 859 722 deaths worldwide. This estimates the current worldwide CFR to be approximately 2.17%. There are limitations to using CFR as a measure of disease mortality. For example, this number is dynamic, because the denominator and numerator are based on documented cases and deaths and can rapidly change. For example, in the earliest stages of

the outbreak, the CFR was much higher: 17.3% across China as a whole and greater than 20% in the center of the outbreak in Wuhan [35]. Underreporting of cases, such as from failure to test individuals with mild disease and asymptomatic infection, can greatly inflate the CFR. Conversely, there are concerns that during the rapid spread of disease during a pandemic, the CFR will underestimate disease, because the death counts do not account for any eventual deaths that may occur in the overall pool of cases. Wide variations (estimates ranging from <0.1% to >25%) in CFR can also arise from country to country as a result of extrinsic or societal factors [36]. CFR, furthermore, does not account for differences in age or sex; it is a cumulative population at-risk metric. Nevertheless, this method, along with others, was used to approximate disease mortality and was consistent with the initial CFR reports released from China in the early stages of the pandemic, outside of Hubei Province [36–38].

Serial Interval

In any infectious disease outbreak, the estimation of transmission dynamics is crucial to contain spread in a new area. Of the tools used in such estimations, the serial interval is one of the significant epidemiological measures that help determine the spread of infectious disease. It is required to understand the turnover of case generation and transmissibility of the disease and is defined as the time between which the infector and the secondarily infected show the symptoms, that is, the time interval between the onset of symptoms in the primary (infector) and secondary cases (infected). The estimated serial interval for SARS-CoV-2 is about 4.5–5 days [39].

Reproduction Number/Reproduction Ratio

Reproduction number (R_0) represents the number of people to whom an infected person passes the disease in its next generation, with length of time determined by the serial interval measure of the disease. This value has had wide variability throughout the pandemic. During the COVID-19 outbreak, the initial estimates of R_0 were between 2.0 and 3.0. However, later studies estimated the R_0 to be 3.82, with a mean reported R_0 range of 1.90–6.49 [40]. Importantly, it is estimated that R_0 is higher for certain variants of concern, such as the alpha or delta variants [40]. This increased transmissibility is of great concern as worldwide spread of variants of concern accelerates and more transmissible variants become the dominant circulating strains.

Excess Mortality

Excess mortality is a measure used by epidemiologists and public health experts to assess the overall impact of pandemic disease. Because not all cases and deaths can realistically be reported, this gives practical insight into overall impact. It is defined as the difference in mortality in a given year compared with the average number of deaths over a given number of previous years. In the United States, data from the National Vital Statistics System of the CDC estimated that 545 600–660 200 excess deaths occurred in the United States from

26 January 2020 to 27 February 2021 (Figure 1.2) [42]. The percentage excess mortality is this difference in mortality for a given time period divided by the average mortality in the same designated time frame during previous years. The estimated number of excess deaths peaked during the weeks ending 11 April 2020, 1 August 2020, and 2 January 2021 (Figure 1.2) [41], with approximately 75–88% of excess deaths directly associated with COVID-19 [42, 43].

Globally, it is difficult to accurately estimate the total number of excess deaths. Not all countries have the infrastructure to report nationwide mortality accurately and expeditiously, and representation from poorer countries is underreported. Keeping in mind these limitations, the WHO estimates, in 2020, a worldwide excess mortality of more than 1.8 million deaths attributed directly to COVID-19, with unofficial total pandemic deaths totaling more than 3 million people [43].

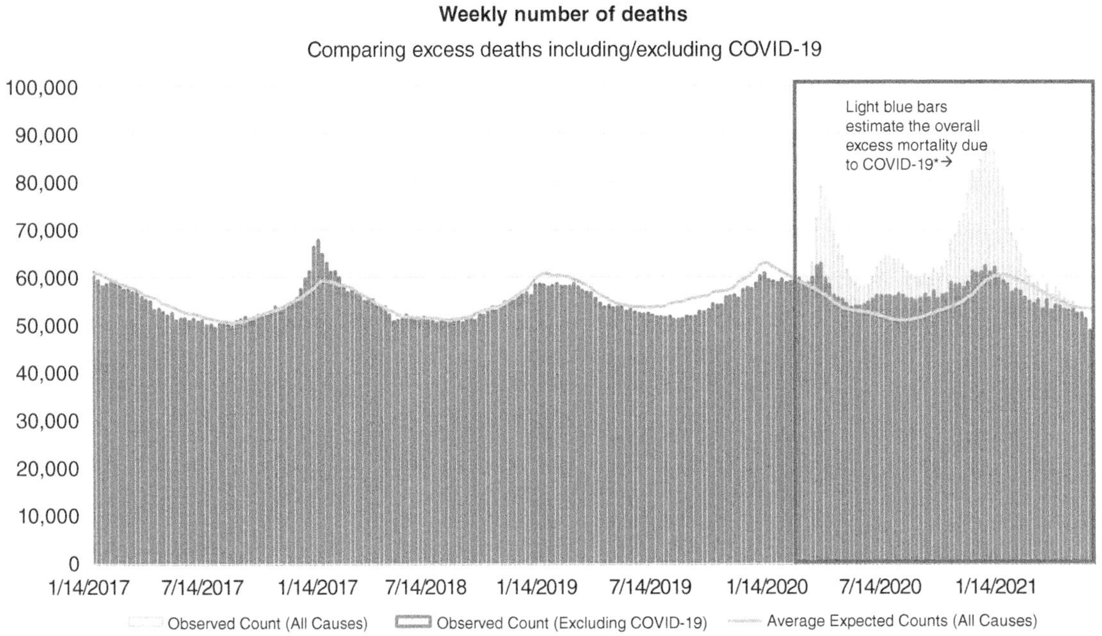

Weekly number of deaths
Comparing excess deaths including/excluding COVID-19

Figure 1.2 Excess mortality counts by week for observed all-cause mortality and observed mortality excluding COVID-19 (1 January 2017 to 1 July 2021). Overlaid trend line is average expected counts based on previous year trends. Red box: Counts may be incomplete because only 60% of death records are submitted to National Center for Health Statistics (NCHS) within 10 days of the date of death, and completeness varied by jurisdiction (1 February 2020 to 26 June 2021). *Number of deaths reported is the total number of deaths received and coded as of the date of analysis and does not represent all deaths that occurred in that period. Data are possibly incomplete because of the lag in time between when the death occurred and when the death certificate was completed, submitted to NCHS, and processed for reporting purposes. *Source:* Data are from the US Centers for Disease Control and Prevention [41].

Demographics

Overview

SARS-CoV-2 has shown the ability to infect all ages, races, and ethnicities across the globe. Notably, COVID-19 disproportionately affected different groups of individuals, with age, race, sex, and medical status all conferring varying levels of morbidity and mortality. In the United States, the virus has infected young adults most often. Elderly individuals (>65 years of age) were among the most vulnerable populations in terms of mortality [44]. Underlying comorbidities, immuno-compromised status, and non-white race all are risk factors for progression of SARS-CoV-2 infection to more serious disease. In the United States, the most frequent comorbidities listed on death certificates of those with COVID-19 are influenza and pneumonia (45.8%), hypertension (19.8%), diabetes (16.0%), Alzheimer disease (13.5% of deaths), and sepsis (9.6%) [44].

Age

Data from the CDC, as well as other public health agencies around the world, demonstrated the ability of SARS-CoV-2 to infect individuals of all ages. Age groups for the CDC were reported in nine categories (Table 1.1). The overall trend showed that young adults make up most cases, with elderly individuals comprising the majority of deaths despite being a smaller percentage of the overall population (Figure 1.3). Most of these deaths occurred in those 85 years and older [45–47].

Sex

Sex demographics reported by the CDC showed that females made up a slight majority (52.2%; males, 47.8%) of COVID-19 cases in the United States (Table 1.2) [45]. Worldwide, there was no significantly observed sex difference in proportion of COVID-19 cases [48]. Interestingly, in the United States, although COVID-19 affected more females than males, mortality disproportionately affected males, who account for approximately 54.2% of all COVID-19 deaths, with females comprising about 45.8% (Figure 1.4) [45]. This trend was also seen in other parts of the world [49]. It is unclear what drives this disparity, but the cause appears to be multifactorial [50–52].

Race and Ethnicity

Sadly, racial and ethnic disparities were apparent throughout the pandemic. Inadequate early prevention measures, testing, and social support and the need to work outside of the home disproportionately affected vulnerable and marginalized populations. This was very well displayed in data obtained from the Los Angeles Department of Public Health in California, where Hispanics were shown to be more than 2.5 times more likely to be infected with COVID-19 (Figure 1.5) than their white peers. Notably, the age-adjusted mortality rate for Hispanics from COVID-19 was more than three times greater than for non-Latino whites (Figure 1.6). For perspective,

Table 1.1 CDC COVID-19 case and death percentages, by age, with respective percentages of the US population (data through July 2021).

Age group	Percent (%) of cases	Percent (%) of deaths	Percent (%) of US population
0–4 yr	2.1	<0.1	6
5–17 yr	10.4	0.1	16.3
18–29 yr	22.5	0.5	16.4
30–39 yr	16.4	1.2	13.5
40–49 yr	14.8	3.0	12.3
50–64 yr	20.2	15.3	19.2
65–74 yr	7.4	21.6	9.6
75–84 yr	3.8	27.4	4.9
≥85 yr	2.2	30.9	2

Of the 27 472 068 cases recorded, age group was available for 27 281 478 (99%) cases. Of the 495 907 deaths recorded, age group was available for 495 867 (99%) deaths.

Table 1.2 CDC data of COVID-19 deaths by sex (all age groups).

Sex	Percent (%) of cases	Percent (%) of deaths	Percent (%) of US population
Female	52.2	45.8	50.75
Male	47.8	54.2	49.25
Other	<0.1	<0.1	Not available

Data as of July 2021. Of the 495 907 deaths recorded, sex was available for 494 710 (99%) deaths.

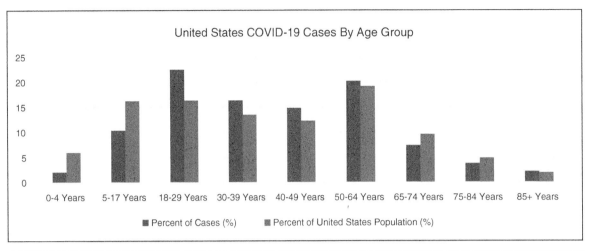

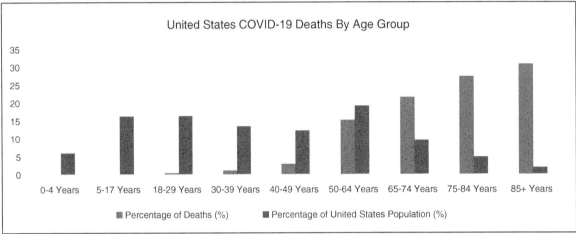

Figure 1.3 Case and death count distribution by age with corresponding percentage of US population for each respective age group. *Source:* Graph data are from the US Centers for Disease Control and Prevention [45].

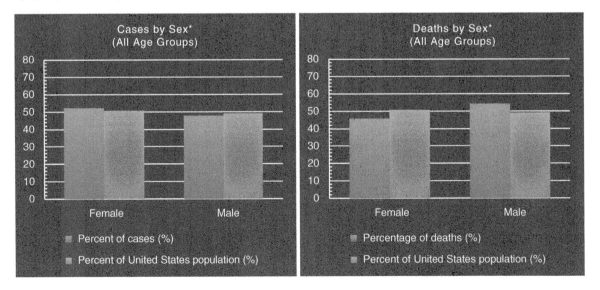

Figure 1.4 US COVID-19 cases and deaths for males and females for all age groups. *Those who were listed as "other" constituted less than 0.001% of cases, and deaths are not graphically represented here. *Source:* Case and mortality data from the US Centers for Disease Control and Prevention [45]. Data are as of July 2021.

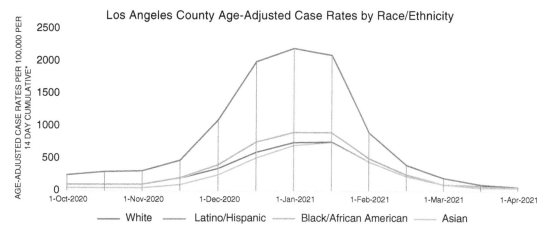

Figure 1.5 Los Angeles County age-adjusted COVID-19 case rate per 100 000 individuals by race/ethnicity, April 2020 to June 2021. *Data are estimated reported data from the Los Angeles County Department of Public Health and do not necessarily reflect exact amounts.

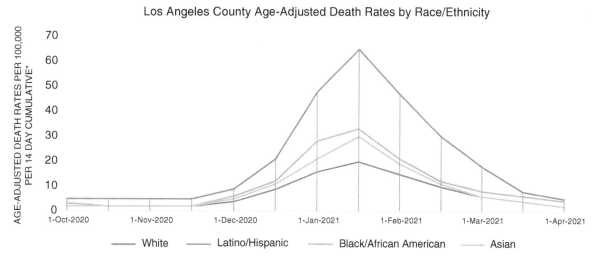

Figure 1.6 Los Angeles County age-adjusted mortality rate per 100 000 individuals by race/ethnicity, April 2020 to June 2021. *Data are estimated reported data from the Los Angeles County Department of Public Health and do not necessarily reflect exact amounts.

in 2020, COVID-19 became the leading cause of death in Los Angeles for Latino/Hispanics (where they account for 49% of the total population), outpacing mortality rates from heart disease, cancer, and diabetes [53].

In terms of the US population overall, crude data demonstrated that non-Hispanic whites accounted for the greatest percentage of morbidity, comprising approximately 50% of cases, with Hispanic and non-Hispanic blacks following at 29% and 11%, respectively (Table 1.3). However, when considering race-respective population percentages, Hispanics and non-Hispanic Blacks have been disproportionately affected in terms of disease morbidity and mortality, with both respective mortalities outpacing their proportions of the population (Figure 1.7) [54–56]. Furthermore, additional studies have reported that American Indian or Alaska Native, non-Hispanic persons were also disproportionately affected and more likely to be infected, hospitalized, or die with COVID-19 in comparison with their white counterparts [55–57].

Table 1.3 CDC data of COVID-19 cases by race/ethnicity.

Race/ethnicity	Percent (%) of cases	Percent (%) of deaths	Percent (%) of US population
Hispanic/Latino	28.7	18.6	18.45
American Indian/Alaska Native non-Hispanic	1	1.2	0.74
Asian non-Hispanic	3.2	3.8	5.76
Black non-Hispanic	11.4	13.7	12.54
Native Hawaiian/Other Pacific Islander non-Hispanic	0.3	0.2	0.182
White non-Hispanic	50.1	58.6	60.11
Multiple/other non-Hispanic	5.3	3.8	2.22

Data as of July 2021. Of the 27 472 068 recorded cases, race/ethnicity was available for 17 382 837 (63%) cases.

Disease Prevention

Vaccinations

One year into the pandemic, vaccination-based prevention was developed and implemented. Numerous vaccines are currently in development, and several have been approved for official use. These largely fall under four technology categories: adenovirus vector vaccines, inactivated viral vaccines, protein subunit vaccines, and messenger RNA (mRNA) vaccines. Following is a brief overview of the more notable vaccines; these and others will be covered in greater detail elsewhere in the text.

Viral vector vaccines use a modified, nonreplicating virus that is taken up and processed by human cells, expressing a viral protein, generating an immune response. Several different viruses have been used as vectors, including influenza, vesicular stomatitis virus, measles virus, and human and nonhuman primate adenoviruses. This technology has been used historically to develop vaccines for many diseases, including malaria, Ebola, leishmaniasis, HIV, tuberculosis, and the common cold [58, 59]. Currently, the adenovirus vector technology has been used to produce publicly available SARS-CoV-2 vaccines, most notably, the Oxford–AstraZeneca and the Johnson & Johnson vaccines [60, 61]. The two-dose Russian Sputnik adenoviral vaccine has shown similar high efficacy [62].

Inactivated or weakened virus vaccines use a form of the virus that has been inactivated or weakened, so it does not replicate or cause disease but still contains sufficient cellular signals to generate an immune response. A caveat to this is that these vaccines typically do not provide as strong an immune response (protection) as live vaccines, so several doses may be required over time (booster shots) to obtain ongoing immunity against diseases [60]. Sinopharm (BBIBP), CoronaVac (Sinovac), and Covaxin are all examples of vaccines that use this technology. These are largely used internationally in countries throughout Asia and Latin America; currently, they have not been approved for use in the United States.

Protein-based vaccines use fragments of proteins or protein shells that mimic viral antigens to generate an immune response, which is enhanced by coformulation with an adjuvant substance. The antigen can be any molecule, such as structural proteins, other peptides, or polysaccharides. Like inactivated vaccines, the vaccine is completely "dead," that is, replication incompetent, and therefore may be less risky [60]. Vaccines that have historically used this technology include the hepatitis B vaccine. Currently, the vaccines against COVID-19 that implement this technology include the Novavax NVX-CoV2373 vaccine, the Sanofi-GSK adjuvanted protein subunit vaccine Vidprevtyn, the Russian EpiVacCorona (Vector), and the Chinese RBD-Dimer (Anhui Zhifei Longcom and the Institute of Medical Biology of the Chinese Academy of Medical Sciences). The latter two are exclusively used in Russia, China, Turkmenistan, and Uzbekistan [60].

mRNA vaccines are a cutting-edge approach that use genetically engineered RNA to synthesize a structural protein and generate an immune response. Although

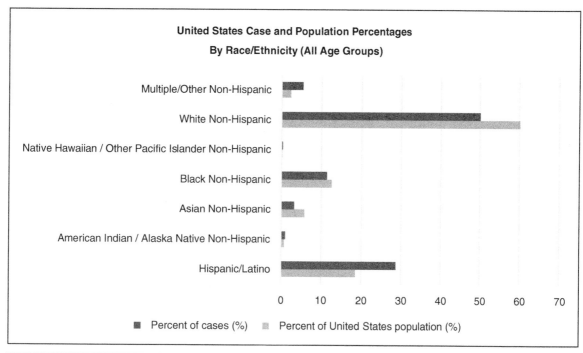

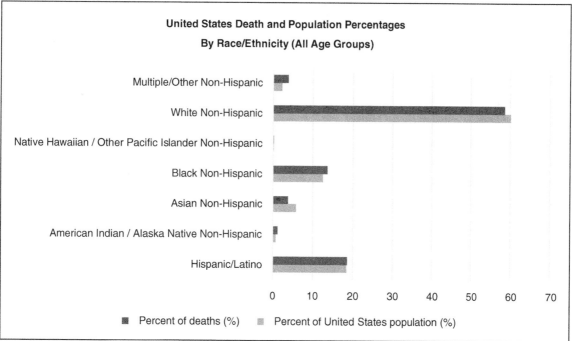

Figure 1.7   Case and death percentages by race/ethnicity with corresponding percentage of US population for each respective group. *Source:* Data are from the US Centers for Disease Control and Prevention [45]. Data are as of July 2021.

this is a relatively new method in the arsenal of vaccine development, this technology has been studied for at least a decade before this specific application, so the science is well understood. mRNA segments coding for the coronavirus spike protein are introduced into the body through an intramuscular injection to trigger an immune response. Using a protective lipid nanoparticle coating, these particles are taken up by cells, processed, coded for synthesis of spike protein, and presented to the immune system, triggering a humoral and a cellular immune response. The Pfizer-BioNTech and Moderna vaccines are examples of this technology and are the main vaccines used by the United States and many countries throughout Europe. These vaccines were approved by the US Food and Drug Administration for Emergency Use Authorization on 11 December 2020 for Pfizer and on 18 December 2020 for Moderna [60, 63]. The Pfizer vaccine received full US Food and Drug Administration approval on 23 August 2021.

The goals of vaccination are grounded on two key concepts: bolstering individual immunity to prevent severe disease and hospitalization and to limit population-wide spread. "Herd immunity" is an indirect form of protection resulting from enough individuals obtaining immunity, via vaccination or infection, to the point where it minimizes further disease circulation within a population. This threshold varies from pathogen to pathogen. Herd immunity to SARS-CoV-2 has been estimated, giving circulating strain considerations, to require immunity in approximately 70–80% of the population. However, this number will increase as newer variants arise with higher R_0 and increased transmissibility [64].

For many viruses, the more it circulates in a population, the more opportunities it has to replicate and/or mutate; SARS-CoV-2 has demonstrated this ability [65]. These mutations have the potential to produce more transmissible and more virulent strains of SARS-CoV-2. For example, the 501Y mutation (present in the B.1.1.7 or alpha variant) and the L452R mutation (present in the B.1.617.2 or delta variant) are both associated with higher levels of transmissibility [66]. Fortunately, preliminary reports of current vaccine effectiveness have demonstrated protection, albeit reduced, to such variants and emphasize their need against more virulent strains [67].

The importance of vaccines cannot be understated. Successful historical examples, such as the polio, measles-mumps-rubella, and smallpox vaccines, have underscored the profound importance of this technology in achieving herd immunity. Vaccine-mediated herd immunity is an essential tool in public health and directly protects vulnerable populations with lesser vaccine responsiveness (i.e. elderly adults, individuals with chronic disease, and immunocompromised persons). The alternative "natural immunity" method would be impractical. Although preventing circulation of virus through naturally acquired herd immunity would occur eventually, it would also result in unnecessary cases and deaths and has possibly been achieved only in close situations such as prisons [68].

Current COVID-19 vaccinations have been shown to not only decrease viral load but also decrease risk for asymptomatic transmission [69–71]. However, emerging variants have the potential to escape some of these benefits of vaccination. Reducing transmission via vaccination carries important implications for reopening and shaping public health guidelines going forward, as the CDC and national governments relax recommended prevention measures for vaccinated individuals [72]. This is a monumental finding because, as mentioned in previous sections, SARS-CoV-2 and its variants carry significant mortality and disproportionately affect the marginalized and the disadvantaged [73]. Given the availability and promising results of this technology, immunity via natural circulation of the virus would be not only medically irresponsible but also potentially morally unacceptable.

Personal Protective Equipment: Respirators and Masks

In the United States, hospitals are required to provide personal protective equipment for staff working with patients with suspected or confirmed COVID-19, which includes the use of a gown, gloves, a respirator or medical mask, and eye or face protection for preventing transmission. N95 masks confer the greatest protection, especially in conditions of greater patient aerosolization, such as during aerosol-generating procedures and certain types of environmental cleaning. However, in the event that N95 masks are not available or are in limited supply, surgical masks are acceptable in many hospital settings [72, 74, 75].

In the community, mask wearing with social distancing as an alternative to widespread lockdown was officially endorsed by the CDC in March 2020. The CDC subsequently issued a mandate requiring masks on public transportation and areas or times of gatherings (including taxis and rideshares) and at transportation hubs (e.g. airports, bus or ferry terminals, railway stations, seaports) [76]. The rationale for community mask wearing is, regardless of symptoms, preventing transmission while maintaining the day-to-day functions for individuals and the country. In the United States, cloth masks or disposable masks (e.g. commercially available surgical masks) were recommended for the general public or in public settings with individuals outside the household to reduce transmission of SARS-CoV-2. In addition, guidance criteria for approved homemade masks were given to the public, stating that masks should be made with several layers, fit snugly over the face, and should not contain respiratory valves [74, 76].

Strategies to improve mask fit include using a mask with an adjustable nose bridge, wearing a cloth mask over a disposable mask, knotting the ear loops of a disposable mask to secure it against the face, using masks with ties rather than ear loops, and using a mask brace. Some individuals may opt to wear commercially available KN95 respirators, but many do not meet the advertised filtration standards. Furthermore, due to necessity in the healthcare setting, N95 respirators are not indicated or necessary for the general public and should generally be reserved for healthcare workers who work in higher-risk environments [74, 75].

Physical Distancing

In the effort against COVID-19 spread, countries across the globe used various physical distancing measures to keep clustering of individuals to a minimum. This included, but was not limited to, limiting the number of individuals in closed spaces, temporarily shutting down schools and universities, and limiting the number of people during indoor shopping, gymnasium use, personal services (e.g. hair cutting, manicures), and dining.

Distancing guidelines were implemented to minimize prolonged close-range contact with an infected individual, which, as previously mentioned, is thought to be the principal risk factor for transmission of SARS-CoV-2. This method was taken from previous data preventing SARS and MERS infections. In a meta-analysis of observational studies evaluating the relationship between physical distance and transmission of SARS-CoV-2, SARS-CoV, and MERS-CoV, proximity and risk for infection were closely associated, and the infection rate was much higher with contact within 3 ft (1 m) compared with contact beyond that distance (12.8% versus 2.6%) [77].

Optimal distance is uncertain, but physical distancing is likely independently associated with a reduced risk for SARS-CoV-2 transmission. Current guidance suggests at least 6 ft. In the United States, the CDC recommends a minimum distance of 6 ft (2 m), whereas the WHO recommends a minimum distance of 1 m. In locations where there is community transmission of SARS-CoV-2 (including throughout the United States), individuals are advised to practice social or physical distancing in both indoor and outdoor spaces by maintaining a minimum distance from other people outside their household.

Widescale shelter-in-place orders and lockdowns were the most aggressive form of these distancing methods. During peak outbreaks, when daily case rates and deaths were the highest, governments strongly encouraged or required individuals to quarantine inside their homes, only leaving for necessities such as food and other items. Although one of the most controversial forms enacted by prevention taskforces, given societal and mental health considerations, studies can speak to the impact of distancing on viral transmission. One such study involving multiple countries showed a significant decrease in viral transmission when individuals were distanced 1 m or more from each other. Moreover, protection was increased as the distance was lengthened [77]. Other studies have shown that, after cases began to emerge, longer time periods for which countries waited to implement quarantine measures were associated with greater CFRs [78].

Hand and Surface Sanitation

Inanimate surfaces may be potential sites for the transmission of COVID-19 infection. Depending on the nature of the surface and conditions of the surrounding environment (temperature, pH, humidity, etc.), the virus can remain viable for several hours [78]. Concern mainly stems from potential contaminated surfaces contacting hands, which then pass the virus to upper respiratory tract mucous membranes (conjunctivae, nose, mouth, etc.) through touch. Although surface contact spread is only theoretical and has not been definitively documented, studies have shown that SARS-CoV-2 has extended longevity on certain surfaces and through skin-to-skin contact [79, 80]. The US Environmental Protection Agency recommends disinfectants that contain quaternary ammonium compounds, hydrogen peroxide, alcohol (ethanol, isopropyl alcohol, phenol), aldehyde, hypochlorous acid, octanoic acid, citric acid conjugate with silver ions, sodium hypochlorite, sodium bicarbonate, etc., all of which contain key virucidal activity. Specifically, alcohols ethanol (78–95%) and isopropanol (70–100%) have been used as reliable and relatively safe disinfectant options because they show potent virucidal activity with a negligible toxic effect on human skin [81]. In autopsy studies, SARS-CoV-2 remained viable on the skin for about nine hours but was completely inactivated within 15 seconds of exposure to 80% alcohol [81].

Adequate Ventilation of Indoor Spaces

A healthy amount of literature emphasizes the importance of air quality and ventilation in the healthcare setting. There is substantial evidence, drawn from prior studies on pandemics, that emphasizes an effective combination of air filtration and circulation can reduce risk for infection. However, much of the data surrounding ventilation and SARS-CoV-2 infection are model based, drawing conclusions from theoretical scenarios and calculated behaviors of similar-size microbes. Using the Wells–Riley equation, a study implementing calculated risk associated with various rates of ventilation concluded a significant theoretical reduction in COVID-19 infection risk with adequate ventilation of an enclosed space. Furthermore, these beneficial effects were compounded by those who concurrently wore a medical-grade mask [82]. A large literature review addressing air recirculation also drew on historical examples and the behavior of similar microorganisms to frame the need for adequate ventilation and concluded that specific filters and air

ventilation flow rates can lead to lower viral air concentrations and a decreased risk for exposure and transmission of virus [83]. Although conclusions of ventilation effects on SARS-CoV-2 transmission are largely drawn from historical and theoretical models, they nonetheless highlight the need for improved air circulation to lower airborne viral concentrations and decrease the risk for transmission.

Use of Outdoor Spaces

Where possible, use of outdoor spaces can further reduce aerosol transmission [84]. Outdoor spaces typically offer greater physical distancing and airflow than indoor spaces. Relatively few SARS-CoV-2 transmissions have been linked to outdoor setting [85]. Although outdoor transmission can occur, and the precise settings in which this can be minimized are still being investigated, the odds of indoor transmission have been shown to be significantly greater [86]. Limiting the duration and frequency of personal contact, using personal protective equipment, and avoiding any indoor contacts may increase the safety of outdoor gatherings [84].

Global Impacts

Distribution

At the time that this was written, the WHO had estimated the total confirmed counts to be more than 200 million cases worldwide, with more than 4 million deaths. As discussed previously, these are confirmed cases only, such that the number of cases (i.e. overall disease burden) has likely been underreported [43]. Geographic distribution is worldwide, as cases have been found in nearly every country. The countries that had the highest disease burden were the United States of America, India, and Brazil. In terms of mortality, the countries with the highest mortality burden were the United States of America, Brazil, India, and Mexico [83].

International Response

This begs the questions, what countries had the most success against the COVID-19 pandemic, and why were they successful? Conversely, what was common among those who were not? There is a public health consensus that limiting the number of contacts between persons can slow COVID-19 transmission in a community and give time for healthcare systems to respond and vaccines to be developed. Factors such as population density, leadership, national wealth, infrastructure, and equitable healthcare resources influence a nation's capacity to do so [87].

Before vaccination, the most meaningful approaches governments took to stop community spread were stay-at-home-orders. These guidelines requested or required people to quarantine in their homes, to leave only for absolute necessities, such as food and healthcare needs [88]. Although there are multiple theoretical and practical models about how stay-at-home orders and travel restrictions slowed COVID-19 transmission, it is clear that consistency in communication and early implementation were key [89]. Retrospective data show that a longer amount of time before implementation of physical distancing measures was associated with worse CFRs [77]. Widespread testing efforts were valuable in the identification of cluster outbreaks. South Korea is a good example of the impact of early and effective measures, in which large-scale testing efforts in combination with contact tracing and social distancing measures led to one of the most successful pandemic responses in the world [90, 91]. Countries such as New Zealand succeeded by enacting strict border control. Of course, having the wealth and resources to accommodate such a large and rapid disease response is crucial to improving individual and population outcomes. Countries with an adequate physician workforce and technological capacity to accommodate pandemic-level crises were able to detect disease earlier and fared better in terms of overall mortality [77].

Future Outbreaks

Global trade, travel, climate change, urbanization, and national wealth all play a part in global infrastructure and the ability to address worldwide pandemics. Lessons learned over the course of the COVID-19 pandemic, compiled from multiple national responses, have created a type of framework, or a "pandemic playbook," in which governments and public health agencies can model policy to stave off future pandemic

emergencies. Such a pandemic playbook has previously been proposed by the CDC to help coordinate pandemic influenza response [92]. This includes, but is not limited to, concepts such as swiftly tightening international borders to travel and trade, supervised traveler isolation and well-coordinated quarantines, early implementation of physical distancing requirements, encouraging good hand hygiene (frequent handwashing, use of alcohol hand sanitizers as an alternative, cough etiquette), and having the infrastructure for quick and widespread testing and contact tracing [91, 93]. In addition to these policies, nations must also possess the capacity to provide social supports in the future, to provide mental health services, adequate resources, and economic assistance to those in need. This is obviously a more attainable goal for wealthier countries, but nevertheless, it is imperative that nations and their leaders come together and offer mutual aid in times of crisis. Sharing of wealth, information, resources, intellectual property, and financial support are all necessary to maximize the safety and well-being of citizens.

Conclusions

This novel SARS-CoV-2 virus was unique in many ways. An insidious, yet defining, characteristic of this disease was its ability for asymptomatic spread. Without efficient widespread testing measures, we saw a virus, seemingly isolated to a limited region of China, stretch to every corner of the globe in a matter of months. In coordination with international leaders, our global health institutions developed guidelines to help contain spread, including isolation, mask wearing, hand hygiene practices, and nationwide shutdowns of business and mass gatherings. However, the aftermath of the outbreak cannot be ignored; shortcomings must be addressed. Hospitals quickly filled to capacity, and we saw our healthcare infrastructure woefully ill-equipped to handle the volume of individuals affected by this disease.

Indeed, the pandemic has revealed shortcomings in our health systems, notably highlighting, in the United States, the systemic racial and economic inequities that plague them. Moreover, this virus has profoundly reshaped how we must think about global public health and emphasizes the magnitude of work needed to be done. This pandemic illness has forced us to reevaluate our approach to disease epidemiology, outbreaks, and how further progress can be made under these new norms. Conversely, we have also seen the capacity for global coordination in an unprecedented time frame. Massive mobilization of manufacturing, testing resources, healthcare workforce, and biomedical engineering allowed us to address the novel challenges of the pandemic. It is essential for us to build on this progress, for the sake of the most affected dense and poor populations around the world. Our institutions, physicians, and healthcare leaders must take the lessons from this unprecedented event to facilitate change with decisive action and prevent any future catastrophes like the COVID-19 pandemic from occurring again.

References

1 World Health Organization (WHO) (2021). COVID-19 – China. WHO. https://www.who.int/emergencies/disease-outbreak-news/item/2020-DON229 (accessed 21 July 2021).

2 World Health Organization (WHO) (2020). Listings of WHO's response to COVID-19 World Health Organization Website. WHO. https://www.who.int/news/item/29-06-2020-covidtimeline (updated 29 June 2020 accessed 21 July 2021).

3 Iroegbu, J.D., Ifenatuoha, C.W., and Ijomone, O.M. (2020). Potential neurological impact of coronaviruses: implications for the novel SARS-CoV-2. *Neurol. Sci.* 41 (6): 1329–1327. https://doi.org/10.1007/s10072-020-04469-4.

4 National Institute of Allergy and Infectious Disease (2021). Coronaviruses. National Institute of Allergy and Infectious Disease https://www.niaid.nih.gov/diseases-conditions/coronaviruses

5 Pooja Jha. (2021). Is the worst of the pandemic over for Europe? *Lancet Reg. Health Eur.* 2: 100077. https://doi.org/10.1016/j.lanepe.2021.100077.

6 Liu, Y.C., Kuo, R.L., and Shih, S.R. (2020). COVID-19: the first documented coronavirus pandemic in history. *Biom. J.* 43 (4): 328–333. https://doi.org/10.1016/j.bj.2020.04.007.

7 Rodriguez-Morales, A.J., Bonilla-Aldana, D.K., Balbin-Ramon, G.J. et al. (2020). History is repeating itself: probable zoonotic spillover as the cause of the 2019 novel coronavirus epidemic. *Infez Med.* 28 (1): 3–5.

8 Reusken, C., Haagmans, B.L., and Koopmans, M.P. (2014). Dromedaris en 'Middle East respiratory syndrome': MERS-coronavirus in het 'schip van de woestijn' [dromedary camels and Middle East respiratory syndrome: MERS coronavirus in the 'ship of the desert']. *Ned. Tijdschr. Geneeskd.* 158: A7806.

9 Wang, L.F. and Eaton, B.T. (2007). Bats, civets and the emergence of SARS. *Curr. Top. Microbiol. Immunol.* 315: 325–344. https://doi.org/10.1007/978-3-540-70962-6_13.

10 Zhang, T., Wu, Q., and Zhang, Z. (2020). Probable pangolin origin of SARS-CoV-2 associated with the COVID-19 outbreak. *Curr. Biol.* 30 (8): 1578. https://doi.org/10.1016/j.cub.2020.03.063. Erratum for: Curr Biol. 2020;30(7):1346–51.e2.

11 Frutos, R., Serra-Cobo, J., Chen, T., and Devaux, C.A. (2020). COVID-19: time to exonerate the pangolin from the transmission of SARS-CoV-2 to humans. *Infect. Genet. Evol.* 84: 104493. https://doi.org/10.1016/j.meegid.2020.104493.

12 Cevik, M., Tate, M., Lloyd, O. et al. (2021). SARS-CoV-2, SARS-CoV, and MERS-CoV viral load dynamics, duration of viral shedding, and infectiousness: a systematic review and meta-analysis. *Lancet Microbe* 2 (1): e13–e22. https://doi.org/10.1016/S2666-5247(20)30172-5.

13 Wölfel, R., Corman, V.M., Guggemos, W. et al. (2020). Virological assessment of hospitalized patients with COVID-2019. *Nature* 581 (7809): 465–469. https://doi.org/10.1038/s41586-020-2196-x.

14 Xu, K., Chen, Y., Yuan, J. et al. (2020). Factors associated with prolonged viral RNA shedding in patients with coronavirus disease 2019 (COVID-19). *Clin. Infect. Dis.* 71 (15): 799–806. https://doi.org/10.1093/cid/ciaa351.

15 Hansen, C.H., Michlmayr, D., Gubbels, S.M. et al. (2021). Assessment of protection against reinfection with SARS-CoV-2 among 4 million PCR-tested individuals in Denmark in 2020: a population-level observational study. *Lancet* 397 (10280): 1204–1212. https://doi.org/10.1016/S0140-6736(21)00575-4.

16 Chagla, Z., Hota, S., Khan, S. et al. (2020). International hospital and community epidemiology group. Airborne transmission of COVID-19. *Clin. Infect. Dis.*: ciaa1118. https://doi.org/10.1093/cid/ciaa1118.

17 Meyerowitz, E.A., Richterman, A., Gandhi, R.T., and Sax, P.E. (2021). Transmission of SARS-CoV-2: a review of viral, host, and environmental factors. *Ann. Intern. Med.* 174 (1): 69–79. https://doi.org/10.7326/M20-5008.

18 Davidson, A.M., Wysocki, J., and Batlle, D. (2020). Interaction of SARS-CoV-2 and other coronavirus with ACE (angiotensin-converting enzyme)-2 as their Main receptor: therapeutic implications. *Hypertension* 76 (5): 1339–1349. https://doi.org/10.1161/HYPERTENSIONAHA.120.15256.

19 Lu, J., Gu, J., Li, K. et al. (2020). COVID-19 outbreak associated with air conditioning in restaurant, Guangzhou, China, 2020. *Emerg. Infect. Dis.* 26 (7): 1628–1631. https://doi.org/10.3201/eid2607.200764.

20 Leung, N.H.L. (2021). Transmissibility and transmission of respiratory viruses. *Nat. Rev. Microbiol.* 19: 528–545. https://doi.org/10.1038/s41579-021-00535-6.

21 Azuma, K., Yanagi, U., Kagi, N. et al. (2020). Environmental factors involved in SARS-CoV-2 transmission: effect and role of indoor environmental quality in the strategy for COVID-19 infection control. *Environ. Health Prev. Med.* 25 (1): 66. https://doi.org/10.1186/s12199-020-00904-2.

22 Cai, J., Sun, W., Huang, J. et al. (2020). Indirect virus transmission in cluster of COVID-19 cases, Wenzhou, China, 2020. *Emerg. Infect. Dis.* 26 (6): 1343–1345. https://doi.org/10.3201/eid2606.200412.

23 World Heath Organization (WHO) (2020). Report of the WHO-China Joint Mission on Coronavirus Disease 2019 (COVID-19) - China. WHO. https://www.who.int/docs/default-source/coronaviruse/who-china-joint-mission-on-covid-19-final-report.pdf

24 Lessells, R., Moosa, Y., de Oliveira, T. (2020). Report into a nosocomial outbreak of coronavirus disease 2019 (COVID-19) at Netcare St. Augustine's Hospital. KwaZulu-Natal Research Innovation and Sequencing Platform (KRISP). https://www.krisp.org.za/news.php?id=421

25 Gu, J., Han, B., and Wang, J. (2020). COVID-19: gastrointestinal manifestations and potential fecal-Oral transmission. *Gastroenterology* 158 (6): 1518–1519. https://doi.org/10.1053/j.gastro.2020.02.054.

26 Abd, E.W., Eassa, S.M., Metwally, M. et al. (2020). SARS-CoV-2 transmission channels: a review of the literature. *MEDICC Rev.* 22 (4): 51–69.

27 Wang, W., Xu, Y., Gao, R. et al. (2020). Detection of SARS-CoV-2 in different types of clinical specimens. *JAMA* 323 (18): 1843–1844. https://doi.org/10.1001/jama.2020.3786.

28 Luzzi, J.R., Navarro, R., and Dinardo, C.L. (2021). COVID-19: further evidence of no transfusion transmission. *Transfus. Apher. Sci.* 60 (1): 102961. https://doi.org/10.1016/j.transci.2020.102961.

29 Li, D., Jin, M., Bao, P. et al. (2020). Clinical characteristics and results of semen tests among men with coronavirus disease 2019. *JAMA Netw. Open* 3 (5): e208292. https://doi.org/10.1001/jamanetworkopen.2020.8292.

30 Qiu, L., Liu, X., Xiao, M. et al. (2020). SARS-CoV-2 is not detectable in the vaginal fluid of women with severe COVID-19 infection. *Clin. Infect. Dis.* 71 (15): 813–817. https://doi.org/10.1093/cid/ciaa375.

31 Johansson, M.A., Quandelacy, T.M., Kada, S. et al. (2021). SARS-CoV-2 transmission from people without COVID-19 symptoms. *JAMA Netw. Open* 4 (1): e2035057. https://doi.org/10.1001/jamanetworkopen.2020.35057. Erratum in: JAMA Netw Open. 2021;4(2):e211383.

32 Zhao, H., Lu, X., Deng, Y. et al. (2020). COVID-19: asymptomatic carrier transmission is an underestimated problem. *Epidemiol. Infect.* 148: e116. https://doi.org/10.1017/S0950268820001235.

33 Li, F., Li, Y.Y., Liu, M.J. et al. (2021). Household transmission of SARS-CoV-2 and risk factors for susceptibility and infectivity in Wuhan: a retrospective observational study. *Lancet Infect. Dis.* 21 (5): 617–628. https://doi.org/10.1016/S1473-3099(20)30981-6.

34 Subramanian, R., He, Q., and Pascual, M. (2021). Quantifying asymptomatic infection and transmission of COVID-19 in New York City using observed cases, serology, and testing capacity. *Proc. Natl. Acad. Sci. U. S. A.* 118 (9): e2019716118. https://doi.org/10.1073/pnas.2019716118.

35 Ritchie H, Ortiz-Ospina E, Beltekian D, Mathieu E, Hasell J, Macdonald B, et al. (2020). Coronavirus

Pandemic (COVID-19). Our World in Data. https://ourworldindata.org/coronavirus

36 Rezaei, N. (2021). *Coronavirus Disease – COVID-19*, Advances in Experimental Medicine and Biology, vol. 1318. Zurich, Switzerland: Springer Nature Switzerland AG https://doi.org/10.1007/978-3-030-63761-3.

37 Global Infectious Hazard Preparedness World Health Organization Headquarters, WHO Worldwide (2020). Estimating mortality from COVID-19. WHO-2019-nCoV-Sci_Brief-Mortality-2020.1. World Health Organization. https://www.who.int/publications/i/item/WHO-2019-nCoV-Sci-Brief-Mortality-2020.1 (published 4 August 2020).

38 Salzberger, B., Glück, T., and Ehrenstein, B. (2020). Successful containment of COVID-19: the WHO-report on the COVID-19 outbreak in China. *Infection* 48 (2): 151–153. https://doi.org/10.1007/s15010-020-01409-4.

39 Rai, B., Shukla, A., and Dwivedi, L.K. (2021). Estimates of serial interval for COVID-19: a systematic review and meta-analysis. *Clin. Epidemiol. Glob. Health* 9: 157–161. https://doi.org/10.1016/j.cegh.2020.08.007.

40 Alimohamadi, Y., Taghdir, M., and Sepandi, M. (2020). Estimate of the basic reproduction number for COVID-19: a systematic review and meta-analysis. *J. Prev. Med. Public Health* 53 (3): 151–157. https://doi.org/10.3961/jpmph.20.076.

41 Centers for Disease Control and Prevention (2021). Excess deaths associated with COVID-19. https://www.cdc.gov/nchs/nvss/vsrr/covid19/excess_deaths.htm (updated 28 July 2021).

42 Rossen, L.M., Branum, A.M., Ahmad, F.B. et al. (2021). Notes from the field: Update on excess deaths associated with the COVID-19 pandemic — United States, January 26, 2020–February 27, 2021. *MMWR Morb. Mortal. Wkly Rep.* 70: 570–571. https://doi.org/10.15585/mmwr.mm7015a4.

43 World Health Organization (2021). The true death toll of COVID-19: estimating global excess mortality. World Health Organization. https://www.who.int/data/stories/the-true-death-toll-of-covid-19-estimating-global-excess-mortality (accessed 24 June 2021).

44 Centers for Disease Control and Prevention (2021). NVSS – provisional death counts for COVID-19: executive summary. https://www.cdc.gov/nchs/covid19/mortality-overview.htm (updated 23 April 2021).

45 Centers for Disease Control and Prevention (CDC) (2021). COVID Data Tracker: Demographic trends of COVID-19 cases and deaths in the US reported to CDC. CDC. https://covid.cdc.gov/covid-data-tracker/#demographics (accessed 24 June 2021).

46 National Center for Health Statistics (2021). COVID-19 provisional counts – weekly updates by select demographic and geographic characteristics. Centers for Disease Control and Prevention. https://www.cdc.gov/nchs/nvss/vsrr/covid_weekly/index.htm#SexAndAge (updated 2 August 2021).

47 Centers for Disease Control and Prevention (CDC) (2021). COVID-19: Risk for COVID-19 infection, hospitalization, and death by age group. National Center for Immunization and Respiratory Diseases (NCIRD), Division of Viral Diseases. https://www.cdc.gov/coronavirus/2019-ncov/covid-data/investigations-discovery/hospitalization-death-by-age.html (accessed 24 June 2021).

48 Peckham, H., de Gruijter, N.M., Raine, C. et al. (2020). Male sex identified by global COVID-19 meta-analysis as a risk factor for death and ITU admission. *Nat. Commun.* 11 (1): 6317. https://doi.org/10.1038/s41467-020-19741-6.

49 Ahrenfeldt, L.J., Otavova, M., Christensen, K., and Lindahl-Jacobsen, R. (2021). Sex and age differences in COVID-19 mortality in Europe. *Wien. Klin. Wochenschr.* 133 (7–8): 393–398. https://doi.org/10.1007/s00508-020-01793-9.

50 Dehingia, N. and Raj, A. (2021). Sex differences in COVID-19 case fatality: do we know enough? *Lancet Glob. Health* 9 (1): e14–e15. https://doi.org/10.1016/S2214-109X(20)30464-2.

51 Pradhan, A. and Olsson, P.E. (2020). Sex differences in severity and mortality from COVID-19: are males more vulnerable? *Biol. Sex Differ.* 11 (1): 53. https://doi.org/10.1186/s13293-020-00330-7.

52 Choi, D. (2020). US Gender/Sex COVID-19 Data Tracker. Harvard T.H. Chan School of Public Health. https://www.hsph.harvard.edu/social-and-behavioral-sciences/2020/07/21/us-gender-sex-covid-19-data-tracker (updated 21 July 2020).

53 Simon, P., Ho, A., Shah, M.D., and Shetgiri, R. (2021). Trends in mortality from COVID-19 and

other leading causes of death among Latino vs white individuals in Los Angeles County, 2011-2020. *JAMA* 326 (10): 973–974. https://doi.org/10.1001/jama.2021.11945.

54 United States Census Bureau (2019). QuickFacts United States https://www.census.gov/quickfacts/fact/table/US/LFE046219.

55 Centers for Disease Control and Prevention (CDC) (2021). NVSS – provisional death counts for COVID-19: executive summary. CDC. https://www.cdc.gov/nchs/covid19/mortality-overview.htm (updated 23 April 2021).

56 Centers for Disease Control and Prevention (CDC) (2020). COVID Data Tracker. CDC. https://covid.cdc.gov/covid-data-tracker (updated 28 March 2020).

57 Centers for Disease Control and Prevention (CDC) (2021). Health disparities: provisional death counts for coronavirus disease 2019 (COVID-19). https://www.cdc.gov/nchs/nvss/vsrr/covid19/health_disparities.htm (updated 28 July 2021).

58 Lauer, K.B., Borrow, R., and Blanchard, T.J. (2017). Multivalent and multipathogen viral vector vaccines. *Clin. Vaccine Immunol.* 24 (1): e00298-16. https://doi.org/10.1128/CVI.00298-16.

59 US Food and Drug Administration (FDA) (2021). Vaccines and related biological products advisory committee February 26, 2021: meeting announcement. FDA. https://www.fda.gov/advisory-committees/advisory-committee-calendar/vaccines-and-related-biological-products-advisory-committee-february-26-2021-meeting-announcement (published 26 February 2021).

60 Kyriakidis, N.C., López-Cortés, A., González, E.V. et al. (2021). SARS-CoV-2 vaccines strategies: a comprehensive review of phase 3 candidates. *NPJ Vaccines* 6 (1): 28. https://doi.org/10.1038/s41541-021-00292-w.

61 Sadoff, J., Gray, G., Vandebosch, A. et al. (2021). ENSEMBLE Study Group. Safety and efficacy of single-dose Ad26.COV2.S vaccine against Covid-19. *N. Engl. J. Med.* 384 (23): 2187–2201. https://doi.org/10.1056/NEJMoa2101544.

62 Logunov, D.Y., Dolzhikova, I.V., Shcheblyakov, D.V. et al. (2021). Gam-COVID-Vac Vaccine Trial Group. Safety and efficacy of an rAd26 and rAd5 vector-based heterologous prime-boost COVID-19 vaccine: an interim analysis of a randomised controlled phase 3 trial in Russia. *Lancet* 397 (10275): 671–681. https://doi.org/10.1016/S0140-6736(21)00234-8. Erratum in: Lancet. 2021;397(10275):670.

63 US Food and Drug Administration (2021). COVID-19 vaccines. FDA. https://www.fda.gov/emergency-preparedness-and-response/coronavirus-disease-2019-covid-19/covid-19-vaccines.

64 Frederiksen, L.S.F., Zhang, Y., Foged, C., and Thakur, A. (2020). The long road toward COVID-19 herd immunity: vaccine platform technologies and mass immunization strategies. *Front. Immunol.* 11: 1817. https://doi.org/10.3389/fimmu.2020.01817.

65 Harvey, W.T., Carabelli, A.M., Jackson, B. et al. (2021). COVID-19 Genomics UK (COG-UK) Consortium. SARS-CoV-2 variants, spike mutations and immune escape. *Nat. Rev. Microbiol.* 19 (7): 409–424. https://doi.org/10.1038/s41579-021-00573-0.

66 Leung, K., Shum, M.H., Leung, G.M. et al. (2021). Early transmissibility assessment of the N501Y mutant strains of SARS-CoV-2 in the United Kingdom, October to November 2020. *Euro Surveill.* 26: 2002106. https://doi.org/10.2807/1560-7917.ES.2020.26.1.2002106.

67 Edara, V.V., Lai, L., Sahoo, M.K. et al. (2021). Infection and vaccine-induced neutralizing antibody responses to the SARS-CoV-2 B.1.617.1 variant. *bioRxiv* https://doi.org/10.1101/2021.05.09.443299.

68 Xu, J., Lim, K., and Rutherford, G.W. (2021). What can we learn about SARS-CoV-2 herd immunity from isolated populations? *J. Correct Health Care* In press.

69 Tande, A.J., Pollock, B.D., Shah, N.D. et al. (2021). Impact of the COVID-19 vaccine on asymptomatic infection among patients undergoing pre-procedural COVID-19 molecular screening. *Clin. Infect. Dis.* 2021: ciab229. https://doi.org/10.1093/cid/ciab229.

70 Levine-Tiefenbrun, M., Yelin, I., Katz, R. et al. (2021). Initial report of decreased SARS-CoV-2 viral load after inoculation with the BNT162b2 vaccine. *Nat. Med.* 27 (5): 790–792. https://doi.org/10.1038/s41591-021-01316-7.

71 Pritchard, E., Matthews, P.C., Stoesser, N. et al. (2021). Impact of vaccination on new SARS-CoV-2 infections in the United Kingdom. *Nat. Med.* 27: 1370–1378. https://doi.org/10.1038/s41591-021-01410-w.

72 Centers for Disease Control and Prevention (CDC) (2021). Interim public health recommendations for

fully vaccinated people. CDC. Available from: https://www.cdc.gov/coronavirus/2019-ncov/vaccines/fully-vaccinated-guidance.html (updated 28 July 2021).

73 Karmakar, M., Lantz, P.M., and Tipirneni, R. (2021). Association of social and demographic factors with COVID-19 incidence and death rates in the US. *JAMA Netw. Open* 4 (1): e2036462. https://doi.org/10.1001/jamanetworkopen.2020.36462.

74 Centers for Disease Control and Prevention (CDC) (2021). Strategies for optimizing the supply of N95 respirators: COVID-19. CDC. https://www.cdc.gov/coronavirus/2019-ncov/hcp/respirators-strategy/index.html (updated 30 July 2021).

75 Centers for Disease Control and Prevention (CDC) (2020). Infection control guidance for healthcare professionals about coronavirus (COVID-19). CDC. https://www.cdc.gov/coronavirus/2019-nCoV/hcp/infection-control.html (updated 18 September 2020).

76 World Health Organization (WHO) (2020). Mask use in the context of COVID-19: WHO. https://www.who.int/publications/i/item/advice-on-the-use-of-masks-in-the-community-during-home-care-and-in-healthcare-settings-in-the-context-of-the-novel-coronavirus-(2019-ncov)-outbreak (published 1 December 2020).

77 Chu, D.K., Akl, E.A., Duda, S. et al. (2020). COVID-19 Systematic Urgent Review Group Effort (SURGE) study authors. Physical distancing, face masks, and eye protection to prevent person-to-person transmission of SARS-CoV-2 and COVID-19: a systematic review and meta-analysis. *Lancet* 395 (10242): 1973–1987. https://doi.org/10.1016/S0140-6736(20)31142-9.

78 Pan, J., St Pierre, J.M., Pickering, T.A. et al. (2020). Coronavirus disease 2019 (COVID-19): a modeling study of factors driving variation in case fatality rate by country. *Int. J. Environ. Res. Public Health* 17 (21): 8189. https://doi.org/10.3390/ijerph17218189.

79 Pradhan, D., Biswasroy, P., Kumar Naik, P. et al. (2020). A review of current interventions for COVID-19 prevention. *Arch. Med. Res.* 51 (5): 363–374. https://doi.org/10.1016/j.arcmed.2020.04.020.

80 Marquès, M. and Domingo, J.L. (2021). Contamination of inert surfaces by SARS-CoV-2: persistence, stability and infectivity. A review. *Environ. Res.* 193: 110559. https://doi.org/10.1016/j.envres.2020.110559.

81 Hirose, R., Ikegaya, H., Naito, Y. et al. (2020). Survival of SARS-CoV-2 and influenza virus on the human skin: importance of hand hygiene in COVID-19. *Clin. Infect. Dis.* 2020: ciaa1517. https://doi.org/10.1093/cid/ciaa1517.

82 Dai, H. and Zhao, B. (2020). Association of the infection probability of COVID-19 with ventilation rates in confined spaces. *Build. Simul.* 13: 1321–1327. https://doi.org/10.1007/s12273-020-0703-5.

83 Mousavi, E.S., Kananizadeh, N., Martinello, R.A., and Sherman, J.D. (2021). COVID-19 outbreak and hospital air quality: a systematic review of evidence on air filtration and recirculation. *Environ. Sci. Technol.* 55 (7): 4134–4147. https://doi.org/10.1021/acs.est.0c03247.

84 Bulfone, T.C., Malekinejad, M., Rutherford, G.W., and Razani, N. (2021). Outdoor transmission of SARS-CoV-2 and other respiratory viruses: a systematic review. *J. Infect. Dis.* 223: 550–561.

85 Qian, H., Miao, T., Liu, L. et al. (2021). Indoor transmission of SARS-CoV-2 [published online ahead of print October 31, 2020]. *Indoor Air* 31: 639–645. https://doi.org/10.1111/ina.12766.

86 Leclerc, Q.J., Fuller, N.M., Knight, L.E. et al. (2020). CMMID COVID-19 Working Group. What settings have been linked to SARS-CoV-2 transmission clusters? *Wellcome Open Res.* 5: 83.

87 Johns Hopkins University & Medicine (2021). Mortality analyses – Johns Hopkins Coronavirus Resource Center. Johns Hopkins University & Medicine. https://coronavirus.jhu.edu/data/mortality.

88 United Nations (2020). UN News: COVID-19 pandemic exposes global "frailties and inequalities": UN deputy chief. UN News Centre. https://news.un.org/en/story/2020/05/1063022 (updated 3 May 2020).

89 Novelli, G., Biancolella, M., Mehrian-Shai, R. et al. (2020). COVID-19 update: the first 6 months of the pandemic. *Hum. Genomics* 14 (1): 48. https://doi.org/10.1186/s40246-020-00298-w.

90 Guest, J.L., Del Rio, C., and Sanchez, T. (2020). The three steps needed to end the COVID-19 pandemic: bold public health leadership, rapid innovations, and courageous political will. *JMIR Public Health Surveill.* 6 (2): e19043. https://doi.org/10.2196/19043.

91 Frieden, T. (January 1, 2021). Which countries have responded best to Covid-19? *Wall Street J.*. https://www.wsj.com/articles/which-countries-have-responded-best-to-covid-19-11609516800.

92 US Department of Health and Human Services (2017). Pandemic influenza plan: 2017 update: US Department of Health and Human Services. https://www.cdc.gov/flu/pandemic-resources/pdf/pan-flu-report-2017v2.pdf.

93 Dighe, A., Cattarino, L., Cuomo-Dannenburg, G. et al. (2020). Response to COVID-19 in South Korea and implications for lifting stringent interventions. *BMC Med.* 18 (1): 321. https://doi.org/10.1186/s12916-020-01791-8.

2

COVID-19: Virology

Saeideh Najafi[1], Salar Tofighi[1], and Juliana Sobczyk[2,3]

[1] Department of Radiology, Keck School of Medicine, University of Southern California, Los Angeles, CA, USA
[2] Department of Pathology, Memorial Satilla Hospital, HCA Healthcare, Waycross, GA, USA
[3] Laboratory Director, St. Augustine Foot & Ankle, Inc., St. Augustine, FL, USA

Abbreviations

ACE2	angiotensin-converting enzyme 2
CoV	coronavirus
ER	endoplasmic reticulum
HE	hemagglutinin esterase
MERS	Middle Eastern respiratory syndrome
MERS-CoV	Middle Eastern respiratory syndrome coronavirus
nsp	nonstructural protein
NTD	N-terminal domain
ORF	open reading frame
RBD	receptor-binding domain
RdRp	RNA-dependent RNA polymerase
SARS	severe acute respiratory syndrome
SARS-CoV-2	severe acute respiratory syndrome coronavirus 2
ssRNA	single-stranded RNA
VoC	variant of concern
VoHC	variant of high consequence
VoI	variant of interest
WHO	World Health Organization

In the 1960s, around the time new methods to grow viruses in laboratories became available, scientists cultivated two previously unknown viruses, 229E and OC43, from patients with symptoms of acute upper respiratory tract infection (Figure 2.1). These viruses had not been detected because the prevalent primary cell types used as culture media were not susceptible to these new viruses. However, brain cell lines derived from neuroblastoma, neuroglioma, and astrocytoma cells demonstrated high susceptibility to infection of these viruses and enabled scientists to grow them in vitro [1]. These viruses were unlike any viruses previously known to cause similar symptoms. These novel viruses had fringe-like projections that resembled solar corona under electron microscopy. Thus, in 1968, these viruses with characteristic surface spikes of 200 Å were proposed to be named coronavirus (CoV) [2]. A study around this time in Italy demonstrated the high prevalence and common occurrence of infection with CoV through detection of antibodies using an indirect immunoperoxidase staining technique, hemagglutination inhibition test, and plaque reduction neutralization assay [3].

Initially, CoV had been deemed to cause only mild symptoms. In 2002, a new CoV emerged that caused symptoms of severe acute respiratory syndrome (SARS) with a high mortality rate. This new strain, named severe acute respiratory syndrome coronavirus (SARS-CoV), is thought to originate from bats as its natural host [4]. Unlike previously known human CoVs that underwent coevolution with humans and therefore caused only minor symptoms, the sudden access of SARS-CoV to a new host led to severe respiratory symptoms and increased mortality. Later, researchers isolated two new strains (NL63 and HKU1) of CoV from patients with pneumonia, although these strains are believed to most commonly cause mild common cold symptoms [5]. In 2012, Middle Eastern respiratory syndrome coronavirus (MERS-CoV)

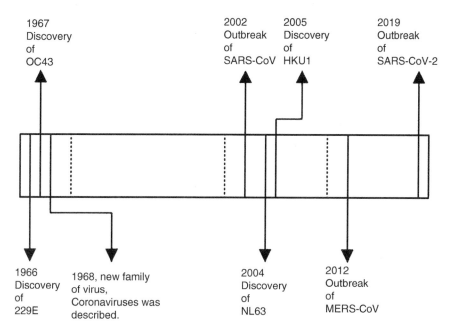

Figure 2.1 Timeline of discoveries of CoVs.

emerged in Saudi Arabia. Similarly, MERS-CoV also rapidly crossed species from bats as reservoirs and camels as intermediate hosts to humans and caused severe respiratory symptoms and high mortality [4]. Nevertheless, prior to 2019, the majority of CoV types known to infect humans (four of six types) primarily caused mild respiratory symptoms.

In early December 2019, an unknown infectious agent caused an outbreak of unusual viral pneumonia in Wuhan in the Hubei province of China. The first cases were linked to a seafood market, but soon widespread person-to-person transmission was observed [6, 7]. Clusters of disease were discovered in families and their close contacts. Many patients presented with fever, cough, and chest discomfort. Some of the infected individuals experienced severe dyspnea and hypoxia with bilateral lung infiltration seen on radiologic imaging. In January 2020, the disease's causative agent was determined to be the seventh CoV to infect humans, SARS-CoV-2, and its genome was sequenced.

In the beginning, the new CoV was known as the 2019-novel coronavirus (2019-nCoV). The disease spread reached epidemic levels in China by February 2020. Although officials worldwide executed rigorous lockdowns as one mean to control the virus spread in and from China, international travelers had already initiated the spread of the virus to other continents. On 31 January 2020, the World Health Organization (WHO) declared a public health emergency of international concern. The International Committee on Taxonomy of Viruses renamed the new virus SARS-CoV-2 and termed the illness sequelae coronavirus disease 2019 (COVID-19) [8]. Rapid worldwide transmission led to the pandemic declaration on 11 March 2020. The number of people infected and the geographical radius of SARS-CoV-2 surpassed those of both MERS and SARS-CoV and caused unprecedented global public health and economic crises.

Coronaviruses

Taxonomy

The Coronavirus family is placed under the order *Nidovirales* and is also known as *Coronaviridae*. *Coronavirinea* is a subfamily under the family *Coronaviridae*. The *Coronavirinae* subfamily is further divided into four genera: *Alphacoronavirus*, *Betacoronavirus*, *Gammacoronavirus*, and *Deltacoronavirus* (Figure 2.2). The second subfamily under *Coronaviridae* is *Torovirinea*. *Torovirus* and

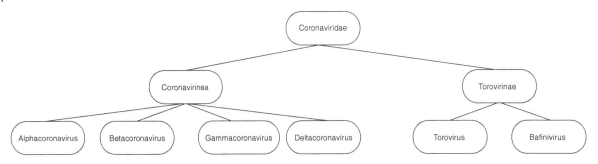

Figure 2.2   Classification of CoVs.

Bafinivirus are two genera under the *Torovirinae* subfamily. *Alphacoronaviruses* and *Betacoronaviruses* replicate in mammal hosts, *Gammacoronaviruses* and *Deltacoronaviruses* in bird hosts, *Toroviruses* in mammal hosts, and *Bafiniviruses* in fish hosts [2].

The four human CoVs that have been known to cause mild symptoms are two *Alphacoronaviruses* (229E and NL63) and two *Betacoronaviruses* (OC43 and HKU1). SARS-CoV-2, SARS-CoV, and MERS-CoV belong to the *Betacoronaviruses*. Most known *Coronavirinea* members have been isolated from bat reservoirs. Bats are believed to be an optimal host among mammals for viral evolution because they live in large colonies with close proximity. SARS-CoV and SARS-related CoVs have been isolated from bats and civets. The closest genetically related species to SARS-CoV-2 have been found in horseshoe bats and pangolins (RmYN02 and RaTG13) [2, 5, 6].

Morphology

Coronaviridae are enveloped viruses with spherical (*Coronaviruses*), bacillar (*Bafinivirus*), or crescentic (*Toroviruses*) shapes (Figure 2.3). Virions are decorated with petal-shaped projections of homotrimeric proteins on their surfaces [2, 5]. These projections, known as protein S, spikes, or peplomers, establish the host range and facilitate the initial steps of infection by binding to host cell receptors and genetic material injection. Another structural protein, protein M, is the most abundant protein in the viral particle. Protein M is a dimeric protein and integrated

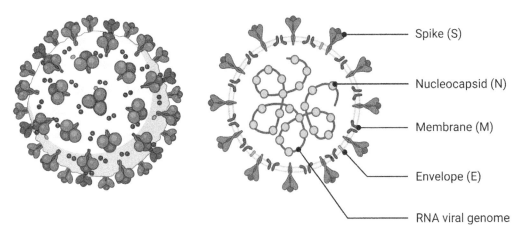

Figure 2.3   Structure of a CoV. *Source:* Created with http://BioRender.com.

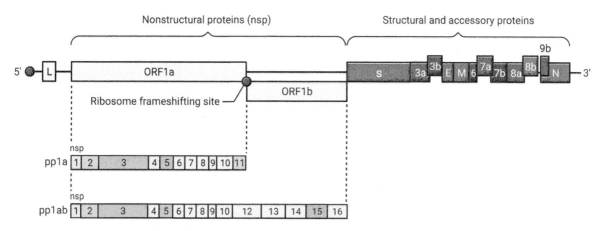

Figure 2.4 Schematic of SARS-CoV-2 genome. ORF, open reading frame. *Source:* Created with http://BioRender.com.

into virion membranes of the *Coronaviridae* family. It plays an essential role in the assembly and morphogenesis of virions. The endodomain of protein M forms a matrix-like lattice that supports the thick membrane of CoVs [5]. The envelope in CoVs (7–7.8 nm) is two times thicker than the average thickness of biologic membranes (4 nm) [2].

The nucleocapsid (protein N) houses the viral genomic RNA. The nucleocapsid forms a helix via attachments to basic phosphoproteins, protein N, and is susceptible to treatment with detergents. In addition to encapsulation, protein N participates in RNA synthesis, translation, and interferon antagonism [2, 5]. Some *Betacoronaviruses* and *Toroviruses* possess hemagglutinin esterase (HE) protein on their surface, which functions in viral attachment. *Coronavirinea* also produce protein E, a small protein on its surface, which acts in virion assembly and morphogenesis.

Nucleic Acid

The family of *Coronaviridae* possesses the largest genetic material among viruses (26–32 kb) that is composed of an unsegmented positive single-stranded RNA (ssRNA) [2]. The RNA molecule is 5′-capped and 3′-polyadenylated, containing multiple open reading frames (ORFs) (Figure 2.4). After the 5′ untranslated region, two thirds of the genome encode replicase proteins (two overlapping ORF1a and ORF1b segments). As a result of ribosomal frameshifting, these segments yield two polyproteins, pp1a and pp1ab. Proteinases further process these polyproteins during and after

translation to produce 15 or 16 nonstructural proteins (nsps), depending on the virus genera. These proteins are named from nsp1 to nsp16 in order of their position from 5′ to 3′. nsps function in viral replication, virus–host interaction, and evasion from the immune system. Distal to the nsp segment, segments for structural proteins S, E, M, and N are positioned. In the *Coronavirinea* subgroup, various numbers of accessory genes, such as HE, are interspersed among structural proteins [2, 4, 5].

Viral-positive ssRNA acts as both a messenger RNA for protein transcription and a template for the synthesis of negative ssRNA. CoVs are RNA viruses and use RNA-dependent RNA polymerase (RdRp) to replicate their genome. Viral RdRp read the genome in a noncontiguous manner, jumping from one region to another to synthesize RNA. A distinguishing feature of CoVs is they synthesize segmented subgenomic messenger RNAs from negative-strand RNA to replicate viral RNA. The nucleocapsid is assembled in the cytoplasm of the host cell and enters the endoplasmic reticulum (ER), whereas the structural proteins are assembled in the ER and Golgi apparatus. Preformed nucleocapsids bud from the ER and Golgi systems and exit the host cell through exocytosis [4].

Antigenicity

The strongest antibody response against CoVs is provoked by exposure to proteins S and N. Production of neutralizing antibodies by the immune system is mainly induced by protein S. These antibodies have been used in some serologic tests for the diagnosis of infections as well. The variability observed in protein genes suggests extensive antigenic drift and shift via mutations and RNA recombination. Cross-reactivity of antibodies is usually limited to viral antigens from the same genera. Protein N is the most abundant protein during cellular replication within the host, but antibodies produced against it do not neutralize the virus. However, these antibodies can be targeted by diagnostic serologic assays to detect immunoglobulins against protein N [9]. Antibodies are also produced against protein M. These antibodies require involvement of the complement system to neutralize the virion. in vivo, virions expressing protein HE on the surface induce production of anti-HE antibodies, which prevents viral attachment. Protein E is the least abundant protein and is required in multiple steps of the viral life cycle, such as assembly, budding, and envelope formation [10]. Virions lacking protein E are a strategy for live attenuated vaccines for MERS and SARS-CoV [11, 12].

SARS-CoV-2

Morphology and Nucleic Acid

The structure and genome of SARS-CoV-2 follows the same principles as other CoVs: a spherical-shaped particle with petal-like spikes. Protein M is the most abundant protein, and protein E is the smallest protein integrated into the envelope. Virion membrane does not possess protein HE. The nucleocapsid resides inside the envelope as a helix attached to protein N. The positive ssRNA contains five major ORFs (ORF1a/1ab, S, N, M, and E) and five accessory ORFs (3a, 6, 7a, 8, and 10). nsp12 is an RdRp that works with nsp7 and nsp8 to replicate the viral genome with the collaboration of the host replicative apparatus [4, 5].

Spike Protein

Because of the role protein S plays in viral infectivity and cellular entry, treatment and prevention strategies for SARS-CoV-2 often target protein S. The ORF related to protein S is the first structural ORF after two replicase ORFs in the viral RNA sequence from 5′ to 3′ and encodes the largest viral structural protein. Protein S is a homotrimeric type 1 transmembrane protein with an N-terminal ectodomain. Each monomer of protein S is subdivided into two subunits, S1 and S2 (Figure 2.5). The S1 subunit interacts with host cell receptor angiotensin-converting enzyme 2 (ACE2), while the S2 subunit runs the fusion machinery. The S1 subunit is composed of the N-terminal domain (NTD), receptor-binding domain (RBD), and

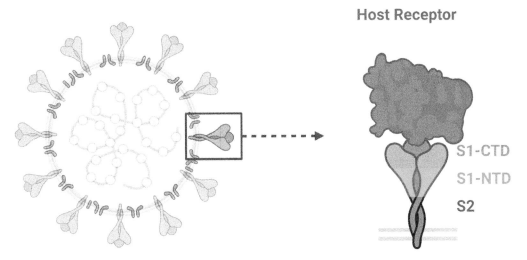

Figure 2.5   Structure of a SARS-CoV-2 spike protein. CTD, C-terminal domain; NTD, N-terminal domain. *Source:* Created with http://BioRender.com.

two conserved subdomains (SD1 and SD2). The S2 subunit is composed of the C-terminal domain, two heptad regions, transmembrane domain, and cytosolic tail [12]. In viral hosts, the ACE2 receptor is expressed in the epithelia of the respiratory system, cardiovascular system, genitourinary system, and gastrointestinal system, as well as the liver, gallbladder, vasculature, and nervous system [13].

In the prefusion state, the S1 shields the S2 subunit and blocks its interaction with the host cell and the resultant fusion. The S1 subunit is cleaved and released by proteases to uncover the S2 subunit and activate the fusion process. The binding of RBD to ACE2 initiates the process of cleaving the S1 subunit. The S1 subunit shows flexibility and undergoes conformational change via a hingelike mechanism between an up (open) state, which hides the RBD from the receptor, and a down (close) state, which exposes the RBD. Monoclonal antibodies used for treatment of COVID-19 may be active against both the up and down states, or may be active against only one of these states [14]. In the up state, the receptor-binding motif within the RBD forms the initial attachment with the carboxypeptidase portion of the ACE2 receptor. After the attachment, host cell proteases initiate two steps of cleavage, priming and activation [15]. Cleavage occurs between S1 and S2, as well as at the S2′ domain, and releases the S1 subunit [16].

In the case of SARS-CoV-2, a polybasic amino acid sequence of PRPP at the junction of S1 and S2 is present, which is susceptible to furin proteases. Furin is found abundantly in the human respiratory system and activates the S protein of viral particles after release from host cells. These preactivated virions do not need to be activated by ACE2 receptors after transmission to another host [17].

Origin

The origin of SARS-CoV-2 is unknown, and proposed theories are controversial. History has demonstrated novel infectious viral agents commonly arise from animal sources. For instance, the H1N1 pdm09 virus responsible for the 2009 H1N1 influenza pandemic resulted from the reassortment of Eurasian avian-like swine H1N1 influenza virus, avian H1N1 virus, classical swine H1N1 virus, and human H3N2 virus [18]. Animal–human contact allows for cross-species transmission (known as spillover), the likelihood of which is increased by increased frequency of contact and proximity between animals and humans. Many factors play a role and must be considered to understand the origin of a virus. The diversity of the virus in animal reservoirs and the complexity of contacts complicate the determination of viral origin. Transmission to humans may also occur multiple times in the evolution of a virus from its animal host, which further complicates the study of viral origin because these early steps may remain undetected. Before the transmission can take place and be sustained, the virus must adapt with the conditions of the new human environment. Adaptation may occur either suddenly or evolve gradually over time. Adaptation may also happen in different steps in viral clusters located in diverse species and geographical sites.

The novel virus's genome is 79% identical to the SARS-CoV genome and 50% identical to MERS-CoV [19]. SARS-CoV-2 structural proteins and nsps share more than 90% and 85% amino acid identity, respectively, with SARS-CoV [13, 19, 20]. Therefore, SARS-CoV-2 was initially assigned to the genus *Betacoronavirus* and subgenus *Sarbecovirus*. However, whole-genome analysis demonstrated a 96.2% similarity between SARS-CoV-2 and bat *Sarbecovirus* RaTG13 [13] and a 93.3% genome identity with novel bat *Sarbecovirus* RmYN02 [6, 21]. In addition, two other bat *Sarbecoviruses* (RshSTT200 and RshSTT182) sampled in 2010 in Cambodia were recently sequenced and demonstrated 92.6% nucleotide similarity with SARS-CoV-2, indicative of the geographical dispersal of related viruses [22]. This indicates that SARS-CoV-2 is more closely related to the bat *Sarbecoviruses* than the previously encountered human viruses of SARS-CoV and MERS-CoV.

One specific feature of SARS-CoV-2 not observed in other CoVs is the insertion of PRRA amino acids at the junction of S1 and S2 domains of spike protein and creation of a polybasic (RRAR) cleavage region for furin proteases, increasing infectivity. Although not a furin cleavage site, a similar three-amino acid insertion (PAA) was seen in RmYN02, indicating the possibility of naturally acquiring this characteristic feature [23]. Amino acid insertions have been discovered in RshSTT200 and RshSTT182 as well.

Recent viral studies found related viruses in Malayan pangolins. One study on viruses isolated from Malayan pangolins (pangolin-CoV-GDC) in 2019 disclosed a 90.1% similarity of genome identity with SARS-CoV-2. The structural protein amino acid sequences were 100% similar for protein E, 98.6% for protein M, 97.8% for protein N, and 90.7% for protein S [24]. In a second study on Malayan pangolins, samples isolated in 2017–2018 (pangolin-CoV-GDC) showed a genomic sequence sharing 85% identity with SARS-CoV-2 [25]. SARS-CoV-2, SARS-CoV, and RaTG13 bind ACE2 receptors in host cells via their RBD, but only one of six critical amino acids in the binding site is shared between SARS-CoV-2 and SARS-CoV and RaTG13. In contrast, all six amino acids are identical between pangolin-CoV-GDC and SARS-CoV-2 [24, 25]. Similarities between pangolin-CoV-GDC and SARS-CoV-2 persuaded some scientists to consider pangolin-CoV-GDC as the most likely reservoir for SARS-CoV-2. However, studies showed that RBD of pangolin-CoV-GDC has a low affinity to ACE2. High affinity to the ACE2 receptor is a feature that is shared by bat viruses [26].

Although studies have suggested bats as natural reservoirs of SARS-CoV-2, the route of transmission to humans remains unknown. In March 2021, a WHO joint team suggested four credible transmission pathways in their latest report: through an intermediate host, through a direct zoonotic introduction, through cold/food chain, or through a laboratory incident. Although pangolin, mink, and bat have been proposed as a potential direct zoonotic source of transmission to humans, the affinity of RBD in the spike protein of related CoVs to ACE2 receptors is lower than SARS-CoV-2, and decades of evolutionary space exist compared with SARS-CoV-2. These facts suggest a missing link between these CoVs and SARS-CoV-2, such as an undiscovered ancestor or an intermediate host. The joint team found no conclusive evidence on the transmission through the cold/food chain, involving the consumption of animal products or the use of containers contaminated with animal wastes, or on the occurrence of a laboratory accident [6].

Viral Transmission

The primary modes of transmission for SARS-CoV-2 include droplets and aerosols [27, 28]. Fomite (contaminated surface) has been suggested as a rare mean of transmission [28]. Although SARS-CoV-2 RNA has been detected in feces and urine, there have been no published reports of transmission. SARS-CoV-2 RNA can be detected in plasma or serum, but the role of bloodborne transmission remains unclear. There is currently no evidence to suggest intrauterine transmission of SARS-CoV-2 or transmission through breastfeeding [28]. Viral particles can access the host via droplet or aerosol inhalation into air spaces or direct deposition (inoculation, touching) of mucous membranes.

Aerosols are particles smaller than 5 μm primarily dispersed during breathing and speaking. They are a significant means of transmission in symptomatic and asymptomatic patients and can travel long distances in the air, which increases transmission. Larger particles, called droplets, are released while talking, coughing, or sneezing and can then be inhaled. Aerosol and droplet emission increases during exercise and loud speech [29]. After reaching the susceptible host, droplets are confined to the upper respiratory tract because of their larger size, whereas aerosols can reach alveolar space and directly infect the lungs [28]. Short-distance (<1 m) transmission is the main transmission route and occurs via aerosols and droplets. Long-distance (≥1 m) transmission mainly occurs as a result of aerosols in poorly ventilated indoor spaces [27]. Droplets may also settle on surfaces to form fomites. Fomites can then be transferred by touching the infective surface and then self-inoculating mucous membranes.

Variants

Mutations take place constantly in viruses, which can change their characteristics. However, the rate of mutations in CoVs is low due to the high proofreading efficacy of RdRp [30]. SARS-CoV-2 variants have emerged because of the extremely high prevalence of SARS-CoV-2. Each variant possesses one or more distinguishing mutations, which separates it from other circulating variants. When a variant confers a selective benefit to the virus, it becomes prevalent. For instance, mutation D614G took place early in the pandemic and essentially replaced the sequence of the original virus. Patients infected with this mutant virus have a higher viral load than the original virus, suggesting increased infectivity that selected for the dominance of this mutation [31, 32]. Nevertheless, numerous other SARS-CoV-2 variants have emerged around the world, most having little clinical significance. Effects on transmissibility, severity of disease, and escape from host immune response or vaccines are possible consequences of new variants that impact the clinical significance, particularly when the mutations arise in the S protein. Changes inside the RBD and NTD of the S protein are most concerning because they are the main target of host antibody production [33].

For rapid characterization of emerging variants and to actively monitor the potential impact on critical SARS-CoV-2 countermeasures (i.e. vaccines, therapeutics, and laboratory diagnostic testing), the Centers for Disease Control and Prevention and WHO classified variants into three groups: variants of interest (VoIs), variants of concern (VoCs), and variants of high consequence (VoHCs). VoIs have been identified to cause multiple clusters of disease and are associated with phenotypic changes that are suspected to negatively modify receptor binding, neutralization by antibodies, efficacy of treatments and diagnostics, and transmissibility or disease severity. VoCs are assigned when comparative studies show evidence of impact on diagnostics, treatments, or vaccines; widespread interference with diagnostic test targets; substantially decreased susceptibility to one or more classes of therapies; significantly decreased neutralization by antibodies generated during previous infection or vaccination; reduced vaccine-induced protection from severe disease; increased transmissibility; or increased disease severity. VoHCs are defined as conferring a negative impact on medical countermeasures, including

failure of diagnostics, a significant reduction in vaccine effectiveness, a disproportionately high number of vaccine breakthrough cases, very low vaccine-induced protection against severe disease, significantly reduced susceptibility to multiple Emergency Use Authorization or approved therapeutics, or more severe clinical disease and increased hospitalizations. As of August 2021, no variant has been assigned to VoHC [6, 34].

Several mutations within the spike protein have been observed among VoCs. The N501Y, E484K, E484Q, and L452R are located inside the RBD. The N501Y and E484K have led to increased affinity to the ACE2 receptor [35, 36]. The E484K, E484Q, and L452R have also caused reduced neutralization [37, 38]. Recently, these mutations have led to four variants that became prevalent and caused public health concerns (Table 2.1). In December 2020, the alpha variant B.1.1.7 (also known as VOC-202012/01) was discovered in the United Kingdom. Also, in December 2020, another variant named B.1.351 (also known as 510Y·V2 or beta) emerged in South Africa. Variant P1 (gamma) was observed in Brazil in January 2021. The mutation in RBD, N501Y, was present in all three variants in which amino acid asparagine (N) is replaced by tyrosine (Y) at position 501. In October 2020, the B.1.617, or delta, variant of SARS-COV-2 was initially detected in India and spread rapidly to become the dominant strain in many other countries, including the United Kingdom and United States. This variant has reduced susceptibility to antibodies produced by vaccines and therapeutic monoclonal antibodies [56]. The variant of B.1.617 is divided into three subgroups: B.1.617.1, B.1.617.2, and B.1.617.3; among them, the B.617.2 variant is assigned as VoC because it drastically enhances infectivity [57]. The B.1.617 variant includes nine spike mutations, two mutations in the RBD, five mutations in the NTD, one mutation in the spike S2 subunit, and one mutation in the furin-cleavage site.

Table 2.1 Characteristics of SARS-CoV-2 variants.

Name	WHO label	Spike protein mutation	Country	Threat level in US	Characteristics
B.1.1.7	Alpha	69del, 70del, 144del, N501Y, A570D, D614G, P681H, T716I, S982A, D1118H	United Kingdom	VoC	• Increased transmission [39] • Potential increased severity based on hospitalizations and case fatality rates [40] • No impact on susceptibility to EUA monoclonal antibody treatments [41, 42] • Minimal impact on neutralization by convalescent and postvaccination sera [43–49]
B.1.351	Beta	D80A, D215G, 241del, 242del, 243del, K417N, E484K, N501Y, D614G, A701V	South Africa	VoC	• Increased transmission [50] • Significantly reduced susceptibility to the combination of bamlanivimab and etesevimab monoclonal antibody treatment [41], but other EUA monoclonal antibody treatments are available [42] • Reduced neutralization by convalescent and postvaccination sera [43, 47, 49, 51, 52]
B.1.617.2	Delta	T19R, T95I, G142D, E156-, F157-, R158G, L452R, T478K, D614G, P681R, D950N	India	VoC	• Potential reduction in neutralization by some EUA monoclonal antibody treatments [41, 42] • Potential reduction in neutralization by postvaccination sera [53]
P.1 P.1.1 P.1.2	Gamma	L18F, T20N, P26S, D138Y, R190S, K417T, E484K, N501Y, D614G, H655Y, T1027I	Japan/Brazil	VoC	• Significantly reduced susceptibility to the combination of bamlanivimab and etesevimab monoclonal antibody treatment [41], but other EUA monoclonal antibody treatments are available [42] • Reduced neutralization by convalescent and postvaccination sera [43]
B.1.525	Eta	A67V, 69del, 70del, 144del, E484K, D614G, Q677H, F888L	United Kingdom/ Nigeria	VoI	• Potential reduction in neutralization by some EUA monoclonal antibody treatments [41, 42] • Potential reduction in neutralization by convalescent and postvaccination sera [54]
B.1.526	Iota	L5F, T95I, D253G, E484K, D614G, A701V	US (New York)	VoI	• Reduced susceptibility to the combination of bamlanivimab and etesevimab monoclonal antibody treatment; however, the clinical implications of this are not known [41, 42]; alternative monoclonal antibody treatments are available [42] • Reduced neutralization by convalescent and postvaccination sera [54, 55]
B.1.617.1	Kappa	(T95I), G142D, E154K, L452R, E484Q, D614G, P681R, Q1071H	India	VoI	• Potential reduction in neutralization by some EUA monoclonal antibody treatments [41, 42] • Potential reduction in neutralization by postvaccination sera [37]
B.1.617.3		T19R, G142D, L452R, E484Q, D614G, P681R, D950N	India	VoI	• Potential reduction in neutralization by some EUA monoclonal antibody treatments [41, 42] • Potential reduction in neutralization by postvaccination sera [37]

EUA, Emergency Use Authorization; US, United States.
Data are from the Centers for Disease Control and Prevention [34].

References

1 Lambert, F., Jacomy, H., Marceau, G., and Talbot, P.J. (2008). Titration of human coronaviruses, HcoV-229E and HCoV-OC43, by an indirect immunoperoxidase assay. *Methods Mol. Biol.* 454: 93–102.

2 de Groot, R.J., Baker, S.C., Baric, R. et al. (2012). Family - Coronaviridae. In: *Virus taxonomy* (eds. A.M.Q. King, M.J. Adams, E.B. Carstens and E.J. Lefkowitz), 806–828. San Diego: Elsevier.

3 Cereda, P.M., Pagani, L., and Romero, E. (1986). Prevalence of antibody to human coronaviruses 229E, OC43 and neonatal calf diarrhea coronavirus (NCDCV) in patients of northern Italy. *Eur. J. Epidemiol.* 2 (2): 112–117.

4 Hu, B., Guo, H., Zhou, P., and Shi, Z.L. (2021). Characteristics of SARS-CoV-2 and COVID-19. *Nat. Rev. Microbiol.* 19 (3): 141–154.

5 Mittal, A., Manjunath, K., Ranjan, R.K. et al. (2020). COVID-19 pandemic: insights into structure, function, and hACE2 receptor recognition by SARS-CoV-2. *PLoS Pathog.* 16 (8): e1008762.

6 World Health Organization (2021). WHO-convened global study of origins of SARS-CoV-2: China part. World Health Organization. https://www.who.int/publications/i/item/who-convened-global-study-of-origins-of-sars-cov-2-china-part.

7 Deng, S.-Q. and Peng, H.-J. (2020). Characteristics of and public health responses to the coronavirus disease 2019 outbreak in China. *J. Clin. Med.* 9 (2): 575.

8 Coronaviridae Study Group of the International Committee on Taxonomy of Viruses (2020). The species severe acute respiratory syndrome-related coronavirus: classifying 2019-nCoV and naming it SARS-CoV-2. *Nat. Microbiol.* 5 (4): 536.

9 Smithgall, M.C., Dowlatshahi, M., Spitalnik, S.L. et al. (2020). Types of assays for SARS-CoV-2 testing: a review. *Lab. Med.* 51 (5): e59–e65.

10 Schoeman, D. and Fielding, B.C. (2019). Coronavirus envelope protein: current knowledge. *Virol. J.* 16 (1): 69.

11 Netland, J., DeDiego, M.L., Zhao, J. et al. (2010). Immunization with an attenuated severe acute respiratory syndrome coronavirus deleted in E protein protects against lethal respiratory disease. *Virology* 399 (1): 120–128.

12 Almazán, F., DeDiego, M.L., Sola, I. et al. (2013). Engineering a replication-competent, propagation-defective Middle East respiratory syndrome coronavirus as a vaccine candidate. *MBio* 4 (5): e00650-13.

13 Zhou, P., Yang, X.L., Wang, X.G. et al. (2020). A pneumonia outbreak associated with a new coronavirus of probable bat origin. *Nature* 579 (7798): 270–273.

14 Corti, D., Purcell, L.A., Snell, G., and Veesler, D. (2021). Tackling COVID-19 with neutralizing monoclonal antibodies. *Cell* 184 (12): 3086–3108.

15 Belouzard, S., Chu, V.C., and Whittaker, G.R. (2009). Activation of the SARS coronavirus spike protein via sequential proteolytic cleavage at two distinct sites. *Proc. Natl. Acad. Sci. U. S. A.* 106 (14): 5871–5876.

16 Pillay, T.S. (2020). Gene of the month: the 2019-nCoV/SARS-CoV-2 novel coronavirus spike protein. *J. Clin. Pathol.* 73 (7): 366–369.

17 Walls, A.C., Park, Y.J., Tortorici, M.A. et al. (2020). Structure, function, and antigenicity of the SARS-CoV-2 spike glycoprotein. *Cell* 181 (2): 281–292.e6.

18 Guo, F., Yang, J., Pan, J. et al. (2020). Origin and evolution of H1N1/pdm2009: a codon usage perspective. *Front. Microbiol.* 11: 1615.

19 Lu, R., Zhao, X., Li, J. et al. (2020). Genomic characterisation and epidemiology of 2019 novel coronavirus: implications for virus origins and receptor binding. *Lancet* 395 (10224): 565–574.

20 Chan, J.F.-W., Kok, K.-H., Zhu, Z. et al. (2020). Genomic characterization of the 2019 novel human-pathogenic coronavirus isolated from a patient with atypical pneumonia after visiting Wuhan. *Emerg. Microbes Infect.* 9 (1): 221–236.

21 Zhou, H., Chen, X., Hu, T. et al. (2020). A novel bat coronavirus closely related to SARS-CoV-2 contains natural insertions at the S1/S2 cleavage site of the spike protein. *Curr. Biol.* 30 (11): 2196–2203.e3.

22 Hul, V., Delaune, D., Karlsson, E.A. et al. (2021). A novel SARS-CoV-2 related coronavirus in bats from Cambodia. *bioRxiv* https://doi.org/10.1101/2021.01.26.428212.

23 Coutard, B., Valle, C., de Lamballerie, X. et al. (2020). The spike glycoprotein of the new coronavirus 2019-nCoV contains a furin-like

cleavage site absent in CoV of the same clade. *Antivir. Res.* 176: 104742.

24 Xiao, K., Zhai, J., Feng, Y. et al. (2020). Isolation of SARS-CoV-2-related coronavirus from Malayan pangolins. *Nature* 583 (7815): 286–289.

25 Lam, T.T., Jia, N., Zhang, Y.W. et al. (2020). Identifying SARS-CoV-2-related coronaviruses in Malayan pangolins. *Nature* 583 (7815): 282–285.

26 Boni, M.F., Lemey, P., Jiang, X. et al. (2020). Evolutionary origins of the SARS-CoV-2 sarbecovirus lineage responsible for the COVID-19 pandemic. *Nat. Microbiol.* 5 (11): 1408–1417.

27 Lv, J., Gao, J., Wu, B. et al. (2021). Aerosol transmission of coronavirus and influenza virus of animal origin. *Front. Vet. Sci.* 8 (109): 572012.

28 Rabaan, A.A., Al-Ahmed, S.H., Al-Malkey, M. et al. (2021). Airborne transmission of SARS-CoV-2 is the dominant route of transmission: droplets and aerosols. *Infez Med.* 29 (1): 10–19.

29 Asadi, S., Wexler, A.S., Cappa, C.D. et al. (2019). Aerosol emission and superemission during human speech increase with voice loudness. *Sci. Rep.* 9 (1): 2348.

30 Nie, Q., Li, X., Chen, W. et al. (2020). Phylogenetic and phylodynamic analyses of SARS-CoV-2. *Virus Res.* 287: 198098.

31 Korber, B., Fischer, W.M., Gnanakaran, S. et al. (2020). Tracking changes in SARS-CoV-2 spike: evidence that D614G increases infectivity of the COVID-19 virus. *Cell* 182 (4): 812–827.e19.

32 Boehm, E., Kronig, I., Neher, R.A. et al. (2021). Geneva Centre for Emerging Viral Diseases. Novel SARS-CoV-2 variants: the pandemics within the pandemic. *Clin. Microbiol. Infect.* 27 (8): 1109–1117.

33 McCallum, M., De Marco, A., Lempp, F.A. et al. (2021). N-terminal domain antigenic mapping reveals a site of vulnerability for SARS-CoV-2. *Cell* 184 (9): 2332–2347.e16.

34 Centers for Disease Control and Prevention (CDC). SARS-CoV-2 variant classifications and definitions. CDC (2021). https://www.cdc.gov/coronavirus/2019-ncov/variants/variant-info.html (updated 14 June 2021 accessed 15 June 2021).

35 Luan, B., Wang, H., and Huynh, T. (2021). Enhanced binding of the N501Y-mutated SARS-CoV-2 spike protein to the human ACE2 receptor: insights from molecular dynamics simulations. *FEBS Lett.* 595 (10): 1454–1461.

36 Nelson, G., Buzko, O., Spilman, P. et al. (2021). Molecular dynamic simulation reveals E484K mutation enhances spike RBD-ACE2 affinity and the combination of E484K, K417N and N501Y mutations (501Y.V2 variant) induces conformational change greater than N501Y mutant alone, potentially resulting in an escape mutant. *bioRxiv* https://doi.org/10.1101/2021.01.13.426558.

37 Greaney, A.J., Loes, A.N., Crawford, K.H.D. et al. (2021). Comprehensive mapping of mutations in the SARS-CoV-2 receptor-binding domain that affect recognition by polyclonal human plasma antibodies. *Cell Host Microbe* 29 (3): 463–476.e6.

38 Zhang, W., Davis, B.D., Chen, S.S. et al. (2021). Emergence of a novel SARS-CoV-2 variant in Southern California. *JAMA* 325 (13): 1324–1326.

39 Davies, N.G., Abbott, S., Barnard, R.C. et al. (2021). Estimated transmissibility and impact of SARS-CoV-2 lineage B.1.1.7 in England. *Science* 372 (6538): eabg3055.

40 Horby, P., Huntley, C., Davies, N., Edmunds, J., Ferguson, N., Medley, G. et al. (2021). NERVTAG paper on COVID-19 variant of concern B.1.1.72021. https://assets.publishing.service.gov.uk/government/uploads/system/uploads/attachment_data/file/961037/NERVTAG_note_on_B.1.1.7_severity_for_SAGE_77__1_pdf (accessed 15 June 2021).

41 Fact sheet for health care providers Emergency Use Authorization (EUA) of bamlanivimab and etesevimab (2021). https://www.fda.gov/media/145802/download (accessed 15 June 2021).

42 Fact sheet for health care providers Emergency Use Authorization (EUA) of REGEN-COVTM (casirivimab and imdevimab) (2021). https://www.fda.gov/media/145611/download (accessed 15 June 2021).

43 Wang, P., Nair, M.S., Liu, L. et al. (2021). Antibody resistance of SARS-CoV-2 variants B.1.351 and B.1.1.7. *Nature* 593 (7857): 130–135.

44 Shen, X., Tang, H., McDanal, C. et al. (2021). SARS-CoV-2 variant B.1.1.7 is susceptible to neutralizing antibodies elicited by ancestral spike vaccines. *Cell Host Microbe* 29 (4): 529–539.e3.

45 Edara, V.V., Floyd, K., Lai, L. et al. Infection and mRNA-1273 vaccine antibodies neutralize SARS-CoV-2 UK variant. *medRxiv*. 2021. doi: https://doi.org/10.1101/2021.02.02.21250799.

46 Collier, D.A., De Marco, A., Ferreira, I.A.T.M. et al. (2021). SARS-CoV-2 B.1.1.7 sensitivity to mRNA vaccine-elicited, convalescent and monoclonal antibodies. *medRxiv* https://doi.org/10.1101/2021.01.19.21249840.

47 Wu, K., Werner, A.P., Moliva, J.I. et al. (2021). mRNA-1273 vaccine induces neutralizing antibodies against spike mutants from global SARS-CoV-2 variants. *bioRxiv* https://doi.org/10.1101/2021.01.25.427948.

48 Emary, K.R.W., Golubchik, T., Aley, P.K. et al. (2021). Efficacy of ChAdOx1 nCoV-19 (AZD1222) vaccine against SARS-CoV-2 variant of concern 202012/01 (B.1.1.7): an exploratory analysis of a randomised controlled trial. *Lancet* 397 (10282): 1351–1362.

49 Novavax COVID-19 vaccine demonstrates 89.3% efficacy in UK phase 3 trial (2021). https://ir.novavax.com/news-releases/news-release-details/novavax-covid-19-vaccine-demonstrates-893-efficacy-uk-phase-3 (published 28 January 2021 accessed 15 June 2021).

50 Pearson CAB, Russell TW, Davies NG, Kucharski AJ. (2021). Estimates of severity and transmissibility of novel SARS-CoV-2 variant 501Y.V2 in South Africa. https://cmmid.github.io/topics/covid19/reports/sa-novel-variant/2021_01_11_Transmissibility_and_severity_of_501Y_V2_in_SA.pdf (accessed 15 June 2021).

51 Madhi, S.A., Baillie, V., Cutland, C.L. et al. Safety and efficacy of the ChAdOx1 nCoV-19 (AZD1222) Covid-19 vaccine against the B.1.351 variant in South Africa. *medRxiv* https://doi.org/10.1101/2021.02.10.21251247.

52 Johnson & Johnson COVID-19 vaccine authorized by U.S. FDA for emergency use - first single-shot vaccine in fight against global pandemic (2021). https://www.jnj.com/johnson-johnson-covid-19-vaccine-authorized-by-u-s-fda-for-emergency-usefirst-single-shot-vaccine-in-fight-against-global-pandemic (accessed 15 June 2021).

53 Deng, X., Garcia-Knight, M.A., Khalid, M.M. et al. (2021). Transmission, infectivity, and neutralization of a spike L452R SARS-CoV-2 variant. *Cell* 184 (13): 3426–3437.e8.

54 Jangra, S., Ye, C., Rathnasinghe, R. et al. (2021). SARS-CoV-2 spike E484K mutation reduces antibody neutralization. *Lancet Microbe* 2 (7): e283–e284.

55 Annavajhala, M.K., Mohri, H., Zucker, J.E. et al. (2021). A novel SARS-CoV-2 variant of concern, B.1.526, identified in New York. *medRxiv* https://doi.org/10.1101/2021.02.23.21252259.

56 Lopez Bernal, J., Andrews, N., Gower, C. et al. (2021). Effectiveness of Covid-19 vaccines against the B.1.617.2 (Delta) variant. *N. Engl. J. Med.* 385 (7): 585–594.

57 Centers for Disease Control and Prevention (CDC). Delta variant: what we know about the science. CDC. https://www.cdc.gov/coronavirus/2019-ncov/variants/delta-variant.html (published 26 August 2021 accessed 1 September 2021).

3

COVID-19: Laboratory/Serologic Diagnostics

Desmond Chin[1], Liesl S. Eibschutz[1], Juliana Sobczyk[2,3], Mobin Azami[4], Michael Jovan Repajic[1], and Michael P. Dube[5]

[1] Department of Radiology, Keck School of Medicine, University of Southern California, Los Angeles, CA, USA
[2] Department of Pathology, Memorial Satilla Hospital, HCA Healthcare, Waycross, GA, USA
[3] Laboratory Director, St. Augustine Foot & Ankle, Inc., St. Augustine, FL, USA
[4] Student Research Committee, Kurdistan University of Medical Sciences, Sanandaj, Iran
[5] Department of Medicine, Division of Infectious Diseases, Keck School of Medicine, University of Southern California, Los Angeles, CA, USA

Abbreviations

ACE2	angiotensin-converting enzyme 2
BALF	bronchoalveolar lavage fluid
CDC	Centers for Disease Control and Prevention
CPE	cytopathic effect
CRISPR	clustered regularly interspaced short palindromic repeats
CSF	cerebrospinal fluid
Ct	cycle threshold
E	envelope
EAU	Emergency Use Authorization
ELISA	enzyme-linked immunosorbent type assay
FDA	US Food and Drug Administration
Ig	immunoglobulin
LFA	lateral flow type assay
LoD	limit of detection
MERS-CoV	Middle East respiratory syndrome coronavirus
MIS-C	multisystem inflammatory syndrome in children
N	nucleocapsid
NAAT	nucleic acid amplification testing
NGS	next generation sequencing
POC	point-of-care
PRNT	plaque reduction neutralization test
RBD	receptor-binding domain
RT-LAMP	reverse transcription loop-mediated isothermal amplification
RT-qPCR	reverse transcription-quantitative real-time polymerase chain reaction
S	spike
SARS	severe acute respiratory syndrome
SARS-CoV-2	severe acute respiratory syndrome coronavirus 2
WHO	World Health Organization

Coronaviruses are positive-sense single-stranded RNA enveloped viruses belonging to the Coronaviridae family. Severe acute respiratory syndrome coronavirus 2 (SARS-CoV-2) is part of the beta-coronavirus genera with a genome size of 29.9 kb [1]. Before the discovery of SARS-CoV-2, six coronaviruses have been shown to infect humans. Four of these coronaviruses (OC43, 229E, NL63, and HKU1) are endemic, causing mild upper respiratory tract infections and accounting for ~30% of common colds [2]. The other two epidemic coronaviruses, called SARS-CoV and Middle East respiratory syndrome coronavirus (MERS-CoV), can cause acute respiratory disease and are transmissible between humans. SARS-CoV (now also referred to as SARS-CoV-1) is responsible for the 2002–2004 severe

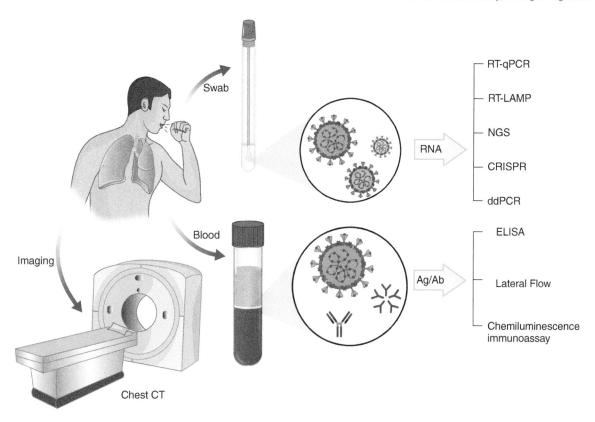

Figure 3.1 Various methods for SARS-CoV-2 detection. Ab, antibody; Ag, antigen; CT, computed tomography. *Source:* Rai et al. [1].

acute respiratory syndrome (SARS) epidemic, and MERS-CoV is responsible for MERS first described in 2012. The SARS-CoV-2 virus, the third epidemic coronavirus proven to infect humans, shares approximately 79% similarity with SARS-CoV and 50% similarity with MERS-CoV [1]. Although the fatality rate of SARS-CoV-2 infection is lower than the first two epidemic coronaviruses in history, this virus is far more transmissible.

Rapid and sensitive detection methods of SARS-CoV-2 have been and continue to be essential for containing the spread of COVID-19 (Figure 3.1). Given the lack of definitive treatments for SARS-CoV-2 infection, disruption of viral transmission through detection and isolation of infected individuals remains critical to limiting further devastation caused by this virus [3]. Notably, widespread vaccination is now becoming a reality, with more than 4.17 billion doses administered worldwide as of 2 August

2021. Apart from mass vaccination, however, breaking the chain of transmission from infected patients to healthy individuals is the best way to manage the COVID-19 pandemic [4]. Not only is it imperative to develop and use diagnostic tests to identify those infected but also to accurately distinguish negative cases, thereby minimizing unnecessary quarantine and subsequent social and economic impact [5]. Moreover, diagnostic testing has been invaluable in characterizing the disease itself: it has and will continue to impact clinical management, assessment of potential therapies, and public health and socioeconomic decisions [6]. The goal of this chapter is to provide up-to-date information on the various diagnostic tests that have been developed and used thus far during the COVID-19 pandemic. This chapter will cover molecular assays and point-of-care (POC) tests of diagnosing COVID-19, plus a particular emphasis on serologic tests.

Molecular Diagnostics for COVID-19

Nucleic Acid Amplification Testing

Within the clinical laboratory for infectious disease testing, nucleic acid amplification testing (NAAT) is a category of molecular techniques used to identify and detect certain organisms, usually a pathogenic virus or bacteria, using genetic material (RNA or DNA) [7]. Nucleic acid amplification tests amplify a small amount of genetic material in a specimen collected from an individual. Detection of amplified genetic material typically allows for earlier identification of disease because small amounts of RNA or DNA are typically present before antigens or antibodies appear in circulation [8]. All nucleic acid amplification techniques rely on the specificity of Watson–Crick base pairing [7]. NAAT techniques have formed the backbone of screening testing during the COVID-19 pandemic, because these tests can identify minute amounts of SARS-CoV-2 RNA in collected specimens, making NAATs highly sensitive for diagnosing COVID-19. However, clinical specimens must be of high quality for accurate detection of SARS-CoV-2 genetic material. Developments and deployment of NAAT technologies have been critical in accurately and rapidly identifying SARS-CoV-2 infection and preventing the further spread of disease. In this section, we discuss the various NAAT techniques that have been used in the diagnosis of COVID-19, including reverse transcription-quantitative real-time polymerase chain reaction (RT-qPCR), reverse transcription loop-mediated isothermal amplification (RT-LAMP)-based assays, and clustered regularly interspaced short palindromic repeats (CRISPR)-based assays [1, 8].

RT-qPCR

Principles of RT-qPCR

RT-qPCR is the gold standard screening test for SARS-CoV-2 infection. RT-qPCR continues to be one of the most ubiquitously used techniques across the world for COVID-19 screening and is the test of choice for COVID-19 screening as recommended by the World Health Organization (WHO) and Centers for Disease Control and Prevention (CDC) [9–11]. Assays have been developed targeting different genes of SARS-CoV-2, including the RNA-dependent RNA polymerase (RdRp) gene, nucleocapsid (N) gene, envelope (E) gene, spike (S) gene, and other open reading frame regions within the viral genome [12]. The process of RT-qPCR involves cycles of temperature changes that allow denaturation, annealing, and polymerization to occur repeatedly to amplify genetic material of interest. Most assays use multiplex RT-PCR, in which multiple regions of the genome are targeted to further improve sensitivity. Fluorescent reporter probes are typically used such that the amplification process can be quantified in real time by measuring fluorescent signal, increasing assay specificity [13].

Specimen Collection for RT-qPCR

RT-qPCR test results depend on several preanalytical factors, primarily proper specimen collection. Additional factors include the specimen type (e.g. nasopharyngeal, oropharyngeal, anterior nares, saliva) and timing of sampling, which are crucial because viral load differs in patients with SARS-CoV-2 infection depending on disease stage and the location of the body where the specimen is obtained [9, 14]. SARS-CoV-2 is a virus that primarily infects the respiratory system, hence why many RT-qPCR assays use respiratory tract specimens [8, 15]. SARS-CoV-2 RNA has been detected in other specimens collected from other sites, including blood, cerebrospinal fluid (CSF), urine, feces, and breast milk [16]. However, testing these other body fluids is currently not recommended because they rarely yield positive results [16–19]. Detection of viral genetic material in a specimen does not necessarily equate to potential for that body fluid to be infectious [20]. Currently, it is unknown whether COVID is transmissible through these nonrespiratory locations [20, 21]. In this section, we discuss the various sites of specimen collection for RT-qPCR tests [13].

Respiratory Tract

Specimen collection sites for the respiratory tract include the upper respiratory tract and lower respiratory tract [22]. Acceptable specimens in the upper respiratory tract include swabs collected from the nasopharyngeal, anterior nares, mid-turbinate, or oropharyngeal regions, or a combination of the above. Specimens in the lower respiratory tract include bronchoalveolar lavage fluid (BALF) and tracheal aspirate [23, 24]. Upper respiratory tract collection is typically easier to perform and less invasive, whereas obtaining lower respiratory tract specimens tends to be more invasive. Lower respiratory collection is ideal for mechanically ventilated patients. Notably, lower respiratory tract testing is reported to have higher sensitivity in comparison with upper respiratory tract testing [9]. This finding has been attributed to higher viral loads in BALF and tracheal aspirates [25–28]. Respiratory tract testing varies according to progression of disease. With later stages of COVID-19, the virus has a predilection for the lower respiratory tract. This shift explains why in later stages of disease, nasopharyngeal swabs often yield negative results, whereas BALF yields positive results. Nevertheless, nasopharyngeal swab remains the gold standard specimen for RT-qPCR detection of SARS-CoV-2 because collection of nasopharyngeal specimens is relatively simple to perform and possesses both high sensitivity and high specificity [29].

Saliva

Saliva is an alternative specimen that is less invasive to obtain in comparison with respiratory specimen collection [30–32]. Salivary testing has certain advantages over respiratory tract testing [31, 33, 34]. Reports suggest that salivary testing has less variability over the disease course in comparison with respiratory tract testing [35]. Salivary testing has also shown great consistency with regard to self-sample collection, likely given the ease of obtaining one's own saliva [34, 36]. However, salivary specimens have been shown to be less sensitive than nasopharyngeal specimens and to produce more invalid test results when compared with swabs. Mucus, which may mix with saliva when coughing, may interfere with assay performance [17, 34, 37]. Many guidelines state that swab testing is preferred over saliva despite certain advantages of salivary testing.

Blood/Plasma

Collection of blood products can be performed readily in the hospital or outpatient setting and is not as invasive as some specimen collection methods. Detection and quantification of SARS-CoV-2 RNA in blood, serum, and plasma have all been reported [16,

38, 39]. However, multiple meta-analyses examining RT-PCR detection profiles of various clinical specimens have reported that blood products (whole blood, plasma, serum) have quite low sensitivity [16, 40]. Instead, the concept of "RNAemia" refers to the detectable presence of viral RNA in blood, serum, or plasma (along the lines of viremia referring to the detectable presence of whole virus in the blood). RNAemia has been observed to occur more readily in clinically severe COVID-19 and has been associated with greater disease severity and mortality [41–43]. Although the positivity rate of SARS-CoV-2 in blood products is low, the association between RNAemia and COVID-19 severity/outcomes have led some to propose plasma RNA testing as a prognostic tool [43]. Nevertheless, viral load determined from RT-PCR of respiratory tract samples appears to be a more robust tool for prognosticating COVID-19 severity given the higher positivity rates of respiratory tract samples [42]. We discuss viral load later in this section.

Cerebrospinal Fluid

Sampling of CSF for the presence of SARS-CoV-2 is an area of interest, particularly because of the growing body of evidence demonstrating neurologic manifestations and sequelae of COVID-19. Detection of SARS-CoV-2 RNA in CSF has been reported in sparse cases, but more robust studies are lacking [16, 21]. Many case series have been unable to demonstrate SARS-CoV-2 RNA positivity in CSF [16]. Moreover, obtaining CSF is an invasive process that requires lumbar puncture. Taken together, CSF samples make for poor RT-qPCR specimens both in terms of SARS-CoV-2 detection and clinical value.

Feces

Sampling of feces for the presence of SARS-CoV-2 is another area that has been investigated, given the involvement of the gastrointestinal system in COVID-19 [44, 45]. Human angiotensin-converting enzyme 2 (ACE2), the cellular entry receptor of SARS-CoV-2, is highly expressed throughout the gastrointestinal tract epithelia. SARS-CoV-2 RNA has been found to be readily detected in stool specimens. Notably, fecal specimens have been shown to remain positive for viral RNA even after negative conversion of pharyngeal swabs. This suggests that SARS-CoV-2 replication in the gastrointestinal tract may not follow the same time course as viral replication in the respiratory tract. Rectal swab RT-qPCR has been reported to remain positive, particularly in pediatric patients [44, 45]. However, fecal–oral transmission of SARS-CoV-2 has yet to be demonstrated. RT-qPCR of stool samples and rectal swabs may provide value above that which nasopharyngeal swabs can provide with regard to monitoring treatment efficacy and/or determining quarantine duration based on duration of viral shedding [46]. Notwithstanding, stool sampling, namely, via rectal swabs, is more invasive, is associated with patient discomfort, and is not preferred for most undergoing screening testing. Fecal sampling can, however, be considered in young children, in whom obtaining reliable nasopharyngeal samples is more difficult [44].

Urine

Although some authors have reported the presence of SARS-CoV-2 RNA in the urine, most meta-analyses have been unable to demonstrate SARS-CoV-2 RNA yield in urogenital specimens [16, 47]. In addition, detection of viral RNA in the urine does not appear to correlate with clinical urinary tract involvement or disease severity, nor does it explain a relationship between SARS-CoV-2 infection and renal injury in COVID-19. Despite the ease of obtaining urine specimens from individuals, these have minimal clinical utility.

Breast Milk

Although some case reports mention the presence of SARS-CoV-2 RNA in breast milk, more comprehensive studies investigating RNA positivity in breast milk are lacking [48, 49]. RT-qPCR using breast milk specimens is an area of particular interest, given the possibility of transmission from infected mothers to neonates through breastfeeding. Notably, detection of SARS-CoV-2 RNA in a body fluid does not equate to infectivity, because at this point in the COVID-19 pandemic, there have been no documented cases of viral transmission from mothers to neonates via breast milk [48, 49]. Further research is necessary regarding the level of infectivity via breast milk and maternal–neonate transmission.

Applications and Obstacles of RT-qPCR

RT-qPCR tests have certain advantages over other diagnostic modalities, especially in the early stages of infection. Because RT-qPCR can detect very small amounts of SARS-CoV-2 RNA through amplification, this highly sensitive technique can identify early infection even when symptoms are not clinically apparent and viral load is low [22, 50]. Over the course of the COVID-19 pandemic, it has been essential to identify infection as early as possible to implement quarantine measures and prevent disease spread [51, 52]. Before widespread vaccination, early identification and prevention was the principal strategy of controlling COVID-19, primarily because of large-scale implementation of RT-qPCR testing.

Another advantage of RT-qPCR testing is its ability to semiquantitively approximate SARS-CoV-2 viral load via cycle threshold (Ct) values [53]. Ct refers to the number of cycles needed to amplify the viral RNA and consider it detectable, and thus is inversely proportional to the level of genetic material present in the specimen. For example, a low Ct indicates a high concentration of viral genetic material in the sample and therefore high risk for infectivity, whereas a high Ct represents a low concentration of genetic material, suggesting a low risk for infectivity [53]. Recent studies have noted the potential utility of Ct values in predicting COVID-19 severity/outcomes, because a high viral load, especially in early disease and in elderly patients, is generally associated with worse disease outcome and greater mortality [54, 55]. Thus, viral load defined by Ct values may represent a prognostic tool to identify patients who may potentially require more aggressive clinical interventions.

However, recent research indicates that the clinical utility of Ct values in patients with COVID-19 is limited. One author highlighted the lack of precision in Ct values, describing vastly different Ct values when using the same sample in separate assays [56]. Although viral load has been demonstrated to be significantly higher in the early and progressive stages of COVID-19 when compared with viral load in the recovery stage, recent studies note that a Ct value taken at a single time point does not provide any information regarding the subsequent course of disease [57–60]. Thus, many authors urge that Ct values be used only on a case-by-case basis when also considering clinical context [53, 56].

False-negative test results have occurred with the commercially developed RT-qPCR test kits. This is because some tests are not reaching the limit of detection (LoD) of that given assay [31, 61]. LoD is defined as the lowest concentration of a molecular target that can reliably be distinguished from a blank sample not containing the target. Thus, if this level is not reached, a false-negative test result will occur. In addition, these false-negative results may also be a consequence of dynamic viral shedding over the course of SARS-CoV-2 infection, because viral load varies depending on the stage of infection, with higher viral loads present in earlier stages [62]. Therefore, the timing at which the specimen is collected affects the Ct value and the performance of RT-qPCR tests. RT-qPCR results also vary depending on the source of the specimen, as well as the quality of genetic material in the specimen. Inadequate collection, inappropriate handling, or delay from collection to performing the assay may result in degradation of the viral material within the sample, leading to null results [17, 52]. False-negative test results are especially problematic for screening tests, where the goal is not to miss potential disease [17–19].

In addition, RT-qPCR tests require dedicated laboratory facilities with expensive equipment, sufficient reagents, and trained personnel capable of executing test protocols. The WHO recommends that SARS-CoV-2 specimens be handled in at least a biosafety level 2 laboratory, which has driven many of these tests to be conducted in centralized laboratories [63]. Although typical turnaround times for RT-qPCR results are 1–3 days, in areas with surging outbreaks, demand for testing may exceed laboratory capacity [22, 64]. Delays in result turnaround hinder the effort to screen early disease and curb the spread of infection. Over the evolution of the pandemic, much effort has been channeled into developing and improving test run time and throughput to address this issue. For example, the Panther Fusion assay developed by Hologic and the Cobas 8800 system developed by Roche are two RT-qPCR assays with Emergency Use Authorization (EUA) status that can process up to 500 and 1056 tests in 8 hours, respectively. Despite its mentioned limitations, RT-qPCR testing has and continues to be the gold standard screening and diagnostic technique for detecting COVID-19. As of 7 December 2021,

there were 270 unique RT-qPCR-based assays approved for use through the US Food and Drug Administration (FDA) EUA [65]. Its widespread implementation has been pivotal in containing the ongoing pandemic.

RT-LAMP

Although RT-PCR has proved itself to be the gold standard for viral load testing, RT-LAMP has recently gained popularity as a faster, more cost-effective amplification technique that does not rely on intricate thermal cycling equipment [66, 67]. Instead, RT-LAMP is a technique that can amplify a target sequence of interest using a single temperature (typically 60–65 °C). Moreover, RT-LAMP produces higher amounts of amplified genetic material, such that a positive test result can be observed visually without the aid of a machine for interpretation [66]. Reactions in RT-LAMP are designed such that the amplified products loop back on their ends, serving as self-primers for a polymerase enzyme [68]. Essentially, the LAMP technique is a chain reaction that runs until the added reagents have been consumed. In some RT-LAMP assays developed for COVID-19, detection of amplified viral material has been coupled to a pH indicator (e.g. phenol red) such that a positive result is signaled by a color change from red to yellow. This color change can be taken as a qualitative positive result using the naked eye or quantified using a spectrophotometer. Ultimately, RT-LAMP has very high amplification efficiency.

The advantages of RT-LAMP are that it is simple to operate, an isothermal reaction, and can return results more rapidly than RT-qPCR [69, 70]. In addition, some studies report that its sensitivity and specificity are comparable with that of the gold standard RT-qPCR technique. LAMP-based amplification has been reported to have a sensitivity of 90–100% and specificity of 95–99%. Like RT-qPCR, LAMP can be performed in a multiplexed fashion (multiple genetic targets) to yield higher specificity. Application of RT-LAMP has strong potential as an alternative screening and diagnostic tool [69, 70]. If scaled up, RT-LAMP assays could provide reliable, rapid, and easy-to-perform SARS-CoV-2 testing that could outcompete conventional RT-qPCR assays. With the development of enclosed near-patient molecular devices, RT-LAMP can serve as an excellent POC testing modality. Yet, much fewer RT-LAMP assays have been granted EUA and commercialized in comparison with RT-qPCR tests, despite multiple proof-of-concept studies. Those that have been granted EUA show great promise to be upscaled and applied in POC testing. For instance, an RT-LAMP-based assay developed by Color Health first received FDA EUA on 20 May 2020 but was initially a prescription-only test. On 19 March 2021, Color Health was granted EUA for an updated direct-to-consumer version of the assay involving anterior nasal swab self-collection. Another RT-LAMP-based test, the BCC19 kit developed by MobileDetect Bio Inc., is one of the most recent RT-LAMP tests to gain FDA EUA as of 17 June 2021 and can return results in 30 minutes. The Abbott ID NOW COVID-19 RT-LAMP-based assay consists of a toaster-size device intended for POC testing that can return results as quickly as 13 minutes. Ultimately, RT-LAMP is a technique still undergoing investigation, with the aim of new RT-LAMP assays being to decrease cross-reactivity and improve sensitivity. LAMP-based diagnostics continue to be developed and improved, showing great promise in the realm of rapid and reliable POC testing.

CRISPR-Based Techniques

Given the search for rapid and reliable diagnostics throughout the pandemic, there has been an increased interest in developing CRISPR-based technology for SARS-CoV-2 detection. Although CRISPR is best known as a technique for genome editing (CRISPR-Cas9 technology), some authors report its utility in diagnostic applications, including detection of Zika virus and *Staphylococcus aureus* [71, 72]. The subsequent discoveries of RNA-targeting effectors Cas13, Cas12, and Cas 14 laid the foundation for single-base specificity nucleic acid detection systems. The majority of CRISPR-Cas systems use either Cas12 or Cas13 effectors, which target DNA and RNA, respectively [22, 73]. In brief, CRISPR systems use guide RNA binding to target sequences in a complementary fashion, which activates a Cas nuclease enzyme that cleaves the target at a specific site. In general, CRISPR-

based systems for SARS-CoV-2 detection begin in a similar fashion to other NAATs with specimen collection (e.g. nasopharyngeal swab). Viral RNA is then extracted from the sample and amplified using RT-PCR or RT-LAMP techniques to increase the LoD. Subsequently, specific regions of the SARS-CoV-2 genome are identified by the CRISPR-Cas RNA complex. Once this identification occurs, the CRISPR-Cas RNA complex carries out a cleavage step, releasing a reporter. The reporter is typically coupled with a fluorescence or colorimetric reaction, which is used for result readout.

CRISPR-Cas technology has strong potential for POC testing. In addition to having rapid turnaround time (some reporting less than 1 hour), it is cost-effective, accurate, and does not require intricate equipment [22]. A CRISPR-Cas13a-based assay developed by Sherlock Biosciences became the first FDA-approved commercially available CRISPR-based detection system for SARS-CoV-2. Another CRISPR-Cas12-based lateral flow assay developed by Mammoth Biosciences, called SARS-CoV-2 DNA Endonuclease-Targeted CRISPR Trans Reporter (DETECTR), received FDA EUA on 31 August 2020 and has a run time of 45 minutes. Although CRISPR-based techniques for detecting SARS-CoV-2 have been developed and show great promise, this field of diagnostics is still in its relative infancy. CRISPR-based methods for detecting SARS-CoV-2 are limited by long sample preparation time, target region constraints, and incompatibility of the assays with multiplexing. Nevertheless, CRISPR-based technologies for SARS-CoV-2 detection show great promise in terms of delivering accurate, rapid, and cost-effective testing that may replace gold standard RT-qPCR assays.

Sequencing Techniques

Next generation sequencing (NGS) technology to sequence the SARS-CoV-2 genome has enabled the development of the primers and probes for the nucleic acid amplification tests that comprise the backbone of COVID-19 testing. NGS, also referred to as massive parallel sequencing, is a technology that has revolutionized the field of genomics research with its high throughput and scalability [74–76]. To put the speed of

NGS into perspective, the Human Genome Project that used traditional Sanger sequencing required more than 10 years to complete; NGS can sequence the entire human genome within a day [77, 78]. NGS consists of sequencing millions of small fragments of genetic material in parallel, and its approaches can be further classified into short-read and long-read techniques. In brief, short-read data are generated from genetic fragments <1000 base pairs, while long-read data are generated from genetic fragments >1000 base pairs in size [75]. Illumina sequencing is an example of short-read NGS, whereas Nanopore sequencing is an example of long-read NGS [75, 76, 79, 80]. The sequenced fragments are subsequently reconstructed into the order of the genome using bioinformatics analyses. NGS can be used to perform whole-genome sequencing (WGS) or can sequence certain target regions within a genome. NGS is an unbiased technology that has enabled the identification of novel pathogen outbreaks [81], such as the Ebola outbreak in West Africa from 2014 to 2016 [82].

Adaptation of sequencing technology to the COVID-19 pandemic has been critical in discovery, diagnosis, and surveillance of SARS-CoV-2 infection. NGS was used to initially identify SARS-CoV-2 from BALF collected from patients from Wuhan, China. Subsequently, data obtained from sequencing helped characterize the S protein mutation that enabled SARS-CoV-2 to infect humans [79, 81]. Sequencing data also were used to confirm the first reported case of SARS-CoV-2 reinfection and play a role in making that determination [83, 84].

NGS also has been used as a tool for COVID-19 clinical diagnosis. The COVIDSeq Test developed by Illumina Inc. was the first sequencing assay to receive EUA on 9 June 2020 [65]. Notably, the scale of NGS as a diagnostic modality has been limited in comparison with other testing modalities because of its relatively longer throughput times, higher cost, and requirements of skilled operators and appropriately equipped laboratories. As of 7 December 2021, six sequencing tests had received EUA approval [65].

Sequencing has been a vital technology for tracking geographic origins, transmission routes, and evolution of SARS-CoV-2 over the progression of the pandemic. For instance, NGS has been used to study early undetected transmission of COVID-19 in Washington state, where the first case of COVID-19 in the United States originated [85, 86]. Sequencing data have similarly been used to characterize routes of COVID-19 entry in the state of California and in the Netherlands [87]. In addition, NGS can identify mutations of the SARS-CoV-2 virus variants. This carries considerable epidemiologic implications, with the B.1.1.7 (alpha), B.1.351 (beta), P.1 (gamma), and most recently, B.1.351 (delta) variants of concern now circulating in the United States [88]. The rapid emergence and spread of novel variants highlight the importance of sequencing technology to detect possible virulent mutations and slow the spread of these new variants. Notably, sequencing technology also has been crucial in evaluating SARS-CoV-2 mutations that affect vaccine efficacy, such as with the delta variant, despite widespread vaccination in the United States [88]. Underlying these aims of using NGS technology for real-time COVID-19 surveillance, outbreak mitigation, and vaccine development is the consolidation of and open access to SARS-CoV-2 genomic data in dedicated databases. The GISAID EpiCov database is one of the most extensive of these collections, storing more than 100 000 SARS-CoV-2 genomes [89].

Antigen Testing

There has been great effort over the course of this pandemic to develop and refine POC antigen tests. POC tests avoid sending samples to centralized laboratories, thus allowing for rapid SARS-CoV-2 detection and more immediate isolation measures in communities. Antigen tests detect the presence of SARS-CoV-2 viral proteins within samples of interest [24, 90, 91]. Specifically, the N protein and S surface glycoprotein are used as targets for detection of SARS-CoV-2, with the N protein being the most commonly chosen target [92]. Most commercially available kits involve taking samples from the nasal cavity, nasopharynx, or saliva [24, 93]. Lateral flow immunochromatographic assay is the most common technique used for SARS-CoV-2 antigen detection, although sandwich immunoassays and microfluidic immunofluorescence assays also have been used. The principles of lateral flow immunochromatographic assay will be discussed later in the Antibody Assays for SARS-CoV-2 section [24, 90, 91].

Antigen tests are relatively inexpensive, have rapid turnaround times, and are simple to perform. Antigen test kits typically contain all necessary materials to carry out the tests and can provide results within 15–30 minutes. Results can typically be read directly from the kit used to perform the test. They are particularly useful in instances where NAAT testing capability is limited or delayed to the point of hindering clinical utility. In addition, they play a role as a screening test for high-risk communities. The WHO recommended SARS-CoV-2 antigen tests be used in settings with limited access to NAATs and within 5–7 days after symptom onset.

Antigen tests have limitations. These tests do not amplify protein or genetic material, unlike NAATs. Because no amplification of SARS-CoV-2 viral genetic material is performed for these tests, specimen integrity is critical for the accuracy of detection [8, 10, 23]. Specimen collection and handling can impact the results of these tests dramatically; for example, swabbing too rapidly may result in collecting inadequate amounts of antigenic material. For this reason, antigen tests tend to be less sensitive than NAATs, and false-negative results remain an issue [8, 10, 23]. As of 7 December 2021, 40 antigen tests have received EUA in the United States [65]. Although the initial four antigen assays reviewed by the FDA showed highly variably sensitivities, the more recently developed antigen assays are reported to have both high sensitivity and specificity [94]. Nevertheless, antigen tests are not the screening test of choice for SARS-CoV-2 given their lower sensitivity in comparison with NAATs; use of RT-PCR tests is recommended in conjunction with antigen tests if available. Even so, antigen assays provide diagnostic value in communities with limited NAAT accessibility and to those early in the disease course.

Viral Culture

Before recent technologic advances, viral culture was considered the gold standard for identification of viruses before the advent of molecular assays (Figure 3.2) [95]. Many virology laboratories now use molecular techniques in lieu of viral culture studies, because viral isolation tends to have long turnaround times and lower sensitivity in detection of the virus of interest. Virology laboratories that continue to perform viral culture also may use molecular techniques such as RT-PCR, metagenomics sequencing, or immunofluorescence to confirm viral identity [95, 96]. Despite the rise of various molecular assays, viral isolation remains an important method of characterizing viral infectivity and identifying novel viruses.

Viral cultures tend to use the shell vial technique, which is a modified version of conventional tube culture that leads to more rapid detection of virus in vitro. As opposed to tube culture, shell vial culture involves inoculating a cell monolayer with the viral specimen of interest, then subsequently centrifuging the mixture at low speed. Centrifugation of the viral specimen into the susceptible cell monolayer is thought to enhance viral entry and infectivity. The vial is subsequently incubated and observed for cytopathic effects (CPEs). Using conventional viral culture, one may expect to observe CPEs within days to weeks depending on the virus; with shell vial viral culture, CPEs can be expected as quickly as 1–2 days depending on the virus [97, 98].

In January 2020 in Wuhan, SARS-CoV-2 was isolated for the first time from bronchoalveolar lavage obtained from patients with pneumonia [99]. Viral culture has since been used in laboratories across the world to study SARS-CoV-2. The SARS-CoV-2 virus can be cultured in several cell lines, including human airway epithelial, Vero E6, Vero CCL-81, and Huh-7. Vero E6 cells highly express ACE2, an essential receptor for SARS-CoV-2 viral entry. Current reports suggest that the Vero E6 cell line may be the cell line of choice in terms of viral propagation, quantification, and use in plaque studies for characterizing different SARS-CoV-2 strains [97, 98]. Viral culture has roles in determining viral stability and characterizing pathogenesis and infectivity [100]. Moreover, isolation of SARS-CoV-2 in culture holds value in studies investigating antiviral therapies and vaccine development [101]. Nevertheless, culture-based methods are not recommended for diagnostic/screening purposes because they have lower sensitivity in comparison with other molecular techniques, are time consuming to perform, and require biosafety level 3 laboratories [98, 100].

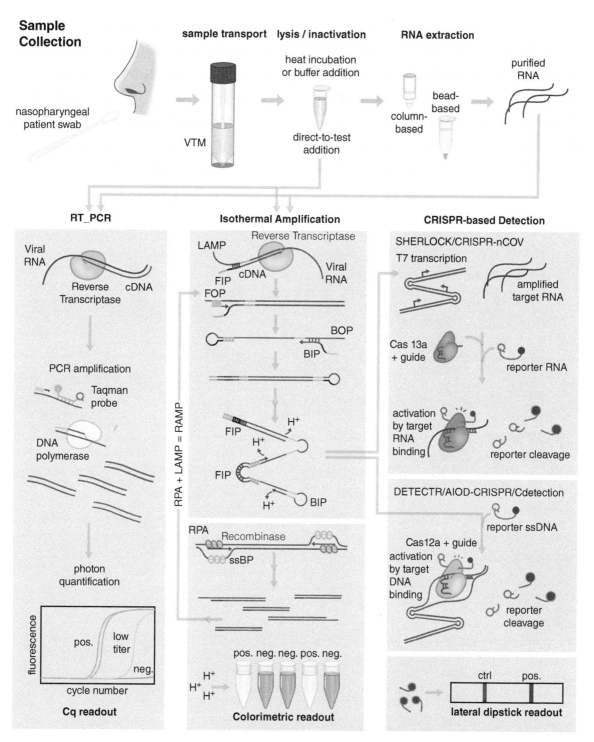

Figure 3.2 Molecular assays for SARS-CoV-2 detection. ctrl, control; neg., negative; pos., positive; BIP, backward inner primer; BOP, backward outer primer; FIP, forward inner primer; FOP, forward outer primer; RAMP, a two-stage isothermal amplification technique combining a primary RPA reaction using the outside LAMP primers with a secondary LAMP reaction including self-complimentary internal primers; RPA, rapid amplification; ssBP, single strand DNA binding protein; VTM, viral transport medium. *Source:* Esbin et al. [69]. A link to the creative commons license: https://creativecommons.org/licenses/by/4.0/legalcode.

Antibody Testing for COVID-19

Antibody tests for COVID-19 are primarily intended for patients at different stages of COVID-19 infection. These tests are used to characterize one's immunologic response to SARS-CoV-2 infection to estimate chronicity and severity of disease [102]. Antibody-based testing is typically not used for diagnosis of acute SARS-CoV-2 infection, but instead it may be used for retrospective diagnosis of patients with suspected COVID-19. Confirmation of infection with a serologic test requires demonstrated seroconversion, which is defined as the recent development of detectable antibodies in serum specific to an invading pathogen. Throughout the COVID-19 pandemic, antibody testing has played a vital role at the epidemiologic level, because serologic surveillance was used to characterize rates of exposure and infection in populations and to subsequently guide public health guidelines. In addition, antibody testing may be used to assess SARS-CoV-2 vaccine efficacy [103].

Principles of Antibody Testing

An antibody is a large Y-shaped glycoprotein produced by the B cells of the humoral immune system in response to an antigen. Each antibody contains sites that recognize one specific antigen to which it can bind. A single antibody contains four protein chains: two heavy and two light chains linked by disulfide bonds. The N-terminal regions of the heavy and light chains comprise the antigen binding site and are where antigenic specificity is determined [104]. Once bound to antigen, antibodies can function to neutralize components of a pathogen (e.g. viral fusion proteins or bacterial toxins), opsonize and subsequently target foreign substances for phagocytosis, or activate the complement system to destroy pathogens via membrane attack complexes.

The terms *antibody* and *immunoglobin* are often used interchangeably. In humans, there are five classes of antibodies: immunoglobulin A (IgA), IgD, IgE, IgG, and IgM. Each of these classes is distinguished by its C-terminal regions. Antibodies are found in blood and mucous secretions. IgM is the first antibody to be produced during an infection and accounts for ~10% of

human Igs. IgG is the most abundant antibody in serum (70–75%), whereas IgA (accounting for 10–15% of human Igs) is the most abundant in mucous membranes and secretions. IgM has a lower affinity for antigens than IgG but has a higher avidity given its pentameric structure. In acute infection, IgM binding to cell surface receptors activates downstream immune cell signaling pathways. IgG generally appears later in the course of an infection but persists longer in circulation; therefore, it is the immunoglobin class largely responsible for long-term immunity after infection or vaccination [104]. An antibody test measures the concentration of IgG and IgM in blood, serum, or plasma to determine whether the body's immune system is reacting to combat a pathogen, for example, an invading virus. In principle, detectable IgM directed against SARS-CoV-2 indicates more recent infection, whereas IgG directed against SARS-CoV-2 indicates more distant exposure to the virus [9].

Antibody Assays for SARS-CoV-2

Assay Target Selection

Although the SARS-CoV-2 genome codes for approximately 27 proteins, 4 structural proteins act as potential targets for antibodies. These structural proteins include S glycoproteins, membrane glycoproteins (M), E proteins, and N phosphoproteins (Figure 3.3). The S protein is the largest structural protein and comprises the distinctive spikes on the surface of the virus; for most coronaviruses, the S protein is cleaved by the host cell into S1 and S2 subunits. The S1 domain functions in receptor binding, whereas the S2 domain functions in viral fusion. The SARS-CoV-2 virus S1 protein binds to the human ACE2 receptor found on human respiratory, renal, and gastrointestinal cells. SARS-CoV-2 binding to ACE2 receptor is a key step in viral entry [105]. The N protein is the most abundant viral protein in SARS-CoV-2, functioning as a component of the helical N and playing a role in pathogenesis, viral replication, and RNA packaging [106]. The N and S2 proteins are highly conserved with SARS-CoV-2 and are important antigenic sites for the development of antibody assays. The S1 subunit and receptor-binding domain (RBD) of the S

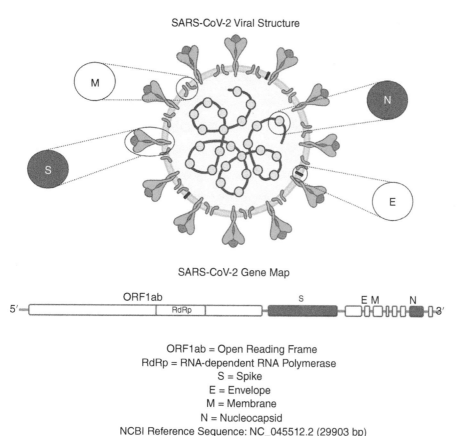

ORF1ab = Open Reading Frame
RdRp = RNA-dependent RNA Polymerase
S = Spike
E = Envelope
M = Membrane
N = Nucleocapsid
NCBI Reference Sequence: NC_045512.2 (29903 bp)

Figure 3.3 SARS-CoV-2 viral structure. Source: Chau et al. [102].

protein are less conserved across coronaviruses and more specific to SARS-CoV-2; therefore, these are more ideal targets for antibody testing. Current and previously studied serologic tests have used antibodies against the N, RBD, S1, S2, and M proteins. No antibodies against E protein have been detected. S1 is proposed as the best protein in differentiating COVID-19 from controls [7, 12].

Binding Assays

Two categories of antibody test are commonly used in the clinical immunology laboratory: binding antibody detection and neutralizing antibody detection. Current antibody tests used for SARS-CoV-2 are primarily binding antibody detection tests, in which the capacity for antibody binding to purified SARS-CoV-2 proteins is measured. However, not all binding antibodies are neutralizing antibodies, which can prevent viral infec-

tion. Therefore, neutralization antibody assays are the ideal gold standard antibody tests in that they provide additional information regarding whether a recovered patient's serum contains antibodies that likely provide immune protection against infection [102]. The most common antibody tests that have been used for SARS-CoV-2 are based on lateral flow type assays (LFAs) (Figure 3.4), enzyme-linked immunosorbent type assays (ELISAs) (Figure 3.5), or chemiluminescent immunoassays (CLIAs) [108]. Although conventional and modified neutralizing antibody assays have been developed for SARS-CoV-2, at the time of writing this section, there are no FDA-approved neutralizing antibody assays [102].

In an antibody LFA test, the molecules of interest are the specific antibodies in the patient's specimen (blood, plasma, or serum). The LFA device typically consists of a cassette enclosing a strip of polymer membrane containing a test line and a control line.

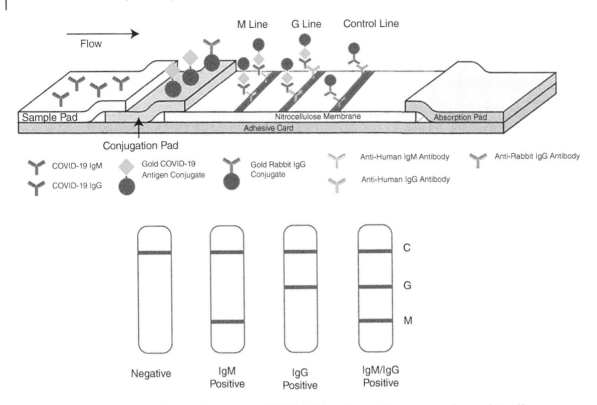

Figure 3.4 Lateral flow assay. *Source:* Augustine et al. [107]. A link to the creative commons license: https://creativecommons.org/licenses/by/4.0/legalcode.

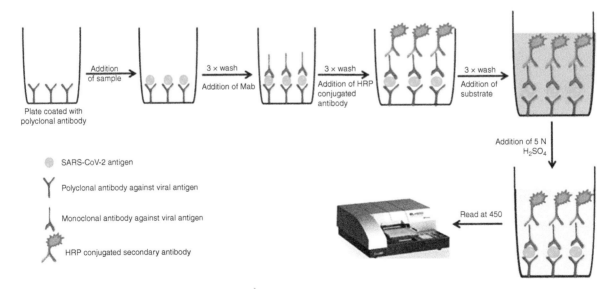

Figure 3.5 An overview of sandwich ELISA assay for the detection of SARS-CoV-2 antigens. HRP, horseradish peroxidase; Mab, monoclonal antibody. *Source:* Rai et al. [1].

The liquid sample is deposited onto the surface of a sample strip, which then moves through the strip via capillary action. When the sample encounters the test line, antibodies labeled with gold nanoparticles bind to the molecules of interest in the sample. As the sample continues to move, the excess gold-labeled antibodies are captured at the control line. Even in the absence of the target molecule in the sample solution, the gold-labeled antibodies must be captured at the control line to ensure test validity. If the test is for a single class of antibody, the window should display either one or two stripes. In this scenario, a negative test should display one stripe only at the control line, whereas a positive test should display two stripes both at the test and control lines. If the test is for two classes of antibodies (e.g. IgG and IgM), the window can display either one, two, or three stripes. In this scenario, a negative test should again display one stripe only at the control line. If the test is positive for both antibodies, three stripes will be displayed (e.g. one at the control line, one at the IgG test line, and one at the IgM test line). In an IgG/IgM test, only one antibody may be present, which serves as an indirect marker of the course of infection [108].

SARS-CoV-2 antibody tests also can be based on ELISA assays, where a recombinant viral antigen is coated onto the surface of a plastic well and acts as the target molecule. The sample (i.e. the patient's blood/serum/plasma) is added to the well. If primary antibodies against the target antigen are present in the sample, binding between recombinant viral antigen and antibodies in the added sample occurs. The excess sample is washed out to ensure all unbound substrate is removed. Next, a second solution containing labeled anti-human secondary antibodies is added and allowed to bind the primary (patient-derived) antibody. If the antibody of interest is absent in the sample, no binding occurs because there are no primary antibodies present to which a secondary antibody can bind. The excess is again washed out, and the binding of target antibodies is confirmed by an enzyme-dependent reaction (e.g. horseradish peroxidase) that usually involves a color change. This color change is measured using a spectrometer. An ELISA can be qualitative, semiquantitative, or quantitative. Qualitative assays provide a binary positive or negative result for a run sample, and the cutoff is determined

by the analyst. A semiquantitative ELISA compares relative levels of antigen within samples. A quantitative assay compares the measured optical density of the run sample with a standard curve of a solution with known concentrations, which is then used to extrapolate the antibody concentration of the analyte [108]. CLIAs are carried out in a similar manner to ELISA tests; however, binding of the secondary antibody is confirmed by a separate chemiluminescent substrate [108]. The detection of antibody binding is based on an immunochemical reaction that produces photons instead of relying on a color change. The emitted photons are measured to quantify the antibody concentration of the analyte.

The rapid evolution of the COVID-19 pandemic, coupled with limited laboratory testing capacity, test reagent shortages, and high demand for diagnostic tests with rapid turnaround time have encouraged the development of POC tests. POC tests provide results at the patient bedside or testing site with rapid turnaround and minimal supplies, without trained laboratory personnel to operate the tests. LFA has the benefit over ELISA or CLIA as potentially being executed as a POC test. ELISA and CLIA are multistep techniques with longer turnaround times, typically on the order of hours, that can be conducted only in laboratories with skilled laboratory personnel and specific equipment. In contrast, LFA tests can return results in a matter of minutes; moreover, operating an LFA is as simple as loading a patient's sample on the test device, which avoids burdening laboratories and consuming resources [1]. This pandemic has led many investigators to focus their efforts on improving the sensitivity and specificity of LFA tests [108].

Neutralization Assays

Although most assays measure antigen-binding antibodies, neutralizing antibody assays have the distinct advantage of measuring the magnitude of effective humoral response, which is important in determining whether those recovered from infection or immunized individuals possess protection from repeat infection (Figure 3.6). Viral neutralization assay is highly sensitive and specific in that it detects only antibodies that inhibit viral replication in cell culture. In a conventional neutralization assay, neutralizing ability is

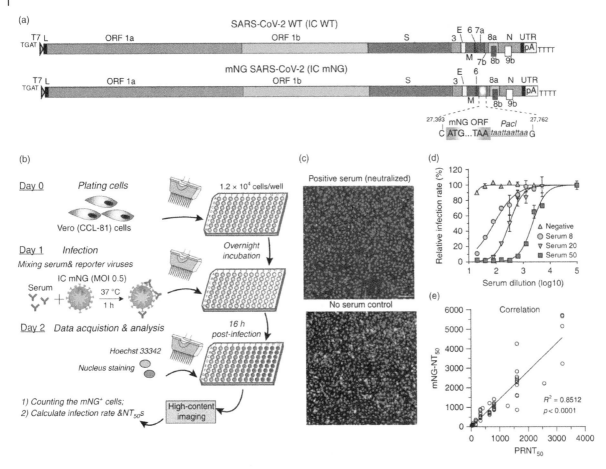

Figure 3.6 A high-throughput neutralizing antibody assay for COVID-19 diagnosis. *Source:* Muruato et al. [109]. A link to the creative commons license: https://creativecommons.org/licenses/by/4.0/legalcode.

measured using a plaque reduction neutralization test (PRNT). In a PRNT, the patient's sample of interest (serum) is diluted and incubated with a viral suspension, allowing antibodies in the serum sample to react with the virus. This mixture is applied over a monolayer of host cells, and agar or carboxymethyl cellulose is subsequently applied to prevent uncontrolled viral spreading. The number of plaques (representing areas of infected cells) that form over time can be used to quantify the concentration of plaque-forming units. The titer of neutralizing antibody is determined by the highest serum dilution required to inhibit infectivity. $PRNT_{50}$ (sometimes denoted NT_{50}) represents the concentration of serum (theoretically containing neutralizing antibodies) required to halve the number of plaques formed when compared with the number of

plaques formed by the viral suspension without incubation with serum. Magnitude of plaque reduction therefore correlates to how effective the serum antibodies are at neutralizing the virus [109].

Neutralization assays are not without their limitations. True neutralization assays require the use of viral culture. Performing these assays poses infectious risk; therefore, these techniques can be conducted only in specially equipped biosafety level 3 laboratories. Moreover, neutralization assays tend to have lower throughput in comparison with enzyme immunoassays, demanding more laboratory resources and run time [109].

The risk for infection can be circumvented by using pseudoviruses. Pseudoviruses are nonpathogenic viruses that are genetically modified to display certain

SARS-CoV-2 proteins. These pseudoviruses may also be modified to include a reporter gene encoding a fluorescent protein, allowing viral entry into host cells to be quantified. Other surrogate tests have been designed, such as a modified ELISA using human ACE2 receptor and horseradish peroxidase–conjugated SARS-CoV-2 RBD protein. In this design, antibodies in patient serum may block the RBD–ACE2 interaction, which serves as a proxy measure of neutralization. These modified techniques can be conducted in biosafety level 2 laboratories. Notably, these nonconventional tests are only surrogate markers for viral neutralization. In the latter design, for example, disruption of the RBD–ACE2 interaction assesses just one of many possible mechanisms through which an antibody may neutralize SARS-CoV-2 entry [108, 110, 111]. Another limitation of neutralization assays is that cell type affects neutralization ability, in that use of the wrong cell line may lead to inaccurate results. Nevertheless, neutralization assays remain the gold standard serologic tests in that they assess an individual's immune protection against infection and may have particular use in evaluating vaccine efficacy [2].

Antibody Assay Sensitivity and Specificity

One of the greatest concerns regarding antibody-based tests is cross-reactivity, potentially leading to false-positive results. Cross-reactivity is the binding of an antibody to an antigen different from the target antigen and is often attributable to similarities in molecular structure. For instance, studies have demonstrated cross-reactivity between SARS-CoV-2 S proteins and MERS-CoV S proteins. No cross-reactivity has yet been shown between the S1 subunit of SARS-CoV-2 and the S1 domain of MERS-CoV S1 domain, suggesting that S1 may be a superior target for antibody testing. For example, a patient previously infected with SARS-CoV or MERS-CoV may inaccurately test positive for SARS-CoV-2. Moreover, a negative antibody test does not confirm that a patient is not infected, because an antibody response does not occur immediately with early SARS-CoV-2 infection. For example, an infected patient may inaccurately test negative for SARS-CoV-2 because the immune system has not yet produced antibodies at detectable levels. Therefore, establishing the clinical sensitivity and specificity

values of serologic tests at different time points is critical in determining their reliability and subsequent applicability in practice [108].

Clinical sensitivity is the ability for an assay to correctly categorize an individual as having a particular disease. Contrast that with analytical sensitivity, which describes the smallest amount/concentration of a target in a sample that an assay can detect. In this respect, analytical sensitivity is often synonymous with LoD. Clinical specificity is the ability for an assay to correctly categorize an individual as not having a particular disease. Contrast that with analytical specificity, which describes the degree to which an assay can exclusively identify the target of interest. Analytical sensitivity and specificity pertain strictly to the performance of the assay itself, whereas clinical sensitivity and specificity are relevant when assays are applied to individuals [112]. Subsequently, in this section, we will be focusing on clinical sensitivity and specificity. The sensitivity of a test can be calculated by dividing the number of true-positive results by the number of true-positive results + false-negative results. In this sense, sensitivity represents the probability of an antibody test being positive when infection with SARS-CoV-2 is present. Conversely, specificity is the ability for a test to correctly categorize an individual as not having a SARS-CoV-2 infection. The specificity of a test can be calculated by dividing the number of true-negative results by the number of true-negative results + false-positive results. Thus, when applied in this sense, specificity represents the probability of an antibody test being negative when infection with SARS-CoV-2 is absent. Sensitivity and specificity are inversely related such that as sensitivity increases, specificity generally decreases, and vice versa. Therefore, selecting the balance of sensitivity and specificity of a test depends on the purpose for which the test is intended. Tests with high specificity rule in disease, whereas tests with high sensitivity rule out disease; therefore, a screening test should aim to be highly sensitive, whereas a confirmatory test should aim to be highly specific. Ideally, screening tests should identify infected patients at an early stage to prevent spread and to allow for monitoring of the development of severe complications in these patients. Conversely, confirmatory tests should aim to identify negative cases to prevent unnecessary isolation and quarantine measures with their associated negative impacts on the economy and social well-being [113].

Humoral Response to SARS-CoV-2 Infection

Kinetics of Antibody Response

As described briefly earlier, immunoglobin isotype profiles change in an infected individual over the course of the disease. A typical response involves early IgM predominance with gradual evolution to IgG predominance to confer long-term immunity. Antibody-based tests take advantage of this principle to surveil and characterize the stage of infection in viral infection. For instance, the presence or absence of certain Igs in hepatitis B is used to distinguish whether an individual is in the acute versus chronic hepatitis B–infected state, recovered state, or immunized state after vaccination. There has been a great effort to characterize the kinetics of antibody response to SARS-CoV-2, in hopes to better understand the immune response to infection and how to apply this information to diagnosis, patient management, public health, and beyond.

Seroconversion is defined as the new development of detectable antibodies in serum specific to an invading pathogen. Current data show that on infection with SARS-CoV-2, seroconversion of IgM, IgG, and IgA take a median of 5–18, 9.5–20, and 5–11 days, respectively [2]. According to the FDA, IgM antibodies to SARS-CoV-2 are detectable in the blood only a few days after initial infection; however, IgM antibody levels are not well characterized over the course of infection. IgG has been noted to be detectable as early as 3 days from symptom onset [10]. Investigators have also examined the antibody kinetics of the SARS-CoV to better predict SARS-CoV-2 disease progression (Figure 3.7). Overall, the kinetics of SARS-CoV-2 seroconversion are similar to that of SARS-CoV infection. In a study of 30 patients with SARS-CoV infection, seroconversion of IgM, IgG, and IgA was reported to occur at a mean of 11, 10, and 11 days, respectively [114].

There has also been an effort to quantify how long different Ig isotypes continue to circulate after infection. In SARS-CoV-2 infection, serum positivity for IgM antibodies initially increases with infection, then decreases over time. IgG positivity tends to peak later but stay elevated for a longer period compared with IgM or IgA. Maximum serum IgG concentration occurs on days 19–21 from symptom onset and has been reported to remain in high concentrations until week 6 of infection. Maximum IgM level is found in weeks 2–4 after disease onset and appears to decline in concentration from the fifth week onward. Peak IgA concentration seems to occur between days 20 and 22 and declines approximately by day 42. Notably, there may be substantial variability among individuals in terms of antibody kinetics. Seroconversion has been shown to occur within less than 1 week of infection to as far out as 6 weeks after symptom onset. Patients with milder SARS-CoV-2 infections tend to seroconvert later (or not at all), and patients with more severe infections tend to seroconvert earlier in the disease course [7, 102].

Characterizing the kinetics of antibody production greatly impacts the role of antibody-based testing in diagnosis. Studies characterizing IgG kinetics, especially those showing the decline of IgG levels in serum after resolution of infection, have called into question whether long-term immunity against SARS-CoV-2 exists. This notion has clear implications with regard to the use of convalescent plasma and vaccinations efforts, which will be discussed later [2].

Antibody Response and Disease Severity

Overall, the more severe an infection is, the more robustly the immune system responds to the infection. In SARS-CoV-2 infection, antibody titers appear to be associated with severity of symptoms: the highest antibody titers are found in patients with the most severe infections. High antibody titer may therefore be considered a risk factor for critical illness [115]. Epidemiologic data have shown disproportionate impacts on populations with regard to age and sex. Notably, age is the most significant predictor of SARS-CoV-2 infection outcome. Patients ≥50 years of age in the United States have the highest mortality rates (representing >94% of total COVID-19 deaths). In contrast, patients 18–29 years of age have a mortality rate of 0.5% but represent the majority of total COVID-19 cases (23.3%). In the United States, 51.7% of COVID-19

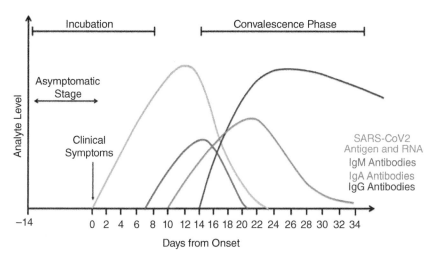

Figure 3.7 Antibody kinetics. *Source:* Younes et al. [10]. A link to the creative commons license: https://creativecommons.org/licenses/by/4.0/legalcode.

cases are female and 48.3% are male; however, only 46% of COVID-19 deaths are female, while 54% are male [116]. Interestingly, the degree of antibody response correlates to age and sex [2]. For instance, one study found that female patients with severe disease exhibited higher IgG levels than male patients. In addition, females generated a more robust IgG response than male patients in the early disease phase [117]. This difference in antibody response may explain the well-described higher clinical severity and mortality rate in males [2, 117].

Conversely, asymptomatic patients develop lower IgG antibody levels compared with symptomatic patients, which suggests that asymptomatic patients do not mount as robust an immune response, and that immunity may diminish sooner after infection than for those with more clinically severe disease [102]. This suggests that antibody-based testing may have more limitations in terms of diagnostic value for those with less severe disease: those with milder infections and associated lower antibody titers may not mount a sufficient humoral response to be detected by antibody-based testing. Further complicating the picture, it has been reported that approximately 5–10% of infected individuals do not develop an antibody response after infection [103]. This suggests that antibody testing may be of limited diagnostic value to a certain percentage of those infected who do not mount a sufficient antibody reaction to SARS-CoV-2 infection.

Duration of Immunity

On 25 August 2020, the first case of SARS-CoV-2 reinfection was reported in an immunocompetent Hong Kong resident. In this patient, the interval between first and second infections was 142 days [84]. The CDC initially released a statement claiming that immunity was thought to last at least 90 days, similar to the immunity duration of other betacoronaviruses. Since the release of that statement, reports of reinfection as early as 45 days after initial infection onset have surfaced, causing many to question the existence of long-term immunity against SARS-CoV-2 [118–123]. Studies investigating SARS-CoV and coronaviruses that cause common colds may provide insight into this question. Studies involving survivors of the 2003 SARS epidemic have reported that neutralizing antibodies are maintained for 2 years, on average, after infection. Other coronaviruses responsible for the common cold show 45 weeks of immunity, on average, implying that if SARS-CoV-2 followed this latter pattern, it could lead to annual outbreaks like the annual seasonal influenza [104]. The duration of antibody response in SARS-CoV-2 infection remains unclear. Some have reported that IgA and IgM antibodies may rapidly decline within 2–3 weeks of development; other studies suggest that IgG may persist in serum for as long as 4 months after SARS-CoV-2 infection. As the pandemic rages on, it will be of particular importance to further characterize the duration of humoral response to SARS-CoV-2 infection, because this has tremendous implications pertaining to long-term immunity.

Many studies demonstrate seroconversion at approximately 7 days after infection; other studies suggest a larger time range during which seroconversion can occur. Asymptomatic patients may seroconvert later in the course of infection or may not seroconvert at all. Patients with more severe disease have been shown to develop antibodies earlier in their course of infection. This variability convolutes the diagnostic certainty of these antibody tests, because one must also consider clinical severity as a factor in characterizing chronicity of antibody response to SARS-CoV-2. It is currently unknown which antibodies, if any, confer immunity to SARS-CoV-2 infection and the duration of this plausible conferred immunity. Given the variation in response among infected patients and delay in serologic positivity from onset of disease, antibody-based tests are mostly intended for monitoring later stages of disease. Recent studies have suggested that an individual's antibody profile has the potential to be used to stage COVID-19 progression and to possibly help guide management of the disease [102]. However, with very little data beyond 35 days postsymptom onset at this time, there is limited utility of antibody tests for individualized disease staging or clinical management, as well as limited utility in public health applications [124]. Results from antibody-based testing should not be used in isolation, but rather should be taken in conjunction with results from the gold standard PCR-based tests [102].

Current and Potential Applications of Antibody-Based Tests in SARS-CoV-2

Management of Individual Disease and Sequelae Monitoring

Ultimately, SARS-CoV-2 antibody testing may play a role in postinfection medical management. There is an increasing appreciation that SARS-CoV-2 causes postinfectious medical sequelae in all age groups, regardless of initial infection severity [5]. These patients suffering from persistent or new symptoms after recovery from acute illness have been referred to as "long haulers" or experiencing "long COVID" [125]. It has been suggested that 50–80% of patients with COVID-19 will experience mild symptoms months after infection, and 10% may experience more severe, prolonged symptoms after recovery from acute infection [126]. Many of the symptoms long haulers experience have been attributed to one of the hallmark features of SARS-CoV-2 infection: inflammatory dysregulation. In the body's normal response to viral invasion, inflammation is a key defense mechanism against infection; however, unregulated inflammation can lead to systemic and indiscriminate self-damage by immune cells. Antibody assays have been proposed as a diagnostic tool for identifying past disease and monitoring for postinfectious sequelae.

In children, SARS-CoV-2 infection is associated with an entity known as multisystem inflammatory syndrome in children (MIS-C) and is characterized by inflammation of two or more organ systems. Heart, lungs, kidneys, brain, skin, eyes, or the gastrointestinal organs have all been shown to be systems affected in MIS-C [5]. Clinical features of MIS-C resemble those of Kawasaki disease (mucocutaneous lymph node syndrome), a rare vasculitis of unknown cause suspected to result from viral infection triggering an unregulated immune response. The pathogenesis of MIS-C is therefore hypothesized to involve a similar postinfectious immune dysregulation [127]. Notably, children presenting with MIS-C have a high seroprevalence. Moreover, pediatric patients with MIS-C have demonstrated significantly higher titers of SARS-CoV-2 binding and neutralizing antibodies compared with children with COVID-19 infection alone. In MIS-C, antibody titer has also been correlated with hospital and intensive care unit length of stay. SARS-CoV-2 antibody assays therefore can provide both diagnostic and prognostic value in MIS-C. In fact, the CDC includes serologic evidence of SARS-CoV-2 as one component in the MIS-C diagnostic criteria [128–130].

In the adult population, however, immune dysregulation is thought to be responsible for the severe manifestations and sequelae of the disease. Severe SARS-CoV-2 infection can result in cytokine storm, in which hyperexpression of circulating inflammatory cytokines and chemokines results in systemic immune cell infiltration and macrophage/neutrophil-mediated tissue destruction. Post-COVID myocarditis, interstitial lung disease, as well as neuronal injury leading to anosmia, headache, anxiety, depression, chronic fatigue, autonomic dysfunction, and even demyelinating or neurodegenerative disorders are among the sequelae reported [5, 126]. Because the majority of those with long COVID have resolved the acute infection and should be PCR negative, antibody-based tests help in determining past infection. Because long-term sequelae can develop even in those with asymptomatic SARS-CoV-2 infection, serologic evidence helps indicate past exposure to the virus.

Contact Tracing

Antibody-based tests have been used in conjunction with PCR testing to identify origin cases. The principle of contact tracing involves the interruption of infection transmission through quarantine measures for contacts of those suspected to be exposed to infectious individuals (termed "cases"). Contact tracing is performed when individuals at risk for infection based on exposure to cases (termed "contacts") take self-quarantine measures.

Antibody-based testing can be of use in contact tracing for SARS-CoV-2 because a large proportion of those infected are asymptomatic. Those without symptoms potentially evade detection and can propagate the spread of infection [131]. Antibody testing has been used to trace the initial cases responsible for outbreaks within families, workplaces, and cities and countries. If contact tracing decisions were based solely on recall of clinical symptoms or qRT-PCR, contacts may not receive adequate quarantining directives [2].

Vaccine Efficacy

Another role of antibody-based testing in COVID-19 is in the assessment of vaccine efficacy. Assessing sensitivity of SARS-CoV-2 (or typically SARS-CoV-2 pseudoviruses displaying certain epitopes) to vaccine-elicited antibodies can also help determine vaccine efficacy against variants of SARS-CoV-2, which are continually undergoing mutations that allow them to evade neutralization by antibodies present in those who have received vaccines [109, 132]. For instance, the BNT162b2 (BioNTech-Pfizer) vaccine, which has

demonstrated 95% efficacy in a phase II/III trial to protect against symptomatic COVID-19, has been shown to generate neutralizing antibodies effective against 22 pseudoviruses displaying different S proteins from various SARS-CoV-2 variants [133, 134]. Neutralizing antibody assays also play a key role in assessing the duration of immunity conferred by vaccines. Neutralization assays performed using serum collected from individuals at different time points after vaccination can indicate when vaccine-induced immunity begins to wane, which subsequently informs public health decisions.

The topic of assessing vaccine efficacy is particularly timely given the emergence of the highly transmissible B.1.617.2 delta variant [88]. There are reports demonstrating the delta variant escaping neutralizing antibodies generated in sera of individuals who received only one dose of the BioNTech-Pfizer vaccine or the AstraZeneca vaccine; however, vaccine efficacy reportedly remains in those who have received both doses of the Pfizer vaccine [135–140]. In addition, the Johnson & Johnson vaccine induces significant neutralizing antibody activity against the delta variant [88, 141]. The results of neutralizing antibody assays in evaluating vaccine efficacy may have major implications regarding the need for vaccine developers to devise booster strategies. As of this writing, however, there are no accepted thresholds of antibody levels that can differentiate protection versus susceptibility of individuals to infection.

Conclusions and Future Directions

The COVID-19 pandemic has wreaked havoc across the world, overwhelming healthcare systems worldwide and causing extensive economic and social disruption. There are currently no proven curative treatments for COVID-19, so control of the pandemic's spread has been geared heavily toward prevention. Aside from the tremendous ongoing vaccination efforts, diagnostic technologies have constituted one of the most important tools in combating the COVID-19 pandemic. Given that SARS-CoV-2 is a highly transmissible respiratory virus that often presents with nonspecific clinical manifestations and is frequently transmissible by asymptomatic carriers, there has been a pressing need for the development of accurate, fast, and accessible diagnostic technologies for detecting SARS-CoV-2 infection. Disruption of the infectious chain through quarantine measures has been paramount to quelling the spread of COVID-19, and diagnostic testing has enabled these measures via timely identification of infected individuals.

As covered in this chapter, many techniques have been developed for the diagnosis of COVID-19. Rapid isolation and genetic sequencing of SARS-CoV-2 enabled the development of NAAT, which continues to be the gold standard diagnostic approach. Antibody-based tests have enabled the characterization of the human immune response to SARS-CoV-2 infection and continue to play a role in epidemiology and public health. There is an increasing demand now for the development of POC tests, which are ideally accurate, accessible, rapid, and cost-effective. POC diagnostic techniques have been generated using newer technologies, which rely less on sophisticated laboratory equipment. These techniques will be particularly important in geographies with limited laboratory infrastructure. The rapid and unprecedented emergence of SARS-CoV-2, as well as the tremendous feats of scientists worldwide to rapidly develop techniques to detect COVID-19, underscores the importance of investing in diagnostic testing technologies so we can be prepared for pandemics to come.

Disclosure statement: The authors declare they have no conflict of interest in this study.

References

1 Rai, P., Kumar, B.K., Deekshit, V.K. et al. (2021). Detection technologies and recent developments in the diagnosis of COVID-19 infection. *Appl Microbiol Biotechnol.* (105): 441–455.

2 Jiang, J.C. and Zhang, Y. (2020). Serological antibody testing in the COVID-19 pandemic: their molecular basis and applications. *Biochem Soc Trans.* 48 (6): 2851–2863.

3 Hellewell, J., Abbott, S., Gimma, A. et al. (2020). Feasibility of controlling COVID-19 outbreaks by isolation of cases and contacts. *Lancet Glob Health* 8 (4): e488–e496.

4 Anderson, R.M., Heesterbeek, H., Klinkenberg, D., and Hollingsworth, T.D. (2020). How will country-based mitigation measures influence the course of the COVID-19 epidemic? *Lancet* 395 (10228): 931–934.

5 West, R., Kobokovich, A., Connell, N., and Gronvall, G.K. (2020). COVID-19 antibody tests: a valuable public health tool with limited relevance to individuals. *Trends Microbiol.* 29 (3): 214–223.

6 Moghadas, S.M., Fitzpatrick, M.C., Sah, P. et al. (2020). The implications of silent transmission for the control of COVID-19 outbreaks. *Proc Natl Acad Sci USA* 117 (30): 17513–17515.

7 Ejazi, S.A., Ghosh, S., and Ali, N. (2021). Antibody detection assays for COVID-19 diagnosis: an early overview. *Immunol Cell Biol.* 99 (1): 21–33.

8 Udugama, B., Kadhiresan, P., Kozlowski, H.N. et al. (2020). Diagnosing COVID-19: the disease and tools for detection. *ACS Nano* 14 (4): 3822–3835.

9 El Jaddaoui, I., Allali, M., Raoui, S. et al. (2021). A review on current diagnostic techniques for COVID-19. *Expert Rev Mol Diagn.* 21 (2): 141–160.

10 Younes, N., Al-Sadeq, D.W., Al-Jighefee, H. et al. (2020). Challenges in laboratory diagnosis of the novel coronavirus SARS-CoV-2. *Viruses* 12 (6): 582.

11 Dramé, M., Teguo, M.T., Proye, E. et al. (2020). Should RT-PCR be considered a gold standard in the diagnosis of Covid-19? *J Med Virol.* 92 (11): 2312–2313.

12 Ward, S., Lindsley, A., Courter, J., and Assa'ad, A. (2020). Clinical testing for COVID-19. *J Allergy Clin Immunol.* 146 (1): 23–34.

13 Li, Y., Yao, L., Li, J. et al. (2020). Stability issues of RT-PCR testing of SARS-CoV-2 for hospitalized patients clinically diagnosed with COVID-19. *J Med Virol.* 92 (7): 903–908.

14 Gao, J. and Quan, L. (2020). Current status of diagnostic testing for SARS-CoV-2 infection and future developments: a review. *Med Sci Monit.* 26: e928552-1.

15 Pfefferle, S., Reucher, S., Nörz, D., and Lütgehetmann, M. (2020). Evaluation of a quantitative RT-PCR assay for the detection of the

emerging coronavirus SARS-CoV-2 using a high throughput system. *Euro Surveill.* 25 (9): 2000152.

16 Bwire, G.M., Majigo, M.V., Njiro, B.J., and Mawazo, A. (2021). Detection profile of SARS-CoV-2 using RT-PCR in different types of clinical specimens: a systematic review and meta-analysis. *J Med Virol.* 93 (2): 719–725.

17 Hanson, K.E., Caliendo, A.M., Arias, C.A. et al. (2021). The Infectious Diseases Society of America Guidelines on the diagnosis of COVID-19: molecular diagnostic testing. *Clin Infect Dis.* https://doi.org/10.1093/cid/ciab048.

18 Hanson, K.E., Caliendo, A.M., Arias, C.A. et al. (2020). Infectious Diseases Society of America Guidelines on the diagnosis of COVID-19: serologic testing. *Clin Infect Dis.* https://doi.org/10.1093/cid/ciaa1343.

19 Hanson, K.E., Altayar, O., Caliendo, A.M. et al. (2021). The Infectious Diseases Society of America Guidelines on the diagnosis of COVID-19: antigen testing. *Clin Infect Dis.* https://doi.org/10.1093/cid/ciab557.

20 Zhang, W., Du, R.H., Li, B. et al. (2020). Molecular and serological investigation of 2019-nCoV infected patients: implication of multiple shedding routes. *Emerg Microbes Infect.* 9 (1): 386–389.

21 Destras, G., Bal, A., Escuret, V. et al. (2020). Systematic SARS-CoV-2 screening in cerebrospinal fluid during the COVID-19 pandemic. *Lancet Microbe* 1 (4): e149.

22 Li, C., Zhao, C., Bao, J. et al. (2020). Laboratory diagnosis of coronavirus disease-2019 (COVID-19). *Clin Chim Acta.* 510: 35.

23 Ji, T., Liu, Z., Wang, G. et al. (2020). Detection of COVID-19: a review of the current literature and future perspectives. *Biosens Bioelectron.* 166: 112455.

24 Lai, C.K. and Lam, W. (2021). Laboratory testing for the diagnosis of COVID-19. *Biochem Biophys Res Commun.* 538: 226–230.

25 Yang, Y., Yang, M., Yuan, J. et al. (2020). Comparative sensitivity of different respiratory specimen types for molecular diagnosis and monitoring of SARS-CoV-2 shedding in COVID-19 patients. *Innovation (New York, NY)* 1 (3): 100061.

26 Torres, A. and El-Ebiary, M. (2000). Bronchoscopic BAL in the diagnosis of ventilator-associated pneumonia. *Chest* 117 (4): S198.

27 Abid, M.B., Chhabra, S., Buchan, B. et al. (2021). Bronchoalveolar lavage-based COVID-19 testing in patients with cancer. *Hematol Oncol Stem Cell Ther.* 14 (1): 65–70.

28 van Grootveld, R., van Paassen, J., de Boer, M.G. et al. (2021). Systematic screening for COVID-19 associated invasive aspergillosis in ICU patients by culture and PCR on tracheal aspirate. *Mycoses* 64 (6): 641–650.

29 Tu, Y.P., Jennings, R., Hart, B. et al. (2020). Patient-collected tongue, nasal, and mid-turbinate swabs for SARS-CoV-2 yield equivalent sensitivity to health care worker collected nasopharyngeal swabs. *MedRxiv* https://doi.org/10.1101/2020.04.0 1.20050005.

30 Lin, C., Xiang, J., Yan, M. et al. (2020). Comparison of throat swabs and sputum specimens for viral nucleic acid detection in 52 cases of novel coronavirus (SARS-Cov-2)-infected pneumonia (COVID-19). *Clin Chem Lab Med.* 58 (7): 1089–1094.

31 Jamal, A.J., Mozafarihashjin, M., Coomes, E. et al. (2021). Sensitivity of nasopharyngeal swabs and saliva for the detection of severe acute respiratory syndrome coronavirus 2. *Clin Infect Dis.* 72 (6): 1064–1066.

32 Dawes, C. and Wong, D.T.W. (2019). Role of saliva and salivary diagnostics in the advancement of oral health. *J Dent Res.* 98 (2): 133–141.

33 Czumbel, L.M., Kiss, S., Farkas, N. et al. (2020). Saliva as a candidate for COVID-19 diagnostic testing: a meta-analysis. *Front Med.* 7: 465.

34 Williams, E., Bond, K., Zhang, B. et al. (2020). Saliva as a noninvasive specimen for detection of SARS-CoV-2. *J Clin Microbiol.* 58 (8): e00776-20.

35 Kojima, N., Turner, F., Slepnev, V. et al. (2020). Self-collected oral fluid and nasal swabs demonstrate comparable sensitivity to clinician collected nasopharyngeal swabs for Covid-19 detection. *medRxiv* https://doi.org/10.1101/2020.04.11.20062372.

36 Wehrhahn, M.C., Robson, J., Brown, S. et al. (2020). Self-collection: an appropriate alternative during the SARS-CoV-2 pandemic. *J Clin Virol.* 128: 104417.

37 Varga, G. (2015). Physiology of the salivary glands. *Surgery (Oxford)* 33 (12): 581–586.

38 Yu, F., Yan, L., Wang, N. et al. (2020). Quantitative detection and viral load analysis of SARS-CoV-2 in infected patients. *Clin Infect Dis.* 71 (15): 793–798.

39 Chen, L., Wang, G., Long, X. et al. (2021). Dynamics of blood viral load is strongly associated with clinical outcomes in coronavirus disease 2019 (COVID-19) patients: a prospective cohort study. *J Mol Diagn.* 23 (1): 10–18.

40 Wang, W., Xu, Y., Gao, R. et al. (2020). Detection of SARS-CoV-2 in different types of clinical specimens. *JAMA* 323 (18): 1843–1844.

41 Richter, E., Al Arashi, D., Schulte, B. et al. (2021). Detectable SARS-CoV-2 RNAemia in critically ill patients, but not in mild and asymptomatic infections. *Transfus Med Hemother.* 48 (3): 154–160.

42 Eberhardt, K.A., Meyer-Schwickerath, C., Heger, E. et al. (2020). RNAemia corresponds to disease severity and antibody response in hospitalized COVID-19 patients. *Viruses* 12 (9): 1045.

43 Hogan, C.A., Stevens, B.A., Sahoo, M.K. et al. (2021). High frequency of SARS-CoV-2 RNAemia and association with severe disease. *Clin Infect Dis.* 72 (9): e291–e295.

44 Xu, Y., Li, X., Zhu, B. et al. (2020). Characteristics of pediatric SARS-CoV-2 infection and potential evidence for persistent fecal viral shedding. *Nat Med.* 26 (4): 502–505.

45 Chen, Y., Chen, L., Deng, Q. et al. (2020). The presence of SARS-CoV-2 RNA in the feces of COVID-19 patients. *J Med Virol.* 92 (7): 833–840.

46 Yang, Y., Yang, M., Yuan, J. et al. (2020). Laboratory diagnosis and monitoring the viral shedding of SARS-CoV-2 infection. *Innovation* 1 (3): 100061.

47 de Souza, S.P., Silveira, M.A.D., de Freitas Souza, B.S. et al. (2021). Evaluation of urine SARS-COV-2 RT-PCR as a predictor of acute kidney injury and disease severity in critical COVID-19 patients. *medRxiv* https://doi.org/10.1101/2021.01.13.21249576.

48 Chambers, C., Krogstad, P., Bertrand, K. et al. (2020). Evaluation for SARS-CoV-2 in breast milk from 18 infected women. *JAMA* 324 (13): 1347–1348.

49 Bastug, A., Hanifehnezhad, A., Tayman, C. et al. (2020). Virolactia in an asymptomatic mother with COVID-19. *Breastfeed Med.* 15 (8): 488–491.

50 Kim, J.Y., Ko, J.H., Kim, Y. et al. (2020). Viral load kinetics of SARS-CoV-2 infection in first two patients in Korea. *J Korean Med Sci.* 35 (7): e86.

51 Hong, K.H., Lee, S.W., Kim, T.S. et al. (2020). Guidelines for laboratory diagnosis of coronavirus disease 2019 (COVID-19) in Korea. *Ann Lab Med.* 40 (5): 351–360.

52 Centers for Disease Control and Prevention (2019). Interim Guidelines for Collecting. Handling, and Testing Clinical Specimens from Persons for Coronavirus Disease. https://www.cdc.gov/coronavirus/2019-ncov/lab/guidelines-clinical-specimens.html (accessed 15 February 2022).

53 Public Health England (2020). Understanding cycle threshold (Ct) in SARS-CoV-2 RT-PCR. https://assets.publishing.service.gov.uk/government/uploads/system/uploads/attachment_data/file/926410/Understanding_Cycle_Threshold__Ct__in_SARS-CoV-2_RT-PCR_.pdf (accessed 15 February 2022).

54 Tan, W., Lu, Y., Zhang, J. et al. (2020). Viral kinetics and antibody responses in patients with COVID-19. *medRxiv* https://doi.org/10.1101/2020.03.24.20042382.

55 Zou, L., Ruan, F., Huang, M. et al. (2020). SARS-CoV-2 viral load in upper respiratory specimens of infected patients. *N Engl J Med.* 382 (12): 1177–1179.

56 Binnicker, M.J. (2020). Challenges and controversies to testing for COVID-19. *J Clin Microbiol.* 58 (11): e01695–e01620. https://doi.org/10.1128/jcm.01695-20.

57 Pujadas, E., Chaudhry, F., McBride, R. et al. (2020). SARS-CoV-2 viral load predicts COVID-19 mortality. *Lancet Respir Med.* 8 (9): e70.

58 Argyropoulos, K.V., Serrano, A., Hu, J. et al. (2020). Association of initial viral load in severe acute respiratory syndrome coronavirus 2 (SARS-CoV-2) patients with outcome and symptoms. *Am J Pathol.* 190 (9): 1881–1887.

59 Tsukagoshi, H., Shinoda, D., Saito, M. et al. (2021). Relationships between viral load and the clinical course of COVID-19. *Viruses* 13 (2): 304.

60 Zheng, S., Fan, J., Yu, F. et al. (2020). Viral load dynamics and disease severity in patients infected with SARS-CoV-2 in Zhejiang province, China, January-March 2020: retrospective cohort study. *BMJ* 369: m1443.

61 Winichakoon, P., Chaiwarith, R., Liwsrisakun, C. et al. (2020). Negative nasopharyngeal and oropharyngeal swabs do not rule out COVID-19. *J Clin Microbiol.* 58 (5): e00297-20.

62 Wölfel, R., Corman, V.M., Guggemos, W. et al. (2020). Virological assessment of hospitalized patients with COVID-2019. *Nature* 581 (7809): 465–469.

63 Yan, Y., Chang, L., and Wang, L. (2020). Laboratory testing of SARS-CoV, MERS-CoV, and SARS-CoV-2 (2019-nCoV): current status, challenges, and countermeasures. *Rev Med Virol.* 30 (3): e2106.

64 Fields, B.K.K., Demirjian, N.L., and Gholamrezanezhad, A. (2020). Coronavirus disease 2019 (COVID-19) diagnostic technologies: a country-based retrospective analysis of screening and containment procedures during the first wave of the pandemic. *Clin Imaging.* 67: 219–225. https://doi.org/10.1016/j.clinimag.2020.08.014.

65 US Food and Drug Administration. FAQs on Testing for SARS-CoV-2. Coronavirus Disease 2019 (COVID-19) Emergency Use Authorizations for Medical Devices. (2021). https://www.fda.gov/medical-devices/coronavirus-disease-2019-covid-19-emergency-use-authorizations-medical-devices/faqs-emergency-use-authorizations-euas-medical-devices-during-covid-19-pandemic (accessed 15 February 2022).

66 Huang, W.E., Lim, B., Hsu, C.C. et al. (2020). RT-LAMP for rapid diagnosis of coronavirus SARS-CoV-2. *J Microbial Biotechnol.* 13 (4): 950–961.

67 Thi, V.L.D., Herbst, K., Boerner, K. et al. (2020). A colorimetric RT-LAMP assay and LAMP-sequencing for detecting SARS-CoV-2 RNA in clinical samples. *Sci Transl Med.* 12 (556): eabc7075.

68 Yang, W., Dang, X., Wang, Q. et al. (2020). Rapid detection of SARS-CoV-2 using reverse transcription RT-LAMP method. *medRxiv* https://doi.org/10.1101/2020.03.02.20030130.

69 Esbin, M.N., Whitney, O.N., Chong, S. et al. (2020). Overcoming the bottleneck to widespread testing: a rapid review of nucleic acid testing approaches for COVID-19 detection. *RNA* 26 (7): 771–783.

70 Oliveira, B.A., Oliveira, L.C.D., Sabino, E.C., and Okay, T.S. (2020). SARS-CoV-2 and the COVID-19 disease: a mini review on diagnostic methods. *Rev Inst Med Trop Sao Paulo* 62: e44.

71 Broughton, J.P., Deng, X., Yu, G. et al. (2020). CRISPR–Cas12-based detection of SARS-CoV-2. *Nat Biotechnol.* 38 (7): 870–874.

72 Nouri, R., Tang, Z., Dong, M. et al. (2021). CRISPR-based detection of SARS-CoV-2: a review from sample to result. *Biosens Bioelectron.* 178: 113012.

73 Guo, L., Sun, X., Wang, X. et al. (2020). SARS-CoV-2 detection with CRISPR diagnostics. *Cell Discov.* 6 (1): 34.

74 Takenouchi, T., Iwasaki, Y.W., Harada, S. et al. (2021). Clinical utility of SARS-CoV-2 whole genome sequencing in deciphering source of infection. *J Hosp Infect.* 107: 40–44.

75 Harilal, D., Ramaswamy, S., Loney, T. et al. (2020). SARS-CoV-2 whole genome amplification and sequencing for effective population-based surveillance and control of viral transmission. *Clin Chem.* 66 (11): 1450–1458.

76 Pillay, S., Giandhari, J., Tegally, H. et al. (2020). Whole genome sequencing of SARS-CoV-2: adapting Illumina protocols for quick and accurate outbreak investigation during a pandemic. *Genes* 11 (8): 949.

77 Chiara, M., D'Erchia, A.M., Gissi, C. et al. (2021). Next generation sequencing of SARS-CoV-2 genomes: challenges, applications and opportunities. *Brief Bioinform.* 22 (2): 616–630.

78 Behjati, S. and Tarpey, P.S. (2013). What is next generation sequencing? *Arch Dis Child Educ Pract Ed.* 98 (6): 236–238.

79 Jayamohan, H., Lambert, C.J., Sant, H.J. et al. (2021). SARS-CoV-2 pandemic: a review of molecular diagnostic tools including sample collection and commercial response with associated advantages and limitations. *Anal Bioanal Chem.* 413: 49–71.

80 McNaughton, A.L., Roberts, H.E., Bonsall, D. et al. (2019). Illumina and Nanopore methods for whole genome sequencing of hepatitis B virus (HBV). *Sci Rep.* 9 (1): 7081.

81 Rahimi, A., Mirzazadeh, A., Tavakolpour, S. et al. (2020). Genetics and genomics of SARS-CoV-2: a review of the literature with the special focus on genetic diversity and SARS-CoV-2 genome detection. *Genomics* 113: 1221–1232.

82 Pollock, N.R. and Wonderly, B. (2017). Evaluating novel diagnostics in an outbreak setting: lessons learned from Ebola. *J Clin Microbiol.* 55 (5): 1255–1261. https://doi.org/10.1128/JCM.00053-17.

83 Lu, R., Zhao, X., Li, J. et al. (2020). Genomic characterisation and epidemiology of 2019 novel coronavirus: implications for virus origins and receptor binding. *Lancet* 395 (10224): 565–574.

84 To, K.K., Hung, I.F., Ip, J.D. et al. (2021). Coronavirus disease 2019 (COVID-19) re-infection by a phylogenetically distinct SARS-coronavirus-2 strain confirmed by whole genome sequencing. *Clin Infect Dis.* 73: e2946–e2951.

85 Bedford, T., Greninger, A.L., Roychoudhury, P. et al. (2020). Cryptic transmission of SARS-CoV-2 in Washington state. *Science* 370 (6516): 571–575.

86 Holshue, M.L., DeBolt, C., Lindquist, S. et al. (2020). First case of 2019 novel coronavirus in the United States. *N Engl J Med.* 382: 929–936.

87 Munnink, B.B.O., Nieuwenhuijse, D.F., Stein, M. et al. (2020). Rapid SARS-CoV-2 whole-genome sequencing and analysis for informed public health decision-making in the Netherlands. *Nat Med.* 26 (9): 1405–1410.

88 Centers for Disease Control and Prevention (2019). Genomic Surveillance for SARS-CoV-2. SARS-CoV-2 Variant Classifications and Definitions. https://www.cdc.gov/coronavirus/2019-ncov/variants/variant-info.html#print. (access 24 Jul 2021).

89 Shu, Y. and McCauley, J. (2017). GISAID: global initiative on sharing all influenza data–from vision to reality. *Euro Surveill.* 22 (13): 30494.

90 Mertens, P., De Vos, N., Martiny, D. et al. (2020). Development and potential usefulness of the COVID-19 Ag Respi-Strip diagnostic assay in a pandemic context. *Front Med.* 7: 225.

91 Porte, L., Legarraga, P., Vollrath, V. et al. (2020). Evaluation of a novel antigen-based rapid detection test for the diagnosis of SARS-CoV-2 in respiratory samples. *Int J Infect Dis.* 99: 328–333.

92 Dinnes, J., Deeks, J.J., Adriano, A. et al. (2020). Rapid, point-of-care antigen and molecular-based tests for diagnosis of SARS-CoV-2 infection. *Cochrane Database Syst Rev.* 3 (3): CD013705. https://doi.org/10.1002/14651858.CD013705.pub2.

93 Lambert-Niclot, S., Cuffel, A., Le Pape, S. et al. (2020). Evaluation of a rapid diagnostic assay for detection of SARS-CoV-2 antigen in nasopharyngeal swabs. *J Clin Microbiol.* 58 (8): e00977-20.

94 Weitzel, T., Legarraga, P., Iruretagoyena, M. et al. (2020). Head-to-head comparison of four antigen-based rapid detection tests for the diagnosis of SARS-CoV-2 in respiratory samples. *bioRxiv* https://doi.org/10.1101/2020.05.27.119255.

95 da Silva, S.J.R., Silva, C.T.A.D., Guarines, K.M. et al. (2020). Clinical and laboratory diagnosis of SARS-CoV-2, the virus causing COVID-19. *ACS Infect Dis.* 6 (9): 2319–2336.

96 Mak, G.C., Cheng, P.K., Lau, S.S. et al. (2020). Evaluation of rapid antigen test for detection of SARS-CoV-2 virus. *J Clin Virol.* 129: 104500.

97 Perera, R.A., Tso, E., Tsang, O.T. et al. (2020). SARS-CoV-2 virus culture and subgenomic RNA for respiratory specimens from patients with mild coronavirus disease. *Emerg Infect Dis.* 26 (11): 2701.

98 Centers for Disease Control and Prevention. SARS-CoV-2 viral culturing at CDC, 2020. https://www.cdc.gov/coronavirus/2019-ncov/lab/grows-virus-cell-culture.html.

99 Zhou, P., Yang, X.L., Wang, X.G. et al. (2020). A pneumonia outbreak associated with a new coronavirus of probable bat origin. *Nature* 579 (7798): 270–273.

100 Van Doremalen, N., Bushmaker, T., Morris, D.H. et al. (2020). Aerosol and surface stability of SARS-CoV-2 as compared with SARS-CoV-1. *N Engl J Med.* 382 (16): 1564–1567.

101 Sheahan, T.P., Sims, A.C., Zhou, S. et al. (2020). An orally bioavailable broad-spectrum antiviral inhibits SARS-CoV-2 in human airway epithelial cell cultures and multiple coronaviruses in mice. *Sci Transl Med.* 12 (541): eabb5883.

102 Chau, C.H., Strope, J.D., and Figg, W.D. (2020). COVID-19 clinical diagnostics and testing technology. *Pharmacotherapy* 40 (8): 857–868.

103 Gulholm, T., Basile, K., Kok, J. et al. (2020). Laboratory diagnosis of severe acute respiratory syndrome coronavirus 2. *Pathology* 52 (7): 745–753.

104 Jacofsky, D., Jacofsky, E.M., and Jacofsky, M. (2020). Understanding antibody testing for COVID-19. *J Arthroplasty* 35 (7): S74–S81.

105 Lan, J., Ge, J., Yu, J. et al. (2020). Structure of the SARS-CoV-2 spike receptor-binding domain bound to the ACE2 receptor. *Nature* 581 (7807): 215–220.

106 Tang, Y.W., Schmitz, J.E., Persing, D.H., and Stratton, C.W. (2020). Laboratory diagnosis of COVID-19: current issues and challenges. *J Clin Microbiol.* 58 (6): e00512–e00520.

107 Augustine, R., Das, S., Hasan, A. et al. (2020). Rapid antibody-based COVID-19 mass surveillance: relevance, challenges, and prospects in a pandemic and post-pandemic world. *J Clin Med.* 9 (10): 3372.

108 Yüce, M., Filiztekin, E., and Özkaya, K.G. (2020). COVID-19 diagnosis – a review of current methods. *Biosens Bioelectron.* 172: 112752.

109 Muruato, A.E., Fontes-Garfias, C.R., Ren, P. et al. (2020). A high-throughput neutralizing antibody assay for COVID-19 diagnosis and vaccine evaluation. *Nat Commun.* 11 (1): 4059.

110 Elshabrawy, H.A., Coughlin, M.M., Baker, S.C., and Prabhakar, B.S. (2012). Human monoclonal antibodies against highly conserved HR1 and HR2 domains of the SARS-CoV spike protein are more broadly neutralizing. *PLoS One* 7 (11): e50366.

111 Duan, J., Yan, X., Guo, X. et al. (2005). A human SARS-CoV neutralizing antibody against epitope on S2 protein. *Biochem Biophys Res Commun.* 333 (1): 186–193.

112 Saah, A.J. and Hoover, D.R. (1997). "Sensitivity" and "specificity" reconsidered: the meaning of these terms in analytical and diagnostic settings. *Ann Intern Med.* 126 (1): 91–94.

113 Parikh, R., Mathai, A., Parikh, S. et al. (2008). Understanding and using sensitivity, specificity and predictive values. *Indian J Ophthalmol.* 56 (1): 45.

114 Hsueh, P.R., Huang, L.M., Chen, P.J. et al. (2004). Chronological evolution of IgM, IgA, IgG and neutralisation antibodies after infection with SARS-associated coronavirus. *Clin Microbiol Infect.* 10 (12): 1062–1066.

115 Zhao, J., Yuan, Q., Wang, H. et al. (2020). Antibody responses to SARS-CoV-2 in patients with novel coronavirus disease 2019. *Clin Infect Dis.* 71 (16): 2027–2034.

116 Pollard, C.A., Morran, M.P., and Nestor-Kalinoski, A.L. (2020). The COVID-19 pandemic: a global health crisis. *Physiol Genomics* 52 (11): 549–557.

117 Zeng, F., Dai, C., Cai, P. et al. (2020). A comparison study of SARS-CoV-2 IgG antibody between male and female COVID-19 patients: a possible reason underlying different outcome between sex. *J Med Virol.* 92 (10): 2050–2054.

118 Centers for Disease Control and Prevention (2019). Interim Guidance on Ending Isolation and Precautions for Adults with COVID-19.

119 Abu-Raddad, L.J., Chemaitelly, H., Malek, J.A. et al. (2021). Assessment of the risk of SARS-CoV-2 reinfection in an intense re-exposure setting. *Clin Infect Dis.* 73: e1830–e1840. https://doi.org/10.1093/cid/ciaa1846.

120 Larson, D., Brodniak, S.L., Voegtly, L.J. et al. (2021). A case of early reinfection with severe acute respiratory syndrome coronavirus 2 (SARS-CoV-2). *Clin Infect Dis.* 73: e2827–e2828.

121 Mulder, M., van der Vegt, D.S., Oude Munnink, B.B. et al. (2021). Reinfection of severe acute respiratory syndrome coronavirus 2 in an immunocompromised patient: a case report. *Clin Infect Dis.* 73: e2841–e2842.

122 Prado-Vivar, B., Becerra-Wong, M., Guadalupe, J.J. et al. (2021). A case of SARS-CoV-2 reinfection in Ecuador. *Lancet Infect Dis.* 21 (6): e142.

123 Shastri, J., Parikh, S., Agarwal, S. et al. (2020). Whole genome sequencing confirmed SARS-CoV-2 reinfections among healthcare workers in India with increased severity in the second episode. *Lancet* http://doi.org/10.2139/ssrn.3688220.

124 Deeks, J.J., Dinnes, J., Takwoingi, Y. et al. (2020). Antibody tests for identification of current and past infection with SARS-CoV-2. *Cochrane Database Syst Rev.* 6 (6): CD013652. https://doi.org/10.1002/14651858.CD013652.

125 Raveendran, A.V., Jayadevan, R., and Sashidharan, S. (2021). Long COVID: an overview. *Diabetes Metab Syndr.* 15 (3): 869–875.

126 Jason, L.A., Islam, M.F., Conroy, K. et al. (2021). COVID-19 symptoms over time: comparing long-haulers to ME/CFS. *Fatigue* 9: 59–68.

127 Nakra, N.A., Blumberg, D.A., Herrera-Guerra, A., and Lakshminrusimha, S. (2020). Multi-system inflammatory syndrome in children (MIS-C) following SARS-CoV-2 infection: review of clinical presentation, hypothetical pathogenesis, and proposed management. *Children.* 7 (7): 69.

128 Rostad, C.A., Chahroudi, A., Mantus, G. et al. (2020). Serology in children with multisystem inflammatory syndrome (MIS-C). *Pediatrics* 146: e2020018242.

129 Feldstein, L.R., Rose, E.B., Horwitz, S.M. et al. (2020). Multisystem inflammatory syndrome in US children and adolescents. *N Engl J Med.* 383 (4): 334–336.

130 Zhou, M.Y., Xie, X.L., Peng, Y.G. et al. (2020). From SARS to COVID-19: what we have learned about children infected with COVID-19. *Int J Infect Dis.* 96: 710–714.

131 Mbunge, E. (2020). Integrating emerging technologies into COVID-19 contact tracing: opportunities, challenges and pitfalls. *Diabetes Metab Syndr.* 14 (6): 1631–1636. https://doi.org/10.1016/j.dsx.2020.08.029.

132 Jalkanen, P., Kolehmainen, P., Häkkinen, H.K. et al. (2021). COVID-19 mRNA vaccine induced antibody responses against three SARS-CoV-2 variants. *Nat Commun.* 12 (1): 3991.

133 Polack, F.P., Thomas, S.J., Kitchin, N. et al. (2020). Safety and efficacy of the BNT162b2 mRNA Covid-19 vaccine. *N Engl J Med.* 383 (27): 2603–2615.

134 Sahin, U., Muik, A., Vogler, I. et al. (2021). BNT162b2 vaccine induces neutralizing antibodies and poly-specific T cells in humans. *Nature* 595: 572–577.

135 Planas, D., Veyer, D., Baidaliuk, A. et al. (2021). Reduced sensitivity of SARS-CoV-2 variant Delta to antibody neutralization. *Nature* 596: 276–280.

136 Hoffmann, M., Hofmann-Winkler, H., Krüger, N. et al. (2021). SARS-CoV-2 variant B. 1.617 is resistant to Bamlanivimab and evades antibodies induced by infection and vaccination. *Cell Rep.* 36: 109415.

137 Tada, T., Zhou, H., Dcosta, B.M. et al. (2021). The spike proteins of SARS-CoV-2 B.1.617 and B.1.618 variants identified in India provide partial resistance to vaccine-elicited and therapeutic monoclonal antibodies. *bioRxiv* https://doi.org/10.1101/2021.05.14.444076.

138 Liu, J., Liu, Y., Xia, H. et al. (2021). BNT162b2-elicited neutralization of B. 1.617 and other SARS-CoV-2 variants. *Nature* 596: 273–275.

139 Edara, V.V., Lai, L., Sahoo, M. et al. (2021). Infection and vaccine-induced neutralizing antibody responses to the SARS-CoV-2 B.1.617.1 variant. *bioRxiv* https://doi.org/10.1101/2021.05.09.443299.

140 Bernal, J.L., Andrews, N., Gower, C. et al. (2021). Effectiveness of COVID-19 vaccines against the B.1.617.2 (Delta) variant. *N Engl J Med.* 385: 585–594.

141 Positive new data for Johnson & Johnson single-shot COVID-19 vaccine on activity against delta variant and long-lasting durability of response. Johnson & Johnson. (2021). https://www.jnj.com/positive-new-data-for-johnson-johnson-single-shot-covid-19-vaccine-on-activity-against-delta-variant-and-long-lasting-durability-of-response (accessed 15 February 2022).

4

COVID-19: Radiologic Diagnosis

Brian P. Pogatchnik[1], Wakana Murakami[2,3], and Shabnam Mortazavi[4]

[1]Clinical Instructor in Radiology, Stanford University School of Medicine, Stanford, CA, USA
[2]Visiting Researcher of Radiological Sciences, David Geffen School of Medicine at UCLA, Los Angeles, CA, USA
[3]Department of Radiology, Showa University Graduate School of Medicine, Tokyo, Japan
[4]Assistant Professor of Radiology, David Geffen School of Medicine at UCLA, Los Angeles, CA, USA

Abbreviations

ACR	American College of Radiology
ARDS	acute respiratory distress syndrome
ASER	American Society of Emergency Radiology
CDC	Centers for Disease Control and Prevention
CI	confidence interval
CO-RADS	COVID-19 Reporting and Data System
COVID-RADS	COVID-19 Imaging Reporting and Data System
CT	computed tomography
CTPA	computed tomography pulmonary angiography
CXR	chest x-ray
DAH	diffuse alveolar hemorrhage
DECT	dual-energy computed tomography
FDG	fluorodeoxyglucose
ICU	intensive care unit
LU	lung ultrasound
MRI	magnetic resonance imaging
NSIP	nonspecific interstitial pneumonia
PE	pulmonary embolism
PET	positron emission tomography
PPE	personal protective equipment
PUI	person under investigation
RSNA	Radiological Society of North America
RT-PCR	reverse transcriptase–polymerase chain reaction
SARS-CoV-2	severe acute respiratory syndrome coronavirus 2
WHO	World Health Organization

Current Guidelines on When to Image

Fleischner Society

The Fleischner Society is an international, multidisciplinary organization that was developed in 1969 by a group of radiologists focusing on chest radiology. On 7 April 2020, the Fleischner Society published guidelines on the role of chest imaging in the management of patients with coronavirus disease 2019 (COVID-19) [1]. This document reflects the expert opinion from a broad range of specialties related to diseases of the chest, including thoracic radiology, pulmonary medicine, intensive care, emergency medicine, and other related sciences. The experts are from 10 different countries that have been heavily affected by COVID-19.

- The Summary of the Imaging Recommendations is as follows:
  - Recommended against the routine use of chest imaging as a screening tool for COVID-19 in patients who are asymptomatic and even for patients who have mild symptoms (unless they have risk factors that make them more likely to have disease progression).
  - Chest imaging is recommended for patients with moderate-to-severe features of COVID-19, regardless of the COVID-19 laboratory test results.
  - Chest imaging is recommended for patients who have been diagnosed with COVID-19 and who demonstrate clinical deterioration.

- Interim Developments
  - Imaging is not recommended as the initial test for establishing the diagnosis of COVID-19. Instead, laboratory testing for COVID-19 is the preferred diagnostic test, especially with increasing availability of reverse transcriptase–polymerase chain reaction (RT-PCR) testing.
  - By comparing the patient's symptoms by the severity scoring, along with associated chest x-ray (CXR) and computed tomography (CT) scan findings, we can determine the patient's anticipated hospitalization course and risk of requiring endotracheal intubation, determine the need for intensive care unit (ICU) admission, and determine risk of death.
  - There is an association of COVID-19 infection with systemic thromboembolism, which contributes to the morbidity and mortality of COVID-19.

- Definitions and criteria for key components of common clinical scenarios are as follows:
  Severity of respiratory disease
  Mild: no evidence of significant pulmonary dysfunction or damage (e.g. absence of hypoxemia, no or mild dyspnea)
  Moderate to severe: evidence of significant pulmonary dysfunction or damage (e.g. hypoxemia, moderate-to-severe dyspnea)
  Pretest probability: Based on background prevalence of disease as estimated by observed transmission patterns. May be further modified by the individual's exposure risk. Subcategorized as follows:

Low: sporadic transmission
Medium: clustered transmission
High: community transmission
Risk factors for disease progression
Present: clinical judgment regarding combination of age 65 years or older and presence of comorbidities (e.g. cardiovascular disease, diabetes, chronic respiratory disease, hypertension, immunocompromised)
Absent: defined by the absence of risk factors for disease progression
Disease progression: progression of mild disease to moderate-to-severe disease as defined earlier, or progression of moderate-to-severe disease with worsening objective measures of hypoxemia
Resource constraints: limited access to personnel, personal protective equipment (PPE), COVID-19 testing ability (including swabs, reagent, or personnel), hospital beds, and/or ventilators with the need to rapidly triage patients
- Clinical utility of chest imaging: benefits and costs/harms

Benefits
Clinically actionable results
- Triage
- Management
- Prognostication

Cost/Harms

- Radiation exposure
- Risk for infection transmission
- Consumption of PPE
- Other resource impacts (e.g. room downtime)

The guidelines did not prescribe the specific imaging modality to be used by the clinician (CXR versus chest CT) and left the choice of imaging modality to the discretion of the treatment provider. Depending on the practice setting, varying expertise and resources may lead to different preferences and availability of imaging equipment.

Scenario 1: Mild features of COVID-19
If a patient presents with mild respiratory features that are consistent with COVID-19, imaging should be considered in the following situations:

1) The patient has risk factors for disease progression, in addition to a positive COVID-19 laboratory test (or negative COVID-19 testing but a high pretest probability)
2) The patient has mild symptoms but has clinical deterioration (regardless of COVID-19 test results)

Scenario 2: Moderate-to-severe features of COVID-19

For patients with moderate to severe respiratory features that are consistent with COVID-19 (regardless of the test results), imaging should be performed. The benefits of such testing include obtaining a baseline evaluation, risk stratification, and assessment of underlying cardiopulmonary disease and also potentially identifying an alternative pulmonary diagnosis in patients who had a negative COVID-19 test result. If CT scan findings demonstrate typical features of COVID-19, repeat laboratory testing should be performed, especially if the pretest probability is high.

Scenario 3: Moderate-to-severe features of COVID-19 in a resource-constrained environment

If COVID-19 testing is not available or the results are negative, imaging should be used to assist with patient triage. If there is a high pretest probability and imaging findings are consistent with COVID-19, the panel recommends that the patient should be diagnosed and appropriately treated for COVID-19. This recommendation uniquely differs from other published guidelines and is based on the expert panelists' direct experience under such a clinical scenario.

Other additional recommendations include:

- Daily use of CXR is not required if an intubated patient with COVID-19 is clinically stable.
- In patients who recover from COVID-19 but continue to suffer from pulmonary symptoms, a chest CT should be obtained for further evaluation.

World Health Organization

In early 2020, the World Health Organization (WHO) received requests from several countries to provide guidelines on the use of chest imaging in the diagnosis and management of COVID-19. Up until that point, there was wide variation in imaging practices, which led to multiple diverging guidelines developed by multiple institutions. This was seen in surveys administered by the International Society of Radiology and the European Society of Radiology.

To make uniform guidelines effective for practical use as soon as possible, the WHO put together these guidelines rather quickly, over the course of 10 weeks. In preparation of the guidelines, a systematic review team performed a literature search including published data up to the end of May 2020. At that time, relatively early in the pandemic, they acknowledged that there was limited evidence available, so the recommendations were considered conditional. In the setting of relative weak evidence, expert opinion was involved in the development of these guidelines [2–5]. A total of 28 studies were identified as meeting the eligibility requirements. Each recommendation refers to the supporting evidence, which was made available on an online Web Annex.

The recommendations do take into account resource availability depending on the practice setting (low- vs. middle- vs. high-income countries). Patient risk factors are considered as well, including age, comorbidities, immunosuppressive conditions, smoking, and special groups. Potential harm from ionizing radiation is considered, especially to children and pregnant women.

In developing the recommendations for chest imaging, there was no distinction made on the modality of the chest imaging (x-ray, ultrasound, CT scan). However, in their guidelines, they do discuss the benefits of CXR with portable equipment, and chest ultrasound with portable scanners can provide point-of-care data without the need for patient transfers. In general, chest imaging is recommended for patients with mild, moderate, and severe symptoms, but in specific circumstances. For patients with mild symptoms, chest imaging can be one of the factors used to decide on hospital admission versus home discharge. For patients with moderate-to-severe disease, chest imaging was recommended as a factor to decide on admission triage, whether to admit the patient to a regular ward or to the ICU. Further, chest imaging was recommended to assist in the decision on therapeutic management.

If patients are hospitalized and no longer symptomatic, chest imaging was not recommended to determine the decision for discharge. Rather, decisions for discharge should be based more on clinical stability and RT-PCR testing (with two negative results at least 24 hours apart).

Practical Points

Do Not Use Imaging to Diagnose Cases Unless RT-PCR Is Unavailable

Imaging features of COVID-19 mostly by CT have become widely available, because that was the primary imaging tool initially used in China [6–9]. Sensitivity and specificity of CT findings have been compared with those of RT-PCR. There are many studies that demonstrated the significant roles of chest CT for the diagnosis of COVID-19 with high sensitivity [8, 10–12]. In February 2020, Chinese studies revealed that chest CT achieved a higher sensitivity for the diagnosis of COVID-19 compared with RT-PCR tests [8, 10]. Subsequently, the National Health Commission of China briefly accepted chest CT findings of viral pneumonia as COVID-19 diagnoses [13]. However, given the advantages and disadvantages of each of these modalities, the major radiologic societies generally advise taking a cautious approach to screening or diagnostic use of imaging in cases of suspected COVID-19. In addition to the WHO recommendations, the Radiological Society of North America (RSNA), together with the American College of Radiology (ACR), Society of Thoracic Radiology (STR), and American Society of Emergency Radiology (ASER), issued a consensus statement that although CT should not be used to diagnose COVID-19, radiologists must be prepared to interpret CT performed on patients suspected of having COVID-19. Furthermore, interpreting radiologists must also understand incidental pulmonary findings that are consistent with COVID-19 infection. These organizations recommended against using CT as a routine screening or first-line tool in the diagnosis of COVID-19 (ACR 2020 recommendations for the use of CXR and CT for suspected COVID-19 infection [14]):

- CT should not be used to screen for or as a first-line test to diagnose COVID-19.
- CT should be used sparingly and reserved for hospitalized, symptomatic patients with specific clinical indications for CT. Appropriate infection-control procedures should be followed before scanning subsequent patients.
- Facilities may consider deploying portable radiography units in ambulatory care facilities for use when CXRs are considered medically necessary.

The surfaces of these machines can be easily cleaned, avoiding the need to bring patients into radiography rooms.

- Radiologists should familiarize themselves with the CT appearance of COVID-19 infection to be able to identify findings consistent with infection in patients imaged for other reasons.
- (Updated 22 March 2020) As an interim measure, until more widespread COVID-19 testing is available, some medical practices are requesting chest CT to inform decisions on whether to test a patient for COVID-19, admit a patient, or provide other treatment. The ACR strongly urges caution in taking this approach. A normal chest CT does not mean a person does not have COVID-19 infection, and an abnormal CT is not specific for COVID-19 diagnosis. A normal CT should not dissuade a patient from being quarantined or provided other clinically indicated treatment when otherwise medically appropriate. Clearly, locally constrained resources may be a factor in such decision making.

The ACR position was updated on March 22 acknowledging the need for performing imaging studies to guide patient management in the setting of insufficient testing capabilities, although with urgent caution in taking this approach.

To encourage use of point-of-care imaging and to discourage unnecessary imaging that would lead to potential spread of COVID-19, the ACR made the following recommendations:

- A portable CXR could be performed in ambulatory care facilities.
- Nuclear medicine ventilation scans should not be used unless absolutely necessary. If deemed necessary, the appropriate infection-control precautions should be conducted.
- Any elective magnetic resonance imaging (MRI) studies should be postponed.

The STR/ASER issued a similar joint statement as follows (STR/ASER COVID-19 Position Statement [March 11, 2020] [15]):

> "At this time, the STR and ASER do not recommend routine CT screening for the diagnosis of patients under investigation for COVID-19.

Chest CT can be restricted to patients who test positive for COVID-19 and who are suspected of having complicating features such as abscess or empyema."

The ASER also announced the following (ASER COVID-19 Task Force: FAQs [16]):

"It needs to be stated that imaging should not replace clinical screening or preclude laboratory confirmation of the disease. CT should not be used on asymptomatic patients. A negative CT also does not exclude the disease."

Dissemination of information and guidelines from other organizations also took place during the start of the COVID-19 worldwide pandemic. The Society of Advanced Body Imaging developed a webinar entitled "COVID-19: Thoracic Imaging Findings and Recommendations," providing important concepts of COVID-19 and the impact on imaging findings. In line with Centers for Disease Control and Prevention (CDC) guidelines at the time, the Society of Cardiovascular Computed Tomography recommended rescheduling nonurgent imaging studies. The North American Society for Cardiovascular Imaging issued an official statement in May 2020 that provided recommendations to preserve healthcare resources during the pandemic. In general, these recommendations involved substitution of invasive tests for noninvasive tests, as well as consolidating diagnostic imaging. For example, in patients with known or suspected COVID-19, one should consider performing a cardiac CT (noninvasive study) instead of performing a transesophageal echocardiogram (a more invasive study) [17].

Imaging Is of Little Utility in Asymptomatic/Mild Cases Unless Multiple Comorbidities Exist

All of the guidelines recommended against the routine use of imaging in asymptomatic/mild cases unless the patients with COVID-19 also had multiple comorbidities [1]. A stand-alone screening tool should have near-perfect sensitivity, because a false-negative result could have significant implications for patient safety, as well as the safety of the patient's close contacts and treatment team. Unfortunately, chest CT findings can often be negative early in the course of COVID-19 respiratory disease, so a negative result does not necessarily exclude the diagnosis. Furthermore, increasing the use of CT scans will lead to an increase in incidentalomas that would lead to potentially unnecessarily medical workup [18].

Imaging Is Useful in Risk Stratification in Moderate-to-Severe Symptomatic Cases

For patients with moderate-to-severe symptoms of respiratory COVID-19, chest imaging is useful for stratification and triage purposes. This is consistent with the consensus statement issued by the Fleischner Society, as well as the ACR guidelines [1, 14]. Furthermore, chest imaging can be considered as a stand-alone tool for situations whereby COVID-19 RT-PCR testing is not readily available. Regarding imaging modality (CXR vs. chest CT), no specific recommendations were made by the Fleischner Society. The benefits of chest imaging include the ability to see features that may be consistent with COVID-19 or to visualize findings that may be more suggestive of a different diagnosis. In performing imaging, it is important to keep in mind the pretest probability of COVID-19 infection, because this would guide the performance of repeat testing.

Technical Considerations to Limit Spread While Imaging

Severe acute respiratory syndrome coronavirus 2 (SARS-CoV-2) is primarily transmitted via droplets and aerosols, which can pose several challenges to imaging patients. The virus has been shown to remain viable in aerosols for up to 3 and 72 hours on surfaces such as plastic and stainless steel [19]. Furthermore, there is evidence to suggest that the virus can spread as an aerosol through central ventilation systems and disperse up to 10 m without ventilation [20, 21]. In light of this, several measures may be taken to help prevent unnecessary exposure to other patients and radiology staff members.

Disease prevention can begin before the patient even arrives at the scanner. Screening for symptomatic patients can help stratify those who require extra isolation. Furthermore, requiring patients to wear a surgical mask while in the imaging department can reduce both symptomatic and asymptomatic transmission [21]. While in the waiting area, patients should be encouraged to maximize distance between themselves and others. Typically, a minimum distance of 2 m is recommended between patients. Installing the appropriate high-efficiency particulate air filters in ventilation systems and even on portable air filters can significantly reduce aerosol spread of the virus among a department [22]. These benefits can be compounded by increasing the air exchange rate, further reducing the number of virus particles circulating in the room.

Radiology personnel can also take several precautions to prevent infection and disease transmission. Daily screening for COVID-19 symptoms has become common across medicine, although it is ineffective at detecting asymptomatic or presymptomatic individuals who are still capable of spreading the disease [23]. Symptomatic staff members should be further risk-stratified by the appropriate medical personnel (typically in the occupational health department of a hospital) and potentially be tested for SARS-CoV-2 before returning to work. If positive, guidelines from the CDC as of January 2021 recommend healthcare providers with mild-to-moderate illness can return to work if it has been at least 10 days since symptoms first appeared, at least 24 hours since the last fever, and their symptoms have improved [24]. Healthcare providers with severe or critical illness may require up to 20 days since symptom onset. Finally, a person who has had a significant exposure to someone with known COVID-19 (defined by the CDC as having spent greater than 15 minutes less than 6 feet apart from a person suspected or confirmed to have COVID-19) is expected to self-quarantine for 14 days after the exposure according to CDC guidelines [25].

Appropriate use of PPE is critical to prevent infection of radiology staff, as well as potential spread to patients. Proper technique is critical for donning and doffing PPE, and adequate training should be available to all necessary personnel. When working with patients with known COVID-19 or persons under investigation (PUIs), airborne precautions may be necessary to limit spread, particularly during aerosolizing procedures. This includes the use of N95 respirators, gowns, and gloves. For patients who are not symptomatic or PUIs, wearing surgical masks is sufficient. The use of eye protection from goggles or face shields varies from site to site, although there is evidence that

this may reduce the risk of spread. Time spent in close proximity (less than 2-m distance) should be limited, ideally to less than 15 minutes.

Once the patient is ready to be imaged, best practices to limit virus spread largely depend on the type of imaging performed.

Chest Radiography

In modern radiology departments, radiographs are acquired with both stationary and portable machines. In both techniques, it is critical to adequately clean the equipment between patients, typically with disinfection wipes. Although cleaning the equipment helps with limiting transmission, stationary equipment requires the patient to travel to it to image the patient. Conversely, portable machines allow for the patient to be imaged in their isolation room or ward. Thus, portable imaging is generally preferred in PUIs and confirmed COVID-19 cases to limit their travel and potential spread of the virus outside their room.

Traditional portable techniques do offer a decreased risk for transmission compared with stationary devices in the radiology department; however, the traditional techniques still place the technician near the patient and require a thorough cleaning of all components of the machine. Early in the pandemic, it became apparent that adjustments could be made without substantially degrading image quality. The most basic method of this is to take the image at an extended distance through the door (typically 10–15 feet). However, a more popular technique involves taking an image through the glass of a door or window of an isolation room. A retrospective review of this technique found no significant change in image quality or radiation dose to the patient compared with the standard technique before implementing it [26]. To accomplish this, the cassette is double bagged and given to a nurse already in the appropriate PPE in the patient's room. The head of the patient's bed is raised, and the cassette is placed behind the patient's back. With the help of hand signaling or a phone call with the nurse in the room, proper alignment is achieved, and the radiograph is taken. The nurse then brings the cassette to the door and opens the outer bag, and the technologist takes the cassette and wipes it down with antimicrobial wipes. Then the cassette is removed and processes the image. By doing so, only one person is required to don full airborne PPE, saving PPE for other providers, and only the cassette requires cleaning between patients.

Cross-Sectional Imaging

Unlike x-ray machines, most CT, MRI, and positron emission tomography (PET) scanners are not portable. For this reason, techniques for limiting transmission fall into two categories: minimizing time spent at the scanner and disinfecting the room after a patient is scanned.

Several techniques can be used to decrease time at the scanner. First, technologists, nurses, and transportation staff must work together to ensure timely transport to and from the scanner. The scanner room should be ready for the patient on arrival, and transportation staff should be on hand to transport the patient out of the room immediately after. Peripheral intravenous lines should be placed before transport to radiology if the study is to be performed with contrast. The study should be protocolled, and any technologist questions regarding the protocol should be addressed before arrival in the radiology department. As with any study, CT should only be ideally performed when there is an important clinical question that can require a CT for an accurate diagnosis.

Ensuring the scanner room is adequately disinfected before scanning the next patient may require multiple methods. A deep clean of all equipment that was in close proximity to patients with or suspected to have COVID-19 can be accomplished with antimicrobial wipes, although multiple other techniques are available, including ultraviolet lights and LED (light-emitting diode) lights, and ultrasonic devices are being investigated [27]. Installing high-efficiency particulate air filters in the scanner room will help filter out the virus from the air, and increasing the air exchange rate can augment this. Various groups have recommended allowing 30–60 minutes between examinations to allow for adequate air filtration and air exchange. Although these measures can reduce throughput in the department, they can also reduce the likelihood of spread within the department.

Ultrasound

Ultrasound machines are inherently portable and can easily be brought into the patient's room. The major drawback of imaging patients with confirmed or suspected COVID-19 is that it necessitates the operator be within 2 m of the patient. Consequentially, adequate PPE is necessary for the operator, and patients should be wearing a mask if able. The ultrasound machine should be positioned at least 2 m from the patient. Special care should be taken to only use a single hand to touch the patient and transducer if possible, to avoid cross-contamination of the machine. Disposable machine covers may provide an additional barrier to spreading the virus, although the machine should still be wiped down with antimicrobial wipes after each use [28]. Finally, obtaining diagnostic images can be a time-consuming process in the best of times. In PUIs or patients with confirmed COVID-19, limited ultrasounds to answer specific clinical questions can be performed on a case-by-case basis to minimize the operator's time spent near the patient [29].

Imaging by Modality

X-Ray

CXR has a limited value in the diagnosis of early stages of COVID-19, especially in mild disease courses. CXR has a lower sensitivity than initial RT-PCR testing (69% vs. 91%, respectively) [30].

Although the chest CT is more sensitive compared with CXR in the detection of pulmonary manifestation of COVID-19, in some countries, CXR has been used as a first-line triage tool mainly because of long turnaround times for RT-PCR to diagnose COVID-19 infection [31].

The role of CXR in clinical monitoring of these patients, especially in the ICU, is still debated: The Fleischner Society does not recommend daily CXR in stable intubated patients [1, 32]. Borghesi and Maroldi [33] recommend that in the emergency setting of COVID-19 pandemic, CXR can be a useful diagnostic tool for monitoring the rapid progression of lung abnormalities in COVID-19, particularly in the ICU setting.

There have been several scoring methods to determine the intensity of COVID-19 in CXR images. The severe acute respiratory infection CXR severity scoring system was created in the pre-COVID era for the nonradiologist clinician to assess acute respiratory disease [34]. Radiographic Assessment of Lung Edema (RALE) classification was presented by Wong et al. [30] to describe the course and severity of CXR findings in COVID-19 and correlate them with RT-PCR results. CXR score by Borghesi and Maroldi (Brixia score) [33] was designed specifically for patients with confirmed COVID-19.

The main feature of parenchymal abnormality in COVID-19 on CXR is consolidation followed by groundless opacity. The distribution pattern is basal, peripheral, and bilateral lung involvement [30, 35–37]. Pleural effusions have been reported as exceedingly rare on CXR and CT in patients with COVID-19 infection [38]. Pleural effusion could serve as an indicator for severe inflammation and poor clinical outcomes in COVID-19 infection. In a retrospective study on 476 inpatients with COVID-19 (involving 153 patients with pleural effusion and 323 without pleural effusion), patients with pleural effusion had a higher incidence of severe or critical illness and mortality rate and had a longer hospital stay time compared with their counterparts without pleural effusion [39]. The temporal pulmonary manifestation of COVID-19 infection in CXR is shown in Figure 4.1.

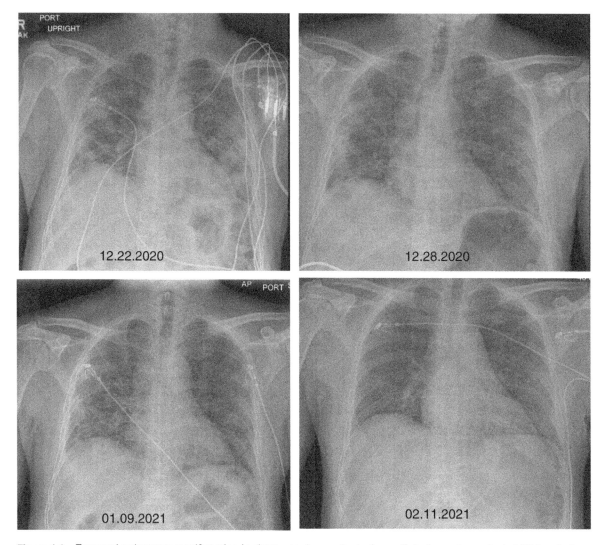

Figure 4.1 Temporal pulmonary manifestation in chest x-ray in a patient whose clinical symptoms started 18 days before the first radiograph.

Pneumothorax was detected in only 2 of 350 patients in one study and was iatrogenic due to mechanical ventilation in intubated patients [40].

Autopsy findings in patients with COVID-19 reveal bilateral diffuse alveolar damage with cellular fibromyxoid exudates, which may cause a ball-valve effect when impacted in bronchioles, resulting in cystic changes; therefore, it has been hypothesized that because of the extensive parenchymal damage caused by COVID-19, some patients may develop cystic changes, especially late into the course of the disease, which are at risk for rupture and subsequent pneumothorax even from the minimal transpulmonary pressures generated from high-flow nasal cannula [41–43].

Computed Tomography

Imaging Protocol

Thoracic CT imaging in COVID-19 is typically performed using one of two protocols depending on the clinical scenario. Noncontrast examinations should be performed when the primary goal is to characterize the pulmonary disease, while computed tomography pulmonary angiography (CTPA) is performed to evaluate for coexistent pulmonary emboli (PEs) [44]. The suspicion for PEs should be raised when there is evidence of hemodynamic compromise or gas exchange is disproportionate to the extent of disease [45]. Routine contrast-enhanced chest CTs are generally not indicated in the evaluation of uncomplicated COVID-19.

Noncontrast chest CTs are acquired with the same technique as used for the evaluation of other thoracic pathology [46]. Patients are placed supine in the scanner with arms above their head. The scan is performed during a breath hold at maximum inspiration to minimize the presence of passive atelectasis. Images are acquired from the thoracic inlet through the inferior margins of the costophrenic angles. The data should be reconstructed in a sharp kernel for better evaluation of the lung parenchyma and bone, while a separate reconstruction should be made with a soft kernel to evaluate the mediastinal structures and soft tissues. Volumetric acquisitions with slice thickness less than 2 mm are generally preferable to best delineate the anatomy and pathology, minimizing partial volume averaging effects.

CTPA studies cover a similar scan range to the standard chest CT but have several notable differences in how they are performed. First, contrast administration is required for the opacification of the pulmonary arteries [47]. Typically, 60 ml of nonionic contrast is injected via a peripheral intravenous line followed by a normal saline bolus of up to 100 ml to ensure a cohesive bolus. However, there is a degree of site-to-site variability regarding the exact contrast dose and saline bolus. Determining the peak contrast enhancement in the main pulmonary artery may be performed using a bolus tracker or test bolus techniques. The examination may be performed with an inspiratory breath hold or during shallow breathing to minimize the risk for an interrupted bolus from influx of unopacified blood from the inferior vena cava during a deep inspiration. Depending on the scanner available, high-pitch scanning or dual-energy imaging may offer increased sensitivity and specificity in the detection of PEs [48, 49]. The scan range remains from the thoracic inlet through the costophrenic angles. In addition, lowing the kVp to 100 or 80 can result in better visualization of the contrast material while lowering the radiation dose. Alternate imaging techniques may be warranted to avoid contrast in patients with acute kidney injury or those with stage IV or V chronic kidney disease (glomerular filtration rate less than 30 ml/min/1.73 m^2).

As the average patient's annual radiation dose from medical imaging has increased over time, so has an increased interest in keeping patient radiation doses As Low As Reasonably Achievable (ALARA). This is of particular concern in patients with COVID-19, because they will typically undergo several imaging studies throughout the course of their hospital admission. The typical noncontrast chest CT is performed at 150 mA. Because of improved scanner technology and iterative and deep learning reconstruction techniques, multiple studies have investigated the possibility of lowering the dose in chest CTs without sacrificing image quality. These studies have found that low-dose (~50 mA) and even ultra-low-dose (~20 mA) techniques provide a similar diagnostic performance as standard-dose protocols [50, 51]. These techniques typically perform well with ground-glass opacities (GGOs) and consolidative pulmonary opacities, although the ultra-low-dose technique can make the detection of low-attenuation abnormalities such as emphysema more difficult. Not surprisingly, a prospective study found the opacities of COVID-19 pneumonias were detectable at the same rate with low-dose and standard-dose techniques [52]. Therefore, adopting low-dose protocols may benefit patients through reduced dose while still obtaining images of diagnostic quality.

Diagnostic Performance of CT in Detecting Infection by SARS-CoV-2

Early in the pandemic, radiologists in Wuhan began noticing that patients with COVID-19 had a characteristic, and radiologists were able to suggest the diagnosis as other forms of testing were frequently unavailable. Indeed, early studies did show CT had a strong sensitivity and specificity (>90%) for detecting COVID-19 in places of high prevalence [53]. However, the positive predictive value was expectedly lower in areas of low disease prevalence, ranging from 1.5% to 30.7% [54]. More recent meta-analyses have shown that although chest CT demonstrates a sensitivity of approximately 94% in detecting COVID-19, the specificity is suboptimal, with a pooled specificity of 46% [55]. Conversely, modern RT-PCR has a sensitivity of at least 90% and a specificity of 100% [56]. With repeated testing, the sensitivity closely approaches 100%. Therefore, although CT demonstrates a high sensitivity, its lack of specificity combined with cost and radiation dose mean that RT-PCR is the current gold standard for the diagnosis of COVID-19.

Pulmonary Parenchymal Manifestations of COVID-19 on CT

Early in the pandemic, CT came to the forefront in the diagnosis of COVID-19. Laboratory testing had to be developed and refined to achieve the high degree of accuracy necessary to be clinically useful. Given the preponderance of respiratory symptoms in this new virus, chest imaging became increasingly used for diagnosis. CT was often selected for its increased sensitivity over radiographs, with CT having approximately 30% higher sensitivity than radiographs [57]. Characteristic patterns on CT became evident (Table 4.1), with a pattern similar to that seen in SARS-CoV-1 and, to a lesser extent, Middle East respiratory syndrome infections [58]. These studies demonstrated a high level of sensitivity and modest

Table 4.1 Chest computed tomography findings in COVID-19.

- Common findings:
  - Ground-glass opacities
  - Consolidation
  - Interlobular septal thickening and intralobular lines
  - Crazy paving
  - Peripheral pulmonary vascular enlargement
- Uncommon findings:
  - Airways dilation
  - Bronchial wall thickening
  - Halo sign
  - Atoll sign/reverse halo sign
  - Pulmonary embolism
  - Lymphadenopathy

specificity for CT in the detection of COVID-19 in symptomatic patients. One meta-analysis found the sensitivity and specificity of chest CT to be 94.6% and 46%, respectively, with RT-PCR positivity as the gold standard [55]. As laboratory testing improved in speed, availability, and accuracy, much of the burden was shifted from radiology for diagnosis of COVID-19 and toward using imaging for risk stratification and diagnosis of complications [59].

Ground-Glass Opacities GGO is the most common parenchymal abnormality in COVID-19 on CT, appearing in more than 80% of confirmed cases on CT [38, 60]. The term GGO refers to confluent opacities that are more dense than normal lung parenchyma on CT, but not so dense that they obscure the pulmonary vasculature on a noncontrast CT, similar to how the translucent ground glass on a shower door obscures the fine details of objects on the other side but still can reveal the coarse details (Figure 4.2) [61]. In any given CT, GGOs can represent regions of interstitial thickening, partial filling of the alveoli, partial collapse of the alveoli, or capillary engorgement. Unsurprisingly, radiologic–pathologic correlation has found that virtually every histopathologic entity associated with COVID-19, from diffuse alveolar damage to interstitial edema, can cause GGOs on CT [62]. The GGOs associated with COVID-19 tend to be round in

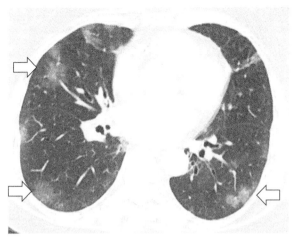

Figure 4.2 Ground-glass opacities (*arrows*) in a peripheral distribution, a pattern typical of COVID-19. Note the visualization of the pulmonary vessels in the regions of pulmonary opacification. Several of these opacities are round in morphology, which was consistent with early-phase disease in this patient presenting with 2 days of cough.

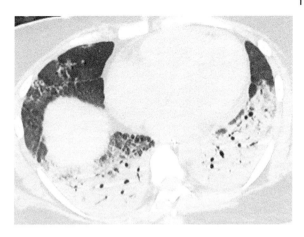

Figure 4.3 The lower lobes exhibit consolidation with air bronchograms. Unlike ground-glass opacities, the pulmonary vessels are not visualized in the regions of opacification.

morphology, often exhibit indistinct boundaries initially, and become more confluent and subpleural toward the progressive stage. Furthermore, they tend to be more frequently seen in isolation in earlier stages of the disease [63].

Consolidation Consolidation is the next most common form of pulmonary parenchymal abnormality seen in COVID-19, manifesting itself in 30–45% of cases [38, 60]. According to the Fleischner lexicon (the standard lexicon used in thoracic imaging), consolidation is a confluent opacity that makes the lungs appear solid, obscuring the underlying vasculature and interstitium (Figure 4.3) [61]. Histologically, consolidation represents alveoli completely filled with material, be it blood, pus, water, or cellular debris. Frequently, the bronchi remain unopacified, termed the "air bronchogram sign." In COVID-19, it can represent any of the typical histologic pathologies typically seen in the disease, similar to GGOs [62]. Consolidation is frequently seen in conjunction with or preceding GGOs, potentially reflecting more severely affected regions of lung. These opacities are more common later in the disease, typically at least one week after symptom onset [7, 63]. Patients older than 50 years also tend to more frequently have consolidation, potentially

because they more frequently experience severe symptoms [64].

Interlobular Septal Thickening and Intralobular Lines Interlobular septal thickening and intralobular lines are also frequently seen; nearly 50% of cases will exhibit these findings [60]. Due to their similarities, they are often confused for one another or lumped into the same finding, although they do represent separate entities radiographically and histologically (Figure 4.4). Interlobular septal thickening (referred to as Kerley B lines on radiography) is defined as linear subpleural opacities arising at 90° angles from the pleural surface according to the Fleischner lexicon [61]. These lines represent dilated lymphatics along the periphery of the secondary pulmonary lobule. In contrast, intralobular lines are defined as fine linear opacities within a secondar pulmonary lobule and can be manifestations of any interstitial abnormality within the lobule [61]. Despite their differences, they can both manifest in the setting of interstitial edema, as well as lymphatic congestion from inflammation or stasis. These features are typically absent in early disease but are frequently seen in the later stages [7, 63].

Crazy Paving Less common than its constituent components on patients with COVID-19, crazy paving is seen in 5–35% of cases [7, 55, 65]. Crazy paving is defined as interlobular septal thickening and/or

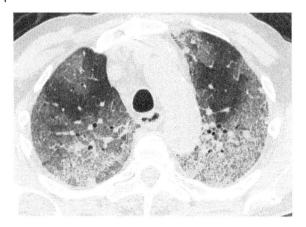

Figure 4.4 Ground-glass opacities with superimposed intralobular lines and interlobular septal thickening, a combination of opacities termed "crazy paving."

intralobular lines superimposed on GGOs (Figure 4.4). Typically, these regions represent areas of severe interstitial abnormalities, often with a superimposed alveolar component. CTs of patients with severe symptoms seem to reveal crazy paving more often [65]. Similarly, during the first SARS pandemic, patients with more severe symptoms more frequently exhibited crazy paving on CT [66]. In addition, crazy paving tends to be a feature seen with increasing frequency as the disease progresses to later stages [7, 63].

Airways Dilation Acute airways dilation is seen in 5–24% of cases. Whether these regions of dilated airways will result in true bronchiectasis is unclear. The airways are typically considered dilated when the inner diameter of the bronchus is larger in diameter than the adjacent pulmonary artery (Figure 4.5). *Bronchiectasis* is most precisely defined as abnormal, permanently dilated airways [67]. This term is source of confusion throughout the literature because it is frequently and incorrectly applied to acute and potentially reversible disease [60, 68]. In a series detailing six-month follow-up CTs in patients with severe COVID-19, 10% of patients exhibited airways dilation, and it was seen in 20% of those with fibrotic-like findings [69]. This indeed shows that some patients will likely experience bronchiectasis, although more study is needed to establish the likelihood of regions with acute dilation resulting in permanent bronchiectasis.

Bronchial Wall Thickening Although bronchopneumonia is one of the most common histopathologic findings in

regions of opacified lung at autopsy, bronchial wall thickening is uncommonly seen in COVID-19 (Figure 4.6) [62]. Pathologically, airways thickening can represent bronchial inflammation and/or secretions coating the airways. When the alveoli and terminal

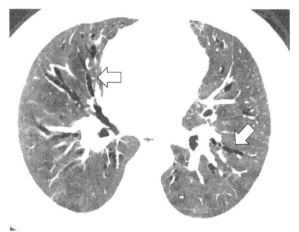

Figure 4.5 Diffuse varicoid bronchial dilation (*arrows*) in the organizing phase of COVID-19 pneumonia. Note the airways are significantly larger than their adjacent pulmonary arteries. Airways dilation tends to be a later finding that is associated with areas of pulmonary opacities.

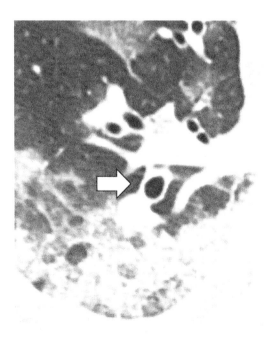

Figure 4.6 Bronchial wall thickening seen in the right lower lobe bronchi (*arrow*). Although there is no standard definition on computed tomography, the bronchial walls are typically thin, measuring 1 mm or less.

bronchioles are thickened and/or filled with debris, the characteristic tree-in-bud pattern is seen, named as it resembles a tree budding in spring [61]. Bronchial wall thickening is seen much more commonly than tree-in-bud, approximately 14% and 4%, respectively [55]. In fact, these opacities seen in isolation may suggest alternate diagnoses [70].

Halo Sign An infrequent finding in COVID-19 is the halo sign, seen in up to 35% of cases [68]. The halo sign describes an opacity with nodular central consolidation surrounded by GGOs (Figure 4.7) [61]. Classically, this was described in angioinvasive fungal infections, but it can be seen in numerous other acute lung injuries. In COVID-19, it likely represents the same findings seen in its constituent parts, GGOs and consolidation.

Atoll Sign/Reverse Halo Sign A less common sign, reported in ~11% of cases, is the atoll sign/reverse halo sign. This sign is defined as peripheral consolidation surrounding GGOs (Figure 4.8) [61]. Classically, it is reported with organizing pneumonia, although it can be seen in numerous acute and subacute lung injuries. It is more typically seen later in the course of

COVID-19 [7]. Histologically, it likely represents regions of organizing pneumonia as a pathologic reaction to the infection [71]. Additional findings of organizing pneumonia are frequently reported mid to late in the acute phase of COVID-19, such as perilobular sparing/subpleural bands and nodular GGOs [70]. A variant of the atoll sign has been described where there is a nodular region of GGO surrounded by a lucent ring and then a GGO ring, called the "bull's-eye sign" [72]. More investigation is necessary to establish whether this sign is indeed specific to COVID-19.

Air Bubble Sign Another proposed sign in COVID-19, the air bubble sign is defined as an ovoid lucency surrounded by consolidation or GGO (Figure 4.9) [73]. It is unclear whether this represents a variant of the atoll sign with unopacified lung tissue surrounded by consolidation, cystic changes, or emphysema [74]. Furthermore, the exact relation of this sign with regard to COVID-19 or any other disease remains unclear because the majority of studies on CT findings in COVID-19 did not specify this finding.

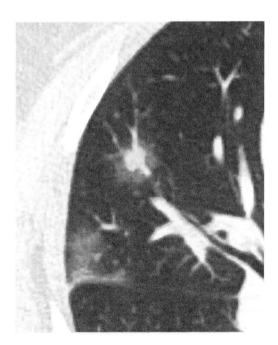

Figure 4.7 A small, consolidative nodular opacity is seen surrounded by ground-glass opacities, termed the "halo sign." Originally described in angioinvasive fungal infections, this finding is infrequently seen in COVID-19 pneumonia.

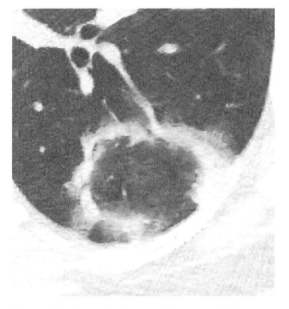

Figure 4.8 A ground-glass opacity surrounded by consolidation is seen in the left lower lobe, referred to as the "atoll sign" and "reverse halo sign." Originally described in cryptogenic organizing pneumonia, this finding can be seen in numerous other entities, including COVID-19.

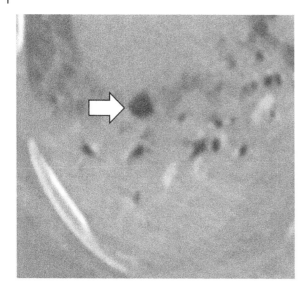

Figure 4.9 The air bubble sign is a proposed sign in COVID-19 pneumonia describing a small, lobular hyperlucency surrounded by pulmonary opacities. Further investigation is needed to establish how well it is correlated with COVID-19 pneumonias versus other pulmonary diseases.

Pulmonary Vascular Manifestations of COVID-19 on CT

Pulmonary Embolism Before the pandemic, PE was, on average, responsible for 40 000 deaths per year in the United States [75]. Because SARS-CoV-2 targets vascular endothelial cells throughout the body and type I and II pulmonary epithelial cells, in addition to promoting a prothrombotic inflammatory state in the body, an increased number of thromboembolic events are seen in COVID-19, particularly in the lungs. Whether these constitute true thromboembolic events or in situ thrombosis within the pulmonary arteries has been debated [76]. A meta-analysis of 3342 patients by Suh et al. [77] found that more than half of patients with PE in the setting of COVID-19 did not have a concurrent deep venous thrombosis. They found the overall rate of deep venous thrombosis and PE to be 14.8% and 16.5%, respectively. In addition, they found the incidence of PE in ICU patients to be twice that of those not requiring ICU care. Other studies have found mortality rates to be higher in patients with COVID-19 and PE, with a 23% mortality rate in those with both COVID-19 and PE, but only a 13% mortality rate in those with only COVID-19 [78]. Consequently, groups

such as the American Society of Hematology recommend the use of prophylactic anticoagulation in the setting of COVID-19 severe enough to warrant hospitalization [79].

The decision on when to suspect PE in patients with COVID-19 can be challenging. Because COVID-19 commonly results in pneumonia, patients are often hypoxemic. Traditional risk-stratification tools, such as the Wells score, can be used to help determine whether a PE may be present in the patient, although there is often a degree of subjectivity involved. Serum D-dimer levels are also routinely used when PE is in the differential, because a level less than 500 ng/ml has a high negative predictive value for PE [77]. The utilization of this is complicated in the setting of COVID-19 because infections can also be a cause of an elevated D-dimer. That said, several studies have found a correlation between death in patients with COVID-19 and serum D-dimer levels [80]. Another meta-analysis found that D-dimer maintained its high negative predictive value in COVID-19 but an overall decreased specificity compared with pre-COVID studies [77]. Thus, it appears reasonable to continue using D-dimer to rule out PE in patients suspected to have PE, as well as potentially for risk stratification.

On CT, the appearance of acute PE is not different from that seen in patients without COVID-19 (Figure 4.10). Non-contrast CT has a very low sensitivity in detecting PE [81]. Features that may suggest a PE on a noncontrast study include focal hyperdensities within the pulmonary arteries, focal dilation of a pulmonary artery, peripheral wedge-shaped opacities (often with a central lucency) as a result of infarctions, or a unilateral pleural effusion. Conversely, CTPA studies are highly sensitive and specific for acute PE. Acute PEs appear as tubular or curvilinear defects in the opacified pulmonary arteries [82]. They can be occlusive or nonocclusive; the former with higher rates of complications, including pulmonary infarcts. When seen en face, an acute PE can appear as a central hypodensity surrounded by contrast within a pulmonary artery, often referred to as the "polo mint sign" [83]. If an embolus is seen draping over the main pulmonary bifurcation, it is referred to as a "saddle embolus." These often pertain to a worse prognosis, because more embolus burden centrally is associated with worse out-

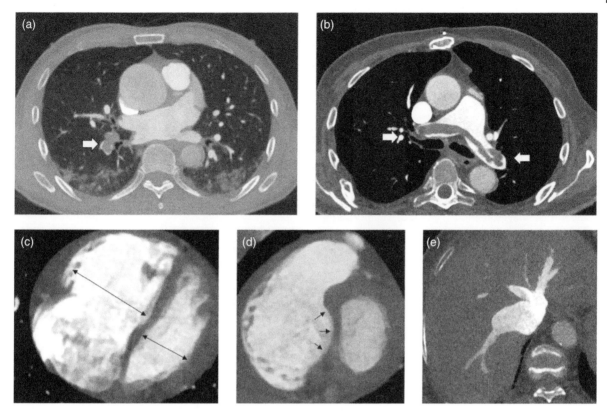

Figure 4.10   Axial and cardiac short-axis reconstruction images from various computed tomography (CT) pulmonary angiograms in the setting of COVID-19. (a) Nonocclusive lobar emboli (*white arrow*) in the right lower lobe with basal and peripheral ground-glass opacities in the lungs in a typical COVID-19 pneumonia pattern. (b) Saddle embolus (*white arrows*) in a patient with bilateral lower extremity deep venous thrombosis and chest pain. The patient tested positive for severe acute respiratory syndrome coronavirus 2 by polymerase chain reaction but had minimal pulmonary findings. (c) Axial CT images show significant right ventricular enlargement relative to the left ventricle, suggesting heart strain. (d) Deviation of the interventricular septum toward the left ventricle on reconstructed short-axis images on the same patient, also indicative of right-heart strain. (e) Significant reflux of contrast into the hepatic veins on the same patient providing further evidence of right-heart dysfunction.

comes [84]. Many techniques for directly assessing the PE burden have been proposed, although they are often too cumbersome for routine clinical work.

Clinically, PEs are divided into low-risk, submassive, and massive PE, with worsening prognoses between each grade. The defining feature between low-risk and submassive/massive PE is evidence of cardiac dysfunction [84]. This can be manifested in hypotension, myocardial necrosis (resulting in an elevated serum troponin), or right ventricular dysfunction (by imaging, electrocardiogram, or elevated serum B-natriuretic peptide). Massive PE is characterized by sustained hypotension (systolic blood pressure <90 mmHg) or need for inotropic support. CT features suggestive of right-heart dysfunction include right ventricular dilation defined as right ventricular-to-left ventricular chamber diameter ratio of more than 0.9 on axial images, interventricular septal straightening/inversion, and significant reflux into the hepatic veins.

Recently, dual-energy CT (DECT) and spectral CT have shown promise in the evaluation of PE [85]. These technologies use beams with different energies to extract information about the tissue composition based on the k-edge of their components. Different vendors have specific ways in which they achieve this, but largely with the same result. One particular advantage with DECT in the evaluation for PE is that DECT allows for the creation of an iodine map based on the k-edge of iodine. In other words, the scanner can derive images based on the iodine density. This allows for a reduction in the contrast dose necessary for adequate opacification of the pulmonary vessels. This results in better delineation of the pulmonary vasculature, although studies do not show improved detection of clinically relevant PEs by iodine maps alone [86]. Furthermore, DECT allows for the creation of virtual noncontrast images, making it easier to troubleshoot if a lesion is enhancing or intrinsically high density on CT. As discussed previously, the primary disadvantage of DECT is longer acquisition, increasing the likelihood of respiratory motion artifact.

Peripheral Pulmonary Vascular Enlargement Early in the pandemic, reports began describing peripheral pulmonary vascular enlargement in the setting of COVID-19 pneumonia [87]. The vascular enlargement was referred to by many names, including "vascular enhancement," "vascular thickening," and "microvascular enlargement," among others [88]. Although each report offered a slightly different description and explanation for the phenomenon, it typically describes enlarged subsegmental blood vessels within or in close proximity to the pulmonary opacities seen in COVID-19 pneumonia (Figure 4.11). The vessels can be deemed enlarged if they are dilated relative to similar generation vessels in the same lobe or changed in diameter compared with a prior or subsequent examination [89]. Multiple explanations have been given for the potential pathophysiology behind this, including capillary congestion, vasculitis, microthrombi, angiogenesis, and dysregulation of the normal pulmonary hypoxic vasoconstriction [78, 88–90].

Vascular enlargement is commonly seen in COVID-19 pneumonia, affecting nearly 70% of patients with parenchymal findings of COVID-19 on CT [88]. In contrast, in patients with pneumonia from influenza, vascular enlargement is less common, affecting around 20% of patients [89]. Li et al. [89] found larger opacities (>5 cm) tend to have higher rates of vascular enlargement, 97% versus 52% in lesions <3 cm. The

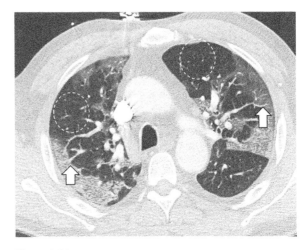

Figure 4.11 Axial computed tomography image showing peripheral vascular dilation associated with pulmonary opacities in COVID-19 (*white arrows*). Regions of unopacified lung demonstrate normal caliber of the pulmonary vessels (*dashed circles*).

vessels traveling through the opacities tended to be more dilated than those outside the opacities. They also noted that vascular enlargement was present in 100% of patients requiring admission to the ICU. On follow-up examinations, the vessels tended to stay the same or decrease in caliber. Although other diseases, such as pulmonary hypertension or hepatopulmonary syndrome, can cause peripheral vascular enlargement, one study by Lang et al. [90] found no patients in their cohort with any potentially confounding diseases despite showing a very high percentage of patients with COVID-19 with peripheral vascular enlargement. That said, more study is necessary on the presence of vascular enlargement in other diseases to better understand its true significance in COVID-19.

Central Pulmonary Artery Enlargement The central pulmonary arteries are more compliant than the central systemic arteries. Consequently, the pulmonary arteries can become distended from increased pressures in both the acute and chronic settings (Figure 4.12). The most commonly cited definition of dilation of the main pulmonary artery, ≥29 mm for men and ≥27 mm for women, is based on the Framingham Trial, although other studies have suggested a cutoff of 32 mm [91, 92]. Another

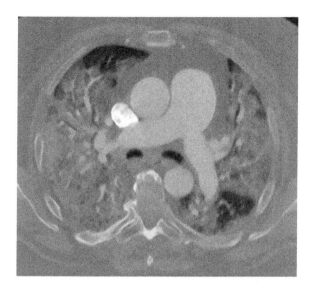

Figure 4.12 Enlargement of the main pulmonary artery in the setting of severe COVID-19 pneumonia with diffuse alveolar damage. Note the caliber of the main pulmonary artery is greater than that of the ascending aorta at the same level.

measure involves taking the ratio of the main pulmonary artery diameter to the diameter of the ascending aorta at the same level. A ratio greater than 1 is considered positive. These measures have specificities of 70–96% in the detection of pulmonary hypertension [91]. Because elevated pulmonary arterial pressures often have nonspecific symptoms but can result in right-heart dysfunction, arrythmias, and death, CT may be the first test to suggest pulmonary hypertension.

Enlargement of the central pulmonary arteries has been shown in COVID-19 to be a marker of disease severity and mortality. A study of 1461 patients by Esposito et al. [93] in Italy found that a main pulmonary artery ≥31 mm to have a hazard ratio of 1.6 for mortality. This was true even after taking into account numerous comorbidities, and it was consistent with other disease states, such as aortic stenosis, connective tissue diseases, and even the general population [94–96]. Furthermore, another study found that change in caliber of the main pulmonary artery and the ratio of the main pulmonary artery to aorta were significantly correlated with mortality, but not extent of pulmonary opacities, in patients with COVID-19 [97]. Thus, assessment for enlargement of the central

pulmonary arteries can help with prognostication in COVID-19.

Perfusional Changes Multiple perfusion abnormalities have been reported in COVID-19 using DECT. Using DECT, iodine, and pulmonary blood volume maps can give a static picture of blood flow at the specific moment scanned. These maps allow for qualitative and quantitative assessments of the pulmonary blood flow and have been validated against perfusion scintigraphy with good correlation [98]. One primary difference is that there tends to be greater perfusion to the dependent portions of lung by CTPA because iodinated contrast material tends to be denser than blood.

Increased perfusion surrounding pulmonary opacities is commonly reported, occurring in approximately 39% of patients in one study [90]. This peripheral hyperemia is thought to represent shunting of blood away from areas of alveolar abnormalities due to the Euler–Liljestrand mechanism (hypoxic vasoconstriction). Similarly, the opacities were associated with oligemia in 96%. These findings are consistent with pneumonias caused by other organisms [99]. Unlike other causes of pneumonia, mosaic perfusion was seen in 52% of patients, suggesting regions of vasoconstriction outside of areas with discrete pulmonary opacities. This is potentially explained by downregulation of angiotensin-converting enzyme 2 and the Angiotensin II receptor leading to regions of vasoconstriction [100]. Interestingly, a study by Lins et al. [101] found that pulmonary blood volumes in vessels <5 mm were decreased in patients with COVID-19, arguing against a commonly held viewpoint that results in dysfunctional hypoxic vasoconstriction [64]. Furthermore, regions of wedge-shaped perfusion defects correlate with vascular territories affected by PE, aiding in their detection as well [102].

Other Noncardiac Thoracic Manifestations of COVID-19
Lymphadenopathy Mediastinal and hilar lymph nodes may rarely become enlarged in the setting of COVID-19, affecting approximately 5% of patients [103]. Lymphadenopathy in the hilum and mediastinum is defined as ≥10 mm in short axis at all nodal stations except the subcarinal station, in which ≥15 mm in short axis is enlarged. The

lymphadenopathy in COVID-19 is presumably reactive to the active inflammation in the pulmonary parenchyma. Interestingly, although most CT data published on patients with COVID-19 were obtained on admission, a study investigating patients in the ICU with COVID-19 demonstrated lymphadenopathy in 66% of patients [104]. However, there were only nine patients in this study. Another study examining the changes over time had 0 of 21 patients showing lymphadenopathy [63]. This could therefore reflect that lymphadenopathy may be caused by the severity of disease versus other causes. Finally, unilateral axillary adenopathy has been reported in the setting of recent vaccination against COVID-19 [105, 106].

Temporal Evolution of the CT Findings in COVID-19

Just as the clinical symptoms of COVID-19 tend to follow a characteristic temporal evolution, largely determined by the severity of disease, the CT findings also follow a classic pattern of progression based on disease severity (Figure 4.13). Several studies have

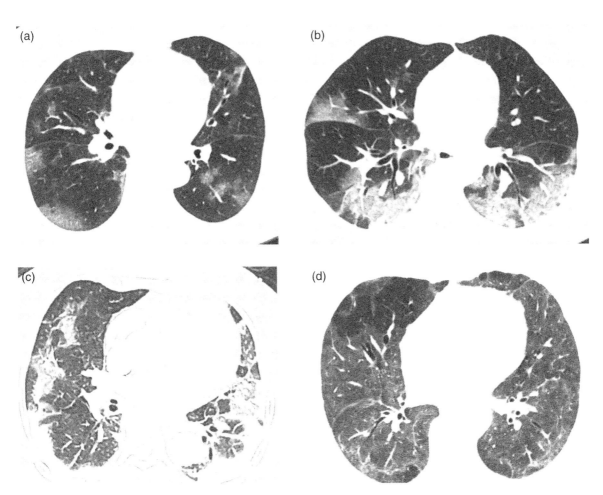

Figure 4.13 Stages of COVID-19 pneumonia across multiple patients. (a) Early stage: multifocal ground-glass opacities (GGOs) are seen, several with a round morphology and indistinct borders in this patient presenting with two days of cough. (b) Progressive stage: crazy paving and increasingly confluent opacities with a peripheral predominance are demonstrated. The patient reported a week of malaise and shortness of breath. (c) Peak stage: approximately 10 days into the patient's symptoms, predominantly consolidative opacities are seen with architectural distortion and organizational changes. (d) Absorption stage: one month after a patient's presentation, their CT demonstrates predominantly GGOs with regions of airways dilation and mild reticulation.

investigated this, largely based on Chinese datasets early in the pandemic. Generally, the extent and density of pulmonary opacities tend to peak late in the second week of symptoms (days 10–13) in patients with symptoms warranting imaging or medical attention, whereas patients with severe symptoms often continue to progress into the third week or longer [107]. Four stages have been described in the evolution of the acute pulmonary manifestations of COVID-19: early, progressive, peak, and absorption stages (Table 4.2) [63, 108].

Early Stage   The early stage typically represents days 0–4 after initiation of symptoms (Figure 4.13a). This phase is characterized by the rapid onset of GGOs occasionally with superimposed consolidation, often with round morphologies located in peripheral and basilar regions [109]. Often the GGOs even precede the onset of symptoms. The next most common opacity seen is superimposed intralobular lines on GGOs, the pattern often described as crazy paving, seen in around a quarter of patients. Peripheral vascular dilation can be seen in up to half of cases at this point [110]. Purely consolidative opacities, architectural distortion, and airways enlargement are uncommon. This is frequently the stage with the most extent of parenchymal abnormalities in mild or asymptomatic patients [107].

Table 4.2   The imaging stages of COVID-19 pneumonia.

Stage	Timing (days)	Imaging features
Early	0–4	Round GGOs with a peripheral and basilar predominance
Progressive	5–8	Crazy paving and consolidation replace regions of GGOs; opacities begin to affect more central lung zones
Peak	9–13	Dense consolidation peaks with regions of adjacent GGOs and airways dilation; crazy paving becomes rare
Absorption	14+	Opacities are largely ground glass, bandlike, and/or reticular with associated airways dilation

GGO, ground-glass opacity.

Progressive Stage   The progressive stage encompasses days 5–8 after symptom onset (Figure 4.13b). This stage is typified by increasing density and volume of pulmonary opacities [63]. Crazy paving and consolidation begin to replace regions of pure GGOs and become the most common opacity types. Peripheral vascular enlargement peaks in this phase [110]. Patients with moderate and severe symptoms may begin to see decreased lung volumes [107]. Furthermore, patients with moderate and severe symptoms begin to exhibit opacities in regions beyond the peripheral lung bases, often involving the posterior upper lungs, peripheral anterior lungs, and central lungs.

Peak Stage   The peak stage is described as days 9–13 after the onset of symptoms (Figure 4.13c). In this phase, crazy-paving patterns become rare, and dense consolidation peaks in frequency [109], although some regions of prior crazy paving may revert to pure GGOs, particularly in more mild cases. More evidence of architectural distortion becomes prevalent with subpleural bands, bronchial dilation, and subsegmental atelectasis. Although described as the "peak" stage, this is only true for patients with moderate disease, typically peaking around day 13 [107]. Mild cases may have completely resolved at this point, whereas severe cases may continue to progress beyond day 14, in line with the typical progression of diffuse alveolar damage. This phase will see pleural effusions develop in approximately 12% of people, although it is unclear if this is due to the infection itself or due to noninfectious entities, such as heart failure or the use of intravenous fluids in the hospital setting [110].

Absorption Stage   The absorption stage is often seen from day 14 onward without a clearly defined end (Figure 4.13d). This phase is characterized by the absorption of the pulmonary opacities. These opacities typically transition from consolidation to GGOs and reticular opacities, likely representing organizational changes. Architectural distortion becomes more common. Pathologically, these organizational changes can represent both organizing pneumonia and the organizational phase of diffuse alveolar damage [62, 71].

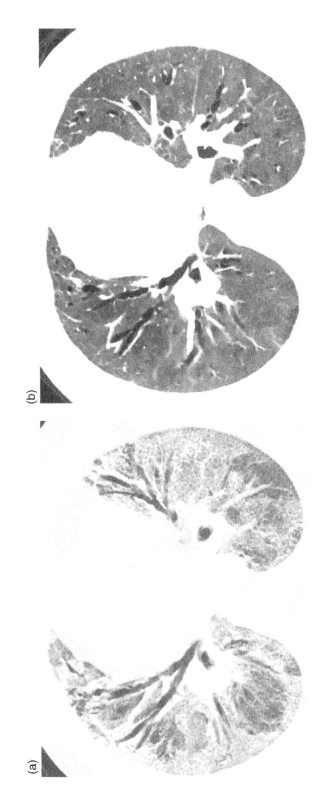

Figure 4.14 Axial computed tomography (CT) images of the same patient at one (a) and four (b) months after the onset of symptoms due to COVID-19. Between examinations the density of pulmonary opacities notably decreased with near-complete resolution of the reticular opacities. However, diffuse airways dilation and diffuse ground-glass opacities remain. The patient was symptomatic at the time of CT with significant functional limitations caused by exertional dyspnea.

As the pandemic has progressed, it has become apparent that many patients remain symptomatic long after the acute phase of their illness. To date, few studies have evaluated the radiographic changes beyond the acute phase of COVID-19, no doubt in part because of the novelty of this disease. One observational study from China found that around 8% of patients had complete resolution of pulmonary parenchymal abnormalities on CT by time of discharge, which increased to 53% by three weeks postdischarge [111]. They found younger patients (<44 years old) and patients with mild disease were the most likely to experience complete resolution by three weeks. Another study found roughly one-third of patients had complete resolution on CT by days 30–53, although their population was slightly older, and they did not evaluate for differences in resolution based on age [112]. They did find that patients with milder disease tended to completely resolve more frequently.

To date, the study with the longest-term follow-up was published by Han et al. [69]. They followed up 114 patients who experienced a severe COVID-19 infection with a CT scan six months after symptom onset. The majority (65%) did not have fibrotic-like findings (Figure 4.14), with 38% of all patients exhibiting complete resolution. Approximately 35% of these patients had fibrotic-like findings at six months, defined as the presence of traction bronchiectasis/airways enlargement, parenchymal bands, or honeycombing. Patients older than 50 years comprised 77% of those with fibrotic-like changes. Furthermore, patients who met a clinical diagnosis of acute respiratory distress syndrome (ARDS) during their hospitalization or required mechanical ventilation had much higher rates of fibrotic-like opacities at six months (63% versus 8% and 55% versus 8%, respectively). The extent of disease was also positively correlated with likelihood of developing fibrotic-like findings. Although only 14% of all patients reported dyspnea on exertion at six months, 50% of those with fibrotic-like findings on CT had abnormally low pulmonary diffusion (diffusing capacity of the lungs for carbon monoxide <80%) compared with only 6% of those without fibrotic-like findings. Overall, these findings raise the question of permanent fibrosis potentially developing as a result of severe COVID-19 pneumonia.

Our current best insight into the expected long-term changes to the lungs on CT may come from the literature from other causes of ARDS. Both severe COVID-19 pneumonia and other causes of ARDS are most commonly associated with diffuse alveolar damage on histology, so direct comparison between the two may be reasonable [62]. Around 50% of patients are expected to show a degree of fibrotic findings at six months, with the majority of those showing abnormally decreased diffusing capacity of the lungs for carbon monoxide [113]. In a study performed using CT at five years after ARDS, 59% of post-ARDS patients had fibrotic findings, but these were generally less extensive than those seen at six months or earlier [114]. In addition, there was no correlation with radiologic extent of disease and any measure by pulmonary function test. Thus, although the effects of COVID-19 on the lungs may extend beyond six months, there is room for optimism that these findings may continue to slowly regress based on reports from other causes of ARDS.

Pulmonary Parenchymal Findings Suggestive of an Alternative Diagnosis to COVID-19

Isolated Segmental or Lobar Consolidation Isolated consolidation, particularly those adhering to a segmental or lobar pattern, most commonly reflect other forms of pneumonia or aspiration (Table 4.3 and Figure 4.15) [115]. Although the exact organism cannot be determined by imaging, this pattern is most commonly seen in community-acquired pneumonias from species such as *Streptococcus pneumoniae*. In contrast, COVID-19 pneumonia tends to be bilateral and does not adhere to a bronchial branching pattern.

Centrilobular Nodules These are defined as nodular opacities occurring centrally in the secondary pulmonary lobules [61]. These opacities typically

Table 4.3 Findings that suggest an alternative diagnosis to COVID-19.

- Isolated segmental or lobar consolidation
- Centrilobular/tree-in-bud nodules
- Cavitation
- Smooth interlobular septal thickening with pleural effusions

(a)

(b)

(c)

(d)

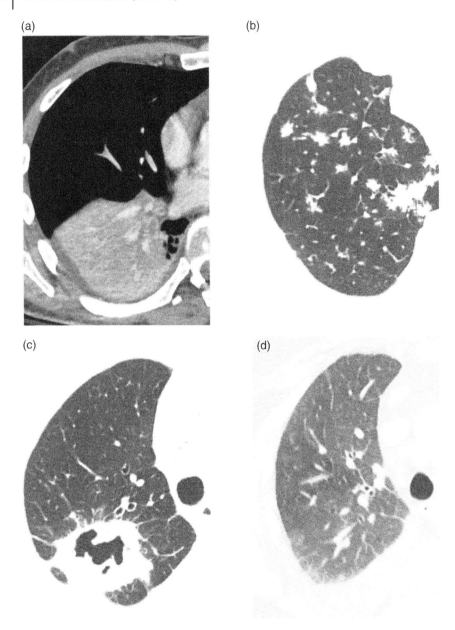

Figure 4.15   Computed tomography findings suggestive of alternative diagnoses to COVID-19. (a) Dense right lower lobe consolidation with bronchial enhancement consistent with aspiration pneumonitis in the setting of polytrauma. (b) Centrilobular/tree-in-bud nodules in the right upper lobe in a patient with active pulmonary tuberculosis. (c) Cavitation in the right upper lobe due to granulomatosis with polyangiitis. (d) Smooth interlobular septal thickening, diffuse ground-glass opacities, and pleural effusions in the setting of cardiogenic pulmonary edema.

occur with pathologic filling of respiratory bronchioles and/or alveoli. Tree-in-bud nodules are a subtype of centrilobular nodules with spread of debris into the terminal bronchioles causing a branching pattern between the nodules. Centrilobular opacities typically indicate a cellular bronchiolitis, most commonly from a bronchopneumonia or aspiration, although numerous other infectious, inflammatory, and neoplastic processes can cause centrilobular nodules. Although COVID-19 can cause nodular opacities, these often span multiple secondary pulmonary lobules and rarely result in debris within the terminal bronchioles (Table 4.3 and Figure 4.15).

Lung Cavitation Lung cavitation occurs when a central gas density is seen within consolidation or a mass/nodule. Typically, cavitation is due to infectious (e.g. tuberculosis or pulmonary abscesses) or neoplastic processes, although numerous other entities may result in cavitation. Cavitation is rare in the setting of COVID-19 pneumonia and may suggest cavitary changes in an infarct or a superinfection resulting in a pulmonary abscess or necrotic pneumonia (Table 4.3 and Figure 4.15).

Smooth Interlobular Septal Thickening with Pleural Effusions Although interlobular septal thickening is relatively common in COVID-19, pleural effusions are rarely seen at presentation. When seen in combination, the findings are indicative of pulmonary edema. In the setting of alveolar pulmonary edema, GGOs may be superimposed with a perihilar and gravity-dependent gradient (Table 4.3 and Figure 4.15).

Pulmonary Complications of COVID-19 on CT
ARDS

ARDS is a clinical diagnosis as defined by the Berlin criteria, although radiographic severity is described as an ancillary variable [116]. ARDS usually results from a pulmonary insult leading to a rapid respiratory decline and need for mechanical respiratory support. There is debate in the pulmonology literature as to whether COVID-19–related ARDS behaves similar to other causes of ARDS or if there are different pheno-types [117–119]. Histologically, it is identical to other forms of ARDS, typified by diffuse alveolar damage, similar to what is seen in severe cases of COVID-19 [62]. With regard to imaging, no features clearly separate ARDS from severe COVID-19 pneumonia, although the extent of pulmonary disease by imaging may be greater than what would be expected for the symptoms [120].

Superinfection A small number of patients will acquire a secondary infection in the setting of COVID-19 pneumonia. The presence of a viral pneumonia can alter the innate and adaptive immune systems, resulting in an increased susceptibility to superimposed bacterial, viral, or fungal infections [121]. Incidence rate of superimposed community- or hospital-acquired infections range from 8% to 22% [122, 123]. Common organisms from community-acquired pneumonias include *S. pneumoniae* and *Staphylococcus aureus*, while hospital-acquired infections were more commonly seen from *Pseudomonas aeruginosa* and *Escherichia coli*. Although the exact pathogens cannot be determined by imaging, findings of segmental/lobar consolidation, tree-in-bud nodules, or cavitation may herald the presence of a superinfection (Figure 4.16). As such, these are important features to note, because a superinfection will require additional treatment.

Pneumothorax/Pneumomediastinum Pneumothorax and pneumomediastinum are seen with increased frequency in the setting of COVID-19 pneumonia (Figure 4.17). Spontaneous pneumothoraces are seen in less than 1% of cases presenting to the emergency department but are seen with increasing frequency in those requiring mechanical ventilation [124, 125]. Similarly, pneumomediastinum is uncommonly seen outside the setting of mechanical ventilation. It has even been reported that there is a sevenfold increase in the cases of ARDS caused by COVID-19 over ARDS from other causes [126]. Barotrauma, decreased lung compliance, and lung frailty are all proposed mechanisms for their increased incidences. Imaging plays a critical role in the diagnosis of both pneumomediastinum and pneumothorax, although often plain films are sufficient. It is important to note evidence of tension physiology, because this requires urgent treatment because the increased pressures in the pleural space can impede blood flow to the heart and cause cardiopulmonary compromise. Signs include flattening or inversion of a hemidiaphragm, mediastinal shift, or increased ipsilateral intercostal spaces.

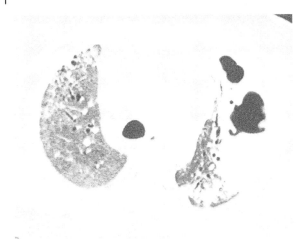

Figure 4.16 Development of a necrotizing pneumonia, presumed to be bacterial, in the setting of severe COVID-19 pneumonia. The thick-walled cavity with air–fluid levels is highly suggestive of an acute infectious process in this setting.

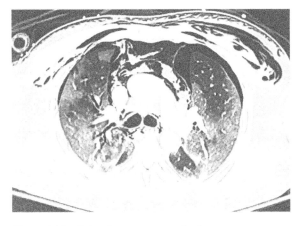

Figure 4.17 Extensive pneumomediastinum, subcutaneous emphysema, and bilateral pneumothoraxes in the setting of barotrauma in acute respiratory distress syndrome from COVID-19.

Differential Diagnosis of COVID-19 on CT

Organizing Pneumonia Organizing pneumonia is a pathologic response to injury by the lungs typified by fibroblastic foci depositing the terminal airways and alveoli. This can be caused by numerous entities that determine the clinical symptoms, including drug reactions, infections (including COVID-19), and toxic inhalants [71, 127]. Consequently, the findings on CT mirror what is seen in COVID-19 pneumonias, includ-

ing peripheral opacities, subpleural and perilobular sparing, as well as halo and reverse halo/atoll signs (Figure 4.18a). As a result, the RSNA consensus reporting guidelines stipulate that any appearance consistent with organizing pneumonia should be considered a "typical appearance" for a COVID-19 pneumonia [70]. In addition, they recommended including the differential diagnosis of organizing pneumonia in all cases with a "typical appearance" on CT (Table 4.4).

Other Viral Pneumonias Other viral pneumonias feature significant overlap in imaging features among themselves, as well as COVID-19 pneumonia [70]. As such, many clinical guidelines recommend against using imaging to diagnose COVID-19 versus other viral pneumonias when RT-PCR is available. These pathogens include influenza, rhinovirus, cytomegalovirus (particularly in those with impaired immune systems), among others. Common imaging features include consolidation, GGOs and/or crazy paving in a peripheral or bronchovascular pattern (Figure 4.18b) [128]. Investigation into using CT to differentiate between pneumonia caused by influenza and SARS-CoV-2 have shown that the imaging overlap is substantial and often it is impossible to do so. However, COVID-19 had a greater predilection for subpleural opacities, while influenza resulted in more mucous plugging and pleural effusions [129].

Aspiration Aspiration occurs when material from the oropharynx or gastrointestinal tract below the protective mechanisms of the larynx leak into the respiratory tract. This may result in a chemical pneumonitis from the aspirate itself or a bacterial pneumonia from gut flora. Like COVID-19, aspiration tends to affect the lung bases more than the apices [130]. The opacities can be a mix of consolidation, GGOs, and tree in bud, typically in a dependent distribution (Figure 4.18c). The tree-in-bud opacities, as well as the endoluminal debris commonly seen in aspiration, are rare in COVID-19 and can help distinguish between these entities. Furthermore, aspiration may affect only one lobe, also uncommon in COVID-19. Ancillary findings such as a hiatal hernia, patulous esophagus, prior stroke, or head and neck malignancies may suggest this diagnosis because they can predispose the patient to aspiration.

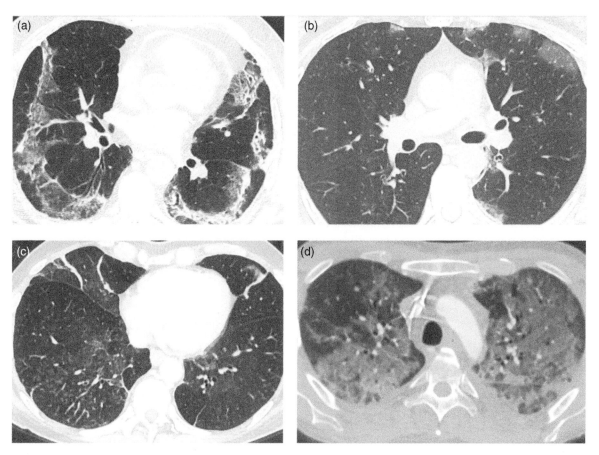

Figure 4.18 (a) Peripheral ground-glass opacities (GGOs) and consolidation with regions of lobular sparing and atoll signs in the setting of cryptogenic organizing pneumonia. This pattern is frequently seen in COVID-19. (b) In this patient with H1N1 influenza pneumonia, subpleural GGOs are seen similar to what is often visualized in COVID-19. Notably, there are fine centrilobular nodules in the anterior right upper lobe, a finding not usually seen in COVID-19, which can occasionally help suggest an alternate infectious cause to these opacities. (c) GGOs and tree-in-bud opacities with a bronchovascular predominance in the right lower lobe. This patient had a history of a head and neck cancer status after several operations resulting in chronic aspiration. (d) Diffuse GGOs seen in the setting of *Pneumocystis jirovecii* pneumonia in a patient with AIDS; note the significant central component of the opacities rather than the typical peripheral distribution in COVID-19.

Atypical Pneumonias Atypical pneumonias are those that behave in a pattern not typically seen in pneumonias. They are often multifocal on imaging and may exhibit a more insidious course clinically. One particular entity in this category, *Pneumocystis jirovecii* pneumonia (PJP), can have a considerable overlap in appearance on CT (Figure 4.18d). *P. jirovecii* pneumonia is most commonly seen in immunocompromised patients, particularly in patients infected by the human immunodeficiency virus. Diffuse GGOs are commonly seen throughout the lungs, although they tend to affect the lung apices more frequently in contrast with COVID-19. Over time, these opacities may evolve to a crazy-paving pattern, with nodular consolidation and cysts, another finding unusual in COVID-19.

Nonspecific Interstitial Pneumonia Nonspecific interstitial pneumonia (NSIP) is an interstitial lung disease most frequently seen in collagen vascular diseases such as systemic sclerosis, although it can also be seen in entities such as drug toxicities and hypersensitivity pneumonitis [131]. Symptoms are typically more insidious with slowly progressive

Table 4.4 Differential diagnosis of COVID-19 on CT.

Diagnosis	Imaging features that may help discriminate from COVID-19
Organizing pneumonia	None. Imaging and even pathologic features can be identical
Other viral pneumonias	No reliable features, but significant mucous plugging or a central predominance to the opacities may favor other viral pneumonias
Atypical pneumonia	Significant nodularity, tree-in-bud opacities, and/or cystic changes
Aspiration	Endobronchial debris or tree-in-bud opacities with a dependent distribution
Nonspecific interstitial pneumonia	Evidence of a connective tissue disease or increasing reticular opacities or GGOs over time with a basilar, subpleural, or bronchovascular predominance
Pulmonary edema	Smooth interlobular septal thickening is a dominant feature; GGOs tend to be more central in location; pleural effusions are common
Diffuse alveolar hemorrhage	The distribution of the opacities tends to be more variable rather than basilar/peripheral, although there can be significant overlap
Eosinophilic pneumonias	Acute eosinophilic pneumonia tends to have more diffuse opacities; chronic eosinophilic pneumonia typically progresses over months rather than days

dyspnea and dry cough. The disease progress usually follows the clinical course of the underlying etiology. These patients exhibit peripheral, basilar, and peribronchovascular reticular and GGOs with traction bronchiectasis. Frequently the opacities demonstrate a degree of subpleural sparing. Late in the disease, the patient may even develop honeycombing. Consequently, NSIP would be most frequently confused with the absorption stage of COVID-19. Distinction between the two can usually be by the clinical history. Radiographically, distinction can most easily be made with serial imaging; symptoms of NSIP will typically progress over time, while COVID-19 should improve over time. Ancillary findings suggestive of collagen vascular diseases or drug toxicity (such as a

hyperdense liver in the setting of amiodarone use) can also suggest a diagnosis of NSIP over COVID-19 (Figure 4.19).

Pulmonary Edema Pulmonary edema refers to abnormal fluid accumulation within the interstitial and air spaces of the lungs. Clinically, pulmonary edema is divided into cardiogenic and noncardiogenic causes based on whether an elevated pulmonary capillary wedge pressure is present, although there are substantial imaging overlaps between these. Pulmonary edema typically exhibits diffuse smooth interlobular septal thickening often with a superimposed ground-glass component (crazy paving) with a hilar or dependent pattern [130]. Pleural effusions are frequently seen in cardiogenic edema. Lymphadenopathy may also be present as a result of venolymphatic congestion. Ancillary findings suggesting particular causes such as left-heart enlargement from heart failure or renal cortical atrophy from end-stage renal disease may be present. The perihilar/dependent nature of the GGOs and pleural effusions can help distinguish pulmonary edema from COVID-19.

Diffuse Alveolar Hemorrhage Diffuse alveolar hemorrhage (DAH) is when there is diffuse bleeding into the alveoli, resulting in progressively bloody washings on bronchoalveolar lavage. DAH has numerous causes, including vasculitides, coagulation disorders, and drug reactions. Patients frequently report hemoptysis, which is rare in COVID-19. Diffuse GGOs (not necessarily sparing the central lung zones, unlike COVID-19 tends to) and smooth interlobular septal thickening are the two most common CT manifestations [130]. As such, DAH may appear quite similar radiographically to severe COVID-19, and differentiating between the two may only be possible with clinical history and laboratory testing.

Eosinophilic Pneumonias Eosinophilic pneumonias are a group of rare diseases characterized by eosinophilic infiltrates in the pulmonary parenchyma [132]. Patients with acute eosinophilic pneumonia present frequently with acute febrile illnesses and hypoxemia, like COVID-19. The exact cause is unknown but has been reported in association with toxic inhalation. The diagnosis typically requires

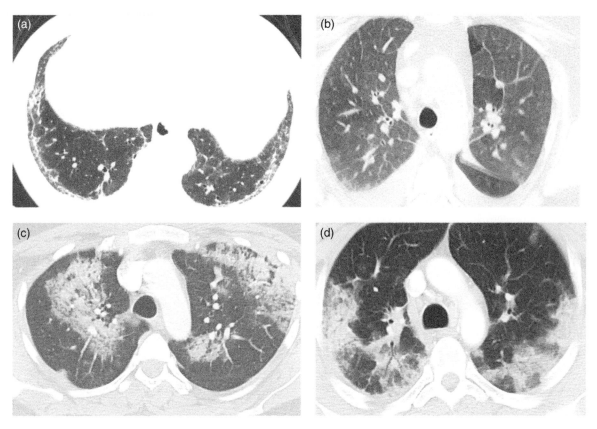

Figure 4.19 (a) In this case of biopsy-proven nonspecific interstitial pneumonia, peripheral reticular and ground-glass opacities (GGOs) can be seen with immediate subpleural sparing. NSIP can mimic the absorption stage of COVID-19. Although COVID-19 pneumonia should regress over time, NSIP typically will progress over time. (b) Diffuse smooth interlobular septal thickening, GGOs, and pleural effusions can be seen in this patient with cardiogenic pulmonary edema. The presence of pleural effusions in the setting of prominent interlobular septal thickening can help differentiate pulmonary edema from COVID-19, which typically does not feature pleural effusions. (c) Diffuse alveolar hemorrhage characterized on CT by patchy consolidation and GGOs, often with crazy paving. Although COVID-19 is typically basal and peripheral predominant, the distribution in diffuse alveolar hemorrhage is random. (d) Subpleural GGOs and consolidation with perilobular sparing in chronic eosinophilic pneumonia. This entity cannot be distinguished radiographically from COVID-19 pneumonia.

a bronchoalveolar lavage showing >25% eosinophils. On CT, the findings often resemble COVID-19, with diffuse patchy regions of GGOs intermixed with smooth interlobular septal thickening and consolidation. In contrast, chronic eosinophilic pneumonia typically manifests with a more indolent course, usually an asthmatic with months of progressive shortness of breath often with a dry cough, helping to clinically distinguish it from COVID-19. However, the imaging appearance can be remarkably similar to COVID-19, with peripheral GGOs (called the "photographic negative of pulmonary edema"), and sometimes with

crazy paving or consolidation. The opacities are frequently seen with an upper lobe predilection, unlike COVID-19.

Using CT to Risk-Stratify Patients

From early in the pandemic, it became apparent that clinicians needed tools to help triage patients for appropriate levels of care and prognosticate which patients are at greatest risk for development of severe symptoms. It rapidly became apparent that extent of disease on imaging correlated with severity of symptoms, and various groups, such as the Fleischner

Society, began recommending imaging be obtained in patients with COVID-19 to help with risk stratification [59]. Various semiquantitative, quantitative, and artificial intelligence-based models were developed, showing incremental benefit in risk-stratifying patients over clinical methods alone [133–137]. These models largely focused on the presence and extent of opacification of the lung parenchyma as a marker for disease severity, invariably showing greater extent of the pulmonary opacities was more correlated with likelihood of having severe clinical disease. Patients with denser opacities (consolidation versus GGOs) had worse outcomes [133]. CT also allows for characterization of other risk factors for disease progression, including coronary artery calcium, emphysema, and pulmonary artery diameter [97, 134, 138]. Finally, CT can assess the long-term sequela of COVID-19 better than plain film.

All this considered, at this time there are no standardized widely accepted models to use CT for risk stratification. The majority of studies have used techniques developed in-house retrospectively and have not been validated in other centers. One particular model, the Chest CT Severity Score, has been validated by an outside center [134, 137]. In this semiquantitative model, the lungs are divided into 20 segments and given a score of 0 if no opacities are present, 1 if opacities are present and occupy less than 50% of the segment, and 2 if opacities occupy more than 50% of a segment. Patients with higher scores had more severe disease, although the optimal cutoff was different between the initial and validation cohorts (19.5 vs. 15.5). The cumbersome nature of obtaining the scores required by these models have also impeded widespread use, because it can be time consuming and delay the care of other patients for incremental gains made by the scoring system. Thus, more research is required to further validate these models and their efficacy in clinical use.

Ultrasound

The utility of lung ultrasound (LU) has been reported as an imaging tool for diagnosis and monitoring of pulmonary manifestation of COVID-19 [139]. In contrast with other imaging modalities, who performs and interprets LU is heterogenous across centers. Most commonly it is used in the bedside setting to answer specific questions, such as severity of lung involvement or assessment of pleural effusions. Furthermore, when used in this fashion, LU could reduce spread through the hospital by limiting need for patient transport outside the COVID ward, and a single device can be designated to remain in the ward [140]. Another benefit of LU is the lack of ionizing radiation used to make diagnostic images, thereby reducing the patient's medical radiation doses. However, many limitations of LU hold back its clinical utility, including variations in scanners, operators and techniques, scan time, and inability to penetrate the central portions of lung [141].

Despite this, the sensitivity of LU to detect pulmonary manifestation of COVID-19 has been reported as high and comparable with that of chest CT, likely because of the fact that pulmonary parenchymal involvement tends to be predominantly peripheral in COVID-19 [142]. The ability of LU to detect pulmonary pathology is consistent with prior work done on LU during the pre-COVID-19 era. Bedside lung ultrasound had been used in the imaging of patients with other infectious diseases, such as Ebola and hemorrhagic fever, as well as noninfectious entities, such as cardiogenic pulmonary edema and ARDS [143, 144]. Imaging protocols range from limited point-of-care evaluations of focal abnormalities, such as pleural effusions, to full standardized evaluation of the lungs by dividing the chest into regions and obtaining cine sweeps across each. Typically, convex or microconvex probes are used to better evaluate both pleural and parenchymal abnormalities.

In normal LU, an "A line" demonstrates repetition of the pleural line at the same distance from skin to pleural line, which represents air below the pleural line. In contrast, "B lines" are hyperechoic laser-like artifacts resembling a comet tail, arise from the pleural line, and move in concert with lung sliding, which is caused by the reverberation of the ultrasound beam between slightly decreased alveolar air and increased interstitial fluids. B lines are seen in most patients with COVID-19 pulmonary involvement and are often coalescent and compacted in cases of more severe involvement [142, 144]. Thus, B lines are frequently used to monitor disease extent and progression to anticipate which patients will clinically deteriorate. Pulmonary consolidation in the ultrasound manifests as hypoechogenic regions and mimics hepatic ecotecture (hepatization of the lung parenchyma). Detecting pulmonary consolidation may serve as an indicator for progression of the disease and allow clinicians to assess the severity and clinical spectrum of COVID-19-associated lung injury [142]. Combining the degree of consolidation and B lines has proven useful in stratifying which patients with ARDS are ready for extubation [144].

LU also can be used to detect pleural abnormalities [145]. If normal sliding of the pleura is lost, the diagnosis of a pneumothorax can be suggested. Pleural effusions are usually detected in dependent locations as hypoechoic collections. Pleural effusions are typically small when present in the setting of COVID-19. LU also has excellent sensitivity in looking for identifying septations and pleural thickening that suggest the pleural fluid is exudative and may need further intervention.

Although the sensitivity for COVID-19 with LU is reported to be high, specificity can be variable because of its similar imaging appearance with other pulmonary pathologies [144]. For example, other viral pneumonias can have an identical appearance on LU and are not specific for COVID-19 [146, 147]. Pulmonary edema also can result in a large number of B lines simulating COVID-19, with both pathologies typically most pronounced in the dependent portions of lung. However, in pulmonary edema, the B lines tend to be more evenly spaced and usually lack interspersed regions of normal lung. In addition, diffuse alveolar damage as a result of COVID-19 and other causes can appear identical with mixed consolidation and B lines throughout the lungs. Therefore, LU may not be appropriate for the initial diagnosis of COVID-19 because multiple other entities can have a similar sonographic appearance.

PET

^{18}F-fluorodeoxyglucose (FDG) PET/CT is a commonly used modality that uses a glucose analogue to target metabolically active tissues. Its primary use remains oncologic imaging, although it has been shown to be useful in several infectious processes. To date, several cases have been described with findings of COVID-19 infection on ^{18}F-FDG PET/CT.

One early study by Qin et al. [148] described ^{18}F-FDG PET/CT results in four patients with COVID-19 infection in early 2020. They noted the presence of peripheral GGOs and/or consolidative opacities in more than two pulmonary lobes that showed a high FDG uptake, showing that these regions of lung are indeed metabolically active. However, FDG uptake in pneumonia is not unique to COVID-19 and can have nearly any cause. Although lymphadenopathy is not a common manifestation of COVID-19, their findings revealed an increase in FDG uptake in the otherwise normal-appearing lymph nodes, also a finding commonly seen in other causes of pneumonia [149].

Alavi et al. [150] suggested that FDG-PET imaging can be used to determine the systemic effects of COVID-19 infection on the entire body, which leads to better characterization of systemic complication throughout the body. They also hypothesized that whole-body PET scan will be of a great value in the assessment of experimental drugs to treat COVID-19 infection [150].

A systematic review assessing the diagnostic value of detecting COVID-19 on PET imaging confirmed that the primary findings are those typical on CT with superimposed FDG uptake where there are pulmonary opacities [151]. The regions had standardized uptake values ranging from 2.2 to 18, which can mask malignancy in those regions. This analysis included primarily patients imaged for cancer staging or follow-up. The authors suggested that these regions should be followed to resolution, particularly in the setting of known malignancy.

Thus, ^{18}F-FDG PET/CT has been shown to be abnormal in patients with SARS-CoV-2 infections beyond what is seen only on the CT portion. However, ^{18}F-FDG PET/CT is not used by any major guidelines in the evaluation of COVID-19, and it remains to be seen whether these additional data from PET will lead to meaningful changes in clinical outcomes.

Pulmonary manifestation in two asymptomatic patients with COVID-19 reported in PET imaging with 68Ga-DOTATATE and 68Ga-PSMA-11 tracers demonstrated hypermetabolic bilateral peripheral GGOs and consolidation [152].

MRI

MRI has been reported as the alternative, nonionizing method for patients with pulmonary manifestation of

COVID-19 [153, 154]. Vasilev et al. [155] reported a case series showing the findings of peripheral and basal predominant opacities with crazy-paving signs on chest MRI were visually similar to CT. Another study by Torkian et al. [153] was able to demonstrate atoll signs with MRI. The majority of patients showed consolidation and GGOs in distributions that match typical findings of COVID-19 by the RSNA consensus criteria. These case series generally found the opacities to be most clearly depicted on T2-weighted images, potentially because of the increased water content in the inflamed lung (Figure 4.20).

Despite this, pulmonary imaging with MRI is limited to a few centers worldwide because of the many technical challenges imaging the lungs on MRI presents. The primary challenge lies in the fact that the lungs are primarily air, while MRI obtains its signal from hydrogen atoms in water molecules [156]. Thus, the relatively sparse distribution of water/lung parenchyma relative to air compounded by the susceptibility effects of oxygen often result in poor signal from the lungs on MRI. Experimental techniques, such as ultrashort echo time sequences, have been developed to minimize this, although this sequence is not widely available [157]. Furthermore, respiratory and cardiac motion can degrade images, often necessitating the use of respiratory and cardiac gating techniques, both of which can drastically increase the imaging time.

The ACR statement recommends minimizing MRI use in COVID-19 pandemic because of the prolonged time spent in the scanner relative to other tests [158]. Given the aforementioned limitations of chest MRI, it is unlikely to become an imaging technique commonly used to evaluate COVID-19 pneumonia. However, lung parenchyma is partially visible in MRI performed for a reason other than lung, such as cardiac, thoracic spine, and abdomen MRI, and thus it is important to recognize the potential findings on MRI.

Guidelines for Reporting

RSNA

In March 2020, the RNSA published an expert consensus document providing guidelines on reporting chest CT findings related to COVID-19 [70]. The statement was developed by experts from nine different US-based academic medical centers.

There was anticipation that chest CT examinations would increase as a result of the ongoing pandemic. Incidental lung findings on CT scan concerning for COVID-19 were also expected. Thus, the consensus document sought to provide guidelines to radiologists reporting on CT scans performed for both when COVID-19 was suspected for PUI and when identified incidentally.

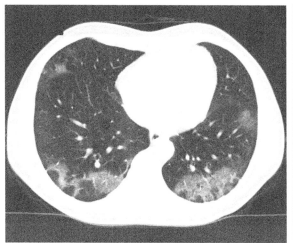 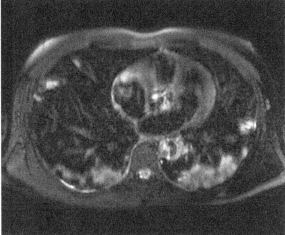

Figure 4.20 An axial T2-weighted magnetic resonance image with peripheral hyperintense opacities corresponding to chest computed tomography finding of ground-glass opacities. *Source:* Courtesy of Shahram Akhlaghpoor, MD, at Pardis Noor Medical Imaging Center, Tehran, Iran.

They provided four distinct categories for reporting chest CT scan findings with respect to COVID-19: (i) typical appearance, (ii) indeterminate appearance, (iii) atypical appearance, and (iv) negative for pneumonia.

The details of the four-tier system for reporting as it relates to COVID-19 pneumonia imaging classification are as follows:

i) *Typical appearance:* Typical CT findings are found in COVID-19 pneumonia, including peripheral GGOs and nodular or masslike GGO involvement in multiple lobes bilaterally, especially in the lower lobes. The suggested reporting language was: "Commonly reported imaging features of (COVID-19) pneumonia are present. Other processes such as influenza pneumonia and organizing pneumonia, as can be seen with drug toxicity and connective pneumonia, as can be seen with drug toxicity and connective tissue disease, can cause a similar imaging pattern."

ii) *Indeterminate appearance:* There are nonspecific imaging features of COVID-19 pneumonia. The suggested reporting language was, "Imaging features can be seen with (COVID-19) pneumonia, though are non-specific and can occur with a variety of infectious and noninfectious processes."

iii) *Atypical appearance:* Uncommonly or not reported features of COVID-19 pneumonia are present. The suggested reporting language was, "Imaging features are atypical or uncommonly reported for (COVID-19) pneumonia. Alternative diagnoses should be considered."

iv) *Negative for pneumonia:* No features of pneumonia are present. The suggested reporting language was, "No CT findings present to indicate pneumonia. (Note: CT may be negative in the early stages of COVID-19.)"

There were certain caveats provided in the suggested reporting language. One of those caveats includes the potential false-negative findings seen early in the disease course. Due to negative CT scans during the first two days of symptom onset, a negative chest CT does not entirely exclude COVID-19 as a diagnosis. Furthermore, the authors do comment that the report does not necessarily have to include the terminology "COVID19

pneumonia," and that the term "viral pneumonia" would be a reasonable and inclusive alternative.

Use of standardized reporting language in the CT scan radiology report was an emphasis of the RSNA recommendations. Multiple benefits were identified in the use of the earlier standardized language, including:

- Improvement in guidance and confidence to radiologists
- Decrease in the variability in reporting and aiding the referring provider's understanding of the CT findings
- Promotion of education, research, and quality improvement
- Provision of some guidance on which patients should be prioritized for RT-PCR testing if such testing is limited in availability
- Typical findings may encourage use of repeat RT-PCR testing

It is well-known that imaging for a particular indication has the potential to identify other incidental findings. How would radiologists handle situations whereby typical features of COVID-19 are found on CT scanning performed for other purposes, that is, when observed as an incidental finding? The RSNA offered some practical suggestions to deal with such situations.

- The RSNA recommended direct communication with the referring provider to determine likelihood of viral infection. This avoids surprising both the patient and referring provider.
- Notifying the referring provider allows them to initialize standard operating procedures to minimize exposure and spread.
- The term "viral pneumonia" can be used instead of specifically COVID-19. This is especially true if indeterminate or atypical features are identified incidentally.
- Other findings (i.e. emphysema and diffuse parenchymal disease) that may increase morbidity should be described.

In their efforts to stratify the findings into four discrete categories, the guidelines do acknowledge that there may be situations where CT scan findings have mixed findings, that is, both typical and atypical features of COVID-19. Certainly, it is possible for patients to have COVID-19 with superimposed lung pathology. For example, patients with COVID-19 pneumonia can develop bacterial pneumonia as well.

The RSNA has created a standardized reporting template to improve communication with providers for efficient patient care [70].

COVID-19 Reporting and Data System

In March 2020, as the world continued to witness an exponential rise in the number of COVID-19 cases, the Dutch Radiological Society established a COVID-19 network to promote dissemination of information and tools to combat the pandemic. A working group was formed to develop a standardized reporting system meant for use by radiologists when interpreting chest CT scan findings. This COVID-19 Reporting and Data System became known as CO-RADS.

This system is akin to the reporting system seen in Lung Imaging Reporting and Data System (LI-RADS), Prostate Imaging Reporting and Data System (PI-RADS), and Breast Imaging Reporting and Data System (BI-RADS). Like these previously described standardized reporting systems, CO-RADS provides seven discrete categories (from zero to six) that establish degrees of suspicion for pulmonary involvement of COVID-19 [159].

To assess the reliability of the CO-RADS system, eight radiologists evaluated 105 chest CT scans of patients admitted because of suspicion of COVID-19 respiratory disease. Overall, there was moderate-to-substantial interobserver agreement (Fleiss k value of 0.47). The discriminatory power of CO-RADS for diagnosing COVID-19 was high, with a mean area under the receiver operating characteristic curve of 0.91 (95% confidence interval [CI]: 0.85–0.97) for positive RT-PCR results.

COVID-19 Imaging Reporting and Data System

The COVID-19 Imaging Reporting and Data System (COVID-RADS) scoring system was developed based on 37 published studies with 3467 patients [160]. The study demonstrates the summary of the typical chest CT findings, atypical features, and temporal changes of chest CT. The developers of COVID-RADS compiled a comprehensive lexicon including the most pertinent terms and can be used for documentation and reporting of typical and atypical imaging findings. They also proposed the COVID-RADS, which is a grading system of CT findings with five categories (0, 1, 2A, 2B, and 3), corresponding to a low, moderate, or high level of suspicion for pulmonary COVID-19 involvement. The implementation of COVID-RADS grading and a structured reporting system would enable consistent, rapid, and efficient communication and decrease the rate of missed diagnosis.

The study of Sushentsev et al. [161] regarding a comparison of the intraobserver and interobserver agreement of COVID-RADS and CO-RADS grading systems with 200 studies demonstrated that the median intraobserver agreement of CO-RADS was considerably higher compared with COVID-RADS. The interobserver agreement became substantial with κ values of 0.74 (95% CI: 0.66–0.82) for COVID-RADS and 0.73 (95% CI: 0.65–0.81) for CO-RADS. The median intraobserver agreement was considerably higher for CO-RADS, reaching 0.81 (95% CI: 0.43–0.76) compared with 0.60 (95% CI: 0.43–0.76) for COVID-RADS.

References

1 Rubin, G.D., Ryerson, C.J., Haramati, L.B. et al. (2020). The role of chest imaging in patient management during the COVID-19 pandemic: a multinational consensus statement from the Fleischner Society. *Radiology* 296 (1): 172–180. doi:10.1148/radiol.2020201365.

2 World Health Organization (2020). *Use of Chest Imaging in COVID-19*. WHO Reference Number: WHO/2019-nCoV/Clinical/Radiology_imaging/2020.1. Geneva: WHO https://www.who.int/publications/i/item/use-of-chest-imaging-in-covid-19.

3 Chou, R., Pappas, M., Buckley, D. et al. (2020). *Use of Chest Imaging in COVID-19: a Rapid Advice Guide Web Annex A. Imaging for COVID-19: a Rapid Review*. Geneva: WHO https://apps.who.int/iris/handle/10665/332326.

4 World Health Organization (2020). *Use of Chest Imaging in COVID-19: a Rapid Advice Guide: Web Annex B: GRADE Evidence-to-Decision Tables*. Geneva: WHO https://apps.who.int/iris/handle/10665/332327.

5 Akl, E.A., Blazic, I., Yaacoub, S. et al. (2020). Use of chest imaging in the diagnosis and management of COVID-19: a WHO rapid advice guide. *Radiology* 298: 203173. doi:10.1148/radiol.2020203173.

6 Chung, M., Bernheim, A., Mei, X. et al. (2020). CT imaging features of 2019 novel coronavirus (2019-nCoV). *Radiology* 295 (1): 202–207. doi:10.1148/radiol.2020200230.

7 Bernheim, A., Mei, X., Huang, M. et al. (2020). Chest CT findings in coronavirus disease 2019 (COVID-19): relationship to duration of infection. *Radiology.* 295 (3): 685–691. doi:10.1148/radiol.2020200463.

8 Ai, T., Yang, Z., Hou, H. et al. (2020). Correlation of chest CT and RT-PCR testing for coronavirus disease 2019 (COVID-19) in China: a report of 1014 cases. *Radiology.* 296 (2): E32–E40. doi:10.1148/radiol.2020200642.

9 Kanne, J.P., Little, B.P., Chung, J.H. et al. (2020). Essentials for radiologists on COVID-19: an update-radiology scientific expert panel. *Radiology* 296 (2): E113–E114. doi:10.1148/radiol.2020200527.

10 Fang, Y., Zhang, H., Xie, J. et al. (2020). Sensitivity of chest CT for COVID-19: comparison to RT-PCR. *Radiology* 296 (2): E115–E117. doi:10.1148/radiol.2020200432.

11 Huang, P., Liu, T., Huang, L. et al. (2020). Use of chest CT in combination with negative RT-PCR assay for the 2019 novel coronavirus but high clinical suspicion. *Radiology* 295 (1): 22–23. doi:10.1148/radiol.2020200330.

12 Zhao, W., Zhong, Z., Xie, X. et al. (2020). Relation between chest CT findings and clinical conditions of coronavirus disease (COVID-19) pneumonia: a multicenter study. *AJR Am J Roentgenol.* 214 (5): 1072–1077. doi:10.2214/AJR.20.22976.

13 Zu, Z.Y., Jiang, M., Di, X.P.P. et al. (2020). Coronavirus disease 2019 (COVID-19): a perspective from China. *Radiology.* 296 (2): E15–E25. doi:10.1148/radiol.2020200490.

14 American College of Radiology (2020). ACR recommendations for the use of chest radiography and computed tomography (CT) for suspected COVID-19 infection. ACR. https://www.acr.org/Advocacy-and-Economics/ACR-Position-Statements/Recommendations-for-Chest-Radiography-and-CT-for-Suspected-COVID19-Infection.

15 Society of Thoracic Radiology (2020). STR/ASER COVID-19 Position Statement (March 11, 2020). Society of Thoracic Radiology. https://thoracicrad.org/?page_id=2879.

16 American Society of Emergency Radiology. ASER COVID-19 Task Force: FAQs. ASER. https://www.aser.org/covid-19-faqs.

17 Kicska, G., Litmanovich, D.E., Ordovas, K.G. et al. (2020). Statement from the North American Society for Cardiovascular Imaging on imaging strategies to reduce the scarcity of healthcare resources during the COVID-19 outbreak. *Int J Cardiovasc Imaging* 36 (8): 1387–1393. doi:10.1007/s10554-020-01861-1.

18 O'Sullivan, J.W., Muntinga, T., Grigg, S., and Ioannidis, J.P.A. (2018). Prevalence and outcomes of incidental imaging findings: umbrella review. *BMJ* 361: k2387. doi:10.1136/bmj.k2387.

19 van Doremalen, N., Bushmaker, T., Morris, D.H. et al. (2020). Aerosol and surface stability of SARS-CoV-2 as compared with SARS-CoV-1. *N Engl J Med.* 382 (16): 1564–1567. doi:10.1056/NEJMc2004973.

20 Setti, L., Passarini, F., De Gennaro, G. et al. (2020). Airborne transmission route of covid-19: why 2 meters/6 feet of inter-personal distance could not be enough. *Int J Environ Res Public Health* 17 (8): 2932. doi:10.3390/ijerph17082932.

21 Mossa-Basha, M., Medverd, J., Linnau, K.F. et al. (2020). Policies and guidelines for COVID-19 preparedness: experiences from the University of Washington. *Radiology* 296 (2): E26–E31. doi:10.1148/radiol.2019201326.

22 Mousavi, E.S., Godri Pollitt, K.J., Sherman, J., and Martinello, R.A. (2020). Performance analysis of portable HEPA filters and temporary plastic anterooms on the spread of surrogate coronavirus. *Build Environ.* 183: 107186. doi:10.1016/j.buildenv.2020.107186.

23 Letizia, A.G., Ramos, I., Obla, A. et al. (2020). SARS-CoV-2 transmission among marine recruits during quarantine. *N Engl J Med.* 383 (25): 2407–2416. doi:10.1056/nejmoa2029717.

24 Centers for Disease Control and Prevention (2020). Criteria for return to work for healthcare personnel with SARS-CoV-2 infection (interim guidance). CDC. https://www.cdc.gov/coronavirus/2019-ncov/hcp/guidance-risk-assesment-hcp.html (accessed 20 April 2021).

25 National Center for Immunization and Respiratory Diseases (NCIRD), Division of Viral Diseases (2020). Public health guidance for community-related exposure. CDC. https://www.cdc.gov/coronavirus/2019-ncov/php/public-health-recommendations.html (accessed 20 April 2021).

26 Gange, C.P., Pahade, J.K., Cortopassi, I. et al. (2020). Social distancing with portable chest radiographs during the COVID-19 pandemic: assessment of radiograph technique and image quality obtained at 6 feet and through glass. *Radiol Cardiothorac Imaging* 2 (6): e200420. doi:10.1148/ryct.2020200420.

27 Centers for Disease Control and Prevention (CDC) (2021). Cleaning and Disinfecting Your Facility: Updated 5 Jan 2021. CDC. https://www.cdc.gov/coronavirus/2019-ncov/community/disinfecting-building-facility.html (accessed 20 April 2021).

28 Wessner, C.E., Nelson, J., Mott, S. et al. (2021). A sonographer's step-by-step approach for preventing transmission of COVID-19. *J Diagn Med Sonogr.* 37 (1): 97–103. doi:10.1177/8756479320959035.

29 Mitchell, C., Collins, K., Hua, L. et al. (2020). Specific considerations for sonographers when performing echocardiography during the 2019 novel coronavirus outbreak: supplement to the American Society of Echocardiography statement. *J Am Soc Echocardiogr.* 33 (6): 654–657. doi:10.1016/j.echo.2020.04.014.

30 Wong, H.Y.F., Lam, H.Y.S., AH-T, F. et al. (2020). Frequency and distribution of chest radiographic findings in patients positive for COVID-19. *Radiology* 296 (2): E72–E78. doi:10.1148/radiol.2020201160.

31 Giovagnoni, A. (2020). Facing the COVID-19 emergency: we can and we do. *Radiol Med.* 125 (4): 337–338. doi:10.1007/s11547-020-01178-y.

32 Fichera, G., Stramare, R., De Conti, G. et al. (2020). It's not over until it's over: the chameleonic behavior of COVID-19 over a six-day period. *Radiol Med.* 125 (5): 514–516. doi:10.1007/s11547-020-01203-0.

33 Borghesi, A. and Maroldi, R. (2020). COVID-19 outbreak in Italy: experimental chest X-ray scoring system for quantifying and monitoring disease progression. *Radiol Med.* 125 (5): 509–513. doi:10.1007/s11547-020-01200-3.

34 Taylor, E., Haven, K., Reed, P. et al. (2015). A chest radiograph scoring system in patients with severe acute respiratory infection: a validation study. *BMC Med Imaging* 15 (1): 61. doi:10.1186/s12880-015-0103-y.

35 Ng, M.-Y., Lee, E.Y.P., Yang, J. et al. (2020). Imaging profile of the COVID-19 infection: radiologic findings and literature review. *Radiol Cardiothorac Imaging.* 2 (1): e200034. doi:10.1148/ryct.2020200034.

36 Yoon, S.H., Lee, K.H., Kim, J.Y. et al. (2020). Chest radiographic and CT findings of the 2019 novel coronavirus disease (COVID-19): analysis of nine patients treated in Korea. *Korean J Radiol.* 21 (4): 494–500. doi:10.3348/kjr.2020.0132.

37 Cozzi, D., Albanesi, M., Cavigli, E. et al. (2020). Chest X-ray in new coronavirus disease 2019 (COVID-19) infection: findings and correlation with clinical outcome. *Radiol Med.* 125 (8): 730–737. doi:10.1007/s11547-020-01232-9.

38 Salehi, S., Abedi, A., Balakrishnan, S., and Gholamrezanezhad, A. (2020). Coronavirus disease 2019 (COVID-19): a systematic review of imaging findings in 919 patients. *Am J Roentgenol.* 215 (1): 87–93. 10.2214/AJR.20.23034.

39 Zhan, N., Guo, Y., Tian, S. et al. (2021). Clinical characteristics of COVID-19 complicated with pleural effusion. *BMC Infect Dis.* 21 (1): 176. doi:10.1186/s12879-021-05856-8.

40 Yasin, R. and Gouda, W. (2020). Chest X-ray findings monitoring COVID-19 disease course and severity. *Egypt J Radiol Nucl Med.* 51: 193. doi:10.1186/s43055-020-00296-x.

41 Wichmann, D., Sperhake, J.-P., Lütgehetmann, M. et al. (2020). Autopsy findings and venous thromboembolism in patients with COVID-19. *Ann Intern Med.* 173 (4): 268–277. doi:10.7326/M20-2003.

42 Liu, K., Zeng, Y., Xie, P. et al. (2020). COVID-19 with cystic features on computed tomography: a case report. *Medicine* 99 (18): e20175. doi:10.1097/MD.0000000000020175.

43 Reyes, S., Roche, B., Kazzaz, F. et al. (2020). Pneumothorax and pneumomediastinum in COVID-19: a case series. *Am J Med Sci.* doi:10.1016/j.amjms.2020.11.024.

44 Rodrigues, J.C.L., Hare, S.S., Edey, A. et al. (2020). An update on COVID-19 for the radiologist – a British society of thoracic imaging statement. *Clin Radiol.* 75 (5): 323–325. doi:10.1016/j.crad.2020.03.003.

45 Rosovsky, R.P., Grodzin, C., Channick, R. et al. (2020). Diagnosis and treatment of pulmonary embolism during the coronavirus disease 2019 pandemic: a position paper from the National PERT Consortium. *Chest* 158 (6): 2590–2601. doi:10.1016/j.chest.2020.08.2064.

46 American College of Radiology (2015). ACR – ASER – SPR practice parameter for the performance of computed tomography (CT). *Am Coll Radiol.* 1076 (Revised 2008): 1–18.

47 Bae, K.T. (2010). Intravenous contrast medium administration and scan timing at CT: considerations and approaches. *Radiology* 256 (1): 32–61. doi:10.1148/radiol.10090908.

48 Doolittle, D.A., Froemming, A.T., and Cox, C.W. (2019). High-pitch versus standard mode CT pulmonary angiography: a comparison of indeterminate studies. *Emerg Radiol.* 26 (2): 155–159. doi:10.1007/s10140-018-1656-1.

49 Weidman, E.K., Plodkowski, A.J., Halpenny, D.F. et al. (2018). Dual-energy CT angiography for detection of pulmonary emboli: incremental benefit of iodine maps. *Radiology* 289 (2): 546–553. doi:10.1148/radiol.2018180594.

50 Kubo, T., Ohno, Y., Nishino, M. et al. (2016). Low dose chest CT protocol (50 mAs) as a routine protocol for comprehensive assessment of intrathoracic abnormality. *Eur J Radiol Open.* 3: 86–94. doi:10.1016/j.ejro.2016.04.001.

51 Kim, Y., Kim, Y.K., Lee, B.E. et al. (2015). Ultra-low-dose CT of the thorax using iterative reconstruction: evaluation of image quality and radiation dose reduction. *AJR Am J Roentgenol.* 204 (6): 1197–1202. doi:10.2214/AJR.14.13629.

52 Tabatabaei, S.M.H., Talari, H., Gholamrezanezhad, A. et al. (2020). A low-dose chest CT protocol for the diagnosis of COVID-19 pneumonia: a prospective study. *Emerg Radiol.* 27 (6): 607–615. doi:10.1007/s10140-020-01838-6.

53 He, J.L., Luo, L., Luo, Z.D. et al. (2020). Diagnostic performance between CT and initial real-time RT-PCR for clinically suspected 2019 coronavirus disease (COVID-19) patients outside Wuhan, China. *Respir Med.* 168: 105980. doi:10.1016/j.rmed.2020.105980.

54 Kim, H., Hong, H., and Yoon, S.H. (2020). Diagnostic performance of CT and reverse transcriptase polymerase chain reaction for coronavirus disease 2019: a meta-analysis. *Radiology* 296 (3): E145–E155. doi:10.1148/radiol.2020201343.

55 Adams, H.J.A., Kwee, T.C., Yakar, D. et al. (2020). Systematic review and meta-analysis on the value of chest CT in the diagnosis of coronavirus disease (COVID-19): Sol Scientiae, Illustra Nos. *AJR Am J Roentgenol.* 215 (6): 1342–1350. doi:10.2214/AJR.20.23391.

56 Giri, B., Pandey, S., Shrestha, R. et al. (2021). Review of analytical performance of COVID-19 detection methods. *Anal Bioanal Chem.* 413 (1): 35–48. doi:10.1007/s00216-020-02889-x.

57 Borakati, A., Perera, A., Johnson, J., and Sood, T. (2020). Diagnostic accuracy of X-ray versus CT in COVID-19: a propensity-matched database study. *BMJ Open.* 10 (11): e042946. doi:10.1136/bmjopen-2020-042946.

58 Chen, X., Zhang, G., Hao, S.Y. et al. (2020). Similarities and differences of early pulmonary CT features of pneumonia caused by SARS-CoV-2, SARS-CoV and MERS-CoV: comparison based on a systemic review. *Chinese Med Sci J* 35 (3): 254–261. doi:10.24920/003727.

59 Rubin, G.D., Ryerson, C.J., Haramati, L.B. et al. (2020). The role of chest imaging in patient management during the COVID-19 pandemic: a multinational consensus statement from the Fleischner Society. *Chest.* 158 (1): 106–116. doi:10.1016/j.chest.2020.04.003.

60 Bao, C., Liu, X., Zhang, H. et al. (2020). Coronavirus disease 2019 (COVID-19) CT findings: a systematic review and meta-analysis. *J Am Coll Radiol.* 17 (6): 701–709. doi:10.1016/j.jacr.2020.03.006.

61 Hansell, D.M., Bankier, A.A., MacMahon, H. et al. (2008). Fleischner Society: glossary of terms for thoracic imaging. *Radiology* 246 (3): 697–722. doi:10.1148/radiol.2462070712.

62 Henkel, M., Weikert, T., Marston, K. et al. (2020). Lethal COVID-19: radiologic-pathologic correlation of the lungs. *Radiol Cardiothorac Imaging* 2 (6): e200406. doi:10.1148/ryct.2020200406.

63 Pan, F., Ye, T., Sun, P. et al. (2020). Time course of lung changes at chest CT during recovery from coronavirus disease 2019 (COVID-19). *Radiology* 295 (3): 715–721. doi:10.1148/radiol.2020200370.

64 Song, F., Shi, N., Shan, F. et al. (2020). Emerging 2019 novel coronavirus (2019-nCoV) pneumonia. *Radiology* 295 (1): 210–217. doi:10.1148/radiol.2020200274.

65 Li, K., Wu, J., Wu, F. et al. (2020). The clinical and chest CT features associated with severe and critical COVID-19 pneumonia. *Invest Radiol.* 55 (6): 327–331. doi:10.1097/RLI.0000000000000672.

66 Wong, K.T., Antonio, G.E., Hui, D.S.C. et al. (2003). Thin-section CT of severe acute respiratory syndrome: evaluation of 73 patients exposed to or with the disease. *Radiology* 228 (2): 395–400. doi:10.1148/radiol.2283030541.

67 Polverino, E., Goeminne, P.C., McDonnell, M.J. et al. (2017). European Respiratory Society guidelines for the management of adult bronchiectasis. *Eur Respir J.* 50 (3): 1700629. doi:10.1183/13993003.00629-2017.

68 Adams, H.J.A., Kwee, T.C., Yakar, D. et al. (2020). Chest CT imaging signature of coronavirus disease 2019 infection: in pursuit of the scientific evidence. *Chest* 158 (5): 1885–1895. doi:10.1016/j.chest.2020.06.025.

69 Han, X., Fan, Y., Alwalid, O. et al. (2021). Six-month follow-up chest CT findings after severe COVID-19 pneumonia. *Radiology* 299 (1): E177–E186. doi:10.1148/radiol.2021203153.

70 Simpson, S., Kay, F.U., Abbara, S. et al. (2020). Radiological Society of North America expert consensus statement on reporting chest CT findings related to COVID-19. Endorsed by the Society of Thoracic Radiology, the American College of Radiology, and RSNA – secondary publication. *J Thorac Imaging* 35 (4): 219–227. doi:10.1097/RTI.0000000000000524.

71 Pogatchnik, B.P., Swenson, K.E., Sharifi, H. et al. (2020). Radiology-pathology correlation in recovered COVID-19, demonstrating organizing pneumonia. *Am J Respir Crit Care Med.* 202 (4): 598–599. doi:10.1164/rccm.202004-1278IM.

72 McLaren, T.A., Gruden, J.F., and Green, D.B. (2020). The Bullseye sign: a variant of the reverse halo sign in COVID-19 pneumonia. *Clin Imaging* 68: 191–196. doi:10.1016/j.clinimag.2020.07.024.

73 Shi, H., Han, X., Jiang, N. et al. (2020). Radiological findings from 81 patients with COVID-19 pneumonia in Wuhan, China: a descriptive study. *Lancet Infect Dis.* 20 (4): 425–434. doi:10.1016/S1473-3099(20)30086-4.

74 Ye, Z., Zhang, Y., Wang, Y. et al. (2020). Chest CT manifestations of new coronavirus disease 2019 (COVID-19): a pictorial review. *Eur Radiol.* 30 (8): 4381–4389. doi:10.1007/s00330-020-06801-0.

75 Barco, S., Valerio, L., Ageno, W. et al. (2021). Age-sex specific pulmonary embolism-related mortality in the USA and Canada, 2000-18: an analysis of the WHO mortality database and of the CDC multiple cause of death database. *Lancet Respir Med.* 9 (1): 33–42. doi:10.1016/S2213-2600(20)30417-3.

76 Price, L.C., McCabe, C., Garfield, B., and Wort, S.J. (2020). Thrombosis and COVID-19 pneumonia: the clot thickens! *Eur Respir J.* 56 (1): E70–E80. 10.1183/13993003.01608-2020.

77 Suh, Y.J., Hong, H., Ohana, M. et al. (2021). Pulmonary embolism and deep vein thrombosis in COVID-19: a systematic review and meta-analysis. *Radiology* 298 (2): E70–E80. doi:10.1148/radiol.2020203557.

78 Malas, M.B., Naazie, I.N., Elsayed, N. et al. (2020). Thromboembolism risk of COVID-19 is high and associated with a higher risk of mortality: a systematic review and meta-analysis. *EClinicalMedicine* 29: 100639. doi:10.1016/j.eclinm.2020.100639.

79 Cuker, A., Tseng, E.K., Nieuwlaat, R. et al. (2021). American Society of Hematology 2021 guidelines on the use of anticoagulation for thromboprophylaxis in patients with COVID-19. *Blood Adv.* 5 (3): 872–888. doi:10.1182/bloodadvances.2020003763.

80 Berger, J.S., Kunichoff, D., Adhikari, S. et al. (2020). Prevalence and outcomes of D-dimer elevation in hospitalized patients with COVID-19. *Arterioscler Thromb Vasc Biol.* 40 (10): 2539–2547. doi:10.1161/ATVBAHA.120.314872.

81 Tatco, V.R. and Piedad, H.H. (2011). The validity of hyperdense lumen sign in non-contrast chest CT scans in the detection of pulmonary thromboembolism. *Int J Cardiovasc Imaging* 27 (3): 433–440. doi:10.1007/s10554-010-9673-5.

82 Wittram, C., Kalra, M.K., Maher, M.M. et al. (2006). Acute and chronic pulmonary emboli: angiography-CT correlation. *AJR Am J Roentgenol.* 186 (6 Suppl 2): S421–S429. doi:10.2214/AJR.04.1955.

83 Moore, A.J.E., Wachsmann, J., Chamarthy, M.R. et al. (2018). Imaging of acute pulmonary embolism: an update. *Cardiovasc Diagn Ther.* 8 (3): 225–243. doi:10.21037/cdt.2017.12.01.

84 Sista, A.K., Kuo, W.T., Schiebler, M., and Madoff, D.C. (2017). Stratification, imaging, and management of acute massive and submassive pulmonary embolism. *Radiology* 284 (1): 5–24. doi:10.1148/radiol.2017151978.

85 Lu, G.-M., Wu, S.-Y., Yeh, B.M., and Zhang, L.-J. (2010). Dual-energy computed tomography in pulmonary embolism. *Br J Radiol.* 83 (992): 707–718. doi:10.1259/bjr/16337436.

86 Monti, C.B., Zanardo, M., Cozzi, A. et al. (2021). Dual-energy CT performance in acute pulmonary embolism: a meta-analysis. *Eur Radiol.* 31: 6248–6258. doi:10.1007/s00330-020-07633-8.

87 Dai, H., Zhang, X., Xia, J. et al. (2020). High-resolution chest CT features and clinical characteristics of patients infected with COVID-19 in Jiangsu, China. *Int J Infect Dis.* 95: 106–112. doi:10.1016/j.ijid.2020.04.003.

88 Lv, H., Chen, T., Pan, Y. et al. (2020). Pulmonary vascular enlargement on thoracic CT for diagnosis and differential diagnosis of COVID-19: a systematic review and meta-analysis. *Ann Transl Med.* 8 (14): 878. doi:10.21037/atm-20-4955.

89 Li, Q., Huang, X.-T., Li, C.-H. et al. (2021). CT features of coronavirus disease 2019 (COVID-19) with an emphasis on the vascular enlargement pattern. *Eur J Radiol.* 134: 109442. doi:10.1016/j.ejrad.2020.109442.

90 Lang, M., Som, A., Carey, D. et al. (2020). Pulmonary vascular manifestations of COVID-19 pneumonia. *Radiol Cardiothorac Imaging* 2 (3): e200277. doi:10.1148/ryct.2020200277.

91 Altschul, E., Remy-Jardin, M., Machnicki, S. et al. (2019). Imaging of pulmonary hypertension: pictorial essay. *Chest.* 156 (2): 211–227. doi:10.1016/j.chest.2019.04.003.

92 Goerne, H., Batra, K., and Rajiah, P. (2018). Imaging of pulmonary hypertension: an update. *Cardiovasc Diagn Ther.* 8 (3): 279–296. doi:10.21037/cdt.2018.01.10.

93 Esposito, A., Palmisano, A., Toselli, M. et al. (2021). Chest CT-derived pulmonary artery enlargement at the admission predicts overall survival in COVID-19 patients: insight from 1461 consecutive patients in Italy. *Eur Radiol.* 31 (6): 4031–4041. doi:10.1007/s00330-020-07622-x.

94 Hossain, R., Chelala, L., Sleilaty, G. et al. (2021). Preprocedure CT findings of right heart failure as a predictor of mortality after transcatheter aortic valve replacement. *AJR Am J Roentgenol.* 216 (1): 57–65. doi:10.2214/AJR.20.22894.

95 Terzikhan, N., Bos, D., Lahousse, L. et al. (2017). Pulmonary artery to aorta ratio and risk of all-cause mortality in the general population: the Rotterdam Study. *Eur Respir J.* 49 (6): 1602168. doi:10.1183/13993003.02168-2016.

96 Li, X., Zhang, C., Sun, X. et al. (2020). Prognostic factors of pulmonary hypertension associated with connective tissue disease: pulmonary artery size measured by chest CT. *Rheumatology* 59 (11): 3221–3228. doi:10.1093/rheumatology/keaa100.

97 Spagnolo, P., Cozzi, A., Foà, R.A. et al. (2020). CT-derived pulmonary vascular metrics and clinical outcome in COVID-19 patients. *Quant Imaging Med Surg.* 10 (6): 1325–1333. doi:10.21037/qims-20-546.

98 Hopkins, S.R., Wielpütz, M.O., and Kauczor, H.-U. (2012). Imaging lung perfusion. *J Appl Phys.* 113 (2): 328–339. doi:10.1152/japplphysiol.00320.2012.

99 Otrakji, A., Digumarthy, S.R., Lo Gullo, R. et al. (2016). Dual-energy CT: spectrum of thoracic abnormalities. *Radiographics* 36 (1): 38–52. doi:10.1148/rg.2016150081.

100 Jain, A., Doyle, D.J., and Mangal, R. (2020). "Mosaic perfusion pattern" on dual-energy CT in COVID-19 pneumonia: pulmonary vasoplegia or vasoconstriction? *Radiol Cardiothorac Imaging* 2 (5): e200433. doi:10.1148/ryct.2020200433.

101 Lins, M., Vandevenne, J., Thillai, M. et al. (2020). Assessment of small pulmonary blood vessels in COVID-19 patients using HRCT. *Acad Radiol.* 27 (10): 1449–1455.

102 Ridge, C.A., Desai, S.R., Jeyin, N. et al. (2020). Dual-energy CT pulmonary angiography (DECTPA) quantifies vasculopathy in severe COVID-19 pneumonia. *Radiol Cardiothorac Imaging* 2 (5): e200428. doi:10.1148/ryct.2020200428.

103 Zhu, J., Zhong, Z., Li, H. et al. (2020). CT imaging features of 4121 patients with COVID-19: a meta-analysis. *J Med Virol.* 92 (7): 891–902. doi:10.1002/jmv.25910.

104 Valette, X., du Cheyron, D., and Goursaud, S. (2020). Mediastinal lymphadenopathy in patients with severe COVID-19. *Lancet Infect Dis.* 20 (11): 1230. doi:10.1016/S1473-3099(20)30310-8.

105 Ahn, R.W., Mootz, A.R., Brewington, C.C., and Abbara, S. (2021). Axillary lymphadenopathy after mRNA COVID-19 vaccination. *Radiol Cardiothorac Imaging* 3 (1): e210008. doi:10.1148/ryct.2021210008.

106 Mortazavi, S. (2021). Coronavirus disease (COVID-19) vaccination associated axillary adenopathy: imaging findings and follow-up recommendations in 23 women. *AJR Am J Roentgenol.* doi:10.2214/AJR.21.25651.

107 Wang, Y.-C., Luo, H., Liu, S. et al. (2020). Dynamic evolution of COVID-19 on chest computed tomography: experience from Jiangsu Province of China. *Eur Radiol.* 30 (11): 6194–6203. doi:10.1007/s00330-020-06976-6.

108 Quispe-Cholan, A., Anticona-De-La-Cruz, Y., Cornejo-Cruz, M. et al. (2020). Tomographic findings in patients with COVID-19 according to evolution of the disease. *Egypt J Radiol Nucl Med.* 51 (1): 215. doi:10.1186/s43055-020-00329-5.

109 Wang, Y., Dong, C., Hu, Y. et al. (2020). Temporal changes of CT findings in 90 patients with COVID-19 pneumonia: a longitudinal study. *Radiology.* 296 (2): E55–E64. doi:10.1148/radiol.2020200843.

110 Zhou, S., Zhu, T., Wang, Y., and Xia, L. (2020). Imaging features and evolution on CT in 100 COVID-19 pneumonia patients in Wuhan, China. *Eur Radiol.* 30 (10): 5446–5454. doi:10.1007/s00330-020-06879-6.

111 Liu, D., Zhang, W., Pan, F. et al. (2020). The pulmonary sequalae in discharged patients with COVID-19: a short-term observational study. *Respir Res.* 21 (1): 125. doi:10.1186/s12931-020-01385-1.

112 Wang, Y., Jin, C., Wu, C.C. et al. (2020). Organizing pneumonia of COVID-19: time-dependent evolution and outcome in CT findings. *PLoS One.* 15 (11): e0240347. doi:10.1371/journal.pone.0240347.

113 Masclans, J.R., Roca, O., Muñoz, X. et al. (2011). Quality of life, pulmonary function, and tomographic scan abnormalities after ARDS. *Chest* 139 (6): 1340–1346. doi:10.1378/chest.10-2438.

114 Wilcox, M.E., Patsios, D., Murphy, G. et al. (2013). Radiologic outcomes at 5 years after severe ARDS. *Chest* 143 (4): 920–926. doi:10.1378/chest.12-0685.

115 Nambu, A. (2014). Imaging of community-acquired pneumonia: roles of imaging examinations, imaging diagnosis of specific pathogens and discrimination from noninfectious diseases. *World J Radiol.* 6 (10): 779. doi:10.4329/wjr.v6.i10.779.

116 ARDS Definition Task Force, Ranieri, V.M., Rubenfeld, G.D. et al. (2012). Acute respiratory distress syndrome: the Berlin definition. *JAMA* 307 (23): 2526–2533. doi:10.1001/jama.2012.5669.

117 Ferrando, C., Suarez-Sipmann, F., Mellado-Artigas, R. et al. (2020). Clinical features, ventilatory management, and outcome of ARDS caused by COVID-19 are similar to other causes of ARDS. *Intensive Care Med.* 46 (12): 2200–2211. doi:10.1007/s00134-020-06192-2.

118 Grasselli, G., Tonetti, T., Protti, A. et al. (2020). Pathophysiology of COVID-19-associated acute respiratory distress syndrome: a multicentre prospective observational study. *Lancet Respir Med.* 8 (12): 1201–1208. doi:10.1016/S2213-2600(20)30370-2.

119 Gattinoni, L., Chiumello, D., and Rossi, S. (2020). COVID-19 pneumonia: ARDS or not? *Crit Care.* 24 (1): 1–3. doi:10.1186/s13054-020-02880-z.

120 Li, X. and Ma, X. (2020). Acute respiratory failure in COVID-19: is it "typical" ARDS? *Crit Care* 24 (1): 198. doi:10.1186/s13054-020-02911-9.

121 Rynda-Apple, A., Robinson, K.M., and Alcorn, J.F. (2015). Influenza and bacterial superinfection: illuminating the immunologic mechanisms of disease. *Infect Immun.* 83 (10): 3764–3770. doi:10.1128/IAI.00298-15.

122 Falcone, M., Tiseo, G., Giordano, C. et al. (2021). Predictors of hospital-acquired bacterial and fungal superinfections in COVID-19: a prospective observational study. *J Antimicrob Chemother.* 76 (4): 1078–1084. doi:10.1093/jac/dkaa530.

123 Garcia-Vidal, C., Sanjuan, G., Moreno-García, E. et al. (2021). Incidence of co-infections and superinfections in hospitalized patients with COVID-19: a retrospective cohort study. *Clin Microbiol Infect.* 27 (1): 83–88. doi:10.1016/j.cmi.2020.07.041.

124 Martinelli, A.W., Ingle, T., Newman, J. et al. (2020). COVID-19 and pneumothorax: a multicentre retrospective case series. *Eur Respir J.* 56 (5): 2002697. doi:10.1183/13993003.02697-2020.

125 Miró, Ò., Llorens, P., Jiménez, S. et al. (2021). Frequency, risk factors, clinical characteristics, and outcomes of spontaneous pneumothorax in patients with coronavirus disease 2019: a case-control, emergency medicine-based multicenter study. *Chest.* 159 (3): 1241–1255. doi:10.1016/j.chest.2020.11.013.

126 Lemmers, D.H.L., Abu Hilal, M., Bnà, C. et al. (2020). Pneumomediastinum and subcutaneous emphysema in COVID-19: barotrauma or lung frailty? *ERJ Open Res.* 6 (4) 00385-2020. doi:10.1183/23120541.00385-2020.

127 Kligerman, S.J., Franks, T.J., and Galvin, J.R. (2013). From the radiologic pathology archives: organization and fibrosis as a response to lung injury in diffuse alveolar damage, organizing pneumonia, and acute fibrinous and organizing pneumonia. *Radiographics* 33 (7): 1951–1975. doi:10.1148/rg.337130057.

128 Koo, H.J., Lim, S., Choe, J. et al. (2018). Radiographic and CT features of viral pneumonia. *Radiographics* 38 (3): 719–739. doi:10.1148/rg.2018170048.

129 Lin, L., Fu, G., Chen, S. et al. (2021). CT manifestations of coronavirus disease (COVID-19) pneumonia and influenza virus pneumonia: a comparative study. *AJR Am J Roentgenol.* 216 (1): 71–79. doi:10.2214/AJR.20.23304.

130 Parekh, M., Donuru, A., Balasubramanya, R., and Kapur, S. (2020). Review of the chest CT differential diagnosis of ground-glass opacities in the COVID era. *Radiology* 297 (3): E289–E302. doi:10.1148/radiol.2020202504.

131 Kligerman, S.J., Groshong, S., Brown, K.K., and Lynch, D.A. (2009). Nonspecific interstitial pneumonia: radiologic, clinical, and pathologic considerations. *Radiographics.* 29 (1): 73–87. doi:10.1148/rg.291085096.

132 Jeong, Y.J., Kim, K.-I., Seo, I.J. et al. (2007). Eosinophilic lung diseases: a clinical, radiologic, and pathologic overview. *Radiographics* 27 (3): 617–637; discussion 637–639. doi:10.1148/rg.273065051.

133 Grodecki, K., Lin, A., Cadet, S. et al. (2020). Quantitative burden of COVID-19 pneumonia on chest CT predicts adverse outcomes: a post-hoc analysis of a prospective international registry. *Radiol Cardiothorac Imaging* 2 (5): e200389. doi:10.1148/ryct.2020200389.

134 Lieveld, A.W.E., Azijli, K., Teunissen, B.P. et al. (2021). Chest CT in COVID-19 at the ED: validation of the COVID-19 reporting and data system (CO-RADS) and CT severity score: a prospective, multicenter, observational study. *Chest* 159 (3): 1126–1135. doi:10.1016/j.chest.2020.11.026.

135 Li, K., Fang, Y., Li, W. et al. (2020). CT image visual quantitative evaluation and clinical classification of coronavirus disease (COVID-19). *Eur Radiol.* 30: 4407–4416. doi:10.1007/s00330-020-06817-6.

136 Lassau, N., Ammari, S., Chouzenoux, E. et al. (2021). Integrating deep learning CT-scan model, biological and clinical variables to predict severity of COVID-19 patients. *Nat Commun.* 12 (1): 1–11. doi:10.1038/s41467-020-20657-4.

137 Yang, R., Li, X., Liu, H. et al. (2020). Chest CT severity score: an imaging tool for assessing severe COVID-19. *Radiol Cardiothorac Imaging* 2 (2): e200047. doi:10.1148/ryct.2020200047.

138 Dillinger, J.G., Benmessaoud, F.A., Pezel, T. et al. (2020). Coronary artery calcification and complications in patients with COVID-19. *JACC Cardiovasc Imaging.* 13 (11): 2468–2470. doi:10.1016/j.jcmg.2020.07.004.

139 Peng, Q.-Y., Wang, X.-T., Zhang, L.-N., and Chinese Critical Care Ultrasound Study Group (CCUSG) (2020). Findings of lung ultrasonography of novel corona virus pneumonia during the 2019-2020 epidemic. *Intensive Care Med.* 46 (5): 849–850. doi:10.1007/s00134-020-05996-6.

140 Buonsenso, D., Pata, D., and Chiaretti, A. (2020). COVID-19 outbreak: less stethoscope, more ultrasound. *Lancet Respir Med.* 8: e27. doi:10.1016/S2213-2600(20)30120-X.

141 Lu, W., Zhang, S., Chen, B. et al. (2020). A clinical study of noninvasive assessment of lung lesions in patients with coronavirus disease-19 (COVID-19) by bedside ultrasound. *Ultraschall Med.* 41 (3): 300–307. doi:10.1055/a-1154-8795.

142 Zhang, Y., Xue, H., Wang, M. et al. (2021). Lung ultrasound findings in patients with coronavirus disease (COVID-19). *AJR Am J Roentgenol.* 216 (1): 80–84. doi:10.2214/AJR.20.23513.

143 Moreno, C.C., Kraft, C.S., Vanairsdale, S. et al. (2015). Performance of bedside diagnostic ultrasound in an Ebola isolation unit: the Emory University Hospital experience. *AJR Am J Roentgenol.* 204 (6): 1157–1159. doi:10.2214/AJR.15.14344.

144 Gargani, L. (2019). Ultrasound of the lungs: more than a room with a view. *Heart Fail Clin.* 15: 297–303. doi:10.1016/j.hfc.2018.12.010.

145 Bugalho, A., Ferreira, D., Dias, S.S. et al. (2014). The diagnostic value of transthoracic ultrasonographic features in predicting malignancy in undiagnosed pleural effusions: a prospective observational study. *Respiration.* 87 (4): 270–278. doi:10.1159/000357266.

146 Tsai, N.W., Ngai, C.W., Mok, K.L., and Tsung, J.W. (2014). Lung ultrasound imaging in avian influenza A (H7N9) respiratory failure. *Crit Ultrasound J.* 6 (1): 6. doi:10.1186/2036-7902-6-6.

147 Tsung, J.W., Kessler, D.O., and Shah, V.P. (2012). Prospective application of clinician-performed lung ultrasonography during the 2009 H1N1 influenza A pandemic: distinguishing viral from bacterial pneumonia. *Crit Ultrasound J.* 4 (1): 16. doi:10.1186/2036-7902-4-16.

148 Qin, C., Liu, F., Yen, T., and Lan, X. (2020). 18F-FDG PET/CT findings of COVID-19: a series of four highly suspected cases. *Eur J Nucl Med Mol Imaging* 47 (5): 1281–1286. doi:10.1007/s00259-020-04734-w.

149 Erdoğan, Y., Özyürek, B.A., Özmen, Ö. et al. (2015). The evaluation of FDG PET/CT scan findings in patients with organizing pneumonia mimicking lung cancer. *Mol Imaging Radionucl Ther.* 24 (2): 60–65. doi:10.4274/mirt.03016.

150 Alavi, A., Werner, T.J., and Gholamrezanezhad, A. (2021). The critical role of FDG-PET/CT imaging in assessing systemic manifestations of COVID-19 infection. *Eur J Nucl Med Mol Imaging* 48 (4): 956–962. doi:10.1007/s00259-020-05148-4.

151 Rafiee, F., Keshavarz, P., Katal, S. et al. (2021). Coronavirus disease 2019 (COVID-19) in molecular imaging: a systematic review of incidental detection of SARS-CoV-2 pneumonia on PET studies. *Semin Nucl Med.* 51 (2): 178–191. doi:10.1053/j.semnuclmed.2020.10.002.

152 Dadgar, H., Norouzbeigi, N., Gholamrezanezhad, A., and Assadi, M. (2021). Incidental detections suggestive of COVID-19 in asymptomatic patients undergoing 68Ga-DOTATATE and 68Ga-PSMA-11 PET-CT scan for oncological indications. *Nuklearmedizin* 60 (2): 106–108. doi:10.1055/a-1311-2856.

153 Torkian, P., Rajebi, H., Zamani, T. et al. (2021). Magnetic resonance imaging features of coronavirus disease 2019 (COVID-19) pneumonia: the first preliminary case series. *Clin Imaging* 69: 261–265. doi:10.1016/j.clinimag.2020.09.002.

154 Ates, O.F., Taydas, O., and Dheir, H. (2020). Thorax magnetic resonance imaging findings in patients with coronavirus disease (COVID-19). *Acad Radiol.* 27 (10): 1373–1378. doi:10.1016/j.acra.2020.08.009.

155 Vasilev, Y.A., Sergunova, K.A., Bazhin, A.V. et al. (2020). Chest MRI of patients with COVID-19. *Magn Reson Imaging.* 2021 (79): 13–19. doi:10.1016/j.mri.2021.03.005.

156 Darçot, E., Delacoste, J., Dunet, V. et al. (2020). Lung MRI assessment with high-frequency noninvasive ventilation at 3 T. *Magn Reson Imaging* 74: 64–73. doi:10.1016/j.mri.2020.09.006.

157 Veldhoen, S., Heidenreich, J.F., Metz, C. et al. (2021). Three-dimensional ultrashort echotime magnetic resonance imaging for combined morphologic and ventilation imaging in pediatric patients with pulmonary disease. *J Thorac Imaging* 36 (1): 43–51. doi:10.1097/RTI.0000000000000537.

158 American College of Radiology (2021). ACR Guidance on COVID-19 and MR Use. ACR. https://www.acr.org/Clinical-Resources/Radiology-Safety/MR-Safety/COVID-19-and-MR-Use.

159 Prokop, M., van Everdingen, W., van Rees Vellinga, T. et al. (2020). CO-RADS: a categorical CT assessment scheme for patients suspected of having COVID-19-definition and evaluation. *Radiology* 296 (2): E97–E104. doi:10.1148/radiol.2020201473.

160 Salehi, S., Abedi, A., Balakrishnan, S., and Gholamrezanezhad, A. (2020). Coronavirus disease 2019 (COVID-19) imaging reporting and data system (COVID-RADS) and common lexicon: a proposal based on the imaging data of 37 studies. *Eur Radiol.* 30 (9): 4930–4942. doi:10.1007/s00330-020-06863-0.

161 Sushentsev, N., Bura, V., Kotnik, M. et al. (2020). A head-to-head comparison of the intra- and interobserver agreement of COVID-RADS and CO-RADS grading systems in a population with high estimated prevalence of COVID-19. *BJR Open* 2 (1): 20200053. doi:10.1259/bjro.20200053.

5

COVID-19: Pathology Perspective

Elham Hatami, Hana Russo, and Grace Y. Lin

Department of Pathology, University of California San Diego Medical Center, San Diego, CA, USA

Abbreviations

ACE-2	angiotensin-converting enzyme 2
ARDS	acute respiratory distress syndrome
EM	electron microscopy
IHC	immunohistochemistry
SARS-CoV-2	severe acute respiratory syndrome coronavirus 2

The outbreak caused by the novel coronavirus, severe acute respiratory syndrome coronavirus 2 (SARS-CoV-2), was first reported in Wuhan, China [1–3]. There are extensive data on the epidemiology and virology of SARS-CoV-2. Although more than 2.8 million people worldwide have died of coronavirus disease 2019 (COVID-19), limited studies reporting the histopathologic findings of COVID-19 have been published [4]. To date, the available histologic data are mostly collected from postmortem and limited antemortem specimens. These reported histopathologic findings represent moderate to severe forms of the disease. No histopathologic findings for mild forms of and only limited histopathologic findings of so-called long-haul COVID-19 have been reported. This chapter reviews histopathologic findings from available studies.

Gross and Histopathologic Findings in the Respiratory System

Acute respiratory distress syndrome (ARDS) is the leading cause of death in patients with COVID-19 infection [5]. Zhong et al. [6] performed a recent meta-analysis of 40 studies on the clinical characteristics of severe or critically ill patients with COVID-19, which revealed that 60.8% of these patients presented with ARDS.

Macroscopically, patients with COVID-19 demonstrated heavy lungs with patchy to diffuse areas of consolidation [7–11]. In some cases, the lungs were edematous or had pleural effusions [8, 9]. Pulmonary thromboemboli have also been identified [7–13].

Microscopic pulmonary findings in patients with COVID-19 are currently based on postmortem lung tissue. The spectrum of pulmonary microscopic findings encompasses the different stages of diffuse alveolar damage (DAD), microvascular injury, including thrombosis and vasculitis, and vascular congestion along with capillary proliferation.

The histopathologic correlate of ARDS is DAD, which has commonly been shown in patients with COVID-19. DAD is characterized by three phases: (i) exudative (acute) phase, (ii) proliferative (organizing) phase, and

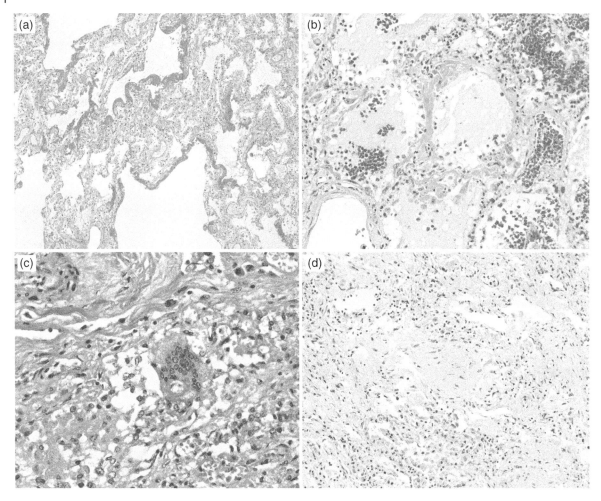

Figure 5.1 Patients with COVID-19 display microscopic features of diffuse alveolar damage (DAD). (a) Exudative phase of DAD with prominent hyaline membranes (hematoxylin and eosin [H&E] stain; original magnification, 100×). (b) Exudative phase of DAD with hyaline membrane deposition, intra-alveolar edema and hemorrhage, and reactive pneumocyte hyperplasia (H&E stain; original magnification, 200×). (c) Multinucleated giant cell (H&E stain; original magnification, 400×). (d) Organizing DAD (H&E stain; original magnification, 200×).

(iii) fibrotic (chronic) phase. A hallmark of the exudative phase that has been identified in patients with COVID-19 is hyaline membrane formation along alveolar air spaces (Figure 5.1a) [7–11, 14–17]. Additional characteristics of the exudative phase that have been seen include capillary congestion and reactive type II pneumocyte hyperplasia, which occurs at the end of the exudative phase and continues into the proliferative phase of DAD (Figure 5.1b) [8–11, 15, 17–19]. Reactive type II pneumocytes demonstrate marked atypia with enlarged nuclei and prominent nucleoli. Multinucleated giant cells also have been identified (Figure 5.1c) [8–11, 15, 17]. Rarely, viral cytopathic inclusions have been reported [9, 12, 18]. Some patients progress to the proliferative (organizing) phase of DAD, which involves

fibroblastic and myofibroblastic proliferation within the interstitium and alveolar air spaces (Figure 5.1d) [8–12, 19]. The final fibrotic phase of DAD is characterized by dense interstitial fibrosis and squamous metaplasia of bronchiolar epithelium. Patients with COVID-19 have demonstrated alveolar septal fibrosis [8, 11, 15] and squamous metaplasia [12, 18].

Evidence of pulmonary microvascular injury in patients with COVID-19 has been described. For example, fibrin microthrombi have been identified within capillaries, arterioles and venules, and small muscular arteries (Figure 5.2a) [12, 20, 21]. Vasculitis also has been identified, which includes lymphocytic and/or neutrophilic vasculitis that is either nonnecrotizing (Figure 5.2b) or with fibrinoid necrosis (Figure 5.2c) [10, 14–17].

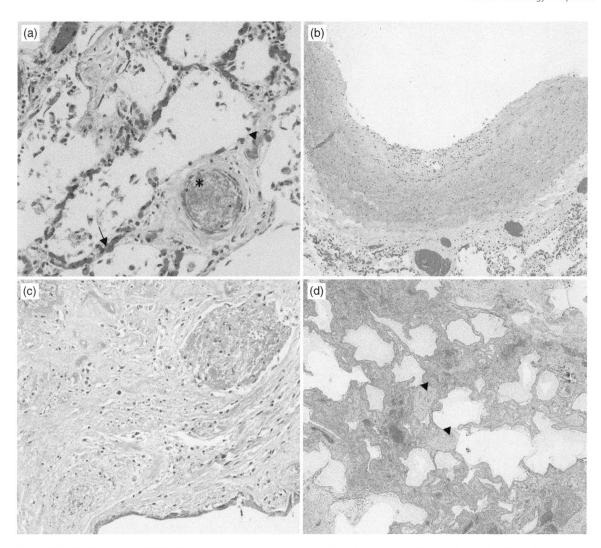

Figure 5.2 Patients with COVID-19 demonstrate pulmonary microthrombi and vasculitis. (a) Fibrin microthrombi in arteriole, venule, and capillary (arteriole: asterisk, venule: arrowheads, capillary: arrow; hematoxylin and eosin [H&E] stain; original magnification, 200×). (b) Larger artery with focal intimal lymphocytic inflammatory infiltrate (H&E stain; original magnification, 40×). (c) Vasculitis with fibrinoid necrosis (H&E stain; original magnification, 200×). (d) Pulmonary infarction with corresponding vessels demonstrating microthrombi (arrowheads; H&E stain; original magnification, 40×).

Specifically, Magro et al. [14] has reported thrombotic microvascular injury that is characterized by neutrophilic infiltrate with fibrinoid necrosis that is complement dependent. Rarely, patients with COVID-19 progress to pulmonary infarction in the setting of thromboembolism, thrombosis, or vasculitis (Figure 5.2d) [11, 17]. Ultrastructural studies have demonstrated evidence of pulmonary microvascular injury, including deformed capillary architecture and endothelial cell injury [12, 20].

A subset of patients with COVID-19 without microscopic DAD have demonstrated evidence of vascular congestion and hemangiomatosis-like change, along with microthrombi [21]. Vascular congestion and

hemangiomatosis-like change are characterized by a proliferation of congested capillaries along the alveolar septal wall [21].

Patients with COVID-19 may also present with superimposed acute pneumonia (Figure 5.3a) [7–11, 14]. Their microscopic presentation ranges from patchy neutrophilic alveolar infiltrate to bronchopneumonia. Lansbury et al. [22] performed a systematic review and meta-analysis on patients with COVID-19 with coinfection to show that 7% of hospitalized patients with COVID-19 had a bacterial coinfection. It is unclear whether acute pneumonia is a result of SARS-CoV-2-induced lung damage versus

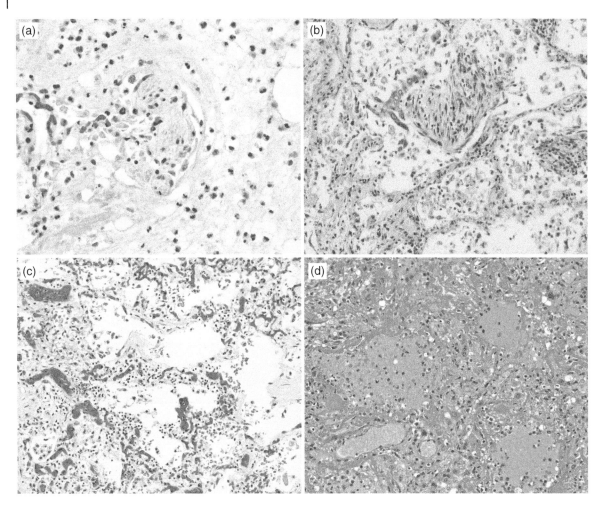

Figure 5.3 Additional pulmonary microscopic findings in patients with COVID-19. (a) Acute and organizing pneumonia (hematoxylin and eosin [H&E] stain; original magnification, 400×). (b) Organizing pneumonia, lymphocytic interstitial inflammation, and reactive pneumocyte hyperplasia (H&E stain; original magnification, 200×). (c) Lymphocytic interstitial infiltrate and capillary congestion (H&E stain; original magnification, 200×). (d) Exudative phase of DAD with intra-alveolar hemorrhage and reactive pneumocyte hyperplasia (H&E stain; original magnification, 200×).

secondary to mechanical ventilator–associated pneumonia. Organizing pneumonia also has been identified (Figure 5.3b) [12, 19].

Additional microscopic findings include acute and chronic tracheobronchitis [10, 12] and interstitial lymphocytic infiltration, involving both perivascular areas and alveolar septal walls (Figure 5.3c) [7–10, 15–17, 23]. Intra-alveolar edema [7, 8, 17] and hemorrhage (Figure 5.3d) [8–11, 14, 15], intra-alveolar accumulation of macrophages and lymphocytes [18], and megakaryocytes [9, 24] also have been identified.

SARS-CoV-2 has been detected using electron microscopy (EM), immunohistochemistry (IHC), and RNA in situ hybridization studies [12, 18]. IHC and RNA in situ hybridization studies have been performed to detect the viral spike protein and spike RNA, respectively, in tracheal epithelium and type II pneumocytes [12]. Ultrastructural examination has demonstrated viral particles located within type II pneumocytes and bronchial epithelial cells [12, 18]. Viral particles also have been identified within pulmonary endothelial cells [12, 20].

Gross and Histopathologic Findings in the Cardiovascular System

Acute cardiac injury, which is marked by elevated high-sensitivity troponin levels, is a common manifestation in severely ill patients with COVID-19 and associated with a higher mortality [25]. Zhong et al. [6] also indicated that 37.1% of severe or critically ill patients demonstrate acute cardiac injury.

On gross evaluation, patients with COVID-19 commonly demonstrated underlying cardiovascular disease. This included cardiomegaly [7–11, 17], varying degrees of coronary artery disease [7, 8, 10, 11] and systemic atherosclerosis [10, 11], and prior myocardial infarctions [11]. Right ventricular dilatation also has been shown [17, 26].

Microscopic cardiovascular findings in patients with COVID-19 are currently based on a few case reports of endomyocardial biopsy findings but predominantly from autopsy series [7–11, 15–17, 26–30]. Patients have demonstrated chronic inflammation within different regions of the heart. For example, a rare but notable finding is lymphocytic myocarditis (Figure 5.4a) [8, 11, 17, 27–29, 31]. In some cases, lymphocytic myocarditis included myocyte damage (Figure 5.4b) [8, 27, 30]. Increased interstitial macrophage accumulation also has been shown [27, 29]. Lymphocytic myocarditis could be directly attributed to SARS-CoV-2 viral infection; however, it could also be secondary to a postviral autoimmune response. Ultrastructural studies have revealed viral particles within the interstitial cells of the myocardium [29] and within cardiac endothelial cells [26]. Within the epicardium, a predominantly lymphocytic infiltrate has been reported (Figure 5.4c) [27, 30, 31], and Tavazzi et al. [29] have shown endocardial inflammation. Chronic inflammation within atherosclerotic coronary arteries also has been identified (Figure 5.4d).

Myocyte injury in the absence of myocarditis has been reported. Fox et al. [26] demonstrated scattered individual myocyte necrosis without associated lymphocytic infiltrate. In addition, Basso et al. [27] showed acute myocyte injury characterized by coagulative necrosis primarily along the subendocardium that was likely attributed to right ventricular strain/overload.

Additional microscopic cardiac findings consist of small vessel fibrin microthrombi [27, 28] and underlying background microscopic disease, including cardiomyocyte hypertrophy [8, 10, 17], cardiac amyloidosis [8, 10, 28, 31], and old myocardial infarction [31].

Histopathologic Findings in Kidney

In patients with COVID-19, clinical manifestations of acute kidney injury with new-onset proteinuria have been reported from 0.9% to 29% of cases; however, histopathologic data of the kidneys are still scarce [15]. Histologic evaluation of the kidney in antemortem and postmortem specimens reveals diverse kidney pathology in SARS-CoV-2-infected patients [8, 32–39]. Acute tubular injury is the most common finding and likely multifactorial (Figure 5.1a) [32–35, 37, 39]. Features of acute tubular injury that have been identified include luminal ectasia, irregular luminal contours, loss of brush border, epithelial necrosis, vacuolization, nuclear enlargement, and prominent nucleoli [32–35, 37, 39], in addition to occasional cellular swelling and edematous expansion of the interstitial spaces in distal collecting tubules and collecting ducts [32]. However, interpretation of histopathologic features of renal disease in autopsies frequently is limited by autolysis [33].

Another common finding in autopsy kidneys is arteriosclerosis and glomerulosclerosis [32, 33]. Due to the high incidence of underlying hypertension, these findings are likely related to hypertensive arterionephrosclerosis. In addition, pigmented casts, along with high serum levels of creatine phosphokinase in both postmortem and antemortem specimens, have been identified; these findings suggest rhabdomyolysis [32–34].

Limited segmental fibrin thrombus in glomerular capillary loops and/or vascular fibrin thrombi (Figure 5.5c and d) are less common histologic findings that in some cases are associated with severe injury of the endothelium [32, 33].

Occasional findings include podocyte vacuolation, focal segmental glomerulosclerosis, and shrinkage of capillary loops with accumulation of plasma in Bowman's space (ischemic changes) (Figure 5.5b) [32]. Collapsing focal segmental glomerulosclerosis is a rare finding that raises the possibility that individuals of African descent with high-risk APOL1 genotype could

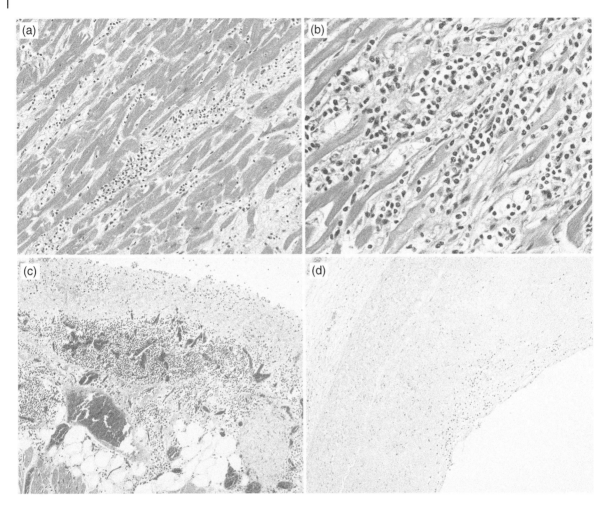

Figure 5.4 Microscopic cardiovascular findings in patients with COVID-19. (a) Lymphocytic myocarditis in the left ventricle (hematoxylin and eosin [H&E] stain; original magnification, 200×). (b) Lymphocytic myocarditis with myocardial damage in the left ventricle (H&E stain; original magnification, 400×). (c) Epicardial surface of the left ventricle with chronic inflammation (H&E stain; original magnification, 100×). (d) Right coronary artery with chronic inflammation and atherosclerosis (H&E stain; original magnification, 100×).

be at increased risk for kidney disease in the setting of COVID-19 [33, 38].

An EM study identified vacuoles in the podocyte cytoplasm, containing numerous spherical particles that may correspond to viral inclusion bodies reported with SARS-CoV-2, although these findings do not provide definite proof of the presence of SARS-CoV-2 in podocytes (32). Also, EM demonstrated spherical virus-like particles with distinctive spikes in proximal tubular epithelium and rarely in endothelium [8, 32]. Overall, the ultrastructural identity of viral particles remains controversial [33]. Immunohistochemical staining (of

SARS-CoV-2 nucleocapsid protein) and reverse transcriptase-polymerase chain reaction of kidney tissues mostly fail to detect SARS-CoV-2 [34, 37]; however, positive IHC results were seen in some studies [8].

In addition, some studies have found that the pathologic findings of acute tubular injury may not fully correlate with clinical findings (in a similar manner with sepsis-associated kidney injury), because for most of the cases, the degree of clinical acute kidney injury is more severe than histologic manifestations [33, 35]. Although several ultrastructural findings have suggested virus infection has been found,

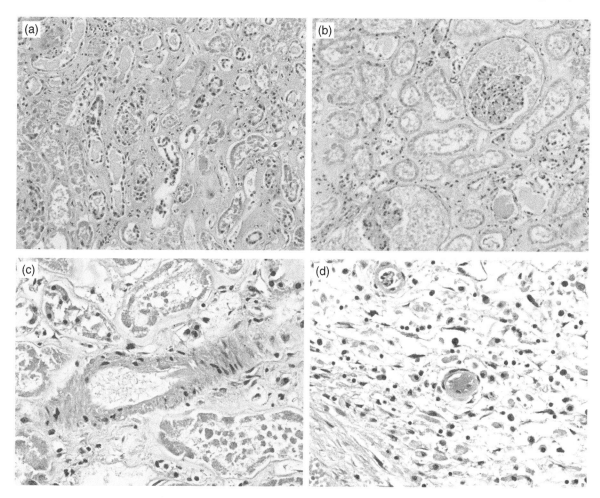

Figure 5.5 Patients with COVID-19 display a spectrum of renal pathologic findings. (a) Acute tubular necrosis (hematoxylin and eosin [H&E] stain; original magnification, 200×). (b) Accumulation of leaked plasma in Bowman's space (H&E stain; original magnification, 200×). (c) Fibrin thrombus in the lumen of an arteriole (H&E stain; original magnification, 400×). (d) Fibrin thrombus in the lumen of a venule (H&E stain; original magnification, 400×).

such as spherical virus particles, the overall findings highlight the potential other secondary insults, especially ischemia, hypoxia, sepsis-associated factors, and secondary infection in addition to the direct virulence of SARS-CoV-2 [32, 33, 38].

Histopathologic Findings in the Gastrointestinal Tract and Liver

Common gastrointestinal manifestations in patients with COVID-19 include diarrhea, abdominal pain, and nausea and vomiting [40–42]. In addition to endothelium of vessels, angiotensin-converting enzyme 2 (ACE-2) has been detected in enterocytes of the small intestine, as well as smooth muscle cells of muscularis mucosa and propria [43]. The pathologic findings in the gastrointestinal tract essentially show normal biopsies, although viral polymerase chain reaction was positive [44]. However, the histologic data remain limited because most studies are postmortem, and autolysis quickly and severely damages the gastrointestinal tract.

Overall, liver injury is mild, manifesting in liver function test abnormalities with an incidence rate of 16–53% and is mostly seen in severely ill patients

[41, 42, 45]. Although the liver sinusoids may be negative for ACE-2, the level of expression of ACE-2 on the cell surface of cholangiocytes is similar to type 2 pneumocytes; further, the expression of ACE-2 on cholangiocytes is higher than in hepatocytes [46]. Hence the liver could be a target for SARS-CoV-2 infection. The majority of histopathologic changes are reported in postmortem patients with moderate to severe illness [8, 15, 47]. The most common microscopic findings are sinusoidal dilatation in zone 3 (a common nonspecific autopsy finding), hepatic cell degeneration and patchy necrosis, and mild lymphocytic infiltration in centrilobular areas and portal triads (Figure 5.6a–c) [8, 47, 48]. Patchy hepatocellular necrosis in both periportal and centrilobular areas without significant inflammation raises the possibility of direct viral infection of

hepatocytes; however, further investigation is required [47]. Mild steatosis also has been reported (Figure 5.6d) [15, 47] but may be related to patients' underlying conditions, such as obesity or diabetes. The hepatic injury seen in patients with SARS-CoV-2 infection could be multifactorial, including hepatotoxic medications, underlying chronic liver disease, and hypoxic state caused by the impact of COVID-19 on the respiratory system [47].

Histopathologic Findings in Brain

Neurologic manifestations in patients with COVID-19 have frequently been observed; however, the extent of histopathologic investigation has

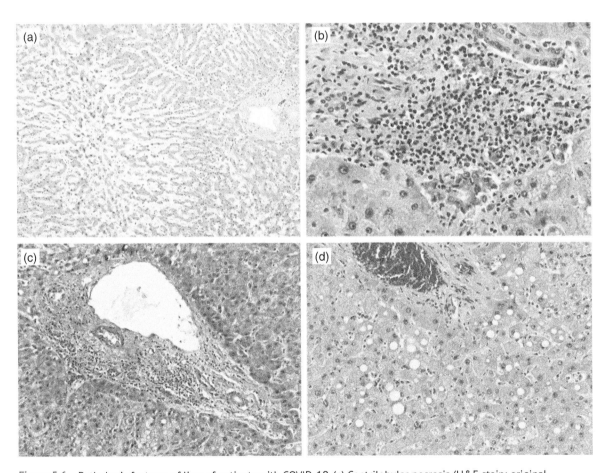

Figure 5.6 Pathologic features of liver of patients with COVID-19. (a) Centrilobular necrosis (H&E stain; original magnification, 100×). (b) Portal inflammation (H&E; original magnification, 400×). (c) Portal inflammation (H&E; original magnification, 200×). (d) Steatosis (H&E; original magnification, 200×).

remained limited. Common neurologic symptoms include headache and dizziness, as well as anosmia and ageusia [49]. Less common neurologic manifestations are encephalopathy, convulsions, stroke, and consciousness deterioration [49, 50]. Microscopically, one of the common findings is acute hypoxic changes in the cerebrum and cerebellum, manifesting as nuclear and cytoplasmatic condensation of neurons in addition to edema and neuronal degeneration [51, 52].

Another histologic finding that has been observed is an extensive inflammatory response in both gray and white matter with formation of nodules by massive activation of microglia, astrogliosis, and perivascular T cell infiltration [51]. The inflammatory reaction is mostly prominent in the medulla oblongata (including respiratory center) and olfactory bulbs; the latter may explain anosmia in many patients [51].

Histopathologic Findings in Skin

Like other viral infections, nonspecific dermatologic signs can be seen in patients with COVID-19, such as an erythematous rash, macular/maculopapular exanthems, urticaria, petechiae, painful purpuric papulovesicular rash, and livedo reticularis lesions [43, 53, 54]. Viral injury of the skin tissue may be caused by an interaction with ACE-2 on endothelial cells [46]; however, ACE-2 is also expressed in the stratum basale of the epidermis, smooth muscle cells around the hair follicle, and cells of sebaceous glands and eccrine glands [43]. Antemortem biopsy results include an inflammatory response causing vasculitis, including dense perivascular lymphocytic and plasmocytic infiltration with extravasation of red blood cells and intraluminal thrombi [53, 55]. Additional cutaneous findings are parakeratosis, acanthosis, necrotic keratinocytes, and acantholytic clefts [53].

References

1 Wong, H.Y.F., HYS, L., Fong, A.H.-T. et al. (2020). Frequency and distribution of chest radiographic findings in patients positive for COVID-19. *Radiology* 296 (2): E72–E78.

2 Phelan, A.L., Katz, R., and Gostin, L.O. (2020). The novel coronavirus originating in Wuhan, China: challenges for Global Health governance. *JAMA* 323 (8): 709–710.

3 Li, Q. et al. (2020). Early transmission dynamics in Wuhan, China, of novel coronavirus-infected pneumonia. *N. Engl. J. Med.* 382 (13): 1199–1207.

4 Johns Hopkins University and Medicine (2021). Coronavirus resource center global map. https://coronavirus.jhu.edu/map.html (accessed April 5, 2021).

5 Ruan, Q. et al. (2020). Clinical predictors of mortality due to COVID-19 based on an analysis of data of 150 patients from Wuhan, China. *Intensive Care Med.* 46 (5): 846–848.

6 Zhong, Z. et al. (2021). Clinical characteristics of 2,459 severe or critically ill COVID-19 patients: a meta-analysis. *Medicine (Baltimore)* 100 (5): e23781.

7 Barton, L.M. et al. (2020). COVID-19 autopsies, Oklahoma, USA. *Am. J. Clin. Pathol.* 153 (6): 725–733.

8 Bradley, B.T. et al. (2020). Histopathology and ultrastructural findings of fatal COVID-19 infections in Washington state: a case series. *Lancet* 396 (10247): 320–332.

9 Fox, S.E. et al. (2020). Pulmonary and cardiac pathology in African American patients with COVID-19: an autopsy series from New Orleans. *Lancet Respir. Med.* 8 (7): 681–686.

10 Menter, T. et al. (2020). Postmortem examination of COVID-19 patients reveals diffuse alveolar damage with severe capillary congestion and variegated findings in lungs and other organs suggesting vascular dysfunction. *Histopathology* 77 (2): 198–209.

11 Wichmann, D. et al. (2020). Autopsy findings and venous thromboembolism in patients with COVID-19: a prospective cohort study. *Ann. Intern. Med.* 173 (4): 268–277.

12 Borczuk, A.C. et al. (2020). COVID-19 pulmonary pathology: a multi-institutional autopsy cohort from Italy and New York City. *Mod. Pathol.* 33 (11): 2156–2168.

13 Edler, C. et al. (2020). Dying with SARS-CoV-2 infection-an autopsy study of the first

consecutive 80 cases in Hamburg, Germany. *Int. J. Legal Med.* 134 (4): 1275–1284.

14 Magro, C. et al. (2020). Complement associated microvascular injury and thrombosis in the pathogenesis of severe COVID-19 infection: a report of five cases. *Transl. Res.* 220: 1–13.

15 Tian, S. et al. (2020). Pathological study of the 2019 novel coronavirus disease (COVID-19) through postmortem core biopsies. *Mod. Pathol.* 33 (6): 1007–1014.

16 Varga, Z. et al. (2020). Endothelial cell infection and endotheliitis in COVID-19. *Lancet* 395 (10234): 1417–1418.

17 Yan, L. et al. (2020). COVID-19 in a Hispanic woman. *Arch. Pathol. Lab. Med.* 144 (9): 1041–1047.

18 Deshmukh, V. et al. (2021). Histopathological observations in COVID-19: a systematic review. *J. Clin. Pathol.* 74 (2): 76–83.

19 Zhang, H. et al. (2020). Histopathologic changes and SARS-CoV-2 immunostaining in the lung of a patient with COVID-19. *Ann. Intern. Med.* 172 (9): 629–632.

20 Ackermann, M. et al. (2020). Pulmonary vascular endothelialitis, thrombosis, and angiogenesis in Covid-19. *N. Engl. J. Med.* 383 (2): 120–128.

21 De Michele, S. et al. (2020). Forty postmortem examinations in COVID-19 patients. *Am. J. Clin. Pathol.* 154 (6): 748–760.

22 Lansbury, L. et al. (2020). Co-infections in people with COVID-19: a systematic review and meta-analysis. *J. Infect.* 81 (2): 266–275.

23 Xu, Z. et al. (2020). Pathological findings of COVID-19 associated with acute respiratory distress syndrome. *Lancet Respir. Med.* 8 (4): 420–422.

24 Roncati, L. et al. (2020). A proof of evidence supporting abnormal immunothrombosis in severe COVID-19: naked megakaryocyte nuclei increase in the bone marrow and lungs of critically ill patients. *Platelets* 31 (8): 1085–1089.

25 Madjid, M. et al. (2020). Potential effects of coronaviruses on the cardiovascular system: a review. *JAMA Cardiol.* 5 (7): 831–840.

26 Fox, S.E. et al. (2020). Unexpected features of cardiac pathology in COVID-19 infection. *Circulation* 142 (11): 1123–1125.

27 Basso, C. et al. (2020). Pathological features of COVID-19-associated myocardial injury: a multicentre cardiovascular pathology study. *Eur. Heart J.* 41 (39): 3827–3835.

28 Bois, M.C. et al. (2021). COVID-19-associated nonocclusive fibrin microthrombi in the heart. *Circulation* 143 (3): 230–243.

29 Tavazzi, G. et al. (2020). Myocardial localization of coronavirus in COVID-19 cardiogenic shock. *Eur. J. Heart Fail.* 22 (5): 911–915.

30 Falasca, L. et al. (2020). Postmortem findings in Italian patients with COVID-19: a descriptive full autopsy study of cases with and without comorbidities. *J. Infect. Dis.* 222 (11): 1807–1815.

31 Halushka, M.K. and Vander Heide, R.S. (2021). Myocarditis is rare in COVID-19 autopsies: cardiovascular findings across 277 postmortem examinations. *Cardiovasc. Pathol.* 50: 107300.

32 Su, H. et al. (2020). Renal histopathological analysis of 26 postmortem findings of patients with COVID-19 in China. *Kidney Int.* 98 (1): 219–227.

33 Santoriello, D. et al. (2020). Postmortem kidney pathology findings in patients with COVID-19. *J. Am. Soc. Nephrol.* 31 (9): 2158–2167.

34 Sharma, P. et al. (2020). COVID-19-associated kidney injury: a case series of kidney biopsy findings. *J. Am. Soc. Nephrol.* 31 (9): 1948–1958.

35 Golmai, P. et al. (2020). Histopathologic and ultrastructural findings in postmortem kidney biopsy material in 12 patients with AKI and COVID-19. *J. Am. Soc. Nephrol.* 31 (9): 1944–1947.

36 Yao, X.H. et al. (2020). Pathological evidence for residual SARS-CoV-2 in pulmonary tissues of a ready-for-discharge patient. *Cell Res.* 30 (6): 541–543.

37 Xia, P. et al. (2020). Clinicopathological features and outcomes of acute kidney injury in critically ill COVID-19 with prolonged disease course: a retrospective cohort. *J. Am. Soc. Nephrol.* 31 (9): 2205–2221.

38 Larsen, C.P. et al. (2020). Collapsing Glomerulopathy in a patient with COVID-19. *Kidney Int. Rep.* 5 (6): 935–939.

39 Kudose, S. et al. (2020). Kidney biopsy findings in patients with COVID-19. *J. Am. Soc. Nephrol.* 31 (9): 1959–1968.

40 Huang, C. et al. (2020). Clinical features of patients infected with 2019 novel coronavirus in Wuhan, China. *Lancet* 395 (10223): 497–506.

41 Chen, N. et al. (2020). Epidemiological and clinical characteristics of 99 cases of 2019 novel coronavirus pneumonia in Wuhan, China: a descriptive study. *Lancet* 395 (10223): 507–513.

42 Guan, W.J. et al. (2020). Clinical characteristics of coronavirus disease 2019 in China. *N. Engl. J. Med.* 382 (18): 1708–1720.

43 Sachdeva, M. et al. (2020). Cutaneous manifestations of COVID-19: report of three cases and a review of literature. *J. Dermatol. Sci.* 98 (2): 75–81.

44 Gaebler, C. et al. (2021). Evolution of antibody immunity to SARS-CoV-2. *Nature* 591 (7851): 639–644.

45 Shi, H. et al. (2020). Radiological findings from 81 patients with COVID-19 pneumonia in Wuhan, China: a descriptive study. *Lancet Infect. Dis.* 20 (4): 425–434.

46 Hamming, I. et al. (2004). Tissue distribution of ACE2 protein, the functional receptor for SARS coronavirus. A first step in understanding SARS pathogenesis. *J. Pathol.* 203 (2): 631–637.

47 Li, Y. and Xiao, S.Y. (2020). Hepatic involvement in COVID-19 patients: pathology, pathogenesis, and clinical implications. *J. Med. Virol.* 92 (9): 1491–1494.

48 Yao, X.H. et al. (2020). A pathological report of three COVID-19 cases by minimal invasive autopsies. *Zhonghua Bing Li Xue Za Zhi* 49 (5): 411–417.

49 Mao, L. et al. (2020). Neurologic manifestations of hospitalized patients with coronavirus disease 2019 in Wuhan, China. *JAMA Neurol.* 77 (6): 683–690.

50 Zubair, A.S. et al. (2020). Neuropathogenesis and neurologic manifestations of the coronaviruses in the age of coronavirus disease 2019: a review. *JAMA Neurol.* 77 (8): 1018–1027.

51 Schurink, B. et al. (2020). Viral presence and immunopathology in patients with lethal COVID-19: a prospective autopsy cohort study. *Lancet Microbe* 1 (7): e290–e299.

52 Solomon, I.H. et al. (2020). Neuropathological features of Covid-19. *N. Engl. J. Med.* 383 (10): 989–992.

53 Gianotti, R., Zerbi, P., and Dodiuk-Gad, R.P. (2020). Clinical and histopathological study of skin dermatoses in patients affected by COVID-19 infection in the northern part of Italy. *J. Dermatol. Sci.* 98 (2): 141–143.

54 Recalcati, S. (2020). Cutaneous manifestations in COVID-19: a first perspective. *J. Eur. Acad. Dermatol. Venereol.* 34 (5): e212–e213.

55 Kolivras, A. et al. (2020). Coronavirus (COVID-19) infection-induced chilblains: a case report with histopathologic findings. *JAAD Case Rep.* 6 (6): 89–492.

6

COVID-19: Immunology

Yasaswi V. Vengalasetti[1], Niyousha Naderi[2], Christian Vega[2], Akhilesh Kumar[3], and Andrew T. Catanzaro[4]

[1] Department of Epidemiology and Population Health, Stanford University School of Medicine, Stanford, CA, USA
[2] Keck School of Medicine, University of Southern California, Los Angeles, CA, USA
[3] Ochsner Clinical School, University of Queensland, New Orleans, LA, USA
[4] Adventist Healthcare, Gaithersburg, MD, USA

Abbreviations

ACE2	angiotensin-converting enzyme 2
ARDS	acute respiratory distress syndrome
CCL	CC chemokine ligand
CXCL10	chemokine (C-X-C motif) ligand 10
GM-CSF	granulocyte-macrophage colony-stimulating factor
HLA-DR	human leukocyte antigen D–related
IFN	interferon
IgG	immunoglobulin G
IL-1	interleukin-1
NK	natural killer
RBD	receptor-binding domain
S	spike
SARS-CoV-2	severe acute respiratory syndrome coronavirus 2
TNF-α	tumor necrosis factor-α

Although coronaviruses have infected humans in the past, mutations in several regions have increased viral infectivity, resulting in widespread human morbidity and mortality. Studies suggest the immune system plays a major role in controlling infection. In general, the immune response to pathogens (including viruses) can be innate or adaptive. The innate response is non-specific to the pathogen, composed of barriers such as enzymes, epithelial cells, and cytokines, including interferon (IFN) and interleukin-1 (IL-1). The adaptive immune system is critical to control most viral infections, including severe acute respiratory syndrome coronavirus 2 (SARS-CoV-2). The effector cells, including CD4$^+$ T cells, CD8$^+$ T cells, and B cells, mount a cellular and antibody response. This chapter will cover the adaptive immune response to this virus and outline some of the immune-based therapies to mitigate morbidity and mortality from SARS-CoV-2.

Anatomic Progression of COVID-19

At a molecular level, the engagement of angiotensin-converting enzyme 2 (ACE2) receptor with the viral spike (S) protein and the activity of the transmembrane protease serine subtype 2 allows SARS-CoV-2 to infect the host cell. Studies have demonstrated that these initial targets of the nasal epithelium are epithelial cells [1]. After that initial invasion, the upper respiratory tract epithelium, ciliated bronchial epithelial cells, and type 1 and 2 pneumocytes become heavily infected [2]. Once the nasal epithelium is infected, the innate immune response is nonspecifically activated. Natural killer (NK) cells, neutrophils, and monocytes express host defense programs, including IFNs, pathogen-associated molecular patterns, and damage-associated molecular patterns. The virus evades the innate response, begins to propagate, and then spreads to the respiratory tract, where it is faced with a more powerful adaptive immune response. Clinically, up to 80% of infected individuals experience mild illness limited to the upper airways most likely because of rapid immunologic control (see Table 6.1) [3–5].

Adaptive Immune Response in the Nasal Passages and the Lungs

Respiratory dendritic cells are the primary cell that functions to present viral antigens to the immune system. Dendritic cells inside tissue nodes deliver the antigen via major histocompatibility complex class I to naive T cells and cause activation of stimulatory signals. T cells, when activated, multiply rapidly and move to the infection site. Activated virus-specific CD4$^+$ T cells release IFN-γ and chemokines to attract more immune cells to the infection site. CD8$^+$ T cells interact with virally infected cells, through cytotoxic chemicals like perforins and granzyme B, to kill affected epithelial cells and improve defense function [6].

Postinfection with SARS-CoV-2, more than 90% of patients develop immunoglobulin G (IgG) and IgM antibodies against the virus antigens, including S protein, receptor-binding domain (RBD), and nucleocapsid (N protein) [7].

Studies from China evaluated the humoral immune response to patients with SARS-CoV-2 who were never exposed before to the novel coronavirus. Long et al. [8] report that in 285 individuals with coronavirus disease 2019 (COVID-19) who were studied, virus-specific IgG and IgM antibody titers increased within the first three weeks after symptom onset. IgG was detected in 100% of patients about 17–19 days after initial symptoms, and patients with severe disease had higher titers of IgG. In addition, IgM was reported in 94% of individuals by 20–22 days after symptoms [8].

A Wuhan study by Zhang et al. [9] identified 112 patients with COVID-19 symptoms who were assessed for serum antibodies: 52% tested positive for both IgM and IgG, while 41% tested positive for only IgG. IgM and IgG antibodies were produced approximately 7 and 10 days after the onset of symptoms, respectively, and IgG lasted longer than IgM [9].

Immune Response to Immunization

The immune response to viruses and immunization includes the development of antibodies and of a long-lived memory response. Both SARS-CoV-2 infection and vaccination immune responses in patients with COVID-19 were distinguished by a significant increase in the IFN response. In addition, evaluation of B and T cells showed that most of the clonal lymphocytes in patients with COVID-19 were effector cells, whereas clonal proliferation in vaccinated individuals was mostly restricted to circulating memory cells [10].

After vaccination, an immunologic response through activation of virus-specific CD4$^+$ (mostly T helper 1) cells, CD8$^+$ T cells, and production of cytokines, as well as a B cell response with the development of neutralizing antibodies were observed [11]. Long-term immunity to coronaviruses may be provided by B cells, CD4$^+$ T cells, and CD8$^+$ T cells [12].

Immune Correlates of Protection from Infection

Defining immunologic correlates of protection is an important part of vaccine development to extend vaccine utilization and identify potential protective mechanisms. Nonhuman primates have proved a viable model for clinical application in evaluating vaccine immunogenicity and efficacy against SARS-CoV-2. Corbett et al. [13], in their recent study on mRNA-1273 (Moderna) vaccine-induced immune responses in nonhuman primates, observed that lower serum antibody concentrations were required for protection in the lower respiratory tract than in the upper tract [13, 14]. Circulating S protein–specific antibodies are associated with limited SARS-CoV-2 airway replication, implicating antibodies as mechanistic correlates. These findings help to explain why vaccination efficacy is higher against severe lower respiratory tract disease than mild upper tract disease [13], and it may also help us predict the durability of developing pipeline therapeutics [15]. See Table 6.2 for COVID-19-relevant therapeutics.

Multiple vaccines were rapidly developed for use in the general population based on the clinical

Table 6.1 COVID-19 anatomical progression.

Anatomy	Nose	Throat	Lungs	Systemic
Stage	Early	Middle	Late	Critical
Symptoms	Rhinorrhea		Cough, dyspnea	
Immune response	Neutrophils, antibodies, IgG, IgM	CD4, CD8	CD4, CD8	CD4, CD8 cytokine storm: IL-6, TNF
Current treatments	Anti-SARS-CoV-2 monoclonal antibodies	Anti-SARS-CoV-2 monoclonal antibodies	Remdesivir, dexamethasone	Tocilizumab, JAK inhibitors

IgG, immunoglobulin G; IgM, immunoglobulin M; IL-6, interleukin-6; JAK, Janus kinase; SARS-CoV-2, severe acute respiratory syndrome coronavirus 2; TNF, tumor necrosis factor.

Sources: Bösmüller et al. [3], Chowdhury et al. [4], and Salian et al. [5].

Table 6.2   COVID-19 therapeutics.

Name	Class	Authorized/Approved for COVID-19 in United States	Basic effect	References
BNT16b2 (Pfizer-BioNTech) vaccine	mRNA vaccine	Approved	mRNA teaches cell to make copies of spike protein of coronavirus; 2 doses separated by 21 days	[56]
mRNA-1273 (Moderna) vaccine	mRNA vaccine	Approved	mRNA teaches cell to make copies of spike protein of coronavirus; 2 doses separated by 28 days	[57]
JNJ-78436735 (J&J Janssen) vaccine	Adenovirus vaccine	Approved	Uses disabled virus to deliver DNA that encodes a characteristic viral protein; 1 dose	[58, 59]
Bamlanivimab + etesevimab	Recombinant human monoclonal antibody	Authorized	Passive immunotherapy	[60]
Casirivimab + imdevimab	Recombinant human monoclonal antibody	Authorized	Passive immunotherapy	[61, 62]
Sotrovimab	Recombinant human monoclonal antibody	Authorized	Passive immunotherapy	[63]
Tocilizumab	IL-6 inhibitor	Authorized	Blocks signaling of IL-6 May interrupt cytokine storm	[52]
Baricitinib	Janus kinase inhibitor	Authorized	Prevents phosphorylation of the proteins involved in signal transduction	[64]
Acalabrutinib	BTK inhibitor	Unapproved	Covalently binds BTK blocking B cell proliferation, trafficking, chemotaxis, and adhesion May interrupt cytokine storm	[65, 66]
Rapamycin	mTOR inhibitor	Unapproved	Inhibits mTOR and protein synthesis and prevents activation of lymphocytes; also blocks expression of proinflammatory cytokines May interrupt cytokine storm	[67]
Cyclosporine	Calcineurin inhibitor	Unapproved	Inhibits calcineurin, an enzyme that activates the T cells in the immune system May have antiviral effect	[68–70]
Auranofin	Metal-based agent	Unapproved	Reduces expression of SARS-CoV-2-induced cytokines in human cells	[71–73]
Etanercept	TNF-α blocker	Unapproved	Suppresses TNF-α and autoinflammation	[70, 74, 75]
Remdesivir	Broad-spectrum antiviral	Approved	Nucleoside analogue	[76–79]
Dexamethasone	Corticosteroid	Approved	Anti-inflammatory for cellular immune system and suppresses expression of inflammatory mediators, including cytokines and chemokines	[78, 80]

BTK, Bruton's tyrosine kinase; IL-6, interleukin-6; mRNA, messenger RNA; mTOR, mammalian target of rapamycin; TNF-α, tumor necrosis factor-α.

endpoint of vaccine efficacy against hospitalization and death. However, recent studies of COVID-19 illness after infection indicate further refinement of the two-dose vaccine is necessary. Most breakthrough infections were mild, and they were not always associated with an absence of vaccine-induced immunity. Therefore, further study into the immune response, specifically in regard to the development of milder variants of disease and particularly the correlates of protection, is necessary [16, 17].

Higher anti-S IgG, anti-RBD IgG, and neutralizing antibody titers might be linked to a decreased chance of developing symptomatic disease and correlate with vaccine efficacy [18–20]. In patients with severe immunosuppression, such as hematologic malignancy, solid organ transplant, or treatment with immune checkpoint modulators, the elderly, or other similarly hampered immune systems demonstrate moderately impaired vaccine immune response [21]. In these patients with immunologic comorbidities, a third dose may be required to ensure clinical efficacy. Healthy adults also experience a waning of peak titers after two doses of the COVID vaccine [22]. These data suggest that the immunization series may require three or more doses to achieve long-lasting immunity even in healthy hosts.

In vaccination, functional results are determined by the quality and quantity of antibody responses. Antibodies with a strong affinity for a certain viral epitope can induce neutralization. So far according to the published clinical reports, COVID-19 immunization exhibited equivalent efficacy and safety in those with comorbidities and those without any underlying medical disorders. The most comorbidities that were studied are body mass index $\geq 30\,\mathrm{kg/m}^2$, hypertension, type 2 diabetes mellitus, and HIV infection [23]. In contrast, Thuluvath et al. [24] uncovered poor antibody responses in patients with chronic liver disease (CLD) and liver transplant (LT) after vaccination.

Given these disparate responses, it would be imperative for future vaccine efforts to develop an international standard as proposed by the World Health Organization [17] for these neutralizing antibodies.

Decline in Vaccine-Induced Immune Responses over Time

Tartof et al. [25] found that the overall and variant-specific effectiveness of BNT162b2 (Pfizer-BioNTech mRNA COVID-19 vaccine) against SARS-CoV-2 infection waned over a six-month study period in fully vaccinated adults. Researchers identified that effectiveness against non-delta variants within one month of being fully vaccinated was 97%, declining to as low as 67% after five months. For the delta variant, effectiveness at one month after full vaccination was 93%, but declined to 53% after five months. It is unclear if the decreased efficacy of coronavirus vaccines is due to viral escape or decreases in immune response. These data suggest that the decline in vaccine effectiveness against the SARS-CoV-2 delta variant is likely due to waning neutralizing antibodies over time rather than an inherent susceptibility to the delta variant. Naaber et al. [26] examined the dynamics of BNT162b2-induced antibody responses after six months, finding deterioration of the antibody and memory T cell responses at six months postvaccination. Anti-S and anti-RBD IgG levels declined to a median of 7% of their peak levels after six months, comparable with the anti-S and anti-RBD antibody levels in patients who had recovered from COVID-19. The neutralization potency of the vaccine-induced antibodies showed a similar decline at 12 weeks after the second dose, with significantly weaker ACE2–Spike interactions for all variant domains between anti-S/anti-RBD IgG antibodies. The findings of both studies indicate that the early effectiveness of vaccination with BNT162b2 may wane over a six-month time period, with diminished numbers and lowered neutralization potency of anti-S protein and anti-RBD IgG antibodies.

Immune Consequences of Virologic Dissemination

The variable clinical course of pneumonia after infection in patients with COVID-19 and abrupt deterioration of the clinical status about a week after the onset of symptoms suggests some individuals have a distinct pattern of cytokine response after viral dissemination. This is further supported by lymphopenia and elevated blood levels of C-reactive protein, erythrocyte sedimentation rate, and D-dimer in severe cases [27]. Unregulated inflammatory innate response and defective adaptive immunity may cause extensive local and systemic tissue injury.

In the lungs, inflammatory recruitment of immune cells in conjunction with a direct viral invasion leads to extensive tissue damage because of the enhanced protease and reactive oxygen species release. Desquamation of alveolar cells, hyaline membrane formation, development of pulmonary edema, and lung fibrosis are all signs of diffuse alveolar injury.

The innate immune system is the primary line of antiviral defense. Due to the shared sequence homology among coronaviruses and conserved immune pathways, many of the interactions between the innate immune system and COVID-19 are like other coronaviruses. These mechanisms are activated by interactions of RNA viruses with the pattern recognition receptors via cytosolic retinoic acid–inducible gene I-like receptors and extracellular and endosomal Toll-like receptors. Subsequently, cytokine release is triggered by secondary signaling cascades. Various cytokines such as proinflammatory tumor necrosis factor-α (TNF-α), IL-1, IL-6, and IL-18 are released, but type I/III IFNs are released as a part of the antiviral defense [27, 28].

Autoantibodies Against Type I IFN

Individuals deficient in certain IFNs may be more prone to severe infection [28–30]. In addition, the autoantibody system suppresses IFN activity and tips the scales in favor of the pathogen, resulting in the absence of appropriate innate immune response and severe illness.

About 10% of individuals who suffered from life-threatening COVID-19 pneumonia exhibited type I IFN-neutralizing autoantibodies in the blood [31]. The autoantibodies were not detected in patients with asymptomatic or mild SARS-CoV-2 infection. B cells produce neutralizing IgG autoantibodies against IFN-ω, IFN-α, and all its subtypes. In the laboratory, the autoantibodies impede the capacity of type I IFNs to prevent SARS-CoV-2 infection and impair the natural antiviral immune response [31].

Viral Evasion

Pattern recognition receptors are specialized units that identify viruses. These are located on the surface and inside of antigen-presenting cells such as macrophages and dendritic cells. Interactions between PRPs and pathogen-associated molecular patterns activate transcription and regulatory factors, which leads to the release of proinflammatory cytokines and type I IFN [32, 33].

IFN suppression is a common technique for viruses to sabotage the innate host response. It has been discovered that viral proteins affect different elements of IFN synthesis and signaling [34]. The coronavirus that causes SARS (SARS-CoV) has devised a way to evade the host's innate immune systems. Kopecky-Bromberg et al. [34] investigated IFN synthesis that was interrupted by viral gene products such as open reading frame 3b, open reading frame 6, and N protein. These three proteins all work as IFN inhibitors and decrease the IFN production by phosphorylation and inactivation of the IFN regulatory factor. Therefore, the virus's ability to entirely block the IFN response is increased by encoding several antagonist proteins contributing to its significant disease.

Neutralizing potency of humoral immunity has also been shown to correlate with infection and severity of COVID-19 [35]. Although all cases of COVID-19 result in increased development of IgG and IgA anti-RBD and anti-S proteins, those with severe illness, including patients who were intubated or died, had the highest levels of these antibodies. To understand the difference in humoral response, researchers used live virus neutralization assays to determine the potency of the RBD and S protein antibodies toward neutralization of SARs-CoV-2. This method of measuring the quality of antibodies rather than the quantities demonstrated that severely ill patients had high levels of anti-RBD IgG with poor neutralization potency. Following these results, researchers stratified patients by neutralization potency, finding that those in the high index group (high anti-RBD IgG neutralization potency) had a 100% 30-day survival, while a low index of diminished neutralization potency was associated with 87% 30-day survival. With severe disease, the increased quality of anti-RBD IgG with low neutralization potency may thereby be associated with increased mortality and can provide a clinical marker for worse outcomes.

Immune Dysregulation

The purpose of the immune system is to control infection, yet for patients with severe infection there is a pattern of multiorgan dysfunction most notably in the lungs. Clinically, patients develop dyspnea, develop infiltrates seen on CT scan, require supplemental oxygen, and their condition may progress to acute respiratory distress syndrome (ARDS) needing mechanical ventilation [36].

Patients with severe disease can have higher circulating levels of early-response proinflammatory cytokines (including IL-6, TNF-α, and chemokine (C-X-C motif) ligand 10 [CXCL10]) that are sustained several weeks into the course of infection. However, despite the increased activity of the innate response, the adaptive immune system fails to adequately resolve the inflammation in patients with severe disease. The prolonged activity of proinflammatory cytokines results in insufficient T cell and B cell activation [8, 37]. In patients with severe disease, both NK cells and CD8+ T cells had patterns of gene expression demonstrating decreased cytotoxic function in comparison with patients with mild disease [37]. Altered cytotoxic pathways and profound lymphopenia can increase the severity of COVID-19 symptoms and result in the development of ARDS.

Immune cell profiling of bronchoalveolar lavage samples from patients with mild and severe COVID-19 can also provide insight into the lung immune responses. Lung epithelial cells of infected patients showed significantly increased expression of ACE2 and transmembrane protease serine subtype 2 compared with healthy controls, resulting in host cell alterations in club and ciliated cells and activation of the IFN pathway and cytokine recruitment [38]. The extent of cytokine signaling was attenuated in patients with mild disease. Patients with severe COVID-19 showed significantly elevated neutrophil infiltration with marked depletion of alveolar macrophages and enrichment of chronic hyperinflammatory monocytes as compared with patients with milder disease [39]. Retention and activity of alveolar macrophages may allow for more efficient clearance of dead epithelial cells and reduce viral load in patients with mild disease. All individuals with ARDS showed macrophage activation syndrome or very low human leukocyte antigen D–related (HLA-DR) expression on CD14+ monocytes [40], which is similar to immunologic dysregulation in sepsis caused by other pathogens [41].

Significant reduction in CD4+ lymphocytes, CD19+ lymphocytes, and NK cells is another characteristic of immune system malfunction. The production of TNF-α and IL-6 by plasma monocytes was preserved. Immune dysregulation and macrophage activation syndrome are suggested to be driven by IL-6 and IL-1b, respectively. The key features for immune dysregulation, overproduction of proinflammatory cytokines by monocytes and dysregulation of lymphocytes, result in CD4 lymphopenia followed by B cell lymphopenia. In addition, the absolute number of NK cells was decreased, likely a result of the virus's rapid spread [40].

IL-6 is one of the factors that contribute to the reduction of HLA-DR presence on CD14+ monocytes because HLA-DR expression is negatively proportional to IL-6 concentrations in the blood.

Antibody-Dependent Cellular Cytotoxicity

Recent literature has shown that hyperimmunoglobulin neutralized SARS-CoV-2 viral particles through a myriad of neutralization methods: plaque reduction, virus-induced cytotoxicity, $TCID_{50}$ (tissue culture infectious dose for 50% of the culture to get infected) reduction, and immunofluorimetry. It has also triggered antibody-dependent cellular cytotoxicity and phagocytosis, and the authors report this therapy may be a key to the neutralization-resistant emerging viral variants given its success across the different methodologies [42].

Cytokine Storm

Cytokine storm can be described as an aberrant host immune response to SARS-CoV-2. It is marked by excessive elevated levels of circulating proinflammatory mediators: IL-1β, IL-1 receptor antagonist, IL-2, IL-6, IL-7, IL-10, TNF-α, IFN-γ, granulocyte-macrophage colony-stimulating factor (GM-CSF), granulocyte colony-stimulating factor, fibroblast growth factor, platelet-derived growth factor, vascular endothelial growth factor, CC chemokine ligand 2 (CCL2), CCL3, CCL4, CXCL10, CCL8, CXCL2, CXCL8, CXCL9, and CXCL16 [43]. An unregulated host immune response can permit an auto-amplifying cytokine cascade. Patients with severe COVID-19 have been found to exhibit greater levels of IL-2, IL-6, IL-7, IL-10, monocyte chemoattractant protein-1 (MCP-1), TNF-α, and granulocyte colony-stimulating factor than patients with mild disease presentation. It is believed to be a key step in the development of severe infection, but the precise mechanism has been difficult to establish. The cytokine storm is consequential: vascular leakage, apoptosis of epithelial and endothelial cells, and ARDS are all potential outcomes [44].

Pathogenic T helper 1 cells begin to secrete IL-6 and GM-CSF, which in turn can further activate monocytes to produce more IL-6, TNF-α, and other cytokines [45]. The anti–GM-CSF monoclonal antibody lenzilumab has shown benefit in severe COVID-19 [46]. Also, elevation of D-dimers, C-reactive protein, ferritin, and other acute-phase reactants may be elevated in this syndrome. These elevated reactants tend to be higher in intensive care unit patients than in non–intensive care unit patients [47, 48].

SARS-CoV has the capacity to phase macrophages and dendritic cells beyond just affecting epithelial lung cells [49]. Although the virus can infect the cell, what is interesting is the virus is then contained and cannot further replicate. However, its capacity to instigate damage is not hampered because it can trigger proinflammatory chemokine secretions by the dendritic and macrophages cells [50]. All of this is not limited to an in vitro setting, because patients with SARS-CoV exhibit elevated serum levels of cytokines and chemokines [41, 51]. Building on this, we observe that postinfection, there was an impaired immune-defensive IFN-β response, while also a simultaneous bolster of proinflammatory cytokines (e.g. IL-6 and TNF-α) and inflammatory chemokines (e.g. CXCL10, CCL3, CCL5, and CCL2). This ties back to the viral evasion mechanism discussed earlier in this chapter [34].

Muting these inflammatory cytokines has been addressed as a viable treatment option. Tocilizumab, a monoclonal antibody against the IL-6 receptor, has been used as a treatment for rheumatoid arthritis. Due to its activity against IL-6, and the role of this cytokine in inflammation, it was studied as a treatment for cytokine storm [52]. A meta-analysis found tocilizumab used in the treatment of moderate to severe COVID-19 infection was associated with a reduction in mortality; 11% in randomized controlled trials (risk ratio, 0.89; 95% confidence interval: 0.82–0.96) and 31% in observational studies (risk ratio, 0.69; 95% confidence interval: 0.58–0.83). Tocilizumab also reduced invasive mechanical ventilation by 19% in randomized controlled trials, but not significantly in observational studies [53].

Cell surface signaling may also play a role in the development of cytokine storm. SARS-CoV-2 activation of nuclear factor-κB and occupation of ACE2 receptors can active an IL-6 amplifier to further induce proinflammatory cytokines and chemokines, including vascular endothelial growth factor, MCP-1, IL-8, and IL-6. Progressive increases in cytokine signaling can subsequently result in decreased lymphocyte counts, particularly for CD8$^+$ cytotoxic T cells, and increases in neutrophil counts. Increased neutrophil-to-lymphocyte ratios in combination with dynamic proinflammatory cytokine monitoring can potentially allow identification of patients at risk for cytokine storm development. This immune response may present other targets for immune therapy [54] to prevent deterioration in patients with severe COVID-19 [55].

Conclusions

Although the COVID-19 pandemic has mostly caught all of public health and the medical establishment by surprise, it also culminated in many novel therapies designed to hamper its morbidity and mortality. The mRNA vaccine, steroids, and monoclonal antibodies were rapidly deployed and are trailblazing therapies brought to the forefront thanks to unprecedented international cooperation and collaboration. These therapeutics, born of desperation, are likely to guide how we think about treating novel viral infections in the future. As our studies into immunology progress, this foundational knowledge will lead us to emerging treatment regimens for viral illnesses in the future.

Acknowledgments

The authors thank Gunakaushik Vengalasetti for his artistic contributions to this chapter.

References

1 Sungnak, W., Huang, N., Bécavin, C. et al. (2020). SARS-CoV-2 entry factors are highly expressed in nasal epithelial cells together with innate immune genes. *Nat. Med.* 26 (5): 681–687. https://doi.org/10.1038/s41591-020-0868-6.

2 Flerlage, T., Boyd, D.F., Meliopoulos, V. et al. (2021). Influenza virus and SARS-CoV-2: pathogenesis and host responses in the respiratory tract. *Nat. Rev. Microbiol.* 19 (7): 425–441. https://doi.org/10.1038/s41579-021-00542-7.

3 Bösmüller, H., Matter, M., Fend, F., and Tzankov, A. (2021). The pulmonary pathology of COVID-19. *Virchows Arch.* 478 (1): 137–150. https://doi.org/10.1007/s00428-021-03053-1.

4 Chowdhury, M.A., Hossain, N., Kashem, M.A. et al. (2020). Immune response in COVID-19: a review. *J. Infect. Public Health.* 13 (11): 1619–1629. https://doi.org/10.1016/j.jiph.2020.07.001.

5 Salian, V.S., Wright, J.A., Vedell, P.T. et al. (2021). COVID-19 transmission, current treatment, and future therapeutic strategies. *Mol. Pharm.* 18 (3): 754–771. https://doi.org/10.1021/acs.molpharmaceut.0c00608.

6 Channappanavar, R., Zhao, J., and Perlman, S. (2014). T cell-mediated immune response to respiratory coronaviruses. *Immunol. Res.* 59 (1–3): 118–128. https://doi.org/10.1007/s12026-014-8534-z.

7 Seow, J., Graham, C., Merrick, B. et al. (2020). Longitudinal observation and decline of neutralizing antibody responses in the three months following SARS-CoV-2 infection in humans. *Nat. Microbiol.* 5 (12): 1598–1607. https://doi.org/10.1038/s41564-020-00813-8.

8 Long, Q.X., Liu, B.Z., Deng, H.J. et al. (2020). Antibody responses to SARS-CoV-2 in patients with COVID-19. *Nat. Med.* 26 (6): 845–848. https://doi.org/10.1038/s41591-020-0897-1.

9 Zhang, G., Nie, S., Zhang, Z., and Zhang, Z. (2020). Longitudinal change of severe acute respiratory syndrome coronavirus 2 antibodies in patients with coronavirus disease 2019. *J. Infect. Dis.* 222 (2): 183–188. https://doi.org/10.1093/infdis/jiaa229.

10 Ivanova, E.N., Devlin, J.C., Buus, T.B. et al. (2021). Discrete immune response signature to SARS-CoV-2 mRNA vaccination versus infection. *medRxiv* https://doi.org/10.1101/2021.04.20.21255677.

11 Sahin, U., Muik, A., Derhovanessian, E. et al. (2020). COVID-19 vaccine BNT162b1 elicits human antibody and T(H)1 T cell responses. *Nature* 586 (7830): 594–599. https://doi.org/10.1038/s41586-020-2814-7.

12 Ganji, A., Farahani, I., Khansarinejad, B. et al. (2020). Increased expression of CD8 marker on T-cells in COVID-19 patients. *Blood Cells Mol. Dis.* 83: 102437. https://doi.org/10.1016/j.bcmd.2020.102437.

13 Corbett, K.S., Nason, M.C., Flach, B. et al. (2021). Immune correlates of protection by mRNA-1273 vaccine against SARS-CoV-2 in nonhuman primates. *Science* 373 (6561): eabj0299. https://doi.org/10.1126/science.abj0299.

14 Huang, A.T., Garcia-Carreras, B., Hitchings, M.D.T. et al. (2020). A systematic review of antibody mediated immunity to coronaviruses: kinetics, correlates of protection, and association with severity. *Nat. Commun.* 11 (1): 4704. https://doi.org/10.1038/s41467-020-18450-4.

15 Roozendaal, R., Solforosi, L., Stieh, D.J. et al. (2021). SARS-CoV-2 binding and neutralizing antibody levels after Ad26.COV2.S vaccination predict durable protection in rhesus macaques. *Nat Commun.* 12 (1): 5877. https://doi.org/10.1038/s41467-021-26117-x.

16 Duarte, L.F., Gálvez, N.M.S., Iturriaga, C. et al. (2021). Immune profile and clinical outcome of breakthrough cases after vaccination with an inactivated SARS-CoV-2 vaccine. *Front. Immunol.* 12: 742914. https://doi.org/10.3389/fimmu.2021.742914.

17 Knezevic, I., Mattiuzzo, G., Page, M. et al. (2022). WHO international standard for evaluation of the antibody response to COVID-19 vaccines: call for urgent action by the scientific community. *Lancet Microbe* 3: e235–e240. https://doi.org/10.1016/s2666-5247(21)00266-4.

18 Feng, S., Phillips, D.J., White, T. et al. (2021). Correlates of protection against symptomatic and asymptomatic SARS-CoV-2 infection. *Nat. Med.* 27: 2032–2040. https://doi.org/10.1038/s41591-021-01540-1.

19 Gilbert, P.B., Montefiori, D.C., McDermott, A. et al. (2021). Immune correlates analysis of the mRNA-1273

COVID-19 vaccine efficacy trial. *medRxiv* https://doi.org/10.1101/2021.08.09.21261290.

20 Sui, Y., Bekele, Y., and Berzofsky, J.A. (2021). Potential SARS-CoV-2 immune correlates of protection in infection and vaccine immunization. *Pathogens* 10 (2): 138. https://doi.org/10.3390/pathogens10020138.

21 Naranbhai, V., Pernat, C.A., Gavralidis, A. et al. (2022). Immunogenicity and reactogenicity of SARS-CoV-2 vaccines in patients with cancer: the CANVAX cohort study. *J. Clin. Oncol.* 40: 12–23. https://doi.org/10.1200/jco.21.01891.

22 Goldberg, Y., Mandel, M., Bar-On, Y.M. et al. (2021). Waning immunity after the BNT162b2 vaccine in Israel. *N. Engl. J. Med.* 385: e85. https://doi.org/10.1056/NEJMoa2114228.

23 Choi, W.S. and Cheong, H.J. (2021). COVID-19 vaccination for people with comorbidities. *Infect. Chemother.* 53 (1): 155–158. https://doi.org/10.3947/ic.2021.0302.

24 Thuluvath, P.J., Robarts, P., and Chauhan, M. (2021). Analysis of antibody responses after COVID-19 vaccination in liver transplant recipients and those with chronic liver diseases. *J. Hepatol.* 75 (6): 1434–1439. https://doi.org/10.1016/j.jhep.2021.08.008.

25 Tartof, S.Y., Slezak, J.M., Fischer, H. et al. (2021). Effectiveness of mRNA BNT162b2 COVID-19 vaccine up to 6 months in a large integrated health system in the USA: a retrospective cohort study. *Lancet* 398: 1407–1416. https://doi.org/10.1016/s0140-6736(21)02183-8.

26 Naaber, P., Tserel, L., Kangro, K. et al. (2021). Dynamics of antibody response to BNT162b2 vaccine after six months: a longitudinal prospective study. *Lancet Reg Health Eur.* 10: 100208. https://doi.org/10.1016/j.lanepe.2021.100208.

27 Vabret, N., Britton, G.J., Gruber, C. et al. (2020). Immunology of COVID-19: current state of the science. *Immunity* 52 (6): 910–941. https://doi.org/10.1016/j.immuni.2020.05.002.

28 Channappanavar, R., Fehr, A.R., Vijay, R. et al. (2016). Dysregulated type I interferon and inflammatory monocyte-macrophage responses cause lethal pneumonia in SARS-CoV-infected mice. *Cell Host Microbe* 19 (2): 181–193. https://doi.org/10.1016/j.chom.2016.01.007.

29 Hadjadj, J., Yatim, N., Barnabei, L. et al. (2020). Impaired type I interferon activity and inflammatory responses in severe COVID-19 patients. *Science* 369 (6504): 718–724. https://doi.org/10.1126/science.abc6027.

30 Zhang, Q., Bastard, P., Liu, Z. et al. (2020). Inborn errors of type I IFN immunity in patients with life-threatening COVID-19. *Science* 370 (6515): eabd4570. https://doi.org/10.1126/science.abd4570.

31 Bastard, P., Rosen, L.B., Zhang, Q. et al. (2020). Autoantibodies against type I IFNs in patients with life-threatening COVID-19. *Science* 370 (6515): eabd4585. https://doi.org/10.1126/science.abd4585.

32 Bonjardim, C.A., Ferreira, P.C., and Kroon, E.G. (2009). Interferons: signaling, antiviral and viral evasion. *Immunol. Lett.* 122 (1): 1–11. https://doi.org/10.1016/j.imlet.2008.11.002.

33 Pichlmair, A. and Reis e Sousa, C. (2007). Innate recognition of viruses. *Immunity* 27 (3): 370–383. https://doi.org/10.1016/j.immuni.2007.08.012.

34 Kopecky-Bromberg, S.A., Martínez-Sobrido, L., Frieman, M. et al. (2007). Severe acute respiratory syndrome coronavirus open reading frame (ORF) 3b, ORF 6, and nucleocapsid proteins function as interferon antagonists. *J. Virol.* 81 (2): 548–557. https://doi.org/10.1128/jvi.01782-06.

35 Garcia-Beltran, W.F., Lam, E.C., Astudillo, M.G. et al. (2021). COVID-19-neutralizing antibodies predict disease severity and survival. *Cell* 184 (2):476–488.e11. https://doi.org/10.1016/j.cell.2020.12.015.

36 Wang, J., Zheng, X., and Chen, J. (2021). Clinical progression and outcomes of 260 patients with severe COVID-19: an observational study. *Sci. Rep.* 11 (1): 3166. https://doi.org/10.1038/s41598-021-82943-5.

37 Yao, C., Bora, S.A., Parimon, T. et al. (2021). Cell-type-specific immune dysregulation in severely ill COVID-19 patients. *Cell Rep.* 34 (1): 108590. https://doi.org/10.1016/j.celrep.2020.108590.

38 Chen, H., Liu, W., Wang, Y. et al. (2021). SARS-CoV-2 activates lung epithelial cell proinflammatory signaling and leads to immune dysregulation in COVID-19 patients. *EBioMedicine* 70: 103500. https://doi.org/10.1016/j.ebiom.2021.103500.

39 Wauters, E., Van Mol, P., Garg, A.D. et al. (2021). Discriminating mild from critical COVID-19 by

innate and adaptive immune single-cell profiling of bronchoalveolar lavages. *Cell Res.* 31 (3): 272–290. https://doi.org/10.1038/s41422-020-00455-9.

40 Giamarellos-Bourboulis, E.J., Netea, M.G., Rovina, N. et al. (2020). Complex immune dysregulation in COVID-19 patients with severe respiratory failure. *Cell Host Microbe* 27 (6): 992–1000.e3. https://doi.org/10.1016/j.chom.2020.04.009.

41 Bellinvia, S., Edwards, C.J., Schisano, M. et al. (2020). The unleashing of the immune system in COVID-19 and sepsis: the calm before the storm? *Inflamm. Res.* 69 (8): 757–763. https://doi.org/10.1007/s00011-020-01366-6.

42 Díez, J.M., Romero, C., Cruz, M. et al. (2021). Anti-SARS-CoV-2 hyperimmune globulin demonstrates potent neutralization and antibody-dependent cellular cytotoxicity and phagocytosis through N and S proteins. *J. Infect. Dis.* 2021: jiab540. https://doi.org/10.1093/infdis/jiab540. Accessed 6 Nov 2021.

43 Ricci, D., Etna, M.P., Rizzo, F. et al. (2021). Innate immune response to SARS-CoV-2 infection: from cells to soluble mediators. *Int. J. Mol. Sci.* 22 (13): 7017. https://doi.org/10.3390/ijms22137017.

44 Channappanavar, R. and Perlman, S. (2017). Pathogenic human coronavirus infections: causes and consequences of cytokine storm and immunopathology. *Semin. Immunopathol.* 39 (5): 529–539. https://doi.org/10.1007/s00281-017-0629-x.

45 Hu, B., Huang, S., and Yin, L. (2021). The cytokine storm and COVID-19. *J. Med. Virol.* 93 (1): 250–256. https://doi.org/10.1002/jmv.26232.

46 Temesgen, Z., Burger, C.D., Baker, J. et al. (2021). Lenzilumab efficacy and safety in newly hospitalized COVID-19 subjects: results from the live-air phase 3 randomized double-blind placebo-controlled trial. *medRxiv* https://doi.org/10.1101/2021.05.01.21256470.

47 Wang, D., Hu, B., Hu, C. et al. (2020). Clinical characteristics of 138 hospitalized patients with 2019 novel coronavirus-infected pneumonia in Wuhan, China. *JAMA* 323 (11): 1061–1069. https://doi.org/10.1001/jama.2020.1585.

48 Chen, G., Wu, D., Guo, W. et al. (2020). Clinical and immunological features of severe and moderate coronavirus disease 2019. *J. Clin. Invest.* 130 (5): 2620–2629. https://doi.org/10.1172/JCI137244.

49 Spiegel, M., Schneider, K., Weber, F. et al. (2006). Interaction of severe acute respiratory syndrome-associated coronavirus with dendritic cells. *J. Gen. Virol.* 87 (Pt 7): 1953–1960. https://doi.org/10.1099/vir.0.81624-0.

50 Law, H.K.W., Cheung, C.Y., Ng, H.Y. et al. (2005). Chemokine up-regulation in SARS-coronavirus-infected, monocyte-derived human dendritic cells. *Blood* 106 (7): 2366–2374. https://doi.org/10.1182/blood-2004-10-4166.

51 Lau, Y.L. and Peiris, J.S.M. (2005). Pathogenesis of severe acute respiratory syndrome. *Curr. Opin. Immunol.* 17 (4): 404–410. https://doi.org/10.1016/j.coi.2005.05.009.

52 Rosas, I.O., Bräu, N., Waters, M. et al. (2021). Tocilizumab in hospitalized patients with severe Covid-19 pneumonia. *N. Engl. J. Med.* 384 (16): 1503–1516. https://doi.org/10.1056/NEJMoa2028700.

53 Kyriakopoulos, C., Ntritsos, G., Gogali, A. et al. (2021). Tocilizumab administration for the treatment of hospitalized patients with COVID-19: a systematic review and meta-analysis. *Respirology* 26 (11): 1027–1040. https://doi.org/10.1111/resp.14152.

54 Tang, Y., Liu, J., Zhang, D. et al. (2020). Cytokine storm in COVID-19: the current evidence and treatment strategies. *Front. Immunol.* 11: 1708–1708. https://doi.org/10.3389/fimmu.2020.01708.

55 Choudhary, S., Sharma, K., and Silakari, O. (2021). The interplay between inflammatory pathways and COVID-19: a critical review on pathogenesis and therapeutic options. *Microb. Pathog.* 150: 104673. https://doi.org/10.1016/j.micpath.2020.104673.

56 Polack, F.P., Thomas, S.J., Kitchin, N. et al. (2020). Safety and efficacy of the BNT162b2 mRNA Covid-19 vaccine. *N. Engl. J. Med.* 383 (27): 2603–2615. https://doi.org/10.1056/NEJMoa2034577.

57 Meo, S.A., Bukhari, I.A., Akram, J. et al. (2021). COVID-19 vaccines: comparison of biological, pharmacological characteristics and adverse effects of Pfizer/BioNTech and Moderna vaccines. *Eur. Rev. Med. Pharmacol. Sci.* 25 (3): 1663–1669. https://doi.org/10.26355/eurrev_202102_24877.

58 Sadoff, J., Gray, G., Vandebosch, A. et al. (2021). Safety and efficacy of single-dose Ad26.COV2.S vaccine against Covid-19. *N. Engl. J. Med.* 384 (23): 2187–2201. https://doi.org/10.1056/NEJMoa2101544.

59 Sadoff, J., De Paepe, E., Haazen, W. et al. (2021). Safety and immunogenicity of the Ad26.RSV.preF investigational vaccine coadministered with an influenza vaccine in older adults. *J. Infect. Dis.* 223 (4): 699–708. https://doi.org/10.1093/infdis/jiaa409.

60 Gottlieb, R.L., Nirula, A., Chen, P. et al. (2021). Effect of bamlanivimab as monotherapy or in combination with etesevimab on viral load in patients with mild to moderate COVID-19: a randomized clinical Trial. *JAMA* 325 (7): 632–644. https://doi.org/10.1001/jama.2021.0202.

61 Weinreich, D.M., Sivapalasingam, S., Norton, T. et al. (2021). REGN-COV2, a neutralizing antibody cocktail, in outpatients with Covid-19. *N. Engl. J. Med.* 384 (3): 238–251. https://doi.org/10.1056/NEJMoa2035002.

62 Baum, A., Fulton, B.O., Wloga, E. et al. (2020). Antibody cocktail to SARS-CoV-2 spike protein prevents rapid mutational escape seen with individual antibodies. *Science* 369 (6506): 1014–1018. https://doi.org/10.1126/science.abd0831.

63 Gupta, A., Gonzalez-Rojas, Y., Juarez, E. et al. (2021). Early treatment for Covid-19 with SARS-CoV-2 neutralizing antibody sotrovimab. *N. Engl. J. Med.* 385: 1941–1950. https://doi.org/10.1056/NEJMoa2107934.

64 Owji, H., Negahdaripour, M., and Hajighahramani, N. (2020). Immunotherapeutic approaches to curtail COVID-19. *Int. Immunopharmacol.* 88: 106924. https://doi.org/10.1016/j.intimp.2020.106924.

65 Owen, C., Berinstein, N.L., Christofides, A., and Sehn, L.H. (2019). Review of Bruton tyrosine kinase inhibitors for the treatment of relapsed or refractory mantle cell lymphoma. *Curr. Oncol.* 26 (2): e233–e240. https://doi.org/10.3747/co.26.4345.

66 Stebbing, J., Phelan, A., Griffin, I. et al. (2020). COVID-19: combining antiviral and anti-inflammatory treatments. *Lancet Infect. Dis.* 20 (4): 400–402. https://doi.org/10.1016/S1473-3099(20)30132-8.

67 Zheng, Y., Li, R., and Liu, S. (2020). Immunoregulation with mTOR inhibitors to prevent COVID-19 severity: a novel intervention strategy beyond vaccines and specific antiviral medicines. *J. Med. Virol.* 92 (9): 1495–1500. https://doi.org/10.1002/jmv.26009.

68 Devaux, C.A., Melenotte, C., Piercecchi-Marti, M.D. et al. (2021). Cyclosporin A: a repurposable drug in the treatment of COVID-19? *Front. Med. (Lausanne)* 8: 663708. https://doi.org/10.3389/fmed.2021.663708.

69 Poulsen, N.N., von Brunn, A., Hornum, M., and Blomberg, J.M. (2020). Cyclosporine and COVID-19: risk or favorable? *Am. J. Transplant.* 20 (11): 2975–2982. https://doi.org/10.1111/ajt.16250.

70 Russell, B., Moss, C., George, G. et al. (2020). Associations between immune-suppressive and stimulating drugs and novel COVID-19-a systematic review of current evidence. *Ecancermedicalscience* 14: 1022. https://doi.org/10.3332/ecancer.2020.1022.

71 Cirri, D., Pratesi, A., Marzo, T., and Messori, L. (2021). Metallo therapeutics for COVID-19. Exploiting metal-based compounds for the discovery of new antiviral drugs. *Expert Opin. Drug Discov.* 16 (1): 39–46. https://doi.org/10.1080/17460441.2020.1819236.

72 Rothan, H.A., Stone, S., Natekar, J. et al. (2020). The FDA-approved gold drug auranofin inhibits novel coronavirus (SARS-COV-2) replication and attenuates inflammation in human cells. *Virology* 547: 7–11. https://doi.org/10.1016/j.virol.2020.05.002.

73 de Paiva, R.E.F., Marçal Neto, A., Santos, I.A. et al. (2020). What is holding back the development of antiviral metallodrugs? A literature overview and implications for SARS-CoV-2 therapeutics and future viral outbreaks. *Dalton Trans.* 49 (45): 16004–16033. https://doi.org/10.1039/d0dt02478c.

74 Chen, Y.F., Jobanputra, P., Barton, P. et al. (2006). A systematic review of the effectiveness of adalimumab, etanercept and infliximab for the treatment of rheumatoid arthritis in adults and an economic evaluation of their cost-effectiveness. *Health Technol. Assess.* 10 (42):iii–iv, xi–xiii, 1–229. https://doi.org/10.3310/hta10420.

75 Chen, X.Y., Yan, B.X., and Man, X.Y. (2020). TNFα inhibitor may be effective for severe COVID-19: learning from toxic epidermal necrolysis. *Ther. Adv. Respir. Dis.* 14: 1753466620926800. https://doi.org/10.1177/1753466620926800.

76 Jin, Y.H., Zhan, Q.Y., Peng, Z.Y. et al. (2020). Chemoprophylaxis, diagnosis, treatments, and discharge management of COVID-19: an evidence-based clinical practice guideline (updated version). *Mil. Med. Res.* 7 (1): 41. https://doi.org/10.1186/s40779-020-00270-8.

77 Rochwerg, B., Agarwal, A., Siemieniuk, R.A. et al. (2020). A living WHO guideline on drugs for covid-19. *BMJ* 370: m3379. https://doi.org/10.1136/bmj.m3379.

78 Raju, R., Prajith, V., and Biatris, P.S., J SJUC.(2021). Therapeutic role of corticosteroids in COVID-19: a systematic review of registered clinical trials. *Future J. Pharm. Sci.* 7 (1): 67–67. https://doi.org/10.1186/s43094-021-00217-3.

79 Chen, R.C., Tang, X.P., Tan, S.Y. et al. (2006). Treatment of severe acute respiratory syndrome with glucosteroids: the Guangzhou experience. *Chest* 129 (6): 1441–1452. https://doi.org/10.1378/chest.129.6.1441.

80 Horby, P., Lim, W.S., Emberson, J.R. et al. (2021). Dexamethasone in hospitalized patients with Covid-19. *N. Engl. J. Med.* 384 (8): 693–704. https://doi.org/10.1056/NEJMoa2021436.

7

COVID-19: Presentation and Symptomatology

Jacek Czubak[1], Karolina Stolarczyk[1], Marcin Frączek[1], Katarzyna Resler[1], Anna Orzeł[2], Wojciech Flieger[2], and Tomasz Zatoński[1]

[1] *Department and Clinic of Otolaryngology, Head and Neck Surgery, Wroclaw Medical University, Wrocław, Poland*
[2] *School of Medicine, Medical University of Lublin, Lublin, Poland*

Abbreviations

ACE2	angiotensin-converting enzyme 2
AKI	acute kidney injury
CI	confidence interval
GI	gastrointestinal
ICU	intensive care unit
OT	olfactory training
SARS-CoV-2	severe acute respiratory syndrome coronavirus 2
SNHL	sensorineural hearing loss
URI	upper respiratory tract infection

Coronavirus disease 2019 (COVID-19) is caused by severe acute respiratory syndrome coronavirus 2 (SARS-CoV-2). First observed at the end of 2019, COVID-19 was declared a pandemic in March 2020. Since then, the entire world has made efforts to stop the spread of the pathogen and to find and define prodromal symptoms, as well as those predisposing to a severe course of infection. Multicenter observations of infected patients have indicated that the virus affects not only the lung tissue but also other vital organs. Olfactory symptoms, which are currently considered to be one of the pathognomonic symptoms of COVID-19, were of particular importance. Other affected organs include the gastrointestinal (GI) tract, liver, and urinary tract. In addition, the symptoms that occur during pregnancy and the impact of infection on fertility are very important for the clinician. This chapter presents the clinical aspects of infection in pulmonology, otolaryngology, gastroenterology, gynecology, and urology.

Pulmonary Manifestations of COVID-19

Pulmonary presentations and severity of SARS-CoV-2 infection differ considerably among patients, ranging from no symptoms or mild pneumonia in most cases (81%) to critical conditions, such as respiratory failure, septic shock, and/or multiple organ dysfunction or failure [1]. SARS-CoV-2 primarily targets the pneumocytes, immune cells, and vascular endothelial cells [2].

The pathogenesis of COVID-19 pulmonary disease involves key molecular interactions between the SARS-CoV-2 spike protein receptor-binding domain and its host receptor angiotensin-converting enzyme 2 (ACE2) on pneumocytes and endothelial cells. This leads to development of acute lung injury that manifests as diffuse alveolar damage. The inflammatory reaction involves endothelial cell damage, capillary leak, activation of type II pneumocytes, and involvement of polarized pulmonary macrophages [3, 4]. Moreover, another cause of acute lung injury in COVID-19 is pulmonary microvascular thrombosis that leads to alveolar damage [2].

Among individuals with COVID-19, the most frequently reported respiratory symptoms were cough (63.1%), expectoration (41.8%), and dyspnea (33.9%). Minor symptoms included chest tightness, chest pain, hemoptysis, and wheezes [5–7] (Table 7.1).

Clinical classification divides COVID-19 into four types based on severity of the symptoms. The mild type involves mild clinical symptoms without pneumonia on radiography, which can be asymptomatic or imitating the common cold. The moderate type presents with fever and/or respiratory symptoms, plus pneumonia in radiography, which may resemble influenza. The severe type is diagnosed based on dyspnea (respiratory rate [RR] $\geq$ 30 breaths/min), resting oxygen saturation $\leq$ 93%, or arterial blood oxygen partial pressure/fraction of inspired oxygen (PaO_2/FiO_2) $\leq$300 mmHg (1 mmHg = 0.133 kPa). The critical type is defined as respiratory failure with shock and multiple organ failure, requiring mechanical ventilation and intensive care unit (ICU) admission [8, 9].

A typical trait of COVID-19 pneumonia is impaired pulmonary diffusion that eventually leads to gradual decline in oxygen saturation. Despite progressive development of respiratory failure, many patients show no signs of pulmonary distress. Such a condition is referred to as silent hypoxemia [10]. Patients tend to have better compliance of the respiratory system that is discrepant to the amount of shunt [11].

Atypical Acute Respiratory Distress Syndrome

Apart from severe hypoxemia, clinical symptoms of acute respiratory distress syndrome in COVID-19 may be differentiated. Two primary phenotypes are distinguished: type L and type H. Type L, often observed in early stages, is characterized by low elastance (i.e.

Table 7.1 Clinical symptoms of acute respiratory distress syndrome.

Major	Minor
• Cough:	• Chest pain
– Productive	• Chest tightness
– Nonproductive	• Hemoptysis
• Dyspnea	• Wheeze

high compliance), low ventilation-to-perfusion ratio, low lung weight, and low lung recruitability. Type L can remain stable, improve, or transform into type H. Typical features of type H involve high elastance, high right-to-left shunt, high lung weight, and high lung recruitability [12]. Only 25.8% of patients had lesions involving a single lung, and 75.7% of patients had lesions involving bilateral lungs [5].

Otolaryngologic Manifestations of COVID-19

Sense of Smell

A properly functioning sense of smell is extremely important for humans [13]. Odors convey information about ourselves and our environment. Its essential role is to warn about danger and to enable the assessment of the intensity of a harmful stimulus and its location [14]. This is applicable both in the event of toxic gases, burnt food, or fire and in assessing the freshness and quality of consumed food. The sense of smell stimulates the appetite and closely influences the taste sensations [15]. It enables the assessment of one's own hygienic condition and at the same time constitutes an important code of social communication and regulates social interactions [16].

Olfactory dysfunction has been noted as a common symptom of viral infection of the upper respiratory airway tract [17]. Postinfectious olfactory disorders are estimated to account for 11–40% of cases [18, 19]. Respiratory viruses are believed to be the pathologic factors responsible for postinfectious loss of smell. These include rhinovirus (30–50%), parainfluenza virus (5%), influenza virus (5–15%), coronavirus (10–15%), Coxsackie virus (<5%), adenovirus (<5%), and respiratory syncytial viruses (10%). However, there are more than 200 viruses that can cause upper respiratory tract infections (URIs) [20]. Because all URI-related inflammation should resolve after the initial infection, postinfectious disorders are considered to be a neurosensory olfactory disorder and are not the result of nasal, olfactory cleft, or paranasal sinuses pathology [21]. Parosmia (distorted olfactory sensation; usually unpleasant) occurs together with hyposmia/anosmia in about two thirds of patients.

Conversely, 40–80% of patients with parosmia have viral URI as the primary cause. This symptom causes a significant daily life disturbance and a reduction in quality of life in more than half of the patients, often resulting in depression and reduced productivity at work [21–24]. These patients often emphasize their fears about the threat they pose to themselves and their families [25, 26].

Early reports have suggested that chemosensory loss may be an early, potential screening symptom associated with COVID-19 [27–29]. Although olfactory disorders are quite common after viral URI, loss of smell is becoming more and more prominent in patients with COVID-19, even in otherwise asymptomatic cases [27, 30–32]. Moreover, it is observed that 10% of patients do not spontaneously recover their olfactory functions after the end of the illness [33]. The British Rhinology Society and the American Academy of Otolaryngology–Head and Neck Surgery have identified loss of smell as a marker of COVID-19 infection [34–36]. Olfactory dysfunction is the reduced or distorted ability to smell when sniffing through the orthonasal or retronasal route [37]. The complete absence of the smell is called anosmia, whereas its diminished sensitivity is hyposmia.

The analysis of available studies (>50 publications; >11 000 cases) of olfactory disorders in COVID-19 indicates the overall prevalence of "loss of smell" at 52.0% [38]. However, there are significant differences in reporting the incidence of this disorder across studies ranging from 5.1% to 98% [39, 40]. One multicenter study reported qualitative olfactory disorders such as phantosmia (smelling an odor that is not actually there) and parosmia at 12.6% and 32.4% incidence, respectively. Smell disorders may precede (11.8–73%), accompany (22.8%), or occur after (65.4%) general or ear, nose, and throat symptoms [30, 41]. It is assumed that the loss of smell in COVID-19 may be associated with a milder clinical course of the infection [38, 42]. Observations in Italy among hospitalized patients with COVID-19 indicate that olfactory disorders were more commonly observed in younger patients and in women [9]. Other sinonasal symptoms included runny nose and nasal congestion. Nevertheless, it has been shown that only 25% of patients reported nasal congestion before the onset of anosmia, while only 18% of them observed nasal discharge [41]. Another analysis reported a significantly lower incidence of rhinorrhea and nasal obstruction of 2–7% and 2–12%, respectively [43].

The duration of an olfactory disorder varies in different reports. One study based on patient-reported symptoms demonstrated 18% return of olfaction in less than one week, 37.5% in one to two weeks, and 18% at two to four weeks [44]. According to other authors, 25.5% of patients regained both sense of smell and taste within 2 weeks of general symptom resolution [42]. Further data suggest a high rate of early recovery, within four to six weeks after the onset of infection [33]. Rates of spontaneous recovery of olfaction, in the absence of treatment, range from 32% to 67% [34]. The reports that the sense of smell does not return at all in about 10% of patients are also concerning [33].

In view of such a diverse manifestation of olfactory disorders and the incomplete known etiology of this disorder, its treatment is quite problematic. The treatment proposed by some authors, consisting of the use of corticosteroid nasal spray, oral steroids, and irrigation with saline solution, did not contribute to a significant regeneration of the sense of smell in long-term observation [45, 46]. According to the British Rhinology Society Consensus, Omega-3 supplements and olfactory training (OT) should be included in the treatment of olfactory disorders [33]. An increasing body of literature shows that the human olfactory system exhibits plasticity, and that its performance can be enhanced as a function of exposure to odors [47]. OT comprises a regular stimulation of the olfactory system by multiple daily exposures to a set of carefully selected odorants. After at least three months of regular sniffing of odors, a significant improvement of olfactory abilities is observed [48–50]. OT involves repeating and deliberately sniffing for 20 seconds, at least twice a day, a set of fragrances (usually lemon, rose, cloves, and eucalyptus). OT should last a minimum of three months. This therapy is low cost with negligible side effects [37] (Figure 7.1).

Voice Disorders

Otolaryngologic symptoms are more common than previously reported in Asia. Recent epidemiologic studies have shown the presence of dysphonia in some patients with COVID-19, and some patients also had aphonia.

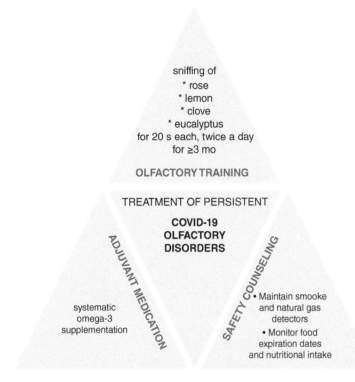

Figure 7.1   Treatment of persistent COVID-19 olfactory disorders in own modification according to Katherine Whitcroft and Thomas Hummel [37].

Acute infectious laryngitis is one of the most common diseases of the larynx and is often associated with URIs. Laryngitis can cause hoarseness or muffled voice, dry, barking cough, odynophagia, sore throat, and difficulty swallowing. Mild-to-moderate epiglottitis, swelling of the vocal folds, and subglottic edema may constrict the upper airway, resulting in inspiratory stridor and dyspnea. These symptoms usually disappear within three weeks. Viral laryngitis can be caused by many pathogens, including the influenza virus, adenovirus, and even varicella zoster virus [51, 52].

Reports from 19 European centers analyzing the course of the disease in 702 patients with mild-to-moderate COVID-19 indicate the presence of dysphonia in more than 26%. Aphonia was found in 3.7%. Sex predilection was observed, as more than 70% of patients were women. The severity of dysphonia was significantly associated with the intensity of dysphagia and cough [53]. Researchers from Lombardy indicate a higher percentage (43.7%) of dysphonia observed among 160 patients with mild-to-moderate COVID-19

and aphonia in just a single patient. This difference in incidence may be because of the difference in study protocols. In the first study, the data were based on self-report, and in the second, medical interview. They did not observe any sex predilection. The voice disturbance positively corresponded to voice fatigue, cough, rhinitis, and dyspnea. During follow-up, the duration of dysphonia was longer than two weeks in 44.1% of patients, including more than 15% lasting longer than a month. Dysphonia was more severe and its duration was longer in patients with cough and rhinitis [54].

Dysphonia may be caused by an inflammatory process involving the upper respiratory tract or may be caused by the swelling or inflammation of the vocal folds themselves. Epithelial cells of the vocal folds had high expression of ACE2, which is recognized as the COVID-19 receptor [55]. Other etiologic factors associated with dysphonia and COVID-19 include postviral vagal neuropathy, damage to the vocal cords as a result of severe coughing or vomiting, intubation trauma leading to granuloma of the vocal cords, vocal cord palsy, cricoarytenoid joint dislocation, and dysphonia secondary to poor lung function [56]. Postviral vagal neuropathy is a group of symptoms resulting from vagal neuropathy after URI [57]. This disorder affects both the sensory and the motor branches of the vagus nerve, which manifest as dysphonia, voice fatigue, dysphagia, odynophagia, neuropathic pain, cough, excessive throat clearing, and symptoms of laryngopharyngeal reflux [56]. Italian researchers point to the psychosomatic background of dysphonia, which may be related to the stress resulting from the ongoing pandemic in some individuals, especially among healthcare workers [58].

Voice acoustic analysis between healthy people and patients with COVID-19 demonstrated significant differences between various acoustic parameters, which confirms the influence of COVID-19 on voice quality. These changes are explained by insufficient airflow resulting from laryngeal and lung involvement [56, 59].

Hearing, Tinnitus, and Facial Nerve

SARS-CoV-2 is transmitted by airborne droplets, which are present in the nasopharynx from where, like other viruses and bacteria, they can pass through the Eustachian tube to the middle ear, where they can cause inflammation under favorable conditions. The cases of acute otitis media with otalgia, ear fullness, conductive hearing loss, and tinnitus in a patient with confirmed COVID-19 have already been documented [60]. According to a systematic review, otalgia can be seen in 13.1% (95% confidence interval [CI]: 7.9–19.3%) of patients with confirmed, probable, or suspected COVID-19 [61]. The presumed mechanism of conductive hearing loss in those cases is a middle ear effusion secondary to an ascending nasopharyngeal infection [62]. In some cases, ear symptoms may precede the onset of lower respiratory symptoms. Therefore, otitis media can be the initial manifestation of COVID-19. A patient with middle ear inflammation requires anti-inflammatory drugs and nasal decongestants treatment, which are sufficient to control viral otitis media. An important element is a follow-up otoscopy to exclude bacterial superinfection that requires antibiotic therapy or drainage.

Currently, no evidence supports the presence of SARS-CoV-2 in the middle ear, but the earlier findings implicate the virus as a potential source of otologic disorders. Cases of external ear infection caused by COVID-19 infection are rare [63].

It is well known that several viruses can damage the inner ear structures; therefore, audiovestibular symptoms are a known complication of a number of such infections [64]. SARS-CoV-2 can reach the inner ear both directly from the middle ear through the round window and through the crossing of the blood–labyrinth or through the cochlear aqueduct that links the scala tympani to the subarachnoid space and has also been proposed as a route of invasion. ACE2 receptors, the key for intracellular invasion, were seen to be expressed in epithelial cells of the middle ear, as well as the stria vascularis, spiral ganglion, and cochlea in mice [65].

The mechanisms underlying post-COVID-19 inner ear impairment may be related to damage not only of inner ear structures but also viral-related inflammation of the vestibulocochlear nerve or ischemia of the hearing center secondary to thrombogenic phenomena related to SARS-CoV-2 infection [66]. COVID-19 is associated with several neurologic manifestations, including Guillain-Barré syndrome, which has been associated with auditory neuropathy spectrum disorder [67, 68].

There have been several case reports of sensorineural hearing loss (SNHL) in patients with COVID-19, some of which were documented to be sudden in onset [69–71]. In most cases, SNHL is limited to one ear, but bilateral hearing loss has also been reported [72]. Hearing loss in the course of COVID-19 can affect both young and old. Hearing loss can also vary in severity. Apart from total bilateral deafness, cases with hearing loss in selected frequencies (mainly high) are also described. SARS-CoV-2 may have deleterious effects on cochlear hair cell functions, despite the patient being asymptomatic. High-frequency hearing impairment may relate to the finding that the number of ACE2 receptors is probably twice as high in the basal gyrus of mice cochlea [65].

It is currently difficult to reliably judge how many SARS-CoV-2–infected patients have a hearing impairment and whether the hearing loss is permanent. The prevalence of hearing loss in patients with confirmed, probable, and suspected COVID-19 is 7.6% (95% CI: 2.5–15.1%) [61].

These data should be interpreted with caution because they were obtained from studies that used mostly self-reported questionnaires without appropriate audiologic testing. There are currently no histologic studies that would confirm the presence of the virus in the cochlea of patients infected with SARS-CoV-2. Examination of convalescent patients did not show any permanent hearing loss [73]. On the contrary, there were 50% more manifestations of sudden-onset SNHL in the COVID-19 pandemic interval compared with the same interval before the pandemic [74].

The generally accepted method of SNHL treatment is systemic steroid therapy and/or intratympanic injections. Progressive clinical improvement in hearing can be expected after oral corticoid therapy with or without intratympanic dexamethasone injections in COVID-19-related SNHL [75–77]. If there is no improvement, a cochlear implant should be considered. However, the inflammatory process in the cochlea caused by SARS-CoV-2 can lead to soft tissue formation or even ossification, making the insertion of a cochlear implant electrode impossible. This is especially true in patients with underlying meningitis. Therefore, timely magnetic resonance imaging scans to confirm cochlear fibrosis/ossification and urgent cochlear implantation should be considered in these cases.

The harmful effect on hair cells of the cochlea caused by SARS-CoV-2 may also result in tinnitus. Tinnitus was the most commonly documented audiovestibular symptom, with an estimated prevalence of 14.8% (95% CI: 6.3–26.1%) in patients with confirmed, probable, or suspected COVID-19 [61]. Post-COVID-19 tinnitus can be an isolated symptom or it can be accompanied by hearing loss [71]. Although tinnitus often results from damage to the hair cells in the cochlea, the mental and emotional stress of the pandemic also may be the trigger. The tinnitus in patients with COVID-19 was described as nonpulsatile or as white noise, intermittent to continuous; others matched the tinnitus to 4-kHz and 10-dB sensation level [61]. Most studies reported tinnitus as an early-onset symptom during COVID-19 infection. The tinnitus was reported as generally lasting from a few days to a few weeks, but it may also persist.

SARS-CoV-2 infection leading to inflammatory changes of the VIIIth cranial nerve also can cause vestibular neuritis associated with symptoms such as sudden, severe vertigo, dizziness, balance problems, and nausea and vomiting [78]. In the case of vestibular neuritis, patients experience labyrinth complaints without tinnitus and without hearing loss. Dizziness and vertigo worsen on any head movement and would improve while lying still. Previous studies showed DNA fragments of the herpes simplex virus in the vestibular nerves of patients with vertigo in the course of vestibular neuritis [78]. A similar mechanism can be expected in patients with post-COVID-19 vestibular neuritis.

Notably, dizziness was among the most typical neurologic manifestations of COVID-19, although it is not necessarily of vestibular origin [79]. The estimated prevalence of vertigo is only 7.2% according to a systematic review [61]. A study from Wuhan reports that as many as 16.8% of confirmed cases of COVID-19 had vestibular symptoms [80]. Unfortunately, these reports lack detailed information on the nature and cause of the ailments. Dizziness and imbalance might simply be the result of the profound asthenia and fatigue often experienced by patients with COVID-19. A study of convalescent patients suggested that no clinically relevant signs of vestibular impairment occurred [81].

A few cases of the inflammation of labyrinth have been reliably documented during the COVID-19 pandemic. Acute labyrinthitis was described as an unusual presentation of COVID-19 with vomiting associated with rotational vertigo, peripheral vestibular nystagmus, and sudden SNHL as the initial symptoms of viral infection [76]. An inflammatory process can be proved by magnetic resonance imaging where vestibule and semicircular canals appear hyperintense on fluid-attenuated inversion recovery and on diffusion-weighted images with normal T1 sequences.

Oral corticosteroid therapy with physiotherapy rehabilitation has proven efficacy in acute COVID-19-related labyrinthitis and neuronitis vestibularis [77]. On the contrary, symptomatic management with anticholinergic, anti-emetics, and antihistamines to reduce the severity of symptoms may often not bring the expected improvement.

Vestibular symptoms usually appear one to four weeks after the beginning of infection but sometimes also weeks after testing negative for COVID-19. Occasionally, it appeared as the initial symptoms of COVID-19 infection [82]. Dizziness, tinnitus, and

OTOLARYNGOLOGIC MANIFESTATION OF COVID-19		
symptom	occurence	
HEARING, TINNITUS AND BALANCE DISORDERS		
SENSORINEURAL HEARING LOSS	7.6%	Almufarrij & Munro (2021)
OTALGIA	13.1%	Almufarrij & Munro (2021)
TINNITUS	14.8%	Almufarrij & Munro (2021)
VERTIGO	7.2%	Almufarrij & Munro (2021)
	16.8%	Mao (2020)
RHINOLOGIC SYMTPOM		
NASAL CONGESTION	2-12%	Czubak (2021)
	25.0%	Kaye (2020)
RHINORRHEA	2-7%	Czubak (2021)
	18.0%	Kaye (2020)
SENS OF SMELL		
LOSS OF SMELL	52.0%	Aziz (2021)
PHANTOSMIA	12.6%	J.R. Lechien (2020)
PAROSMIA	32.4%	J.R. Lechien (2020)
VOICE DISORDERS		
DYSPHONIA	26.0%	J.R. Lechien (2020)
	43.7%	Giovanna Cantarella (2021)
APHONIA	3.7%	J.R. Lechien (2020)

Figure 7.2   Otolaryngologic manifestation of COVID-19.

otalgia can persist from 4 to even more than 12 weeks and are referred to as "long COVID" symptoms [83].

COVID-induced peripheral nerve injury also can involve the facial nerve [84, 85]. It is certain that SARS-CoV-2 infection can involve several cranial nerves. This is evidenced by a case with overlapping manifestations from facial and vestibulocochlear nerve damage, including bilateral facial palsy, vertigo, nausea, vomiting, and SNHL [86]. The postulated pathogenesis of facial palsy includes direct infection injury, ischemia of the vasa nervorum, and local inflammation causing demyelination [87]. Complete facial nerve recovery can be achieved after treatment with intravenous steroids and immunoglobulins therapy.

It is difficult to judge which COVID-19-positive patients are predisposed to developing symptoms of the ear and facial nerve. The available information does not allow for linking the occurrence of ear symptoms with the presence of systemic comorbidities or with the severity of the course of COVID-19.

Whether in the inpatient or outpatient setting, COVID-19 should be considered in the differential diagnosis for patients presenting with these symptoms, irrespective of the presence of respiratory symptoms or hypoxia (Figure 7.2).

Gastrointestinal Manifestation of COVID-19

The pathophysiology of digestive system symptoms is not entirely clear, and few mechanisms have been suggested [88]. SARS-CoV-2 enters cells through the ACE2 receptor and may induce a cytopathic response [88]. ACE2 receptors are expressed in gastric and intestinal epithelial cell cytoplasm, in contrast with the esophagus epithelium [89]. Infiltration of SARS-CoV-2 by ACE2 receptors in the GI tract is confirmed by finding virus nucleocapsid protein in the gastric, duodenal, and rectal glandular cytoplasm [89].

Virus affinity to ACE2 receptors present on cells leads to a cytopathic effect, resulting in GI manifestations [88]. Another mechanism that plays a key role in the pathophysiology of SARS-CoV-2 is an inflammatory cytokine storm. Infection can lead to an inflammatory overreaction, with cytokines and chemokine release. The main inflammatory mediators in Sars-CoV-2 infections are interleukin-1B, interferon-т, interferon-γ inducible protein 10, and monocyte chemotactic protein 1 [90]. An inflammatory cytokine storm may lead to multiple organ insufficiency, including the digestive system. Damage of the gut–lung axis may lead to altered GI microbiota and drug-related harm. The intestinal microbiota produce butyric acid, which can inhibit cytokine storms. Some studies report dysbiosis (decreased *Lactobacillus*

and *Bifidobacterium*) during SARS-CoV-2 infections [88]. Disturbances in this area may reduce beneficial effects of intestinal microbiota, which could also decrease COVID-19 complications (Figure 7.3).

Liver damage in the course of COVID-19 is related with inflammatory immune response, drug cytotoxicity, and viral infection [88]. Direct viral infection is mediated by ACE2 receptors present on hepatocytes (2.6%), bile duct cells (59.7%), and liver endothelial cells [91, 92]. Direct infection of liver cells is confirmed by the presence of SARS genetic material in liver tissue. That direct infection leads to hepatic impaired function without fibrosis. Other causes could be hypoxic hepatitis and complications during mechanical ventilation (positive end-expiratory pressure) that cause hepatic congestion [93] (Figure 7.4).

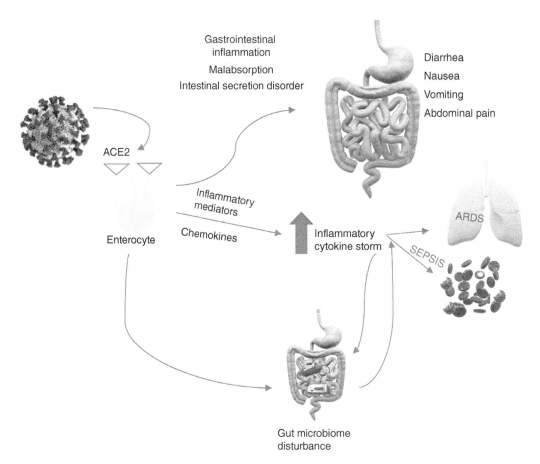

Figure 7.3 Mechanisms of gastrointestinal tract damage by SARS-CoV-2. ARDS, acute respiratory distress syndrome. Data are from Almufarrij and Munro [61], Mao et al. [39], Czubak et al. [43], Kaye et al. [41], Aziz et al. [38], Lechien et al. [30], and Cantarella et al. [54].

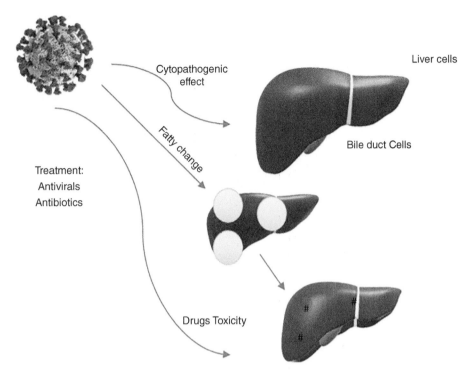

Figure 7.4 Hepatic injury by SARS-CoV-2.

GI symptoms are present in almost 50% of patients with SARS-CoV-2 as their chief complaint [94, 95]. Fewer than 10% of patients have only digestive symptoms without respiratory symptoms [94]. Therefore, clinicians must know that digestive symptoms may be the first indication of COVID-19, before respiratory symptoms, or may be the only presenting symptom of COVID-19 [94].

The main GI manifestations of COVID-19 include the following:

- Diarrhea (1.3–33.98%) [90, 94–103]
- Anorexia (1–83.8%) [90, 94–103]
- Nausea (1–10%) [89, 93–102]
- Vomiting (1–5%) [90, 94–103]
- Abdominal pain (1.94%) [90, 94–103]
- Possible upper or lower GI hemorrhage

Invasion of intestinal cells with SARS-CoV-2 can cause malabsorption and activation of the enteric nervous system [104]. Drugs used in treatment during SARS-CoV-2 infections may also provoke symptoms [105]. Antibiotics used for treating bacterial coinfection during COVID more often cause GI symptoms, especially diarrhea, than does no antibiotic therapy [105]. Antiviral treatment also may cause GI manifestations [105]. Patients who suffer GI symptoms have a worse prognosis and stay longer in the hospital than those without GI manifestations. This is probably the result of viral replication in the GI tract, which can promote severity of infection [106].

Hepatic injury is reported in 58–78% patients during SARS-CoV-2 infections with various degrees [107]. Laboratory tests may show the following:

- Increased aspartate aminotransferase and alanine aminotransferase levels
- Increased gamma-glutamyl transferase level
- Increased total bilirubin levels
- Decreased serum albumin
- Thrombocytopenia
- Prolonged prothrombin time

Ultrasonography may show the following:

- Hepatomegaly
- Fatty liver

There are associations between COVID-19 and prior liver disease [88]. Patients with hepatitis B virus infection and SARS-CoV-2 infection have worse clinical outcomes. This coinfection contributes to an increase of hepatitis B virus replication, and thus faster development of viral hepatitis and liver damage [96]. Other preexisting liver diseases, such as nonalcoholic fatty liver disease, steatohepatitis, and cirrhosis, significantly worsen SARS-CoV-2 infection [108]. Elevated alanine aminotransferase levels, thrombocytopenia, and decreased serum albumin concentration were correlated with a higher mortality rate [105]. Based on published data, it is not clear whether patients who are taking immunosuppressive medication for liver transplantation are more predisposed to development of severe COVID-19 [88, 109]. Others report that liver transplant recipients had worse COVID-19 symptoms than healthy patients [110]. The greatest risk may result from pretransplant and posttransplant comorbidities (e.g. renal insufficiency, asthma, hyperlipidemia, hypertension) [87, 102]. The American Association for the Study of Liver Diseases includes patients receiving immunosuppressant therapy as a high-risk group for severe COVID-19 [111].

GI infection with SARS-CoV-2 may provide a new fecal–oral transmission route [89]. More than 20% of patients with SARS-CoV-2 showed positive results for viral RNA in feces, even in those whose real-time reverse transcriptase-polymerase chain reaction from the respiratory tract had negative results. Testing for SARS-CoV-2 from feces can be considered for hospitalized patients, especially to exclude the risk for virus transmission to healthy patients with negative respiratory tract results [89].

Coronavirus and Pregnancy

Physiologic Changes and Effect of SARS-CoV-2 Infection

Physiologic and immunologic changes during pregnancy make women more vulnerable to infections of the respiratory tract. These adaptations include increased consumption of oxygen, decreased chest compliance, and immunologic alterations, especially related to T lymphocytes and that might exacerbate the transmission and clinical presentation of the virus [112]. Enhanced inflammatory symptoms and easier transmission of the virus during pregnancy can also be explained by a shift in T cell CD4$^+$ population toward Th2 lymphocytes over Th1 cells, resulting in a decrease of cellular immune response. In contrast, hormonal changes, such as increases in progesterone levels, may have beneficial effects on the response to SARS-CoV-2. Immunomodulatory properties of progesterone enable enhanced repair of lung tissue and may contribute to faster recovery after viral lung infections. Further studies are needed to confirm these traits [113].

COVID-19 infection creates the risk for not only respiratory failure but also of venous and arterial thromboembolic events. The mechanism includes previously mentioned dysregulation of the renin–angiotensin–aldosterone system, ACE2 activity, and oxidative stress damage. These components include overexpression of lectin-like oxidized low-density lipoprotein receptor 1, cyclooxygenase-2, and vascular endothelial growth factor in the endothelium, causing endothelial damage that is directly related to vascular coagulopathy [113]. During gestation, physiologic adaptation increases production of coagulative factors, such as thrombin, as well as fibrinolytic factors, including plasmin.

Because of the synergistic activity of the aforementioned factors, pregnant women infected with COVID-19 may need specific medical and prophylactic interventions [112].

General Symptoms of COVID-19 in Obstetric Patients

Clinical presentation of COVID-19 symptoms differs among obstetric patients. Based on the National Institute of Health Classification, the severity scale of COVID-19 includes:

- Asymptomatic infection (positive COVID-19 test result with no symptoms)
- Mild disease (flu-like symptoms)
- Moderate disease (lower respiratory disease tract with clinical assessment and oxygen saturation > 93%)
- Severe disease (increased RR, hypoxia, oxygen saturation < 93%, >50% of lung involvement on imaging)
- Critical disease (multiorgan failure, shock, respiratory failure) [114]

A majority of pregnant patients did not have symptoms of COVID-19. A cross-sectional systematic analysis, "Universal Screening for SARS-CoV-2 Infection Among Pregnant Women at Elmhurst Hospital Center" and PregCOV-19 Living Systematic Review, reported that the range of asymptomatic cases varies from 72% to 74% [115–117]. Figueiro-Filho et al. [118] reported that 74.1% of patients with symptoms manifested only mild signs of infection. An even higher percentage of pregnant patients with mild symptoms was observed in the work of Elshafeey et al. [119] – 95.6% (368/385) of infected patients – with only 3.6% (14) presenting with severe symptoms and 0.8% (3) assessed as critical cases. Finally, the study of Breslin et al. [120] demonstrated that the general pattern in symptom distribution was similar in groups of pregnant and nonpregnant women.

Clinical manifestations of maternal COVID-19 correspond to symptoms observed in the general population. Results of the PregCOV-19 Living Systematic Review, presented in the guidance of Royal College of Obstetricians and Gynaecologists, showed that the most common symptoms in a group of 64 000 pregnant women were as follows: cough (41%), fever (40%), dyspnea (21%), myalgia (19%), loss of sense of taste (14%), and diarrhea (8%) (Table 7.2) [121]. In this study, fever and myalgia were observed at a lower rate than in nonpregnant women [122].

Fox and Melka [123] reported emergence of anosmia in 27% of pregnant women. Evaluation of the excess frequency of vomiting, nausea, or fatigue may be limited in this group because pregnancy is also associated with these symptoms.

Despite similarities in clinical symptoms, frequency of hospital admission was significantly higher in pregnant (31.5%) than in nonpregnant (5.8%) women [124]. The risk for severe COVID-19 pneumonia in pregnant patients may be additionally enhanced by other comorbidities. Galang et al. [125] indicated that any one condition (underlying medical or pregnancy-related condition) escalates the risk for moderate-to-severe or critical COVID-19 infection by 25%. With the increasing number of accompanying factors, the risk for development of severe COVID-19 further increases – for two conditions by 52% and for three or more conditions by 200% [125]. Factors associated with increased risk for moderate-to-severe or critical COVID-19 are presented in Table 7.3.

Obstetric patients were more likely to be admitted to ICUs and receive ventilation, intubation, or extracorporeal membrane oxygenation [124, 126]. Pierce-Williams et al. [127] reported, in a group of females with critical disease, that 95% required intubation, 70% had acute respiratory distress syndrome, and 20% needed prone positioning.

As mentioned in the earlier discussion of pathophysiology, both infection with SARS-CoV-2 and time of gestation increase the risk for coagulation and thromboembolic events. Additional concerns include maternal mortality caused by thrombotic complications [128]. Although some studies minimize the increased risk for thrombosis in pregnant women in comparison with a nonpregnant group, current guidelines underline the role of thromboprophylaxis [129]. Low-molecular-weight heparin should be supplied to obstetric patients hospitalized because of

Table 7.2 Clinical manifestations of COVID infection: most common symptoms in pregnant patients.

Clinical manifestations	% of pregnant patients
Fever	40%
Cough	41%
Dyspnea	21%
Myalgia	19%
Loss sense of taste	14%
Diarrhea	8%

Source: Royal College of Obstetricians and Gynaecologists [121].

Table 7.3 Risk factors of moderate-to-severe or critical COVID-19 during pregnancy.

Age of 30–34 or 35–39 yr
Prepregnancy obesity
Chronic lung disease
Chronic hypertension
Cardiovascular disease
Pregestational diabetes mellitus
Gestational diabetes
Black/non-Hispanic race/ethnicity

Source: Galang et al. [125].

COVID-19 infection until 10 days after discharge. Moreover, during self-isolation, pregnant women should be investigated for the risk for venous thromboembolism and may require thromboprophylaxis on an individual basis [130]. Women with confirmed or suspected COVID-19 within six weeks of postpartum also should be considered for thromboprophylaxis.

Impact of COVID-19 on Gestation: Maternal and Neonatal Outcomes

Complications of maternal COVID-19 influence both the patient and the fetus. One of the adverse effects associated with the infection is increased risk for preterm labor in patients [121]. As per a national cohort study using the UK Obstetric Surveillance System, one in five symptomatic women had preterm birth, whereas in the case of asymptomatic patients, the rate was lower at 9%. Its cause is typically iatrogenic rather than spontaneous, so prophylactic cervical-length measurement is not necessary. Rodrigues et al. [131] provided similar results: from 2059 published pregnant cases, 2015 were live births and 23% of these occurred as preterm birth (<37 weeks). The number of abortions and stillbirths was significantly lower, 42 and 21 cases, respectively [131]. One adverse effect of maternal COVID-19 infection connected to preterm birth is low birthweight (<2500 g). Occurrence of low birthweight may derive from preplacental hypoxia as a result of infection of the mothers' lower respiratory tract. This may promote antiangiogenic and proinflammatory activity that eventually leads to placenta insufficiency and consequently fetal hypoxia and distress [132].

Altered placental function was observed in even asymptomatic or mildly symptomatic obstetric patients, possibly indicating an independent effect of COVID-19 on subclinical placenta injury. Changes included maternal vascular malperfusion with retroplacental hematomas, hyperplasia of distal villi, atherosis/fibrinoid necrosis, or vessel ectasia. Furthermore, histopathologic evaluation indicated features of fetal vascular malperfusion: chorioangiosis, intramural fibrin deposition, or thrombi in the fetal vessels [133].

Earlier-mentioned injury of placenta and ACE2 expression caused by SARS-CoV-2 predispose to pre-eclampsia independently of COVID-19 symptoms appearance. As presented in the study, 80% of patients with pre-eclampsia were asymptomatic, whereas the rest presented mild symptoms. Seventy percent (14/20) of the examined pregnant women met criteria of severe hypertensive disorders of pregnancy, including patients with severe pre-eclampsia (9/14), eclampsia (2/14), and HELLP syndrome (5/14) [134]. In addition, severe SARS-CoV-2 infection may contribute to occurrence of a pre-eclampsia-like syndrome that can be misdiagnosed as pre-eclampsia because of overlapping symptoms. Differentiation between the conditions might be challenging yet possible by assessment of uterine artery pulsatility index, lactate dehydrogenase, and angiogenic factors (soluble fms-like tyrosine kinase-1/placental growth factor). Unlike pre-eclampsia, patients with pre-eclampsia-like syndrome recover after respiratory function improves, and the condition may not result in early delivery [135].

Vertical Transmission and Possible Fetal Complications

Evidence for possible vertical transmission remains unclear and needs further investigation. In an analysis of 31 COVID-19-positive pregnant women, no nucleic acid of SARS-CoV-2 was present in RT-PCR tests of placenta and neonatal throats [136]. Similarly, the study of Schwartz [137] supported no vertical transmission of COVID because no offspring of 38 obstetric patients were COVID-19 positive. In contrast, Rodrigues et al. [131] presented 67 intrauterine samples with 11.9% of placentas, 1.8% of amniotic fluid, and 2.4% umbilical cord blood samples positive for COVID-19. Regarding neonates, positive RT-PCR for SARS-CoV-2 was observed in 3% (n = 61) of cases, whereas of 71 serum samples, 4 (6%) were reactive for IgM and 7 (10%) for IgG antibodies [131]. Complications in newborns resulting from maternal COVID-19 infections included fetal distress (25%) with a low rate of neonatal asphyxia (1.6%). General outcome of neonates was favorable as 95% were born in good health [121]. Admission of newborns to the ICU was estimated to be 11.3%, yet the indications of the admissions were not identified [138]. A minority of neonates presented mild COVID-19-related symptoms, yet the explanation of their emergence remained unclear [139].

COVID-19 and Delivery

While planning delivery of pregnant woman with SARS-CoV-2 infection, multiple factors, such as clinical symptoms, age of gestation, and fetal condition, should be evaluated. If maternal oxygenation is sustained at an optimal level, COVID-19 should not indicate a need for termination of pregnancy [121]. In stable patients, mode of delivery is optional because choice between cesarean section and vaginal delivery does not increase the risk for mother or neonate. For symptomatic patients, cardiotocography monitoring should be used during the birth [140]. In contrast, worsening of clinical symptoms, including respiratory distress (with an RR ≥ 30 breaths/min), decrease in oxygen saturation (≤93%) or PaO_2/FiO_2 (≤300 mmHg), and critical illness with respiratory failure or shock, require early delivery without regard to the gestational age via cesarean section. Epidural anesthesia may be used, whereas for intubated patients with severe pneumonia, general anesthesia may be applied [141].

Breastfeeding

Undoubtedly, the best form of nourishing a baby is breastfeeding. Currently, there is no evidence that breastfeeding could pose a threat to the child because it has not been proved that the virus passes into breast milk. Milk tests were carried out both in the acute phase of the patient's infection and in convalescence [142, 143]. However, it has been proved that milk contains beneficial IgM and IgG antibodies in mothers with COVID-19, as well as macrophages, immunoglobulins, and complement, which additionally provide antiviral protection [144]. Breastfeeding protects the newborn against respiratory tract infection, the main route of infection for SARS-CoV-2. In the first six months of life, the number of feverish illnesses is significantly reduced in breastfed infants [145]. There is a high probability that infants can obtain passive immunization through this type of nutrition. However, protective measures should be taken for the newborn. During the infectious period, mothers should use a protective mask during feeding and thoroughly wash her hands and the areas of contact with the baby [146].

Vaccination

Vaccination during pregnancy is safe and may prevent both mother and the fetus from serious consequences of COVID-19. Pregnant women should consult with a gynecologist for assessment of infection risk [147]. Pregnant females were not included in vaccine licensing trials. Yet, in the Pfizer trial, 23 pregnant women were inadvertently exposed (12 vaccine and 11 placebo). In Moderna trials with 13 exposed females (6 vaccine and 7 placebo), all pregnancies have proceeded without a proven negative effect of vaccination. Importantly, IgG antibodies produced during vaccination pass into breast milk [148].

Despite obvious beneficial effects of vaccination, postvaccination menstrual irregularities have been reported, including vaginal hemorrhages. Moreover, symptoms appeared in twice as many of those vaccinated with the AstraZeneca vaccine than with the Pfizer vaccine (643 vs. 315, respectively) [149]. Considerable blood loss may result from thrombocytopenia and eventually increase the risk for hemorrhages and clots. Physicians should encourage women to report any adverse effects of vaccination [149].

Urologic Manifestations of COVID-19

Kidneys

With SARS-CoV-2 infection, disturbances in renal function are frequently observed. Depending on the series, the incidence of acute kidney injury (AKI) ranges from 0.1% to 46% in infected individuals. The highest percentages of AKI are for those who required an ICU stay. This is a significant problem due to the worse prognosis for these patients and the approximately three times higher risk for death [102, 150, 151].

In COVID-19 infection, renal tubules are most often damaged, causing acute kidney damage. Altered renal parameters include increased blood creatinine, increased levels of urea in urine, and proteinuria. The mechanism of kidney damage is not fully understood. It is not known whether the kidney damage is caused by a systemic inflammatory process or by direct infection by the virus.

Due to the high expression of ACE2 and TMPRSS2 receptors in kidney cells, they are a potential target of the virus, which needs these factors to enter cells. Notably, the expression level is 100 times higher than in lung tissue. Postmortem microscopy, which was performed on 26 patients with confirmed AKI during the course of infection, showed that microscopic lesions characterized kidney damage in most cases, and viral RNA particles were detected in both the glomerular and the tubular compartments [152].

During the course of the infection, some patients suffer from respiratory failure or heart failure associated with insufficient oxygenation of the body and its organs. The kidneys are extremely susceptible to damage in the event of hypoxia or ischemia [153].

Another reason may be the systemic immune response induced by viruses during septic shock, when immune cells in tissues and organs secrete proinflammatory cytokines in response to the infection. A cytokine storm can cause endothelial damage, apoptosis, damage to the cytoskeleton of podocytes, or changes in renal tubules.

In addition, a state of hypercoagulability occurs and frequently also rhabdomyolysis, which can also impair kidney function. All of these factors, either individually or together, can contribute to high rates of AKI [154].

Kidney transplantation is a risky procedure in the era of a pandemic. High rates of AKI have been observed in transplant patients who contracted COVID-19. It has been observed that immunosuppressive therapy taken by this group of patients may contribute to the body's impaired response to infection and persistent viral replication [155].

Genital and Lower Urinary Tract Infection

There are many reports on the emergence of symptoms of lower urinary tract infections and the reproductive system in men infected with SARS-CoV-2. At the end of 2020, in a study of 575 hospitalized patients with a positive PCR test result, both in the acute phase of viral infection and in the convalescence phase, as many as 50 patients had lower urinary tract symptoms (de novo). The most common signs were pain, swelling, or discomfort in the scrotal area. Ultrasound examination showed 10 cases of acute epididymitis, 7 cases of acute epididymitis, and 16 cases of acute testicular

inflammation, including epididymis. It is not entirely clear whether these conditions were caused directly by viral infection or by a systemic reaction [156–158].

Outside of type II alveolar epithelial cells, renal tubular and intestinal epithelial cells, smooth muscle cells of blood vessels and cardiomyocytes, significant ACE2 receptor expression occurs in the cells of the lower urinary tract and the male reproductive system, especially in the testes. Higher ACE2 expression may be responsible for a higher level of infection severity; therefore, acute lung and heart muscle damage is often observed in patients during COVID-19 infection [159, 160]. It can be assumed that both urinary and genital systems in men are at risk for viral entry, which may lead to local infection and damage within the cells and, as a consequence, disruption of the functioning of the relevant organs.

Disorders of Genital Organ Function

Erectile dysfunction, as well as priapism, may occur as complications of SARS-CoV-2 infection. Male erectile dysfunction may be short term or long lasting. There is currently no information on how long the virus might affect erectile function and whether it acts directly in the tissue of the reproductive organs through disrupted endothelial function. In two individuals who had COVID-19, virus particles were detected in tissues taken from the sexual organ during surgery. In addition, reduced concentrations of endothelial nitric oxide synthase 3, which is responsible for the synthesis of vascular nitric oxide, was detected [161, 162].

Nitric oxide is one of the factors responsible for the erectile process, and it has many functions, but the most important seems to be the regulation of smooth muscle tone and blood flow in blood vessels. Thus, the reduced amount of nitric oxide may account for the observed dysfunctions of this organ [163, 164].

There are also instances when priapism has occurred during infection with the SARS-CoV-2 virus; that is, a long-lasting, painful erection lasting at least four hours, which is not related to sexual arousal. It is a rare condition that is an emergency and requires immediate care. Tissue ischemic changes begin as early as 12 hours after the onset of symptoms, and after approximately 48 hours, irreversible tissue necrosis and the development of permanent impotence develops [165, 166]. The reported cases of this rare disease are most likely related to thromboembolic events caused by the prothrombotic state during SARS-CoV-2 infection [167–169].

Infertility

Any systemic infection with fever may affect spermatogenesis and reduce its efficiency. In SARS-CoV-2 infection, there are more mechanisms that are likely to disrupt this process. It is currently unknown whether this is a short-term problem or a potentially permanent one [170]. This question requires more research, but also increased attention to the problem of infertility after infection.

The testis is one of the organs in whose cells there is a significant expression of ACE2 and TMPRSS2, which are receptors for SARS-CoV-2. Importantly, the degree of expression in the testis is higher than that of type 2 pneumocytes found in lung tissue [171]. There are many potential points where spermatogenesis may be disrupted in the event of COVID-19. Cells directly responsible for spermatogenesis, that is, spermatogonia and Sertoli cells, as well as Leydig cells, which produce testosterone and thus may have an indirect effect on fertility, can be attacked by the virus [172, 173]. SARS-CoV-2 interferes with the expression of ACE2, which regulates sperm motility and function [174]. In patients with infection, there is a high probability that in the early stage of the disease, the luteinizing hormone–testosterone gonadal axis was disturbed as a result of reduced testosterone secretion by the testes, which suggests an influence of the infection directly on Leydig cells [175].

Generalized infection during which proinflammatory cytokine release occurs may disrupt spermatogenesis. The sperm production process is protected against cytotoxic or autoimmune factors by Sertoli cells, which are involved in the formation of the so-called epithelial barrier between the nucleus and the circulating blood. Damage to Sertoli cells occurs during COVID-19, potentially disrupting spermatogenesis [176, 177].

Along with the earlier-described cell changes, formation of anti-sperm antibodies (ASAs) occurs. Both the damaged blood–nucleus barrier and the testicular inflammation can cause the immune system to produce ASAs, which can negatively affect fertility. Individuals with positive ASA results have a significantly reduced concentration of sperm in the ejaculate and reduced sperm mobility [178]. Taking into account all these mechanisms, in a male patient after SARS-CoV-2 infection, it may be useful to assess the sperm DNA fragmentation index, an indicator of damage to the sperm genetic material. Many of the diseases that trigger systemic inflammatory reactions also affect DNA fragmentation index. In the case of COVID-19, this indicator can also be used to evaluate infertility [179, 180].

References

1 Wu, Z. and McGoogan, J.M. (2020). Characteristics of and important lessons from the coronavirus disease 2019 (COVID-19) outbreak in China: summary of a report of 72 314 cases from the Chinese Center for Disease Control and Prevention. *JAMA* 323 (13): 1239–1242. https://doi.org/10.1001/jama.2020.2648.

2 Iba, T., Connors, J.M., and Levy, J.H. (2020). The coagulopathy, endotheliopathy, and vasculitis of COVID-19. *Inflamm. Res.* 69: 1181–1189. https://doi.org/10.1007/s00011-020-01401-6.

3 Shang, J., Ye, G., Shi, K. et al. (2020). Structural basis of receptor recognition by SARS-CoV-2. *Nature* 581: 221–224. https://doi.org/10.1038/s41586-020-2179-y.

4 Buja, L.M., Wolf, D.A., Zhao, B. et al. (2020). The emerging spectrum of cardiopulmonary pathology of the coronavirus disease 2019 (COVID-19): report of 3 autopsies from Houston, Texas, and review of autopsy findings from other United States cities. *Cardiovasc. Pathol.* 48: 107233. https://doi.org/10.1016/j.carpath.2020.107233.

5 Zhu, J., Ji, P., Pang, J. et al. (2020). Clinical characteristics of 3062 COVID-19 patients: a meta-analysis. *J. Med. Virol.* 92 (10): 1902–1914. https://doi.org/10.1002/jmv.25884.

6 Grant, M.C., Geoghegan, L., Arbyn, M. et al. (2020). The prevalence of symptoms in 24,410 adults infected by the novel coronavirus (SARS-CoV-2; COVID-19):

a systematic review and meta-analysis of 148 studies from 9 countries. *PLoS One* 15: e0234765. https://doi.org/10.1371/journal.pone.0234765.

7 Wang, D., Hu, B., Hu, C. et al. (2020). Clinical characteristics of 138 hospitalized patients with 2019 novel coronavirus-infected pneumonia in Wuhan, China. *JAMA* 323: 1061–1069. https://doi.org/10.1001/jama.2020.1585.

8 Lovato, A. and de Filippis, C. (2020). Clinical presentation of COVID-19: a systematic review focusing on upper airway symptoms. Ear Nose *Throat J.* 99: 569–576. https://doi.org/10.1177/0145561320920762.

9 Giacomelli, A., Pezzati, L., Conti, F. et al. (2020). Self-reported olfactory and taste disorders in patients with severe acute respiratory coronavirus 2 infection: a cross-sectional study. *Clin. Infect. Dis.* 71 (15): 889–890. https://doi.org/10.1093/cid/ciaa330.

10 Ottestad, W., Seim, M., and Mæhlen, J.O. (2020). COVID-19 with silent hypoxemia. *Tidsskr. Nor. Laegeforen.* 140 (7) https://doi.org/10.4045/tidsskr.20.0299.

11 Gattinoni, L., Chiumello, D., Caironi, P. et al. (2020). COVID-19 pneumonia: different respiratory treatments for different phenotypes? *Intensive Care Med.* 46: 1099–1102. https://doi.org/10.1007/s00134-020-06033-2.

12 Bos, L.D.J. (2020). COVID-19-related acute respiratory distress syndrome: not so atypical. *Am. J. Respir. Crit. Care Med.* 202 (4): 622–624. https://doi.org/10.1164/rccm.202004-1423LE.

13 Hoskison, E.E. (2013). Olfaction, pheromones and life. *J. Laryngol. Otol.* 127: 1156–1159.

14 Landis, B.N., Stow, N.W., Lacroix, J.-S. et al. (2009). Olfactory disorders: the patients' view. *Rhinology* 47: 454–459.

15 Croy, I., Nordin, S., and Hummel, T. (2014). Olfactory disorders and quality of life – an updated review. *Chem. Senses* 39: 185–194.

16 Oleszkiewicz, A., Walliczek-Dworschak, U., Klötze, P. et al. (2016). Developmental changes in Adolescents' olfactory performance and significance of olfaction. *PLoS One* 11 (6): e0157560.

17 Seiden, A.M. (2004). Postviral olfactory loss. *Otolaryngol. Clin. N. Am.* 37 (6): 1159–1166. https://doi.org/10.1016/j.otc.2004.06.007.

18 Welge-Lüssen, A. and Wolfensberger, M. (2006). Olfactory disorders following upper respiratory tract infections. *Adv. Otorhinolaryngol.* 63: 125–132. https://doi.org/10.1159/000093758.

19 Damm, M., Temmel, A., Welge-Lüssen, A. et al. (2004). Riechstörungen. Epidemiologie und therapie in Deutschland, Österreich und der Schweiz. *HNO* 52 (2): 112–120. https://doi.org/10.1007/s00106-003-0877-z.

20 Eccles, R. (2005). Understanding the symptoms of the common cold and influenza. *Lancet Infect. Dis.* 5 (11): 718–725. https://doi.org/10.1016/S1473-3099(05)70270-X.

21 Welge-Leusen, A. and Hummel, T. (2014). *Management of smell and taste disorders.* Stuttgart: Thieme.

22 Portier, F., Faulcon, P., Lamblin, B., and Bonfils, P. (2000). Signs and symptoms, etiologies and clinical course of parosmia + in a series of 84 patients. *Ann. Otolaryngol. Chir. Cervicofac.* 117 (1): 12–18.

23 Dewa, C.S., Hoch, J.S., Nieuwenhuijsen, K. et al. (2019). Toward effective work accommodations for depression: examining the relationship between different combinations of depression symptoms and work productivity losses. *J. Occup. Environ. Med.* 61 (1): 75–80. https://doi.org/10.1097/JOM.0000000000001486.

24 Lerner, D. and Henke, R.M. (2008). What does research tell us about depression, job performance, and work productivity? *J. Occup. Environ. Med.* 50 (4): 401–410. https://doi.org/10.1097/JOM.0b013e31816bae50.

25 Philpott, C.M. and Boak, D. (2014). The impact of olfactory disorders in the United Kingdom. *Chem. Senses* 39 (8): 711–718.

26 Blomqvist, E.H., Brämerson, A., Stjärne, P., and Nordin, S. (2004). Consequences of olfactory loss and adopted coping strategies. *Rhinology* 42 (4): 189–194.

27 Parma, V., Ohla, K., Veldhuizen, M.G. et al. (2020). More than smell-COVID-19 is associated with severe impairment of smell, taste, and Chemesthesis. *Chem. Senses* 45 (7): 609–622. https://doi.org/10.1093/chemse/bjaa041.

28 Menni, C., Valdes, A.M., Freidin, M.B. et al. (2020). Real-time tracking of self-reported symptoms to predict potential COVID-19. *Nat. Med.* 26 (7):

1037–1040. https://doi.org/10.1038/
s41591-020-0916-2.

29 Gerkin, R.C., Ohla, K., Veldhuizen, M.G. et al. (2020).
Recent smell loss is the best predictor of COVID-19: a
preregistered, cross-sectional study. *medRxiv* https://
doi.org/10.1101/2020.07.22.20157263.

30 Lechien, J.R., Chiesa-Estomba, C.M., De Siati, D.R.
et al. (2020). Olfactory and gustatory dysfunctions
as a clinical presentation of mild-to-moderate
forms of the coronavirus disease (COVID-19): a
multicenter European study. *Eur. Arch.
Otorhinolaryngol.* 277 (8): 13. https://doi.
org/10.1007/s00405-020-05965-1.

31 Lechien, J.R., Chiesa-Estomba, C.M., Place, S. et al.
(2020). Clinical and epidemiological characteristics
of 1420 European patients with mild-to-moderate
coronavirus disease 2019. *J. Intern. Med.* 288:
335–344. https://doi.org/10.1111/joim.13089.

32 Eliezer, M., Hautefort, C., Hamel, A.L. et al. (2020).
Sudden and complete olfactory loss of function as a
possible symptom of COVID-19. *JAMA Otolaryngol.
Head Neck Surg.* 146 (7): 674–675. https://doi.
org/10.1001/jamaoto.2020.0832.

33 Hopkins, C., Alanin, M., Philpott, C. et al. (2021).
Management of new onset loss of sense of smell
during the COVID-19 pandemic – BRS consensus
guidelines. *Clin. Otolaryngol.* 46: 16–22. https://doi.
org/10.1111/coa.13636.

34 Hopkins, C., Surda, P., and Nirmal, K.B. (2020).
Presentation of new onset anosmia during the
covid-19 pandemic. *Rhinology* 58 (3): 295–298.
https://doi.org/10.4193/Rhin20.116.

35 Lechien, J.R., Hopkins, C., and Saussez, S. (2020).
Sniffing out the evidence; It's now time for public
health bodies recognize the link between COVID-19
and smell and taste disturbance. *Rhinology* 48:
402–403. https://doi.org/10.4193/Rhin20.159.

36 AAO-HNS: Anosmia, hyposmia, and dysgeusia
symptoms of coronavirus disease. American
Academy of Otolaryngology-Head and Neck Surgery
(2020). https://www.entnet.org/content/aao-hns-
anosmia-hyposmia-and-dysgeusia-symptoms-
coronavirus-disease (accessed 18 May 2021).

37 Whitcroft, K.L. and Hummel, T. (2020). Olfactory
dysfunction in COVID-19: diagnosis and
management. *JAMA* 323 (24): 2512–2514. https://
doi.org/10.1001/jama.2020.8391.

38 Aziz, M., Goyal, H., Haghbin, H. et al. (2021). The
association of "loss of smell" to COVID-19: a
systematic review and meta-analysis. *Am J Med Sci*
361 (2): 216–225. https://doi.org/10.1016/j.
amjms.2020.09.017.

39 Mao, L., Jin, H., Wang, M. et al. (2020). Neurologic
manifestations of hospitalized patients with
coronavirus disease 2019 in Wuhan, China. *JAMA
Neurol.* 77: 683–690. https://doi.org/10.1001/
jamaneurol.2020.1127.

40 Moein, S.T., Hashemian, S.M.R., Mansourafshar, B.
et al. (2020). Smell dysfunction: a biomarker for
COVID-19. *Int. Forum Allergy Rhinol.* 10 (8):
944–950. https://doi.org/10.1002/alr.22587.

41 Kaye, R., Chang, C.W.D., Kazahaya, K. et al. (2020).
COVID-19 anosmia reporting tool: initial findings.
Otolaryngol. Neck Surg. 163: 132–134. https://doi.
org/10.1177/0194599820922992.

42 Marchese-Ragona, R., Restivo, D.A., De Corso, E.
et al. (2020). Loss of smell in covid-19 patients: a
critical review with emphasis on the use of
olfactory tests. *Acta Otorhinolaryngol. Ital.* 40 (4):
241–247. https://doi.
org/10.14639/0392-100X-N0862.

43 Czubak, J., Stolarczyk, K., Orzeł, A. et al. (2021).
Comparison of the clinical differences between
COVID-19, SARS, influenza, and the common cold:
a systematic literature review. *Adv. Clin. Exp. Med.*
30 (1): 109–114. doi:10.17219/acem/129573.

44 Yan, C.H., Faraji, F., Prajapati, D.P. et al. (2020).
Association of chemosensory dysfunction and
Covid-19 in patients presenting with influenza-like
symptoms. *Int. Forum Allergy Rhinol.* 10: 806–813.
https://doi.org/10.1002/alr.22579.

45 Chiesa-Estomba, C.M., Lechien, J.R., Radulesco, T.
et al. (2020). Patterns of smell recovery in 751
patients affected by the COVID-19 outbreak. *Eur. J.
Neurol.* 27 (11): 2318–2321. https://doi.org/10.1111/
ene.14440.

46 World Health Organization (WHO) (2020). Clinical
management of severe acute respiratory infection
(SARI) when COVID-19 disease is suspected.
https://www.who.int/docs/default-source/
coronaviruse/clinical-management-of-novel-cov.
pdf (accessed 22 May 2021).

47 Al Aïn, S., Poupon, D., Hétu, S. et al. (2019). Smell
training improves olfactory function and alters

brain structure. *NeuroImage* 189: 45–54. https://doi.org/10.1016/j.neuroimage.2019.01.008.

48 Croy, I., Olgun, S., Mueller, L. et al. (2015). Peripheral adaptive filtering in human olfaction? Three studies on prevalence and effects of olfactory training in specific anosmia in more than 1600 participants. *Cortex* 73: 180–187. https://doi.org/10.1016/j.cortex.2015.08.018.

49 Hummel, T., Rissom, K., Reden, J. et al. (2009). Effects of olfactory training in patients with olfactory loss. *Laryngoscope* 119 (3): 496–499. https://doi.org/10.1002/lary.20101.

50 Oleszkiewicz, A., Hanf, S., Whitcroft, K.L. et al. (2018). Examination of olfactory training effectiveness in relation to its complexity and the cause of olfactory loss. *Laryngoscope* 128 (7): 1518–1522. https://doi.org/10.1002/lary.26985.

51 Dworkin, J.P. (2008). Laryngitis: types, causes, and treatments. *Otolaryngol. Clin. N. Am.* 41 (2): 419–436. https://doi.org/10.1016/j.otc.2007.11.011.

52 Jaworek, A.J., Earasi, K., Lyons, K.M. et al. (2018). Acute infectious laryngitis: a case series. *Ear Nose Throat J.* 97 (9): 306–313. https://doi.org/10.1177/014556131809700920.

53 Lechien, J.R., Chiesa-Estomba, C.M., Cabaraux, P. et al. (2020). Features of mild-to-moderate COVID-19 patients with dysphonia. *J. Voice* https://doi.org/10.1016/j.jvoice.2020.05.012.

54 Cantarella, G., Aldè, M., Consonni, D. et al. (2021). Prevalence of dysphonia in non hospitalized patients with COVID-19 in Lombardy, the Italian epicenter of the pandemic. *J. Voice* https://doi.org/10.1016/j.jvoice.2021.03.009.

55 Descamps, G., Verset, L., Trelcat, A. et al. (2020). Ace2 protein landscape in the head and neck region: the conundrum of SARS-CoV-2 infection. *Biology (Basel)* 9 (8): 235. https://doi.org/10.3390/biology9080235.

56 Saniasiaya, J., Kulasegarah, J., Narayanan, P. et al. (2021). New-onset dysphonia: A silent manifestation of COVID-19. *Ear Nose Throat J.* https://doi.org/10.1177/0145561321995008.

57 Amin, M.R. and Koufman, J.A. (2001). Vagal neuropathy after upper respiratory infection: a viral etiology? *Am. J. Otolaryngol.* 22 (4): 251–256. https://doi.org/10.1053/ajot.2001.24823.

58 Buselli, R., Corsi, M., Necciari, G. et al. (2020). Sudden and persistent dysphonia within the framework of COVID-19: the case report of a nurse. *Brain Behav. Immun. Heal.* 9: 100160. https://doi.org/10.1016/j.bbih.2020.100160.

59 Asiaee, M., Vahedian-azimi, A., Atashi, S.S. et al. (2020). Voice quality evaluation in patients with COVID-19: an acoustic analysis. *J. Voice* https://doi.org/10.1016/j.jvoice.2020.09.024.

60 Ye, W. and Xianyang, L. (2020). A novel coronavirus pneumonia case report from an ear, nose and throat clinic. *Laryngoscope* 130: 1106–1107.

61 Almufarrij, I. and Munro, K.J. (2021). One year on: an updated systematic review of SARS-CoV-2, COVID-19 and audio-vestibular symptoms. *Int. J. Audiol.* https://doi.org/10.1080/14992027.2021.1896793.

62 Fidan, V. (2020). New type of corona virus induced acute otitis media in adult, 102487. *Am. J. Otolaryngol.* 41: 102487.

63 Cui, C., Yao, Q.I., Zhang, D.I. et al. (2020). Approaching otolaryngology patients during the COVID-19 pandemic. *Otolaryngol. Head Neck Surg.* 163 (1): 121–131.

64 Cohen, B.E., Durstenfeld, A., and Roehm, P.C. (2014). Viral causes of hearing loss: a review for hearing health professionals. *Trends Hear.* 18:233121651454136.

65 Uranaka, T., Kashio, A., Ueha, R. et al. (2021). Expression of ACE2, TMPRSS2, and furin in mouse ear tissue, and the implications for SARS-CoV-2 infection. *Laryngoscope* 131: e2013–e2017.

66 Kilic, O., Kalcioglu, M.T., Cag, Y. et al. (2020). Could sudden sensorineural hearing loss be the sole manifestation of COVID-19? An investigation into SARS-COV-2 in the aetiology of sudden sensorineural hearing loss. *Int. J. Infect. Dis.* 97: 208–211.

67 Sedaghat, Z. and Karimi, N. (2020). Guillain Barre syndrome associated with COVID-19 infection: a case report. *J. Clin. Neurosci.* 76: 233–235.

68 Wong, V. (1997). A neurophysiological study in children with miller fisher syndrome and Guillain-Barre syndrome. *Brain and Development* 19 (3): 197–204.

69 Degen, C., Lenarz, T., and Willenborg, K. (2020). Acute profound sensorineural hearing loss after COVID-19 pneumonia. *Mayo Clin. Proc.* 95: 1801–1803.

70 Lang, B., Hintze, J., and Conlon, B. (2020). Coronavirus disease 2019 and sudden sensorineural hearing loss. *J. Laryngol. Otol.* 134: 1026–1028.

71 Karimi-Galougahi, M., Naeini, A.S., Raad, N. et al. (2020). Vertigo and hearing loss during the COVID-19 pandemic – is there an association? *Acta Otorhinolaryngol. Ital.* 40: 463–465.

72 Chern, A., Famuyide, A.O., Moonis, G., and Lalwani, A.K. (2021). Bilateral sudden sensorineural hearing loss and Intralabyrinthine hemorrhage in a patient with COVID-19. *Otol. Neurotol.* 42 (1): e10–e14.

73 Dror, A.A., Kassis-Karayanni, N., Oved, A. et al. (2021). Auditory performance in recovered SARS-COV-2 patients. *Otol. Neurotol.* 42: 666–670. https://doi.org/10.1097/MAO.0000000000003037.

74 Fidan, V., Akin, O., and Koyuncu, H. (2021). Rised sudden sensorineural hearing loss during COVID-19 widespread. *Am. J. Otolaryngol.* 42 (5): 102996.

75 Koumpa, F.S., Forde, C.T., and Manjaly, J.G. (2020). Sudden irreversible hearing loss post COVID-19. *BMJ Case Rep.* 13: e238419. https://doi.org/10.1136/bcr-2020-238419.

76 Rhman, S.A. and Wahid, A.A. (2020). COVID-19 and sudden sensorineural hearing loss: a case report. *Otolaryngol. Case Rep.* 16: 100198.

77 Perret, M., Bernard, A., Rahmani, A. et al. (2021). Acute labyrinthitis revealing COVID-19. *Diagnostics (Basel)* 11 (3): 482.

78 Goddard, J.C. and Fayad, J.N. (2011). Vestibular neuritis. *Otolaryngol. Clin. N. Am.* 44: 361–365.

79 Saniasiaya, J. and Kulasegarah, J. (2021). Dizziness and COVID-19. *Ear Nose Throat J.* 100: 2930.

80 Mao, L., Jin, H., Wang, M. et al. (2020). Neurologic manifestation of hospitalized patients with coronavirus disease 2019 un Wuhan, China. *JAMA Neurol.* 77 (60): 683–690.

81 Gallus, R., Melis, A., Rizzo, D. et al. (2021). Audiovestibular symptoms and sequelae in COVID-19 patients. *J. Vestib. Res.* 31: 381–387.

82 Malayala, S.V., Mohan, G., Vasireddy, D., and Atluri, P. (2021). A case series of vestibular symptoms in positive or suspected COVID-19 patients. *Infez Med.* 29 (1): 117–122.

83 National Institute for Health and Care Excellence (2020). COVID-19 rapid guideline: Managing the long-term effects of COVID-19. www.nice.org.uk/guidance/ng188/resources/covid19-rapid-guideline-managing-the-longterm-effects-of-covid19-pdf-66142028400325.

84 Dinkin, M., Gao, V., and Kahan, J. (2020). COVID-19 presenting with ophthalmoparesis from cranial nerve palsy. *Neurology* 95 (5): 221–223.

85 Goh, Y., Beh, D., and Makmur, A. (2020). Pearls and oy-sters: facial nerve palsy as a neurological manifestation of Covid-19 infection. *Neurology* 95: 364–367.

86 Aasfara, J., Hajjij, A., Bensouda, H. et al. (2021). A unique association of bifacial weakness, paresthesia and vestibulocochlear neuritis as post-COVID-19 manifestation in pregnant women: a case report. *Pan. Afr. Med. J.* 38: 30.

87 Lima, M.A., Silva, M.T.T., Soares, C.N. et al. (2020). Peripheral facial nerve palsy associated with COVID-19. *J. Neurovirol.* 26: 941–944.

88 Lei, H.Y., Ding, Y.H., Nie, K. et al. (2021). Potential effects of SARS-CoV-2 on the gastrointestinal tract and liver. *Biomed. Pharmacother.* 133: 111064. https://doi.org/10.1016/j.biopha.2020.111064.

89 Xiao, F., Tang, M., Zheng, X. et al. (2020). Evidence for gastrointestinal infection of SARS-CoV-2. *Gastroenterology* 158 (6): 1831–1833.e3. doi:https://doi.org/10.1053/j.gastro.2020.02.055.

90 Huang, C., Wang, Y., Li, X. et al. (2020). Clinical features of patients infected with 2019 novel coronavirus in Wuhan, China. *Lancet* 395 (10223): 497–506. https://doi.org/10.1016/S0140-6736(20)30183-5.

91 Zhou, F., Yu, T., Du, R. et al. (2020). Clinical course and risk factors for mortality of adult inpatients with COVID-19 in Wuhan, China: a retrospective cohort study. *Lancet* 395 (10229): 1054–1062. https://doi.org/10.1016/S0140-6736(20)30566-3.

92 Chai, X., Hu, L., Zhang, Y. et al. (2020). Specific ACE2 expression in cholangiocytes may cause liver damage after 2019-nCoV infection. *bioRxiv* https://doi.org/10.1101/2020.02.03.931766M.

93 Kukla, M., Skonieczna-Zydecka, K., Kotfis, K. et al. (2020). COVID-19, MERS and SARS with concomitant liver injury-systematic review of the existing literature. *J. Clin. Med.* 9 (5): 1420. https://doi.org/10.3390/jcm9051420.

94 Pan, L., Mu, M., Yang, P. et al. (2020). Clinical characteristics of COVID-19 patients with digestive symptoms in Hubei, China: a descriptive, cross-sectional, multicenter study. *Am. J. Gastroenterol.* 115 (5): 766–773. https://doi.org/10.14309/ajg.0000000000000620.

95 Lee, I.C., Huo, T.I., and Huang, Y.H. (2020). Gastrointestinal and liver manifestations in patients with COVID-19. *J. Chin. Med. Assoc.* 83 (6): 521–523. https://doi.org/10.1097/JCMA.0000000000000319.

96 Xu, L., Liu, J., Lu, M. et al. (2020). Liver injury during highly pathogenic human coronavirus infections. *Liver Int.* 40 (5): 998–1004. https://doi.org/10.1111/liv.14435.

97 Chen, N., Zhou, M., Dong, X. et al. (2020). Epidemiological and clinical characteristics of 99 cases of 2019 novel coronavirus pneumonia in Wuhan, China: a descriptive study. *Lancet* 395 (10223): 507–513. https://doi.org/10.1016/S0140-6736(20)30211-7.

98 Xu, X.W., Wu, X.X., Jiang, X.G. et al. (2020). Clinical findings in a group of patients infected with the 2019 novel coronavirus (SARS-Cov-2) outside of Wuhan, China: retrospective case series. *BMJ* 368: m606. https://doi.org/10.1136/bmj.m606.

99 Wu, J., Liu, J., Zhao, X. et al. (2020). Clinical characteristics of imported cases of coronavirus disease 2019 (COVID-19) in Jiangsu Province: a multicenter descriptive study. *Clin. Infect. Dis.* 71 (15): 706–712. https://doi.org/10.1093/cid/ciaa199.

100 Wang, D., Hu, B., Hu, C. et al. (2020). Clinical characteristics of 138 hospitalized patients with 2019 novel coronavirus-infected pneumonia in Wuhan, China. *JAMA* 323 (11): 1061–1069. https://doi.org/10.1001/jama.2020.1585.

101 Shi, H., Han, X., Jiang, N. et al. (2020). Radiological findings from 81 patients with COVID-19 pneumonia in Wuhan, China: a descriptive study. *Lancet Infect. Dis.* 20 (4): 425–434. https://doi.org/10.1016/S1473-3099(20)30086-4.

102 Yang, X., Yu, Y., Xu, J. et al. (2020). Clinical course and outcomes of critically ill patients with SARS-CoV-2 pneumonia in Wuhan, China: a single-centered, retrospective, observational study. *Lancet Respir. Med.* 8 (5): 475–481. https://doi.org/10.1016/S2213-2600(20)30079-5.

103 Mo, P., Xing, Y., Xiao, Y. et al. (2020). Clinical characteristics of refractory COVID-19 pneumonia in Wuhan, China. *Clin. Infect. Dis.* https://doi.org/10.1093/cid/ciaa270.

104 Lin, L., Jiang, X., Zhang, Z. et al. (2020). Gastrointestinal symptoms of 95 cases with SARS-CoV-2 infection. *Gut* 69 (6): 997–1001. https://doi.org/10.1136/gutjnl-2020-321013.

105 Hamming, I., Timens, W., Bulthuis, M.L. et al. (2004). Tissue distribution of ACE2 protein, the functional receptor for SARS coronavirus. A first step in understanding SARS pathogenesis. *J. Pathol.* 203 (2): 631–637. https://doi.org/10.1002/path.1570.

106 Zhou, J., Li, C., Zhao, G. et al. (2017). Human intestinal tract serves as an alternative infection route for Middle East respiratory syndrome coronavirus. *Sci. Adv.* 3 (11): eaao4966. https://doi.org/10.1126/sciadv.aao4966.

107 Guan, W., Ni, Z., Hu, Y. et al. (2020). Clinical characteristics of coronavirus disease 2019 in China. *N. Engl. J. Med.* 382 (18): 1708–1720. https://doi.org/10.1056/nejmoa2002032.

108 Singh, S. and Khan, A. (2020). Clinical characteristics and outcomes of coronavirus disease 2019 among patients with preexisting liver disease in the United States: a multicenter research network study. *Gastroenterology* 159 (2): 768–771. e3. doi:https://doi.org/10.1053/j.gastro.2020.04.064.

109 Bhoori, S., Rossi, R.E., Citterio, D., and Mazzaferro, V. (2020). COVID-19 in long-term liver transplant patients: preliminary experience from an Italian transplant Centre in Lombardy. *Lancet Gastroenterol. Hepatol.* 5 (6): 532–533. https://doi.org/10.1016/S2468-1253(20)30116-3.

110 Huang, J.F., Zheng, K.I., George, J. et al. (2020). Fatal outcome in a liver transplant recipient with COVID-19. *Am. J. Transplant.* 20 (7): 1907–1910. https://doi.org/10.1111/ajt.15909.

111 Fix, O.K., Hameed, B., Fontana, R.J. et al. (2020). Clinical best practice advice for hepatology and liver transplant providers during the COVID-19 pandemic: AASLD expert panel consensus statement. *Hepatology* 72 (1): 287–304. https://doi.org/10.1002/hep.31281.

112 Wenling, Y., Junchao, Q., Xiao, Z., and Ouyang, S. (2020). Pregnancy and COVID-19: management and challenges. *Rev. Inst. Med. Trop. Sao Paulo* 62: e62.

113 Wastnedge, E.A.N., Reynolds, R.M., van Boeckel, S.R. et al. (2021). Pregnancy and COVID-19. *Physiol. Rev.* 101 (1): 303–318. https://doi.org/10.1152/physrev.00024.2020.

114 Ali, M.A.M. and Spinler, S.A. (2021). COVID-19 and thrombosis: from bench to bedside. *Trends Cardiovasc. Med.* 31 (3): 143–160.

115 Society for Maternal-Fetal Medicine. Management considerations for pregnant patients with COVID-19 (2021). https://s3.amazonaws.com/cdn.smfm.org/media/2336/SMFM_COVID_Management_of_COVID_pos_preg_patients_4-30-20_final.pdf (accessed 13 May 2021).

116 Geng, M.J., Wang, L.P., Ren, X. et al. (2021). Risk factors for developing severe COVID-19 in China: an analysis of disease surveillance data. *Infect. Dis. Poverty* 10 (1): 48.

117 Maru, S., Patil, U., Carroll-Bennett, R. et al. (2020). Universal screening for SARS-CoV-2 infection among pregnant women at Elmhurst hospital center, Queens, New York. *PLoS One* 15 (12): e0238409.

118 Figueiro-Filho, E.A., Yudin, M., and Farine, D. (2020). COVID-19 during pregnancy: an overview of maternal characteristics, clinical symptoms, maternal and neonatal outcomes of 10,996 cases described in 15 countries. *J. Perinat. Med.* 48 (9): 900–911.

119 Elshafeey, F., Magdi, R., Hindi, N. et al. (2020). A systematic scoping review of COVID-19 during pregnancy and childbirth. *Int. J. Gynaecol. Obstet.* 150 (1): 47–52.

120 Breslin, N., Baptiste, C., Gyamfi-Bannerman, C. et al. (2020). Coronavirus disease 2019 infection among asymptomatic and symptomatic pregnant women: two weeks of confirmed presentations to an affiliated pair of New York City hospitals. *Am. J. Obstet. Gynecol. MFM* 2 (2): 100118.

121 Royal College of Obstetricians and Gynaecologists. Coronavirus (COVID-19) infection in pregnancy (2021). https://www.rcog.org.uk/globalassets/documents/guidelines/2021-11-02-coronavirus-covid-19-infection-in-pregnancy-v14.1.pdf (accessed 22 May 2021).

122 Allotey, J., Stallings, E., Bonet, M. et al. (2020). Clinical manifestations, risk factors, and maternal and perinatal outcomes of coronavirus disease 2019 in pregnancy: living systematic review and meta-analysis. *BMJ* 370: m3320.

123 Fox, N.S. and Melka, S. (2020). COVID-19 in pregnant women: case series from one large New York City obstetrical practice. *Am. J. Perinatol.* 37 (10): 1002–1004.

124 Ellington, S., Strid, P., Tong, V.T. et al. (2020). Characteristics of women of reproductive age with laboratory-confirmed SARS-CoV-2 infection by pregnancy status – United States, January 22 June 7, 2020. *MMWR Morb. Mortal. Wkly Rep.* 69 (25): 769–775.

125 Galang, R.R., Newton, S.M., Woodworth, K.R. et al. (2021). Risk factors for illness severity among pregnant women with confirmed SARS-CoV-2 infection – surveillance for emerging threats to mothers and babies network, 22 state, local, and territorial health departments, March 29, 2020 -March 5, 2021. *Clin. Infect. Dis.* 73 (Suppl 1): 17–23.

126 Collin, J., Byström, E., Carnahan, A., and Ahrne, M. (2020). Public Health Agency of Sweden's brief report: Pregnant and postpartum women with severe acute respiratory syndrome coronavirus 2 infection in intensive care in Sweden. *Acta Obstet. Gynecol. Scand.* 99 (7): 819–822.

127 Pierce-Williams, R.A.M., Burd, J., Felder, L. et al. (2020). Clinical course of severe and critical coronavirus disease 2019 in hospitalized pregnancies: a United States cohort study. *Am. J. Obstet. Gynecol. MFM* 2 (3): 100134.

128 Ahmed, I., Azhar, A., Eltaweel, N., and Tan, B.K. (2020). First COVID-19 maternal mortality in the UK associated with thrombotic complications. *Br. J. Haematol.* 190 (1): e37–e38.

129 D'Souza, R., Malhamé, I., Teshler, L. et al. (2020). A critical review of the pathophysiology of thrombotic complications and clinical practice recommendations for thromboprophylaxis in pregnant patients with COVID-19. *Acta Obstet. Gynecol. Scand.* 99 (9): 1110–1120.

130 Khodamoradi, Z., Boogar, S., Shirazi, F. et al. (2020). COVID-19 and acute pulmonary embolism in postpartum patient. *Emerg. Infect. Dis.* 26 (8): 1937–1939.

131 Rodrigues, C., Baía, I., Domingues, R., and Barros, H. (2020). Pregnancy and breastfeeding during

COVID-19 pandemic: a systematic review of published pregnancy cases. *Front. Public Health* 8: 558144.

132 Smith, V., Seo, D., Warty, R. et al. (2020). Maternal and neonatal outcomes associated with COVID-19 infection: a systematic review. *PLoS One* 15 (6): e0234187.

133 Jaiswal, N., Puri, M., Agarwal, K. et al. (2021). COVID-19 as an independent risk factor for subclinical placental dysfunction. *Eur. J. Obstet. Gynecol. Reprod. Biol.* 259: 7–11.

134 Coronado-Arroyo, J.C., Concepción-Zavaleta, M.J., Zavaleta-Gutiérrez, F.E., and Concepción-Urteaga, L.A. (2021). Is COVID-19 a risk factor for severe preeclampsia? Hospital experience in a developing country. *Eur. J. Obstet. Gynecol. Reprod. Biol.* 256: 502–503.

135 Mendoza, M., Garcia-Ruiz, I., Maiz, N. et al. (2020). Pre-eclampsia-like syndrome induced by severe COVID-19: a prospective observational study. *BJOG* 127 (11): 1374–1380.

136 Karimi-Zarchi, M., Neamatzadeh, H., Dastgheib, S.A. et al. (2020). Vertical transmission of coronavirus disease 19 (COVID-19) from infected pregnant mothers to neonates: a review. *Fetal Pediatr. Pathol.* 39 (3): 246–250.

137 Schwartz, D.A. (2020). An analysis of 38 pregnant women with COVID-19, their newborn infants, and maternal-fetal transmission of SARS-CoV-2: maternal coronavirus infections and pregnancy outcomes. *Arch. Pathol. Lab. Med.* 144 (7): 799–805.

138 Diriba, K., Awulachew, E., and Getu, E. (2020). The effect of coronavirus infection (SARS-CoV-2, MERS-CoV, and SARS-CoV) during pregnancy and the possibility of vertical maternal-fetal transmission: a systematic review and meta-analysis. *Eur. J. Med. Res.* 25 (1): 39.

139 Shalish, W., Lakshminrusimha, S., Manzoni, P. et al. (2020). COVID-19 and neonatal respiratory care: current evidence and practical approach. *Am. J. Perinatol.* 37 (8): 780–791.

140 Ryan, G.A., Purandare, N.C., McAuliffe, F.M. et al. (2020). Clinical update on COVID-19 in pregnancy: a review article. *J. Obstet. Gynaecol. Res.* 46 (8): 1235–1245.

141 Qi, H., Luo, X., Zheng, Y. et al. (2020). Safe delivery for pregnancies affected by COVID-19. *BJOG* 127 (8): 927–929.

142 Wu, Y., Liu, C., Dong, L. et al. (2020). Coronavirus disease 2019 among pregnant Chinese women: case series data on the safety of vaginal birth and breastfeeding. *BJOG* 127 (9): 1109–1115.

143 Lackey, K.A., Pace, R.M., Williams, J.E. et al. (2020). SARS-CoV-2 and human milk: what is the evidence? *Matern. Child Nutr.* 16 (4): e13032.

144 Gao, X., Wang, S., Zeng, W. et al. (2020). Clinical and immunologic features among COVID-19-affected mother-infant pairs: antibodies to SARS-CoV-2 detected in breast milk. *New Microbes New Infect.* 37: 100752.

145 Maertens, K., De Schutter, S., Braeckman, T. et al. (2014). Breastfeeding after maternal immunisation during pregnancy: providing immunological protection to the newborn: a review. *Vaccine* 32 (16): 1786–1792.

146 Demers-Mathieu, V., Do, D.M., Mathijssen, G.B. et al. (2021). Difference in levels of SARS-CoV-2 S1 and S2 subunits- and nucleocapsid protein-reactive SIgM/IgM, IgG and SIgA/IgA antibodies in human milk. *J. Perinatol.* 41 (4): 850–859.

147 Zambrano, L.D., Ellington, S., Strid, P. et al. (2020). Update: characteristics of symptomatic women of reproductive age with laboratory-confirmed SARS-CoV-2 infection by pregnancy status – United States, January 22 October 3, 2020. *MMWR Morb. Mortal. Wkly Rep.* 69 (44): 1641–1647.

148 Rasmussen, S.A., Kelley, C.F., Horton, J.P., and Jamieson, D.J. (2021). Coronavirus disease 2019 (COVID-19) vaccines and pregnancy: what obstetricians need to know [published correction appears in Obstet Gynecol. 2021;137(5):962]. *Obstet. Gynecol.* 137 (3): 408–414.

149 Hunter, P.R. (2021). Thrombosis after covid-19 vaccination. *BMJ* 373: n958.

150 Malberti, F., Pecchini, P., Marchi, G., and Foramitti, M. (2020). When a nephrology ward becomes a COVID-19 ward: the Cremona experience. *J. Nephrol.* 33 (4): 625–628. https://doi.org/10.1007/s40620-020-00743-y.

151 Hassanein, M., Radhakrishnan, Y., Sedor, J. et al. (2020). COVID-19 and the kidney. *Cleve. Clin. J. Med.* 87 (10): 619–631. https://doi.org/10.3949/ccjm.87a.20072.

152 Su, H., Yang, M., Wan, C. et al. (2020). Renal histopathological analysis of 26 postmortem findings of patients with COVID-19 in China.

Kidney Int. 98 (1): 219–227. https://doi. org/10.1016/j.kint.2020.04.003.

153 Han, X. and Ye, Q. (2021). Kidney involvement in COVID-19 and its treatments. *J. Med. Virol.* 93: 1387–1395. https://doi.org/10.1002/jmv.26653.

154 Chong, W.H. and Saha, B.K. (2021). Relationship between severe acute respiratory syndrome coronavirus 2 (SARS-CoV-2) and the etiology of acute kidney injury (AKI). *Am J Med Sci* 361 (3): 287–296. https://doi.org/10.1016/j. amjms.2020.10.025.

155 Farouk, S.S., Fiaccadori, E., Cravedi, P., and Campbell, K.N. (2020). COVID-19 and the kidney: what we think we know so far and what we don't. *J. Nephrol.* 33 (6): 1213–1218. https://doi.org/10.1007/ s40620-020-00789-y.

156 Creta, M., Sagnelli, C., Celentano, G. et al. (2021). SARS-CoV-2 infection affects the lower urinary tract and male genital system: a systematic review. *J. Med. Virol.* 93 (5): 3133–3142. https://doi. org/10.1002/jmv.26883.

157 Bourgonje, A.R., Abdulle, A.E., Timens, W. et al. (2020). Angiotensin-converting enzyme 2 (ACE2), SARS-CoV-2 and the pathophysiology of coronavirus disease 2019 (COVID-19). *J. Pathol.* 251 (3): 228–248. https://doi.org/10.1002/path.5471.

158 Chen, Y., Guo, Y., Pan, Y., and Zhao, Z.J. (2020). Structure analysis of the receptor binding of 2019-nCoV. *Biochem. Biophys. Res. Commun.* 525 (1): 135–140. https://doi.org/10.1016/j. bbrc.2020.02.071.

159 Zou, X., Chen, K., Zou, J. et al. (2020). Single-cell RNA-seq data analysis on the receptor ACE2 expression reveals the potential risk of different human organs vulnerable to 2019-nCoV infection. *Front. Med.* 14 (2): 185–192. https://doi. org/10.1007/s11684-020-0754-0.

160 Kashi, A.H., De la Rosette, J., Amini, E. et al. (2020). Urinary viral shedding of COVID-19 and its clinical associations: a systematic review and meta-analysis of observational studies. *Urol. J.* 17 (5): 433–441. https://doi.org/10.22037/uj.v16i7.6248.

161 Kresch, E., Achua, J., Saltzman, R. et al. (2021). COVID-19 endothelial dysfunction can cause erectile dysfunction: histopathological, immunohistochemical, and ultrastructural study of the human penis. *World J. Mens Health* 39: 466–469. https://doi.org/10.5534/wjmh.210055.

162 Barbosa, L.C., Gonçalves, T.L., de Araujo, L.P. et al. (2021). Endothelial cells and SARS-CoV-2: an intimate relationship. *Vasc. Pharmacol.* 137: 106829. https://doi.org/10.1016/j. vph.2021.106829.

163 Förstermann, U. and Münzel, T. (2006). Endothelial nitric oxide synthase in vascular disease: from marvel to menace. *Circulation* 113 (13): 1708–1714. https://doi.org/10.1161/ CIRCULATIONAHA.105.602532.

164 Dean, R.C. and Lue, T.F. (2005). Physiology of penile erection and pathophysiology of erectile dysfunction. *Urol. Clin. North Am.* 32 (4): 379-v. https://doi.org/10.1016/j.ucl.2005.08.007.

165 Podolej, G.S. and Babcock, C. (2017). Emergency department management of priapism. *Emerg. Med. Pract.* 19 (1): 1–16.

166 Silverman, M.L., VanDerVeer, S.J., and Donnelly, T.J. (2021). Priapism in COVID-19: a thromboembolic complication. *Am. J. Emerg. Med.* 45: 686.e5–686.e6. https://doi.org/10.1016/j. ajem.2020.12.072.

167 Lamamri, M., Chebbi, A., Mamane, J. et al. (2021). Priapism in a patient with coronavirus disease 2019 (COVID-19). *Am. J. Emerg. Med.* 39: 251.e5–251.e7. https://doi.org/10.1016/j.ajem.2020.06.027.

168 Addar, A., Al Fraidi, O., Nazer, A. et al. (2021). Priapism for 10 days in a patient with SARS-CoV-2 pneumonia: a case report. *J. Surg. Case Rep.* 2021 (4):rjab020. doi:https://doi.org/10.1093/jscr/ rjab020.

169 Lam, G., McCarthy, R., and Haider, R. (2020). A peculiar case of priapism: the hypercoagulable state in patients with severe COVID-19 infection. *Eur. J. Case Rep. Intern. Med.* 7 (8): 001779. https://doi. org/10.12890/2020_001779.

170 Bendayan, M., Robin, G., Hamdi, S. et al. (2021). COVID-19 in men: with or without virus in semen, spermatogenesis may be impaired. *Andrologia* 53 (1): e13878. https://doi.org/10.1111/ and.13878.

171 Fan, C., Lu, W., Li, K. et al. (2021). ACE2 expression in kidney and testis may cause kidney and testis infection in COVID-19 patients. *Front. Med. (Lausanne)* 7: 563893. https://doi.org/10.3389/ fmed.2020.563893.

172 Illiano, E., Trama, F., and Costantini, E. (2020). Could COVID-19 have an impact on male fertility?

Andrologia 52 (6): e13654. https://doi.org/10.1111/and.13654.

173 Zirkin, B.R. and Papadopoulos, V. (2018). Leydig cells: formation, function, and regulation. *Biol. Reprod.* 99 (1): 101–111. https://doi.org/10.1093/biolre/ioy059.

174 Pan, P.P., Zhan, Q.T., Le, F. et al. (2013). Angiotensin-converting enzymes play a dominant role in fertility. *Int. J. Mol. Sci.* 14 (10): 21071–21086. https://doi.org/10.3390/ijms141021071.

175 Ma, L., Xie, W., Li, D. et al. (2020). Effect of SARS-CoV-2 infection upon male gonadal function: a single center-based study. *medRxiv* https://doi.org/10.1101/2020.03.21.20037267.

176 Yang, M., Chen, S., Huang, B. et al. (2020). Pathological findings in the testes of COVID-19 patients: clinical implications. *Eur. Urol. Focus* 6 (5): 1124–1129. https://doi.org/10.1016/j.euf.2020.05.009.

177 Archana, S.S., Selvaraju, S., Binsila, B.K. et al. (2019). Immune regulatory molecules as modifiers of semen and fertility: a review. *Mol. Reprod. Dev.* 86 (11): 1485–1504. https://doi.org/10.1002/mrd.23263.

178 Cui, D., Han, G., Shang, Y. et al. (2015). Antisperm antibodies in infertile men and their effect on semen parameters: a systematic review and meta-analysis. *Clin. Chim. Acta* 444: 29–36. https://doi.org/10.1016/j.cca.2015.01.033.

179 Lewis, S.E., Agbaje, I., and Alvarez, J. (2008). Sperm DNA tests as useful adjuncts to semen analysis. *Syst Biol Reprod Med* 54 (3): 111–125. https://doi.org/10.1080/19396360801957739.

180 Shen, Q., Xiao, X., Aierken, A. et al. (2020). The ACE2 expression in Sertoli cells and germ cells may cause male reproductive disorder after SARS-CoV-2 infection. *J. Cell. Mol. Med.* 24 (16): 9472–9477. https://doi.org/10.1111/jcmm.15541.

8

COVID-19: Risk Stratification

Dominique Duncan, Rachael Garner, and Yujia Zhang

Laboratory of Neuro Imaging, USC Stevens Neuroimaging and Informatics Institute, Keck School of Medicine of USC, University of Southern California, Los Angeles, CA, USA

Abbreviations

ACE2	angiotensin I–converting enzyme 2
BNP	B-type natriuretic peptide
CDC	Centers for Disease Control and Prevention
CNN	convolutional neural network
COVID-19	coronavirus disease 2019
CRP	C-reactive protein
CT	computed tomography
ICU	intensive care unit
IL-6	interleukin-6
ML	machine learning
NT	N-terminal
S	Spike
SAA	serum amyloid A
SARS-CoV-2	severe acute respiratory syndrome coronavirus 2
SNN	Siamese neural network
TMPRSS2	transmembrane protease serine 2
VEGF-D	vascular endothelial growth factor-D

On 31 December 2019, unidentified pneumonia cases from Wuhan, China, were reported to the World Health Organization. On 7 January 2020, the cause of those cases was found to be the 2019 novel coronavirus. Later, the virus was named severe acute respiratory syndrome coronavirus 2 (SARS-CoV-2) and the illness coronavirus disease 2019 (COVID-19) [1]. As of 11 November 2021, the total death count is up to 5 093 833, and the pandemic has impacted people's living and working conditions worldwide [2, 3].

The goal of this chapter is to summarize key findings of risk factors, including age, ethnicity, sex, medical conditions, socioeconomic status, occupations, pregnancy, blood type, as well as some biomarkers for disease detection, severity, and mortality. Also, various machine learning (ML) methods that have been applied to x-ray and computed tomography (CT) image classification will be discussed.

The first section focuses on clinical biomarkers for COVID-19 detection, severity, and mortality. The second section concentrates on host risk factors listed by the Centers for Disease Control and Prevention (CDC). The third section includes blood type as an additional risk factor and explains the genetic association and underlying molecular mechanisms. The last section introduces some ML methods, such as convolutional neural networks (CNNs) and transfer learning, which can be useful tools for CT or x-ray image classification and prediction.

Potential Biomarkers for COVID-19 Detection, Severity, and Mortality

The transmembrane protease serine 2 (TMPRSS2) is the cellular serine protease for Spike (S) protein priming, facilitating viral entry and activation [4, 5]. TMPRSS2 has been shown to be an important enzyme for disease spread and pathogenesis in the infected host [6]. For example, the genetic polymorphisms rs2070788 and rs383510 of the TMPRSS2 gene are associated with severe influenza from H1N1 and H7N9, and they also increase the expression of TMPRSS2 in lungs [7] (Figure 8.1).

The angiotensin I–converting enzyme 2 (ACE2) is the cellular receptor for SARS-CoV-2, and it can regulate the susceptibility for infections [4, 8, 9]. Both ACE2 and TMPRSS2 are modulated by sex-related effects, because ACE2 is located in the X chromosome

and TMPRSS2 is responsive to androgen/estrogen stimulations [10]. SARS-COV-2 relies on the host cell ACE2 for entry and the host transmembrane serine protease TMPRSS2 for SARS-COV-2 S protein for priming. Then fusion of the virus and host membranes through the S protein allows host cell entry [6] (Figure 8.2).

Based on a CDC report, there is an observed sex difference in clinical outcomes for patients with COVID-19; data suggest that men have a greater risk for severe illness and death from COVID-19 than

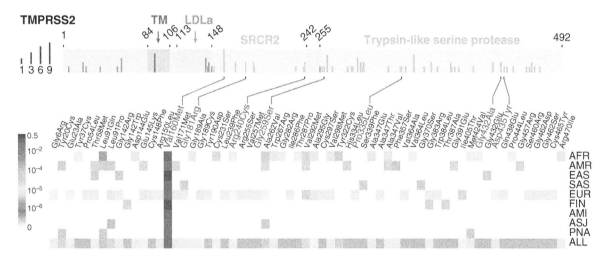

Figure 8.1 Distributions of deleterious variants in the TMPRSS2 coding region. *Source:* Hou et al. [6], under a Creative Commons Attribution 4.0 international (CC BY 4.0) license (https://creativecommons.org/licenses/by/4.0).

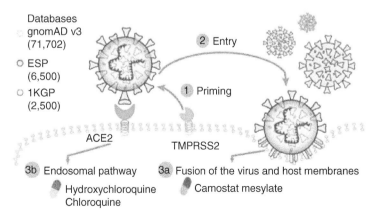

Figure 8.2 ACE2 and TMPRSS2 across human genome databases. *Source:* Hou et al. [6], under a Creative Commons Attribution 4.0 international (CC BY 4.0) license (https://creativecommons.org/licenses/by/4.0).

women [11]. A recent study has shown that TMPRSS2 can be a contributing factor for COVID-19 outcomes [5, 12]. TMPRSS2 is expressed in kidneys, cardiac endothelium, and digestive tract, which may be important target organs for SARS-CoV-2 [5]. TMPRSS2 is also expressed in microvascular endothelial cells, and it may cause endothelial dysfunction after infection with SARS-CoV-2, which can lead to thrombosis and associated complications, such as stroke or heart attack [5].

Serum amyloid A (SAA) concentrations and D-dimer are also clinical biomarkers for COVID-19 severity and mortality. SAA genes are highly activated during the acute-phase response and might contribute to increased temperature and hormonal and metabolic alterations [13]. SAA is typically reported as 20–50 mg/L under physiologic circumstances but can increase up to 1000-fold within the first 24–48 hours of the acute-phase response. Notably, the acute increase in SAA concentrations in patients with COVID-19 is not only represented in the acute-phase response but also is associated with the development of multiorgan failure or severe outcomes [13]. Studies have mentioned that SAA concentrations can be considered as a biomarker, although there are inconclusive reports: it may be a protective factor for severe outcomes and may be significantly and highly associated with COVID-19 severity and mortality [13–16].

D-dimer is a protein fragment that is made when blood clots dissolve in the body [17] and is also highly associated with COVID-19 severity and in-hospital mortality. In one study, patients with D-dimer greater than 2.0 mg/L at admission had increased mortality (odds ratio, 10.17; 95% confidence interval: 1.10–94.38; $P = 0.041$), and the D-dimer level is higher in severe cases and can be used as a biomarker for COVID-19 prognosis [18].

Vascular endothelial growth factor-D (VEGF-D) is identified as an important indicator related to the severity and mortality of COVID-19, followed by D-dimer, age, and other factors (Figure 8.3) [19]. Also the level of VEGF-D is highly associated with sequential organ failure assessment scores, and critical patients had a higher level of VEGF-D [19, 20].

Proteinuria may also be a biomarker for COVID-19 severity [21–24]. Researchers have found that 93.3% of patients had renal involvement, and significant proteinuria by the urinary protein-to-creatine ratio

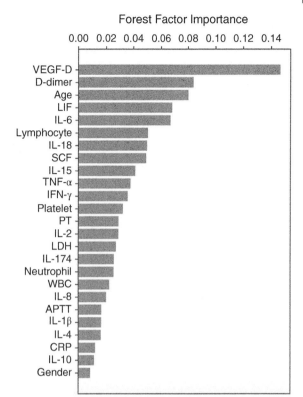

Figure 8.3 Clinical indicators for severity and mortality of COVID-19. APTT, activated partial thromboplastin time; IFN-γ, interferon-γ; LDH, lactate dehydrogenase; LIF, leukemia inhibitory factor; PT, prothrombin time; SCF, stem cell factor; TNF-α, tumor necrosis factor-α; WBC, white blood cell count. *Source:* Kong et al. [19], under a Creative Commons Attribution 4.0 international (CC BY 4.0) license (https://creativecommons.org/licenses/by/4.0).

occurs in 60% of patients. Patients who required intensive care unit (ICU) admission had higher proteinuria, and a level greater than 0.3 g/g was related to the higher prevalence of ICU admission and a longer inpatient hospital stay [23]. Another study has reported that serum calcium levels are associated with COVID-19 severity and prognosis. Patients with lower serum calcium levels, especially ≤2.0 mmol/L, had worse outcomes, such as higher incidence of organ injuries and septic shock and higher 28-day mortality [24].

Calprotectin, a heterodimer involved in neutrophil-related inflammatory processes, is a potential serologic biomarker for COVID-19 [25, 26]. Calprotectin levels are associated with severe clinical outcomes, such as significantly reduced survival time for patients with severe pulmonary disease. Compared with mild cases, calprotectin levels increased among severe cases [25, 26].

Some scientists suggest that levels of B-type natriuretic peptide (BNP) can help discriminate the level of risk for patients with COVID-19 [27]. A recent study showed that the N-terminal (NT)-proBNP levels are associated with COVID-19 severity with the mean of NT-proBNP levels of 791 pg/ml for fatal or severe cases and 161 pg/mL for patients who recovered or have only mild symptoms [27]. Also, it has been found that the NT-proBNP levels increased significantly in critically ill or fatal cases compared with other nonsevere cases [27].

Serum C-reactive protein (CRP), a type of protein produced by the liver, has been found to be an important clinical biomarker that increases in patients with COVID-19 with severe conditions [28]. Other studies also suggested this by reporting increased levels of CRP in patients with COVID-19 [29–31]. Another study also mentioned that a level of CRP ≥40 mg/L was associated with mortality in patients with COVID-19 [32].

Furthermore, some immune-based biomarkers, such as interleukin-6 (IL-6), IL-10, and IL-15, are associated with mortality in patients with COVID-19 [33, 34]. It has been suggested that these biomarkers are independently associated with mortality when the levels increased [33, 34]. Also, IL-10 and IL-15 were higher in hospitalized patients who died than those who recovered, which shows that these clinical biomarkers may provide an early indicator of outcomes [33].

The clinical biomarker platelets are colorless blood cells that help blood clot, and lower blood platelet counts may cause thrombocytopenia [35]. Studies have found that patients with thrombocytopenia had significantly higher mortality after COVID-19 infection [36]. Other studies also suggested that platelet changes were associated with mortality in patients with COVID-19 [37, 38].

One limitation to some of these factors is that because most of them fluctuate daily, it is challenging to use them to inform clinical decision making. Furthermore, some of these factors (i.e. VEGF-D, SAA, CRP) are not able to be collected in normal laboratory settings, so it is useful to consider biomarkers that can be routinely acquired.

Host Risk Factors for COVID-19

In general, there are two types of risk factor: modifiable and nonmodifiable [39]. Modifiable risk factors can be controlled or manipulated through intervention or lifestyle change. However, nonmodifiable risk factors are innate traits, such as ethnicity or blood type.

Based on a CDC report, some groups of people may be at increased risk for severe outcomes of COVID-19 infection, such as older adults, people with medical conditions, pregnant and postpartum women, and certain races, such as American Indians [40].

Age is a risk factor for severe outcomes, and older adults are more likely to have more severe outcomes from COVID-19. People 85 years or older are most likely to get very sick [40]. Also, a study focused on elderly patients older than 80 years has shown that those elderly patients had a higher mortality rate because of multiple comorbidities [41]. A report by the CDC shows the rate ratio of different age groups, setting individuals aged 18–29 years as the reference [42] (Table 8.1).

Age is not associated with acquisition of COVID-19 but is highly related to some severe outcomes, such as hospitalization or death (considering all cases reported to the CDC by state and territorial jurisdictions) [42]. Also, adults of any age with certain medical conditions may become severely ill from COVID-19 [40]. The most common medical conditions were asthma, hypertension, chronic kidney disease, neurodevelopmental disorders, anxiety and fear-related disorders, depressive disorders, and obesity [43, 44]. Also, more than 70% of hospitalized cases had at least one medical condition excluding hypertension [44].

Pregnant or recently pregnant women are also at higher risk for severe outcomes from COVID-19 compared with nonpregnant women [40]. A CDC report has shown that pregnant women are more likely to be admitted to the ICU, receive ventilation, or receive extracorporeal membrane oxygenation compared with nonpregnant women [45].

Ethnicity is a risk factor as well. Hispanic or Latinx people had the highest number of cases, while American Indian or Alaska natives had the highest number of hospitalizations and deaths after COVID-19 infection [42] (Table 8.2).

Other factors, such as certain occupations, sex, and socioeconomic status, can also impact the outcomes of

Table 8.1 The rate ratio of different age groups.

	0–4 yr old	5–17 yr old	18–29 yr old	30–39 yr old	40–49 yr old	50–64 yr old	65–74 yr old	75–84 yr old	85+ yr old
Cases	<1×	1×	Reference group	1×	1×	1×	1×	1×	1×
Hospitalization	<1×	<1×	Reference group	2×	2×	4×	6×	9×	15×
Death	<1×	<1×	Reference group	4×	10×	35×	95×	230×	600×

Source: Centers for Disease Control and Prevention [42].

Table 8.2 Association of COVID-19 infection, hospitalization, and death by ethnicity.

Rate ratios compared with White, non-Hispanic persons	Cases	Hospitalization	Death
American Indian or Alaska Native, non-Hispanic persons	1.6×	3.3×	2.4×
Asian, non-Hispanic persons	0.7×	1.0×	1.0×
Black or African American, non-Hispanic persons	1.1×	2.9×	2.0×
Hispanic or Latinx persons	2.0×	2.8×	2.3×

Source: Data are from Centers for Disease Control and Prevention [42].

COVID-19 [40]. Healthcare workers, social and education workers, and other essential workers had a higher risk for COVID-19 infection or severe outcomes compared with other nonessential workers because of greater exposure to COVID-19 [46, 47].

Sex is also a COVID-19 risk factor. Studies have shown that both women and men have the same prevalence of becoming infected with COVID-19, but males may develop more severe outcomes, such as death or ICU admission [11, 48–50]. Although the reason for this sex gap is still unknown, there are several potential reasons. For example, some psychosocial and behavioral factors are significant for the progression of diseases. The level of smoking and alcohol use among males is higher than for females [48]. Also, the expression of ACE2, a receptor of SARS-CoV-2, was higher in men compared with women [48]. Finally, differences in sex hormones may impact the outcomes of infection [11].

Poverty and health inequality are prevalent worldwide, and people with lower socioeconomic status have higher susceptibility to COVID-19 infection or severe outcomes [51, 52]. People with low income often live in overcrowded housing, are unable to

reduce their mobility during lockdown periods, or do not have access to testing as needed [51, 52] (Figure 8.4). Some people with low income have limited knowledge regarding COVID-19, which may make them more susceptible to acquiring infection.

ABO Blood Type as an Additional Risk Factor

ABO Blood Group and Rh Factor

The ABO blood group consists of four antigens – A, B, AB, and O – and it has been found that the gene of the ABO blood group is at chromosome locus 9 [53]. The Rhesus (Rh) antigen is another key compound that is present or absent on the erythrocyte surfaces; hence the Rh protein determines whether the person is Rh positive or Rh negative [54]. The percentage of people with A-positive blood type is about 30%; however, the percentage of people with AB-negative type is only 1% [55].

For blood type A, the surface of red blood cells contains only A antigens; the surface of red blood cells for

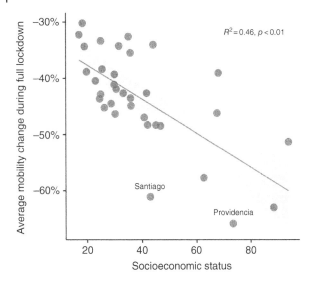

Figure 8.4 The association between socioeconomic status and the average reduction in mobility during a full lockdown period in Chile. Higher socioeconomic status was associated with a greater capacity to reduce personal mobility. *Source:* Mena et al. [52], under a Creative Commons Attribution 4.0 international (CC BY 4.0) license (https://creativecommons.org/licenses/by/4.0).

blood type B contains only B antigens. The surface of red blood cells for blood type AB contains both A and B antigens, while blood type O contains neither antigen [56].

Association of Blood Group with Viral Respiratory Diseases

SARS is a respiratory disease caused by a member of the Coronaviridae family known as SARS-associated coronavirus [54]. It was first reported in February 2003 and then quickly spread globally. The primary spread is by close contact and is transmitted by respiratory droplets when patients cough or sneeze [57]. According to the World Health Organization, 8098 people were infected with SARS, and 774 of them died [57]. Researchers later found that individuals with blood type O were at lower risk to contract SARS compared with all non-O blood-type individuals [58].

Influenza (flu) is a respiratory viral infection caused by the influenza virus. People infected may have mild to severe symptoms, such as fever, cough, and sore throat [59]. There are two influenza viruses: type A and type B. Both can be transmitted by droplets when patients cough, sneeze, or talk [59]. Studies have found that people with blood type O were less susceptible to become infected compared with blood type A and B patients with H1N1, a subtype of the type A flu virus [60]. Researchers also found that people with blood type B were at increased risk to contract H3N2, a subtype of type A flu virus [61].

Association of Blood Type with Higher Susceptibility to COVID-19 Infection and Outcomes

Several studies have suggested that blood types are associated with SARS-COV-2 infection (Table 8.3). Blood groups are not only associated with COVID-19 infection rates but also with severe outcomes, such as requiring mechanical ventilation, longer ICU stay, or death (Table 8.4). Because blood type can be characterized as positive or negative depending on the presence of the Rh factor, it is important to investigate the association between Rh and COVID-19 infection and outcomes (Table 8.5 and Figure 8.5).

Genetic Association and Underlying Molecular Mechanisms

Genetics plays a significant role in susceptibility to infection and disease pathogenesis [83]. Scientists have found that chromosome 3p21.31 gene cluster is a susceptibility locus with outcome severity, especially for respiratory failure [83]. Moreover, an association was identified at chromosome 9q34.2 with index single-nucleotide polymorphism rs9411378. This single-nucleotide polymorphism is in linkage disequilibrium with a functional variant in the ABO gene, which usually confers to blood type O. Hence it is believed that blood type O appears to be more protective than other blood types [83].

Due to glycosylation, blood type O has downregulated immunoglobulin M activity, while types A, B, and AB have upregulated immunoglobulin M activity. Hence blood types A, B, and AB are preferential targets because they possess A/B phenotypic-determining enzymes, whereas blood type O lacks these enzymes and binds the virus only via H-type antigen formation [84].

Although the molecular mechanisms of ABO blood type in COVID-19 susceptibility have not been

Table 8.3 Studies on associations between blood type and higher susceptibility of testing positive for COVID-19.

References	Number of patients	Selection criteria	Major findings
Fan et al. [62]	Cases: n = 105 Controls: n = 103	Patients tested positive at Zhongnan Hospital of Wuhan University in Wuhan, China, from 1 January 2020 to 5 March 2020	Blood type A patients had higher risk and blood type O patients had lower risk of becoming infected with SARS-CoV-2
Zhao et al. [63]	N = 2173	Patients from Jinyintan Hospital in Wuhan, China; Renmin Hospital of Wuhan University in Wuhan, China; and Shenzhen Third People's Hospital, in Shenzhen, China	Blood type A patients had higher risk and blood type O patients had lower risk of becoming infected with SARS-CoV-2
Golinelli et al. [64]	Cases: n = 7503 Controls: n = 2962160	Data in MEDLINE [65] and LitCovid [66] databases from studies published until 15 July 2020	Blood type A patients had higher risk and blood type O patients had lower risk of becoming infected with SARS-CoV-2
Zietz et al. [67]	N = 14112	Patients >18 years old who tested positive for SARS-CoV-2 with known blood types in the New York Presbyterian hospital system	Blood type O was protective against SARS-CoV-2 infection compared with non-O blood type
Wu et al. [68]	N = 31100	Studies extracted from five databases: PubMed, medRxiv, bioRxiv, Web of Science, and China National Knowledge Infrastructure (CNKI)	Blood type A patients had higher risk and blood type O patients had lower risk of becoming infected with SARS-CoV-2
Wu et al. [69]	N = 187	Patients with COVID-19 recorded between 20 January 2020 and 5 March 2020 at the First Hospital of Changsha	Blood type A patients had higher risk and blood type O patients had lower risk of becoming infected with SARS-CoV-2
Barnkob et al. [70]	SARS-CoV-2 positive: n = 7422 SARS-CoV-2 negative: n = 466232	Danish people who were tested for SARS-CoV-2 between 27 February 2020 and 30 July 2020 with known blood group	Blood type O was protective against SARS-CoV-2 infection compared with non-O blood type
Latz et al. [71]	N = 1289	Patients tested positive for SARS-CoV-2 with a known blood type	Blood types B and AB were associated with higher risk of testing positive for COVID-19; blood type O was associated with lower risk of testing positive; no correlation was found between blood type A and positive test rates
Padhi et al. [72]	N = 277649	COVID-19 patient data collected from Ministry of Health and Family Welfare of India	Blood type O may be protective against COVID-19 infection
Majeed et al. [73]	N = 5668	Patients were admitted to Al-Hussein Teaching Hospital, Thi-Qar and Alkarama Teaching Hospital, Wasit in Iraq from March to June 2020	Blood type O is partially protective against COVID-19 infection
Yilmaz et al. [74]	N = 1316676	From Turkish Red Crescent (TRC) whole blood donors	Blood types A and AB are associated with increased risk for infection, while blood types O and B are at decreased risk
Bhandari et al. [75]	Cases: n = 825 Controls: n = 396	All patients aged ≥18 yr admitted to Elmhurst Hospital Center (EHC) from 1 March 2020 to 24 June 2020	Blood type is not significantly associated with susceptibility for COVID-19
Araç et al. [76]	Cases: n = 392 Controls: n = 127091	Patients admitted to Diyarbakır Gazi Yasargil Training and Research Hospital from 16 March 2020 to 20 May 2020	There is no association between ABO blood types and COVID-19 infection

COVID-19, coronavirus disease 2019; SARS-CoV-2, severe acute respiratory syndrome coronavirus 2.

Table 8.4 Summary of findings for ABO blood type and COVID-19 clinical outcomes of severity.

References	Number of patients	Selection criteria	Major outcomes
Zietz et al. [67]	N = 14 112	Patients ≥18 yr old who tested positive for SARS-CoV-2 with known blood types in the New York Presbyterian hospital system	Blood type A patients had lower risk for intubation and death compared with blood type O patients, whereas blood type AB had higher risk for both intubation and death.
Wu et al. [68]	N = 31 100	Studies extracted from five databases: PubMed, medRxiv, bioRxiv, Web of Science, and CNKI	There is no correlation between blood type and COVID-19 severity or mortality.
Latz et al. [71]	N = 1289	Patients tested positive for SARS-CoV-2 with a known blood type	There is no correlation between blood type and COVID-19 intubation or death.
Padhi et al. [72]	N = 277 649	COVID-19 patient data collected from Ministry of Health and Family Welfare of India	Blood type O was protective against COVID-19 death, whereas blood type B was more strongly correlated with death.
Ray et al. [77]	N = 225 556	People who had ABO blood group assessed between January 2007 and December 2019 and who also had SARS-CoV-2 testing conducted between 15 January 2020 and 30 June 2020 in Ontario, Canada	Blood type A and AB had higher risk for severe illness or death.
Hoiland et al. [78]	N = 125	ICU patients in six metropolitan Vancouver hospitals between 21 February 2020 and 28 April 2020	Blood type A and AB patients are at higher risk for requiring mechanical ventilation and experience more severe outcomes.
Hultström et al. [79]	N = 64	Data were collected from a Swedish critical care center	Blood type A has higher risk for requiring critical care and death.
Nasiri et al. [80]	N = 329	Patients were from Kamkar-Arab Nia Hospital, Qom, Iran from 1 March 1 2020 to 31 June 2020	Blood type was not associated with COVID-19 severity, death rate, or admission duration. However, blood type B did show a significant association with the time interval to return to normal oxygen levels.
Szymanski et al. [81]	N = 4968	Positive COVID-19 patients hospitalized or with an emergency department visit from 10 March 2020 to 8 June 2020	Blood type A was associated with increased risk for in-hospital death.
Majeed et al. [73]	N = 5668	Patients were admitted to Al-Hussein Teaching Hospital, Thi-Qar and Alkarama Teaching Hospital, Wasit in Iraq from March to June 2020	Blood type was not associated with COVID-19 death rate.
Bhandari et al. [75]	Cases: n = 825 Controls: n = 396	All patients aged ≥18 yr admitted to Elmhurst Hospital Center (EHC) from 1 March 2020 to 24 June 2020	Blood type is not significantly associated with mortality for COVID-19.

COVID-19, coronavirus disease 2019; ICU, intensive care unit; SARS-CoV-2, severe acute respiratory syndrome coronavirus 2.

Table 8.5 Summary of findings for association of Rh with susceptibility to COVID-19 and outcomes.

References	Number of patients	Selection criteria	Major outcomes
Zietz et al. [67]	N = 14112	Patients ≥18 yr old who tested positive for SARS-CoV-2 with known blood types in the New York Presbyterian hospital system	Rh− patients had a 2.7% lower risk for initial infection after adjustment and also a lower risk for both intubation and death.
Latz et al. [71]	N = 1289	Patients tested positive for SARS-CoV-2 with a known blood type	Individuals with Rh− blood type were less susceptible to infection by SARS-CoV-2.
Ray et al. [77]	N = 225556	People who had ABO blood group assessed between January 2007 and December 2019 and who also had SARS-CoV-2 testing conducted between 15 January 2020 and 30 June 2020 in Ontario, Canada	B-positive was associated with higher odds of testing positive, whereas O-negative was associated with lower infection rate; Rh+ had higher risk for severe illness or death.
Taha et al. [82]	N = 557	Individuals surveyed online	O-positive blood group has the lowest risk of having severe symptoms, and A-positive individuals were the most vulnerable when exposed to the virus.
Majeed et al. [73]	N = 5668	Patients were admitted to Al-Hussein Teaching Hospital, Thi-Qar and Alkarama Teaching Hospital, Wasit in Iraq from March to June 2020	Individuals with RhD− blood type were more susceptible than RhD+ to infection by SARS-CoV-2.
Yilmaz et al. [74]	N = 1316676	From Turkish Red Crescent (TRC) whole blood donors	RhD+ individuals are associated with increased risk for infection, while RhD− individuals are at decreased risk for infection.
Bhandari et al. [75]	Cases: n = 825 Controls: n = 396	All patients aged ≥18 yr admitted to Elmhurst Hospital Center (EHC) from 1 March 2020 to 24 June 2020	Rh blood type is not significantly associated with susceptibility to and mortality from COVID-19.
Araç et al. [76]	Cases: n = 392 Controls: n = 127091	Patients admitted to Diyarbakır Gazi Yasargil Training and Research Hospital from 16 March 2020 to 20 May 2020	RhD+ individuals are associated with increased risk for infection, while RhD− individuals are at decreased risk for infection.

SARS-CoV-2, severe acute respiratory syndrome coronavirus 2.

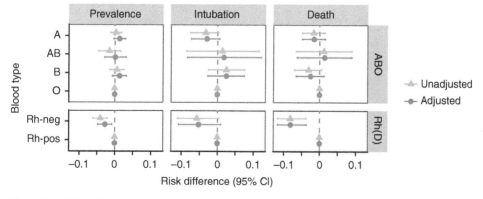

Figure 8.5 Risk differences for each blood type. CI, confidence interval. *Source:* Zietz et al. [67], under a Creative Commons Attribution 4.0 international (CC BY 4.0) license (https://creativecommons.org/licenses/by/4.0).

discovered yet, some scientists have considered potential molecular mechanisms underlying the susceptibility. It has been suggested that blood type O has a Rosette-disrupting effect to prevent severe *Plasmodium falciparum* malaria, so researchers speculated that blood type O has a similar effect on SARS-COV-2 [68]. Cellular models have also suggested that S protein/ACE2-dependent adhesion to the ACE2-expressing cell line was specifically inhibited by monoclonal or natural human anti-A antibodies, so patients with non-A blood types, especially O or B blood types, may be less susceptible to COVID-19 infection [54]. Several researchers also proposed that TMPRSS2, located at chromosome 21q22.3, has been found to be significant for S protein priming and subsequent infection of COVID-19 [54].

ML Methods for X-Ray and CT Image Classification and Prediction

ML is a rapidly growing field and has emerged as a useful method to study COVID-19 and understand the disease progression [85]. Furthermore, the growing number of publicly available datasets [86] make applying ML algorithms to these data more appropriate and widely used. ML can provide helpful tools for intelligent data analysis, especially in medical diagnosis [87]. Many hospitals collect, gather, and share large amounts of imaging data, and ML methods can be useful for analyzing those data, particularly with data that are annotated, curated, and harmonized [86, 87].

CNNs are a type of deep learning algorithm with multiple hidden layers that are important for feature learning ability because of their high accuracy [86, 88]. Each layer is composed of multiple two-dimensional planes in the network, and each plane consists of multiple compositions [89]. CNNs can analyze thousands of images within a day even with limited hardware resources [90]. The capacity of CNN models can be adjusted by changing the depth and breadth of the network. CNNs can be effectively used to reduce the learning complexity of a network model and have fewer network connections and weight parameters so that they are more likely to be trained with considerable size than fully connected networks [89].

Transfer learning is another ML method that has been used to predict COVID-19 infection using chest CT or x-ray images. Regions such as ground-glass opacities (GGO), consolidation, and other imaging features in patients with COVID-19 are identified and labeled. Pretrained CNN architectures (i.e. DenseNet, ResNet18, DarkNet) are loaded and retrained with the original images. Before training, the final layers of the pretrained model are replaced to learn data-specific features and predict or classify COVID-19 images and normal images (Figure 8.6) [91].

In one study, transfer learning was applied to six pretrained CNN models on one dataset to compare their performance in classifying patients with COVID-19 using chest CT images [86]. Transfer learning that uses a pretrained CNN model has shown promise in this COVID-19 application: a pretrained InceptionV3 Model yielded 98.71% accuracy when applied to a dataset of 489 subjects from Sao Paulo, Brazil (Figure 8.7). Data were split into 80% for training and 20% for validation. Each model was trained and tested using five rounds of cross-validation

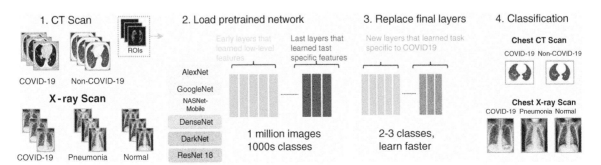

Figure 8.6 COVID-19 prediction using CT and x-ray images with deep transfer learning models. *Source:* Chaddad et al. [91].

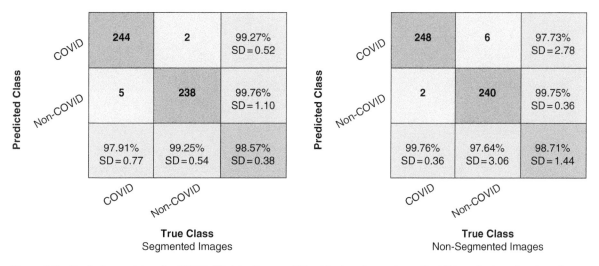

Figure 8.7 Confusion matrices for COVID-19 detection on 489 subjects using an InceptionV3 transfer learning-based architecture. Classification was performed using both segmented images, in which lungs were first segmented from CT, and nonsegmented images. Both classifications yielded >98% accuracy. SD, standard deviation.

on augmented segmented and nonsegmented training classes; it was found that training on segmented images is statistically comparable with training on nonsegmented images.

Deep learning is a promising, low-cost, and reliable way to determine whether patients are infected with COVID-19 from examining their lung CT scans. However, the commonly used CNNs risk overfitting to hospital-specific data because of the lack of publicly available CT data. The performance of Siamese neural networks (SNNs) [92] was tested; these are networks that learn to determine the similarity between two images rather than label them as COVID-19 positive or negative. SNNs have previously demonstrated state-of-the-art performance even when applied to test data that have little resemblance to their training data. Four different SNNs were trained on CT images collected from Sari, Iran. The SNN models in one recent study [86] achieved higher accuracy than other ML

models and lay the groundwork to create a model that correctly discriminates COVID-19-positive and -negative CT images collected from any hospital.

Saliency maps can be used to highlight potentially novel patterns and locations in the lower lobes that are related to COVID-19 infection. SNNs are useful for tasks where labeled data are difficult to acquire, as is the case with many COVID-19 imaging datasets, so SNNs may be a promising tool to use with ML methods to study COVID-19 in patients using CT images while having only a small number of reference images available.

ML methods are a powerful tool to study COVID-19 in an automated and efficient way. Various ML methods have been shown to be promising tools to identify the disease and understand its progression. As more COVID-19 data become available, these ML analytic tools will become even more useful in studying this disease.

References

1 Salehi, S., Abedi, A., Balakrishnan, S., and Gholamrezanezhad, A. (2020). Coronavirus disease 2019 (COVID-19): a systematic review of imaging findings in 919 patients. *Am. J. Roentgenol.* 215 (1): 87–93. https://doi.org/10.2214/AJR.20.23034.

2 Johns Hopkins Coronavirus Resource Center. (2021). COVID-19 Map. https://coronavirus.jhu.edu/map.html. Accessed 25 Aug 2021.

3 Bick A, Blandin A, Mertens K. (2020). Work from home after the COVID-19 outbreak. *Federal Reserve*

Bank of Dallas Working Papers. 2020. doi:10.24149/wp2017r1.

4 Hoffmann, M., Kleine-Weber, H., Schroeder, S. et al. (2020). SARS-CoV-2 cell entry depends on ACE2 and TMPRSS2 and is blocked by a clinically proven protease inhibitor. *Cell* 181 (2): 271–280.e8. https://doi.org/10.1016/j.cell.2020.02.052.

5 Strope, J.D., Chau, C.H., and Figg, W.D. (2020). TMPRSS2: potential biomarker for COVID-19 outcomes. *J. Clin. Pharmacol.* 60: 801–807. https://doi.org/10.1002/jcph.1641.

6 Hou, Y., Zhao, J., Martin, W. et al. (2020). New insights into genetic susceptibility of COVID-19: an *ACE2* and *TMPRSS2* polymorphism analysis. *BMC Med.* 18: 216.

7 Cheng, Z., Zhou, J., To, K.K.W. et al. (2015). Identification of TMPRSS2 as a susceptibility gene for severe 2009 pandemic A(H1N1) influenza and A(H7N9) influenza. *J. Infect. Dis.* 212 (8): 1214–1221. https://doi.org/10.1093/infdis/jiv246.

8 Gómez, J., Albaiceta, G.M., García-Clemente, M. et al. (2020). Angiotensin-converting enzymes (ACE, ACE2) gene variants and COVID-19 outcome. *Gene* 762: 145102. https://doi.org/10.1016/j.gene.2020.145102.

9 Yan, R., Zhang, Y., Li, Y. et al. (2020). Structural basis for the recognition of SARS-CoV-2 by full-length human ACE2. *Science* 367: 1444–1448.

10 Asselta, R., Paraboschi, E.M., Mantovani, A., and Duga, S. (2020). ACE2 and TMPRSS2 variants and expression as candidates to sex and country differences in COVID-19 severity in Italy. *Aging* 12 (11): 10087–10098. https://doi.org/10.18632/aging.103415.

11 Griffith, D.M. (2020). Men and COVID-19: a biopsychosocial approach to understanding sex differences in mortality and recommendations for practice and policy interventions. *Prev. Chronic Dis.* 17: 200247. https://doi.org/10.5888/pcd17.200247.

12 Stopsack, K.H., Mucci, L.A., Antonarakis, E.S. et al. (2020). TMPRSS2 and COVID-19: serendipity or opportunity for intervention? *Can. Discov.* 10 (6): 779–782. https://doi.org/10.1158/2159-8290.CD-20-0451.

13 Zinellu, A., Paliogiannis, P., Carru, C., and Mangoni, A.A. (2021). Serum amyloid A concentrations, COVID-19 severity and mortality: an updated systematic review and meta-analysis. *Int. J. Infect. Dis.* 105: 668–674. https://doi.org/10.1016/j.ijid.2021.03.025.

14 Li, H., Xiang, X., Ren, H. et al. (2020). Serum amyloid A is a biomarker of severe coronavirus disease and poor prognosis. *J. Infect.* 80 (6): 646–655. https://doi.org/10.1016/j.jinf.2020.03.035.

15 Fu, J., Huang, P.P., Zhang, S. et al. (2020). The value of serum amyloid A for predicting the severity and recovery of COVID-19. *Exp. Ther. Med.* 20 (4): 3571–3577. https://doi.org/10.3892/etm.2020.9114.

16 Mo, X., Su, Z., Lei, C. et al. (2020). Serum amyloid A is a predictor for prognosis of COVID-19. *Respirol.* 25: 764–765. https://doi.org/10.1111/resp.13840.

17 National Library of Medicine. (2021). D-Dimer test. MedlinePlus Medical Test. https://medlineplus.gov/lab-tests/d-dimer-test Accessed 20 Aug 2021.

18 Yao, Y., Cao, J., Wang, Q. et al. (2020). D-dimer as a biomarker for disease severity and mortality in COVID-19 patients: a case control study. *J. Intensive Care* 8 (1): 49. https://doi.org/10.1186/s40560-020-00466-z.

19 Kong, Y., Han, J., Wu, X. et al. (2020). VEGF-D: a novel biomarker for detection of COVID-19 progression. *Crit. Care* 24 (1): 373. https://doi.org/10.1186/s13054-020-03079-y.

20 Zhang, L., Yan, X., Fan, Q. et al. (2020). D-dimer levels on admission to predict in-hospital mortality in patients with Covid-19. *J. Thromb. Haemost.* 18 (6): 1324–1329. https://doi.org/10.1111/jth.14859.

21 Karras, A., Livrozet, M., Lazareth, H. et al. (2021). Proteinuria and clinical outcomes in hospitalized COVID-19 patients: a retrospective single-center study. *Clin. J. Am. Soc. Nephrol.* 16 (4): 514–521. https://doi.org/10.2215/CJN.09130620.

22 Huart, J., Bouquegneau, A., Lutteri, L. et al. (2021). Proteinuria in COVID-19: prevalence, characterization and prognostic role. *J. Nephrol.* 34 (2): 355–364. https://doi.org/10.1007/s40620-020-00931-w.

23 Ouahmi, H., Courjon, J., Morand, L. et al. Proteinuria as a biomarker for COVID-19 severity. *Front. Physiol.* https://www.frontiersin.org/articles/10.3389/fphys.2021.611772/full. Accessed 20 Aug 2021.

24 Sun, J.K., Zhang, W.H., Zou, L. et al. (2020). Serum calcium as a biomarker of clinical severity and

prognosis in patients with coronavirus disease 2019. *Aging* 12 (12): 11287–11295. https://doi. org/10.18632/aging.103526.

25 Mahler, M., Meroni, P.L., Infantino, M. et al. (2021). Circulating calprotectin as a biomarker of COVID-19 severity. *Expert. Rev. Clin. Immunol.* 17 (5): 431–443. https://doi.org/10.1080/1744666X.2021.1905526.

26 Udeh, R., Advani, S., de Guadiana Romualdo, L.G., and Dolja-Gore, X. (2021). Calprotectin, an emerging biomarker of interest in COVID-19: a systematic review and meta-analysis. *J. Clin. Forensic Med.* 10 (4): 775. https://doi.org/10.3390/jcm10040775.

27 Sorrentino, S., Cacia, M., Leo, I. et al. (2020). B-type natriuretic peptide as biomarker of COVID-19 disease severity – a meta-analysis. *J. Clin. Forensic Med.* 9 (9): 2957. https://doi.org/10.3390/jcm9092957.

28 Ali, N. (2020). Elevated level of C-reactive protein may be an early marker to predict risk for severity of COVID-19. *J. Med. Virol.* 92: 2409–2411. https://doi.org/10.1002/jmv.26097.

29 Chen, N., Zhou, M., Dong, X. et al. (2020). Epidemiological and clinical characteristics of 99 cases of 2019 novel coronavirus pneumonia in Wuhan, China: a descriptive study. *Lancet. Lond. Engl.* 395 (10223): 507–513. https://doi.org/10.1016/S0140-6736(20)30211-7.

30 Gao, Y., Li, T., Han, M. et al. (2020). Diagnostic utility of clinical laboratory data determinations for patients with the severe COVID-19. *J. Med. Virol.* 92: 791–796. https://doi.org/10.1002/jmv.25770.

31 Smilowitz, N.R., Kunichoff, D., Garshick, M. et al. (2021). C-reactive protein and clinical outcomes in patients with COVID-19. *Eur. Heart J.* 42 (23): 2270–2279. https://doi.org/10.1093/eurheartj/ehaa1103.

32 Stringer, D., Braude, P., Myint, P.K. et al. (2021). The role of C-reactive protein as a prognostic marker in COVID-19. *Int. J. Epidemiol.* 50 (2): 420–429. https://doi.org/10.1093/ije/dyab012.

33 Abers, M.S., Delmonte, O.M., Ricotta, E.E. et al. (2021). An immune-based biomarker signature is associated with mortality in COVID-19 patients. *JCI Insight.* 6 (1): e144455. https://doi.org/10.1172/jci.insight.144455.

34 Frisoni, P., Neri, M., D'Errico, S. et al. (2022). Cytokine storm and histopathological findings in 60 cases of COVID-19-related death: from viral load research to immunohistochemical quantification of major players IL-1β, IL-6, IL-15 and TNF-α. *Foren. Sci. Med. Pathol.* 18: 4–19. https://doi.org/10.1007/s12024-021-00414-9.

35 Mayo Clinic. (2021). Thrombocytopenia (low platelet count). https://www.mayoclinic.org/diseases-conditions/thrombocytopenia/symptoms-causes/syc-20378293. Accessed 5 Nov 2021

36 Zhu, Y., Zhang, J., Li, Y. et al. (2021). Association between thrombocytopenia and 180-day prognosis of COVID-19 patients in intensive care units: a two-center observational study. *PLoS One* 16 (3): e0248671. https://doi.org/10.1371/journal.pone.0248671.

37 Zhao, X., Wang, K., Zuo, P. et al. (2020). Early decrease in blood platelet count is associated with poor prognosis in COVID-19 patients – indications for predictive, preventive, and personalized medical approach. *EPMA J.* 11 (2): 139–145. https://doi.org/10.1007/s13167-020-00208-z.

38 Liu, Y., Sun, W., Guo, Y. et al. (2020). Association between platelet parameters and mortality in coronavirus disease 2019: retrospective cohort study. *Platelets* 31 (4): 490–496. https://doi.org/10.1080/09537104.2020.1754383.

39 Sacco, R.L., Benjamin, E.J., Broderick, J.P. et al. (1997). Risk factors. *Stroke* 28 (7): 1507–1517. https://doi.org/10.1161/01.STR.28.7.1507.

40 Centers for Disease Control and Prevention. 2020. COVID-19 and your health. https://www.cdc.gov/coronavirus/2019-ncov/your-health/index.html. Accessed 20 Aug 2021.

41 D'ascanio, M., Innammorato, M., Pasquariello, L. et al. (2021). Age is not the only risk factor in COVID-19: the role of comorbidities and of long staying in residential care homes. *BMC Geriatr.* 21 (1): 63. https://doi.org/10.1186/s12877-021-02013-3.

42 Centers for Disease Control and Prevention. 2020. Cases, data, and surveillance. https://www.cdc.gov/coronavirus/2019-ncov/covid-data/investigations-discovery/hospitalization-death-by-age.html. Accessed 20 Aug 2021.

43 Kompaniyets, L., Agathis, N.T., Nelson, J.M. et al. (2021). Underlying medical conditions associated with severe COVID-19 illness among children. *JAMA Net. Open.* 4 (6): e2111182. https://doi.org/10.1001/jamanetworkopen.2021.11182.

44 Ko, J.Y., Danielson, M.L., Town, M. et al. (2021). Risk factors for coronavirus disease 2019 (COVID-19)–associated hospitalization: COVID-19–associated hospitalization surveillance network and behavioral risk factor surveillance system. *Clin. Infect. Dis.* 72 (11): e695–e703. https://doi.org/10.1093/cid/ciaa1419.

45 Zambrano, L.D. (2020). Update: characteristics of symptomatic women of reproductive age with laboratory-confirmed SARS-CoV-2 infection by pregnancy status – United States, January 22–October 3, 2020. *MMWR Morb. Mortal. Wkly Rep.* 69: 1641–1647. https://doi.org/10.15585/mmwr. mm6944e3.

46 Mutambudzi, M., Niedwiedz, C., Macdonald, E.B. et al. (2021). Occupation and risk of severe COVID-19: prospective cohort study of 120 075 UK Biobank participants. *Occup. Environ. Med.* Published online December 9 78: 307–314. https://doi.org/10.1136/oemed-2020-106731.

47 Zhang, M. (2021). Estimation of differential occupational risk of COVID-19 by comparing risk factors with case data by occupational group. *Am. J. Ind. Med.* 64 (1): 39–47. https://doi.org/10.1002/ajim.23199.

48 Bwire, G.M. (2020). Coronavirus: why men are more vulnerable to Covid-19 than women? *Sn Compr. Clin. Med.* 2: 874–876. https://doi.org/10.1007/s42399-020-00341-w.

49 Jin, J.M., Bai, P., He, W. et al. (2020). Gender differences in patients with COVID-19: focus on severity and mortality. *Front. Pub. Health.* 8: 152. https://doi.org/10.3389/fpubh.2020.00152.

50 Peckham, H., de Gruijter, N.M., Raine, C. et al. (2020). Male sex identified by global COVID-19 meta-analysis as a risk factor for death and ITU admission. *Nat. Commun.* 11 (1): 6317. https://doi.org/10.1038/s41467-020-19741-6.

51 Patel, J.A., Nielsen, F.B.H., Badiani, A.A. et al. (2020). Poverty, inequality and COVID-19: the forgotten vulnerable. *Pub. Health.* 183: 110–111. https://doi.org/10.1016/j.puhe.2020.05.006.

52 Mena, G.E., Martinez, P.P., Mahmud, A.S. et al. (2021). Socioeconomic status determines COVID-19 incidence and related mortality in Santiago, Chile. *Science* 372 (6545): eabg5298. https://doi.org/10.1126/science.abg5298.

53 Hosoi, E. (2008). Biological and clinical aspects of ABO blood group system. *J. Med. Investig.* 55 (3–4): 174–182. https://doi.org/10.2152/jmi.55.174.

54 Zhang, Y., Garner, R., Salehi, S. et al. (2021). Association between ABO blood types and coronavirus disease 2019 (COVID-19), genetic associations, and underlying molecular mechanisms: a literature review of 23 studies. *Ann. Hematol.* 100 (5): 1123–1132. https://doi.org/10.1007/s00277-021-04489-w.

55 Association for the Advancement of Blood & Biotherapies (AABB). (2021) Home page. www.aabb.org. Accessed 7 Jul 2021.

56 Blood types: what are they and what do they mean? (2021). *Medical News Today.* June 3, 2020. https://www.medicalnewstoday.com/articles/218285. Accessed 7 Jul 2021.

57 Centers for Disease Control and Prevention. (2021). Severe Acute Respiratory Syndrome. https://www.cdc.gov/sars/index.html. Accessed 7 Jul 2021.

58 Cheng, Y., Cheng, G., Chui, C.H. et al. (2005). ABO blood group and susceptibility to severe acute respiratory syndrome. *JAMA* 293 (12): 1447–1451. https://doi.org/10.1001/jama.293.12.1450-c.

59 Centers for Disease Control and Prevention. (2021). About flu. https://www.cdc.gov/flu/about/index.html. Accessed 7 Jul 2021.

60 Lebiush, M., Rannon, L., and Kark, J.D. (1981). The relationship between epidemic influenza A(H1N1) and ABO blood group. *J. Hyg. (Lond.)* 87 (1): 139–146.

61 Mackenzie, J.S. and Fimmel, P.J. (1978). The effect of ABO blood groups on the incidence of epidemic influenza and on the response to live attenuated and detergent split influenza virus vaccines. *J. Hyg. (Lond.)* 80 (1): 21–30.

62 Fan, Q., Zhang, W., Li, B. et al. (2020). Association between ABO blood group system and COVID-19 susceptibility in Wuhan. *Front. Cell. Infect. Microbiol.* 10: 404. https://doi.org/10.3389/fcimb.2020.00404.

63 Zhao, J., Yang, Y., Huang, H. et al. (2021). Relationship between the ABO Blood Group and the COVID-19 Susceptibility. *Clin. Infect. Dis.* 73: 328–331. https://doi.org/10.1093/cid/ciaa1150.

64 Golinelli, D., Boetto, E., Maietti, E., and Fantini, M.P. (2020). The association between ABO blood group and SARS-CoV-2 infection: a meta-analysis. *PLoS*

One 15 (9): e0239508. https://doi.org/10.1371/journal.pone.0239508.

65 MEDLINE: description of the database. https://www.nlm.nih.gov/bsd/medline.html. Accessed 18 Dec 2020.

66 LitCovid. National Center for Biotechnology Information. https://www.ncbi.nlm.nih.gov/research/coronavirus. Accessed 18 Dec 2020.

67 Zietz, M., Zucker, J.E., and Tatonetti, N.P. (2020). Associations between blood type and COVID-19 infection, intubation, and death. *Nat. Commun.* 11: 5761. https://doi.org/10.1101/2020.04.08.20058073.

68 Wu, B.B., Gu, D.Z., Yu, J.N. et al. (2020). Association between ABO blood groups and COVID-19 infection, severity and demise: a systematic review and meta-analysis. *Infect. Genet. Evol. J. Mol. Epidemiol. Evol. Genet. Infect. Dis.* 84: 104485. https://doi.org/10.1016/j.meegid.2020.104485.

69 Wu, Y., Feng, Z., Li, P., and Yu, Q. (2020). Relationship between ABO blood group distribution and clinical characteristics in patients with COVID-19. *Clin. Chim. Acta Int. J. Clin. Chem.* 509: 220–223. https://doi.org/10.1016/j.cca.2020.06.026.

70 Barnkob, M.B., Pottegård, A., Støvring, H. et al. (2020). Reduced prevalence of SARS-CoV-2 infection in ABO blood group O. *Blood Adv.* 4 (20): 4990–4993. https://doi.org/10.1182/bloodadvances.2020002657.

71 Latz, C.A., DeCarlo, C., Boitano, L. et al. (2020). Blood type and outcomes in patients with COVID-19. *Ann. Hematol.* 99 (9): 2113–2118. https://doi.org/10.1007/s00277-020-04169-1.

72 Padhi, S., Suvankar, S., Dash, D. et al. (2020). ABO blood group system is associated with COVID-19 mortality: an epidemiological investigation in the Indian population. *Transfus. Clin. Biol. J. Soc. Francaise Transfus. Sang.* 27 (4): 253–258. https://doi.org/10.1016/j.tracli.2020.08.009.

73 Majeed KR, Al-Fahad D, Jalood HH, et al. RhD blood type significantly influences susceptibility to contract COVID-19 among a study population in Iraq. *F1000Research* 2021;10:38.

74 Yilmaz, M., Karaca, A., Sozmen, N.N. et al. (2021). Association between COVID-19 and ABO blood groups: an analysis on convalescent plasma donors in Turkey. *Med. Bull. Haseki.* 59 (1): 7–14. https://doi.org/10.4274/haseki.galenos.2021.7235.

75 Bhandari, P., Durrance, R.J., Bhuti, P., and Salama, C. (2020). Analysis of ABO and Rh blood type association with acute COVID-19 infection in hospitalized patients: a superficial association among a multitude of established confounders. *J. Clin. Med. Res.* 12 (12): 809–815. https://doi.org/10.14740/jocmr4382.

76 Araç, E., Solmaz, I., Akkoc, H. et al. (2020). Association between the Rh blood group and the Covid-19 susceptibility. *Uluslararasi. Hematoloji. Onkoloji. Dergisi.* 30: 81–86.

77 Ray, J.G., Schull, M.J., Vermeulen, M.J., and Park, A.L. (2021). Association between ABO and Rh blood groups and SARS-CoV-2 infection or severe COVID-19 illness: a population-based cohort study. *Ann. Intern. Med.* 174: 308–315. https://doi.org/10.7326/M20-4511.

78 Hoiland, R.L., Fergusson, N.A., Mitra, A.R. et al. (2020). The association of ABO blood group with indices of disease severity and multiorgan dysfunction in COVID-19. *Blood Adv.* 4 (20): 4981–4989. https://doi.org/10.1182/bloodadvances.2020002623.

79 Hultström, M., Persson, B., Eriksson, O. et al. (2020). Blood type A associates with critical COVID-19 and death in a Swedish cohort. *Crit. Care* 24 (1): 496. https://doi.org/10.1186/s13054-020-03223-8.

80 Nasiri, M., Khodadadi, J., Hajrezaei, Z., and Bizhani, N. (2021). The probable association between blood groups and prognosis of COVID-19. *Iran. J. Public Health* 50 (4): 825–830. https://doi.org/10.18502/ijph.v50i4.6009.

81 Szymanski, J., Mohrmann, L., Carter, J. et al. (2021). ABO blood type association with SARS-CoV-2 infection mortality: a single-center population in New York City. *Transfus. (Paris)* 61 (4): 1064–1070. https://doi.org/10.1111/trf.16339.

82 Taha, S.A.H., Osman, M.E.M., Abdoelkarim, E.A.A. et al. (2020). Individuals with a Rh-positive but not Rh-negative blood group are more vulnerable to SARS-CoV-2 infection: demographics and trend study on COVID-19 cases in Sudan. *New Microb. New Infect.* 38: 100763. https://doi.org/10.1016/j.nmni.2020.100763.

83 Shelton, J.F., Shastri, A.J., Ye, C. et al. (2021). Trans-ancestry analysis reveals genetic and nongenetic associations with COVID-19

susceptibility and severity. *Nat. Genet.* 53 (6): 801–808. https://doi.org/10.1038/s41588-021-00854-7.

84 Arend, P. (2021). Why blood group A individuals are at risk whereas blood group O individuals are protected from SARS-CoV-2 (COVID-19) infection: a hypothesis regarding how the virus invades the human body via ABO(H) blood group-determining carbohydrates. *Immunobiol.* 226 (3): 152027. https://doi.org/10.1016/j.imbio.2020.152027.

85 Jordan, M.I. and Mitchell, T.M. (2015). Machine learning: trends, perspectives, and prospects. *Science* 349 (6245): 255–260. https://doi.org/10.1126/science.aaa8415.

86 Duncan, D. (2021). COVID-19 data sharing and collaboration. *Commun. Inf. Syst.* 21 (3): 325–340.

87 Kononenko, I. (2001). Machine learning for medical diagnosis: history, state of the art and perspective. *Artif. Intell. Med.* 23 (1): 89–109. https://doi.org/10.1016/S0933-3657(01)00077-X.

88 Zheng, W., Zhang, X., Kim, J.J. et al. (2019). High accuracy of convolutional neural network for evaluation of helicobacter pylori infection based on endoscopic images: preliminary experience. *Clin. Transl. Gastroenterol.* 10 (12): e00109. https://doi.org/10.14309/ctg.0000000000000109.

89 Al-Saffar AAM, Tao H, Talab MA. (2017). Review of deep convolution neural network in image classification. *2017 International Conference on Radar, Antenna, Microwave, Electronics, and Telecommunications (ICRAMET)*. New York: IEEE; 2017:26–31. doi:10.1109/ICRAMET.2017.8253139

90 Polsinelli, M., Cinque, L., and Placidi, G. (2020). A light CNN for detecting COVID-19 from CT scans of the chest. *Pattern Recognit. Lett.* 140: 95–100. https://doi.org/10.1016/j.patrec.2020.10.001.

91 Chaddad, A., Hassan, L., and Desrosiers, C. (2021). Deep CNN models for predicting COVID-19 in CT and x-ray images. *J. Med. Imag.* 8 (Suppl. 1): 014502. https://doi.org/10.1117/1.JMI.8.S1.014502.

92 Koch G, Zemel R, Salakhutdinov R. 2015. Siamese neural networks for one-shot image recognition. Proceedings of the 32nd International Conference on Machine Learning. Lille, France: JMLR https://www.cs.cmu.edu/~rsalakhu/papers/oneshot1.pdf

9

COVID-19: Outpatient Management in Adults

Michael P. Dubé

Department of Medicine, Division of Infectious Diseases, Keck School of Medicine, University of Southern California, Los Angeles, CA, USA

Abbreviations

ACE	angiotensin-converting enzyme
CI	confidence interval
EUA	Emergency Use Authorization
FDA	US Food and Drug Administration
IMPROVE	International Medical Prevention Registry on Venous Thromboembolism
mAb	monoclonal antibody
NHC	*N*-hydroxycytidine
NIH	National Institutes of Health
RBD	receptor binding domain
RCT	randomized controlled trial
SARS-CoV-2	severe acute respiratory syndrome coronavirus 2
SSRI	selective serotonin reuptake inhibitor
WHO	World Health Organization

Potential Conflicts of Interest

Dr. Dubé has received grant support to his institution for an Astra-Zeneca COVID-19 vaccine clinical trial.

Initial Diagnosis

Diagnostic methods for confirming infection caused by severe acute respiratory syndrome coronavirus 2 (SARS-CoV-2) are covered elsewhere in this textbook.

Patients everywhere should be encouraged to seek diagnostic testing when they experience symptoms of coronavirus disease 2019 (COVID-19), even if very mild. This testing will facilitate disease and variant tracking in the community, as well as allow the initiation of isolation to reduce spread of the virus. Moreover, early testing allows early diagnosis, and early diagnosis is key to being able to benefit most from emerging early treatments. Benefit from various treatments among high-risk patients is likely maximal among those treated early in the course of disease [1–10]. That said, with many medications, delayed therapy will not have been studied in clinical trials, leaving open the possibility of some benefit when treatment is initiated past the entry criteria used in studies.

Prognosis and Choice of Admission Versus Outpatient Management

General criteria that would favor either initial inpatient or outpatient management of COVID-19 are summarized in Table 9.1.

Before the availability of vaccines, anti-SARS-CoV-2 monoclonal antibodies (mAbs), or other successful interventions for reducing the severity of COVID-19, the US Centers for Disease Control and Prevention estimated that 14% of people with confirmed

Coronavirus Disease 2019 (COVID-19): A Clinical Guide, First Edition. Edited by Ali Gholamrezanezhad and Michael P. Dube.

Table 9.1 Criteria that would favor inpatient care over outpatient care.

	Favors inpatient care	Favors outpatient care
Structural	Homelessness High-risk household member Unavailability of home isolation Lack of support person(s) No method of contact (phone, email)	Availability of home isolation away from other household members Adequate access to food and water
Illness characteristics	Oxygen saturation ≤ 94% on room air Requirement for supplemental O_2 or increase in chronic home O_2 Respiratory rate ≥ 24/min Persistent heart rate ≥ 120/min Systolic blood pressure ≤ 100 mmHg Hypothermia	Oxygen saturation > 94% on room air No need for supplemental O_2 Able to consume adequate food and water
Comorbidities	Serious ongoing, unstable medical conditions Need for ongoing parenteral therapies Advanced age Moderate to severe cognitive disorder Advanced chronic obstructive pulmonary disease Unstable congestive heart failure Uncontrolled asthma Major concurrent acute illness Rapidly progressing respiratory illness Uncontrolled HIV infection	Well-controlled medical comorbidities Ongoing engagement with care teams for chronic conditions

COVID-19 required hospitalization at some point during their illness [11]. Presumably, this 14% figure is considerably higher than the true proportion, because asymptomatic and mildly infected persons often do not get tested, particularly when access to testing is limited. A modeling study estimated the true prevalence rate of hospitalization was closer to 2% using data from the US state of Indiana [12].

Certainly, no single criterion or combination of criteria can substitute for clinical judgment and consideration of local norms and resources. The "HOME-CoV Rule" has been proposed as an evidence-based algorithm to assist in hospitalization decisions [13]. The presence of one or more of the following criteria corresponds to a greater risk for adverse outcomes and should lead the provider to consider hospitalization:

- Peripheral oxygen saturation ≤ 94% on room air
- Respiratory rate ≥ 25/min
- Ability to talk without breathing < 8 seconds
- Systolic blood pressure ≤ 90 mmHg
- Heart rate ≥ 120 beats/min
- Confusion or impaired consciousness
- Clinically significant worsening within the last 24 hours
- Severe comorbidity and inadequate living conditions

These criteria were then tested in a pragmatic clinical setting in France during April and May 2020 [14]. Patients with negative HOME-CoV Rule findings represented 41% of patients (1239/3000) seeking treatment at their emergency department with probable or confirmed COVID-19. Only 4 of 1239 (0.3%) experienced a serious adverse outcome (invasive ventilation or death) within the ensuing seven days. HOME-CoV represents a useful tool to identify a subgroup of patients likely to have a favorable outcome at the time of an emergency department visit.

Home Monitoring

Telehealth Diagnosis and Follow-up

The expanded use of telehealth has been encouraged during the pandemic [15]. In many cases, particularly with mild outpatient disease, the need for in-person evaluation has been obviated by liberal use of telehealth visits for both COVID-19 and general medical care. Specifically regarding COVID-19 care, telehealth provides added protection for healthcare workers and spares the infected individual the need to be transported to a medical facility, with subsequent possible exposure of others during private or public transport [16, 17]. There is evidence that telehealth has improved outcomes during the pandemic [18].

Pulse Oximetry Monitoring

Home use of pulse oximetry [19] has been suggested by World Health Organization (WHO) [20] and the National Institutes of Health (NIH) guidelines panel [21]. The WHO Living Guidelines include a conditional recommendation for use of pulse oximetry monitoring at home as part of a package of care, including patient and provider education and appropriate follow-up, in symptomatic patients with COVID-19 and risk factors for progression to severe disease who are not hospitalized [20]. Specific recommendations for implementing home pulse oximetry have been published [19, 22]. Key caveats for the use of home oximetry include the following:

- It is useful for high-risk patients, particularly those with dyspnea.
- Finger pulse oximeters are preferred, using a warm finger with the patient seated.
- Symptoms are at least as important as an oxygen saturation reading in isolation.
- Black and brown-skinned individuals may have falsely high SpO_2 readings by pulse oximetry.
- In those with chronic lung disease, oxygen saturation at baseline may be depressed.
- Home pulse oximetry is not a substitute for conventional forms of clinical monitoring.
- Trends over time should be followed and documented; single low readings should not necessarily be interpreted as clinical worsening unless supported by symptomatic decline.
- In the setting of limited resources, consideration should be given to prioritizing the highest risk individuals for home pulse oximetry.

Post–Hospital Discharge Care

Once patients improve to the point where hospital discharge can be considered, the trajectory of illness improvement typically continues in a favorable direction. Potential reasons for worsening in the short term (days to weeks after discharge) include thromboembolic disease, including deep vein thrombosis and pulmonary embolism, bacterial or fungal superinfection [23], and worsening chronic comorbidities, such as congestive heart failure, diabetes mellitus, and COPD [24]. Clinical worsening should prompt repeat medical evaluation, which may include in-person physical examination consisting of pulse oximetry, screening laboratory testing, and chest radiography.

General Management Issues

Isolation

Wherever possible, individuals receiving home care for COVID-19 should follow local guidance for isolation, such as the US Centers for Disease Control and Prevention guidelines [25]. If supplies are available locally, personal protective equipment can be provided by providers to increase the safety of household contacts. Where necessary and available, patients from multigenerational households or who are homeless and who cannot self-isolate but have lower risk for serious illness may be provided temporary housing units.

Hydration and Nutrition

Initial evaluation of patients with confirmed or suspected COVID-19 should include ascertainment of food security. This is particularly important for areas with known preexisting food insecurity, which has been projected to increase during the pandemic [26].

Continuation of Ongoing Therapies

Ongoing pharmacologic management for comorbidities should generally continue during COVID-19 illness. Specifically, angiotensin-converting enzyme (ACE) inhibitors and angiotensin receptor blockers should be continued [21]. Initially, there was concern for both beneficial and deleterious effects from ACE/angiotensin receptor blocker drugs by modulating interactions with the ACE2 receptor. A systematic meta-analysis concluded that there were no positive or negative effects with these agents [27].

Similarly, although studies have shown divergent results regarding benefits from continuing statins during COVID-19 [28–30], none has suggested a deleterious effect. It is recommended to continue statins in this setting [21].

Nonsteroidal anti-inflammatory drugs have not been found to have negative effects during COVID-19 [31–33] and need not be limited [21].

Nutritional Supplements

A wide variety of micronutrients have been advocated for COVID-19 [34–36]. Among the most widely used have been zinc, vitamin C, and vitamin D. Certainly, any ongoing supplementation for specific indications, such as malabsorption, osteoporosis, or pregnancy, should be continued. At the time of this writing, the NIH guidelines panel has not recommended for or against use of zinc, vitamin C, and vitamin D [21].

Among 214 participants who received high-dose zinc (zinc gluconate 50 mg daily), high-dose ascorbic acid (8000 mg daily), or both, there was no improvement in COVID-19 symptoms compared with routine care in an open-label randomized trial [37]. Although this trial was likely underpowered with approximately 50 participants per group, it did not provide support for supplementation. If clinicians choose to prescribe zinc, it is suggested that the dose should not exceed the recommended daily allowance [21].

Vitamin D insufficiency and deficiency are common in COVID-19 [38]. Both infection acquisition and severe disease appear to be greater with lower vitamin D levels [39]. One meta-analysis has suggested improved outcomes among individuals initiating vitamin D after COVID-19 diagnosis. A randomized clinical trial examined a single high dose of vitamin D_3 of 200 000 units compared with placebo in 240 hospitalized participants with moderate to severe COVID-19 [40]. Serum 25-hydroxyvitamin D levels more than doubled in treated patients, but there was no effect on length of hospital stay or any secondary endpoint. In another trial focused on inflammatory markers, mild to moderately ill inpatients with COVID-19 and serum 25-hydroxyvitamin D levels less than 30 ng/ml were randomized in an open-label fashion to high-dose oral vitamin D_3 versus standard of care [41]. The vitamin D group had 25-hydroxyvitamin D levels increase into the 80–100 ng/ml range and had greater reductions in C-reactive protein, lactate dehydrogenase, and ferritin. These results suggest a potential benefit with vitamin D supplementation among deficient individuals that deserves further study. Currently, there is little to support the routine use of vitamin D supplementation in COVID-19.

Anticoagulation

At the time of this writing, the NIH panel has recommended that hospitalized patients with COVID-19 should not be routinely discharged while receiving venous thromboembolism prophylaxis, unless they have another indication or are participating in a clinical trial [21], but other groups have recommended this for higher risk patients [42]. A recent trial of rivaroxaban 10 mg/day in participants at increased risk for venous thromboembolism who received heparin during hospitalization [43] reports a reduction in the composite outcome consisting of symptomatic or fatal venous thromboembolism, asymptomatic venous thromboembolism on bilateral lower-limb venous ultrasound and computed tomography pulmonary angiogram, symptomatic arterial thromboembolism, and cardiovascular death at day 35. This primary efficacy outcome occurred in 5 (3%) of 159 patients assigned to rivaroxaban and 15 (9%) of 159 patients assigned to no anticoagulation (relative risk, 0.33; 95% confidence interval [CI]: 0.12–0.90; $P = 0.0293$), without any major bleeding events [43]. Importantly, the difference was driven mainly by a lower incidence of pulmonary embolism (one symptomatic and one asymptomatic pulmonary embolism detected by computed tomography pulmonary angiogram) in the treatment group compared with the control group (four asymptomatic, three symptomatic, and three fatal).

These results provide strong support for the use of rivaroxaban 10 mg/day in patients being discharged with a modified International Medical Prevention Registry on Venous Thromboembolism (IMPROVE) venous thromboembolism score [44] of 2–3 plus increased D-dimer levels or an IMPROVE score ≥ 4.

Use of Home Supplemental Oxygen

Home use of supplemental oxygen can be considered for both initial outpatient management and following hospital discharge [45]. The ability to avoid inpatient hospitalization is particularly important when institutional resources are scarce. In addition, it may become necessary to discharge an adult patient and provide an advanced level of home care to free up hospital resources for more acutely ill individuals [21, 46]. One retrospective cohort described 621 patients who were discharged with at least 3 L/min of supplemental oxygen supporting an oxygen saturation of at least 92%, including 149 (24%) who were discharged from an emergency department who had not had inpatient stays [47]. Patients received daily telephone follow-up starting within 18 hours of discharge. Although outcomes were not reported separately for inpatient discharges and emergency department discharges, the overall mortality rate of 1.3% for the full cohort was thought to support the feasibility of this home oxygen approach in select individuals during pandemic surge conditions.

Antivirals and Anti-inflammatory Treatments

A variety of antiviral interventions have become available or are in late stages of clinical development for treatment of mild to moderate COVID-19. Anti-SARS-CoV-2 mAbs have taken a lead role in the management of outpatient illness in higher risk patients. These highly active treatments are limited, however, by the need for parenteral (intravenous or, in some instances, subcutaneous) administration and requirement for at least one hour of close observation after administration. Oral antivirals and anti-inflammatory treatments are somewhat less well-proven and effective interventions at the time of this writing. However, oral drugs hold great promise to provide much greater treatment accessibility both in high- and low-income countries. The requirement to administer these mAbs and oral drugs early in the course of disease underscores the need to have a robust testing and outpatient clinical care infrastructure for these to succeed.

Anti-SARS-CoV-2 mAbs

Anti-SARS-CoV-2 mAbs have been shown to be of benefit in reducing the need for hospitalization [3, 48, 49]. Several mAbs, including the combination of bamlanivimab and etesevimab, the combination of casirivimab and imdevimab, and the single agent sotrovimab (Table 9.2), have received Emergency Use Authorization (EUA) in the United States and are recommended by the NIH guidelines panel [21] for outpatient use in certain clinical situations. At the time of this writing, only casirivimab plus imdevimab has been recommended by the WHO for outpatient use [20]. Clinicians in all countries should always consult their local guidelines and the latest regulatory information, which are expected to be in considerable ongoing flux over time. Ultimately, the emergence of new variants of concern may rapidly shift these considerations.

Selection of Outpatients to Receive Anti-SARS-CoV-2 mAbs

These agents currently are recommended for mild-to-moderate outpatient COVID-19 in adults and pediatric patients (≥12 years of age and weighing at least 40 kg) who are at high risk for progression to severe COVID-19 [50–52]. These conditions or other factors that may place individuals at higher risk for progression to severe illness and are quite broad, for example:

- Older age (e.g. ≥65 years)
- Obesity or being overweight (e.g. adults with body mass index > 25 kg/m^2, or if 12–17 years of age, have body mass index ≥ 85th percentile for their age and sex)
- Pregnancy
- Chronic kidney disease

Table 9.2   Anti-SARS-CoV-2 monoclonal antibodies for outpatient treatment of COVID-19.

	Bamlanivimab plus etesevimab [50]	Casirivimab and imdevimab [51]	Sotrovimab [52]	Bebtelovimab [ref see below*]
Manufacturer	Lilly	Regeneron	GSK	Lilly
Brand name	–	REGEN-COV	Xevudy	–
Dose	BAM 700 mg ETE 1400 mg	CAS 600 mg IMD 600 mg	500 mg	175 mg
Mode of administration	IV	IV or subcutaneous (IV preferred)	IV	IV
Half-life (days)	BAM 20.9 ETE 32.6	CAS 31.8 IMD 26.9	49	27
Target	Different, but overlapping, epitopes in SARS-CoV-2 RBD	Nonoverlapping epitopes in SARS-CoV-2 spike RBD	Spike RBD epitopes conserved in both SARS-CoV and SARS-CoV-2	Spike RBD epitope of SARS-CoV-2
Major published efficacy trials	BLAZE-1 (ClinicalTrials.gov: NCT04427501)	COV-2067 (ClinicalTrials.gov: NCT04425629)	COMET-ICE (ClinicalTrials.gov: NCT04545060)	–
Reduction in need for inpatient hospitalization	70% [2] to 87% [50]	70–71% [5]	85% [3]	–
Notes	Only where resistant variants are unlikely			Active *in vitro* against Omicron variants BA.2, BA.2.12.1, BA.4, BA.5

BAM, bamlanivimab; CAS, casirivimab; ETE, etesevimab; IMD, imdevimab; IV, intravenous; RBD, receptor binding domain; SARS-CoV-2, severe acute respiratory syndrome coronavirus 2.
REF for above: (Eli Lilly and Co., FACT SHEET FOR HEALTHCARE PROVIDERS: EMERGENCY USE AUTHORIZATION FOR BEBTELOVIMAB, June 2022)

- Diabetes mellitus
- Immunosuppressive disease or immunosuppressive treatment
- Cardiovascular disease (including congenital heart disease) or hypertension
- Chronic lung diseases (chronic obstructive pulmonary disease, moderate-to-severe asthma, interstitial lung disease, cystic fibrosis, and pulmonary hypertension)
- Sickle cell disease
- Neurodevelopmental disorders (e.g. cerebral palsy) or other conditions that confer medical complexity (e.g. genetic or metabolic syndromes and severe congenital anomalies)
- Having a medical-related technologic dependence (e.g. tracheostomy, gastrostomy, or positive pressure ventilation [not related to COVID-19])

In settings with varying degrees of limited resources and availability, individual entities are expected to use more narrow selection criteria. In addition to outpatient illness, patients who are hospitalized for reasons other than COVID-19 and do not require supplemental oxygen are also candidates for mAbs if other criteria for administration are also met. All three of these agents can be used in persons as young as 12 years old weighing at least 40 kg.

Bamlanivimab Plus Etesevimab

This combination mAb product targets two different but overlapping epitopes in the SARS-CoV-2 spike protein receptor binding domain (RBD) [53]. Early enthusiasm about bamlanivimab alone was tempered by the recognition that common SARS-CoV-2 variants carrying mutations such as the E484K mutation can render bamlanivimab alone ineffective against variants such as beta (B.1.351) and gamma (P.1) [54, 55], as well as the combination product. However, in the setting of minimal to no circulation of variants with resistance to bamlanivimab plus etesevimab in the second half of 2021 during the Delta variant surge, the use of this combination was resumed in the United States.

Using the currently approved dose, there was an 87% reduction in the risk for hospitalization or death among high-risk individuals treated in the BLAZE-1 trial [50]. Importantly, there were four deaths with placebo and none with bamlanivimab 700 mg plus etesevimab 1400 mg ($P = 0.01$).

Casirivimab Plus Imdevimab

This combination mAb product targets two different, nonoverlapping epitopes in the SARS-CoV-2 spike protein RBD [4, 51]. This feature has the potential to reduce the likelihood of a single mutation to result in resistance to both antibodies. The use of casirivimab plus imdevimab is supported by a clinical trial in high-risk outpatients involving two different doses, with comparable results from both 600/600 mg and 1200/1200 mg levels approximating 70% reduction in the incidence of hospitalization or death [51]. Few deaths occurred in the trial. Symptom duration was shortened by four days with casirivimab plus imdevimab. In addition to randomized controlled trial (RCT) data, there is supportive real-world evidence for efficacy of the combination [56].

Sotrovimab

Sotrovimab targets spike RBD epitopes that are highly conserved in both SARS-CoV (the causative agent of the 2003 SARS outbreak) and SARS-CoV-2, and thus is considered a pan-sarbecovirus mAb. This characteristic increases the likelihood that its use may make it more difficult for escape mutants to develop, with the mAb targeting an area that would be functionally retained as SARS-CoV-2 evolves. The COMET-ICE trial established a high degree of efficacy with an 85% reduction (1% vs. 7%) in the risk for hospitalization or death among participants with at least one risk factor for disease progression [3]. Preliminary data suggest that activity is maintained with sotrovimab against the omicron variant [57], although real-world efficacy against omicron has not been documented for any of the anti-SARS-CoV-2 mAbs as of this writing.

Bebtelovimab

The mAb bebtelovimab is the only mAb recommended for use in the US as of March 2022 when the BA.2 Omicron variant became dominant (https://covid.cdc. gov/covid-data-tracker/#variant-proportions. Accessed 29 June 2022). It is administered as a single 175 mg IV injection, administered over ≥30 seconds. Although efficacy data are lacking, bebtelovimab retains in vitro activity against BA.2 and other recent Omicron variants including BA.2.12, BA.4, and BA.5 (Eli Lilly and Co., FACT SHEET FOR HEALTHCARE PROVIDERS: EMERGENCY USE AUTHORIZATION FOR BEBTELOVIMAB, June 2022). The NIH panel recommends use of bebtelovimab within 7 days of symptom onset only when ritonavir-boosted nirmatrelvir and remdesivir are not available, feasible to use, or clinically appropriate (https://www.covid19treatmentguidelines.nih.gov/management/clinical-management/nonhospitalized-adults--therapeutic-management/. Accessed 25 June 2022).

Side Effects of Anti-SARS-CoV-2 mAbs

These agents have been universally well tolerated among COVID-19-affected outpatients, with serious adverse events being similar or more common in the placebo arms of trials [2, 3, 5, 50–52]. Anti-SARS-CoV-2 mAbs should be administered by intravenous infusion or subcutaneous injections and should be administered only in healthcare settings by qualified healthcare providers who have immediate access to emergency medical services and medications that treat severe infusion-related reactions [21]. Patients should be monitored during and for at least one hour after the infusion or injections are completed because of the low risk for hypersensitivity reactions, which include anaphylaxis.

Distribution of mAbs

Data regarding how many individuals for whom anti-SARS-CoV-2 mAbs are indicated who actually have been able to receive them have not been available. In the United States, distribution to local hospitals and clinics of these mAbs has shifted to individual state/territories as of September 2021 [58]. The amount distributed to each state is determined centrally by the US government based on weekly reports of new COVID-19 cases and hospitalizations in addition to data on inventories and use submitted to the federal government. Individual State/Territorial Health Departments will then determine where product goes within their jurisdictions.

Administration of mAbs requires the capacity to provide intravenous infusions and monitor patients for at least one hour after infusion. Many hospitals have been able to establish the capacity for outpatient infusion centers, as have some home health agencies, pharmacies, and chronic care facilities. Anti-SARS-CoV-2 mAbs have been effectively used in US inner-city populations [59]. The WHO provided a conditional recommendation for the outpatient use of casirivimab plus imdevimab among patients at very high risk (>10%) for adverse outcomes [60].

Oral Antivirals

Molnupiravir

Molnupiravir is an oral prodrug of an antiviral nucleoside [61–64]. After absorption, molnupiravir is converted to N-hydroxycytidine (NHC), which is taken up by cells, where it is phosphorylated to the active moiety NHC-triphosphate. NHC-triphosphate successfully competes with native nucleotides, resulting in transition errors (i.e. mutations) in the replicating viral RNA strand that escape proofreading functions and impair viral infectivity and replication [63].

Initial efficacy data were highly promising for molnupiravir at the time of the MOVe-OUT trial interim analysis (Table 9.3) [9], with a relative risk reduction for hospitalization or death of 50% among adult participants with five or fewer days of symptoms and one risk factor for severe disease. Based on these favorable results, an independent data safety and monitoring board recommended study termination. However, the final analysis of this trial showed only a 30% overall reduction in the risk for hospitalization or death. The relative risk with molnupiravir compared with placebo of 0.70 (95% CI: 0.49–0.99) barely achieved statistical significance. Notably, in the postinterim analysis population (those participants who had not reached day 29 by the interim analysis data cutoff date of 18 September 2021, N = 646), there was no apparent benefit to molnupiravir with hospitalization or death in 6.2% compared with 4.7% for placebo. The reasons for this attenuation in efficacy are unclear at this time, but it is possible that a greater prevalence of the Delta variant during the postinterim analysis contributed. Indeed, in a post hoc analysis of 237 molnupiravir recipients and 221 placebo recipients with confirmed Delta infection, the incidence of hospitalization or death was only 2.7% lower with molnupiravir (95% CI: −7.8 to 2.9), which was not statistically significant [9]. These disappointing efficacy data contributed to the US Food and Drug Administration (FDA) Advisory Committee's 13 to 10 vote marginally recommending approval of the drug [65].

Short-term safety data for molnupiravir are encouraging [9], with no remarkable acute toxicities. Because of a finding of bone marrow toxicity in dogs, hematologic parameters were assessed (leukocytes, lymphocytes, platelets, and hemoglobin) and were no different with molnupiravir compared with placebo.

However, concerns for human mutagenicity of molnupiravir have been voiced [65–67]. Although the primary mechanism of action of molnupiravir is introducing errors in viral RNA synthesis, the compound NHC can be metabolized in the host cell to a deoxyribonucleoside and incorporated into the host cell DNA [67]. A mutagenic effect was demonstrated in a mammalian cell culture model and suggests the possibility of molnupiravir promoting carcinogenesis and adverse consequences on fetal development or spermatogenesis [67]. Ultimately, this should limit its use in persons of reproductive potential, during pregnancy, and in children. This limitation may favor alternative therapies having similar efficacy but less concern for long-term adverse events. The short duration of treatment could partially mitigate these concerns.

New viral mutations induced by molnupiravir have the potential to generate evolution of new SARS-CoV-2 variants of concern. In data presented by the manufacturer to the FDA [9], treatment-emergent amino acid changes in spike protein occurred more often with molnupiravir than with placebo (in 34% and 23%, respectively) with a much greater absolute number of changes (72 vs. 9, respectively), including two instances of emergence of the troublesome E484K mutation among 113 analyzed molnupiravir recipients. Unquestionably, very close monitoring for molnupiravir-induced variants will be essential in the postmarketing period. Moreover, concern for promoting new variants has led some to suggest that molnupiravir should not be given to people with significant immunocompromise in whom prolonged viral evolution is likely [65, 68].

Table 9.3   Selected outpatient oral therapies for COVID-19.

	Fluvoxamine	Molnupiravir	Nirmatrelvir (PF-07321332)/ Ritonavir
Manufacturer	Jazz, generics	Merck	Pfizer
Brand name	Luvox	Lagevrio	Paxlovid
Drug class	SSRI	Antiviral nucleoside	Protease inhibitor
1° mechanism of action	Anti-inflammatory; S1R agonist (modulates ER stress response and ↓ proinflammatory cytokines)	Prodrug→NHC →NHC-triphosphate incorporated into viral RNA inducing multiple RNA errors	Inhibition of viral 3C-like protease
Dose	100 mg b.i.d. × 10 days	4 × 200 mg capsules b.i.d. × 5 days	2 × 150 mg tablets nirmatrelvir plus 1 × 100 mg tablet ritonavir, each b.i.d. for 5 days
Half-life (h)	15.6	3.3	Not available at time of this writing
Cost/course	US$16 (GoodRx)	US$700 (licensing planned for low-income countries	US$529 (licensing planned for low-income countries)
Trial entry criteria	≤7 days of symptoms, 1 risk factor for severe	≤5 days of symptoms, 1 risk factor for severe	≤5 days of symptoms, 1 risk factor for severe
N	1497 (TOGETHER-Brazil) [7]	1433 (final MOVe-OUT) [9]	774 (EPIC-HR Study, Pfizer press release) [10]
Hospitalization or death	RR, 0.68 (0.52–0.88) 32% ↓	RR, 0.70 (0.49–0.99) 30% ↓	85% ↓
Deaths (drug/placebo)	17/25	1/9	0/10
Death rate placebo group	3.3%	1.3%	1.6%
Drug–drug interactions	Potent inhibitor CYP1A2 (do not use tizanidine, thioridazine, alosetron, pimozide, monoamine oxidase inhibitors); ↓ warfarin, theophylline, benzodiazepines, omeprazole, phenytoin	None expected	Multiple major CYP3A4 inhibition issues expected from ritonavir

ER, endoplasmic reticulum; NHC, N-hydroxycytidine; RR, relative risk; SSRI, selective serotonin reuptake inhibitor. The largest randomized clinical trials of each drug are summarized in the table, as well as general characteristics of the agents.

Nirmatrelvir (PF-07321332)/Ritonavir

The compound PF-07321332 inhibits the viral 3-chymotrypsin-like protease of SARS-CoV-2 [69]. It is coadministered with the HIV-1 protease inhibitor ritonavir, which acts as a pharmacokinetic enhancer by its potent inhibition of CYP3A4. Thus, it is anticipated that PF-07321332/ritonavir will have multiple major drug–drug interactions that will complicate its use. At the time of this writing, no drug–drug interaction studies have been published with PF-07321332/ritonavir. The publicly available information for PF-07321332/ritonavir is presently limited, with the only clinical data available via a press release from the sponsor [10].

The aforementioned press release reports a substantial 85% decrease in the risk for hospitalization or death among adult outpatients with five or fewer days of symptoms and one risk factor for severe disease. Ten deaths were reported with placebo versus none with PF-07321332/ritonavir (Table 9.3). If full peer-reviewed results show similar efficacy and a favorable safety profile is confirmed, then it is likely that PF-07321332/ritonavir will be able to play a major role in management of early (≤5 days of symptoms) disease in higher risk individuals. Access remains a major concern, particularly in developing countries and other settings where anti-SARS-CoV-2 mAbs are difficult to administer and timely testing is not generally available. The United States has pledged to purchase 10 million treatment courses for US$5.29 billion. The manufacturer Pfizer, Inc. has stated that "a tiered pricing approach based on the income level of each country to promote equity of access across the globe" is planned [10]. Details about this plan were not available at the time of this writing. If PF-07321332/ritonavir becomes widely available at a reasonable cost, it has the potential to have a tremendous impact on the global pandemic. Activity against the emerging SARS-CoV-2 variant of concern omicron may be needed for PF-07321332/ritonavir to have a lasting impact on the pandemic.

Outpatient Anti-inflammatory Interventions

Inhaled Budesonide

Budesonide is a topical steroid with anti-inflammatory properties; it has been approved for topical asthma treatment [70], has minimal systemic absorption, and is widely available. Budesonide may also have intrinsic antiviral activity against SARS-CoV-2 [71].

Two open-label RCTs have suggested some benefit of inhaled budesonide in mild to moderate outpatient COVID-19 [8, 72]. In the smaller STOIC trial, budesonide 800 μg inhaled b.i.d. until symptom resolution was given to adults with ≤7 days of symptoms and mild disease. Mean age was 45 years with a low rate of comorbidities. There was a marked 91% reduction in the number of participants requiring urgent care visits or hospitalization, with 10 of 70 (14%) participants in the usual care group and 1 of 69 (1%) participants in the budesonide group meeting the primary endpoint (difference in proportions, 0.131; 95% CI: 0.043–0.218; $P = 0.004$). Significant adverse reactions were not reported.

PRINCIPLE was a larger open-label trial in 1856 outpatients with COVID-19 at higher risk for disease progression than in STOIC, requiring age ≥65 years or ≥50 years with comorbidities [73]. In this trial,

inhaled budesonide 800 μg b.i.d. for 14 days did not affect the rate of hospitalization or death but did reduce time to self-reported recovery. The relevance of improved self-reported recovery, a secondary endpoint, in this open-label trial should be interpreted with caution. At the time of this writing, the NIH guidelines panel has opined that there is insufficient evidence for the panel to recommend either for or against the use of budesonide in COVID-19 [21]. At present, the authors prefer the use of anti-SARS-CoV-2 mAbs (see earlier) for symptomatic outpatient COVID-19 in patients at increased risk for disease progression. For patients with mild disease at low risk for disease progression who are not candidates for mAb treatment, inhaled budesonide represents a reasonable option to reduce the need for urgent care visits or hospitalization. Additional trials of inhaled corticosteroids are needed, particularly in combination with antiviral interventions.

Fluvoxamine

Fluvoxamine is a selective serotonin reuptake inhibitor (SSRI) approved for use in obsessive compulsive disorder but is chemically unrelated to other SSRIs [74]. The approved starting dosage for adults is 50 mg once daily. The primary mechanism of action has not been established but is most likely an anti-inflammatory effect related to sigma-1 receptor agonism with consequent reduction in endoplasmic reticulum stress and proinflammatory cytokines [75, 76]. In a large observational retrospective matched case–control study of COVID-19, SSRI use was associated with lower mortality [77]. In that study, specifically fluoxetine and fluvoxamine appeared to mediate much of the observed overall SSRI effect.

In the largest randomized placebo-controlled trial to date, the Brazilian TOGETHER trial (https://www.togethertrial.com/flv) used fluvoxamine 100 mg b.i.d. for 10 days in outpatients with COVID-19 and at least one risk factor for a poor outcome with seven or fewer days of symptoms [7]. Fluvoxamine use was associated with a 32% reduction in the risk for death or hospitalization/prolonged emergency department visit (relative risk, 0.68; 95% CI: 0.52–0.88) and was well tolerated, in spite of the dosage at four times the usual starting adult dose. At the time of this writing, the NIH guidelines panel does not recommend routine use of fluvoxamine outside of a clinical trial [21]. However, this author recommends considering the use of fluvoxamine in outpatients with increased risk for a poor outcome who are not candidates for **oral antivirals or** anti-SARS-CoV-2 mAb treatment, with seven or fewer days of symptoms. A course of treatment is estimated to cost as little as US$16. Importantly, clinicians should carefully review the fluvoxamine prescribing information before prescribing with particular attention to drug–drug interactions because fluvoxamine is a potent inhibitor of CYP1A2 (Table 9.3). Future trials of fluvoxamine should investigate combination therapies, in particular fluvoxamine in combination with a primary antiviral intervention, such as an anti-SARS-CoV-2 mAb or one of the emerging oral antivirals.

Dexamethasone

Dexamethasone should not be used in individuals who do not require supplemental oxygen or an increase in supplemental oxygen because of COVID-19. In the RECOVERY trial, there was no benefit, and there was a signal for possible harm with dexamethasone in those participants who did not require supplemental oxygen [78]. However, it is recommended to finish a course of dexamethasone among individuals for whom it was initiated during an inpatient stay where supplemental oxygen was required [21].

Drugs That Are Not Recommended for Outpatient Use

Janus Kinase Inhibitors/Anti-IL-6 Therapies

Janus kinase inhibitors (baricitinib, tofacitinib) have not been studied in outpatients and are not recommended. Similarly, anti-IL-6 mAbs (tocilizumab, sarilumab) are indicated only for severe disease.

Chloroquine and Hydroxychloroquine

These agents increase the endosomal pH and may have an antiviral effect [79–81]. However, clinical trials fail to suggest any role for hydroxychloroquine in COVID-19 in outpatients [82, 83]. The FDA revoked the EUA for hydroxychloroquine and chloroquine in June 2020.

Ivermectin

Ivermectin has been a controversial potential treatment for COVID-19. It is well tolerated as an antiparasitic treatment for a broad range of infections [84], has antiviral effects in vitro [85, 86], and may have anti-inflammatory properties [87]. However, there is no reliable randomized clinical trial data showing relevant benefit from its use at the time of this writing. Existing data on ivermectin have been extensively summarized by the NIH guidelines panel [21]. In the largest RCT to date, ivermectin 300 μg/kg body weight per day for five days was compared with placebo in 400 participants with mild disease [88]. There was no benefit seen with ivermectin on time to illness resolution. Further data are needed to better define the role of ivermectin in management of outpatient illness. At this time, the clear benefits of anti-SARS-CoV-2 mAb treatment or the promise of benefit from fluvoxamine or the emerging oral antivirals are much more compelling than the limited and problematic ivermectin data available as of this writing.

Azithromycin

This macrolide antibiotic possesses anti-inflammatory properties. In the largest trial to date, azithromycin 500 mg once daily for three days plus standard of care (n = 500) was compared with standard of care alone (n = 823) in outpatient high-risk, older adults [89]. There was no benefit of azithromycin for either time to self-reported recovery or hospitalization or death as a result of COVID-19. Until further supportive data are available, we do not recommend azithromycin for outpatient illness [21].

Lopinavir/Ritonavir

Lopinavir/ritonavir did not demonstrate a clinical or virologic benefit in hospitalized patients with COVID-19 in several randomized clinical trials [90, 91]. In a large randomized trial in the United Kingdom involving 1616 patients allocated to receive lopinavir/ritonavir and 3424 patients to receive usual care, there was no benefit for mortality or any key secondary endpoints [91]. Although data on outpatient treatment are lacking, these negative results among hospitalized patients suggest that lopinavir/ritonavir is unlikely to have beneficial effects for outpatients.

Convalescent Plasma

The largest trial of convalescent plasma in outpatients (C3PO) evaluated convalescent plasma in patients with seven or fewer days of mild to moderate COVID-19 symptoms and at least one risk factor for severe COVID-19. An interim analysis indicated no benefit of convalescent plasma after 511 of the planned 900 participants were enrolled [92]. Disease progression occurred in 77 patients (30.0%) in the convalescent-plasma group and in 81 patients (31.9%) in the placebo group, and a preplanned interim analysis halted the trial for futility. There is currently insufficient evidence to recommend high-titer convalescent plasma for outpatients, and it is not authorized for nonhospitalized patients with COVID-19 under the EUA [21].

Colchicine

Colchicine is an anti-inflammatory drug that is used for gout and other inflammatory conditions. The large COLCORONA randomized trial evaluated colchicine 0.5 mg b.i.d. for 3 days and then once daily for 27 days in outpatients with outpatient COVID-19 who had at least one risk factor for an adverse COVID-19 outcome [93]. Compared with placebo, the primary endpoint of hospitalization or death was not improved by colchicine, but a secondary analysis of those participants with a positive SARS-CoV-2 PCR showed a modest benefit, with the primary endpoint occurring in 4.6% and 6.0% of patients in the colchicine and placebo groups, respectively (odds ratio, 0.75; 95% CI: 0.57–0.99; $P = 0.04$). Colchicine recipients experienced more gastrointestinal adverse events and serious adverse events [93]. Due to this modest benefit seen in only a subgroup analysis, we do not recommend the use of colchicine for outpatient illness [21]. It is possible that combination of the anti-inflammatory colchicine with an antiviral intervention may result in synergistic benefits, but this has not been reported.

Summary

Most patients who contract COVID-19 are appropriate for outpatient management. In this chapter, we outline strategies for home care and monitoring. Outpatient management will help reduce the inpatient hospital burden of disease, resulting in the maintenance of bed capacity for severe and critical COVID-19 in addition to the community's ongoing non-COVID needs.

For patients at increased risk for an adverse outcome from COVID-19, the anti-SARS-CoV-2 mAbs represent a major milestone that can dramatically reduce the need for hospitalization, further freeing up healthcare resources. However, availability of oral therapies will help expand treatment in areas where mAbs are unavailable or difficult to administer. At the time of this writing, there are adequate data to support the use of fluvoxamine where **oral antivirals or** mAbs cannot be given. The marginal efficacy of molnupiravir is disappointing, but this agent may provide some benefit, although mutagenicity and induction of new SARS-CoV-2 variants will need to be considered and monitored intensively. The promise of PF-07321332/ritonavir is potentially massive, if approved, and has real-world efficacy that approaches the data reported in press release form. Crucially, universal access to rapid testing for COVID-19 is an essential component of any strategy for early intervention with any of the emerging antiviral interventions.

References

1 Kreuzberger, N., Hirsch, C., Chai, K.L. et al. (2021). SARS-CoV-2-neutralising monoclonal antibodies for treatment of COVID-19. *Cochrane Database Syst. Rev.* 9: CD013825.

2 Dougan, M., Nirula, A., Azizad, M. et al. (2021). Bamlanivimab plus etesevimab in mild or moderate Covid-19. *N. Engl. J. Med.* 385 (15): 1382–1392.

3 Gupta, A., Gonzalez-Rojas, Y., Juarez, E. et al. (2021). Early treatment for Covid-19 with SARS-CoV-2 neutralizing antibody sotrovimab. *N. Engl. J. Med.* 385 (21): 1941–1950. https://doi.org/10.1056/NEJMoa2107934.

4 Taylor, P.C., Adams, A.C., Hufford, M.M. et al. (2021). Neutralizing monoclonal antibodies for treatment of COVID-19. *Nat. Rev. Immunol.* 21 (6): 382–393. https://doi.org/10.1038/s41577-021-00542-x.

5 Weinreich, D.M., Sivapalasingam, S., Norton, T. et al. (2021). REGEN-COV antibody combination and outcomes in outpatients with Covid-19. *N. Engl. J. Med.* 385 (23): e81. https://doi.org/10.1056/NEJMoa2108163.

6 Pfizer. (2021). Pfizer Announces Additional Phase 2/3 Study Results Confirming Robust Efficacy of Novel COVID-19 Oral Antiviral Treatment Candidate in Reducing Risk of Hospitalization or Death. Business Wire. 2021. https://www.businesswire.com/news/home/20211214005548/en. Accessed 14 Dec 2021.

7 Reis, G., dos Santos Moreira-Silva, E.A., Silva, D.C.M. et al. (2022). Effect of early treatment with fluvoxamine on risk of emergency care and hospitalisation among patients with COVID-19: the TOGETHER randomised, platform clinical trial. *Lancet Glob. Health* 10: e42–e51. https://doi.org/10.1016/S2214-109X(21)00448-4.

8 Agusti, A., Torres, F., and Faner, R. (2021). Early treatment with inhaled budesonide to prevent clinical deterioration in patients with COVID-19. *Lancet Respir. Med.* 9 (7): 682–683. https://doi.org/10.1016/s2213-2600(21)00171-5.

9 US Food and Drug Administration. (2021): Antimicrobial Drugs Advisory Committee Meeting Announcement. 2021. https://www.fda.gov/advisory-committees/advisory-committee-calendar/november-30-2021-antimicrobial-drugs-advisory-committee-meeting-announcement-11302021-11302021#event-materials. Accessed 30 Nov 2021

10 Pfizer, Inc. 2021. Pfizer seeks Emergency Use Authorization for novel COVID-19 oral antiviral candidate.https://www.pfizer.com/news/press-release/press-release-detail/pfizer-seeks-emergency-use-authorization-novel-covid-19. Accessed 26 Nov 2021.

11 Stokes, E., Zambrano, L., and Anderson, K. (2020). Coronavirus disease 2019 case surveillance – United States, January 22–May 30, 2020. *MMWR Morb. Mortal. Wkly Rep.* 69: 759–765. https://doi.org/10.15585/mmwr.mm6924e2.

12 Menachemi, N., Dixon, B.E., Wools-Kaloustian, K.K. et al. (2021). How many SARS-CoV-2-infected people require hospitalization? Using random sample testing to better inform preparedness efforts. *J. Public Health Manag. Pract.* 27 (3): 246–250. https://doi.org/10.1097/phh.0000000000001331.

13 Douillet, D., Mahieu, R., Boiveau, V. et al. (2020). Outpatient management or hospitalization of patients with proven or suspected SARS-CoV-2 infection: the HOME-CoV rule. *Intern. Emerg. Med.* 15 (8): 1525–1531. https://doi.org/10.1007/s11739-020-02483-0.

14 Douillet, D., Penaloza, A., Mahieu, R. et al. (2021). Outpatient management of patients with COVID-19. *Chest* 160 (4): 1222–1231. https://doi.org/10.1016/j.chest.2021.05.008.

15 US Department of Health and Human Services. 2021. Telehealth: delivering care safely during COVID-19. https://www.hhs.gov/coronavirus/telehealth/index.html. Accessed 14 Dec 2021.

16 Centers for Disease Control and Prevention. (2021). Using telehealth to expand access to essential health services during the COVID-19 pandemic. 2021. https://www.cdc.gov/coronavirus/2019-ncov/hcp/telehealth.html.

17 US Department of Health and Human Services. 2021. Telehealth and COVID-19. https://telehealth.hhs.gov/patients/telehealth-and-covid. Accessed 14 Dec 2021.

18 Monaghesh, E. and Hajizadeh, A. (2020). The role of telehealth during COVID-19 outbreak: a systematic review based on current evidence. *BMC Public Health* 20 (1): 1193. https://doi.org/10.1186/s12889-020-09301-4.

19 Greenhalgh, T., Knight, M., Inada-Kim, M. et al. (2021). Remote management of covid-19 using home pulse oximetry and virtual ward support. *BMJ* 372: n677. https://doi.org/10.1136/bmj.n677.

20 World Health Organization. (2021). Therapeutics and COVID-19: living guideline. https://www.who.int/publications/i/item/WHO-2019-nCoV-therapeutics-2021.3. Accessed 3 Dec 2021

21 National Institutes of Health. (2021). COVID-19 Treatment Guidelines Panel. Coronavirus disease 2019 (COVID-19) treatment guidelines. https://www.covid19treatmentguidelines.nih.gov. Accessed 3 Dec 2021.

22 Luks, A.M. and Swenson, E.R. (2020). Pulse oximetry for monitoring patients with COVID-19 at home. Potential pitfalls and practical guidance. *Ann. Am. Thorac. Soc.* 17 (9): 1040–1046. https://doi.org/10.1513/annalsats.202005-418fr.

23 Garcia-Vidal, C., Sanjuan, G., Moreno-García, E. et al. (2021). Incidence of co-infections and superinfections in hospitalized patients with COVID-19: a retrospective cohort study. *Clin. Microbiol. Infect.* 27 (1): 83–88. https://doi.org/10.1016/j.cmi.2020.07.041.

24 Romero-Duarte, Á., Rivera-Izquierdo, M., Guerrero-Fernández De Alba, I. et al. (2021). Sequelae, persistent symptomatology and outcomes after COVID-19 hospitalization: the ANCOHVID multicentre 6-month follow-up study. *BMC Med.* 19 (1): 129. https://doi.org/10.1186/s12916-021-02003-7.

25 Centers for Disease Control and Prevention. (2021). Quarantine and isolation. https://www.cdc.gov/coronavirus/2019-ncov/your-health/quarantine-isolation.html Accessed 14 Dec 2021

26 Feeding America. (2020). The impact of the coronavirus on local food insecurity in 2020 and 2021. https://www.feedingamerica.org/research/coronavirus-hunger-research. Accessed 1 Dec 2021.

27 Flacco, M.E., Acuti Martellucci, C., Bravi, F. et al. (2020). Treatment with ACE inhibitors or ARBs and risk of severe/lethal COVID-19: a meta-analysis. *Heart* 106 (19): 1519–1524. https://doi.org/10.1136/heartjnl-2020-317336.

28 Tan, W.Y.T., Young, B.E., Lye, D.C. et al. (2020). Statin use is associated with lower disease severity in COVID-19 infection. *Sci. Rep.* 10 (1): 17458. https://doi.org/10.1038/s41598-020-74492-0.

29 Zhang, X.J., Qin, J.J., Cheng, X. et al. (2020). In-hospital use of statins is associated with a reduced risk of mortality among individuals with COVID-19. *Cell Metab.* 32 (2): 176-187.e4. https://doi.org/10.1016/j.cmet.2020.06.015.

30 Grasselli, G., Greco, M., Zanella, A. et al. (2020). Risk factors associated with mortality among patients with COVID-19 in intensive care units in Lombardy, Italy. *JAMA Intern Med.* 180 (10): 1345–1355. https://doi.org/10.1001/jamainternmed.2020.3539.

31 Lund, L.C., Kristensen, K.B., Reilev, M. et al. (2020). Adverse outcomes and mortality in users of non-steroidal anti-inflammatory drugs who tested positive for SARS-CoV-2: a Danish nationwide cohort study. *PLoS Med.* 17 (9): e1003308. https://doi.org/10.1371/journal.pmed.1003308.

32 Abu Esba, L.C., Alqahtani, R.A., Thomas, A. et al. (2021). Ibuprofen and NSAID use in COVID-19 infected patients is not associated with worse outcomes: a prospective cohort study. *Infect. Dis. Ther.* 10 (1): 253–268. https://doi.org/10.1007/s40121-020-00363-w.

33 Wong, A.Y., MacKenna, B., Morton, C.E. et al. (2021). Use of non-steroidal anti-inflammatory drugs and risk of death from COVID-19: an OpenSAFELY cohort analysis based on two cohorts. *Ann. Rheum. Dis.* 80 (7): 943–951. https://doi.org/10.1136/annrheumdis-2020-219517.

34 Gasmi, A., Tippairote, T., Mujawdiya, P.K. et al. (2020). Micronutrients as immunomodulatory tools for COVID-19 management. *Clin. Immunol.* 220: 108545. https://doi.org/10.1016/j.clim.2020.108545.

35 McAuliffe, S., Ray, S., Fallon, E. et al. (2020). Dietary micronutrients in the wake of COVID-19: an appraisal of evidence with a focus on high-risk groups and preventative healthcare. *BMJ Nutr. Prev. Health* 3 (1): 93–99. https://doi.org/10.1136/bmjnph-2020-000100.

36 Keflie, T.S. and Biesalski, H.K. (2021). Micronutrients and bioactive substances: their potential roles in combating COVID-19. *Nutrition* 84: 111103. https://doi.org/10.1016/j.nut.2020.111103.

37 Thomas, S., Patel, D., Bittel, B. et al. (2021). Effect of high-dose zinc and ascorbic acid supplementation vs usual care on symptom length and reduction among ambulatory patients with SARS-CoV-2 infection. *JAMA Netw. Open* 4 (2): e210369. https://doi.org/10.1001/jamanetworkopen.2021.0369.

38 Ghasemian, R., Shamshirian, A., Heydari, K. et al. (2021). The role of vitamin D in the age of COVID-19: a systematic review and meta-analysis. *Int. J. Clin. Pract.* 75 (11): e14675. https://doi.org/10.1111/ijcp.14675.

39 Pereira, M., Dantas Damascena, A., Galvão Azevedo, L.M. et al. (2022). Vitamin D deficiency aggravates COVID-19: systematic review and meta-analysis. *Crit. Rev. Food Sci. Nutr.* 62: 1308–1316. https://doi.org/10.1080/10408398.2020.1841090.

40 Murai, I.H., Fernandes, A.L., Sales, L.P. et al. (2021). Effect of a single high dose of vitamin D3 on hospital length of stay in patients with moderate to severe COVID-19. *JAMA* 325 (11): 1053. https://doi.org/10.1001/jama.2020.26848.

41 Lakkireddy, M., Gadiga, S.G., Malathi, R.D. et al. (2021). Impact of daily high dose oral vitamin D therapy on the inflammatory markers in patients with COVID 19 disease. *Sci. Rep.* 11 (1): 10641. https://doi.org/10.1038/s41598-021-90189-4.

42 Gerotziafas, G.T., Catalano, M., Colgan, M.-P. et al. (2020). Guidance for the management of patients with vascular disease or cardiovascular risk factors and COVID-19: position paper from VAS-European Independent Foundation in Angiology/Vascular Medicine. *Thromb. Haemost.* 120 (12): 1597–1628.

43 Ramacciotti, E., Barile Agati, L., Calderaro, D. et al. (2021). Rivaroxaban versus no anticoagulation for post-discharge thromboprophylaxis after hospitalisation for COVID-19 (MICHELLE): an open-label, multicentre, randomised, controlled trial. *Lancet* 399: 50–59. https://doi.org/10.1016/S0140-6736(21)02392-8.

44 Raskob, G.E., Spyropoulos, A.C., Zrubek, J. et al. (2016). The MARINER trial of rivaroxaban after hospital discharge for medical patients at high risk of VTE. Design, rationale, and clinical implications. *Thromb. Haemost.* 115 (6): 1240–1248. https://doi.org/10.1160/th15-09-0756.

45 Sardesai, I., Grover, J., Garg, M. et al. (2020). Short term home oxygen therapy for COVID-19 patients: the COVID-HOT algorithm. *J. Family Med. Prim. Care Rev.* 9 (7): 3209–3219. https://doi.org/10.4103/jfmpc.jfmpc_1044_20.

46 Borgen, I., Romney, M.C., Redwood, N. et al. (2021). From hospital to home: an intensive transitional care management intervention for patients with COVID-19. *Popul. Health Manag.* 24 (1): 27–34.

47 Banerjee, J., Canamar, C.P., Voyageur, C. et al. (2021). Mortality and readmission rates among patients with COVID-19 after discharge from acute care setting with supplemental oxygen. *JAMA Netw. Open* 4 (4): e213990. https://doi.org/10.1001/jamanetworkopen.2021.3990.

48 Esmaeilzadeh, A., Rostami, S., Yeganeh, P.M. et al. (2021). Recent advances in antibody-based immunotherapy strategies for COVID-19. *J. Cell. Biochem.* 122 (10): 1389–1412.

49 Hammarstrom, L., Marcotte, H., Piralla, A. et al. (2021). Antibody therapy for COVID-19. *Curr. Opin. Allergy Clin. Immunol.* 21 (6): 553–558.

50 Eli Lilly and Company. (2021). Fact Sheet for Health Care Providers Emergency Use Authorization (EUA) of Bamlanivimab and Etesimab. https://www.fda.gov/media/145802/download. Accessed 3 Dec 2021

51 Regeneron Pharmaceuticals, Inc. (2021). Fact Sheet for Health Care Providers Emergency Use Authorization (EUA) of REGEN-COV® (casirivimab and imdevimab). https://www.fda.gov/media/143891/download. Accessed 21 Nov 2021

52 GlaxoSmithKline. (2021). Fact Sheet for Healthcare Providers Emergency Use Authorization (EUA) of Sotrovimab https://www.fda.gov/media/149534/download

53 Chigutsa, E., O'Brien, L., Ferguson-Sells, L. et al. (2021). Population pharmacokinetics and pharmacodynamics of the neutralizing antibodies bamlanivimab and etesevimab in patients with mild to moderate COVID-19 infection. *Clin. Pharm. Therap.* 110 (5): 1302–1310.

54 Laurini, E., Marson, D., Aulic, S. et al. (2021). Molecular rationale for SARS-CoV-2 spike circulating mutations able to escape bamlanivimab and etesevimab monoclonal antibodies. *Sci. Rep.* 11 (1): 20274.

55 Tuccori, M., Convertino, I., Ferraro, S. et al. (2021). An overview of the preclinical discovery and development of bamlanivimab for the treatment of novel coronavirus infection (COVID-19): reasons for limited clinical use and lessons for the future. *Expert Opin. Drug Discovery* 16 (12): 1403–1414.

56 Razonable, R.R., Pawlowski, C., O'Horo, J.C. et al. (2021). Casirivimab–Imdevimab treatment is associated with reduced rates of hospitalization among high-risk patients with mild to moderate coronavirus disease-19. *EClinicalMedicine* 40: 101102. https://doi.org/10.1016/j.eclinm.2021.101102.

57 Cathcart, A.L., Havenar-Daughton, C., Lempp, F.A. et al. (2021). The dual function monoclonal antibodies VIR-7831 and VIR-7832 demonstrate potent in vitro and in vivo activity against SARS-CoV-2. *bioRxiv* 2021.03.09.434607. https://doi.org/10.1101/2021.03.09.434607.

58 Public Health Emergency. (2021). HHS announces state/territory-coordinated distribution system for

monoclonal antibody therapeutics. US Department of Health and Human Services. https://www.phe. gov/emergency/events/COVID19/investigation-MCM/Bamlanivimab-etesevimab/Pages/Update-13Sept21.aspx. Accessed 10 Dec 2021

59 Chilimuri S, Mantri N, Gurjar H, et al. Implementation and outcomes of monoclonal antibody infusion for COVID-19 in an inner-city safety net hospital: a South-Bronx experience. *J. Natl. Med. Assoc.* 2022;113:701–705.

60 Agarwal, A., Rochwerg, B., Siemieniuk, R.A. et al. (2020). A living WHO guideline on drugs for covid-19. *BMJ* 370: m3379. https://doi.org/10.1136/bmj.m3379.

61 Bakowski, M.A., Beutler, N., Wolff, K.C. et al. (2021). Drug repurposing screens identify chemical entities for the development of COVID-19 interventions. *Nat. Commun.* 12 (1): 3309. https://doi.org/10.1038/s41467-021-23328-0.

62 Gordon, C.J., Tchesnokov, E.P., Schinazi, R.F., and Götte, M. (2021). Molnupiravir promotes SARS-CoV-2 mutagenesis via the RNA template. *J. Biol. Chem.* 297 (1): 100770. https://doi.org/10.1016/j.jbc.2021.100770.

63 Kabinger, F., Stiller, C., Schmitzová, J. et al. (2021). Mechanism of molnupiravir-induced SARS-CoV-2 mutagenesis. *Nat. Struct. Mol. Biol.* 28 (9): 740–746. https://doi.org/10.1038/s41594-021-00651-0.

64 Miller, S.R., McGrath, M.E., Zorn, K.M. et al. (2021). Remdesivir and EIDD-1931 interact with human equilibrative nucleoside transporters 1 and 2: implications for reaching SARS-CoV-2 viral sanctuary sites. *Mol. Pharmacol.* 100 (6): 548–557. https://doi.org/10.1124/molpharm.121.000333.

65 US Food and Drug Administration. 2021. Antimicrobial Drugs Advisory Committee Meeting. YouTube. https://www.youtube.com/watch?v=fR9FNSJT64M. Accessed 30 Nov 2021.

66 Menéndez-Arias, L. (2021). Decoding molnupiravir-induced mutagenesis in SARS-CoV-2. *J. Biol. Chem.* 297 (1): 100867–100867. https://doi.org/10.1016/j.jbc.2021.100867.

67 Zhou, S., Hill, C.S., Sarkar, S. et al. (2021). β-d-N4-hydroxycytidine inhibits SARS-CoV-2 through lethal mutagenesis but is also mutagenic to mammalian cells. *J. Infect. Dis.* 224 (3): 415–419. https://doi.org/10.1093/infdis/jiab247.

68 Karim, F., Moosa, M., Gosnell, B. et al. (2021). Persistent SARS-CoV-2 infection and intra-host evolution in association with advanced HIV infection. *medRxiv* 2021.06.03.21258228. https://doi.org/10.1101/2021.06.03.21258228.

69 Ahmad, B., Batool, M., Ain, Q.U. et al. (2021). Exploring the binding mechanism of PF-07321332 SARS-CoV-2 protease inhibitor through molecular dynamics and binding free energy simulations. *Int. J. Mol. Sci.* 22 (17): 9124. https://doi.org/10.3390/ijms22179124.

70 AstraZeneca. 2000.Pulmicort Respules Prescribing Information. https://www.accessdata.fda.gov/drugsatfda_docs/label/2000/20929lbl.pdf.

71 Heinen, N., Meister, T.L., Klöhn, M. et al. (2021). Antiviral effect of budesonide against SARS-CoV-2. *Viruses* 13 (7): 1411. https://doi.org/10.3390/v13071411.

72 Ramakrishnan, S., Nicolau, D.V. Jr., Langford, B. et al. (2021). Inhaled budesonide in the treatment of early COVID-19 (STOIC): a phase 2, open-label, randomised controlled trial. *Lancet Respir. Med.* 9 (7): 763–772. https://doi.org/10.1016/s2213-2600(21)00160-0.

73 Yu, L.M., Bafadhel, M., Dorward, J. et al. (2021). Inhaled budesonide for COVID-19 in people at high risk of complications in the community in the UK (PRINCIPLE): a randomised, controlled, open-label, adaptive platform trial. *Lancet* 398 (10303): 843–855. https://doi.org/10.1016/s0140-6736(21)01744-x.

74 Jazz Pharmaceuticals. 2021. LUVOX® prescribing information. https://www.accessdata.fda.gov/drugsatfda_docs/label/2007/021519lbl.pdf. Accessed 3 Dec 2021.

75 Sukhatme, V.P., Reiersen, A.M., Vayttaden, S.J., and Sukhatme, V.V. (2021). Fluvoxamine: a review of its mechanism of action and its role in COVID-19. *Front. Pharmacol.* 12: 652688. https://doi.org/10.3389/fphar.2021.652688.

76 Narita, N., Hashimoto, K., Tomitaka, S., and Minabe, Y. (1996). Interactions of selective serotonin reuptake inhibitors with subtypes of sigma receptors in rat brain. *Eur. J. Pharmacol.* 307 (1): 117–119. https://doi.org/10.1016/0014-2999(96)00254-3.

77 Oskotsky, T., Marić, I., Tang, A. et al. (2021). Mortality risk among patients with COVID-19 prescribed selective serotonin reuptake inhibitor

antidepressants. *JAMA Netw. Open* 4 (11): e2133090. https://doi.org/10.1001/jamanetworkopen.2021.33090.

78 RECOVERY Collaborative Group (2021). Dexamethasone in hospitalized patients with Covid-19 — preliminary report. *N. Engl. J. Med.* 384: 693–704. https://doi.org/10.1056/NEJMoa2021436.

79 Wang, M., Cao, R., Zhang, L. et al. (2020). Remdesivir and chloroquine effectively inhibit the recently emerged novel coronavirus (2019-nCoV) in vitro. *Cell Res.* 30 (3): 269–271. https://doi.org/10.1038/s41422-020-0282-0.

80 Liu, J., Cao, R., Xu, M. et al. (2020). Hydroxychloroquine, a less toxic derivative of chloroquine, is effective in inhibiting SARS-CoV-2 infection in vitro. *Cell Discov.* 6: 16. https://doi.org/10.1038/s41421-020-0156-0.

81 Zhou, D., Dai, S.M., and Tong, Q. (2020). COVID-19: a recommendation to examine the effect of hydroxychloroquine in preventing infection and progression. *J. Antimicrob. Chemother.* 75: 1667–1670.

82 Mitjà, O., Corbacho-Monné, M., Ubals, M. et al. (2021). Hydroxychloroquine for early treatment of adults with mild coronavirus disease 2019: a randomized, controlled trial. *Clin. Infect. Dis.* 73 (11): e4073–e4081. https://doi.org/10.1093/cid/ciaa1009.

83 Skipper, C.P., Pastick, K.A., Engen, N.W. et al. (2020). Hydroxychloroquine in nonhospitalized adults with early COVID-19: a randomized trial. *Ann. Intern. Med.* 173 (8): 623–631. https://doi.org/10.7326/m20-4207.

84 Kircik, L.H., Del Rosso, J.Q., Layton, A.M., and Schauber, J. (2016). Over 25 years of clinical experience with ivermectin: an overview of safety for an increasing number of indications. *J. Drugs Dermatol.* 15 (3): 325–332.

85 Yang, S.N.Y., Atkinson, S.C., Wang, C. et al. (2020). The broad spectrum antiviral ivermectin targets the host nuclear transport importin $\alpha/\beta 1$ heterodimer. *Antivir. Res.* 177: 104760. https://doi.org/10.1016/j.antiviral.2020.104760.

86 Lehrer, S. and Rheinstein, P.H. (2020). Ivermectin docks to the SARS-CoV-2 spike receptor-binding domain attached to ACE2. *in vivo* 34 (5): 3023–3026. https://doi.org/10.21873/invivo.12134.

87 Zhang, X., Song, Y., Ci, X. et al. (2008). Ivermectin inhibits LPS-induced production of inflammatory cytokines and improves LPS-induced survival in mice. *Inflamm. Res.* 57 (11): 524–529. https://doi.org/10.1007/s00011-008-8007-8.

88 López-Medina, E., López, P., Hurtado, I.C. et al. (2021). Effect of ivermectin on time to resolution of symptoms among adults with mild COVID-19: a randomized clinical trial. *JAMA* 325 (14): 1426–1435. https://doi.org/10.1001/jama.2021.3071.

89 PRINCIPLE Trial Collaborative Group (2021). Azithromycin for community treatment of suspected COVID-19 in people at increased risk of an adverse clinical course in the UK (PRINCIPLE): a randomised, controlled, open-label, adaptive platform trial. *Lancet* 397 (10279): 1063–1074. https://doi.org/10.1016/s0140-6736(21)00461-x.

90 Cao, B., Wang, Y., Wen, D. et al. (2020). A trial of lopinavir-ritonavir in adults hospitalized with severe Covid-19. *N. Engl. J. Med.* 18: 1787–1799.

91 RECOVERY Collaborative Group (2020). Lopinavir-ritonavir in patients admitted to hospital with COVID-19 (RECOVERY): a randomised, controlled, open-label, platform trial. *Lancet* 396 (10259): 1345–1352. https://doi.org/10.1016/s0140-6736(20)32013-4.

92 Korley, F.K., Durkalski-Mauldin, V., Yeatts, S.D. et al. (2021). Early convalescent plasma for high-risk outpatients with Covid-19. *N. Engl. J. Med.* 385 (21): 1951–1960. https://doi.org/10.1056/NEJMoa2103784.

93 Tardif, J.-C., Bouabdallaoui, N., L'Allier, P.L. et al. (2021). Efficacy of colchicine in non-hospitalized patients with COVID-19. *medRxiv* 2021.01.26.21250494. https://doi.org/10.1101/2021.01.26.21250494.

10

COVID-19: Inpatient Management

Angelena Lopez*, Yuri Matusov, Isabel Pedraza, Victor Tapson, Jeremy Falk, and Peter Chen

Department of Medicine, Division of Pulmonary and Critical Care Medicine, Cedars-Sinai Medical Center, Los Angeles, CA, USA
*Angelena Lopez and Yuri Matusov contributed equally to this work.

Abbreviations

ACE2	angiotensin-converting enzyme 2
ACS	acute coronary syndrome
ACTIV-3	Accelerating COVID-19 Therapeutic Interventions and Vaccines-3
ACTT	Adaptive COVID-19 Treatment Trial 1
AKI	acute kidney injury
ARDS	acute respiratory distress syndrome
CAPE-COVID	Community-Acquired Pneumonia: Evaluation of Corticosteroids in Coronavirus Disease
CLABSI	central line-associated bloodstream infection
CRP	C-reactive protein
ECMO	extracorporeal membrane oxygenation
FDA	US Food and Drug Administration
FiO_2	fraction of inspired oxygen
HFNC	high-flow nasal cannula
HEPA	high-efficiency particulate air
ICU	intensive care unit
IDSA	Infectious Diseases Society of America
IL-6	interleukin-6
IMV	invasive mechanical ventilation
LOS	length of stay
LV	left ventricular
MERS	Middle East respiratory syndrome
NIH	National Institutes of Health
NIPPV	noninvasive positive pressure ventilation
NIV	noninvasive ventilation
NMBA	neuromuscular blockade agent
PACU	postanesthesia care unit
PAPR	powered air-purifying respirator
PEEP	positive end-expiratory pressure
PPE	personal protective equipment
RCT	randomized controlled trial
REMAP-CAP	Randomized, Embedded, Multi-factorial Adaptive Platform Trial for Community-Acquired Pneumonia
RRT	renal replacement therapy
SARS-CoV-2	severe acute respiratory syndrome coronavirus 2
SOC	standard of care
STEMI	ST elevations myocardial infarction
VTE	venous thromboembolism
WHO	World Health Organization

Patients with more severe manifestations of coronavirus disease 2019 (COVID-19) require hospitalization. In the overwhelming majority of patients, hospitalization is driven by progressive respiratory distress/failure that is largely managed with supportive care.

As such, the management of hospitalized patients with COVID-19 minimally differs from that given to patients without COVID-19 but with respiratory illness. However, COVID-19 created unique challenges, with infection control first and foremost to minimize aerosolization and exposure of healthcare workers and other hospitalized patients to the severe acute respiratory syndrome coronavirus 2 (SARS-CoV-2).

Early in the COVID-19 pandemic, the scientific community quickly mobilized and began testing a number of therapeutics that led to rapid development of antiviral and immunomodulatory treatments for COVID-19. As we gained experience with the care of patients infected with SARS-CoV-2, it was quickly recognized that this respiratory virus also causes many extrapulmonary manifestations that can significantly impact morbidity and mortality.

In this chapter, we will discuss the current best practice for the inpatient management of patients with COVID-19. The chapter is organized into the following sections: Respiratory Support for Hospitalized Patients with COVID-19, Caring for the Critically Ill Patient with COVID-19, Pharmacologic Therapies for Hospitalized Patients with COVID-19, Extrapulmonary Disease in Acutely Ill Patients with COVID-19, Performing Aerosol-Generating Procedures in Patients with COVID-19, and Coordinating Patient Placement and Care in COVID-19 Units.

Respiratory Support for Hospitalized Patients with COVID-19

Approximately 80–85% of patients affected with COVID-19 will be either asymptomatic or have mild disease that does not require hospitalization [1]. However, those hospitalized have respiratory failure that ranges in severity from mild to fulminant acute respiratory distress syndrome (ARDS). Although rates vary among countries and within the United States, some studies reported up to 25% of those who are hospitalized require intensive care unit (ICU) care [2]. Appropriate respiratory support in these patients is central to their care and recovery.

Noninvasive Respiratory Support

Recommendations regarding safe practice and respiratory therapies have evolved as further studies examining these modalities have been completed. Respiratory therapies may be either aerosol generating, aerosol dispersing, or both. Aerosol generating refers to therapies that by their nature promote aerosolization of patients' secretions that contain viable virus. These particles may be dispersed to the environment and potentially inhaled by others. Aerosol-dispersing procedures do not cause de novo generation of particles or droplets but may act to increase the distance these particles travel from a patient. In a study done by Gaeckle et al. [3] and colleagues of healthy volunteers, particle concentrations were measured at a distance of 5 cm from the volunteer's mouth while using different oxygen therapy devices (low-flow nasal cannula, face mask, high-flow nasal cannula (HFNC), and noninvasive positive pressure ventilation [NIPPV]). Measurements were taken with each device while volunteers were breathing normally, talking, breathing deeply, and coughing, and their results showed that although oxygen delivery devices are aerosol dispersing, none was aerosol generating [3]. Thus, initial reluctance to use devices such as HFNC has been attenuated, and even NIPPV has been found to have a role in the management of respiratory failure in certain patients with COVID-19 [4].

Low-Flow Oxygen Devices

Low-flow oxygen systems include nasal cannula, oxygen pendant, simple mask, Venturi mask, and non-rebreather. Both nasal cannula and oxygen pendant can be set as high as 6 l/min flow and achieve approximately 44% fraction of inspired oxygen (FiO_2) at this flow rate. Nasal cannula is typically the first-line therapy for mild hypoxemia because it has few contraindications and is typically well tolerated. Any patient on nasal cannula who is unable to maintain oxygen saturations >90% should be escalated to a higher supplemental oxygen device.

Although a simple mask and Venturi mask are able to deliver FiO_2 up to 60%, a non-rebreather mask can deliver an FiO_2 from 60% to 90% [5, 6]. These masks are indicated in moderate to severe hypoxia. When using a simple mask, a minimal flow rate of 5 L/min is necessary to prevent rebreathing of exhaled carbon dioxide that can be retained in the mask. Although it has been suggested that a non-rebreather mask can deliver up to 100% FiO_2, this is unlikely given the lack of seal between the mask and face that leads to entrainment of room air and because of valve insufficiency between the oxygen reservoir bag and the patient.

Low-flow oxygen delivery systems have not been found to increase aerosol generation from the respiratory tract [3, 7]. Devices such as a simple mask, Venturi mask, and non-rebreather can be used to achieve higher flow rates; however, as flow increases, so too does the risk for dispersion. Notably, aerosol dispersion appears to be less with these devices than with nasal cannula, possibly because of the obstructing mask [3, 7].

All of these devices can cause discomfort, and skin breakdown from the mask can occur when used for longer periods [8]. In addition, eating, drinking, and in some cases, speaking can be impaired. Mispositioning of the mask, which happens frequently with patient speaking, can also affect the function of these devices and increase the amount of entrained room air.

HFNC

HFNC systems have the capability to deliver flow rates up to 60 L/min and FiO_2 from 21% to 100% [9, 10]. These systems deliver heat and humidified air, and the flow and FiO_2 can be independently adjusted. Large nasal prongs are designed to fit snugly into the patient's nares and prevent entrainment of room air. In addition to high supplemental oxygen support, HFNC can effectively wash out dead space and continually replace potentially rebreathed gas with fresh gas [11]. This is particularly important in patients with respiratory failure, such as COVID pneumonia, in which dead space increases.

As previously noted, further studies found that HFNC does affect dispersion distance and does not generate aerosols, which has made this a commonly used modality in patients with COVID-19 with respiratory failure [3, 7, 12]. The heated and humidified air from HFNC has been shown to improve mucociliary clearance in patients with bronchiectasis, and this is thought to be a benefit that extends beyond this patient population [13, 14]. HFNC is typically well tolerated by patients and does not interfere with prone positioning. In addition, there is evidence to suggest that the use of HFNC in patients with COVID-19 is associated with a lower rate of mechanical ventilation [15, 16]. For these reasons, HFNC is the preferred oxygen delivery modality for patients who require support beyond low-flow nasal cannula [4].

NIPPV

NIPPV includes both continuous positive airway pressure and bilevel positive airway pressure. Although the benefit of NIPPV is well documented in respiratory failure caused by decompensated heart failure, in chronic obstructive pulmonary disease exacerbations, and in immunocompromised states, its utility in patients with COVID-19 is unclear. Direct evidence regarding the use of NIPPV in patients with COVID-19 is limited. Indirectly, use of NIPPV in Middle East respiratory syndrome (MERS) was not associated with improved outcomes, and rates of failure with NIPPV were high [17]. During the SARS outbreak in China in 2002–2003, NIPPV was commonly used, and small observational studies demonstrated improvements in oxygenation and tachypnea in patients treated with NIPPV [18, 19].

Current society recommendations vary but have shifted since the beginning of the pandemic, specifically those provided by the World Health Organization (WHO) [20]. Although a small, randomized trial in patients with COVID-19 with respiratory failure found no difference between HFNC and NIPPV in the days free of respiratory support [21], studies from non-COVID respiratory failure have found that HFNC has better outcomes with fewer ventilator-free days and lower mortality at 90 days when compared with NIPPV [22]. Moreover, a meta-analysis of oxygenation strategies before intubation found that compared with NIPPV, HFNC reduced the rate of intubations [23]. As such, HFNC is recommended over the use of NIPPV by the National Institutes of Health (NIH) and Society of Critical Care Medicine [4, 24]. The WHO, however, makes no recommendation of one modality over the other, but rather that either NIPPV or HFNC may be appropriate in select patients with mild ARDS from COVID-19 [20]. When HFNC is unavailable, both the WHO and the NIH recommend use of NIPPV [4, 20]. These guidelines should be weighed accordingly with the clinical scenario. For example, if a patient presents with chronic obstructive pulmonary disease exacerbation or decompensated heart failure (instead of hypoxemic respiratory failure from COVID-19), then NIPPV may have superiority [24–27]. NIPPV also may be indicated in patients with treatment limitations such as "do not intubate" directives.

Given the greater concern for aerosol generation by NIPPV, it is recommended that certain precautions be taken with its use. A full face mask with a good seal should be used, and use of nasal masks or nasal pillows, which have increased leak and droplet dispersion distance, should be avoided [12]. Standard airborne precautions should be applied to minimize risk to healthcare workers with patients placed in negative pressure rooms and use of an inline high-efficiency particulate air (HEPA) filter placed on the exhaust port. A retrospective analysis in Italy of 53 patients with COVID-19 treated with NIPPV used these safety precautions and had a low rate of COVID-19 infection among healthcare workers caring for these patients [28].

Prone Positioning in Awake Patients

In 2015, Scaravilli et al. [29] presented a retrospective case series of 15 nonintubated patients with hypoxemic respiratory failure who were treated with prone positioning. Their findings showed improvements in oxygenation in the subjects and demonstrated tolerability of the procedure. Since the beginning of the COVID-19 pandemic, there has been a renewed interest in the application of prone positioning in nonintubated patients (i.e. awake proning or self-proning). Awake proning is a simple technique that does not require additional supplies or place significant additional strain on staff.

A case series by Caputo et al. [30] that described 50 patients with respiratory failure from COVID-19 in the emergency department found improvement in median oxygen saturations (from 84% to 94%) within five minutes of self-proning. Furthermore, a single-center cohort study in Italy evaluating the use of awake prone positioning with confirmed COVID-19 pneumonia demonstrated significant improvement in oxygenation that reversed on supination. Importantly, self-proning was found to be feasible, with 47 of the 56 patients tolerating the position for the minimum three-hour duration [31]. Although these trials demonstrate better oxygenation (at least transiently) with awake proning [31, 32], the ability to improve outcomes has not been established. A multicenter, prospective trial evaluating the effect of self-proning positioning in conjunction with HFNC in patients with COVID-19 with acute respiratory failure did not find the intervention to reduce the rate of intubation [32]. Nevertheless, awake proning is still being encouraged

at our institution because of its positive effects on oxygenation and tolerability, including pregnant and postpartum patients [33].

Importantly, use of self-proning may delay intubation [32]; thus, care providers must remain vigilant and exercise caution with a clear trend in increasing oxygen requirements because delaying intubation can increase the risk for adverse events. Furthermore, awake proning is contraindicated in patients who are unable to tolerate the prone position, who are unable to change positions on their own, and who are hemodynamically unstable [4].

Caring for the Critically Ill Patient with COVID-19

Despite treatment and supportive care, some patients with COVID-19 will have progressive respiratory failure resulting in the need for intubation and mechanical ventilation. Intubation in patients with COVID-19 presents unique challenges that are exacerbated when the patient is in a non-ICU environment. Unfortunately, predicting which patients with COVID-19 will decline and require ICU care is difficult, and baseline clinical factors do not correlate with eventual need for ICU care [34]. Although many variables, such as provider comfort and available ICU space, will influence transfer guidelines, certain criteria can help guide physicians. At our institution, we recommend transferring any patient with rapidly escalating oxygen requirements. Similarly, any patient with increased work of breathing despite adequate oxygenation or with altered mental status, or absence of improvement in patients on HFNC 40 L or greater with FiO_2 >60% should be considered for transfer to the ICU.

Appropriate timing of intubation in these patients remains unclear. Although debate centers around "early" versus "late" intubation strategies, these are ill-defined and vary between institutions [35, 36]. Early in the pandemic, guidelines from the Chinese Society of Anesthesiology Task Force on Airway Management recommended intubation in those patients with no improvement in respiratory distress (as manifested by respiratory rate > 30) and oxygenation (determined as PaO_2/FiO_2 ratio < 150 mmHg) despite at least two hours of either HFNC or NIPPV [37]. Moreover, the logistical considerations for intubation with COVID-19 make this a unique situation. Significant consideration must be given for the extra setup time required to mobilize the intubation team and don personal protective equipment (PPE). In addition, patients with COVID-19 can deteriorate rapidly, hampering the ability to pre-oxygenate patients with significant desaturations, which is associated with a greater risk for cardiac arrest peri-intubation [38].

Rather than adopting a "late" or "early" strategy for intubation, the timing of intubation should be individualized for each patient. Variables such as trajectory or rapidity of deterioration, increasing work of breathing, and change in mental status provide guidance as to the right time for intubation. For patients whose condition is precipitously declining, it may be prudent to intubate them before they reach maximal settings on HFNC or NIPPV to prevent a higher-risk intubation. Thus, a reasonable approach is to have a low threshold for intubation in any patient whose condition rapidly deteriorates over a few hours; who fails to demonstrate improvement with increased settings on HFNC or NIPPV; and who has increased work of breathing, development of respiratory acidosis, hemodynamic instability, or altered mental status.

Practical Considerations for Intubating Patients

Endotracheal intubation and other airway procedures carry known risks of infection for healthcare workers, especially when dealing with aerosol or droplet transmissible infections. As such, additional precautions should be taken when preforming endotracheal intubation in patients with COVID-19 [39]. PPE recommendations from various societies (American Society of Anesthesiology, Society of Critical Medicine, Infectious Diseases Society of America [IDSA]) stem in part from previous experience with other infectious etiologies, such as SARS, and evolving data from the current pandemic [20, 40–45]. Aerosol-generating procedures increased the risk for infection for healthcare workers with SARS [46, 47]. When involved in aerosol-generating procedures in patients with known or suspected COVID-19, these societies recommend healthcare personal be wearing a gown, gloves, and a fit-tested N95 mask with appropriate eye protection (or alternatively a powered air-purifying respirator

[PAPR] or similar respirator device) [24, 41, 42]. Appropriate donning of PPE cannot be overemphasized, and all personnel should have adequate training on proper donning and doffing to avoid self-contamination [48].

Whenever possible, intubation should be done in a negative pressure room. If negative pressure rooms are not available, portable HEPA filters should be used before the start of the procedure and continued for a period based on the device clean air delivery rate and the size of the room [47, 49]. To facilitate intubation, our institution had premade intubation kits that included oral airways, supraglottic airways devices, various sizes of endotracheal tubes (ETTs), a bougie, and high-efficiency viral filters present in the ICU and frequently restocked. In addition, difficult airway carts with surgical airway kits were readily available.

For the intubation itself, it is recommended that as few personnel as possible are in the room to minimize exposure risk and conserve PPE [50, 51]. Staff with PPE donned should be available outside the room and ready to support any complications (e.g. code). At minimum, the provider performing the intubation, a nurse for administration of medication, and a respiratory therapist need to be present. All medications and intubation equipment should be set up outside the room, before the start of the procedure. If time avails, a preprocedural huddle to go over the intubation plan outside the room should be performed. Using a checklist method for this preprocedure huddle that included verifying all necessary equipment had been obtained and set up, and initial ventilator settings had been determined and reviewed with the respiratory therapist, reviewing induction plan and reviewing initial intubation technique and backup plans in the case of difficult airway, can facilitate the procedure.

When possible, bag mask ventilation should be avoided because studies in SARS found an increased risk for transmission [52]. If unavoidable, bag mask ventilation should be performed with high-efficiency viral filters in place and two-handed bag mask technique to help with efficiency, which improves mask seal and minimizes dispersion. It has been proposed by some to use the lowest flow necessary to achieve adequate preoxygenation [51], although patients are often already on near-maximal support. In the case of NIPPV, the mask should remain in place until laryngoscopy.

HFNC can also be kept in place during the entirety of the intubation procedure to provide apneic oxygenation [53].

Although data on video laryngoscopy versus direct laryngoscopy and first-pass success vary in the setting of respiratory failure from COVID-19, video laryngoscopy has the benefit of allowing the operator to maintain a further distance from the patient without sacrificing laryngeal view [54–56]. Rapid sequence intubation is also recommended to minimize procedural time as well. Given the risk for aerosolization with awake fiberoptic intubation, this method is recommended against unless specifically indicated [39, 40, 50]. A low threshold for surgical airway should be kept and prepared for with suspected difficult airways [39, 57]. After placement of the ETT, the balloon should be inflated before starting ventilation, and the patient should be immediately connected to the ventilator. If a colorimetry device is used to evaluate appropriate tube placement, an ETT clamp should be used when interrupting the ventilator circuit to help minimize aerosolization.

Mechanical Ventilation of Patients with COVID-19

Studies within the United States indicate that between 17% and 26% of hospitalized patients require mechanical ventilation during their hospital course, or approximately 80% of patients admitted to ICU [58–60]. Guidelines for mechanical ventilation stem mainly from ARDSNet protocol and other studies that established evidence-based strategies for management of ARDS [4, 20, 24]. Early in the pandemic, it was proposed that respiratory failure from COVID manifests in two distinct phenotypes, described as L and H. The L phenotype was thought to be characterized by low elastance (nearly normal compliance) and low lung recruitability, and thus minimally responsive to positive end-expiratory pressure (PEEP) [61]. Conversely, the H phenotype was thought to be characterized by high elastance or decreased lung compliance as a result of increased pulmonary edema and significant responsiveness to PEEP [61]. Gattinoni et al. [61] further suggested that patients who fall into the L phenotype should be ventilated with a low PEEP strategy, contrary to ARDSNet

guidelines. However, further studies have not supported this approach [62, 63].

Fundamentally, current management of COVID ARDS does not differ significantly from routine ARDS. One of the mainstays in the ventilation strategy for patients with ARDS is the use of lung protective ventilation or low tidal volume ventilation (tidal volumes ≤6 ml/kg ideal body weight *and* plateau pressures ≤30 cm H_2O), which irrefutability improves survival [64]. Alveolar overdistention with high tidal volumes is thought to contribute to additional lung injury for mechanical ventilation and increased mortality in ARDS, with evidence indicating low tidal volume ventilation mitigates the detrimental volutrauma [64]. For details on the implementation of lung protective ventilation in patients with ARDS, refer to the guideline implementation tools from the American Thoracic Society/European Society of Intensive Care Medicine/Society of Critical Care Medicine: https://www.thoracic.org/statements/guideline-implementation-tools/mechanical-ventilation-in-adults-with-ards.php.

Guidelines suggest targeting an SaO_2 (arterial oxygen saturation) of 88–95% or PaO_2 of 55–88 mmHg [65, 66]. Although minute ventilation should be set to ideally target a pH from 7.30 to 7.45, permissive hypercapnia is acceptable, as is tolerance of a pH as low as 7.15 to accommodate low tidal volume ventilation. Respiratory rate should not be increased to more than 35 because this increases the risk for dynamic air hyperinflation and intrinsic PEEP (auto-PEEP) [67].

PEEP helps minimize repetitive opening and closing of alveoli (i.e. atelectotrauma) that can promote ventilator-induced lung injury [68, 69]. In addition, PEEP improves oxygenation, allowing for a lower FiO_2. There is an additional benefit of recruitment by splinting open the alveoli, which leads to improvement of oxygenation. To date, no trial has established an optimal PEEP level in the ventilation of patients with ARDS. The ALVEOLI study specifically tested the question of the effect of a high versus low PEEP ventilation strategy and found no difference in outcomes [70]. In clinical practice, optimal PEEP is likely dependent on several factors, such as lung compliance and extent of disease, and may change over time as a result of disease progression and patient positioning.

In acute lung injury/ARDS, either direct or indirect lung injury precipitates innate immune cell–mediated damage of the alveolar epithelial–interstitial–endothelial complex [71]. Disruption of this barrier allows protein-rich fluid to accumulate within the interstitium and alveoli [72], while at the same time there may be an inability of alveolar cells to upregulate fluid clearance [73]. The resultant pulmonary edema contributes to the ARDS disease process, which manifests clinically as changes in lung compliance and impaired gas exchange [74]. In 2006, the FACTT trial sought to determine optimal fluid management strategy in ARDS by comparing a liberal fluid management strategy with a conservative strategy [75]. No significant difference in 60-day mortality between the groups was noted; however, the conservative group was found to have not only improved lung function but also a shortened duration of mechanical ventilation [75]. Thus, clinical management guidelines in ARDS recommend following a conservative fluid management strategy [76], which should also be followed in the management of ARDS in COVID-19 [4, 20].

Rescue Therapies for Refractory Hypoxemia of Ventilated Patients

Patients with severe COVID-19 infections often have progressive hypoxemia requiring the use of rescue therapies (Table 10.1). Our general approach has been to use proning as the first-line rescue therapy in patients with COVID-19 with ARDS who have been optimized on lung protective ventilation (Figure 10.1). Prone positioning facilitates recruitment and reduces overinflated lung areas, thereby decreasing ventilator-induced lung injury by evenly distributing stress and strain throughout the lung [77]. In addition, the resultant postural changes during prone therapy have also been shown to facilitate drainage of secretions, which may be an especially important benefit in patients with COVID-19 who may be unable to receive nebulized mucolytics [78]. Prone positioning had been widely adopted into practice in patients with severe ARDS before the COVID-19 pandemic, in large part as a result of findings from the PROSEVA (Proning Positioning in Severe ARDS Patients) study that demonstrated this intervention improved 28-day mortality in patients with severe ARDS [79].

Use of neuromuscular blockade agents (NMBAs) is another rescue therapy that is commonly used in the ICU setting to improve oxygenation by decreasing overall oxygen consumption [80]. In 2010, Papazian et al. [81] randomized patients with early ARDS to paralysis for 48 hours or usual care and demonstrated improved 90-day survival and increased ventilator-free days in the paralysis group. However, given concerns regarding ICU-acquired weakness and adoption of lighter sedation goals in the ICU [82], the Reevaluation of Systemic Early Neuromuscular Blockade (ROSE trial) was conducted in 2019, which showed neuromuscular blockade was not associated with reduced mortality in ARDS but was associated with increased ICU weakness and serious adverse cardiovascular events [83]. Despite this conflicting evidence, The Surviving Sepsis COVID management guidelines suggest use of as needed intermittent NMBA boluses to facilitate lung protective ventilation [24]. Moreover, continuous NMBAs (up to 48 hours) can be used to facilitate mechanical ventilation in patients when persistent ventilator dyssynchrony exists.

Although they have not been directly studied in COVID-19 ARDS, recruitment maneuvers have been evaluated in ARDS. De-recruited alveoli in injured or dependent lung regions are not normally aerated during positive pressure ventilation [84–86], and thus recruitment of collapsed alveoli may increase the number of alveolar lung units participating in ventilation [87]. Varying types of recruitment maneuvers exist; however, most commonly, these are either sustained inflation or incremental or stepwise PEEP increases. A system review and meta-analysis of randomized trials evaluating recruitment maneuvers in patients with ARDS found that lung recruitment maneuvers with high PEEP ventilatory strategy were associated with decreased mortality, improved oxygenation, and decreased need for additional rescue therapies [87]. Contrasting this, a randomized clinical trial evaluated a stepwise (or staircase recruitment maneuver) in moderate-to-severe ARDS and found an increased mortality [88]. In patients with ARDS from COVID-19, recruitment maneuvers can be used for refractory hypoxemia, but the staircase or stepwise recruitment maneuvers should be avoided [4].

Table 10.1   Rescue therapies for acute respiratory distress syndrome.

Rescue therapy	Advantages	Disadvantages/risks	Contraindications

Prone therapy	Evidence based mortality benefit.
	Improved V/Q matching
	Potential postural drainage benefit
	No special equipment required
		Training needed for proning staff
		Labor intensive
		Risk for dislodgement of ETT, lines, and catheters
		Facial edema, facial trauma
		Brachial nerve injury
		Retinal damage
			Absolute:
			  Spinal instability
			  Unstable fractures
			  Increased ICP > 30 mmHg or CPP < 60 mmHg
			  Hemorrhagic shock or massive hemoptysis
			  Tracheal surgery or sternotomy within two weeks
			
			Relative:
			  Recent thoracic or abdominal surgery
			  Anterior chest tube
			  Hemodynamic instability (MAP < 65 mmHg)
			  Pregnancy

Neuromuscular blockade	Improves ventilator desynchrony Decreases oxygen consumption Improves chest wall compliance	No proven mortality benefit Risk for prolonged: • Paralysis • Neuromuscular weakness	No contraindications
Inhaled pulmonary vasodilators	Reduced PVR Improved V/Q matching Short-acting and minimal systemic effects	No proven mortality benefit Potential pulmonary edema in the setting of significant LV dysfunction Antiplatelet effect Hemodynamic deterioration (rare) Methemoglobinemia (iNO) Renal dysfunction (iNO)	LV failure Existing methemoglobinemia
Recruitment maneuvers	Improved oxygenation No special equipment required	No proven mortality benefit Hypotension Barotrauma Staircase maneuver increased mortality	Untreated pneumothorax Presence of subcutaneous emphysema or pneumomediastinum Increased ICP RV failure Shock (MAP < 60) Severe obstructive lung disease Unilateral lung disease

Table 10.1 (Continued)

Rescue therapy	Advantages	Disadvantages/risks	Contraindications
VV ECMO	Oxygenation and ventilation support Ability to use "ultra-lung protective ventilation" Can be used as a bridge to recovery or transplant	Requires a specialized team and equipment Resource intensive Vascular damage Major bleeding Thrombosis Hemolysis Air embolism Infection Neurologic complications Limb ischemia	*Absolute:* Significant neurologic injury Terminal disease with short life expectancy Progressive nonrecoverable lung disease that is not amenable to lung transplant Chronic, severe RV failure Advanced malignancy Aortic dissection *Relative:* Prolonged mechanical ventilation (>7 days) Severe coagulopathy Age > 75 years Body weight > 140 kg Significant immunosuppression Trauma with multiple bleeding sites

CPP, cerebral perfusion pressure; ICP, intracranial pressure; LV, left ventricle; MAP, mean arterial pressure; iNO, inducible nitric oxide; PVR, pulmonary vascular resistance; RV, right ventricle; V/Q, ventilation/perfusion; VV ECMO, venovenous extracorporeal membrane oxygenation.

Inhaled pulmonary vasodilators improves ventilation/perfusion matching by vasodilating areas of better ventilation [89]. Furthermore, pulmonary vasodilation reduces the pulmonary vascular resistance and right ventricular afterload and can potentially improve cardiopulmonary dynamics [90]. Despite the ability to improve oxygenation, no studies have demonstrated any benefits on mortality [91–93]. As such, routine use of inhaled pulmonary vasodilators in ARDS is not recommended, and instead they are primarily reserved for patients with refractory hypoxemia despite the implementation of other rescue therapies [24].

As a final option for those with persistent refractory hypoxemia, extracorporeal membrane oxygenation (ECMO) is offered as an intervention for properly selected candidates. With venovenous ECMO, blood is drained from the venous system, passed through a membrane that oxygenates and removes carbon dioxide from the blood, and then returned to the venous circulation [94]. The CESAR (Conventional ventilation or ECMO for Severe Adult Respiratory failure) trial showed that referral to a specialized ECMO center improved outcomes in ARDS [95]. However, the subsequent EOLIA (ECMO to Rescue Lung Injury in Severe ARDS) study did not find any significant benefit in 60-day mortality with ECMO versus conventional mechanical ventilation in severe ARDS [96]. Nevertheless, early COVID-19 recommendations suggested ECMO use in COVID-19 as a rescue therapy after failure of conventional therapies and interventions [97]. Subsequent data suggest ECMO may have a beneficial role in patients with COVID-19, particularly

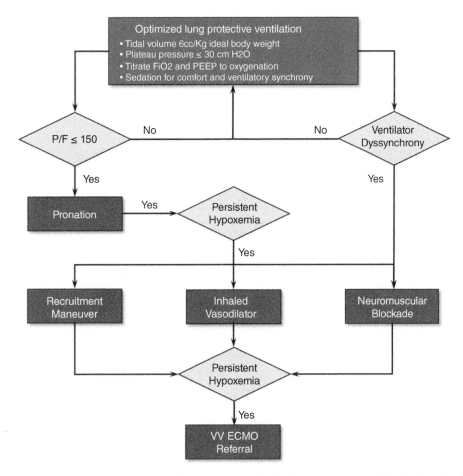

Figure 10.1 Algorithm for initiating rescue therapies in the management of the intubated patient with acute respiratory distress syndrome. PEEP, positive end-expiratory pressure; VV ECMO, venovenous extracorporeal membrane oxygenation.

when performed early, in young patients, and at high-volume centers [98, 99]. Accordingly, younger patients with COVID-19 with progressive hypoxemia despite maximal interventions should have an early referral to an appropriate ECMO center for evaluation [99].

Pharmacologic Therapies for Hospitalized Patients with COVID-19

One of the major unique aspects of the COVID pandemic on the practice of medicine has been the astonishing speed at which therapeutics have been used in clinical practice despite marginal supportive data. An extraordinary variety of medications repurposed from other indications, often on a theoretical basis, quickly

became standard of care (SOC). Not only did this produce profound variability in care depending on medication availability around the world, but it also affected the structure of clinical trial development, creating de facto gold standard untested control groups against which other untested therapies were tried. Other issues related to clinical trial data during the COVID pandemic included failures to control for potentially confounding regimens of other medications in either arm, comparisons with historical controls that may have had different outcomes related to the temporal capacity of the healthcare system in dealing with surges of patients, the inclusion of a wide spectrum of illness in the same trial, and publication bias toward positive trials. Finally, the extraordinary rise of non-peer-reviewed publications as preprints may have led to overemphasis on data that was not as rigidly obtained.

The fundamental basis of many COVID therapies is largely divided into two categories: (i) antiviral therapy to reduce viral load and subsequent injury associated with the infection; and (ii) attenuation of the so-called cytokine storm – a dysregulated host immune response, which precipitated ARDS, shock, renal failure, myocardial damage, and thromboembolic disease [100–103]. The following section provides a summary of peer-reviewed published data on selected antiviral and immunomodulatory medications, emphasizing, where available, prospective, randomized controlled trials (RCTs) as of the time of this writing (April 2021). As a perspective, therapies definitively demonstrated to have no benefit and the associated literature leading to these conclusions will also be reviewed.

Use of Antivirals in Patients Hospitalized for COVID-19

Remdesivir

To date, remdesivir is the only antiviral medication that has been US Food and Drug Administration (FDA) approved for use in hospitalized patients with SARS-CoV-2 infection [104]. Remdesivir is a nucleoside analogue that inhibits RNA-dependent RNA polymerase, thereby preventing the production of viral RNA required for viral proliferation [105]. This mechanism provides broad-spectrum antiviral effects with demonstrable in vitro activity against the MERS and SARS-CoV-1 coronaviruses, among other viruses [106–109]. With the onset of the COVID-19 pandemic, remdesivir was quickly repurposed for use in SARS-CoV-2 [110].

The first large-scale data for benefit of remdesivir emerged from the Adaptive COVID-19 Treatment Trial 1 (ACTT-1) trial, which randomized more than 1000 hospitalized patients (about a quarter of whom were on mechanical ventilation or ECMO, with 87% of the study population requiring at least some supplemental oxygen) to receive 10 days of remdesivir or placebo [111]. The trial found a reduction in median recovery time by five days, a mortality reduction from 11.9% to 6.7% by day 15, a shorter time to discharge, lower hospital length of stay (LOS), fewer days of invasive mechanical ventilation (IMV)/ECMO, and lower need for IMV among the patients receiving remdesivir.

This effect was most pronounced in hospitalized patients receiving supplemental oxygen, although the remdesivir group had overall lower risk than the control group. These results were corroborated by two other smaller trials. In the first, 500 patients with a SpO_2 ≤94% on room air were randomized to receive 10 days of remdesivir, 5 days of remdesivir, or placebo [112]; on day 11, the 5-day group had higher odds of having better clinical status than the standard care group, with no significant difference as compared with the 10-day group (although the median treatment length in the 10-day group was 6 days). The second trial also compared 5 versus 10 days of remdesivir (without a placebo group), in which the 10-day group had significantly worse baseline clinical status; after adjusting for this difference, there was no significant effect in outcomes [113].

Enthusiasm for remdesivir has been tempered by two studies that suggested no significant clinical benefit. The first, a smaller trial of moderately hypoxic hospitalized patients who received 10 days of remdesivir or placebo found no difference in time to clinical improvement, although there was a numerically faster time to improvement in the remdesivir group [114]. In a second larger trial (SOLIDARITY), more than 11 000 inpatients were randomly assigned to receive remdesivir, hydroxychloroquine, lopinavir, or interferon [115]. The trial found no benefit by any regimen, including remdesivir, on mortality, need for IMV, or hospital LOS. The discrepancy in the findings between SOLIDARITY and ACTT-1 may be related partly to the imbalance in the study groups' baseline illness, as noted earlier, and to risk stratification between the trials. In addition, ACTT-1 was a double-blind, placebo-controlled RCT, unlike SOLIDARITY, which had a more standardized control arm (there was more heterogeneity in the usual care arm of SOLIDARITY). Notably, no significant safety issues arose in any of the trials.

Taken together, the IDSA and NIH recommendation for remdesivir use is five days for patients receiving supplemental oxygen and 10 days for patients receiving IMV or ECMO [4, 116]. In contrast, the WHO has taken a different view and conditionally recommends against the use of remdesivir in patients hospitalized for COVID-19 [117]. Our approach has been to follow the IDSA and NIH recommendations particularly in light of the established safety for remdesivir.

Convalescent Plasma

Convalescent plasma was a mainstay of infection treatment before the era of antibiotics more than 100 years ago and is based on principles of using preformed immunity for pathogen neutralization, phagocytosis, and antibody-dependent cytotoxicity [118]. Early studies of convalescent plasma in severely ill patients with COVD-19 suggested faster clinical improvement [119, 120], and one nonrandomized prospective trial of moderately ill patients suggested a mortality benefit [121], leading to an expanded access program in the United States that has treated more than 75 000 patients with moderate-to-severe infection. Two large retrospective studies investigating convalescent plasma in hospitalized patients have suggested a reduction in mortality when high-titer plasma is used earlier in the course of disease, with little or no benefit in critically ill, intubated patients [122, 123]. Another large, retrospective, matched control study demonstrated a significant reduction of 7- and 14-day mortality with no difference at 28 days among hospitalized patients but was limited by a significantly greater use of steroids in the convalescent plasma group, which confounded the findings [124].

Unfortunately, no such mortality benefit has been demonstrated in RCTs. The PlasmAr trial randomized 228 patients with severe disease ($PaO_2 : FiO_2$ [P : F] ratio < 300) to convalescent plasma (median titer, 1 : 3200) or placebo and showed no difference in clinical status or mortality at 30 days [125]. The PLACID trial (phase II multicenter randomized controlled trial) was an open-label trial that randomized 464 patients with a P : F ratio of 200–300 to convalescent plasma (median neutralizing antibody titer, 1 : 40) or usual care and showed no difference in progression to P : F <100 or all-cause mortality at 28 days [126]. Another open-label study randomized 103 severe or critically ill (including intubated) patients to convalescent plasma or usual care and showed no difference in 28-day mortality or time to discharge, although it was stopped early because of inadequate enrollment and may have been underpowered [127]. In another small study, which looked at early (within 7 days of symptom onset) convalescent plasma as compared with convalescent plasma deferred until deterioration (about 13% of "control" group), no difference was found in the composite end point of IMV, hospitalization of >14 days, or death, and in fact had a trend toward increased mortality and need for and duration of IMV with early convalescent plasma [128]. Notably, only one small RCT, which was stopped early because of inadequate enrollment, has demonstrated that high-titer, very early (within 72 hours of symptoms) administration of convalescent plasma may reduce progression to severe disease [129].

Part of the challenge in identifying whether convalescent plasma has a role in treating hospitalized patients with COVID-19 has been establishing the adequate cutoff titers for neutralizing antibodies present in the collected serum; the FDA recommends neutralizing antibody titers of >1 : 160, but these measurements are not always available or used in a standard fashion. The current data indicate that neutralizing activity of convalescent plasma is correlated to higher antibody titers [122, 123, 130, 131], but the optimal cutoffs, timing, and patient population remain unclear. Complicating the situation is the fact that a significant proportion of donors do not have adequate antibody titers for viral neutralization [132]. Convalescent plasma appears to be safe with a transfusion reaction rate of <1% and a mortality rate of about 0.3% related to transfusion among 20 000 patients; other adverse events included transfusion-associated circulatory overload and transfusion-related acute lung injury [133, 134]. Although the FDA continues to provide Emergency Use Authorization for the use of convalescent plasma in COVID-19, both the IDSA and the NIH currently recommend against the use of convalescent plasma in hospitalized patients [4, 116].

Ivermectin

The antiparasitic ivermectin has demonstrated some in vitro activity against SARS-CoV-2, although standard doses of the drug used in humans rarely achieve the necessary serum and lung tissue concentrations [135, 136]. Although two retrospective trials of >250 patients comparing ivermectin versus usual care suggested a mortality benefit [137, 138], this has not been replicated in prospective studies.

To date, four medium-size RCTs (one placebo-controlled) have evaluated ivermectin as a treatment for hospitalized patients with COVID-19. The largest, which randomized 168 patients to chloroquine, hydroxychloroquine, or ivermectin, found no difference in the need for oxygen, IMV, admission to the ICU, or mortality [139]. Similarly, no effect on duration of hospitalization was found in a 72-patient trial testing ivermectin 12 mg once daily for five days versus a single dose of ivermectin plus five days of doxycycline versus placebo [140]. Finally, two small (<65 patients) open-label trials of moderately ill hospitalized patients who received ivermectin or usual care failed to demonstrate any symptomatic improvement with treatment [141, 142]. Better data are needed before making firmer recommendations on the use of ivermectin for hospitalized patients with COVID-19 and, at this time, should be used only in clinical trials [4, 116].

Anti-inflammatory Therapies for Hospitalized Patients with COVID-19

Glucocorticoids

The principle of glucocorticoid use in moderate-to-severe COVID infection is grounded in the attenuation of a hyperinflammatory response. The optimal type and dose of glucocorticoid remains uncertain. The largest prospective RCT to date, RECOVERY, included more than 6000 patients and used a regimen of dexamethasone at a dosage of 6 mg daily for up to 10 days as compared with the SOC; there was a significant 34% reduction in 28-day mortality in patients receiving IMV, a significant 17% reduction in patients receiving supplemental oxygen, and no significant difference in hospitalized patients not receiving oxygen [143]. Additional benefit was seen in a reduction in hospital LOS and lower rates of progression to IMV. Two independent trials compared dexamethasone dosages of 20 mg/d for five days followed by 10 mg/d for five days with SOC in patients receiving IMV, which demonstrated benefit for steroid therapy [144, 145]. The COVID-19 Dexamethasone (CoDEX) trial was limited by a 35% use of steroids in the control group but found a significant reduction in ventilator-free days, sequential organ failure assessment scores, ICU-free days, and duration of IMV. No difference was found in mortality, but this trial was underpowered for this end point, which had a 56.3% mortality rate in the dexamethasone group [144]. In contrast, the trial from Villar et al. [145] found a mortality reduction to 21% from 36% in the control group and a 4.8-day increase in ventilator-free days.

Two medium-size trials, Randomized, Embedded, Multi-factorial Adaptive Platform Trial for Community-Acquired Pneumonia (REMAP-CAP) and Community-Acquired Pneumonia: Evaluation of Corticosteroids in Coronavirus Disease (CAPE-COVID), prospectively evaluated the use of hydrocortisone in critically ill patients [146, 147]. REMAP-CAP was an open-label randomized trial that found a Bayesian probability of superiority (odds of improvement in organ support-free days within 21 days) of 93% and 80% for patients treated with hydrocortisone 50 or 100 mg every six hours for 7 days or while in shock for up to 28 days, respectively, as compared with no hydrocortisone [146]. CAPE-COVID was a double-blind RCT that compared a dosage of hydrocortisone 200 mg/d for seven days followed by a taper versus placebo [147]. Likely underpowered with a trend toward improvement in the study group, this trial was stopped early for futility after no difference was found in 21-day treatment failure, need for IMV, incidence of proning, or need for ECMO.

Two small and one moderately sized trials evaluated the use of methylprednisolone in non-ICU patients. One of the smaller trials, which used dosages of methylprednisolone of 250 mg/d, demonstrated a significant mortality benefit and likelihood of clinical improvement [148]; the other, which used a dosage of 1 mg/kg/d, showed no difference in clinical deterioration [149]. The Methylprednisolone as Adjunctive Therapy for Patients Hospitalized With Coronavirus Disease 2019 (METCOVID) trial, which randomized more than 300 hypoxic (including critically ill) patients to methylprednisolone 0.5 mg/kg twice daily or placebo, overall demonstrated no difference in 28-day mortality with an exception in the subgroup of patients older than 60 years who had better survival [150].

The cumulative data on the use of glucocorticoids in patients with COVID-19 indicate significant benefit in hospitalized patients who require supplemental oxygen or mechanical ventilation. Based on the earlier data, it is reasonable to treat all hypoxemic hospitalized patients with dexamethasone at a dosage of 6 mg daily or its equivalent [4, 116]. Patients receiving IMV may benefit from higher dosages of steroids, potentially up to 20 mg daily of dexamethasone or its equivalent because these dosages may favor a reduction in duration of mechanical ventilation, although this conclusion is limited by trial differences in patient population, design, and power.

Despite initial reservations about the use of corticosteroids early in the days of the pandemic, the data are supportive for steroids in select patients with COVID-19. Recent society guidelines have favored the use of glucocorticoids for hospitalized patients who require supplemental oxygen or mechanical ventilation [4, 116]. Notably, glucocorticoids should not be prescribed for hospitalized patients who are not receiving supplemental oxygen.

Baricitinib

Baricitinib is a Janus kinase 1 and 2 inhibitor, which inhibits the intracellular signaling path of proinflammatory cytokines and may have an added benefit in inhibiting SARS-CoV-2 cellular entry [151, 152]; small studies had suggested improvement in oxygenation and inflammatory marker reduction in treated patients with COVID-19 [151, 153, 154]. The ACTT2 trial tested a regimen of remdesivir (up to 10 days) combined with baricitinib (up to 14 days) versus remdesivir alone in hospitalized patients, of whom 10% were receiving IMV or ECMO [155]. The ACTT-2 trials showed that in the combination group, median time to recovery was reduced by 1 day (to 7 days) overall and by 8 days (to 10 days) in patients who were receiving HFNC or IMV, and also demonstrated a 28-day mortality reduction to 5.1% from 7.8% and lower need for oxygen and IMV/ECMO among patients who had not required these at baseline with fewer adverse events [155].

The findings of this study led to recommendations that baricitinib be added to remdesivir therapy in hospitalized patients who cannot receive steroids [4, 116]. However, this recommendation was made without any data demonstrating superiority of dexamethasone to baricitinib. Accordingly, the ACTT-4 trial was designed to directly compare steroids versus baricitinib in the treatment of hospitalized patients with COVID-19, all of whom were given remdesivir [156]. ACTT-4 was recently stopped for futility, but the results are as yet unpublished. The recently presented COV-BARRIER trial of baricitinib (Randomized, Double-Blind, Placebo-Controlled, Parallel-Group Phase 3 Study of Baricitinib in Patients with COVID-19 Infection) versus placebo as addition to usual care (in which approximately 90% of participants received dexamethasone) demonstrated a significant mortality benefit with baricitinib addition [157]. These findings have led to NIH recommendations for the use of baricitinib in addition to dexamethasone in patients with COVID-19 progressing on HFNC or NIV [4].

Tocilizumab

Early in the COVID-19 pandemic, patients with severe COVID-19 were recognized to have elevated interleukin-6 (IL-6) levels [158], which led to the trials of IL-6 signaling blockade as a potential therapy. Tocilizumab is a monoclonal antibody that antagonizes IL-6 signaling by binding the IL-6 receptor. Originally approved for the treatment of cytokine release syndrome in chimeric antigen receptor T cell therapy and used in several rheumatologic diseases and lung fibrosis from systemic sclerosis [159–161], this biologic (and others with similar mechanisms of action) was tested as a therapeutic for patients with COVID-19 with severe illness. The Evaluating Minority Patients with Actemra (EMPACTA) trial, a double-blind, placebo-controlled RCT, randomized more than 300 hospitalized, moderately ill patients to tocilizumab 8 mg/kg once or twice versus placebo and found a reduction in the composite of IMV and mortality (12% vs. 19%, respectively), as well as a lower median time to hospital discharge and time to improvement in clinical status [162].

The largest published trial, REMAP-CAP, was an open-label study that randomized more than 800 critically ill patients (about 30% on IMV, all on at least HFNC), to tocilizumab 8 mg/kg once, sarilumab 400 mg once (5.5% of study participants), or standard care and found a significantly higher number of organ support-free days, improved in-hospital survival (odds ratio [OR] 1.64 for tocilizumab and 2.01 for sarilumab), improved 90-day survival, decreased time to ICU and hospital discharge, and improvement in clinical status at 14 days in the intervention groups [163]. Data from the open-label RECOVERY trial of more than 4000 patients, currently available as preprint only, likewise suggests mortality benefit and a reduction in progression to mechanical ventilation among patients who receive tocilizumab [164].

However, the data testing the efficacy of tocilizumab have been disparate, with several trials demonstrating conflicting effects. One example is the BACC Bay trial (double-blind, placebo-controlled) that randomized moderately ill patients to receive tocilizumab or placebo and found no significant difference in likelihood of intubation or death, worsening disease, or discontinuation of supplemental oxygen [165]. The Study to Evaluate the Safety and Efficacy of Tocilizumab in Patients With Severe COVID-19 Pneumonia (COVACTA) trial, in which almost 40% of participants were receiving IMV, randomized patients to tocilizumab or placebo and found no difference in clinical status at 28 days and no difference in mortality, ventilator-free days, ICU days, incidence of ICU transfer, and incidence of IMV between the groups [166]. Three other trials (RCT-TCZ-COVID-19 [167], CORIMUNO-TOCI-1 [168], and by Veiga et al. [169]) each randomized moderately ill hospitalized patients to tocilizumab in addition to SOC or SOC alone, and found either no difference in clinical status or were stopped early (Veiga et al. [169]) out of concern for increased mortality in the treatment arm [167–169].

The divergent results between these studies may be related to differences in levels of inflammatory markers, timing of tocilizumab administration in the course of illness, and use of concomitant medications (e.g. dexamethasone) between the study populations [170]. Nevertheless, these data have led to recommendations that in severe or critical illness (patients with C-reactive protein [CRP] ≥ 75 mg/L), tocilizumab be added to treatment [4, 116]. Whether sarilumab is equally efficacious or whether lower-dose or subcutaneous tocilizumab may be used remains unclear with limited data from small, uncontrolled studies [171–173]. Concerns about increased rates of infection with IL-6 inhibition, particularly when combined with steroids [174], have not been borne out in RCTs. Although tocilizumab can be given in addition to dexamethasone, it should not be given in conjunction with baricitinib [4].

Colchicine

Use of colchicine for COVID is founded on its anti-inflammatory action in pericarditis and inflammatory arthritis with a suggestion of reduction of production of IL-1 [175, 176]. GRECCO-19 was an open-label study that randomized 105 patients to colchicine (1.5-mg loading dose followed by 0.5 mg once, then 0.5 mg twice daily for up to three weeks) or usual care and found significant reduction in deterioration of the clinical status in the colchicine group with no difference in troponin levels, CRP levels, or event-free survival time [177]. However, a very low event rate and a slightly sicker control group may have affected the results. The only placebo-controlled trial of colchicine was in 72 patients with moderate hypoxemia with significantly lower median time of need for supplemental oxygen and hospital LOS in the colchicine group [178]. Another case–control study evaluated colchicine in moderately to severely ill hospitalized patients and found that colchicine use correlated with lower mortality, lower likelihood of intubation, and higher discharge rate; however, this trial was limited by a significantly higher rate of renal failure and higher rates of hypertension and diabetes mellitus in the control group, which are known risk factors for severe COVID-19 and likely confounded these outcomes [179]. Similarly, an observational cohort study, which suggested a lower mortality with colchicine, was limited by significantly higher use of azithromycin and hydroxychloroquine in the control group [180].

Although these initial studies in the use of colchicine are promising, the small nature of the trials to date cannot fully support its use in hospitalized patients with COVID-19. Two large trials testing colchicine in nonhospitalized (COLCORONA) and hospitalized (RECOVERY) patients with COVID-19 have pending results, but the current recommendation is that colchicine not be used in hospitalized patients outside of clinical trials [4].

Therapies that Have No Benefit in Hospitalized Patients with COVID-19

Hydroxychloroquine with or without Azithromycin

One of the first combinations to be widely used in hospitalized patients with COVID-19 was hydroxychloroquine and azithromycin. The impetus was predicated on the principle that hydroxychloroquine, an antimalarial, had antiviral effects and activity against IL-1 and IL-6 [181–184], and that azithromycin had been shown in vitro to have antiviral activity against RNA viruses [185–187]. Initial excitement arose after the publication of a small, nonrandomized series of 20 patients compared with contemporaneous controls, which showed improved virologic clearance [188]. The initial excitement for this cocktail was quickly tempered after multiple RCTs showed, at best, no clinical benefit of hydroxychloroquine for SARS-CoV-2 infection and, in some cases, even suggested a detrimental effect [115, 189–196].

The largest trial testing the efficacy of hydroxychloroquine in patients with COVID-19 comes from the RECOVERY group. The RECOVERY study of hydroxychloroquine randomized more than 4000 hospitalized patients (of whom 23% were not receiving oxygen and 17% were receiving IMV) to receive hydroxychloroquine or usual care. Not only was there no difference in 28-day mortality rate (27% vs. 25% in usual care), the hydroxychloroquine group had a lower likelihood of hospital discharge alive, longer duration of hospitalization, higher likelihood of initiation of mechanical ventilation, and a trend toward increased cardiac death [194]. Similarly, the RECOVERY study of azithromycin, which randomized more than 7700 patients to azithromycin or usual care, found no difference in hospital LOS, proportion of patients discharged alive from the hospital, or a composite of IMV and death [189]. Significant safety concerns for these medications alone or in combination raised the specter of the harmful effects of this unproven therapy, with some studies showing hydroxychloroquine treatment to have a statistical increase in QTc prolongation and arrhythmias, as well as overall mortality [191, 197–200]. The lack of efficacy coupled with the risk for arrythmias and death have led to recommendations against the use of these medications in hospitalized patients [4, 20, 116].

Lopinavir/Ritonavir

The combination of lopinavir and ritonavir, approved for the treatment of HIV in 2000, consists of a protease inhibitor (lopinavir) coupled with a booster (inhibitor of CYP3A metabolism of lopinavir) and has been shown to have in vitro activity in SARS-CoV-1 inhibition [201]. Small studies of lopinavir/ritonavir combined with ribavirin in patients with SARS-CoV-1 and MERS led to interest in its use for COVID-19 [202, 203].

Early in the pandemic, a trial of 127 patients randomized to lopinavir/ritonavir, ribavirin, and interferon beta-1b versus lopinavir/ritonavir alone showed a reduction in time to negative viral swab and in time to clinical improvement in the combination group [204]. However, a subsequent trial testing lopinavir/ritonavir against usual care in almost 200 hospitalized patients with moderate hypoxemia found no significant difference in time to clinical improvement, 28-day mortality, or viral RNA clearance [205]. Two large trials, SOLIDARITY and RECOVERY, which in total had a study population of more than 16 000 patients, randomized moderately to severely ill patients to lopinavir/ritonavir at a dose of 400 mg/100 mg versus usual care and also found no effect on mortality, time to discharge alive from the hospital, or initiation of IMV [115, 206]. As such, this antiviral therapy was quickly abandoned as a potential treatment in COVID-19 and is not recommended for use for patients with COVID-19 [4, 20, 116].

Interferon

Interferons are important antiviral cytokines that had suggestions of clinical efficacy in SARS-CoV-1, which led to an interest in testing several different interferon formulations in patients with COVID-19 [207, 208]. A placebo-controlled trial of nebulized interferon beta-1a in hospitalized patients, most of whom were receiving supplemental oxygen, found greater odds of improvement on day 15 and increased likelihood of improving clinical status during treatment among the intervention group [209]. Two small studies investigated interferon beta-1a and interferon beta-1b as compared with usual care. The first study of 92 patients that tested interferon beta-1a found improved mortality and increased likelihood of discharge with no difference in time to clinical response [210]. In contrast, in the other study of 80 patients, interferon beta-1b was demonstrated to increase the likelihood of discharge and lower ICU admission rate but had no difference in mortality or hospital or ICU LOS [211]. These trials were limited by both a significant imbalance in the severity of illness and the administration of concomitant medications, including corticosteroids. Finally, a trial of recombinant superinterferon compared with traditional interferon alpha showed reduced time to clinical improvement, time to radiographic improvement, and time to negative conversion [212].

Several trials have also evaluated combination therapies of interferon with an antiviral in COVID-19. A small trial of nebulized interferon alpha-2b alone or in combination with the antiviral, umifenovir, suggested a reduction in proinflammatory markers and increased viral clearance in the combination group [213]. Nebulized interferon beta-1b combined with favipiravir had no effect on mortality, hospital LOS, need for ICU transfer, or inflammatory markers when compared with hydroxychloroquine [214]. Another trial of Novaferon, Novaferon with lopinavir/ritonavir, or lopinavir/ritonavir alone showed greater rates of viral clearance in the Novaferon-containing groups [215].

The NIH-sponsored the ACTT-3 in late 2020, which was a large, double-blind, placebo-controlled RCT comparing remdesivir plus interferon beta-1a to remdesivir plus placebo in severe COVID-19 requiring high-flow oxygen or noninvasive ventilation (NIV)/invasive ventilation [216]. An interim review of safety data found an increase in serious adverse events among patients receiving high-flow oxygen/non-IMV who received interferon beta-1a as compared with those who did not [217]. As such, the NIH guidelines do not recommend using interferon therapy in severely or critically ill patients [4].

Anakinra

Anakinra is an IL-1 antagonist that has been used in hemophagocytic lymphohistiocytosis and other autoimmune inflammatory syndromes. Five small RCTs have tested the use of anakinra as a therapy for patients with COVID-19. The largest of these, CORIMUNO-ANA-1, randomized 116 hospitalized patients to anakinra at 200 mg twice daily intravenously (IV) on days 1–3, then at 100 mg twice daily on day 4, and 100 mg once daily on day 5 or usual care but was stopped early for futility after no difference was found in need for or survival without IMV or NIV [218]. Four other small trials (<70 patients) compared anakinra with historical controls or usual care in hospitalized patients with moderate-to-severe hypoxemia; one of these found no difference in mortality but reduced need for IMV [219]. Another trial found lower mortality with the combination of anakinra and methylprednisolone as compared with historical controls [220]. One trial found a lower likelihood of IMV or mortality with anakinra as

compared with historical controls [221], and one found no difference in duration of IMV or ICU LOS in critically ill patients [222]. Finally, a study of patients with hypoxemia with CRP >50 mg/L whose treatment allocations were stratified by severity of illness (methylprednisolone if 3–5 L of oxygen, methylprednisolone plus anakinra if ≥6 L of oxygen, versus control) demonstrated a reduction in mortality in the treatment arms regardless of whether anakinra was included [223]. The lack of convincing evidence for efficacy of anakinra does not support its use in patients with COVID-19.

Monoclonal Antibody

Monoclonal antibodies that can bind and neutralize the SARS-CoV-2 virus were identified early in the COVID-19 pandemic and quickly shuttled into clinical trials to test as a therapy in COVID-19 [224, 225]. By binding the spike protein of the coronavirus, these monoclonal antibodies provide passive immunity by effectively working as an antiviral therapy and blocking viral attachment to cells and facilitating viral clearance [226]. Preliminary results for neutralizing monoclonal antibody use in mild-to-moderate COVID-19 (i.e. nonhospitalized patients) demonstrated a decrease in viral load and had an intriguing trend in decreasing the secondary end point of hospitalization and emergency department visits [227–229]. However, the efficacy for monoclonal antibody in severely ill hospitalized patients with COVID-19 did not follow the same pattern as for nonhospitalized patients. Indeed, bamlanivimab was tested in the Accelerating COVID-19 Therapeutic Interventions and Vaccines-3 (ACTIV-3)/TICO double-blind, placebo-controlled RCT and was stopped early for futility [230].

Several issues may have led to the lackluster effect of monoclonal antibodies in hospitalized patients. Bamlanivimab was tested in addition to remdesivir, which may limit the antiviral effect. More importantly, hospitalized patients with COVID-19 tend to present later in their disease course, and the window in which effective antiviral therapy will have an impact on the clinical outcome may be diminished (or passed). Ongoing studies as part of the ACTIV-3 trials continue to study the possible utility of monoclonal antibodies for severe COVID-19 illness. Nevertheless, monoclonal antibodies are currently

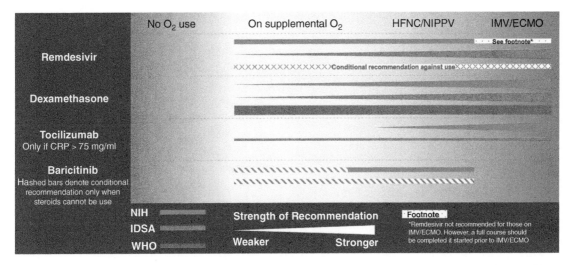

Figure 10.2 Summary of treatment recommendations from the National Institutes of Health (NIH), Infectious Diseases Society of America (IDSA), and World Health Organization (WHO) for hospitalized patients with COVID-19. Current recommendations from the NIH (blue), IDSA (green), and WHO (burnt orange) for remdesivir, dexamethasone, tocilizumab, and baricitinib (accessed 2 June 2021). Treatment is defined for hospitalized patients with COVID-19 across a spectrum of disease severity. The WHO currently has no recommendations for tocilizumab and baricitinib. CRP, C-reactive protein; ECMO, extracorporeal membrane oxygenation; HFNC, high-flow nasal cannula; IMV, invasive mechanical ventilation; NIPPV, noninvasive positive pressure ventilation.

not recommended in patients hospitalized for COVID-19 [4, 116].

Conclusions

The field of therapeutics for hospitalized patients with COVID-19 continues to evolve (Figure 10.2). As an aggregate of data, the best practice at the time of this writing is the administration of dexamethasone at a dosage of 6 mg daily (or equivalent) to all hospitalized patients who require supplemental oxygen and to consider higher doses in patients who are receiving IMV. Remdesivir should be given to all inpatients who require supplemental oxygen who do not have contraindications, with a 5-day course for acutely ill patients and a 10-day course for critically ill patients. Baricitinib should be considered for all patients in conjunction with remdesivir who would otherwise receive corticosteroids but have contraindications. For patients receiving HFNC or NIV who are progressing, either baricitinib or tocilizumab can be used in addition to dexamethasone. Furthermore, tocilizumab should be considered in all patients with severe or critical illness and elevated markers of inflammation (i.e. CRP ≥ 75 mg/L). At this time, all inpatients should receive prophylactic-dose anticoag-

ulation with a low threshold for investigation of thromboembolic disease, or when not possible, empiric-dose escalation to intermediate or therapeutic dose. These practices will likely change as further evidence becomes available.

Extrapulmonary Disease in Acutely Ill Patients with COVID-19

As COVID has now infected an estimated 137 million people worldwide and caused nearly 3 million deaths, more is known about the many complications outside the respiratory system that are associated with the disease [231]. Early in the COVID-19 pandemic, it became clear that those infected experienced multiorgan disease, and some have postulated that diffuse vascular injury may be a common mechanism responsible for the observed protean manifestations of COVID infection [232]. Therefore, those caring for patients with COVID-19 must maintain vigilance to monitor for potential complications that oftentimes cause respiratory symptoms that may be confounded by those of the underlying viral pneumonia.

Thromboembolic Disease

Acutely ill patients are known to be at increased risk for thromboembolic complications, which roughly correlate with severity of disease [233, 234]. Similar to other respiratory viral pathogens, such as influenza, MERS, and SARS, the incidence of thrombotic complications observed with COVID-19 is increased [235]. Therefore, thrombosis must be promptly recognized in patients with COVID-19 because data suggest mortality rate increases with its presence [236].

Numerous risk factors for the development of venous thromboembolism (VTE) in COVID have been identified, including male sex, advanced age, coronary artery disease, Hispanic ethnicity, obesity, prior myocardial infarction, hypertension, and diabetes [236, 237]. Given the rapidly evolving knowledge base regarding COVID infection, as well as significant changes in disease management, the true incidence of VTE associated with COVID is unknown. A recent systematic review estimated an overall incidence of 17% with a fourfold higher rate in ICU compared with non-ICU patients (28% vs. 7%, respectively) [238]. Numerous autopsy studies have also identified frequent occurrence of microvascular thrombosis, which may explain many of the systemic manifestations of COVID illness [239, 240].

Although hospitalized patients, particularly those in the ICU, are at risk for thrombosis as a result of stasis, hypoxemia, central venous catheters, and sepsis, it appears that SARS-CoV-2 infections may trigger unique pathways that lead to clinical clot formation [241]. Severe lung injury in COVID-19 not only causes endothelial injury, but also direct vascular injury from the SARS-CoV-2 spike protein may contribute to activation of the coagulation cascade [242–246]. Indeed, elevations in D-dimer, fibrinogen, platelet count, von Willebrand factor (VWF) activity, and factor VIII activity are observed in severe COVID-19 illness [247–249]. In addition, SARS-CoV-2 infection produces a highly inflammatory state as marked by elevations in CRP, IL-6, and ferritin, which have been postulated as causative factors for clot formation, although the precise mechanism is still unknown [241, 250, 251].

Although not SOC, inpatients and those in the ICU routinely undergo one-time or serial serologic measures of coagulation, including complete blood count, prothrombin time/partial thromboplastin time, fibrinogen, and D-dimer. Although therapeutic decisions may not be initiated based on these results, clues may be obtained suggesting the diagnosis of VTE or other coagulation disorders. Moreover, prognostic information can be obtained, including risk for mortality, as is the case with D-dimer [252]. Routine use of screening imaging modalities to diagnose VTE is generally not recommended because there are insufficient data that it alters outcomes and unnecessarily exposes healthcare workers to COVID-19 [4].

Given the multiple published reports of higher-than-expected incidence of VTE in patients admitted to the hospital with COVID, numerous treatment trials were initiated to determine whether nonstandard thresholds should be implemented to initiate anticoagulation therapy. A recent meta-analysis from the American Society of Hematology found a reduction in the incidence of pulmonary embolism in critically ill patients (OR 0.09; 95% confidence interval, 0.02–0.57) was counterbalanced by a significant increase in bleeding complications (OR 3.84; 95% confidence interval, 1.44–10.21) and accordingly recommended against the use of intermediate- or treatment-dose anticoagulation over prophylaxis dose, citing a lack of benefit in preventing VTE [253]. Three recently published prospective clinical trials examined the appropriate level of prophylactic anticoagulation in patients with COVID-19: Antithrombotic Therapy to Ameliorate Complications of COVID-19 (ATTACC), ACTIV-4, and the REMAP-CAP. Although these three international trials were independent studies, they were part of a multiplatform RCT that instituted "harmonized protocols." By using common combined superiority and futility end points, the trials allowed for more rapid patient enrollment. All three studies randomized patients to receive either treatment-dose low-molecular-weight or unfractionated heparin compared with usual-care pharmacologic VTE prophylaxis. Interim analysis of these studies revealed futility in critically ill patients [254] with an increased need for ongoing organ support for patients receiving full-dose anticoagulation and no mortality benefit [255, 256]. Finally, a recently reported prospective trial comparing intermediate-dosage (enoxaparin 1 mg/kg daily) versus standard prophylactic anticoagulation (enoxaparin 40 mg daily) in COVID-infected patients admitted to the ICU found no benefit [257]. The INSPIRATION trial's primary efficacy outcome was a composite of venous or arterial thrombosis, treatment with ECMO, or mortality within 30 days, with the treatment arm and control group reaching the combined end point in 45.7% and 44.1% of enrolled patients (OR, 1.06). At the current state, the most recent guidelines recommend against the use of full anticoagulation for COVID-infected individuals in the absence of known or suspected VTE [4].

If VTEs are identified, the treatment algorithm is very much the same as it is for hospitalized patients without COVID-19. In the absence of a contraindication, treatment-dose anticoagulation should be initiated for all known or suspected VTE patients because it improves mortality [258–264]. Because anticoagulation carries a chance for bleeding complications, this risk must be weighed against the potential benefit, and in cases in which anticoagulation cannot be safely initiated, consideration should be made for placement of an inferior vena cava filter [262, 263]. In cases associated with hemodynamic instability, severe tachycardia, or refractory hypoxemia, more aggressive treatment approaches should be considered, including thrombolytics, catheter-directed thrombolysis, or mechanical retrieval [265]. Currently, no data favor the use of one particular anticoagulant agent over another for the treatment of known or suspected VTE in patients with COVID infection, and the choice of agent should be determined based on half-life, route of administration, and bleeding risk [266].

Cardiac Complications

Numerous manifestations of cardiac disease have been described in association with COVID infection. Patients with preexisting cardiac disease have consistently been identified as being at high risk for mortality [267]. A proposed mechanism for this association includes limited physiologic reserve, impaired immunity, heightened inflammatory state, direct endothelial injury caused by the COVID-19 virus itself, and dysfunctional angiotensin-converting enzyme 2 (ACE2) receptor [268].

Acute Coronary Syndromes

Acute coronary syndromes (ACSs) comprise a spectrum of cardiac dysfunction, including angina, non-ST elevations myocardial infarction (non-STEMI), and STEMI. A common thread among ACSs is that all are consequences of either partial or complete obstruction of blood flow of the coronary arteries as a result of thrombus formation and endothelial injury. Given COVID-19 creates a degree of endothelial damage or dysfunction, it is not surprising that ACS is a recognized complication [269]. As previously discussed, COVID-19 is associated with a robust inflammatory response in many infected individuals that may have a detrimental effect on endothelial structure and function [242–246]. In addition, it has been postulated that the virus itself may cause direct injury to the endothelium, perhaps mediated by the ACE2 receptor, although evidence of this is still lacking [270]. Several small studies evaluating patients with acute COVID-19 with ACS found a high rate of normal coronary angiography, suggesting either direct myocyte injury or microvascular disease [271–273]. Because elevations in troponin have been consistently described in acute COVID infection, it becomes difficult to distinguish acute macrovascular cardiac injury evident on angiogram as opposed to a systemic inflammatory state leading to myocarditis or microvascular cardiac injury [274].

The general management of ACS in patients with COVID-19 is not dissimilar to uninfected patients. For low-risk non-STEMI patients, medical management is generally recommended, with invasive testing (angiography) reserved for those with high suspicion for acute coronary occlusion [275]. For patients with COVID-19 with STEMI, percutaneous coronary intervention should be pursued with haste given its superiority to systemic fibrinolysis and conservative medical therapy, when feasible [276]. Because COVID-infected individuals commonly have multiorgan dysfunction, decisions to take patients to the cardiac catheterization lab need to be individually weighed against expected survival, risk of procedure, and in times of overwhelming volume, allocation of resources [277].

Myocarditis and Heart Failure

Patients with preexisting heart failure have a worse prognosis if infected with COVID [277–280].

However, acute myocarditis with new-onset heart failure (sometimes fulminant) associated with elevations in cardiac biomarkers (troponin, creatine kinase-MB, and brain natriuretic peptide) and nonischemic in origin has been described [281–283]. Despite suspicion that SARS-CoV-2 infection directly causes myocarditis, the viral genome is only rarely identified in endomyocardial biopsies, leaving the mechanism of myocardial damage an open debate [284]. Microvascular injury and clotting have been identified, which could be another possible cause of myocardial injury [273, 284]. Finally, stress-induced (takotsubo) cardiomyopathy has been described as a cause of heart failure in patients with COVID-19, which at times can be difficult to distinguish from myocarditis because cardiac biomarkers are elevated in both diseases [285–295].

Arrythmias

A recent meta-analysis found that 10.3% of hospitalized patients had evidence of cardiac arrhythmias [296]. The same study also identified supraventricular tachycardia as the most commonly observed arrythmia, followed by ventricular tachyarrhythmias, and lastly bradyarrhythmias. Patients admitted to the ICU have a higher incidence of arrythmias with a relative risk of 12.1 compared with non-critically ill patients [296–298]. Indeed, a single-center study from New York reported an incidence of atrial arrythmias in the ICU to be much higher than those admitted to a general medical ward (17.7% vs 1.9%) [297]. Moreover, an early report from Wuhan found that patients in the ICU were significantly more likely to experience arrythmias of all types when compared with non-ICU patients (44.4% vs. 6.9%) [298].

Clearly, COVID-19 increases the risk for cardiac arrhythmias, but the impact on mortality from cardiac arrest is conflicting [299–301]. Two single-center reports described the occurrence of cardiac arrest in 5.6% and 11% of hospitalized patients with COVID-19 [299, 300]. Notably, most of these events were unshockable rhythms and could have been a secondary consequence (e.g. caused by hypoxemia from respiratory failure) rather than a primary cardiac event. More recently, a prospective, observational study of 143 patients in a single center identified sustained ventricular tachycardia or ventricular fibrillation occurring in approximately 2% of hospitalized patients with COVID-19, supporting the notion that malignant ventricular arrythmias are rare events [301].

Assessment for Cardiac Disease

Because COVID-19 frequently presents with nonspecific symptoms or as multiorgan disease, an electrocardiogram may be the only clue of an ongoing ACS and should be obtained on all patients admitted to the hospital. In addition, underlying electrocardiogram abnormalities may be able to help with risk stratification because a multivariate analysis found statistically significant increased OR for death with the presence of one or more atrial premature contractions (OR 2.57), a right bundle branch or intraventricular block (OR 2.61), ischemic T-wave inversion (OR 3.49), or nonspecific repolarization (OR 2.31) [302].

Numerous inflammatory markers have been observed to be elevated in patients with acute COVID-19 infection [303]. Cardiac biomarkers were among the first reported serologic markers that seemed to potentially correlate with outcomes [304]. Abnormal values of cardiac biomarkers may be evidence of a primary cardiac disease and aid in predicting mortality and other clinical end points [4]. For example, cardiac troponin levels correlate with increased severity of illness and are predictive of poor outcomes [267]. Troponin elevations are common in patients with acute COVID-19 infection, making it a less reliable marker of cardiac dysfunction or ischemia and necessitates abnormalities being interpreted with caution and in concert with other testing so as not to miss ACSs or other cardiac disease.

Elevations in natriuretic peptide levels are known to occur both in patients with known cardiovascular disease and with acute hemodynamic or hypoxemic stress [278, 305–308]. However, natriuretic peptides also increase both in inflammatory states and with acute respiratory disease [309]. Both brain natriuretic peptide and N-terminal pro-B-type natriuretic peptide have been noted to be elevated in acute COVID-19 infection in a pattern similar to that of troponin [310]. As with troponin, natriuretic peptide levels in acute COVID-19 infection provide important prognostic information but infrequently alter management decisions.

The routine use of echocardiography has varied in patients with acute COVID-19 infection [311]. A large international survey study of 1216 patients hospitalized with COVID-19 found patients with abnormal echocardiograms (55%) were older and had a higher prevalence of preexisting cardiovascular disease [312]. Moreover, 39% of patients had left ventricular (LV) dysfunction, with biventricular dysfunction noted in 14.3% of patients. Several smaller prospective observational studies noted LV dysfunction in 10–27% of patients [313–315]. Interestingly, little correlation was found between disease severity and severity of LV dysfunction. Another retrospective study of 305 hospitalized patients with COVID-19 from seven hospitals in New York City and Milan reported a 31.7% mortality rate for patients with both troponin elevation and abnormal echocardiograms, which contrasted the respective mortality rates of 5.2% and 18.6% for those with normal troponin/normal echo and elevated troponin/normal echo [316].

Renal Complications

Despite initial infection of the respiratory tract, the incidence of acute kidney injury (AKI) in hospitalized patients has been reported in a recent meta-analysis at 17%, with 5% requiring renal replacement therapy (RRT) [317]. Risk factors for the development of AKI include advanced age, diabetes mellitus, coronary artery disease, Black race, hypertension, mechanical ventilation, and vasopressor use [318]. Moreover, mechanical ventilation and the use of vasopressors were particularly strong predictors for the development of AKI (OR 10.7 and 4.53, respectively).

Whether the incidence of AKI observed in COVID-19 infection is a by-product of generalized inflammation and hemodynamic compromise as opposed to a direct effect on the kidney by the virus is not clear [319]. In addition, preexisting kidney dysfunction likely plays a role. The proximal tubule epithelium expresses ACE2, which SARS-CoV-2 uses to bind with the spike protein to facilitate cellular uptake and could contribute to detrimental effects such as increased vasoconstriction, inflammation, fibrosis, coagulation, and sodium retention [319–321]. In fact, autopsy studies have confirmed the presence of

COVID viral particles in the kidney [322, 323] and in the urine of patients with AKI, but no definite causation has been proved [100, 324–327].

Unfortunately, no specific therapy exists to minimize or reverse AKI associated with COVID-19 infection. Supportive care, including hemodynamic support, and appropriate volume management are recommended, although there is disagreement about how to optimize these strategies in patients with COVID-19, particularly when critically ill [4]. Standard indications, such as to correct acidosis and volume overload, should be used to determine the appropriate timing to initiate RRT. Furthermore, RRT may have additional therapeutic benefits in the treatment of severely ill patients with COVID-19. Experience with prior infection (SARS, MERS, and sepsis) has suggested that use of high-volume hemofiltration can significantly reduce IL-6 levels and is associated with improved sequential organ failure assessment scores [17, 328, 329]. However, it remains to be seen whether high-volume hemofiltration or other RRT modalities on COVID-19-associated AKI improve outcomes.

Infectious Complications

Secondary infections contributing to the morbidity and mortality of patients initially infected with a respiratory virus is well established [330–334]. Similarly, patients with COVID-19 have been found to acquire secondary bacterial and fungal infections [335–340]. Numerous factors exist that may increase the risk for superinfections, including prolonged hospitalizations with high rates of ICU care, high rate of mechanical intubation, liberal use of immunosuppressing medications, need for central venous access, and frequent use of prone positioning [341, 342].

Central Line-Associated Bloodstream Infection
A recent publication from an academic center in Detroit noted an increased central line-associated bloodstream infection (CLABSI) rate in patients with COVID-19 (1.7 CLABSI per 1000 central line days) compared with prepandemic rates (0.4 CLABSI per 1000 central line days). Interestingly, the rate of CLABSIs correlated with the numbers of hospitalized patients with COVID-19 [343]. Another single-center

study of patients with refractory hypoxemia undergoing extended prone positioning found a 4.9% incidence rate of CLABSI [344]. Another study performed in several hospitals in Saudi Arabia reported an increased CLABSI rate of 9.2 CLABSIs per 1000 line days during the height of their patient load compared with 0 before COVID-19 [345]. A much larger study reviewed 78 hospitals from a single healthcare system before and after the COVID pandemic and found a 51% increase in CLABSI rate from 0.56 to 0.85 CLABSIs per 1000 line days [346]. Lastly, a recent publication using data from the Centers for Disease Control and Prevention National Healthcare Safety Network analyzed CLASBI data from the second quarter of 2019 and the second quarter of 2020 during the first US peak of COVID cases [347]. The analysis included data from 2986 acute-care hospitals and found a 28% increase in the standard infection ratio in 2020 for CLABSI and a 39% increase in the standard infection ratio for patients admitted to the ICU. These studies highlight the need to maintain vigilance and evaluate for secondary infections, such as CLABSIs, in hospitalized patients with COVID-19 who may have persistent or worsening sepsis.

Evidenced-based prevention measures against CLABSI specifically in patients with COVID-19 are generally not available. Extrapolating from prior experience, the use of critical care bundles, limited use of central lines, hand washing with sterile insertion technique, internal jugular/subclavian as opposed to femoral placement, antiseptic impregnated catheters, avoidance of prolonged use of unnecessary antibiotics, and insertion done by experienced personnel may all help reduce CLABSI in the patient population [348–350].

Fungal Infections

A recent large, systematic review of hospitalized patients with COVID-19 in six countries found the incidence of *Candida* infections ranged from 0.7% to 23.5% [351]. The authors postulated that increased broad-spectrum antibiotic use, increased use of central venous catheters, use of immunosuppressants (glucocorticoids and tocilizumab), and ECMO were all likely culprit risk factors. Similarly, there have been numerous reports describing invasive aspergillus infections, likely from similar risk factors [337–340, 352].

Secondary Bacterial Infections

Secondary bacterial superinfections complicating COVID-19 infections are no surprise based on experience with other respiratory viral pathogens [353]. Most studies describing an infection pattern associated with COVID-19 have made the distinction between coinfection (infected at the time of admission) and secondary or superinfections in which signs or symptoms do not develop until several days into hospitalization [354]. The rate of coinfection in patients admitted to the hospital with COVID-19 infection has been reported to be quite low, with rates consistently around 3% [342, 354, 355]. Superinfections, primarily bacterial, have been reported in the range of 9% to 35%, with rates directly correlating with severity of disease and occurring despite the fact that the majority of patients received broad-spectrum antibiotics [278, 341, 354–356]. One study using highly sensitive polymerase chain reaction on 257 hospitalized patients with COVID found that 94% had evidence of superinfection, which was primarily bacterial [357].

Performing Aerosol-Generating Procedures in Patients with COVID-19

Urgent (and emergent) procedures required by hospitalized patients should proceed with haste and can be safely performed with proper precautions. Intubation of patients was already discussed within the earlier section Caring for the Critically Ill Patient with COVID-19. Therefore, this section provides guidelines on safely performing bronchoscopy, tracheostomy, and cardiopulmonary resuscitation in patients with COVID-19.

Bronchoscopy in COVID-19

Bronchoscopy is an essential tool that can assist in diagnosis of respiratory disease, in management of respiratory secretions, and with emergent airway management and can be safely undertaken provided appropriate measures are taken to ensure safety of the staff. Although elective procedures should probably be deferred if patients are actively infected with SARS-CoV-2, delays for more urgent and emergent situations cannot be tolerated, as is often the case in critically ill, intubated patients. Indeed, bronchoscopic clearance of airway secretions in mechanically ventilated patients has been a mainstay of traditional ICU care. In particular, patients with COVID-19 have been noted to have tenacious and occasionally hardened mucous plugs obstructing or occluding their airways [358]. A precipitating factor was surges of critically ill patients that stretched existing ventilator resources necessitating the use of transport and anesthesia ventilators, which are not designed for long-term ventilation and lack the ability for humidifying the airways during ventilation [359, 360]. Humidification is required for appropriate secretion management and can be delivered through different modalities. Although heated humidification provides superior airways humidification, current recommendations favor using a heat–moisture exchanger instead to prevent nosocomial transmission in COVID-19 [361, 362].

Critically ill patients with COVID-19 also have a significant risk for bacterial superinfections, including fungal infections, which may require lower airway sampling [352, 363, 364]. Lower respiratory specimens are more likely to be positive for SARS-CoV-2 than upper respiratory specimens [358]. As such, bronchoscopic sampling is indicated in patients who have high clinical suspicion for COVID-19 but persistently negative tests by nasopharyngeal swab [365]. Moreover, bronchoalveolar lavage is more sensitive than tracheal aspirates in identifying bacterial and fungal pathogens to facilitate the care of intubated patients with COVID-19 [366].

Indisputably, bronchoscopy is a vital clinical tool in the care of patients with COVID-19. However, as an aerosol-generating procedure, a legitimate fear existed about the ability to protect healthcare workers from exposure to and infection by the SARS-CoV-2 virus [367]. Throughout the COVID-19 pandemic, bronchoscopies continued to be used for the management of intubated patients, and data now support the safety of this procedure [366, 368, 369]. Importantly, certain modifications should be adopted to minimize healthcare worker exposure [352, 358, 370]. Bronchoscopies should be done in a negative pressure room whenever possible, with at least 12 air changes per hour and control direction of airflow [358, 371]. If negative pressure rooms are unavailable, a HEPA filter should be placed in the room before the procedure and

for several hours after procedure completion [358]. Several studies have used disposable bronchoscopes as part of their protocol to minimize healthcare worker transmission [366, 368, 369]. Intubated patients should be adequately preoxygenated before the procedure and paralyzed to prevent coughing during the procedure that could increase risk for aerosolization [368]. Only essential staff should be present in the room during the procedure; whenever possible, the bedside nurse and respiratory therapist should be immediately available outside the room. All participating staff should be in full PPE to minimize exposure, which at minimum includes gloves, a fluid-impermeable or resistant gown, and an N95 mask with eye protection (goggles or face shield that extends beyond the brow line) or a PAPR [370, 372]. For prolonged procedures, consideration should be given to wearing an N95 mask with a PAPR, because battery life may be limited and lead to equipment malfunction [373, 374].

Tracheostomy in Patients with COVID-19

Placement of a tracheostomy tube has many benefits, including facilitating safe ventilator weaning, optimizing patient comfort, and reducing sedation requirement, complications from prolonged intubation and ventilator-related pneumonia. Optimal timing of tracheostomy is unknown, and the procedure itself presents a unique challenge in this patient population [375]. In one cohort study out of Italy, early tracheostomy (performed within 10 days of intubation) was found to be associated with more ventilator-free days, shorter ICU stay, and lower mortality than delay tracheostomy [376]. However, many patients with COVID ARDS have been successfully extubated after prolonged intubation (two to three weeks), and the fact that a tracheostomy is not without risk counterbalances the potential benefits of early tracheostomy. Some have suggested evaluation for tracheostomy between 10 and 21 days of mechanical ventilation [377], but oftentimes, a limiting factor to early tracheostomy is persistently high oxygenation needs (FiO_2 and/or PEEP) that is prohibitive for the procedure.

The current data have not established an advantage for percutaneous or surgical tracheostomy approaches in COVID-19 [378–380]. However, the percutaneous approach has been the favored approach at our institution because of the ability to be performed at the bedside with fewer healthcare personnel being exposed to an actively infected patient with COVID-19. It is not necessary for the SARS-CoV-2 polymerase chain reaction to be negative before tracheostomy, and routine testing is not recommended [381]. In fact, several case series have demonstrated safety and low risk of COVID-19 transmission to the involved personnel [377–380, 382]. A bedside percutaneous tracheostomy can typically be accomplished with four providers in the room, which include two proceduralists (one providing bronchoscopic guidance and one for tracheostomy insertion), one respiratory therapist, and one ICU nurse. Additional staff outside the room should be available to provide assistance and additional equipment, and also act as a spotter for those performing the procedure. Given the risk of exposure to providers and minimal pulmonary reserve in patients, minimizing the duration of the procedure is important, and it is recommended that providers most experienced with percutaneous tracheostomy perform the procedure.

Ideally, the procedure should be performed in a negative pressure room, but at our institution, we have used portable, medical-grade HEPA filters in nonnegative pressure rooms as an alternative. Patients should be sedated and paralyzed to minimize the cough reflex and aerosolization [377, 381]. To mitigate potential aerosolization when interrupting the ventilator circuit, we temporarily pause ventilation (i.e. apnea) at these points during the procedure. Such events include adding the bronchoscope adaptor to the circuit (we also recommend use of an ETT clamp with this step), insertion of the bronchoscope into the ETT, repositioning of the ETT with the balloon deflated, needle and guidewire insertion, dilation, and insertion of the tracheostomy tube. Alternatively, one study found that aerosolization can be minimized by covering the stoma with gauze rather than pausing ventilation with no evidence of viral transmission to staff [383]. Due to the difference in procedural technique and increased coordination required, it is recommended that those who will be in the room during tracheostomy perform a pre-procedure huddle and review the plan before entering the patient room. During open or surgical tracheostomy, apneas should also be instituted during

incision into the anterior tracheal wall, and the use of diathermy and suction should be avoided or minimized [381]. A fenestrated technique whereby immediate suturing of the skin to the edges of the tracheotomy window occurs after tracheal incision forms a tight seal between the tracheostomy tube and stoma has been described and may decrease aerosolization [384].

Cardiopulmonary Resuscitation of the Patient with COVID-19

Cardiac arrest, unfortunately, occurs in critically ill patients with COVID-19. Before COVID-19, in a single-center study from Wuhan, China, only 3% of patients with in-hospital cardiac arrest were alive at 30 days [299]. In addition, a multicenter cohort study of more than 5000 patients admitted to the ICU with COVID-19 in the United States found the prevalence rate of cardiac arrest at 14%. Of these patients, approximately half received cardiopulmonary resuscitation, with only 12% surviving to discharge [385]. Not surprisingly, mortality with cardiac arrest increased with age. These studies seem to emphasize the need for early discussion about the goals of care for critically ill patients with COVID-19. Although it is recommended these conversions be done at admission, they should be updated throughout the hospitalization, especially with changes in clinical condition. It is especially helpful to determine a patient's minimal acceptable outcome early on in their clinical course.

Cardiopulmonary resuscitation is an aerosol-generating procedure and, as such, poses an increased risk for transmission to healthcare workers [71]. Therefore, as with most other aspects of health care, it poses unique considerations with COVID-19. First and foremost, because cardiac arrest can quickly become a disorderly and crowded event, it is important to emphasize that all persons entering the patient room be wearing appropriate PPE. This should include a gown, gloves, and a fit-tested N95 with face shield or goggles (PAPR is an excellent alternative if available). Limiting the number of personnel in the room is critical for infection control, and many centers recommend no more than seven healthcare providers in the room and utilization of mechanical chest compression devices when available [386]. Additional providers should remain outside of the room to act as spotters, provide assistance, obtain additional needed equipment, and maintain crowd control and keep additional personnel from entering the room unless indicated. Communication between the code leader and personnel outside the room can be facilitated by intercom, phone, two-way radio, or writing on a white board. Equipment, including the code cart and medications, should be kept outside of the room and only that which is needed passed into the room. To minimize risk for infection, the door should remain closed except when passing medications or equipment into the room.

Because awake proning therapy is widely used in nonintubated patients with COVID-19, providers may encounter a patient in cardiac arrest in the prone position. It is recommended to supinate the patient at the earliest feasible opportunity. However, until sufficient help arrives and can safely enter the room, compressions may need to be performed in the prone position. To do so, a two-handed technique over the midthoracic spine at the inferior boarder of the scapulae can be performed [387].

Patients who go into cardiac arrest may or may not already have an established airway. In patients not yet intubated, an advanced or secure airway should be obtained at the earliest feasible opportunity (previously discussed in Pharmacologic Therapies for Hospitalized Patients with COVID-19 section). Pause chest compressions during airway management and intubation to decrease aerosolization and increase success. If there is difficulty or delay in endotracheal intubation, strong consideration should be given to laryngeal mask airway placement [39, 386].

Coordinating Patient Placement and Care in COVID-19 Units

Several medical centers across the United States are part of the Regional Ebola and Special Pathogens Treatment Centers that contained high-level isolation units, referred to as biocontainment units. This network was created as a response to the 2014 Ebola virus disease outbreak in West Africa and was undertaken to enhance readiness to respond to highly infectious pathogens. This network included our hospital, and members of our ICU team had undergone training and readiness drills as members of the Special Pathogens team. With assistance from the Special Pathogens nurse educator, the ICU staff was able to apply many of the biocontainment principles learned and adapt them for SARS-CoV-2 patient management.

Similar to many hospitals, our institution cohorted COVID-19 hospitalized patients away from patients without COVID-19 in medical-surgical units and in the ICU. Ideally, patients are housed within individual rooms to minimize cross-contamination, which allows for each room to become a self-contained "dirty" zone where full PPE is required during patient care activities. Movable equipment and furniture (e.g. curtains, chairs, bedside tables) that are not essential for the immediate care of patients are removed from rooms to reduce tripping hazards and prevent inadvertent contamination of staff. An Ambu bag with a HEPA filter attachment in place, should be positioned at the head wall for emergent needs. Each room should have a workstation to allow for chart access and documentation while in PPE. The door of each room should have posted a visual instruction card describing proper donning and doffing techniques, a healthcare worker sign-in sheet, a COVID-19 isolation sign, and a list of nurse server supplies for purposes of daily inventory.

"Clean" areas are reserved for nondirect clinical care activities that can be performed in the absence of PPE. These areas include workstations for the healthcare staff, conference rooms, bathrooms, medication rooms and dispensers, and supply rooms. Donning stations are also within this area, and only PPE (face shields, PAPRs, etc.) that have been properly decontaminated should be allowed to be stored within the clean zone. High-touch areas, such as counter surfaces and computer monitors, should be cleaned with disinfectant every four hours. The "dirty" zones are direct patient care areas that include the patient rooms and adjacent desks and workstations.

The transition between the "dirty" and "clean" zones should be tightly regulated to prevent cross-contamination. To facilitate transfer of clinical samples, staff within "dirty" zones placed the samples in clean biohazard bags held by staff in the "clean" zone ensuring containment of the biohazardous material. Immediately outside the room and within the "dirty" zone should be a cleaning station with disinfectant solutions and clean gloves for decontamination of reused PPE (e.g. PAPRs) and other equipment. Foot-operated containers need to be clearly labeled for disposal of contaminated PPE or trash.

If the floorplan allows, "dirty" and "clean" zones can be created to encompass multiple rooms to facilitate the care of patients (Figure 10.3). For example, if a nurse is caring for several patients within the same "dirty" zone, they can move more freely between rooms, which improves efficiency and reduces the strain on the healthcare worker. Our institution created "dirty" and "clean" zones within the ICU to facilitate care and was particularly helpful in emergent situations (i.e. codes) by reducing the response time by eliminating the need for donning because staff who were already in full PPE can immediately intervene [388, 389]. To facilitate the visual recognition of the appropriate zones, we placed red tape to denote dirty areas and green tape to identify clean zones.

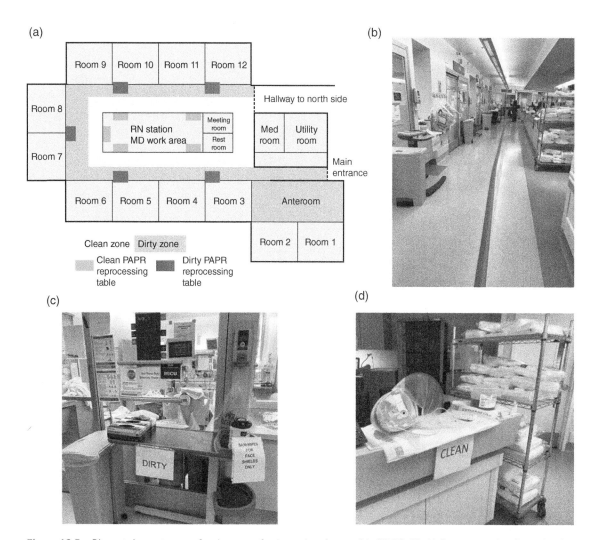

Figure 10.3   Biocontainment zones for the care of cohorted patients with COVID-19. (a) Representative floorplan for dividing "clean" and "dirty" zones within a COVID-19 cohort unit. The patient rooms are all within the "dirty zone" (pink shading). "Clean" zones (green shade) contain areas that are not used for direct patient care. (b) Green and red tape provide a visual for healthcare staff on the "clean" and "dirty" zones, respectively. (c) "Dirty" zones have doffing areas. (d) "Clean" zones have donning areas. PAPR, powered air-purifying respirator.

From an infection-control standpoint, we still recommend changing gloves and gowns between rooms within a "dirty" zone to reduce healthcare-associated infections (e.g. methicillin-resistant *Staphylococcus aureus*, vancomycin-resistant enterococcus, *Clostridium difficile*). However, the establishment of a "dirty" zone allows caregivers to access multiple rooms without having to don and doff their respiratory PPE. Our experience found that the doffing of the respiratory PPE was not only time consuming but is also a common point of accidental exposure. Indeed, trained healthcare workers often incorrectly doff contaminated PPE, which can be mitigated through proper training and competency assessment [390, 391]. Furthermore, the intensity of care of critically ill patients required frequent donning and doffing of PPE, which increases the chance of self-contamination, particularly in weary ICU staff. As a matter of fact, the study by Phan et al. [390] directly observing doffing practices among healthcare workers found proper PPE for droplet precautions was used in only 64% of the observations. More concerning were the numerous errors observed during doffing, with only 10% of the observations properly performed. Safety officers should be available to assist with the safe donning and doffing of staff working in COVID-19 units. Non-ICU staff providing care at the bedside, such as dialysis nurses, should be provided just-in-time training, which has been shown to be effective in limiting the likelihood of healthcare worker exposure to infectious disease [392]. Using a "doffing buddy" to observe removal of PPE may assist in ensuring proper doffing technique and reduce risk for self-contamination and is recommended by both the Centers for Disease Control and Prevention and the National Institute for Occupational Safety and Health [392, 393]. In our institution, we used the expertise of our Special Pathogens nurse educator to mirror several of these processes and to ensure ongoing PPE training of staff.

Increasing ICU Capacity

Hospitalized patients with COVID-19 are incredibly ill, and between 14% and 32% end up in the ICU, which can be extremely taxing on this limited resource [58, 394–396]. In areas of the world where patient influx outpaced ICU bed availability, hospitals have been forced to develop strategies to rapidly increase their ICU capacity and staffing capabilities by modifying standard practices [397–399]. This poses particular challenges in regard to ICU bed capacity, which requires specially trained staff and equipment that is often in limited supply. The Society of Critical Care Medicine, the NIH, the WHO, and others published guidelines to assist institutions in implementing these modifications [392, 397, 400, 401]. To increase ICU bed capacity, one of the first requirements is to increase the number of available ICU-grade rooms, which can be done by appropriating patient care areas commonly used for other purposes, such as medical wards, postanesthesia care units (PACUs), operating rooms, and even open areas of the hospital [392, 400]. Each of these areas has different benefits and challenges when converting it into an ICU space.

One of the areas that can be converted to ICU space is the medical ward. These areas typically have single patient rooms with a core infrastructure, including gas access and physiologic monitoring capabilities that can support ICU care. Ideally, each room should be converted to a negative pressure room if not already as such. For example, the flow of air can be directed outside by using a preconstructed window adapter though which a HEPA machine and flex duct can be placed [402].

COVID-19 care also requires a direct line of sight into the patient room from the outside, which may require the placement of a window into a solid door. Additional monitoring can be achieved by placing a webcam in the room. Physiologic monitors with alarms should be placed in the patient room, in addition to remote monitoring. Workstations should be placed inside the room to allow for patient charting while in PPE at the bedside. There should also be a nursing station set up nearby with workstations and a display of physiologic monitoring. Ventilator alarms should also be made audible outside the room, either through a baby monitor or through an EMR informatics solution. Hand sanitizer dispensers should be immediately outside each room, as well as a PPE cleaning station and clearly marked waste bins. Full PPE should be readily available, and there should be a "clean" area where processed PPE can be placed in keeping with biocontainment needs.

The use of PACUs as ICU spaces poses particular problems when being used for patients with COVID-19. Although they contain all the infrastructure required to operate critical care devices, they are typically open spaces with beds separated by only a curtain, which is problematic when trying to implement droplet or airborne isolation. One solution has been to cohort patients, all of which have COVID-19, into the open space, maintaining at least 6 feet of separation [392]. However, this method requires all staff within the open area to maintain full PPE at all times. Creative solutions to this problem have been developed, such as building an enclosure for common core areas within which positive pressure is applied so that staff have the ability to continuously monitor patients and perform nondirect clinical care work (e.g. charting) without having to stay in full PPE [392]. Alternatively, barriers around each bed can be constructed with transparent materials, such as plastic or plexiglass, and a HEPA filter is sealed into the barrier with the output vented outside the enclosure to maintain negative flow within each "room" [392, 399].

In some hard-hit areas during the COVID-19 pandemic, the conversion of operating rooms to ICUs was undertaken [399, 403]. Operating rooms have the infrastructure required to house ICU patients, although they have certain limitations. The primary positive feature of the operating room is the ability to use anesthesia machines as ventilators. Operating room beds must be exchanged for a hospital or ICU bed, and workstations may need to be added to the rooms. One particular limitation is that most operating rooms are positive pressured, which makes the performance of aerosol-generating procedures such as intubation problematic. Standard hospital infection-prevention and -control policies recommend that operating room doors remain closed for at least 14–18 minutes after aerosol-generating procedures to allow for the high-particulate air filters to remove most of the particulate air matter [402, 404]. Operating rooms can also be engineered to provide negative pressure, but this typically requires significant alterations to the existing air management systems that can present a significant challenge.

A final option of last resort is the use of open spaces (e.g. auditoriums, cafeterias, tents). Clearly, this is not a step that would be taken unless there was a dire need to create ICU space because it requires the incorporation of infrastructure including sufficient power, gases, wired and wireless communication, data ports, water, and appropriate drainage systems [392]. If these infrastructure challenges are overcome, the layout will be very similar to what was described for using a PACU as an alternative area for critically ill patients.

Physical space is only one consideration in the face of disasters such as the COVID-19 pandemic that generate large numbers of critically ill patients. An equally important challenge is the staffing of these ICU beds with physicians, nurses, respiratory therapist, among other healthcare staff. Truth be told, adequate staffing with a suitably trained workforce was probably the greatest challenge when faced with a surge of critically ill patients. Because all hospitals had similar issues, hiring new or temporary staff was no easy feat as the demand outstripped the supply. Accordingly, alternative staffing models were proposed using a tiered approach where noncritically trained healthcare staff were redeployed to operate as part of a team working together to provide patient care under the direction of a critical-care-trained provider [397].

This tiered strategy sets up pyramids with the most experienced staff at the apex of the triangle and staff with progressively less critical care experience at the base of the pyramid to expand the caretaking capacity [392, 405]. Our institution, like most academic programs, already had these structures in place with an attending and pulmonary and critical care fellow at the top, and with residents, interns, and medical students at the base of the pyramid. However, to meet the demands of a large ICU COVID-19 population that grew our ICU census to four to five times the norm, we develop other pyramids using nonmedical ICU attendings (e.g. anesthesia critical care, neurocritical care), fellows (e.g. cardiology, gastroenterology, etc.), hospitalists, and physician extenders.

This strategy can also be used with nurses, respiratory therapists, pharmacists, or any ICU specialty-trained care staff who may be in short supply. In fact, this tiered strategy for ICU bedside nurses is not a new concept. "Team nursing" staffing model was first described in 1957 by Eleanor C. Lambertsen [406] in her dissertation, "Nursing Team Organization and Functioning," where she outlined a model where nurses would work closer with doctors and support staff to oversee patient care. Adapted to the needs of surge staffing, a structure was created where critical-care-trained nurses supervised non-critical-care nurses, Certified Nursing Assistants, Licensed Practical Nurse, or nurses' aides, thus allowing for expansion of the typical ICU nurse-to-patient ratios. It is recommended that an educational program be developed to serve as a primer in critical care for any non-ICU staff who will be participating in a tiered staffing model [392, 405].

A final consideration in the face of a surging ICU census is the availability of sufficient numbers of traditional ICU ventilators, which may necessitate the use of anesthesia and transport ventilators or conversion of NIPPV systems into ventilators. As less-than-ideal alternatives that lack humidification and have limitations in the ventilatory support, they are used because of the dire situation in the face of an overwhelming surge of critically ill patients.

One obvious resource is anesthesia machines, especially considering the reduced number of surgical cases during the height of the COVID-19 pandemic. Although anesthesia machines are designed to provide ventilatory support, several features make them suboptimal for use in ICU patients. Anesthesia machines allow for rebreathing of exhaled gas through the ventilator circuit and thus increase the risk for ventilator contamination unless a breathing system filter is placed [359]. They also differ in their abilities to deliver consistent tidal volume depending on the model of machine. Normally not approved for use in ICU patients, the FDA, at the onset of the COVID-19 pandemic, granted temporary approval of the use of anesthesia machines for patients who required mechanical ventilation [359]. If used, it should be operated only by experienced anesthesiology staff.

Transport ventilators can also be used for ICU patients when traditional resources have been depleted. Two of the most commonly used transport ventilators are pneumatic models and turbine-driven models [360]. Pneumatic transport ventilators are gas-driven pumps that can provide up to 100% oxygen and a set respiratory rate and tidal volume, and some models can also provide pressure support ventilation. Turbine-driven transport ventilators

require a pressurized gas source of oxygen to reach high FiO_2 values. Both have limitations in terms of the consistency and accuracy of the delivered tidal volumes and pressures when used for prolonged periods. HEPA filtration attachments should be placed on the exhaust port of some models to prevent aerosolization of exhaled secretions.

Certain NIPPV models can also be modified for use as ICU ventilators [407]. NIV with bilevel positive airway pressure capability can deliver a set tidal volume at a set respiratory rate and provide PEEP. Current models also contain oxygen blenders for precise delivery of supplemental oxygen concentrations. Most will require a HEPA filter to be applied to the exhaust port tubing to minimize the risk for aerosolization.

The splitting of ventilators was also described by a group at New York Presbyterian Hospital [408]. Their detailed protocol stressed the importance of matching patients and required the use of pressure-cycled ventilation to avoid deleterious interactions between patients. Ventilator splitting also requires controlled ventilation at a set rate with the patient unable to trigger a breath, again to ensure the safety of both patients. The FDA has issued a letter to healthcare providers detailing the risks inherent to this technique and recommend its use only when there are no other alternatives for invasive ventilation [409].

As a final point, guidelines have been established on the best approach for ICU bed triage in the face of an overwhelming number of patients that outstrips the hospital ICU capacity. A prescient publication released in October 2018 estimated that an influenza pandemic similar to that of 1918 would require ICU and ventilator capacity greater than what was currently available [410]. They described a framework to assist with statewide allocation of resources in such an event that could be used to determine how best to apportion the available ICU beds. This framework was based on a scoring system that took into account the likelihood of a patient's short-term and long-term survival. The scores for each component were added together to produce a triage score that determined the patient priority for ICU bed admission. Since the onset of the COVID-19 pandemic, numerous publications have outlined similar recommendations [397, 400, 411].

Additional Management Considerations

Any patient activities that required presence at the bedside, including laboratory draws, suctioning, patient cleaning, dressing changes, routine airway management, tubing changes, blood draws, routine assessments, and verification of patient identification bracelets should be completed in bundled tasks whenever possible.

One of the more time-consuming responsibilities of the bedside nurse involves IV medication administration and adjustment. PPE must be used with every entry into the room, and IV pump alarms are less detectible through a closed door. In a study from Mt. Sinai Hospital in New York, modifications were made to infusion pumps to place them outside the room to minimize nursing time at the bedside [412]. This allowed nursing staff to titrate continuous infusions and administer IV push and intermittent IV piggyback medications without entering the room. IV infusion pumps were secured on a rolling pole and were moved immediately outside the patient room. Because the tubing extensions add volume to the circuitry of the system, this modification is most appropriate for continuous IV fluid administration and requires priming of greater than 20 ml (depending on the length of tubing) to prevent medication delays through the tubing to the patient's IV site. In addition, a carrier line was attached to the end of the manifold with crystalloid running at a rate of 10–50 ml/hr to assist with infusion delivery. The additional tubing was smaller in caliber causing increased resistance requiring occlusion limits being raised from 300 to 500 mmHg to prevent occlusion-related alarms. Nursing staff must routinely inspect the tubing, insertion sites, connections, and manifold junctures (bihourly is recommended). Two sets of patient identification bracelets are allotted to ensure proper patient identification, with one band placed on the patient's wrist as standard procedure and the other band taped to the inside of the glass door for scanning of medications.

The placement of IV infusion pumps outside the room provides significant benefits: a decrease in exposure of nursing staff, a reduction in the consumption of PPE, and the ability to more immediately hear pump alarms. However, several notable limitations must be considered before initiating this modification. Placing the IV pumps outside the room may not be practical when patients are housed in a very large ward or room because of the significant length of tubing required to reach from the pump to the patient. The use of extension tubing can increase the tubing resistance, which can affect the accuracy of the infusion rate. If multiple patients are housed in one room, space outside the room for all the required pumps may be insufficient and also increase the risk for patient/pump misidentification. There is also a risk for unintentionally dislodging catheters if the tubing is pulled by accident when performing another patient care task. In addition, the administration of medications that are prepared as lipid emulsions may pose an infectious risk with the additional lengths of tubing and require more frequent changes in tubing per manufacturer recommendations and infection-prevention guidelines [412, 413]. Therefore, the decision to place IV pumps outside the room must be individualized to the needs of the unit and considerations for availability of PPE and level of risk to the nursing staff.

The numerous monitoring devices that are part of the core elements of ICU care pose another challenge in patients with COVID-19. Monitors following blood pressure, heart rate, respiratory rate, and pulse oximetry have alarms to alert the medical staff against possible decompensations, which conflicts with infection-control measures in COVID-19 requiring a closed door through which an alarm may not be audible. Moreover, mechanical ventilators often require frequent adjustments, and alarms can be difficult to hear behind closed doors. To compensate for these challenges, some hospitals made adjustments, such as placing baby monitors in the patient room. One group also described a process by which they connected cable extensions to make ventilators' control panel usable outside patients' rooms allowing the anesthesiologists to interpret ventilator waveforms, adjust ventilation settings, ensure lung protective ventilation, and hear alarms while outside the patient room [414, 415]. Another group of clinicians and computer scientists at Johns Hopkins have also been working to develop robotic systems to operate ventilators and other bedside monitors and machines [416]. These innovative technologies offer the promise of a safer work environment for staff caring for patients with COVID-19 and other highly infectious diseases.

References

1 Stokes, E.K., Zambrano, L.D., Anderson, K.N. et al. (2020). Coronavirus disease 2019 case surveillance – United States, January 22-May 30, 2020. *MMWR Morb. Mortal. Wkly Rep.* 69 (24): 759–765.

2 Guan, W.J., Ni, Z.Y., Hu, Y. et al. (2020). Clinical characteristics of coronavirus disease 2019 in China. *N. Engl. J. Med.* 382 (18): 1708–1720.

3 Gaeckle, N.T., Lee, J., Park, Y. et al. (2020). Aerosol generation from the respiratory tract with various modes of oxygen delivery. *Am. J. Respir. Crit. Care Med.* 202 (8): 1115–1124.

4 COVID-19 Treatment Guidelines Panel. (2021). Coronavirus disease 2019 (COVID-19) treatment guidelines. National Institutes of Health. http://www.covid19treatmentguidelines.nih.gov. (accessed 22 April 2021).

5 Bateman, N.T. and Leach, R.M. (1998). ABC of oxygen. Acute oxygen therapy. *BMJ* 317 (7161): 798–801.

6 Farias, E. (1991). Delivery of high inspired oxygen by face mask. *J. Crit. Care* 6 (3): 119–124.

7 Hui, D.S., Chan, M.T., and Chow, B. (2014). Aerosol dispersion during various respiratory therapies: a risk assessment model of nosocomial infection to health care workers. *Hong Kong Med. J.* 20 (Suppl 4): 9–13.

8 Yamaguti, W.P., Moderno, E.V., Yamashita, S.Y. et al. (2014). Treatment-related risk factors for development of skin breakdown in subjects with acute respiratory failure undergoing noninvasive ventilation or CPAP. *Respir. Care* 59 (10): 1530–1536.

9 Spoletini, G., Alotaibi, M., Blasi, F., and Hill, N.S. (2015). Heated humidified high-flow nasal oxygen in adults: mechanisms of action and clinical implications. *Chest* 148 (1): 253–261.

10 Sharma, S., Danckers, M., Sanghavi, D., and Chakraborty, R.K. (2021). *High Flow Nasal Cannula*. Treasure Island, FL: StatPearls.

11 Moller, W., Feng, S., Domanski, U. et al. (2017). Nasal high flow reduces dead space. *J. Appl. Physiol.* 122 (1): 191–197.

12 Hui, D.S., Chow, B.K., Lo, T. et al. (2019). Exhaled air dispersion during high-flow nasal cannula therapy versus CPAP via different masks. *Eur. Respir. J.* 53 (4): 1802339.

13 Hasani, A., Chapman, T.H., McCool, D. et al. (2008). Domiciliary humidification improves lung mucociliary clearance in patients with bronchiectasis. *Chron. Respir. Dis.* 5 (2): 81–86.

14 Kilgour, E., Rankin, N., Ryan, S., and Pack, R. (2004). Mucociliary function deteriorates in the clinical range of inspired air temperature and humidity. *Intensive Care Med.* 30 (7): 1491–1494.

15 Demoule, A., Vieillard Baron, A., Darmon, M. et al. (2020). High-flow nasal cannula in critically Ill patients with severe COVID-19. *Am. J. Respir. Crit. Care Med.* 202 (7): 1039–1042.

16 Bonnet, N., Martin, O., Boubaya, M. et al. (2021). High flow nasal oxygen therapy to avoid invasive mechanical ventilation in SARS-CoV-2 pneumonia: a retrospective study. *Ann. Intensive Care* 11 (1): 37.

17 Arabi, Y.M., Arifi, A.A., Balkhy, H.H. et al. (2014). Clinical course and outcomes of critically ill patients with Middle East respiratory syndrome coronavirus infection. *Ann. Intern. Med.* 160 (6): 389–397.

18 X-q, L., S-b, C., He, G.-q. et al. (2003). Management of critical severe acute respiratory syndrome and risk factors for death. *Zhonghua Jie He He Hu Xi Za Zhi* 26 (6): 329–333.

19 Han, F., Jiang, Y.Y., Zheng, J.H. et al. (2004). Noninvasive positive pressure ventilation treatment for acute respiratory failure in SARS. *Sleep Breath.* 8 (2): 97–106.

20 World Health Organization. (2000). Clinical management of COVID-19: interim guidance, 27 May 2020. World Health Organization. https://apps.who.int/iris/handle/10665/332196 (accessed 10 April 2021).

21 Grieco, D.L., Menga, L.S., Cesarano, M. et al. (2021). Effect of helmet noninvasive ventilation vs high-flow nasal oxygen on days free of respiratory support in patients with COVID-19 and moderate to severe hypoxemic respiratory failure: the HENIVOT randomized clinical trial. *JAMA* 325 (17): 1731–1743.

22 Frat, J.P., Thille, A.W., Mercat, A. et al. (2015). High-flow oxygen through nasal cannula in acute hypoxemic respiratory failure. *N. Engl. J. Med.* 372 (23): 2185–2196.

23 Ni, Y.N., Luo, J., Yu, H. et al. (2018). The effect of high-flow nasal cannula in reducing the mortality and the rate of endotracheal intubation when used before mechanical ventilation compared with conventional oxygen therapy and noninvasive positive pressure ventilation. A systematic review and meta-analysis. *Am. J. Emerg. Med.* 36 (2): 226–233.

24 Alhazzani, W., Evans, L., Alshamsi, F. et al. (2021). Surviving sepsis campaign guidelines on the management of adults with coronavirus disease 2019 (COVID-19) in the ICU: first update. *Crit. Care Med.* 49 (3): e219–e234.

25 Dobler, C.C., Murad, M.H., and Wilson, M.E. (2020). Noninvasive positive pressure ventilation in patients with COVID-19. *Mayo Clin. Proc.* 95 (12): 2594–2601.

26 Rochwerg, B., Brochard, L., Elliott, M.W. et al. (2017). Official ERS/ATS clinical practice guidelines: noninvasive ventilation for acute respiratory failure. *Eur. Respir. J.* 50 (2): 1602426.

27 Brochard, L., Mancebo, J., Wysocki, M. et al. (1995). Noninvasive ventilation for acute exacerbations of chronic obstructive pulmonary disease. *N. Engl. J. Med.* 333 (13): 817–822.

28 Faraone, A., Beltrame, C., Crociani, A. et al. (2020). Effectiveness and safety of noninvasive positive pressure ventilation in the treatment of COVID-19-associated acute hypoxemic respiratory failure: a single center, non-ICU setting experience. *Intern. Emerg. Med.* https://doi.org/10.1007/ s11739-020-02562-2.

29 Scaravilli, V., Grasselli, G., Castagna, L. et al. (2015). Prone positioning improves oxygenation in spontaneously breathing nonintubated patients with hypoxemic acute respiratory failure: a retrospective study. *J. Crit. Care* 30 (6): 1390–1394.

30 Caputo, N.D., Strayer, R.J., and Levitan, R. (2020). Early self-proning in awake, non-intubated patients in the emergency department: a single ED's experience during the COVID-19 pandemic. *Acad. Emerg. Med.* 27 (5): 375–378.

31 Coppo, A., Bellani, G., Winterton, D. et al. (2020). Feasibility and physiological effects of prone positioning in non-intubated patients with acute respiratory failure due to COVID-19 (PRON-COVID): a prospective cohort study. *Lancet Respir. Med.* 8 (8): 765–774.

32 Ferrando, C., Mellado-Artigas, R., Gea, A. et al. (2020). Awake prone positioning does not reduce the risk of intubation in COVID-19 treated with high-flow nasal oxygen therapy: a multicenter, adjusted cohort study. *Crit. Care* 24 (1): 597.

33 Society for Maternal Fetal Medicine. (2020). Management considerations for pregnant patients with COVID-19. https://s3.amazonaws.com/cdn. smfm.org/media/2336/SMFM_COVID_ Management_of_COVID_pos_preg_patients_4-30-20_final.pdf. (accessed 14 April 2021).

34 Hashmi, M.D., Alnababteh, M., Vedantam, K. et al. (2020). Assessing the need for transfer to the intensive care unit for coronavirus-19 disease: epidemiology and risk factors. *Respir. Med.* 174: 106203.

35 Rola, P., Farkas, J., Spiegel, R. et al. (2020). Rethinking the early intubation paradigm of COVID-19: time to change gears? *Clin. Exp. Emerg. Med.* 7 (2): 78–80.

36 Matta, A., Chaudhary, S., Bryan Lo, K. et al. (2020). Timing of intubation and its implications on outcomes in critically ill patients with coronavirus disease 2019 infection. *Crit. Care Explor.* 2 (10): e0262.

37 Zuo, M.Z., Huang, Y.G., Ma, W.H. et al. (2020). Expert recommendations for tracheal intubation in critically ill patients with noval coronavirus disease 2019. *Chin. Med. Sci. J.* 35 (2): 105–109.

38 De Jong, A., Rolle, A., Molinari, N. et al. (2018). Cardiac arrest and mortality related to intubation procedure in critically ill adult patients: a multicenter cohort study. *Crit. Care Med.* 46 (4): 532–539.

39 Cook, T.M., El-Boghdadly, K., McGuire, B. et al. (2020). Consensus guidelines for managing the airway in patients with COVID-19: guidelines from the difficult airway society, the Association of Anaesthetists the Intensive Care Society, the Faculty of Intensive Care Medicine and the Royal College of Anaesthetists. *Anaesthesia* 75 (6): 785–799.

40 Caputo, K.M., Byrick, R., Chapman, M.G. et al. (2006). Intubation of SARS patients: infection and perspectives of healthcare workers. *Can. J. Anaesth.* 53 (2): 122–129.

41 American Society of Anesthesiologists Committee on Occupational Health. (2021). Coronavirus information for health care professionals (clinical FAQs). https://www.asahq.org/about-asa/

governance-and-committees/asa-committees/ committee-on-occupational-health/coronavirus/ clinical-faqs (accessed 20 April 2021).

42 Lynch, J.B., Davitkov, P., Anderson, D.J., et al. (2020). Infectious Disease Society of America Guidelines on infection prevention in patients with suspected or known COVID-19. Version 1.0.1. Infectious Disease Society of America. https://www.idsociety.org/ practice-guideline/covid-19-guideline-infection-prevention (accessed 14 April 2021).

43 Wang, X., Pan, Z., and Cheng, Z. (2020). Association between 2019-nCoV transmission and N95 respirator use. *J. Hosp. Infect.* 105: 104–105.

44 Offeddu, V., Yung, C.F., Low, M.S.F., and Tam, C.C. (2017). Effectiveness of masks and respirators against respiratory infections in healthcare workers: a systematic review and meta-analysis. *Clin. Infect. Dis.* 65 (11): 1934–1942.

45 Bartoszko, J.J., Farooqi, M.A.M., Alhazzani, W., and Loeb, M. (2020). Medical masks vs N95 respirators for preventing COVID-19 in healthcare workers: a systematic review and meta-analysis of randomized trials. *Influenza Other Respi. Viruses* 14 (4): 365–373.

46 Yam, L.Y., Chen, R.C., and Zhong, N.S. (2003). SARS: ventilatory and intensive care. *Respirology* 8 (Suppl)): S31–S35.

47 Twu, S.J., Chen, T.J., Chen, C.J. et al. (2003). Control measures for severe acute respiratory syndrome (SARS) in Taiwan. *Emerg. Infect. Dis.* 9 (6): 718–720.

48 Kwon, J.H., Burnham, C.D., Reske, K.A. et al. (2017). Assessment of healthcare worker protocol deviations and self-contamination during personal protective equipment donning and doffing. *Infect. Control Hosp. Epidemiol.* 38 (9): 1077–1083.

49 Christopherson, D.A., Yao, W.C., Lu, M. et al. (2020). High-efficiency particulate air filters in the era of COVID-19: function and efficacy. *Otolaryngol. Head Neck Surg.* 163 (6): 1153–1155.

50 Orser, B.A. (2020). Recommendations for endotracheal intubation of COVID-19 patients. *Anesth. Analg.* 130 (5): 1109–1110.

51 Shrestha, G.S., Shrestha, N., Lamsal, R. et al. (2021). Emergency intubation in Covid-19. *N. Engl. J. Med.* 384 (7): e20.

52 Tran, K., Cimon, K., Severn, M. et al. (2012). Aerosol generating procedures and risk of transmission of acute respiratory infections to healthcare workers: a systematic review. *PLoS One* 7 (4): e35797.

53 Oliveira, J.E.S.L., Cabrera, D., Barrionuevo, P. et al. (2017). Effectiveness of apneic oxygenation during intubation: a systematic review and meta-analysis. *Ann. Emerg. Med.* 70 (4): 483–494. e11.

54 Lascarrou, J.B., Boisrame-Helms, J., Bailly, A. et al. (2017). Video laryngoscopy vs direct laryngoscopy on successful first-pass orotracheal intubation among ICU patients: a randomized clinical trial. *JAMA* 317 (5): 483–493.

55 Bhattacharjee, S., Maitra, S., and Baidya, D.K. (2018). A comparison between video laryngoscopy and direct laryngoscopy for endotracheal intubation in the emergency department: a meta-analysis of randomized controlled trials. *J. Clin. Anesth.* 47: 21–26.

56 Brown, C.A. 3rd, Kaji, A.H., Fantegrossi, A. et al. (2020). Video laryngoscopy compared to augmented direct laryngoscopy in adult emergency department tracheal intubations: a National Emergency Airway Registry (NEAR) study. *Acad. Emerg. Med.* 27 (2): 100–108.

57 Sullivan, E.H., Gibson, L.E., Berra, L. et al. (2020). In-hospital airway management of COVID-19 patients. *Crit. Care* 24 (1): 292.

58 Richardson, S., Hirsch, J.S., Narasimhan, M. et al. (2020). Presenting characteristics, comorbidities, and outcomes among 5700 patients hospitalized with COVID-19 in the New York City area. *JAMA* 323 (20): 2052–2059.

59 Cummings, M.J., Baldwin, M.R., Abrams, D. et al. (2020). Epidemiology, clinical course, and outcomes of critically ill adults with COVID-19 in New York City: a prospective cohort study. *Lancet* 395 (10239): 1763–1770.

60 Price-Haywood, E.G., Burton, J., Fort, D., and Seoane, L. (2020). Hospitalization and mortality among black patients and white patients with Covid-19. *N. Engl. J. Med.* 382 (26): 2534–2543.

61 Gattinoni, L., Chiumello, D., Caironi, P. et al. (2020). COVID-19 pneumonia: different respiratory treatments for different phenotypes? *Intensive Care Med.* 46 (6): 1099–1102.

62 Fan, E., Beitler, J.R., Brochard, L. et al. (2020). COVID-19-associated acute respiratory distress syndrome: is a different approach to management warranted? *Lancet Respir. Med.* 8 (8): 816–821.

63 Ziehr, D.R., Alladina, J., Petri, C.R. et al. (2020). Respiratory pathophysiology of mechanically ventilated patients with COVID-19: a cohort study. *Am. J. Respir. Crit. Care Med.* 201 (12): 1560–1564.

64 Acute Respiratory Distress Syndrome Network, Brower, R.G., Matthay, M.A. et al. (2000). Ventilation with lower tidal volumes as compared with traditional tidal volumes for acute lung injury and the acute respiratory distress syndrome. *N. Engl. J. Med.* 342 (18): 1301–1308.

65 Siemieniuk, R.A.C., Chu, D.K., Kim, L.H.-Y. et al. (2018). Oxygen therapy for acutely ill medical patients: a clinical practice guideline. *BMJ* 363: k4169.

66 ARDSNet. (2021). NIH NHLBI ARDS clinical network mechanical ventilation protocol summary. http://www.ardsnet.org/files/ventilator_protocol_2008-07.pdf (accessed 26 April 2021).

67 Kondili, E., Prinianakis, G., and Georgopoulos, D. (2003). Patient-ventilator interaction. *Br. J. Anaesth.* 91 (1): 106–119.

68 Slutsky, A.S. and Ranieri, V.M. (2013). Ventilator-induced lung injury. *N. Engl. J. Med.* 369 (22): 2126–2136.

69 Gaver, D.P. 3rd, Nieman, G.F., Gatto, L.A. et al. (2020). The POOR get POORer: a hypothesis for the pathogenesis of ventilator-induced lung injury. *Am. J. Respir. Crit. Care Med.* 202 (8): 1081–1087.

70 Brower, R.G., Lanken, P.N., MacIntyre, N. et al. (2004). Higher versus lower positive end-expiratory pressures in patients with the acute respiratory distress syndrome. *N. Engl. J. Med.* 351 (4): 327–336.

71 Thompson, B.T., Chambers, R.C., and Liu, K.D. (2017). Acute respiratory distress syndrome. *N. Engl. J. Med.* 377 (19): 1904–1905.

72 Sweeney, R.M. and McAuley, D.F. (2016). Acute respiratory distress syndrome. *Lancet* 388 (10058): 2416–2430.

73 Ware, L.B. and Matthay, M.A. (2001). Alveolar fluid clearance is impaired in the majority of patients with acute lung injury and the acute respiratory distress syndrome. *Am. J. Respir. Crit. Care Med.* 163 (6): 1376–1383.

74 Lee, W.L. and Slutsky, A.S. (2016). *Murray and Nadel's Textbook of Respiratory Medicine*. Philadelphia, PA: Elsevier Saunders.

75 National Heart, Lung, and Blood Institute Acute Respiratory Distress Syndrome (ARDS) Clinical Trials Network, Wiedemann, H.P., Wheeler, A.P. et al. (2006). Comparison of two fluid-management strategies in acute lung injury. *N. Engl. J. Med.* 354 (24): 2564–2575.

76 Dellinger, R.P., Levy, M.M., Rhodes, A. et al. (2013). Surviving sepsis campaign: international guidelines for management of severe sepsis and septic shock: 2012. *Crit. Care Med.* 41 (2): 580–637.

77 Galiatsou, E., Kostanti, E., Svarna, E. et al. (2006). Prone position augments recruitment and prevents alveolar overinflation in acute lung injury. *Am. J. Respir. Crit. Care Med.* 174 (2): 187–197.

78 Mackenzie, C.F. (2001). Anatomy, physiology, and pathology of the prone position and postural drainage. *Crit. Care Med.* 29 (5): 1084–1085.

79 Guerin, C., Reignier, J., Richard, J.C. et al. (2013). Prone positioning in severe acute respiratory distress syndrome. *N. Engl. J. Med.* 368 (23): 2159–2168.

80 Murray, M.J., Cowen, J., DeBlock, H. et al. (2002). Clinical practice guidelines for sustained neuromuscular blockade in the adult critically ill patient. *Crit. Care Med.* 30 (1): 142–156.

81 Papazian, L., Forel, J.-M., Gacouin, A. et al. (2010). Neuromuscular blockers in early acute respiratory distress syndrome. *N. Engl. J. Med.* 363 (12): 1107–1116.

82 Devlin, J.W. and Pandharipande, P.P. (2018). Light sedation is the goal: making the evidence heavier. *Crit. Care Med.* 46 (6): 1003–1004.

83 National Heart, Lung, and Blood Institute PETAL Clinical Trials Network, Moss, M., Huang, D.T. et al. (2019). Early neuromuscular blockade in the acute respiratory distress syndrome. *N. Engl. J. Med.* 380 (21): 1997–2008.

84 Gattinoni, L., D'Andrea, L., Pelosi, P. et al. (1993). Regional effects and mechanism of positive end-expiratory pressure in early adult respiratory distress syndrome. *JAMA* 269 (16): 2122–2127.

85 Gattinoni, L., Pelosi, P., Crotti, S., and Valenza, F. (1995). Effects of positive end-expiratory pressure on regional distribution of tidal volume and recruitment in adult respiratory distress syndrome. *Am. J. Respir. Crit. Care Med.* 151 (6): 1807–1814.

86 Gattinoni, L., Pesenti, A., Avalli, L. et al. (1987). Pressure-volume curve of total respiratory system in acute respiratory failure. Computed

tomographic scan study. *Am. Rev. Respir. Dis.* 136 (3): 730–736.

87 Goligher, E.C., Hodgson, C.L., Adhikari, N.K.J. et al. (2017). Lung recruitment maneuvers for adult patients with acute respiratory distress syndrome. A systematic review and meta-analysis. *Ann. Am. Thorac. Soc.* 14 (Suppl 4): S304–S311.

88 Writing Group for the Alveolar Recruitment for Acute Respiratory Distress Syndrome Trial (ART) Investigators (2017). Effect of lung recruitment and titrated positive end-expiratory pressure (PEEP) vs low PEEP on mortality in patients with acute respiratory distress syndrome: a randomized clinical trial. *JAMA* 318 (14): 1335–1345.

89 Ichinose, F., Roberts, J.D. Jr., and Zapol, W.M. (2004). Inhaled nitric oxide: a selective pulmonary vasodilator: current uses and therapeutic potential. *Circulation* 109 (25): 3106–3111.

90 Griffiths, M.J. and Evans, T.W. (2005). Inhaled nitric oxide therapy in adults. *N. Engl. J. Med.* 353 (25): 2683–2695.

91 Dellinger, R.P., Zimmerman, J.L., Taylor, R.W. et al. (1998). Effects of inhaled nitric oxide in patients with acute respiratory distress syndrome: results of a randomized phase II trial. Inhaled nitric oxide in ARDS study group. *Crit. Care Med.* 26 (1): 15–23.

92 Taylor, R.W., Zimmerman, J.L., Dellinger, R.P. et al. (2004). Low-dose inhaled nitric oxide in patients with acute lung injury: a randomized controlled trial. *JAMA* 291 (13): 1603–1609.

93 Lundin, S., Mang, H., Smithies, M. et al. (1999). Inhalation of nitric oxide in acute lung injury: results of a European multicentre study. The European Study Group of Inhaled Nitric Oxide. *Intensive Care Med.* 25 (9): 911–919.

94 Vuylsteke, A., Brodie, D., Combes, A. et al. (2017). *ECMO in the Adult Patient (Core Critical Care)*. Cambridge, UK: Cambridge University Press.

95 Peek, G.J., Mugford, M., Tiruvoipati, R. et al. (2009). Efficacy and economic assessment of conventional ventilatory support versus extracorporeal membrane oxygenation for severe adult respiratory failure (CESAR): a multicentre randomised controlled trial. *Lancet* 374 (9698): 1351–1363.

96 Combes, A., Hajage, D., Capellier, G. et al. (2018). Extracorporeal membrane oxygenation for severe acute respiratory distress syndrome. *N. Engl. J. Med.* 378 (21): 1965–1975.

97 Rajagopal, K., Keller, S.P., Akkanti, B. et al. (2020). Advanced pulmonary and cardiac support of COVID-19 patients: emerging recommendations from ASAIO-A "living working document". *ASAIO J.* 66 (6): 588–598.

98 Daniela, M., Felipe, S., Van Nicolette, S.J. et al. (2021). Mobile ECMO in COVID-19 patient: case report. *J. Artif. Organs* 24 (2): 287–292.

99 Badulak, J., Antonini, M.V., Stead, C.M. et al. (2021). Extracorporeal Membrane Oxygenation for COVID-19: updated 2021 guidelines from the extracorporeal life support organization. *ASAIO J.* 67 (5): 485–495.

100 Huang, C., Wang, Y., Li, X. et al. (2020). Clinical features of patients infected with 2019 novel coronavirus in Wuhan, China. *Lancet* 395 (10223): 497–506.

101 Moore, J.B.J. and Carl, H. (2020). Cytokine release syndrome in severe COVID-19. *Science* 368 (6490): 473–474.

102 Ruan, Q., Yang, K., Wang, W. et al. (2020). Clinical predictors of mortality due to COVID-19 based on an analysis of data of 150 patients from Wuhan, China. *Intensive Care Med.* 46 (5): 846–848.

103 Yao, C., Bora, S.A., Parimon, T. et al. (2021). Cell-type-specific immune dysregulation in severely ill COVID-19 patients. *Cell Rep.* 34 (1): 108590.

104 US Food and Drug Administration. (2021). Remdesivir (Veklury) approval for the treatment of COVID-19 - the evidence for safety and efficacy. http://fda.gov/drugs/news-evets-human-drugs/ remdesivir-veklury-approval-treatment-covid-19- evidence-safety-and-efficacy (accessed 29 April 2021).

105 Gordon, C.J., Tchesnokov, E.P., Woolner, E. et al. (2020). Remdesivir is a direct-acting antiviral that inhibits RNA-dependent RNA polymerase from severe acute respiratory syndrome coronavirus 2 with high potency. *J. Biol. Chem.* 295 (20): 6785–6797.

106 Sheahan, T.P., Sims, A.C., Graham, R.L. et al. (2017). Broad-spectrum antiviral GS-5734 inhibits both epidemic and zoonotic coronaviruses. *Sci. Transl. Med.* 9 (396): eaal3653.

107 Agostini, M.L., Andres, E.L., Sims, A.C. et al. (2018). Coronavirus susceptibility to the antiviral remdesivir (GS-5734) is mediated by the viral polymerase and the proofreading exoribonuclease. *MBio* 9 (2).

108 Brown, A.J., Won, J.J., Graham, R.L. et al. (2019). Broad spectrum antiviral remdesivir inhibits human endemic and zoonotic deltacoronaviruses with a highly divergent RNA dependent RNA polymerase. *Antiviral Res.* 169: 104541.

109 Sheahan, T.P., Sims, A.C., Leist, S.R. et al. (2020). Comparative therapeutic efficacy of remdesivir and combination lopinavir, ritonavir, and interferon beta against MERS-CoV. *Nat. Commun.* 11 (1): 222.

110 Williamson, B.N., Feldmann, F., Schwarz, B. et al. (2020). Clinical benefit of remdesivir in rhesus macaques infected with SARS-CoV-2. *Nature* 585 (7824): 273–276.

111 Beigel, J.H., Tomashek, K.M., Dodd, L.E. et al. (2020). Remdesivir for the treatment of Covid-19 – final report. *N. Engl. J. Med.* 383 (19): 1813–1826.

112 Spinner, C.D., Gottlieb, R.L., Criner, G.J. et al. (2020). Effect of remdesivir vs standard care on clinical status at 11 days in patients with moderate COVID-19: a randomized clinical trial. *JAMA* 324 (11): 1048–1057.

113 Goldman, J.D., Lye, D.C.B., Hui, D.S. et al. (2020). Remdesivir for 5 or 10 days in patients with severe Covid-19. *N. Engl. J. Med.* 383 (19): 1827–1837.

114 Wang, Y., Zhang, D., Du, G. et al. (2020). Remdesivir in adults with severe COVID-19: a randomised, double-blind, placebo-controlled, multicentre trial. *Lancet* 395 (10236): 1569–1578.

115 WHO Solidarity Trial Consortium, Pan, H., Peto, R. et al. (2021). Repurposed antiviral drugs for Covid-19 – interim WHO solidarity trial results. *N. Engl. J. Med.* 384 (6): 497–511.

116 Bhimraj, A.M., Morgan, R., Shumaker, A.H., et al. (2021). Infectious Diseases Society of America guidelines on the treatment and management of patients with COVID-19. Version 4.4.1. Infectious Diseases Society of America. https://www.idsociety.org/practice-guideline/covid-19-guideline-treatment-and-management/.

117 World Health Organization. (2021). WHO recommends against the use of remdesivir in COVID-19 patients. https://www.who.int/news-room/feature-stories/detail/who-recommends-against-the-use-of-remdesivir-in-covid-19-patients (accessed 29 April 2021).

118 Casadevall, A.S. and Matthew, D. (1995). Return to the past: the case for antibody-based therapies in infectious diseases. *Clin. Infect. Dis.* 21: 150–161.

119 Duan, K., Liu, B., Li, C. et al. (2020). Effectiveness of convalescent plasma therapy in severe COVID-19 patients. *Proc. Natl. Acad. Sci. U. S. A.* 117 (17): 9490–9496.

120 Salazar, E., Perez, K.K., Ashraf, M. et al. (2020). Treatment of coronavirus disease 2019 (COVID-19) patients with convalescent plasma. *Am. J. Pathol.* 190 (8): 1680–1690.

121 Abolghasemi, H., Eshghi, P., Cheraghali, A.M. et al. (2020). Clinical efficacy of convalescent plasma for treatment of COVID-19 infections: results of a multicenter clinical study. *Transfus. Apher. Sci.* 59 (5): 102875.

122 Joyner, M.J., Carter, R.E., Senefeld, J.W. et al. (2021). Convalescent plasma antibody levels and the risk of death from Covid-19. *N. Engl. J. Med.* 384 (11): 1015–1027.

123 Salazar, E., Christensen, P.A., Graviss, E.A. et al. (2021). Significantly decreased mortality in a large cohort of coronavirus disease 2019 (COVID-19) patients transfused early with convalescent plasma containing high-titer anti-severe acute respiratory syndrome coronavirus 2 (SARS-CoV-2) spike protein IgG. *Am. J. Pathol.* 191 (1): 90–107.

124 Shenoy, A.G., Hettinger, A.Z., Fernandez, S.J. et al. (2021). Early mortality benefit with COVID-19 convalescent plasma: a matched control study. *Br. J. Haematol.* 192 (4): 706–713.

125 Simonovich, V.A., Burgos Pratx, L.D., Scibona, P. et al. (2021). A randomized trial of convalescent plasma in Covid-19 severe pneumonia. *N. Engl. J. Med.* 384 (7): 619–629.

126 Agarwal, A., Mukherjee, A., Kumar, G. et al. (2020). Convalescent plasma in the management of moderate covid-19 in adults in India: open label phase II multicentre randomised controlled trial (PLACID trial). *BMJ* 371: m3939.

127 Li, L., Zhang, W., Hu, Y. et al. (2020). Effect of convalescent plasma therapy on time to clinical improvement in patients with severe and life-threatening COVID-19: a randomized clinical trial. *JAMA* 324 (5): 460–470.

128 Balcells, M.E., Rojas, L., Le Corre, N. et al. (2021). Early versus deferred anti-SARS-CoV-2 convalescent plasma in patients admitted for COVID-19: a randomized phase II clinical trial. *PLoS Med.* 18 (3): e1003415.

129 Libster, R., Perez Marc, G., Wappner, D. et al. (2021). Early high-titer plasma therapy to prevent severe Covid-19 in older adults. *N. Engl. J. Med.* 384 (7): 610–618.

130 Salazar, E., Kuchipudi, S.V., Christensen, P.A. et al. (2020). Convalescent plasma anti-SARS-CoV-2 spike protein ectodomain and receptor-binding domain IgG correlate with virus neutralization. *J. Clin. Invest.* 130 (12): 6728–6738.

131 Santiago, L., Uranga-Murillo, I., Arias, M. et al. (2021). Determination of the concentration of IgG against the spike receptor-binding domain that predicts the viral neutralizing activity of convalescent plasma and serum against SARS-CoV-2. *Biology (Basel)* 10 (3): 208.

132 Klein, S.L., Pekosz, A., Park, H.S. et al. (2020). Sex, age, and hospitalization drive antibody responses in a COVID-19 convalescent plasma donor population. *J. Clin. Invest.* 130 (11): 6141–6150.

133 Joyner, M.J., Bruno, K.A., Klassen, S.A. et al. (2020). Safety update: COVID-19 convalescent plasma in 20,000 hospitalized patients. *Mayo Clin. Proc.* 95 (9): 1888–1897.

134 Joyner, M.J., Wright, R.S., Fairweather, D. et al. (2020). Early safety indicators of COVID-19 convalescent plasma in 5000 patients. *J. Clin. Invest.* 130 (9): 4791–4797.

135 Bray, M., Rayner, C., Noel, F. et al. (2020). Ivermectin and COVID-19: a report in antiviral research, widespread interest, an FDA warning, two letters to the editor and the authors' responses. *Antiviral Res.* 178: 104805.

136 Caly, L., Druce, J.D., Catton, M.G. et al. (2020). The FDA-approved drug ivermectin inhibits the replication of SARS-CoV-2 in vitro. *Antiviral Res.* 178: 104787.

137 Khan, M.S.I., Khan, M.S.I., Debnath, C.R. et al. (2020). Ivermectin treatment may improve the prognosis of patients with COVID-19. *Arch. Bronconeumol.* 56 (12): 828–830.

138 Rajter, J.C., Sherman, M.S., Fatteh, N. et al. (2021). Use of ivermectin is associated with lower mortality in hospitalized patients with coronavirus disease 2019: the Ivermectin in COVID Nineteen Study. *Chest* 159 (1): 85–92.

139 Galan, L.E.B., Santos, N.M.D., Asato, M.S. et al. (2021). Phase 2 randomized study on chloroquine, hydroxychloroquine or ivermectin in hospitalized patients with severe manifestations of SARS-CoV-2 infection. *Pathog. Global Health* 115: 235–242.

140 Ahmed, S., Karim, M.M., Ross, A.G. et al. (2021). A five-day course of ivermectin for the treatment of COVID-19 may reduce the duration of illness. *Int. J. Infect. Dis.* 103: 214–216.

141 Podder, C.S., Nandini, C., Ibne Sina, M. et al. (2020). Outcome of ivermectin treated mild to moderate COVID-19 cases: a single-centre, open-label, randomised study. *IMC J. Med. Sci.* 14 (2): 2. https://doi.org/10.3329/imcjms.v14i2.52826.

142 Zeeshan Khan Chachar, A., Ahmad Khan, K., Asif, M. et al. (2020). Effectiveness of Ivermectin in SARS-CoV-2/COVID-19 patients. *Int. J. Sci.* 9 (9): 31–35.

143 RECOVERY Collaborative Group, Horby, P., Lim, W.S. et al. (2021). Dexamethasone in hospitalized patients with Covid-19. *N. Engl. J. Med.* 384 (8): 693–704.

144 Tomazini, B.M., Maia, I.S., Cavalcanti, A.B. et al. (2020). Effect of dexamethasone on days alive and ventilator-free in patients with moderate or severe acute respiratory distress syndrome and COVID-19: the CoDEX randomized clinical trial. *JAMA* 324 (13): 1307–1316.

145 Villar, J., Ferrando, C., Martínez, D. et al. (2020). Dexamethasone treatment for the acute respiratory distress syndrome: a multicentre, randomised controlled trial. *Lancet Respir. Med.* 8 (3): 267–276.

146 Angus, D.C., Derde, L., Al-Beidh, F. et al. (2020). Effect of hydrocortisone on mortality and organ support in patients with severe COVID-19: the REMAP-CAP COVID-19 corticosteroid domain randomized clinical trial. *JAMA* 324 (13): 1317–1329.

147 Dequin, P.F., Heming, N., Meziani, F. et al. (2020). Effect of hydrocortisone on 21-day mortality or respiratory support among critically ill patients with COVID-19: a randomized clinical trial. *JAMA* 324 (13): 1298–1306.

148 Edalatifard, M., Akhtari, M., Salehi, M. et al. (2020). Intravenous methylprednisolone pulse as a treatment for hospitalised severe COVID-19 patients: results from a randomised controlled clinical trial. *Eur. Respir. J.* 56 (6): 2002808.

149 Tang, X., Feng, Y.M., Ni, J.X. et al. (2021). Early use of corticosteroid may prolong SARS-CoV-2 shedding in non-intensive care unit patients with COVID-19 pneumonia: a multicenter, single-blind, randomized control trial. *Respiration* 100 (2): 116–126.

150 Jeronimo, C.M.P., Farias, M.E.L., Val, F.F.A. et al. (2021). Methylprednisolone as adjunctive therapy for patients hospitalized with coronavirus disease 2019 (COVID-19; Metcovid): a randomized, double-blind, phase IIb, placebo-controlled trial. *Clin. Infect. Dis.* 72: e373–e381.

151 Cantini, F., Niccoli, L., Nannini, C. et al. (2020). Beneficial impact of Baricitinib in COVID-19 moderate pneumonia; multicentre study. *J. Infect.* 81 (4): 647–679.

152 Stebbing, J., Krishnan, V., de Bono, S. et al. (2020). Mechanism of baricitinib supports artificial intelligence-predicted testing in COVID-19 patients. *EMBO Mol. Med.* 12 (8): e12697.

153 Rodriguez-Garcia, J.L., Sanchez-Nievas, G., Arevalo-Serrano, J. et al. (2021). Baricitinib improves respiratory function in patients treated with corticosteroids for SARS-CoV-2 pneumonia: an observational cohort study. *Rheumatology* 60 (1): 399–407.

154 Titanji, B.K., Farley, M.M., Mehta, A. et al. (2021). Use of Baricitinib in patients with moderate to severe coronavirus disease 2019. *Clin. Infect. Dis.* 72 (7): 1247–1250.

155 Kalil, A.C., Patterson, T.F., Mehta, A.K. et al. (2021). Baricitinib plus remdesivir for hospitalized adults with Covid-19. *N. Engl. J. Med.* 384 (9): 795–807.

156 National Institute of Allergy and Infectious Diseases (NIAID). (2021). Adaptive COVID-19 Treatment Trial 4 (ACTT-4). ClinicalTrials.gov. https://clinicaltrials.gov/ct2/show/NCT04640168 (accessed 29 April 2021).

157 Marconi, V.C., Ramanan, A.V., de Bono, S. et al. (2021). Efficacy and safety of baricitinib in patients with COVID-19 infection: results from the randomised, double-blind, placebo-controlled, parallel-group COV-BARRIER phase 3 trial. *medRxiv* https://doi.org/10.1101/2021.04.30.21255934.

158 Chen, G., Wu, D., Guo, W. et al. (2020). Clinical and immunological features of severe and moderate coronavirus disease 2019. *J. Clin. Invest.* 130 (5): 2620–2629.

159 Singh, J.A., Beg, S., and Lopez-Olivo, M.A. (2011). Tocilizumab for rheumatoid arthritis: a cochrane systematic review. *J. Rheumatol.* 38 (1): 10–20.

160 Khanna, D., Denton, C.P., Lin, C.J.F. et al. (2018). Safety and efficacy of subcutaneous tocilizumab in systemic sclerosis: results from the open-label period of a phase II randomised controlled trial (faSScinate). *Ann. Rheum. Dis.* 77 (2): 212–220.

161 Le, R.Q., Li, L., Yuan, W. et al. (2018). FDA approval summary: tocilizumab for treatment of chimeric antigen receptor T cell-induced severe or life-threatening cytokine release syndrome. *Oncologist* 23 (8): 943–947.

162 Salama, C., Han, J., Yau, L. et al. (2021). Tocilizumab in patients hospitalized with Covid-19 pneumonia. *N. Engl. J. Med.* 384 (1): 20–30.

163 REMAP-CAP Investigators, Gordon, A.C., Mouncey, P.R. et al. (2021). Interleukin-6 receptor antagonists in critically ill patients with Covid-19. *N. Engl. J. Med.* 384 (16): 1491–1502.

164 Horby, P.W., Pessoa-Amorim, G., Peto, L. et al. (2021). Tocilizumab in patients admitted to hospital with COVID-19 (RECOVERY): preliminary results of a randomised, controlled, open-label, platform trial. *medRxiv* https://doi.org/10.1101/2021.02.11.2 1249258.

165 Stone, J.H., Frigault, M.J., Serling-Boyd, N.J. et al. (2020). Efficacy of tocilizumab in patients hospitalized with Covid-19. *N. Engl. J. Med.* 383 (24): 2333–2344.

166 Rosas, I.O., Brau, N., Waters, M. et al. (2021). Tocilizumab in hospitalized patients with severe Covid-19 pneumonia. *N. Engl. J. Med.* 384 (16): 1503–1516.

167 Hermine, O., Mariette, X., Tharaux, P.L. et al. (2021). Effect of tocilizumab vs usual care in adults hospitalized with COVID-19 and moderate or severe pneumonia: a randomized clinical trial. *JAMA Intern. Med.* 181 (1): 32–40.

168 Salvarani, C., Dolci, G., Massari, M. et al. (2021). Effect of tocilizumab vs standard care on clinical

worsening in patients hospitalized with COVID-19 pneumonia: a randomized clinical trial. *JAMA Intern. Med.* 181 (1): 24–31.

169 Veiga, V.C., Prats, J., Farias, D.L.C. et al. (2021). Effect of tocilizumab on clinical outcomes at 15 days in patients with severe or critical coronavirus disease 2019: randomised controlled trial. *BMJ* 372: n84.

170 Rubin, E.J., Longo, D.L., and Baden, L.R. (2021). Interleukin-6 receptor inhibition in Covid-19 – cooling the inflammatory soup. *N. Engl. J. Med.* 384 (16): 1564–1565.

171 Della-Torre, E., Campochiaro, C., Cavalli, G. et al. (2020). Interleukin-6 blockade with sarilumab in severe COVID-19 pneumonia with systemic hyperinflammation: an open-label cohort study. *Ann. Rheum. Dis.* 79 (10): 1277–1285.

172 Malekzadeh, R., Abedini, A., Mohsenpour, B. et al. (2020). Subcutaneous tocilizumab in adults with severe and critical COVID-19: a prospective open-label uncontrolled multicenter trial. *Int. Immunopharmacol.* 89 (Pt B): 107102.

173 Strohbehn, G.W., Heiss, B.L., Rouhani, S.J. et al. (2021). COVIDOSE: a phase II clinical trial of low-dose tocilizumab in the treatment of noncritical COVID-19 pneumonia. *Clin. Pharmacol. Ther.* 109 (3): 688–696.

174 Guaraldi, G., Meschiari, M., Cozzi-Lepri, A. et al. (2020). Tocilizumab in patients with severe COVID-19: a retrospective cohort study. *Lancet Rheumatol.* 2 (8): e474–e484.

175 Deftereos, S., Giannopoulos, G., Papoutsidakis, N. et al. (2013). Colchicine and the heart: pushing the envelope. *J. Am. Coll. Cardiol.* 62 (20): 1817–1825.

176 Leung, Y.Y., Yao Hui, L.L., and Kraus, V.B. (2015). Colchicine–update on mechanisms of action and therapeutic uses. *Semin. Arthritis Rheum.* 45 (3): 341–350.

177 Deftereos, S.G., Giannopoulos, G., Vrachatis, D.A. et al. (2020). Effect of colchicine vs standard care on cardiac and inflammatory biomarkers and clinical outcomes in patients hospitalized with coronavirus disease 2019: the GRECCO-19 randomized clinical trial. *JAMA Netw. Open* 3 (6): e2013136.

178 Lopes, M.I., Bonjorno, L.P., Giannini, M.C. et al. (2021). Beneficial effects of colchicine for moderate to severe COVID-19: a randomised, double-blinded, placebo-controlled clinical trial. *RMD Open* 7 (1): e001455.

179 Sandhu, T., Tieng, A., Chilimuri, S., and Franchin, G. (2020). A case control study to evaluate the impact of colchicine on patients admitted to the hospital with moderate to severe COVID-19 infection. *Can. J. Infect. Dis. Med. Microbiol.* 2020: 8865954.

180 Brunetti, L., Diawara, O., Tsai, A. et al. (2020). Colchicine to weather the cytokine storm in hospitalized patients with COVID-19. *J. Clin. Med.* 9 (9): 2961.

181 Sperber, K., Quraishi, H., Talb, T. et al. (1993). Selective regulation of cytokine secretion by hydroxychloroquine: inhibition of interleukin 1 alpha (IL-1-alpha) and IL-6 in human monocytes and T cells. *J. Rheumatol.* 20 (5): 803–808.

182 Keyaerts, E., Vijgen, L., Maes, P. et al. (2004). in vitro inhibition of severe acute respiratory syndrome coronavirus by chloroquine. *Biochem. Biophys. Res. Commun.* 323 (1): 264–268.

183 Vincent, M.J., Bergeron, E., Benjannet, S. et al. (2005). Chloroquine is a potent inhibitor of SARS coronavirus infection and spread. *Virol. J.* 2: 69.

184 Ben-Zvi, I., Kivity, S., Langevitz, P., and Shoenfeld, Y. (2012). Hydroxychloroquine: from malaria to autoimmunity. *Clin Rev Allergy Immunol* 42 (2): 145–153.

185 Tyteca, D., Van Der Smissen, P., Mettlen, M. et al. (2002). Azithromycin, a lysosomotropic antibiotic, has distinct effects on fluid-phase and receptor-mediated endocytosis, but does not impair phagocytosis in J774 macrophages. *Exp. Cell Res.* 281 (1): 86–100.

186 Gielen, V., Johnston, S.L., and Edwards, M.R. (2010). Azithromycin induces anti-viral responses in bronchial epithelial cells. *Eur. Respir. J.* 36 (3): 646–654.

187 Li, C., Zu, S., Deng, Y.-Q. et al. (2019). Azithromycin protects against Zika virus infection by Upregulating virus-induced type I and III interferon responses. *Antimicrob. Agents Chemother.* 63 (12): e00394–e00319.

188 Gautret, P., Lagier, J.C., Parola, P. et al. (2020). Hydroxychloroquine and azithromycin as a treatment of COVID-19: results of an open-label non-randomized clinical trial. *Int. J. Antimicrob. Agents* 56 (1): 105949.

189 RECOVERY Collaborative Group (2021). Azithromycin in patients admitted to hospital with COVID-19 (RECOVERY): a randomised, controlled, open-label, platform trial. *Lancet* 397: 605–612.

190 Abd-Elsalam, S., Esmail, E.S., Khalaf, M. et al. (2020). Hydroxychloroquine in the treatment of COVID-19: a multicenter randomized controlled study. *Am. J. Trop. Med. Hyg.* 103 (4): 1635–1639.

191 Cavalcanti, A.B., Zampieri, F.G., Rosa, R.G. et al. (2020). Hydroxychloroquine with or without azithromycin in mild-to-moderate Covid-19. *N. Engl. J. Med.* 383 (21): 2041–2052.

192 Chen, C.P., Lin, Y.C., Chen, T.C. et al. (2020). A multicenter, randomized, open-label, controlled trial to evaluate the efficacy and tolerability of hydroxychloroquine and a retrospective study in adult patients with mild to moderate coronavirus disease 2019 (COVID-19). *PLoS One* 15 (12): e0242763.

193 Furtado, R.H.M., Berwanger, O., Fonseca, H.A. et al. (2020). Azithromycin in addition to standard of care versus standard of care alone in the treatment of patients admitted to the hospital with severe COVID-19 in Brazil (COALITION II): a randomised clinical trial. *Lancet* 396 (10256): 959–967.

194 RECOVERY Collaborative Group, Horby, P., Mafham, M. et al. (2020). Effect of hydroxychloroquine in hospitalized patients with Covid-19. *N. Engl. J. Med.* 383 (21): 2030–2040.

195 Self, W.H., Semler, M.W., Leither, L.M. et al. (2020). Effect of hydroxychloroquine on clinical status at 14 days in hospitalized patients with COVID-19: a randomized clinical trial. *JAMA* 324 (21): 2165–2176.

196 Tang, W., Cao, Z., Han, M. et al. (2020). Hydroxychloroquine in patients with mainly mild to moderate coronavirus disease 2019: open label, randomised controlled trial. *BMJ* 369: m1849.

197 Chorin, E., Wadhwani, L., Magnani, S. et al. (2020). QT interval prolongation and torsade de pointes in patients with COVID-19 treated with hydroxychloroquine/azithromycin. *Heart Rhythm* 17 (9): 1425–1433.

198 Rosenberg, E.S., Dufort, E.M., Udo, T. et al. (2020). Association of treatment with hydroxychloroquine or azithromycin with in-hospital mortality in patients with COVID-19 in New York state. *JAMA* 323 (24): 2493–2502.

199 Fiolet, T., Guihur, A., Rebeaud, M.E. et al. (2021). Effect of hydroxychloroquine with or without azithromycin on the mortality of coronavirus disease 2019 (COVID-19) patients: a systematic review and meta-analysis. *Clin. Microbiol. Infect.* 27 (1): 19–27.

200 O'Connell, T.F., Bradley, C.J., Abbas, A.E. et al. (2021). Hydroxychloroquine/azithromycin therapy and QT prolongation in hospitalized patients with COVID-19. *JACC Clin. Electrophysiol.* 7 (1): 16–25.

201 Chen, F., Chan, K.H., Jiang, Y. et al. (2004). in vitro susceptibility of 10 clinical isolates of SARS coronavirus to selected antiviral compounds. *J. Clin. Virol.* 31 (1): 69–75.

202 Chu, C.M., Cheng, V.C., Hung, I.F. et al. (2004). Role of lopinavir/ritonavir in the treatment of SARS: initial virological and clinical findings. *Thorax* 59 (3): 252–256.

203 Kim, U.J., Won, E.J., Kee, S.J. et al. (2016). Combination therapy with lopinavir/ritonavir, ribavirin and interferon-alpha for middle east respiratory syndrome. *Antiviral Ther.* 21 (5): 455–459.

204 Hung, I.F.-N., Lung, K.-C., Tso, E.Y.-K. et al. (2020). Triple combination of interferon beta-1b, lopinavir–ritonavir, and ribavirin in the treatment of patients admitted to hospital with COVID-19: an open-label, randomised, phase 2 trial. *Lancet* 395 (10238): 1695–1704.

205 Cao, B., Wang, Y., Wen, D. et al. (2020). A trial of lopinavir-ritonavir in adults hospitalized with severe Covid-19. *N. Engl. J. Med.* 382 (19): 1787–1799.

206 Horby, P.W., Mafham, M., Bell, J.L. et al. (2020). Lopinavir–ritonavir in patients admitted to hospital with COVID-19 (RECOVERY): a randomised, controlled, open-label, platform trial. *Lancet* 396 (10259): 1345–1352.

207 Loutfy, M., Blatt, L., Siminovitch, K. et al. (2003). Interferon alfacon-1 plus corticosteroids in severe acute respiratory syndrome. *JAMA* 290 (24): 3222–3228.

208 Wang, B.X. and Fish, E.N. (2019). Global virus outbreaks: interferons as 1st responders. *Semin. Immunol.* 43: 101300.

209 Monk, P.D., Marsden, R.J., Tear, V.J. et al. (2021). Safety and efficacy of inhaled nebulised interferon beta-1a (SNG001) for treatment of SARS-CoV-2 infection: a randomised, double-blind, placebo-controlled, phase 2 trial. *Lancet Respir. Med.* 9 (2): 196–206.

210 Davoudi-Monfared, E.R., Rahmani, H., Khalili, H. et al. (2020). A randomized clinical trial of the efficacy and safety of interferon beta-1a in treatment of severe COVID-19. *Antimicrob. Agents Chemother.* 64 (9): e01061–e01020.

211 Rahmani, H., Davoudi-Monfared, E., Nourian, A. et al. (2020). Interferon beta-1b in treatment of severe COVID-19: a randomized clinical trial. *Int. Immunopharmacol.* 88: 106903.

212 Li, C., Luo, F., Liu, C. et al. (2021). Effect of a genetically engineered interferon-alpha versus traditional interferon-alpha in the treatment of moderate-to-severe COVID-19: a randomised clinical trial. *Ann. Med.* 53 (1): 391–401.

213 Zhou, Q., Chen, V., Shannon, C.P. et al. (2020). Interferon-alpha2b treatment for COVID-19. *Front. Immunol.* 11: 1061.

214 Khamis, F., Al Naabi, H., Al Lawati, A. et al. (2021). Randomized controlled open label trial on the use of favipiravir combined with inhaled interferon beta-1b in hospitalized patients with moderate to severe COVID-19 pneumonia. *Int. J. Infect. Dis.* 102: 538–543.

215 Zheng, F., Zhou, Y., Zhou, Z. et al. (2020). SARS-CoV-2 clearance in COVID-19 patients with novaferon treatment: a randomized, open-label, parallel-group trial. *Int. J. Infect. Dis.* 99: 84–91.

216 National Institute of Allergy and Infectious Diseases (NIAID). (2021). Adaptive COVID-19 Treatment Trial 3 (ACTT-3). https://clinicaltrials.gov/ct2/show/NCT04492475 (accessed 29 April 2021).

217 National Institute of Allergy and Infectious Diseases (NIAID). (2021). NIAID stops enrollment of severely ill COVID-19 participants in clinical trial of investigational treatments. https://www.niaid.nih.gov/news-events/bulletin-niaid-stops-enrollment-severely-ill-covid-19-participants-clinical-trial (accessed 29 April 2021).

218 Tharaux, P.-L., Pialoux, G., Pavot, A. et al. (2021). Effect of anakinra versus usual care in adults in hospital with COVID-19 and mild-to-moderate pneumonia (CORIMUNO-ANA-1): a randomised controlled trial. *Lancet Respir. Med.* 9 (3): 295–304.

219 Balkhair, A., Al-Zakwani, I., Al Busaidi, M. et al. (2021). Anakinra in hospitalized patients with severe COVID-19 pneumonia requiring oxygen therapy: results of a prospective, open-label, interventional study. *Int. J. Infect. Dis.* 103: 288–296.

220 Bozzi, G., Mangioni, D., Minoia, F. et al. (2021). Anakinra combined with methylprednisolone in patients with severe COVID-19 pneumonia and hyperinflammation: an observational cohort study. *J. Allergy Clin. Immunol.* 147 (2): 561–566. e4.

221 Huet, T., Beaussier, H., Voisin, O. et al. (2020). Anakinra for severe forms of COVID-19: a cohort study. *Lancet Rheumatol.* 2 (7): e393–e400.

222 Kooistra, E.J., Waalders, N.J.B., Grondman, I. et al. (2020). Anakinra treatment in critically ill COVID-19 patients: a prospective cohort study. *Crit. Care* 24 (1): 688.

223 Borie, R., Savale, L., Dossier, A. et al. (2020). Glucocorticoids with low-dose anti-IL1 anakinra rescue in severe non-ICU COVID-19 infection: a cohort study. *PLoS One* 15 (12): e0243961.

224 Wu, Y., Wang, F., Shen, C. et al. (2020). A noncompeting pair of human neutralizing antibodies block COVID-19 virus binding to its receptor ACE2. *Science* 368 (6496): 1274–1278.

225 Shi, R., Shan, C., Duan, X. et al. (2020). A human neutralizing antibody targets the receptor-binding site of SARS-CoV-2. *Nature* 584 (7819): 120–124.

226 Taylor, P.C., Adams, A.C., Hufford, M.M. et al. (2021). Neutralizing monoclonal antibodies for treatment of COVID-19. *Nat. Rev. Immunol.* 21: 382–393.

227 Chen, P., Nirula, A., Heller, B. et al. (2021). SARS-CoV-2 neutralizing antibody LY-CoV555 in outpatients with Covid-19. *N. Engl. J. Med.* 384 (3): 229–237.

228 Gottlieb, R.L., Nirula, A., Chen, P. et al. (2021). Effect of bamlanivimab as monotherapy or in combination with etesevimab on viral load in patients with mild to moderate COVID-19: a randomized clinical trial. *JAMA* 325 (7): 632–644.

229 Weinreich, D.M., Sivapalasingam, S., Norton, T. et al. (2021). REGN-COV2, a neutralizing antibody cocktail, in outpatients with Covid-19. *N. Engl. J. Med.* 384 (3): 238–251.

230 ACTIV-3/TICO LY-CoV555 Study Group, Lundgren, J.D., Grund, B. et al. (2021). A neutralizing monoclonal antibody for hospitalized patients with Covid-19. *N. Engl. J. Med.* 384 (10): 905–914.

231 Dong, E., Du, H., and Gardner, L. (2020). An interactive web-based dashboard to track COVID-19 in real time. *Lancet Infect. Dis.* 20 (5): 533–534.

232 Chotirmall, S.H., Leither, L.M., Coruh, B. et al. (2021). Update in COVID-19. *Am. J. Respir. Crit. Care Med.* 203: 1462–1471.

233 Lim, W., Meade, M., Lauzier, F. et al. (2015). Failure of anticoagulant thromboprophylaxis: risk factors in medical-surgical critically ill patients*. *Crit. Care Med.* 43 (2): 401–410.

234 Castellucci, L.A., Wells, P.S., and Duffett, L. (2015). Nonleg venous thrombosis in critically ill adults. *JAMA* 313 (4): 411–412.

235 Bikdeli, B., Madhavan, M.V., Jimenez, D. et al. (2020). COVID-19 and thrombotic or thromboembolic disease: implications for prevention, antithrombotic therapy, and follow-up: JACC state-of-the-art review. *J. Am. Coll. Cardiol.* 75 (23): 2950–2973.

236 Bilaloglu, S., Aphinyanaphongs, Y., Jones, S. et al. (2020). Thrombosis in hospitalized patients with COVID-19 in a New York City health system. *JAMA* 324 (8): 799–801.

237 Lax, S.F., Skok, K., Zechner, P. et al. (2020). Pulmonary arterial thrombosis in COVID-19 with fatal outcome: results from a prospective, single-center, clinicopathologic case series. *Ann. Intern. Med.* 173 (5): 350–361.

238 Jimenez, D., Garcia-Sanchez, A., Rali, P. et al. (2021). Incidence of VTE and bleeding among hospitalized patients with coronavirus disease 2019: a systematic review and meta-analysis. *Chest* 159 (3): 1182–1196.

239 Wichmann, D., Sperhake, J.P., Lutgehetmann, M. et al. (2020). Autopsy findings and venous thromboembolism in patients with COVID-19: a prospective cohort study. *Ann. Intern. Med.* 173 (4): 268–277.

240 Ackermann, M., Verleden, S.E., Kuehnel, M. et al. (2020). Pulmonary vascular endothelialitis, thrombosis, and angiogenesis in Covid-19. *N. Engl. J. Med.* 383 (2): 120–128.

241 Berkman, S.A. and Tapson, V.F. (2020). Methodological issues and controversies in COVID-19 coagulopathy: a tale of two storms. *Clin. Appl. Thromb. Hemost.* 26: 1076029620945398.

242 Magro, C., Mulvey, J.J., Berlin, D. et al. (2020). Complement associated microvascular injury and thrombosis in the pathogenesis of severe COVID-19 infection: a report of five cases. *Transl. Res.* 220: 1–13.

243 Libby, P. and Luscher, T. (2020). COVID-19 is, in the end, an endothelial disease. *Eur. Heart J.* 41 (32): 3038–3044.

244 Yu, J., Yuan, X., Chen, H. et al. (2020). Direct activation of the alternative complement pathway by SARS-CoV-2 spike proteins is blocked by factor D inhibition. *Blood* 136 (18): 2080–2089.

245 Teuwen, L.A., Geldhof, V., Pasut, A., and Carmeliet, P. (2020). COVID-19: the vasculature unleashed. *Nat. Rev. Immunol.* 20 (7): 389–391.

246 Lowenstein, C.J. and Solomon, S.D. (2020). Severe COVID-19 is a microvascular disease. *Circulation* 142 (17): 1609–1611.

247 Maier, C.L., Truong, A.D., Auld, S.C. et al. (2020). COVID-19-associated hyperviscosity: a link between inflammation and thrombophilia? *Lancet* 395 (10239): 1758–1759.

248 Ranucci, M., Ballotta, A., Di Dedda, U. et al. (2020). The procoagulant pattern of patients with COVID-19 acute respiratory distress syndrome. *J. Thromb. Haemost.* 18 (7): 1747–1751.

249 Panigada, M., Bottino, N., Tagliabue, P. et al. (2020). Hypercoagulability of COVID-19 patients in intensive care unit: a report of thromboelastography findings and other parameters of hemostasis. *J. Thromb. Haemost.* 18 (7): 1738–1742.

250 Saghazadeh, A., Hafizi, S., and Rezaei, N. (2015). Inflammation in venous thromboembolism: cause or consequence? *Int. Immunopharmacol.* 28 (1): 655–665.

251 Branchford, B.R. and Carpenter, S.L. (2018). The role of inflammation in venous thromboembolism. *Front. Pediatr.* 6: 142.

252 Zhang, L., Yan, X., Fan, Q. et al. (2020). D-dimer levels on admission to predict in-hospital mortality in patients with Covid-19. *J. Thromb. Haemost.* 18 (6): 1324–1329.

253 Cuker, A., Tseng, E.K., Nieuwlaat, R., et al. (2021). Should DOACs LMWH, UFH, Fondaparinux, Argatroban, or Bivalirudin at intermediate-intensity or therapeutic-intensity vs. prophylactic intensity be used for patients with COVID-19 related critical illness who do not have suspected or confirmed VTE? https://guidelines.ash. gradepro.org/profile/3CQ7J0SWt58 (accessed 22 April 2021).

254 The REMAP-CAP, ACTIV-4a, and ATTACC Investigators (2021). Therapeutic anticoagulation with heparin in critically ill patients with Covid-19. *N. Engl. J. Med.* https://doi.org/10.1056/ NEJMoa2103417.

255 The ATTACC, ACTIV-4a, and REMAP-CAP Investigators (2021). Therapeutic anticoagulation with heparin in noncritically ill patients with Covid-19. *N. Engl. J. Med.* https://doi.org/10.1056/ NEJMoa2105911.

256 National Heart, Lung, and Blood Institute (NHLBI). (2021). ATTACC, ACTIV-4a & REMAP-CAP: multiplatform RCT. https://nhlbi-connects. org/documents/mpRCT%20Interim%20 Presentation.pdf.

257 INSPIRATION Investigators (2021). Effect of intermediate-dose vs standard-dose prophylactic anticoagulation on thrombotic events, extracorporeal membrane oxygenation treatment, or mortality among patients with COVID-19 admitted to the intensive care unit: the INSPIRATION Randomized Clinical Trial. *JAMA* 325 (16): 1620–1630.

258 Raschke, R.A., Reilly, B.M., Guidry, J.R. et al. (1993). The weight-based heparin dosing nomogram compared with a standard care nomogram. *Ann. Intern. Med.* 119 (9): 874–881.

259 Alpert, J.S., Smith, R., Carlson, C.J. et al. (1976). Mortality in patients treated for pulmonary embolism. *JAMA* 236 (13): 1477–1480.

260 Barritt, D.W. and Jordan, S.C. (1960). Anticoagulant drugs in the treatment of pulmonary embolism: a controlled TRIAL. *Lancet* 275 (7138): 1309–1312.

261 Bauer, G. (1959). The introduction of heparin therapy in cases of early thrombosis. *Circulation* 19 (1): 108–109.

262 Kearon, C., Akl, E.A., Ornelas, J. et al. (2016). Antithrombotic therapy for VTE disease: CHEST guideline and expert panel report. *Chest* 149 (2): 315–352.

263 Konstantinides, S.V., Meyer, G., Becattini, C. et al. (2019). 2019 ESC guidelines for the diagnosis and management of acute pulmonary embolism developed in collaboration with the European Respiratory Society (ERS): the task force for the diagnosis and management of acute pulmonary embolism of the European Society of Cardiology (ESC). *Eur. Heart J.* 41 (4): 543–603.

264 Smith, S.B., Geske, J.B., Maguire, J.M. et al. (2010). Early anticoagulation is associated with reduced mortality for acute pulmonary embolism. *Chest* 137 (6): 1382–1390.

265 Tapson, V.F. and Weinberg, A.S. (2020). Overview of management of intermediate- and high-risk pulmonary embolism. *Crit. Care Clin.* 36 (3): 449–463.

266 Schulman, S., Hu, Y., and Konstantinides, S. (2020). Venous thromboembolism in COVID-19. *Thromb. Haemost.* 120 (12): 1642–1653.

267 Figliozzi, S., Masci, P.G., Ahmadi, N. et al. (2020). Predictors of adverse prognosis in COVID-19: a systematic review and meta-analysis. *Eur. J. Clin. Invest.* 50 (10): e13362.

268 Chatterjee, N.A. and Cheng, R.K. (2020). Cardiovascular disease and COVID-19: implications for prevention, surveillance and treatment. *Heart* 106 (15): 1119–1121.

269 O'Gara, P.T., Kushner, F.G., Ascheim, D.D. et al. (2013). 2013 ACCF/AHA guideline for the management of ST-elevation myocardial infarction: executive summary: a report of the American College of Cardiology Foundation/American Heart Association Task Force on Practice Guidelines. *Circulation* 127 (4): 529–555.

270 Altamimi, H., Abid, A.R., Othman, F., and Patel, A. (2020). Cardiovascular manifestations of COVID-19. *Heart Views* 21 (3): 171–186.

271 Bangalore, S., Sharma, A., Slotwiner, A. et al. (2020). ST-segment elevation in patients with covid-19 – a case series. *N. Engl. J. Med.* 382 (25): 2478–2480.

272 Inciardi, R.M., Lupi, L., Zaccone, G. et al. (2020). Cardiac involvement in a patient with coronavirus disease 2019 (COVID-19). *JAMA Cardiol.* 5 (7): 819–824.

273 Hendren, N.S., Drazner, M.H., Bozkurt, B., and Cooper, L.T. Jr. (2020). Description and proposed management of the acute COVID-19 cardiovascular syndrome. *Circulation* 141 (23): 1903–1914.

274 Sandoval, Y., Januzzi, J.L. Jr., and Jaffe, A.S. (2020). Cardiac troponin for assessment of myocardial injury in COVID-19: JACC review topic of the week. *J. Am. Coll. Cardiol.* 76 (10): 1244–1258.

275 Bandyopadhyay, D., Akhtar, T., Hajra, A. et al. (2020). COVID-19 pandemic: cardiovascular complications and future implications. *Am. J. Cardiovasc. Drugs* 20 (4): 311–324.

276 Keeley, E.C., Boura, J.A., and Grines, C.L. (2003). Primary angioplasty versus intravenous thrombolytic therapy for acute myocardial infarction: a quantitative review of 23 randomised trials. *Lancet* 361 (9351): 13–20.

277 Welt, F.G.P., Shah, P.B., Aronow, H.D. et al. (2020). Catheterization laboratory considerations during the coronavirus (COVID-19) pandemic: from the ACC's Interventional Council and SCAI. *J. Am. Coll. Cardiol.* 75 (18): 2372–2375.

278 Zhou, F., Yu, T., Du, R. et al. (2020). Clinical course and risk factors for mortality of adult inpatients with COVID-19 in Wuhan, China: a retrospective cohort study. *Lancet* 395 (10229): 1054–1062.

279 Chen, T., Wu, D., Chen, H. et al. (2020). Clinical characteristics of 113 deceased patients with coronavirus disease 2019: retrospective study. *BMJ* 368: m1091.

280 Alvarez-Garcia, J., Lee, S., Gupta, A. et al. (2020). Prognostic impact of prior heart failure in patients hospitalized with COVID-19. *J. Am. Coll. Cardiol.* 76 (20): 2334–2348.

281 Zeng, J.H., Liu, Y.X., Yuan, J. et al. (2020). First case of COVID-19 complicated with fulminant myocarditis: a case report and insights. *Infection* 48 (5): 773–777.

282 Hu, H., Ma, F., Wei, X., and Fang, Y. (2021). Coronavirus fulminant myocarditis treated with glucocorticoid and human immunoglobulin. *Eur. Heart J.* 42 (2): 206.

283 Kang, Y., Chen, T., Mui, D. et al. (2020). Cardiovascular manifestations and treatment considerations in COVID-19. *Heart* 106 (15): 1132–1141.

284 Escher, F., Pietsch, H., Aleshcheva, G. et al. (2020). Detection of viral SARS-CoV-2 genomes and histopathological changes in endomyocardial biopsies. *ESC Heart Fail.* 7 (5): 2440–2447.

285 Giustino, G., Croft, L.B., Oates, C.P. et al. (2020). Takotsubo cardiomyopathy in COVID-19. *J. Am. Coll. Cardiol.* 76 (5): 628–629.

286 Tsao, C.W., Strom, J.B., Chang, J.D., and Manning, W.J. (2020). COVID-19-associated stress (Takotsubo) cardiomyopathy. *Circ. Cardiovasc. Imaging* 13 (7): e011222.

287 Sang, C.J. 3rd, Heindl, B., Von Mering, G. et al. (2020). Stress-induced cardiomyopathy precipitated by COVID-19 and influenza a coinfection. *JACC Case Rep.* 2 (9): 1356–1358.

288 Bapat, A., Maan, A., and Heist, E.K. (2020). Stress-induced cardiomyopathy secondary to COVID-19. *Case Rep. Cardiol.* 2020: 8842150.

289 Minhas, A.S., Scheel, P., Garibaldi, B. et al. (2020). Takotsubo syndrome in the setting of COVID-19. *JACC Case Rep.* 2 (9): 1321–1325.

290 Roca, E., Lombardi, C., Campana, M. et al. (2020). Takotsubo syndrome associated with COVID-19. *Eur. J. Case Rep. Intern. Med.* 7 (5): 001665.

291 Park, J.H., Moon, J.Y., Sohn, K.M., and Kim, Y.S. (2020). Two fatal cases of stress-induced cardiomyopathy in COVID-19 patients. *J. Cardiovasc. Imaging* 28 (4): 300–303.

292 Nguyen, D., Nguyen, T., De Bels, D., and Castro Rodriguez, J. (2020). A case of takotsubo cardiomyopathy with COVID 19. *Eur. Heart J. Cardiovasc. Imaging* 21 (9): 1052.

293 Meyer, P., Degrauwe, S., Van Delden, C. et al. (2020). Typical takotsubo syndrome triggered by SARS-CoV-2 infection. *Eur. Heart J.* 41 (19): 1860.

294 Faqihi, F., Alharthy, A., Alshaya, R. et al. (2020). Reverse takotsubo cardiomyopathy in fulminant

COVID-19 associated with cytokine release syndrome and resolution following therapeutic plasma exchange: a case-report. *BMC Cardiovasc. Disord.* 20 (1): 389.

295 Singh, S., Desai, R., Gandhi, Z. et al. (2020). Takotsubo syndrome in patients with COVID-19: a systematic review of published cases. *SN Comp. Clin. Med.* 2: 2102–2108.

296 Garcia-Zamora, S., Lee, S., Haseeb, S. et al. (2021). Arrhythmias and electrocardiographic findings in coronavirus disease 2019: a systematic review and meta-analysis. *Pacing Clin. Electrophysiol.* 44: 1062–1074.

297 Goyal, P., Choi, J.J., Pinheiro, L.C. et al. (2020). Clinical characteristics of Covid-19 in New York City. *N. Engl. J. Med.* 382 (24): 2372–2374.

298 Wang, D., Hu, B., Hu, C. et al. (2020). Clinical characteristics of 138 hospitalized patients with 2019 novel coronavirus-infected pneumonia in Wuhan, China. *JAMA* 323 (11): 1061–1069.

299 Shao, F., Xu, S., Ma, X. et al. (2020). In-hospital cardiac arrest outcomes among patients with COVID-19 pneumonia in Wuhan, China. *Resuscitation* 151: 18–23.

300 Bhatla, A., Mayer, M.M., Adusumalli, S. et al. (2020). COVID-19 and cardiac arrhythmias. *Heart Rhythm* 17 (9): 1439–1444.

301 Cho, J.H., Namazi, A., Shelton, R. et al. (2020). Cardiac arrhythmias in hospitalized patients with COVID-19: a prospective observational study in the western United States. *PLoS One* 15 (12): e0244533.

302 McCullough, S.A., Goyal, P., Krishnan, U. et al. (2020). Electrocardiographic findings in coronavirus disease-19: insights on mortality and underlying myocardial processes. *J. Card. Fail.* 26 (7): 626–632.

303 Tjendra, Y., Al Mana, A.F., Espejo, A.P. et al. (2020). Predicting disease severity and outcome in COVID-19 patients: a review of multiple biomarkers. *Arch. Pathol. Lab. Med.* 144 (12): 1465–1474.

304 Aboughdir, M., Kirwin, T., Abdul Khader, A., and Wang, B. (2020). Prognostic value of cardiovascular biomarkers in COVID-19: a review. *Viruses* 12 (5): 527.

305 Mueller, C., Laule-Kilian, K., Frana, B. et al. (2006). Use of B-type natriuretic peptide in the management of acute dyspnea in patients with pulmonary disease. *Am. Heart J.* 151 (2): 471–477.

306 Christ-Crain, M., Breidthardt, T., Stolz, D. et al. (2008). Use of B-type natriuretic peptide in the risk stratification of community-acquired pneumonia. *J. Intern. Med.* 264 (2): 166–176.

307 Mueller, C., McDonald, K., de Boer, R.A. et al. (2019). Heart Failure Association of the European Society of Cardiology practical guidance on the use of natriuretic peptide concentrations. *Eur. J. Heart Fail.* 21 (6): 715–731.

308 Dinort, J. (2019). Medizinische Fakultät der Universität Basel.

309 Mueller, C., Giannitsis, E., Jaffe, A.S. et al. (2021). Cardiovascular biomarkers in patients with COVID-19. *Eur. Heart J. Acute Cardiovasc. Care* 10: 310–319.

310 Shi, S., Qin, M., Shen, B. et al. (2020). Association of cardiac injury with mortality in hospitalized patients with COVID-19 in Wuhan, China. *JAMA Cardiol.* 5 (7): 802–810.

311 Carrizales-Sepulveda, E.F., Vera-Pineda, R., Flores-Ramirez, R. et al. (2021). Echocardiographic manifestations in COVID-19: a review. *Heart Lung Circ.* 30: 1117–1129.

312 Dweck, M.R., Bularga, A., Hahn, R.T. et al. (2020). Global evaluation of echocardiography in patients with COVID-19. *Eur. Heart J. Cardiovasc. Imaging* 21 (9): 949–958.

313 Szekely, Y., Lichter, Y., Taieb, P. et al. (2020). Spectrum of cardiac manifestations in COVID-19. *Circulation* 142 (4): 342–353.

314 van den Heuvel, F.M.A., Vos, J.L., Koop, Y. et al. (2020). Cardiac function in relation to myocardial injury in hospitalised patients with COVID-19. *Netherland Heart J.* 28 (7): 410–417.

315 Rath, D., Petersen-Uribe, A., Avdiu, A. et al. (2020). Impaired cardiac function is associated with mortality in patients with acute COVID-19 infection. *Clin. Res. Cardiol.* 109 (12): 1491–1499.

316 Giustino, G., Croft, L.B., Stefanini, G.G. et al. (2020). Characterization of myocardial injury in patients with COVID-19. *J. Am. Coll. Cardiol.* 76 (18): 2043–2055.

317 Robbins-Juarez, S.Y., Qian, L., King, K.L. et al. (2020). Outcomes for patients with COVID-19 and

acute kidney injury: a systematic review and meta-analysis. *Kidney Int. Rep.* 5 (8): 1149–1160.

318 Hirsch, J.S., Ng, J.H., Ross, D.W. et al. (2020). Acute kidney injury in patients hospitalized with COVID-19. *Kidney Int.* 98 (1): 209–218.

319 Armaly, Z., Kinaneh, S., and Skorecki, K. (2021). Renal manifestations of Covid-19: physiology and pathophysiology. *J. Clin. Med.* 10 (6): 1216.

320 Yan, R., Zhang, Y., Li, Y. et al. (2020). Structural basis for the recognition of SARS-CoV-2 by full-length human ACE2. *Science* 367 (6485): 1444–1448.

321 Hoffmann, M., Kleine-Weber, H., Schroeder, S. et al. (2020). SARS-CoV-2 cell entry depends on ACE2 and TMPRSS2 and is blocked by a clinically proven protease inhibitor. *Cell* 181 (2): 271–280.e8.

322 Braun, F., Lütgehetmann, M., Pfefferle, S. et al. (2020). SARS-CoV-2 renal tropism associates with acute kidney injury. *Lancet* 396 (10251): 597–598.

323 Su, H., Yang, M., Wan, C. et al. (2020). Renal histopathological analysis of 26 postmortem findings of patients with COVID-19 in China. *Kidney Int.* 98 (1): 219–227.

324 Frithiof, R., Bergqvist, A., Järhult, J.D. et al. (2020). Presence of SARS-CoV-2 in urine is rare and not associated with acute kidney injury in critically ill COVID-19 patients. *Crit. Care* 24 (1): 587.

325 Werion, A., Belkhir, L., Perrot, M. et al. (2020). SARS-CoV-2 causes a specific dysfunction of the kidney proximal tubule. *Kidney Int.* 98 (5): 1296–1307.

326 Brönimann, S., Rebhan, K., Lemberger, U. et al. (2020). Secretion of severe acute respiratory syndrome coronavirus 2 in urine. *Curr. Opin. Urol.* 30 (5): 735–739.

327 Remmelink, M., De Mendonça, R., D'Haene, N. et al. (2020). Unspecific post-mortem findings despite multiorgan viral spread in COVID-19 patients. *Crit. Care* 24 (1): 495.

328 Ghani, R.A., Zainudin, S., Ctkong, N. et al. (2006). Serum IL-6 and IL-1-ra with sequential organ failure assessment scores in septic patients receiving high-volume haemofiltration and continuous venovenous haemofiltration. *Nephrology (Carlton)* 11 (5): 386–393.

329 Chu, K.H., Tsang, W.K., Tang, C.S. et al. (2005). Acute renal impairment in coronavirus-associated severe acute respiratory syndrome. *Kidney Int.* 67 (2): 698–705.

330 Wilson, R., Dowling, R.B., and Jackson, A.D. (1996). The biology of bacterial colonization and invasion of the respiratory mucosa. *Eur. Respir. J.* 9 (7): 1523–1530.

331 Rynda-Apple, A., Robinson, K.M., and Alcorn, J.F. (2015). Influenza and bacterial superinfection: illuminating the immunologic mechanisms of disease. *Infect. Immunol.* 83 (10): 3764–3770.

332 Paget, C. and Trottein, F. (2019). Mechanisms of bacterial superinfection post-influenza: a role for unconventional T cells. *Front. Immunol.* 10: 336.

333 Medell, M., Medell, M., Martínez, A., and Valdés, R. (2012). Characterization and sensitivity to antibiotics of bacteria isolated from the lower respiratory tract of ventilated patients hospitalized in intensive care units. *Braz. J. Infect. Dis.* 16 (1): 45–51.

334 Hendaus, M.A., Jomha, F.A., and Alhammadi, A.H. (2015). Virus-induced secondary bacterial infection: a concise review. *Ther. Clin. Risk Manage.* 11: 1265–1271.

335 Rawson, T.M., Moore, L.S.P., Zhu, N. et al. (2020). Bacterial and fungal coinfection in individuals with coronavirus: a rapid review to support COVID-19 antimicrobial prescribing. *Clin. Infect. Dis.* 71 (9): 2459–2468.

336 Sepulveda, J., Westblade, L.F., Whittier, S. et al. (2020). Bacteremia and blood culture utilization during COVID-19 surge in New York City. *J. Clin. Microbiol.* 58 (8): e00875–e00820.

337 Koehler, P., Cornely, O.A., Bottiger, B.W. et al. (2020). COVID-19 associated pulmonary aspergillosis. *Mycoses* 63 (6): 528–534.

338 Blaize, M., Mayaux, J., Nabet, C. et al. (2020). Fatal invasive aspergillosis and coronavirus disease in an immunocompetent patient. *Emerg. Infect. Dis.* 26 (7): 1636–1637.

339 van Arkel, A.L.E., Rijpstra, T.A., Belderbos, H.N.A. et al. (2020). COVID-19-associated pulmonary aspergillosis. *Am. J. Respir. Crit. Care Med.* 202 (1): 132–135.

340 Bartoletti, M., Pascale, R., Cricca, M. et al. (2020). Epidemiology of invasive pulmonary aspergillosis among COVID-19 intubated patients: a prospective study. *Clin. Infect. Dis.* 2020: ciaa1065.

341 Ripa, M., Galli, L., Poli, A. et al. (2021). Secondary infections in patients hospitalized with COVID-19: incidence and predictive factors. *Clin. Microbiol. Infect.* 27 (3): 451–457.

342 Nori, P., Cowman, K., Chen, V. et al. (2021). Bacterial and fungal coinfections in COVID-19 patients hospitalized during the New York City pandemic surge. *Infect. Control Hosp. Epidemiol.* 42 (1): 84–88.

343 LeRose, J., Sandhu, A., Polistico, J. et al. (2020). The impact of COVID-19 response on central line associated bloodstream infections and blood culture contamination rates at a tertiary care center in greater Detroit area. *Infect. Control Hosp. Epidemiol.*: 1–4. https://doi.org/10.1017/ice.2020.1335.

344 Douglas, I.S., Rosenthal, C.A., Swanson, D.D. et al. (2021). Safety and outcomes of prolonged usual care prone position mechanical ventilation to treat acute coronavirus disease 2019 hypoxemic respiratory failure. *Crit. Care Med.* 49 (3): 490–502.

345 Aldawood, F., El-Saed, A., Zunitan, M.A., and Alshamrani, M. (2021). Central line-associated blood stream infection during COVID-19 pandemic. *J. Infect. Public Health* 14 (5): 668–669.

346 Fakih, M.G., Bufalino, A., Sturm, L. et al. (2021). Coronavirus disease 2019 (COVID-19) pandemic, central-line-associated bloodstream infection (CLABSI), and catheter-associated urinary tract infection (CAUTI): the urgent need to refocus on hardwiring prevention efforts. *Infect. Control Hosp. Epidemiol.*: 1–6. https://doi.org/10.1017/ice.2021.70.

347 Patel, P.R., Weiner-Lastinger, L.M., Dudeck, M.A. et al. (2021). Impact of COVID-19 pandemic on central-line-associated bloodstream infections during the early months of 2020, National Healthcare Safety Network. *Infect. Control Hosp. Epidemiol.*: 1–4. https://doi.org/10.1017/ice.2021.108.

348 Pronovost, P., Needham, D., Berenholtz, S. et al. (2006). An intervention to decrease catheter-related bloodstream infections in the ICU. *N. Engl. J. Med.* 355 (26): 2725–2732.

349 Parienti, J.J., Mongardon, N., Megarbane, B. et al. (2015). Intravascular complications of central venous catheterization by insertion site. *N. Engl. J. Med.* 373 (13): 1220–1229.

350 Marschall, J., Mermel, L.A., Fakih, M. et al. (2014). Strategies to prevent central line-associated bloodstream infections in acute care hospitals: 2014 update. *Infect. Control Hosp. Epidemiol.* 35 (Suppl 2)): S89–S107.

351 Arastehfar, A., Carvalho, A., Nguyen, M.H. et al. (2020). COVID-19-associated candidiasis (CAC): an underestimated complication in the absence of immunological predispositions? *J. Fungi (Basel)* 6 (4): 211.

352 Arastehfar, A., Carvalho, A., van de Veerdonk, F.L. et al. (2020). COVID-19 associated pulmonary aspergillosis (CAPA) – from immunology to treatment. *J. Fungi* 6 (2): 91.

353 Vaillancourt, M. and Jorth, P. (2020). The unrecognized threat of secondary bacterial infections with COVID-19. *MBio* 11 (4): e01806–e01820.

354 Langford, B.J., So, M., Raybardhan, S. et al. (2020). Bacterial co-infection and secondary infection in patients with COVID-19: a living rapid review and meta-analysis. *Clin. Microbiol. Infect.* 26 (12): 1622–1629.

355 Garcia-Vidal, C., Sanjuan, G., Moreno-García, E. et al. (2021). Incidence of co-infections and superinfections in hospitalized patients with COVID-19: a retrospective cohort study. *Clin. Microbiol. Infect.* 27 (1): 83–88.

356 Feng, Y., Ling, Y., Bai, T. et al. (2020). COVID-19 with different severities: a multicenter study of clinical features. *Am. J. Respir. Crit. Care Med.* 201 (11): 1380–1388.

357 Zhu, X., Ge, Y., Wu, T. et al. (2020). Co-infection with respiratory pathogens among COVID-2019 cases. *Virus Res.* 285: 198005.

358 Pritchett, M.A., Oberg, C.L., Belanger, A. et al. (2020). Society for Advanced Bronchoscopy Consensus Statement and Guidelines for bronchoscopy and airway management amid the COVID-19 pandemic. *J. Thorac. Dis.* 12 (5): 1781–1798.

359 American Society of Anesthesiologists; Anesthesia Patient Safety Foundation. (2020). APSF/ASA Guidance on Purposing Anesthesia Machines as ICU Ventilators. https://www.asahq.org/in-the-

spotlight/coronavirus-covid-19-information/
purposing-anesthesia-machines-for-ventilators.
(accessed 29 April 2021).

360 Savary, D., Lesimple, A., Beloncle, F. et al. (2020).
Reliability and limits of transport-ventilators to
safely ventilate severe patients in special surge
situations. *Ann. Intensive Care* 10 (1): 166.

361 Branson, R.D. (2007). Secretion management in the
mechanically ventilated patient. *Respir. Care* 52
(10): 1328–1342. discussion 42–47.

362 Respiratory care committee of Chinese Thoracic
Society (2020). Expert consensus on preventing
nosocomial transmission during respiratory care
for critically ill patients infected by 2019 novel
coronavirus pneumonia. *Zhonghua Jie He He Hu Xi
Za Zhi* 17: E020.

363 Lansbury, L., Lim, B., Baskaran, V., and Lim, W.S.
(2020). Co-infections in people with COVID-19: a
systematic review and meta-analysis. *J. Infect.* 81
(2): 266–275.

364 Kim, D., Quinn, J., Pinsky, B. et al. (2020). Rates of
co-infection between SARS-CoV-2 and other
respiratory pathogens. *JAMA* 323 (20): 2085–2086.

365 Wang, W., Xu, Y., Gao, R. et al. (2020). Detection of
SARS-CoV-2 in different types of clinical
specimens. *JAMA* 323 (18): 1843–1844.

366 Chang, S.H., Jiang, J., Kon, Z.N. et al. (2021). Safety
and efficacy of bronchoscopy in critically ill
patients with coronavirus disease 2019. *Chest* 159
(2): 870–872.

367 Jackson, T., Deibert, D., Wyatt, G. et al. (2020).
Classification of aerosol-generating procedures: a
rapid systematic review. *BMJ Open Respir. Res.* 7 (1):
e000730.

368 Gao, C.A., Bailey, J.I., Walter, J.M. et al. (2021).
Bronchoscopy on intubated COVID-19 patients is
associated with low infectious risk to operators.
Ann. Am. Thorac. Soc. 18: 1243–1246.

369 Bruyneel, M., Gabrovska, M., Rummens, P. et al.
(2020). Bronchoscopy in COVID-19 intensive care
unit patients. *Respirology* 25 (12): 1313–1315.

370 Lentz, R.J. and Colt, H. (2020). Summarizing societal
guidelines regarding bronchoscopy during the
COVID-19 pandemic. *Respirology* 25 (6): 574–577.

371 Luo, F., Darwiche, K., Singh, S. et al. (2020).
Performing bronchoscopy in times of the

COVID-19 pandemic: practice statement from an
international expert panel. *Respiration* 99 (5):
417–422.

372 Wahidi, M.M., Shojaee, S., Lamb, C.R. et al. (2020).
The use of bronchoscopy during the coronavirus
disease 2019 pandemic: CHEST/AABIP guideline
and expert panel report. *Chest* 158 (3): 1268–1281.

373 Licina, A. and Silvers, A. (2021). Use of powered
air-purifying respirator (PAPR) as part of protective
equipment against SARS-CoV-2-a narrative review
and critical appraisal of evidence. *Am. J. Infect.
Control* 49 (4): 492–499.

374 Roberge, M.R., Vojtko, M.R., Roberge, R.J. et al.
(2008). Wearing an N95 respirator concurrently
with a powered air-purifying respirator: effect on
protection factor. *Respir. Care* 53 (12):
1685–1690.

375 Miles, B.A., Schiff, B., Ganly, I. et al. (2020).
Tracheostomy during SARS-CoV-2 pandemic:
recommendations from the New York Head and
Neck Society. *Head Neck* 42 (6): 1282–1290.

376 Rosano, A., Martinelli, E., Fusina, F. et al. (2021).
Early percutaneous tracheostomy in coronavirus
disease 2019: association with hospital mortality and
factors associated with removal of tracheostomy
tube at ICU discharge. A cohort study on 121
patients. *Crit. Care Med.* 49 (2): 261–270.

377 McGrath, B.A., Brenner, M.J., Warrillow, S.J. et al.
(2020). Tracheostomy in the COVID-19 era: global
and multidisciplinary guidance. *Lancet Respir. Med.*
8 (7): 717–725.

378 Obata, K., Miyata, R., Yamamoto, K. et al. (2020).
Tracheostomy in patients with COVID-19: a
single-center experience. *in vivo* 34 (6): 3747–3751.

379 Krishnamoorthy, S., Polanco, A., Coleman, N. et al.
(2020). The safety and efficacy of tracheostomy in
patients diagnosed with COVID-19: an analysis of
143 patients at a major NYC Medical Center. *Ann.
Surg.* https://doi.org/10.1097/
SLA.0000000000004612.

380 Mattioli, F., Fermi, M., Ghirelli, M. et al. (2020).
Tracheostomy in the COVID-19 pandemic. *Eur.
Arch. Otorhinolaryngol.* 277 (7): 2133–2135.

381 Lamb, C.R., Desai, N.R., Angel, L. et al. (2020). Use
of tracheostomy during the COVID-19 pandemic:
American College of Chest Physicians/American

Association for Bronchology and Interventional Pulmonology/Association of Interventional Pulmonology Program Directors Expert Panel Report. *Chest* 158 (4): 1499–1514.

382 Freeman, B.D., Isabella, K., Lin, N., and Buchman, T.G. (2000). A meta-analysis of prospective trials comparing percutaneous and surgical tracheostomy in critically ill patients. *Chest* 118 (5): 1412–1418.

383 Kim, E.J., Yoo, E.H., Jung, C.Y., and Kim, K.C. (2020). Experience of percutaneous tracheostomy in critically ill COVID-19 patients. *Acute Crit. Care* 35 (4): 263–270.

384 Okuyemi, O.T., Spinner, A., Elkins, T. et al. (2021). Safe and efficient performance of open tracheostomies in patients with COVID-19-the fenestrated technique. *JAMA Otolaryngol. Head Neck Surg.* 147 (3): 301–302.

385 Hayek, S.S., Brenner, S.K., Azam, T.U. et al. (2020). In-hospital cardiac arrest in critically ill patients with covid-19: multicenter cohort study. *BMJ* 371: m3513.

386 Craig, S., Cubitt, M., Jaison, A. et al. (2020). Management of adult cardiac arrest in the COVID-19 era: consensus statement from the Australasian College for Emergency Medicine. *Med. J. Aust.* 213 (3): 126–133.

387 Mazer, S.P., Weisfeldt, M., Bai, D. et al. (2003). Reverse CPR: a pilot study of CPR in the prone position. *Resuscitation* 57 (3): 279–285.

388 Frost, D.W., Shah, R., Melvin, L. et al. (2020). Principles for clinical care of patients with COVID-19 on medical units. *CMAJ* 192 (26): E720–E726.

389 Mojoli, F., Mongodi, S., Grugnetti, G. et al. (2020). Setup of a dedicated coronavirus intensive care unit: logistical aspects. *Anesthesiology* 133 (1): 244–246.

390 Phan, L.T., Maita, D., Mortiz, D.C. et al. (2019). Personal protective equipment doffing practices of healthcare workers. *J. Occup. Environ. Hyg.* 16 (8): 575–581.

391 Liu, M., Cheng, S.Z., Xu, K.W. et al. (2020). Use of personal protective equipment against coronavirus disease 2019 by healthcare professionals in Wuhan, China: cross sectional study. *BMJ* 369: m2195.

392 Halpern, N., Kaplan, J., Rausen, M., and Yang, J. Configuring ICUs in the COVID-19 Era. Society of Critical Care Medicine. https://www.sccm.org/COVID19RapidResources/Resources/Configuring-ICUs-in-the-COVID-19-Era-A-Collection.

393 Department of Health and Human Services, Centers for Disease Control and Prevention, National Institute for Occupational Safety and Health. (2021). NIOSH fact sheet: the buddy system. National Institute for Occupational Safety and Health. https://www.cdc.gov/vhf/ebola/pdf/buddy-system.pdf (accessed 18 April 2021).

394 Abate, S.M., Ahmed Ali, S., Mantfardo, B., and Basu, B. (2020). Rate of intensive care unit admission and outcomes among patients with coronavirus: a systematic review and meta-analysis. *PLoS One* 15 (7): e0235653.

395 Petrilli, C.M., Jones, S.A., Yang, J. et al. (2020). Factors associated with hospital admission and critical illness among 5279 people with coronavirus disease 2019 in New York City: prospective cohort study. *BMJ* 369: m1966.

396 Argenziano, M.G., Bruce, S.L., Slater, C.L. et al. (2020). Characterization and clinical course of 1000 patients with coronavirus disease 2019 in New York: retrospective case series. *BMJ* 369: m1996.

397 Griffin, K.M., Karas, M.G., Ivascu, N.S., and Lief, L. (2020). Hospital preparedness for COVID-19: a practical guide from a critical care perspective. *Am. J. Respir. Crit. Care Med.* 201 (11): 1337–1344.

398 Fagiuoli, S., Lorini, F.L., Remuzzi, G., and Covid-19 Bergamo Hospital Crisis Unit (2020). Adaptations and lessons in the province of Bergamo. *N. Engl. J. Med.* 382 (21): e71.

399 Peters, A.W., Chawla, K.S., and Turnbull, Z.A. (2020). Transforming ORs into ICUs. *N. Engl. J. Med.* 382 (19): e52.

400 Aziz, S., Arabi, Y.M., Alhazzani, W. et al. (2020). Managing ICU surge during the COVID-19 crisis: rapid guidelines. *Intensive Care Med.* 46 (7): 1303–1325.

401 Harris, G.H., Baldisseri, M.R., Reynolds, B.R. et al. (2020). Design for implementation of a system-level

ICU pandemic surge staffing plan. *Crit. Care Explor.* 2 (6): e0136.

402 Anderson, J., Geeslin, A., and Streifel, A. (2021). Airborne infectious disease management: methods for temporary negative pressure isolation. Office of Emergency Preparedness, Minnesota Department of Health, Healthcare Systems Preparedness Program. https://www.health.state.mn.us/communities/ep/surge/infectious/airbornenegative.pdf (accessed 18 April 2021).

403 Tan, Z., Phoon, P.H.Y., Tien, C.J. et al. (2020). Practical considerations for converting operating rooms and post-anaesthesia care units into intensive care units in the COVID-19 pandemic – experience from a large Singapore Tertiary Hospital. *Ann. Acad. Med. Singapore* 49 (12): 1009–1012.

404 Ong, S. and Khee, T.T. (2020). Practical considerations in the anaesthetic management of patients during a COVID-19 epidemic. *Anaesthesia* 75 (6): 823–824.

405 Anderson, B.R., Ivascu, N.S., Brodie, D. et al. (2020). Breaking silos: the team-based approach to coronavirus disease 2019 pandemic staffing. *Crit Care Explor.* 2 (11): e0265.

406 Lambertsen, E.C. (1953). Nursing team organization and functioning: results of a study. Bureau of Publications, Teachers College, Columbia University.

407 Ferreira, P.C., Oliveira, E.S.T.S., Almeida, D.R. et al. (2021). Conversion of noninvasive mechanical ventilator to provide invasive mechanical ventilation. *Eur. J. Anaesthesiol.* 38 (3): 311–313.

408 Beitler, J.R., Mittel, A.M., Kallet, R. et al. (2020). Ventilator sharing during an acute shortage caused by the COVID-19 pandemic. *Am. J. Respir. Crit. Care Med.* 202 (4): 600–604.

409 US Food and Drug Administration. (2020). Using ventilator splitters during the COVID-19 pandemic – letter to health care providers.https://www.fda.gov/medical-devices/letters-health-care-providers/using-ventilator-splitters-during-covid-19-pandemic-letter-health-care-providers (accessed 20 April 2021).

410 Daugherty Biddison, E.L., Faden, R., Gwon, H.S. et al. (2019). Too many patients. . . A framework to guide statewide allocation of scarce mechanical ventilation during disasters. *Chest* 155 (4): 848–854.

411 Carenzo, L., Costantini, E., Greco, M. et al. (2020). Hospital surge capacity in a tertiary emergency referral centre during the COVID-19 outbreak in Italy. *Anaesthesia* 75 (7): 928–934.

412 Shah, A.G., Taduran, C., Friedman, S. et al. (2020). Relocating IV pumps for critically ill isolated coronavirus disease 2019 patients from bedside to outside the patient room. *Crit. Care Explor.* 2 (8): e0168.

413 King, C.A. and Ogg, M. (2012). Safe injection practices for administration of propofol. *AORN J.* 95 (3): 365–372.

414 Garzotto, F., Comoretto, R.I., Ostermann, M. et al. (2021). Preventing infectious diseases in intensive care unit by medical devices remote control: lessons from COVID-19. *J. Crit. Care* 61: 119–124.

415 Austin, A., Pezzano, C., Lydon, D., and Chopra, A. (2020). Use of external ventilator control panel for mechanical ventilation in patients with severe SARS-CoV-2 infection. *QJM* 2020: hcaa229.

416 Donovan, D. (2020). Remote control for patient ventilators. https://www.hopkinsmedicine.org/news/articles/remote-control-for-patient-ventilators (accessed 29 April 2021).

11

COVID-19: ICU and Critical Care Management

Daniel Crouch, Alexandra Rose, Cameron McGuire, Jenny Yang, Mazen Odish, and Amy Bellinghausen

Division of Pulmonary, Critical Care, and Sleep Medicine, Department of Medicine, University of California San Diego, La Jolla, CA, USA

Abbreviations

AGP	aerosol-generating procedure
ARDS	acute respiratory distress syndrome
CI	confidence interval
CoV	coronavirus
CPR	cardiopulmonary resuscitation
ECMO	extracorporeal membrane oxygenation
FiO$_2$	fraction of inspired oxygen
GI	gastrointestinal
HCW	healthcare worker
HFO	high-flow oxygen
ICU	intensive care unit
IHCA	in-hospital cardiac arrest
MAP	mean arterial pressure
MERS	Middle East respiratory syndrome
NIV	noninvasive ventilation
OR	odds ratio
PaO$_2$	partial pressure of oxygen, arterial
PEEP	positive end-expiratory pressure
PICS	post–intensive care syndrome
PPE	personal protective equipment
PTSD	posttraumatic stress disorder
R$_0$	reproductive value
SARS	severe acute respiratory syndrome
SpO$_2$	oxygen saturation
VAP	ventilator-associated pneumonia
VTE	venous thromboembolism
WHO	World Health Organization

Epidemiology of Critically Ill Patients with COVID-19 Pneumonia

The first report of a new respiratory illness in Wuhan, China, was made on December 31, 2019 [1]. Ninety-two days later, the international case count would top 1 million [2]. The pace at which coronavirus disease 2019 (COVID-19) proliferated remains astounding to contemplate. Early attempts at tracking the spread and attempting to understand the severity of the disease were complicated by limited access to testing, inadequate early point-of-care test characteristics, and inefficient reporting mechanisms, among numerous other problems. As a result, there are widely divergent reports throughout the literature about incidence, prevalence, clinical features of disease, severity of disease, risk factors for severe disease, and clinically significant outcomes such as intensive care unit (ICU) admission, mechanical ventilation, and death.

A review of the overall epidemiology of COVID-19 is beyond the scope of this chapter. We will focus on the epidemiology of severe and critical illness. Severe illness from COVID-19 pneumonia is defined as patients with oxygen saturation (SpO$_2$) < 94% on room air at sea level, a partial pressure of oxygen, arterial/fraction of inspired oxygen (PaO$_2$/FiO$_2$) ratio < 300 mmHg, a respiratory rate > 30 breaths/min, or lung infiltrates in more than 50% of the thorax on imaging. Critical illness is defined as individuals with respiratory failure, septic shock, or multiorgan dysfunction [3].

With the aforementioned limitations and definitions in mind, about 80–85% of patients who tested positive for COVID-19 infection experienced asymptomatic, mild, or moderate disease. In China, 19% of patients with COVID-19 infection were hospitalized (14% with severe disease and 5% with critical disease) [4]. In the United States, 14% of patients with COVID-19 infection were hospitalized with severe or critical disease [5]. Similar rates were observed in other early hard-hit countries such as Italy, Iran, Spain, and the United Kingdom.

Risk Factors for Severe Disease

A number of factors have been associated with the development of severe disease, hospitalization, and mortality, although three in particular require emphasis because of their nonmodifiable nature: age, sex, and the presence of comorbidities. A modeling study from China showed an 18% chance of hospitalization for patients older than 80 years old compared with 1% for patients 20–29 years old and only 4% for those 50–59 years old [6]. In a large US study, patients 80 years and older had 16 times greater mortality when compared with patients 18–34 years old [7]. A large UK study demonstrated a 20-fold increased risk for death in individuals 80 years and older when compared with individuals 50–59 years [8]. Male sex also has been associated with an increased risk for all endpoints, independent of comorbidities. A large meta-analysis of more than 3 million global cases showed an odds ratio (OR) of 2.84 for ICU admission and an OR of 1.39 for mortality when comparing men with women [9]. Numerous comorbidities [10] with varying levels of evidence [11] have been linked to worse outcomes in COVID-19. The most notable comorbidities, because of their global prevalence, include cardiovascular disease (including hypertension), diabetes mellitus, chronic kidney disease, obesity, smoking, chronic lung disease, and cancer. Immunosuppression is also significantly associated with worse outcomes, with the highest rates in solid organ and stem cell transplant patients. In an early report from Italy, of 355 patients who died with COVID-19, only 3 patients had no comorbidities and the average number of

comorbidities was 2.7, with 172 patients (48.5%) having three or more conditions [12]. Similar trends were seen in an early analysis of more than 1.3 million laboratory-confirmed cases of COVID-19 reported to the Centers for Disease Control and Prevention between 22 January 2020 and 20 May 2020. Patients with underlying comorbidities were 6 times as likely to be hospitalized and 12 times as likely to die when compared with patients who reported no underlying conditions; cardiovascular disease, diabetes, and chronic lung disease represent the most frequently reported comorbidities [5].

Mortality

For those patients ill enough to be admitted to the hospital, in-hospital mortality from COVID-19 infection during the pandemic was high. A study from the US Veterans Health Administration system showed a mortality rate fivefold higher for nearly 4000 patients with COVID-19 hospitalized between March and May of 2020 when compared with nearly 5500 patients with influenza hospitalized from October 2018 to February 2020 (21% vs. 3.8% mortality rate, respectively) even after controlling for age, sex, race/ethnicity, and underlying comorbidities [13]. This mortality rate was supported in a large cohort study of 35 302 patients admitted to US hospitals between 1 April 2020 and 31 May 2020, in which there was a 20.3% mortality rate, a 19.4% ICU admission rate, and a 15.9% mechanical ventilation rate [6]. However, as the pandemic progressed, mortality among the critically ill declined, as demonstrated in a large study from England [14]. It is uncertain whether this was due to an initial surge that overwhelmed systems, better resource allocation later, improved understanding of the disease, better therapeutics, or some combination of all of these factors. In contrast with these improvements in resource-rich settings, in resource-limited settings the in-hospital 30-day mortality has remained exceedingly high (48.2%) [15]. However, what proportion of this mortality is from insufficient resources and what proportion is from significant comorbidities known to increase risk for severe and critical disease is unclear.

Although the pandemic has slowed, emerging variants, reduced precautions such as masking, and inadequate global vaccination threaten the ability to control this disease [16]. As such, the epidemiology may continue to change, placing even greater primacy on promising, but as yet unproven, prediction models [17] aimed at improving earlier diagnosis and prognosis in COVID-19.

Infection Prevention and Control of COVID-19 in the ICU

Early during the pandemic, much was written about the basic reproductive value (R_0) of COVID-19. Simplified for the purposes of this review, R_0 is the number of people who are likely to become infected by one positive person (e.g. $R_0 = 4$ means 1 person is likely to infect 4 others) [18]. A virus with an $R_0 > 1$ will continue to spread, while an $R_0 < 1$ will eventually recede. Early accounts of COVID-19's spread had widely divergent R_0 estimates ranging from 1.5 to 5, although the best estimates listed an R_0 of 2.5 [19]. More importantly, nearly 30% of people with COVID-19 were asymptomatic, accounting for nearly 50% of its transmission [20]. Therefore, it stands to reason that impeccable infection-control measures are essential for protection of patients and hospital staff. What follows are recommendations for infection prevention and control in an ICU unburdened by scarce resources or supply chain issues.

Due to the rates of presymptomatic transmission, symptom screening of hospitalized patients and visitors is insufficient [21, 22]. As a result, universal masking of all people entering the hospital is a widespread recommendation by all major public health groups [23, 24]. Additional recommendations regarding what type of mask to wear vary widely among sources and depend largely on context. However, N95 masks have superior filtration efficiency compared with surgical masks with ties or procedural masks with ear loops (98.5% vs. 71.5% vs. 38.1, respectively) [25]. In all cases, the filtration efficiency was contingent on the tightness of the fit of the mask. Based on these differences in filtration efficiency, the Centers for Disease Control and Prevention recommends that all healthcare workers (HCWs) wear N95 masks for direct patient care of anyone who is known to be positive or suspected to be positive for COVID-19 [26]. Conversely, the World Health Organization (WHO) recommends medical-grade masks for HCWs if aerosol-generating procedures (AGPs) are not being performed consistent with standard contact and droplet precautions [27].

Aerosol-Generating Procedures

A partial list of AGPs performed in most ICUs includes bronchoscopy, intubation, extubation, percutaneous tracheostomy, high-flow oxygen (HFO), noninvasive ventilation (NIV), ventilator filter/tubing changes, airway suctioning, sputum induction, and nebulizer treatments, among others [28]. As a result, HCWs in ICUs are at significantly increased risk for infection because of aerosolization of viral particles. From barrier shields during intubation [29] to constant flow canopies for patients on HFO and NIV [30], various solutions have been used to minimize risk for infection to HCWs. Although an overview of all these techniques is beyond the scope of this section, we will discuss a few specific protocols at our institution that we use to mitigate risk from viral aerosolization.

When intubating patients with impending respiratory failure from COVID-19, maximizing first-pass success is fundamental. A failed endotracheal intubation attempt usually requires bag-valve mask oxygenation to be performed before a second attempt, which unnecessarily exposes HCWs to aerosolized virus and potentially increases infection risk. To maximize first-pass success, our institution has a COVID-19 intubation team consisting of the most experienced intubators in the hospital (usually anesthesia) with a dedicated intubation kit and dedicated personal protective equipment (PPE). We prefer to intubate with video laryngoscopy over direct laryngoscopy because it increases the likelihood of first-pass success in some [31–33], but not all, studies [34]. During intubation, we try to minimize the number of staff in the room and have very specific protocols about entering a room after intubation (more on this later). Early in the pandemic, the need for first-pass intubation success was particularly important because we were not routinely preoxygenating patients with HFO or NIV to minimize the risk for aerosolization.

Institutional protocols can also minimize AGPs. Protocols exist for respiratory culture sampling, bronchodilator administration, and ventilator filter/tubing changes. For respiratory culture sampling, we prefer endotracheal aspirates rather than bronchoalveolar lavage in most cases, acknowledging the limitations of this approach [35]. We rarely administer nebulizers and instead rely on metered-dose inhalers consistent with Centers for Disease Control and Prevention [11] and WHO [36] recommendations, especially because data suggest equal efficacy between modalities [37, 38]. For ventilator filter/tubing changes or switching to a transport ventilator, we have cloth-covered clamps to occlude the circuit at the endotracheal tube both to prevent alveolar derecruitment from loss of positive end-expiratory pressure (PEEP) and to avoid accidental aerosolization from a patient cough at an inopportune time.

After intubation, percutaneous tracheostomy is probably the next most common AGP performed in our ICU. Our protocol is largely in line with the October 2020 consensus statement regarding tracheostomy in patients with COVID-19 [39]. In short, we perform percutaneous dilatational tracheostomy at the bedside in the ICU in airborne infection isolation rooms, also known as negative pressure rooms. We favor the use of enhanced PPE over standard PPE, substituting a powered air-purifying respirator or contained air-purifying respirator instead of an N95 mask with a face shield. We maintain a closed circuit for as much of the procedure as possible and pause ventilation for as long as the patient can tolerate during the portion of the procedure with an open airway. After an AGP of any kind is performed, we require at least one hour before an HCW can enter the room without enhanced PPE. This time interval was chosen because our airborne infection isolation rooms have six air changes per hour and 69 minutes is the estimated time necessary for 99.9% air clearance [40].

Visitation

Finally, because the risk for asymptomatic and presymptomatic transmission was exceedingly high before the initiation of vaccinations, we had a very strict ICU visitation policy. Visitors were permitted only for patients at the end of life, to assist with communication, for procedural consent, and to help offset delirium. This policy was informed by two separate considerations. First, although it was highly unlikely, an asymptomatic visitor could expose HCWs to COVID-19 despite a nega-

tive symptom screen, strict social distancing protocols, and universal masking mandates at our institution. Second, and more importantly, the frequency with which AGPs are performed in our ICU had the potential to expose visitors to COVID-19, whereupon they could subsequently become ill and/or potentially expose additional people after leaving the hospital. This was primarily because we had no way of ensuring that visitors had adequate-fitting masks and could not guarantee that N95 masks provided to visitors would work in the absence of certified fit-testing. Similar policies were enacted in ICUs across the country, with many examples of the negative consequences of these policies [41–44]. With the variable uptake of vaccines and the emerging threat of variants, we will continually adjust and update our policies to maintain fastidious infection prevention and control.

Cardiopulmonary Resuscitation in COVID-19

There are approximately 300 000 in-hospital cardiac arrests (IHCAs) annually in the United States, with approximately 25% who survive to hospital discharge [45, 46]. Over the last decade, rate of survival to discharge after IHCA has increased, because it is appreciated that delays in initiation of chest compressions and defibrillations lead to poorer outcomes [47, 48]. The COVID-19 pandemic has led to a resurgence in these discussions as survival rates are anticipated to be poor because of delays in cardiopulmonary resuscitation (CPR) efforts.

Early experiences from Wuhan reported a 30-day survival after IHCA of less than 3%, while a more recent study found 12% survival to discharge after IHCA [49, 50]. Notably, only 57% of patients underwent CPR, while the remainder had a do not resuscitate order in place. Although no details are provided, the pandemic has prompted discussions regarding futility of CPR in patients with COVID-19, especially considering limited resources, potential aerosolization during CPR with high risk for transmission to providers, and the assumption of poor survival and outcomes in these patients. Given these concerns, some have advocated for blanket do not resuscitate orders for all patients with COVID-19 [51, 52]. There remains significant controversy in these decisions, but appropriate goals-of-care conversations should continue as usual for all ICU patients.

In general, IHCAs (i.e. "code blue") tend to attract many individuals, with a host of people both in and directly outside the room. However, for patients with COVID-19, there should be an emphasis on minimizing the number of providers who are at risk for exposure and maximizing skill level of the code blue team. As an example, the COVID-19 code blue protocol at our institution calls for a code leader who is the most senior physician on the ICU team, an attending anesthesiologist for intubation, two respiratory therapists, one pharmacist, one code nurse, one primary nurse, and two additional staff members for chest compressions (if necessary) to be in the room. There are also a limited number of individuals outside the room as well, including a few people who may be substituted for chest compressions if needed.

Most importantly, healthcare providers need to take the time to appropriately don PPE before entering the room. Although this will inherently lead to a delay in initiation of CPR, it is vital that providers take the time to protect themselves [53, 54]. To help expedite this, a cart or box with PPE for three to five individuals should be reserved and available on the unit for emergent situations. In addition to PPE, other delays to CPR may include if the patient is in the prone position. Although it is possible to perform CPR in the prone position, it is likely more effective in the supine position because of provider familiarity [55, 56]. However, a provider may start CPR with the patient prone until adequate personnel are available to position a patient supine.

Cardiac arrest is common in critically ill patients, and there is a heightened awareness in the COVID-19 pandemic. With a systematic approach and well-organized protocols in place, it is possible to balance patient care during IHCA with the safety of healthcare providers.

Hemodynamic Support in COVID-19

Adult patients with shock in the setting of COVID-19 infection should be managed identically to those adult patients with septic shock as previously published in the *Surviving Sepsis Campaign* guidelines [57, 58]. Fluid resuscitation should be guided by dynamic measurements, such as pulse pressure variation, stroke volume variation, and stroke volume changes with straight leg raises or fluid boluses. Other parameters that may also be helpful in assessing fluid responsiveness are lactate levels, skin temperature, and capillary refill time [59, 60]. Balanced crystalloids are recommended over unbalanced crystalloids for acute resuscitation for shock [61]. It is not recommended to use albumin routinely for initial resuscitation.

When vasoactive medications are required, norepinephrine is the first-line vasopressor choice [62]. Vasopressin or epinephrine should be added to norepinephrine if needed to raise mean arterial pressure (MAP) and decrease the norepinephrine dosage. A MAP of 60–65 mmHg should be targeted with vasoactive agent titration, rather than targeting a higher MAP goal [63]. For those patients with refractory shock who have completed a course of corticosteroids for COVID-19 treatment, stress-dose steroids should be used. Hydrocortisone 200 mg intravenously, either as a continuous infusion or divided into bolus dosing, is the typical dosage. If the patient is currently prescribed corticosteroids for COVID-19 treatment, then additional hydrocortisone therapy is not recommended. For those patients with evidence of cardiac dysfunction despite adequate fluid resuscitation and vasopressor titration, the use of dobutamine should be considered. Echocardiogram and mixed venous oxygen saturations, along with the other dynamic measurements, and lactate levels can be helpful in making this determination.

Management of Respiratory Failure from COVID-19

In a non-resource-limited setting, patients admitted to the hospital with rapidly escalating oxygen requirements should be transferred to an ICU setting, where clinical deterioration can be monitored closely. Concerns about aerosolization of viral particles and increased transmission to HCWs via heated high-flow nasal cannula or noninvasive mechanical ventilation has frequently limited the use of these devices in patients with COVID-19. It is increasingly recognized that high-flow nasal cannula and noninvasive positive pressure ventilation may be used safely in patients with COVID-19. Strategies such as the use of negative pressure rooms when available; surgical mask placement over high-flow, high-humidity nasal cannulas; tight-fitting oral masks or full-face masks when using noninvasive mechanical ventilation; and the use of viral filters both with nonrebreather masks and on the expiratory ports of noninvasive ventilators may increase the safety of these devices [64, 65]. Beyond the risk of aerosolization of viral particles, at the time of this publication, there remains insufficient evidence to support routine use of noninvasive positive pressure ventilation and high-flow nasal cannula in patients with COVID-19-associated hypoxemic respiratory failure or acute respiratory distress syndrome (ARDS). Society guidelines variably support the use of these measures in the treatment of respiratory failure from this disease, with some suggesting that the use of noninvasive positive-pressure ventilation may be appropriate in cases of mild COVID-19-associated ARDS or as a trial period before intubation and invasive mechanical ventilation [66].

Intubation

One of the biggest challenges facing critical care providers is determining when to proceed with intubation in a patient with COVID-19. Early and incomplete reports of the outcomes of invasive mechanical ventilation in this patient population deterred both physicians and the public from pursuing invasive mechanical ventilation and remain a challenge to treating physicians today [67]. Patients with ARDS secondary to COVID-19 have prolonged stays in the ICU and an average time of 14 days on mechanical ventilation, similar to other studies in non-COVID-19-associated ARDS [68].

There are a number of very clear reasons to proceed with intubation in a patient with hypoxemic respiratory failure and COVID-19. A patient with rapidly evolving infiltrates on chest imaging and an increased work of breathing is more likely to fail treatment with high-flow nasal cannula or noninvasive positive-pressure ventilation. A ROX index [ratio of SpO_2/FiO_2 (%) to respiratory rate (breaths/min)] may be a useful adjunct in early identification of patients who will

progress to require invasive mechanical ventilation [69]. Physicians should additionally be attentive to patient-reported symptoms of increased dyspnea despite adequate oxygenation and ventilation. Furthermore, indicators of secondary organ damage are critical considerations in the decision to intubate. Patients with signs of cardiovascular failure (i.e. worsening pulmonary edema, electrocardiographic changes, inducible chest pain), progressive renal injury, and neurologic changes, such as increased agitation or delirium, are dynamic changes to be considered in a critically ill patient with COVID-19.

Ventilator Management

Once the decision has been made to intubate, it is ideal to evaluate respiratory mechanics in the first hour after intubation while the patient remains effectively paralyzed to assess optimal ventilator settings. Ventilator management should include strategies to minimize ventilator-induced lung injury: low tidal volume ventilation with tidal volumes approximating 6 cc/kg ideal body weight or occasionally lower [70], plateau pressure of less than 30 cm H_2O, some amount of PEEP [71], and prone positioning [72]. Driving pressure (plateau pressure − PEEP) less than 15 cm H_2O while on a volume-controlled mode of ventilation has been associated with improved survival in ARDS, recognizing that the accuracy of this measurement (plateau pressure) is dependent on a patient who makes no spontaneous respiratory effort [73, 74]. The decision to initiate neuromuscular blockade is patient dependent. Patients in whom ventilator asynchrony persists despite adequate sedation and patients with refractory hypoxemia may benefit from a trial of early neuromuscular blockade [75, 76]. Prone positioning is not an inherent indication to initiate neuromuscular blockade, although in patients in whom there are safety concerns with prone positioning (such as hemodynamic instability or increased ventilator asynchrony), bolus-dose paralytic for the prone positioning may be helpful but rarely indicates a need for continuous neuromuscular blockade.

Although many patients with COVID-19-associated ARDS may require relatively high levels of PEEP to maintain oxygenation early in their disease course, ARDS remains a dynamic disease process. Moderate to high levels of PEEP later in the clinical course may result in alveolar overdistension and worsening gas exchange, perhaps as patients enter the fibroproliferative phase or even progress to the fibrotic phase of ARDS. Frequent bedside assessment is paramount to ensuring that both the patient's ventilator settings remain optimized and the patient–ventilator synchrony promotes a truly lung-protective approach.

Prone Positioning

Prone positioning is a fundamental component of the management of ARDS with PROSEVA (2013), a large multicenter randomized control trial, demonstrating a significant reduction in mortality with prone positioning [72] and subsequent meta-analysis including earlier trials supporting this benefit [77]. Prone positioning improves ventilation–perfusion matching, recruitment of dependent lung regions, and chest wall mechanics, and it enhances postural mucociliary clearance [77, 78]. Ventral displacement of the right atrium in the prone position may additionally increase venous return via gravity, allowing a preload-dependent patient to augment cardiac output in this position [78]. The benefit of prone positioning on ARDS mortality appears to be independent of improvements in gas exchange in the prone position [79], which is an important concept to consider before aborting efforts at prone positioning.

Patients with COVID-19-associated ARDS benefit from prone positioning early and often in their disease course. Based on the data from PROSEVA, many clinicians target prone positioning in patients with a PaO_2/FiO_2 ratio less than 150 while on a minimum FiO_2 of 0.6 and PEEP of 5 cm H_2O in conjunction with low tidal volume ventilation for at least 16 hours daily. Virtually all patients with COVID-19-associated ARDS will meet these criteria after intubation. The length of time in the prone position may be extended beyond 16 hours in a 24-hour period based on patient tolerance (attention to skin breakdown, pressure points, safety) and clinical resources. The decision to stop prone positioning in a patient is typically made when a patient has demonstrated significant and sustained clinical improvement such that ventilator support remains minimal. There are very few relative contraindications to prone positioning in ARDS, with the only absolute contraindication being an unstable spinal fracture [80]. Strategies such as a prone team, a "prone champion," and increased education and collaboration between staff and institutions have been proposed and executed in various settings to overcome barriers to widespread prone positioning of mechanically ventilated patients with COVID-19 [81].

Treatment of COVID-19-Associated ARDS with Corticosteroids

Interest in the use of corticosteroids for the treatment of ARDS long precedes the COVID-19 pandemic and has produced conflicting data to date [82–85]. Most recently, the DEXA-ARDS study, which randomized patients with moderate to severe ARDS to dexamethasone versus placebo, demonstrated both a reduction in duration of mechanical ventilation and a mortality benefit [86]. It remains unclear from available data whether corticosteroids are beneficial in ARDS due to pneumonia from other viruses. In prior severe acute respiratory syndrome (SARS) and Middle East respiratory syndrome (MERS) epidemics, steroids have been associated with delayed coronavirus (CoV) RNA clearance [87, 88], and in influenza, steroids have been associated with higher mortality and increased secondary infections [89].

Corticosteroids remain an attractive therapeutic option to target the proinflammatory-mediated lung injury characteristic of ARDS, and they are an inexpensive, globally available resource. Early case series during the COVID-19 pandemic [90] resulted in robust efforts to clarify the use of steroids in COVID-19 pneumonia and specifically in patients with ARDS. Before publication of the dexamethasone data from the RECOVERY trial, a large, randomized, open-label trial comparing various COVID-19 treatments versus usual care, the WHO and other professional societies did not support the use of steroids in the treatment of COVID-19 pneumonia.

RECOVERY trial data resoundingly support the use of dexamethasone in patients with severe COVID-19 requiring mechanical ventilation with a decreased incidence of death compared with usual care (29.3% vs. 41.4%; rate ratio, 0.64; 95% confidence interval [CI], 0.51–0.81) and in patients with an oxygen requirement not requiring invasive mechanical ventilation (23.3% vs. 26.2%; rate ratio, 0.82; 95% CI, 0.72–0.94) [91]. On 2 September 2020, *JAMA* published three randomized controlled trials [92–94], a prospective meta-analysis of seven randomized trials [95], and an editorial [96]. Based on these results, the WHO updated guidelines to recommend systemic corticosteroids in the treatment of patients with severe and critical COVID-19.

It is now standard of care to use corticosteroids in the treatment of COVID-19 ARDS in both mechanically ventilated patients and patients with an oxygen requirement. Many institutions have adopted protocols using the protocol from the RECOVERY trial: dexamethasone 6 mg once daily (intravenous or oral) for up to 10 days or until hospital discharge if sooner. Adjustments to corticosteroid dosing may be considered in light of individual patient characteristics, such as preceding use of corticosteroids for immunosuppression or chronic lung disease. Patients from areas with endemic fungal or parasitic infections (such as coccidiomycosis or strongyloidiasis) should be treated with caution. The optimal timing of corticosteroid initiation remains to be determined, although data would suggest administration of corticosteroids at any time in the patient's COVID-19 ARDS course would be superior to withholding therapy.

Tocilizumab for Critical COVID-19 Illness

Among other inflammatory cytokines, interleukin-6 has been shown to be elevated in critically ill patients with COVID-19 infection. Tocilizumab is a recombinant humanized anti–interleukin-6 receptor monoclonal antibody that has been studied for the treatment of COVID-19 infection. Two of the largest randomized controlled trials, REMAP-CAP and RECOVERY, evaluated the use of tocilizumab in COVID-19 infections. Both studies reported both a mortality benefit and a reduction in the need for mechanical ventilation in specific subsets of patients who were showing rapid respiratory deterioration and/or an increased inflammatory response [91, 97].

The National Institutes of Health and WHO recommend the use of tocilizumab as a single intravenous dose of 8 mg/kg actual body weight up to 800 mg in combination with dexamethasone in hospitalized patients with COVID-19 who are showing rapid respiratory decompensation [28, 98]. More specifically, physicians should consider treatment with tocilizumab for patients hospitalized within the past three days and admitted to the ICU within the past 24 hours requiring advanced respiratory support, such as mechanical ventilation, noninvasive mechanical ventilation, or high-flow nasal cannula, or recently admitted (within three days) patients not in the ICU requiring NIV or high-flow nasal cannula and who also have elevated markers of inflammation (C-reactive protein > 75 mg/l). There is insufficient evidence to support tocilizumab use in patients receiving conventional oxygen therapy. There is also insufficient evidence to support repeat dosing of tocilizumab. Cases of disseminated strongyloidiasis infection have been reported in patients receiving tocilizumab with dexamethasone [99, 100]. Prophylaxis with ivermectin should be considered in patients from strongyloidiasis-endemic areas, which are typically in the tropics, subtropics, and warm temperature regions [101].

Liver enzymes should be monitored while administering tocilizumab therapy, and the treatment should be avoided in patients with alanine aminotransferase levels more than five times the upper limit of normal. Neutropenia and thrombocytopenia are uncommon. Tocilizumab should also generally be avoided in patients with recent use of biologic immunomodulating drugs other than glucocorticoids; those at high risk for gastrointestinal (GI) perforation; and patients with uncontrolled serious bacterial, fungal, or non-COVID viral infection, an absolute neutrophil count < 500 cells/μl, a platelet count < 50 000 cells/μl, or known hypersensitivity to tocilizumab. Current recommendations are against use of tocilizumab in pregnancy due to paucity of available data [102].

Extracorporeal Membrane Oxygenation for COVID-19 ARDS

Extracorporeal membrane oxygenation (ECMO) may be considered in patients with COVID-19 ARDS with severe and refractory hypoxemic and hypercapnic respiratory failure despite conventional management [103]. ECMO is a type of mechanical circulatory life support that oxygenates and removes carbon dioxide from the patient's blood. Although it was initially used in the pediatric population, adult use has substantially increased after the influenza H1N1 pandemic in 2009 [104].

The inclusion and exclusion ECMO criteria for patients with COVID-19 are similar to other causes of ARDS. ECMO criteria guidelines have been published by the Extracorporeal Life Support Organization (ELSO; see Table 11.1) [105]. The inclusion criteria require a low PaO_2/FiO_2 ratio despite using low tidal volume ventilation, prone positioning, appropriate PEEP titration, and possibly neuromuscular blockade and pulmonary vasodilators. Patients who meet criteria should be referred to a regional ECMO center for consideration. Legal medical decision makers should be appropriately counseled on the risks of ECMO, including the survival rate in patients with COVID-19, which is approximately 55–70% [106].

ECMO is a supportive therapy and is used as a bridge to recovery or even rarely lung transplantation [107]. ECMO allows clinicians to further minimize ventilator pressures and respiratory rate, to ultimately decrease ventilator-induced lung injury [108]. ECMO is not without risks, which include bleeding (i.e. intracranial or cannulation site hemorrhage), infections, hemolysis, and circuit thrombosis or failure [100]. Despite its risks, ECMO may be considered for patients with severe ARDS caused by COVID-19 that is refractory to conventional therapies.

Tracheostomy Placement in COVID-19

For patients with COVID-19 with prolonged need for mechanical ventilation, tracheostomy placement should be considered. The optimal timing of tracheostomy placement is currently unknown, and recommendations vary widely [39]. Some guidelines recommend early tracheostomy, which may be attributed to higher case volumes in those regions. Others recommend waiting for at least 14 days of mechanical ventilation before tracheostomy placement [109]. More recent data have suggested that early tracheostomy tube placement, within 7–12 days, was associated with improved outcomes, including shorter duration of mechanical ventilation and a higher rate of weaning from mechanical ventilation [110]. Routine RT-PCR testing for COVID-19 before tracheostomy is not generally recommended [103], although some

Table 11.1 Indications and contraindications for VV-ECMO for adults with COVID-19.

Indications

$PaO_2/FiO_2 < 60$ mmHg for >6 h

$PaO_2/FiO_2 < 50$ mmHg for >3 h

$pH < 7.2 + PaCO_2 > 80$ mmHg for >6 h

Relative contraindications

Age ≥ 65 yr

Obesity BMI ≥ 40

Immunocompromised status

No legal medical decision maker available

Advanced chronic underlying systolic heart failure

High-dose vasopressor requirement (and not under consideration for VA or V-VA ECMO)

Absolute contraindications

Advanced age

Clinical Frailty Scale category ≥ 3

Mechanical ventilation >10 d

Significant underlying comorbidities: CKD stage ≥ 3

Cirrhosis

Dementia

Baseline neurologic disease that would preclude rehabilitation potential

Disseminated malignancy

Advanced lung disease

Uncontrolled diabetes with chronic end-organ dysfunction

Severe deconditioning

Protein-energy malnutrition

Severe peripheral vascular disease

Other preexisting life-limiting medical condition

Nonambulatory or unable to perform activities

Severe multiple organ failure

Severe acute neurologic injury, e.g. anoxic, stroke

Uncontrolled bleeding

Contraindications to anticoagulation

Inability to accept blood products

Ongoing CPR

BMI, body mass index; CKD, chronic kidney disease; VA, venoarterial; VV, venovenous; V-VA, veno-venous arterial.
Source: Adapted from the ELSO guidelines [105].

institutions opt to wait for negative COVID testing before an elective tracheostomy. Most importantly, tracheostomy placement should not be done during times of increased instability or significant ventilator dependence. General guidance for appropriate ventilator settings would include PEEP at or less than 8 cm H_2O and FiO_2 at or less than 60%.

Tracheostomy tube placement is likely to benefit only those patients who are clinically improving. Tracheostomy tube placement can be done via an open surgical or percutaneous approach. There is no clear advantage to an open surgical tracheostomy over a percutaneous approach, but preference is institution dependent. Many centers have favored routine percutaneous tracheostomies for most patients with positive outcomes, reserving surgical tracheostomies for those patients with more difficult airway anatomy [111]. Techniques minimizing aerosolization of the virus during the procedure are important, regardless of whether the tracheostomy is done via an open surgical or percutaneous approach.

Similar to endotracheal intubations, particular attention should be made to minimize risk for transmission of the virus to HCWs. The most experienced staff and the fewest number of staff needed in the room should be utilized for this procedure. Proper donning and doffing of full PPE should be performed, including N95 or equivalent mask, eye protection, gloves, and gown, because this is an AGP [103]. Some guidelines recommend the use of powered air-purifying respiratory devices for this procedure. When following proper safety guidelines, risk for infection to HCWs is minimal [112, 113]. Tracheostomy placement should be done in a negative-pressure room, if possible, or in an operating room. If available, a disposable bronchoscope should be considered when performing percutaneous tracheostomy placement. A closed ventilatory circuit with in-line suctioning should be used after completion of the tracheostomy tube placement. After tracheostomy placement, standard care and tracheostomy tube replacement procedures should be followed, similar to those placed for non-COVID-related reasons. However, as described earlier, there needs to be an emphasis on safety precautions at all times when manipulating or opening the airway.

Standard ICU Care During COVID-19

Arguably one of the most important aspects of care for patients with COVID-19 admitted to the ICU is standardized, bundled, evidence-based practices. In 2005, this was recognized by Jean-Louis Vincent, MD,

PhD, FCCM, who published the "give fast hug (at least) once a day" [114]. The FASTHUG mnemonic within the next few years would become the ICU standard checklist for general care of all ICU patients. This was updated to the FASTHUGS-BID in 2019 [115]. The Society of Critical Care Medicine created a similar ICU liberation bundle in 2013, ABCDEF, which was updated in 2018 [116, 117]. Both of these checklists are shown in Figure 11.1, and the breakdown of these ICU checklists/bundles will be detailed briefly in this section.

Nutritional support in the ICU is important to help minimize the catabolic state of critically ill patients with COVID-19. Enteral tube feeds should be started within 48 hours on patients who have been appropriately resuscitated, although obtaining full caloric replacement is likely unnecessary for the first seven days [119]. Early nutrition may also decrease infectious complications [120]. Many mechanically ventilated patients require a continuous infusion of propofol for sedation. Due to the lipid emulsion in propofol, these patients may require less overall enteral nutrition, and consultation with a registered dietitian is recommended. Patients with COVID-19 and respiratory failure are frequently placed in the prone position; however, this should not be a contraindication to enteral nutrition [121]. Due to high sedation requirements and critical illness in patients with COVID-19, many may have gut motility alterations, such as constipation, feeding intolerance, or diarrhea. Although there are bundles to prevent constipation, there is little evidence that it improves patient-centric outcomes, such as mortality, ICU days, or ventilator days [122]. Nutrition support is preferably done enterally and early, while ensuring appropriate bowel care.

Nutritional and bowel care goes hand in hand with glucose control in the ICU. Hypoglycemia is an acute and dangerous state that should be corrected quickly. However, hyperglycemia is also common in the ICU and has been associated with poor outcomes [123]. Intensive glucose control (goal 80–110 mg/dl) increases hypoglycemic events and may actually increase ICU mortality [124, 125]. Many patients with COVID-19 are at risk for hyperglycemia due to their predisposing diabetes and obesity, compounded by corticosteroid therapy [126, 127]. Thus, the goal

FAST HUGS BID	ABCDEF		
Feeding/Fluids	**A Element**	: Assess, Prevent, and Manage Pain	
Analgesia	**B Element**	: Both Spontaneous Awakening Trials (SATs) and Spontaneous Breathing Trials (SBTs)	
Sedation	**C Element**	: Choice of Analgesia and Sedation	
Thromboprophylaxis	**D Element**	: Delirium: Assess, Prevent, and Manage	
Head up Position	**E Element**	: Early Mobility and Exercise	
Ulcer prophylaxis	**F Element**	: Family Engagement and Empowerment	
Glycemic Control			
Spontaneous Breathing Trial			
Bowel care			
Indwelling catheter removal			
De-escalation of antibiotics			

Figure 11.1 Standard ICU care during COVID-19. FAST-HUGS-BID mnemonic on the left column and the ABCDEF liberation bundle on the right column [115, 116]. *Sources:* Based on Lim et al. [118] and Mahmood et al. [111].

glucose level in the ICU should be 140–180 mg/dl for the majority of ICU patients, including ones with COVID-19.

Nosocomial bacterial pneumonia is common in patients with ARDS. Ventilator-associated pneumonias (VAPs) can develop after 48 hours of mechanical ventilation and have clinical signs (fevers, tachycardia, increased/purulent secretions), worsening hypoxemia, leukocytosis, decreasing tidal volume or pulmonary compliance, and suggestive infiltrates on imaging. VAPs are the leading cause of death in hospital-acquired infections, with a mortality rate of 10–40% [128]. VAP prevention includes elevating the head of the bed to 30–45 degrees, oral care, peptic ulcer disease prophylaxis, and synchronized spontaneous breathing and awakening trials. Multiple organizations recommend elevating the head of the bed to 30–45° [129–131]. If this is not possible, then the highest degree elevation would be appropriate. Similarly, daily oral care with chlorhexidine gluconate helps decrease oral bacterial burden. Ventilator liberation is a very important goal for all patients. The practice of spontaneous awakening trials coupled with spontaneous breathing trials have increased mechanical ventilator–free days and decreased ICU length of stay [132, 133]. Nursing and respiratory therapist coordination is essential to perform spontaneous breathing trials and spontaneous awakening trials together. Overall, these bundles help decrease ICU mortality, morbidity, and length of stay.

Similar to VAPs, patients who require prolonged intubation are at increased risk for stress-related GI bleeding [134]. Gastric stress ulcers normally develop in the fundus and body of the stomach. Patients with the following are considered high risk for GI bleeding: mechanical ventilation for greater than 48 hours, coagulopathy (platelets $<50\,000\,m^3$, international normalized ratio > 1.5, partial thromboplastin time $>2\times$ control), renal replacement therapy, recent GI bleed, traumatic brain/spinal injury, severe burns (>35%), or two or more minor factors (sepsis, occult GI bleeding ≥6 days, ICU stay >1 week, glucocorticoid administration) [135]. These high-risk patients should be given a histamine (H2) receptor antagonist or proton pump inhibitor. There have been previous concerns of *Clostridium difficile* infections with proton pump inhibitors, although this has not been seen in more recent studies [136]. Overall, because of long intubation times, many patients with COVID-19 will require at least an H2-blocker.

Although adequate and timely empiric broad-spectrum antibiotics are essential in sepsis or septic shock to reduce mortality, the appropriate de-escalation of antibiotics is similarly crucial to minimize drug resistance and *C. difficile* rates [137–139]. De-escalating antibiotics is especially important in patients with COVID-19 because many are empirically started on them at admission. Furthermore, many mechanically ventilated patients will have an ICU course complicated by a VAP, so antibiotic stewardship is necessary to prevent drug-resistant organisms [140]. In addition, preventing urinary catheter and central line infections by removing them as early as clinically possible is important to minimize ICU morbidity and mortality [141].

Venous Thromboembolism and Anticoagulation in COVID-19

Venous thromboembolism (VTE) prophylaxis is part of routine ICU care and is one of the cornerstones of the ICU care bundle. However, despite prophylactic anticoagulation, it has been anecdotally observed that rates of VTE remain high in critically ill patients with COVID-19 [142]. Reports of VTE incidence in patients with COVID-19 are exceedingly variable, ranging between 7% and 70% [136–147], likely reflecting the heterogeneity in protocols for VTE screening, prophylaxis, and patient population.

The underlying pathogenesis of hypercoagulability in COVID-19 is incompletely understood but is thought to be related to dysfunction in all three arms of Virchow's triad. Autopsy studies of patients with COVID-19 have commonly indicated widespread microthrombi in alveolar capillaries, endotheliitis, and angiogenesis [148–150]. Due to the prevalence of microthrombi that have been clinically observed, some have advocated for the use of fibrinolytic therapy for refractory hypoxemia in select patients [151–153]. Although these published case series report optimistic results, thrombolytics (i.e. tissue plasminogen activator) should not be assumed as a standard of care in these patients.

Although there appears to be a strong association with thrombosis in COVID-19, there are reports of devastating hemorrhages as well. One study noted that more than 20% of patients developed a hemorrhagic complication while receiving therapeutic anticoagulation, with only about half of those patients having a documented VTE or other strong indication for full-dose anticoagulation [154]. In a different report of critically ill patients with COVID-19, the incidence of major bleeding in the cohort was just greater than 5%,

which was balanced with a VTE rate of approximately 7% [137]. Many of these bleeding events occurred while the patient was receiving normal prophylactic anticoagulation. Therefore, if empiric intensification of anticoagulation to therapeutic doses or administration of fibrinolytic therapy is being considered, it should be done with caution in select patients and weighed against the risk for bleeding.

Given the lack of robust data, the best course of action regarding anticoagulation is to continue with usual ICU care, which has been well studied for decades. This includes thromboprophylaxis at standard doses for all ICU patients unless there is a contraindication. Low-molecular-weight heparin and fondaparinux may be preferred given once-daily dosing compared with unfractionated heparin. Active surveillance for VTE with routine D-dimer levels and lower extremity dopplers is likely unnecessary. However, if there is clinical concern for VTE, diagnostic imaging and testing should be pursued at that time, and if confirmatory, therapeutic anticoagulation should be started. Limited evidence exists for empiric therapeutic anticoagulation, higher dose prophylactic anticoagulation, and fibrinolytic therapy. Ongoing research is investigating optimal thromboprophylaxis in patients with COVID-19, including the potential role of antiplatelet agents (COVID-PACT; ClinicalTrials.gov: NCT04409834). However, pending these results, as well as those of multiple other studies that are underway, thromboprophylaxis in critically ill patients with COVID-19 should be guided by previous large studies of VTE prophylaxis in the ICU.

After the ICU: Challenges for Survivors of COVID-19 Critical Illness

Post–intensive care syndrome (PICS) is a constellation of deficits in physical, psychosocial and cognitive functioning that persist after a critical illness and often have major impacts on quality of life (see Figure 11.2). Unfortunately, PICS is a common outcome after ICU admission; even 5 years after their index hospitalization, patients with ARDS have reduced quality of life, six-minute walk distance, and physical function compared with population norms [155].

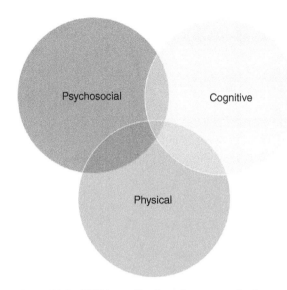

Figure 11.2 PICS is a collection of symptoms in three domains of function, which occurs after ICU discharge and has major impacts on quality of life.

Rates of cognitive dysfunction in ARDS survivors are elevated, and in elderly patients, average cognitive function scores were similar to patients with a diagnosis of Alzheimer dementia [156]. Symptoms of post-traumatic stress disorder (PTSD) and depression are also common after ARDS, with rates of up to 44% and 37%, respectively [150, 157].

Because COVID-19 was only identified in 2019, data on long-term outcomes are very limited. However, it is likely that patients with ARDS secondary to COVID-19 will have some of the same challenges as patients recovering from ARDS as a result of other causes. A recent case series of 488 patients recovering from COVID-19 (including both patients admitted to the ICU and those treated in general wards) showed that at 60 days after discharge, approximately 40% (188/488) were "unable to return to normal activity" [158]. Psychiatric complications are also not uncommon after COVID-19, with Mazza et al. [159] describing a cohort of survivors, 55% of whom had symptoms of at least one mental disorder (including depression, anxiety, PTSD, and insomnia). Cognitive outcomes after COVID-19 are not well studied, but there is reason to believe that patients may struggle with thought clarity and memory impairment [160].

As with cognitive, psychosocial, and physical dysfunction after COVID-19 infection, data on long-term pulmonary outcomes are very limited. However, predictions regarding long-term outcomes can be made based on what is known about long-term outcomes of ARDS and other CoV infections (SARS-CoV-1 and MERS). For survivors of ARDS, although many patients have spirometric and gas-exchange abnormalities at the time of hospital discharge, most will have normal or near-normal pulmonary function testing at five years after their illness. The most frequent long-term change in pulmonary function is reduced diffusing capacity [149]. Fibrotic pulmonary changes were seen not infrequently after SARS-CoV-1 or MERS infection, and it is anticipated that SARS-CoV-2 may have similar consequences [161, 162].

Management of PICS, whether caused by COVID-19 or other critical illness, is directed at reducing symptoms and improving function. For instance, patients struggling with exercise tolerance because of residual pulmonary scarring may benefit from pulmonary rehabilitation. Others with symptoms of anxiety or PTSD may benefit from mental health referral. If available, referral to an ICU recovery clinic (a multidisciplinary, intensivist-led, critical illness follow-up clinic) can be beneficial. These clinics provide not only diagnostic and therapeutic help to patients but also education about and normalization of the symptoms of PICS. Survivor support groups (held either virtually or in person) may also assist patients in the recovery process.

References

1 Center for Infectious Disease Research and Policy, University of Minnesota. Chinese Officials probe unidentified pneumonia outbreak in Wuhan. CIDRAP. 2021. https://www.cidrap.umn.edu/news-perspective/2019/12/news-scan-dec-31-2019 (accessed 27 Jun 2021).

2 Johns Hopkins University & Medicine Coronavirus Resource Center. COVID-19 Dashboard. 2021. https://coronavirus.jhu.edu/map.html (accessed 27 Jun 2021).

3 COVID-19 Treatment Guidelines Panel. Coronavirus Disease 2019 (COVID-19) Treatment Guidelines.

National Institutes of Health. 2021. https://www.covid19treatmentguidelines.nih.gov (accessed 26 Jun 2021).

4 Wu, Z. and McGoogan, J.M. (2020). Characteristics of and important lessons from the coronavirus disease 2019 (COVID-19) outbreak in China: summary of a report of 72 314 cases from the Chinese Center for Disease Control and Prevention. *JAMA* 323 (13): 1239–1242.

5 Stokes, E.K., Zambrano, L.D., Anderson, K.N. et al. (2020). Coronavirus disease 2019 case surveillance – United States, January 22-May 30, 2020. *MMWR Morb Mortal Wkly Rep.* 69 (24): 759–765.

6 Verity, R., Okell, L.C., Dorigatti, I. et al. (2020). Estimates of the severity of coronavirus disease 2019: a model-based analysis. *Lancet Infect Dis.* 20 (6): 669–677.

7 Rosenthal, N., Cao, Z., Gundrum, J. et al. (2020). Risk factors associated with in-hospital mortality in a US National Sample of patients with COVID-19. *JAMA Netw. Open* 3 (12): e2029058.

8 Williamson, E.J., Walker, A.J., Bhaskaran, K. et al. (2020). Factors associated with COVID-19-related death using OpenSAFELY. *Nature* 584: 430–436.

9 Peckham, H., de Gruijter, N.M., Raine, C. et al. (2020). Male sex identified by global COVID-19 meta-analysis as a risk factor for death and ITU admission. *Nat Commun.* 11: 6317.

10 Centers for Disease Control and Prevention. COVID-19 and Underlying Medical Conditions, Information for Healthcare Workers. 2021. https://www.cdc.gov/coronavirus/2019-ncov/hcp/clinical-care/underlyingconditions.html (accessed 29 Jun 2021).

11 Centers for Disease Control and Prevention. Evidence for Conditions that Increase Risk of Severe Illness. 2021. https://www.cdc.gov/coronavirus/2019-ncov/science/science-briefs/underlying-evidence-table.html (accessed 29 Jun 2021).

12 Onder, G., Rezza, G., and Brusaferro, S. (2020). Case-fatality rate and characteristics of patients dying in relation to COVID-19 in Italy. *JAMA.* 323 (18): 1775–1776.

13 Cates, J., Lucero-Obusan, C., Dahl, R.M. et al. (2020). Risk for in-hospital complications associated with COVID-19 and influenza – veterans health administration, United States, October 1, 2018–May 31, 2020. *MMWR Morb Mortal Wkly Rep.* 69: 1528–1534.

14 Dennis, J.M., McGovern, A.P., Vollmer, S.J., and Mateen, B.A. (2021). Improving survival of critical care patients with coronavirus disease 2019 in England: a National Cohort Study, March to June 2020. *Crit Care Med.* 49 (2): 209–214.

15 Biccard, B.M., Gopalan, P.D., Miller, M. et al. (2021). Patient care and clinical outcomes for patients with COVID-19 infection admitted to African high-care or intensive care units (ACCCOS): a multicentre, prospective, observational cohort study. *Lancet* 397 (10288): 1885–1894.

16 Usherwood, T., LaJoie, Z., and Srivastava, V. (2021). A model and predictions for COVID-19 considering population behavior and vaccination. *Sci Rep.* 11: 12015.

17 Wynants, L., Van Calster, B., Collins, G.S. et al. (2020). Prediction models for diagnosis and prognosis of covid-19: systematic review and critical appraisal. *BMJ* 369 (m1328).

18 Diekmann, O., Heesterbeek, J.A., and Metz, J.A. (1990). On the definition and the computation of the basic reproduction ratio R0 in models for infectious diseases in heterogeneous populations. *J Math Biol.* 28 (4): 365–382.

19 Li, Q., Guan, X., Wu, P. et al. (2020). Early transmission dynamics in Wuhan, China, of novel coronavirus–infected pneumonia. *N Engl J Med.* 382: 1199–1207.

20 Subramanian, R., He, Q., and Pascual, M. (2021). Quantifying asymptomatic infection and transmission of COVID-19 in New York city using observed cases, serology, and testing capacity. *Proc Natl Acad Sci USA.* 118 (9): e2019716118.

21 Wei, W.E., Li, Z., Chiew, C.J. et al. (2020). Presymptomatic transmission of SARS-CoV-2 – Singapore, January 23-March 16, 2020. *MMWR Morb Mortal Wkly Rep.* 69 (14): 411–415.

22 Arons, M.M., Hatfield, K.M., Reddy, S.C. et al. (2020). Presymptomatic SARS-CoV-2 infections and transmission in a skilled nursing facility. *N Engl J Med.* 382 (22): 2081–2090.

23 Klompas, M., Morris, C.A., Sinclair, J. et al. (2020). Universal masking in hospitals in the Covid-19 era. *N Engl J Med.* 382 (21): e63.

24 Leung, N.H.L., Chu, D.K.W., Shiu, E.Y.C. et al. (2020). Respiratory virus shedding in exhaled breath and efficacy of face masks. *Nat Med.* 26: 676–680.

25 Sickbert-Bennett, E.E., Samet, J.M., Clapp, P.W. et al. (2020). Filtration efficiency of hospital face mask alternatives available for use during the COVID-19 pandemic. *JAMA Intern Med.* 180 (12): 1607–1612.

26 Centers for Disease Control and Prevention. Strategies for optimizing the supply of N95 respirators. 2021. https://www.cdc.gov/coronavirus/2019-nCoV/hcp/infection-control.html (accessed 12 Jul 2021).

27 World Health Organization. Mask use in the contxt of COVID-19. (2021). https://www.who.int/publications/i/item/advice-on-the-use-of-masks-in-the-community-during-home-care-and-in-healthcare-settings-in-the-context-of-the-novel-coronavirus-(2019-ncov)-outbreak (accessed Jul 12, 2021).

28 National Institutes of Health. COVID-19 treatment guidelines. 2021. https://www.covid19treatmentguidelines.nih.gov/about-the-guidelines/whats-new. (accessed 12 Jul 2021).

29 Canelli, R., Connor, C.W., Gonzalez, M. et al. (2020). Barrier enclosure during endotracheal intubation. *N Engl J Med.* 382: 1957–1958.

30 Adir, Y., Segol, O., Kompaniets, D. et al. (2020). COVID-19: minimising risk to healthcare workers during aerosol-producing respiratory therapy using an innovative constant flow canopy. *Eur Respir J.* 55 (5): 2001017.

31 Liu, D.X., Ye, Y., Zhu, Y.H. et al. (2019). Intubation of non-difficult airways using video laryngoscope versus direct laryngoscope: a randomized, parallel-group study. *BMC Anesthesiol.* 19 (75).

32 Mosier, J.M., Whitmore, S.P., Bloom, J.W. et al. (2013). Video laryngoscopy improves intubation success and reduces esophageal intubations compared to direct laryngoscopy in the medical intensive care unit. *Crit Care.* 17 (R237).

33 Hypes, C.D., Stolz, U., Sakles, J.C. et al. (2016). Video laryngoscopy improves odds of first-attempt success at intubation in the intensive care unit. A propensity-matched analysis. *Ann Am Thorac Soc.* 13 (3): 382–390.

34 Lascarrou, J.B., Boisrame-Helms, J., Bailly, A. et al. (2017). Video laryngoscopy vs direct laryngoscopy on successful first-pass orotracheal intubation among ICU patients: a randomized clinical trial. *JAMA* 317 (5): 483–493.

35 Scholte, J.B., van Dessel, H.A., Linssen, C.F. et al. (2014). Endotracheal aspirate and bronchoalveolar lavage fluid analysis: interchangeable diagnostic modalities in suspected ventilator-associated pneumonia? *J Clin Microbiol.* 52 (10): 3597–3604.

36 World Health Organization. Infection prevention and control during health care when novel coronavirus (nCoV) infection is suspected. 2021. https://www.who.int/publications/i/item/10665-331495. (accessed 3 Jul 2021).

37 Cates, C.J., Welsh, E.J., and Rowe, B.H. (2013). Holding chambers (spacers) versus nebulisers for beta-agonist treatment of acute asthma. *Cochrane Database Syst Rev.* 9: CD000052.

38 Dhuper, S., Chandra, A., Ahmed, A. et al. (2011). Efficacy and cost comparisons of bronchodilatator administration between metered dose inhalers with disposable spacers and nebulizers for acute asthma treatment. *J Emerg Med.* 40 (3): 247–255.

39 Lamb, C.R., Desai, N.R., Angel, L. et al. (2020). Use of tracheostomy during the COVID-19 pandemic: American College of Chest Physicians/American Association for Bronchology and Interventional Pulmonology/Association of Interventional Pulmonology Program Directors Expert Panel Report. *Chest* 158 (4): 1499–1514.

40 Centers for disease Control and Prevention. Infection control – Appendix B: air. 2021. https://www.cdc.gov/infectioncontrol/guidelines/environmental/appendix/air.html (accessed 14 Jul 2021).

41 Griffin, K.M., Karas, M.G., Ivascu, N.S., and Lief, L. (2020). Hospital preparedness for COVID-19: a practical guide from a critical care perspective. *Am J Respir Crit Care Med.* 201 (11): 1337–1344.

42 Wakam, G.K., Montgomery, J.R., Biesterveld, B.E., and Brown, C.S. (2020). Not dying alone – modern compassionate care in the Covid-19 pandemic. *N Engl J Med.* 382 (24): e88.

43 Haziq Siddiqi, B.S. (2020). To suffer alone: hospital visitation policies during COVID-19. *J Hosp Med.* 11: 694–695.

44 Valley, T.S., Schutz, A., Nagle, M.T. et al. (2020). Changes to visitation policies and communication practices in Michigan ICUs during the COVID-19 pandemic. *Am J Respir Crit Care Med.* 202 (6): 883–885.

45 Holmberg, M.J., Ross, C.E., Fitzmaurice, G.M. et al. (2019). Annual incidence of adult and pediatric in-hospital cardiac arrest in the United States. *Circ Cardiovasc Qual Outcomes* 12 (7): e005580. https://doi.org/10.1161/CIRCOUTCOMES.119.005580.

46 Andersen, L.W., Holmberg, M.J., Berg, K.M. et al. (2019). In-hospital cardiac arrest: a review. *JAMA* 321 (12): 1200–1210. https://doi.org/10.1001/jama.2019.1696.

47 Girotra, S., Nallamothu, B.K., Spertus, J.A. et al. (2012). Trends in survival after in-hospital cardiac arrest. *N Engl J Med.* 367 (20): 1912–1920. https://doi.org/10.1056/NEJMoa1109148.

48 Chan, P.S., Krumholz, H.M., Nichol, G., and Nallamothu, B.K. (2008). Delayed time to defibrillation after in-hospital cardiac arrest. *N Engl J Med.* 358 (1): 9–17. https://doi.org/10.1056/NEJMoa0706467.

49 Shao, F., Xu, S., Ma, X. et al. (2020). In-hospital cardiac arrest outcomes among patients with COVID-19 pneumonia in Wuhan, China. *Resuscitation* 151: 18–23. https://doi.org/10.1016/j.resuscitation.2020.04.005.

50 Hayek, S.S., Brenner, S.K., Azam, T.U. et al. (2020). In-hospital cardiac arrest in critically ill patients with covid-19: multicenter cohort study. *BMJ* 371: m3513. https://doi.org/10.1136/bmj.m3513.

51 Chan, P.S., Berg, R.A., and Nadkarni, V.M. (2020). Code blue during the COVID-19 pandemic. *Circ Cardiovasc Qual Outcomes* 13 (5): e006779. https://doi.org/10.1161/CIRCOUTCOMES.120.006779.

52 Mahase, E. and Kmietowicz, Z. (2020). Covid-19: doctors are told not to perform CPR on patients in cardiac arrest. *BMJ* 368: m1282. https://doi.org/10.1136/bmj.m1282.

53 Couper, K., Taylor-Phillips, S., Grove, A. et al. (2020). COVID-19 in cardiac arrest and infection risk to rescuers: a systematic review. *Resuscitation* 151: 59–66. https://doi.org/10.1016/j.resuscitation.2020.04.022.

54 Watson, L., Sault, W., Gwyn, R., and Verbeek, P.R. (2008). The "delay effect" of donning a gown during cardiopulmonary resuscitation in a simulation model. *Can J Emerg Med.* 10 (4): 333–338. https://doi.org/10.1017/S1481803500010332.

55 Bhatnagar, V., Jinjil, K., Dwivedi, D. et al. (2018). Cardiopulmonary resuscitation: unusual techniques for unusual situations. *J Emerg Trauma Shock* 11 (1): 31–37. https://doi.org/10.4103/JETS.JETS_58_17.

56 Ludwin, K., Szarpak, L., Ruetzler, K. et al. (2020). Cardiopulmonary resuscitation in the prone position: a good option for patients with COVID-19. *Anesth Analg.* 131 (3): e172–e173. http://doi.org/10.1213/ANE.0000000000005049.

57 Rhodes, A., Evans, L.E., Alhazzani, W. et al. (2017). Surviving sepsis campaign: international guidelines for management of sepsis and septic shock: 2016. *Crit Care Med.* 45 (3): 486–552.

58 Alhazzani, W., Evans, L., Alshamsi, F. et al. (2021). Surviving sepsis campaign guidelines on the management of adults with coronavirus disease 2019 (COVID-19) in the ICU: first update. *Crit Care Med.* 49 (3): e219–e234.

59 Bednarczyk, J.M., Fridfinnson, J.A., Kumar, A. et al. (2017). Incorporating dynamic assessment of fluid responsiveness into goal-directed therapy: a systematic review and meta-analysis. *Crit Care Med.* 45 (9): 1538–1545.

60 Pan, J., Peng, M., Liao, C. et al. (2019). Relative efficacy and safety of early lactate clearance-guided therapy resuscitation in patients with sepsis: a meta-analysis. *Medicine (Baltimore)* 98 (8): e14453.

61 Semler, M.W., Self, W.H., Wanderer, J.P. et al. (2018). Balanced crystalloids versus saline in critically ill adults. *N Engl J Med.* 378 (9): 829–839.

62 Avni, T., Lador, A., Lev, S. et al. (2015). Vasopressors for the treatment of septic shock: systematic review and meta-analysis. *PLoS One* 10 (8): e0129305.

63 Asfar, P., Meziani, F., Hamel, J.F. et al. (2014). High versus low blood-pressure target in patients with septic shock. *N Engl J Med* 370 (17): 1583–1593.

64 Kaur, R., Weiss, T.T., Perez, A. et al. (2020). Practical strategies to reduce nosocomial transmission to healthcare professionals providing respiratory care to patients with COVID-19. *Crit Care.* 24 (1): 571. https://doi.org/10.1186/s13054-020-03231-8.

65 Li, J., Fink, J.B., and Ehrmann, S. (2020). High-flow nasal cannula for COVID-19 patients: low risk of bio-aerosol dispersion. *Eur Respir J.* 55 (5): 2000892. https://doi.org/10.1183/13993003.00892-2020.

66 Dobler, C.C., Murad, M.H., and Wilson, M.E. (2020). Noninvasive positive pressure ventilation in patients with COVID-19. *Mayo Clin Proc.* 95 (12): 2594–2601. https://doi.org/10.1016/j.mayocp.2020.10.001.

67 Richardson, S., Hirsch, J.S., Narasimhan, M. et al. (2020). Presenting characteristics, comorbidities, and outcomes among 5700 patients hospitalized with COVID-19 in the New York city area. *JAMA* 323 (20): 2052–2059. https://doi.org/10.1001/jama.2020.6775.

68 Ferrando, C., Suarez-Sipmann, F., Mellado-Artigas, R. et al. (2020). Clinical features, ventilatory management, and outcome of ARDS caused by COVID-19 are similar to other causes of ARDS. *Intensive Care Med.* 46 (12): 2200–2211. https://doi.org/10.1007/s00134-020-06192-2.

69 Roca, O., Caralt, B., Messika, J. et al. (2019). An index combining respiratory rate and oxygenation to predict outcome of nasal high-flow therapy. *Am J Respir Crit Care Med.* 199 (11): 1368–1376. https://doi.org/10.1164/rccm.201803-0589OC.

70 Acute Respiratory Distress Syndrome Network, Brower, R.G., Matthay, M.A. et al. (2000). Ventilation with lower tidal volumes as compared with traditional tidal volumes for acute lung injury and the acute respiratory distress syndrome. *N Engl J Med* 342 (18): 1301–1308. https://doi.org/10.1056/nejm200005043421801.

71 Brower, R.G., Lanken, P.N., MacIntyre, N. et al. National Heart, Lung, and Blood Institute ARDS Clinical Trials Network(2004). Higher versus lower positive end-expiratory pressures in patients with the acute respiratory distress syndrome. *N Engl J Med* 351 (4): 327–336. https://doi.org/10.1056/nejmoa032193.

72 Guérin, C., Reignier, J., Richard, J.C. et al. (2013). Prone positioning in severe acute respiratory distress syndrome. *N Engl J Med.* 368 (23): 2159–2168. https://doi.org/10.1056/nejmoa1214103.

73 Amato, M.B.P., Meade, M.O., Slutsky, A.S. et al. (2015). Driving pressure and survival in the acute respiratory distress syndrome. *N Engl J Med.* 372 (8): 747–755. https://doi.org/10.1056/nejmsa1410639.

74 Aoyama, H., Pettenuzzo, T., Aoyama, K. et al. (2018). Association of driving pressure with mortality among ventilated patients with acute respiratory distress syndrome: a systematic review and meta-analysis. *Crit Care Med.* 46 (2): 300–306. https://doi.org/10.1097/CCM.0000000000002838.

75 National Heart, Lung, and Blood Institute PETAL Clinical Trials Network, Moss, M., Huang, D.T. et al. (2019). Early neuromuscular blockade in the acute respiratory distress syndrome. *N Engl J Med.* 380 (21): 1997–2008. https://doi.org/10.1056/nejmoa1901686.

76 Papazian, L., Forel, J.M., Gacouin, A. et al. (2010). Neuromuscular blockers in early acute respiratory distress syndrome. *N Engl J Med.* 363: 1107–1116.

77 Beitler, J.R., Shaefi, S., Montesi, S.B. et al. (2014). Prone positioning reduces mortality from acute respiratory distress syndrome in the low tidal volume era: a meta-analysis. *Intensive Care Med.* 40 (3): 332–41. https://doi.org/10.1007/s00134-013-3194-3.

78 Scholten, E.L., Beitler, J.R., Prisk, G.K., and Malhotra, A. (2017). Treatment of ARDS with prone positioning. *Chest* 151: 215–224. https://doi.org/10.1016/j.chest.2016.06.032.

79 Albert, R.K., Keniston, A., Baboi, L. et al. (2014). Prone position-induced improvement in gas exchange does not predict improved survival in the acute respiratory distress syndrome. *Am J Respir Crit Care Med.* 189 (4): 494–496. https://doi.org/10.1164/rccm.201311-2056LE.

80 Guérin, C., Albert, R.K., Beitler, J. et al. (2020). Prone position in ARDS patients: why, when, how and for whom. *Intensive Care Med.* 46 (12): 2385–2396. https://doi.org/10.1007/s00134-020-06306-w.

81 Cotton, S., Zawaydeh, Q., LeBlanc, S. et al. (2020). Proning during covid-19: challenges and solutions. *Heart Lung.* 49 (6): 686–687. https://doi.org/10.1016/j.hrtlng.2020.08.006.

82 Annane, D., Sébille, V., and Bellissant, E. (2006). Effect of low doses of corticosteroids in septic shock patients with or without early acute respiratory distress syndrome. *Crit Care Med.* 34 (1): 22–30. https://doi.org/10.1097/01.CCM.0000194723.78632.62.

83 Meduri, G.U., Golden, E., Freire, A.X. et al. (2007). Methylprednisolone infusion in early severe ARDS: results of a randomized controlled trial. *Chest* 131 (4): 954–963. https://doi.org/10.1378/chest.06-2100.

84 Tongyoo, S., Permpikul, C., Mongkolpun, W. et al. (2016). Hydrocortisone treatment in early sepsis-associated acute respiratory distress syndrome:

results of a randomized controlled trial. *Crit Care.* 20 (1): 329. https://doi.org/10.1186/s13054-016-1511-2.

85 Steinberg, K.P., Hudson, L.D., Goodman, R.B. et al. National Heart, Lung, and Blood Institute Acute Respiratory Distress Syndrome (ARDS) Clinical Trials Network(2006). Efficacy and safety of corticosteroids for persistent acute respiratory distress syndrome. *N Engl J Med.* 354 (16): 1671–1684. https://doi.org/10.1056/nejmoa051693.

86 Villar, J., Ferrando, C., Martínez, D. et al. (2020). Dexamethasone treatment for the acute respiratory distress syndrome: a multicentre, randomised controlled trial. *Lancet Respir Med.* 8 (3): 267–276. https://doi.org/10.1016/S2213-2600(19)30417-5.

87 Lee, N., Allen Chan, K.C., Hui, D.S. et al. (2004). Effects of early corticosteroid treatment on plasma SARS-associated coronavirus RNA concentrations in adult patients. *J Clin Virol.* 31 (4): 304–309. https://doi.org/10.1016/j.jcv.2004.07.006.

88 Arabi, Y.M., Mandourah, Y., Al-Hameed, F. et al. (2018). Corticosteroid therapy for critically ill patients with middle east respiratory syndrome. *Am J Respir Crit Care Med.* 197 (6): 757–767. https://doi.org/10.1164/rccm.201706-1172OC.

89 Lansbury, L.E., Rodrigo, C., Leonardi-Bee, J. et al. (2020). Corticosteroids as adjunctive therapy in the treatment of influenza: an updated Cochrane systematic review and meta-analysis. *Crit Care Med.* 48 (2): e98–e106. https://doi.org/10.1097/CCM.0000000000004093.

90 Wu, C., Chen, X., Cai, Y. et al. (2020). Risk factors associated with acute respiratory distress syndrome and death in patients with coronavirus disease 2019 pneumonia in Wuhan, China. *JAMA Intern Med* 180 (7): 934–943. https://doi.org/10.1001/jamainternmed.2020.0994.

91 RECOVERY Collaborative Group, Horby, P., Lim, W.S. et al. (2021). Dexamethasone in hospitalized patients with Covid-19. *N Engl J Med.* 384 (8): 693–704. https://doi.org/10.1056/nejmoa2021436.

92 Tomazini, B.M., Maia, I.S., Cavalcanti, A.B. et al. (2020). Effect of dexamethasone on days alive and ventilator-free in patients with moderate or severe acute respiratory distress syndrome and COVID-19: the CoDEX randomized clinical trial. *JAMA* 324 (13): 1307–1316. https://doi.org/10.1001/jama.2020.17021.

93 Dequin, P.F., Heming, N., Meziani, F. et al. (2020). Effect of hydrocortisone on 21-day mortality or respiratory support among critically ill patients with COVID-19: a randomized clinical trial. *JAMA.* 324 (13): 1298–1306. https://doi.org/10.1001/jama.2020.16761.

94 Angus, D.C., Derde, L., Al-Beidh, F. et al. (2020). Effect of hydrocortisone on mortality and organ support in patients with severe COVID-19: the REMAP-CAP COVID-19 corticosteroid domain randomized clinical trial. *JAMA* 324 (13): 1317–1329. https://doi.org/10.1001/jama.2020.17022.

95 WHO Rapid Evidence Appraisal for COVID-19 Therapies (REACT) Working Group, Sterne, J.A.C., Murthy, S. et al. (2020). Association between administration of systemic corticosteroids and mortality among critically ill patients with COVID-19: a meta-analysis. *JAMA* 324 (13): 1330–1341. https://doi.org/10.1001/jama.2020.17023.

96 Prescott, H.C. and Rice, T.W. (2020). Corticosteroids in COVID-19 ARDS: evidence and hope during the pandemic. *JAMA* 324 (13): 1292–1295. http://doi.org/10.1001/jama.2020.16747.

97 REMAP-CAP Investigators, Gordon, A.C., Mouncey, P.R. et al. (2021). Interleukin-6 receptor antagonists in critically ill patients with COVID-19. *N Engl J Med.* 384 (16): 1491–1502.

98 World Health Organization. Therapeutics and COVID-19: living guideline [WHO/2019-nCoV/therapeutics/2021.3]. Geneva: World Health Organization; 2021. https://apps.who.int/iris/bitstream/handle/10665/345356/WHO-2019-nCoV-therapeutics-2021.3-eng.pdf (accessed 24 Sep 2021).

99 Lier, A.J., Tuan, J.L., Davis, M.W. et al. (2020). Case report: disseminated strongyloidiasis in a patient with COVID-19. *Am J Trop Med Hyg.* 103 (4): 1590–1592. https://doi.org/10.4269/ajtmh.20-0699.

100 Marchese, V., Crosato, V., Gulletta, M. et al. (2021). Strongyloides infection manifested during immunosuppressive therapy for SARS-CoV-2 pneumonia. *Infection* 49: 539–542. https://doi.org/10.1007/s15010-020-01522-4.

101 Stauffer, W.M., Alpern, J.D., and Walker, P.F. (2020). COVID-19 and dexamethasone: a potential strategy to avoid steroid-related strongyloides hyperinfection. *JAMA* 324 (7): 623–624. https://doi.org/10.1001/jama.2020.13170.

102 Sammaritano, L.R., Bermas, B.L., Chakravarty, E.E. et al. (2020). 2020 American College of Rheumatology guideline for the management of reproductive health in rheumatic and musculoskeletal diseases. *Arthritis Rheumatol.* 72 (4): 529–556.

103 Brodie, D., Slutsky, A.S., and Combes, A. (2019). Extracorporeal life support for adults with respiratory failure and related indications. *JAMA* 322: 557.

104 Davies, A.R., Jones, D., Bailey, M. et al. (2009). Extracorporeal membrane oxygenation for 2009 influenza a(H1N1) acute respiratory distress syndrome. *JAMA* 302: 1888.

105 Shekar, K., Badulak, J., Peek, G. et al. (2020). Extracorporeal life support organization coronavirus disease 2019 interim guidelines: a consensus document from an International Group of Interdisciplinary Extracorporeal Membrane Oxygenation Providers. *ASAIO J.* 66: 707–721.

106 Barbaro, R.P., MacLaren, G., Boonstra, P.S. et al. (2020). Extracorporeal membrane oxygenation support in COVID-19: an international cohort study of the extracorporeal life support organization registry. *Lancet* 396: 1071–1078.

107 Bharat, A., Querrey, M., Markov, N.S. et al. (2020). Lung transplantation for patients with severe COVID-19. *Sci Transl Med.* 12: eabe4282.

108 Finfer, S.R., Vincent, J.-L., Slutsky, A.S., and Ranieri, V.M. (2013). Critical care medicine ventilator-induced lung injury. *N Engl J Med.* 22369: 2126–2136.

109 Chiesa-Estomba, C.M., Lechien, J.R., Calvo-Henríquez, C. et al. (2020). Systematic review of international guidelines for tracheostomy in COVID-19 patients. *Oral Oncol.* 108: 104844.

110 Angel, L.F., Amoroso, N.E., Rafeq, S. et al. (2021). Percutaneous dilational tracheostomy for coronavirus disease 2019 patients requiring mechanical ventilation. *Crit Care Med.* 49 (7): 1058–1067.

111 Mahmood, K., Cheng, G.Z., Van Nostrand, K. et al. (2021). Tracheostomy for COVID-19 respiratory failure: multidisciplinary, multicenter data on timing, technique, and outcomes. *Ann Surg.* 274 (2): 234–239.

112 Angel, L., Kon, Z.N., Chang, S.H. et al. (2020). Novel percutaneous tracheostomy for critically ill patients with COVID-19. *Ann Thorac Surg.* 110 (3): 1006–1011.

113 Chao, T.N., Harbison, S.P., Braslow, B.M. et al. (2020). Outcomes after tracheostomy in COVID-19 patients. *Ann Surg.* 272: e181–e186.

114 Vincent, J.L. (2005). Give your patient a fast hug (at least) once a day. *Crit Care Med.* 33 (6): 1225–1229. https://doi.org/10.1097/01. ccm.0000165962.16682.46.

115 Vincent, W.R. 3rd and Hatton, K.W. (2009). Critically ill patients need "FAST HUGS BID" (an updated mnemonic). *Crit Care Med.* 37 (7): 2326–2327. author reply 2327. https://doi.org/10.1097/CCM.0b013e3181aabc29.

116 Society of Critical Care Medicine. ICU Liberation. https://www.sccm.org/Clinical-Resources/ICULiberation-Home

117 Pun, B.T., Balas, M.C., Barnes-Daly, M.A. et al. (2019). Caring for critically ill patients with the ABCDEF bundle: results of the ICU liberation collaborative in over 15,000 adults. *Crit Care Med.* 47 (1): 3–14. https://doi.org/10.1097/CCM.0000000000003482.

118 Lim, C.M., Png, L.H., Wen, S.D. et al. Tracheotomy in the era f COVID-19 pandemic. Department of Otorhinolaryngology-Head and Neck Surgery. *Singapore General Hospital Guideline.* https://www.yoifos.com/sites/default/files/covid_tracheotomy_critical_care.pdf.

119 Koretz, R.L. (2009). Enteral nutrition: a hard look at some soft evidence. *Nutr Clin Pract.* 24 (3): 316–324. https://doi.org/10.1177/0884533609335378.

120 Arabi, Y.M., Aldawood, A.S., Haddad, S.H. et al. PermiT Trial Group(2015). Permissive underfeeding or standard enteral feeding in critically ill adults. *N Engl J Med* 372 (25): 2398–2408. https://doi.org/10.1056/NEJMoa1502826.

121 Saez de la Fuente, I., Saez de la Fuente, J., Quintana Estelles, M.D. et al. (2016). Enteral nutrition in patients receiving mechanical ventilation in a prone position. *JPEN J Parenter Enteral Nutr.* 40 (2): 250–255. https://doi.org/10.1177/0148607114553232.

122 Oczkowski, S.J.W., Duan, E.H., Groen, A. et al. (2017). The use of bowel protocols in critically ill adult patients: a systematic review and

meta-analysis. *Crit Care Med.* 45 (7): e718–e726. https://doi.org/10.1097/CCM.0000000000002315.

123 Falciglia, M., Freyberg, R.W., Almenoff, P.L. et al. (2009). Hyperglycemia-related mortality in critically ill patients varies with admission diagnosis. *Crit Care Med.* 37 (12): 3001–3009. https://doi.org/10.1097/CCM.0b013e3181b083f7.

124 NICE-SUGAR Study Investigators, Finfer, S., Chittock, D.R. et al. (2009). Intensive versus conventional glucose control in critically ill patients. *N Engl J Med.* 360: 1283–1297. https://doi.org/10.1056/NEJMoa0810625.

125 Brunkhorst, F.M., Engel, C., Bloos, F. et al. German Competence Network Sepsis (SepNet)(2008). Intensive insulin therapy and pentastarch resuscitation in severe sepsi. *N Engl J Med.* 358: 125–139. https://doi.org/10.1056/NEJMoa070716.

126 Nikniaz, Z., Somi, M.H., Dinevari, M.F. et al. (2021). Diabesity associated with poor COVID-19 outcomes among hospitalized patients. *J Obes Metab Syndr.* 30 (2): 149–154. https://doi.org/10.7570/jomes20121.

127 Ceriello, A. and Prattichizzo, F. (2021). Pharmacological management of COVID-19 in type 2 diabetes. *J Diabetes Complicat* 35: 107927. https://doi.org/10.1016/j.jdiacomp.2021.107927.

128 Kalil, A.C., Metersky, M.L., Klompas, M. et al. (2016). Management of Adults With Hospital-acquired and Ventilator-associated Pneumonia: 2016 Clinical Practice Guidelines by the Infectious Diseases Society of America and the American Thoracic Society. *Clin Infect Dis.* 63 (5): e61–e111. https://doi.org/10.1093/cid/ciw353.

129 Klompas, M., Branson, R., Eichenwald, E.C. et al. (2014). Strategies to prevent ventilator-associated pneumonia in acute care hospitals: 2014 update. *Infect Control Hosp Epidemiol.* 35 (8): 915–936.

130 American Thoracic Society, Infectious Diseases Society of America (2005). Guidelines for the management of adults with hospital-acquired, ventilator-associated, and healthcare-associated pneumonia. *Am J Respir Crit Care Med.* 171 (4): 388–416.

131 Head of bed elevation or semirecumbent positioning literature review. AHRQ Publication No. 16(17)-0018–16-EF. 2017. Agency for Healthcare Research and Quality, Rockville, MD. https://www.ahrq.gov/hai/tools/mvp/modules/technical/head-bed-elevation-lit-review.html.

132 Kress, J.P., Pohlman, A.S., O'Connor, M.F. et al. (2000). Daily interruption of sedative infusions in critically ill patients undergoing mechanical ventilation. *N Engl J Med.* 342 (20): 1471–1477.

133 Blackwood, B., Alderdice, F., Burns, K. et al. (2011). Use of weaning protocols for reducing duration of mechanical ventilation in critically ill adult patients: Cochrane systematic review and meta-analysis. *BMJ* 342: c7237.

134 Cook, D.J., Fuller, H.D., Guyatt, G.H. et al. (1994). Risk factors for gastrointestinal bleeding in critically ill patients. Canadian critical care trials group. *N Engl J Med.* 330: 377–381. https://doi.org/10.1056/NEJM199402103300601.

135 Cook, D. and Guyatt, G. (2018). Prophylaxis against upper gastrointestinal bleeding in hospitalized patients. *N Engl J Med.* 378: 2506–2516. https://doi.org/10.1056/NEJMra1605507.

136 Krag, M., Marker, S., Perner, A. et al. (2018). SUP-ICU trial group. Pantoprazole in patients at risk for gastrointestinal bleeding in the ICU. *N Engl J Med.* 379: 2199–2208. https://doi.org/10.1056/NEJMoa1714919.

137 Whiles, B.B., Deis, A.S., and Simpson, S.Q. (2017). Increased time to initial antimicrobial administration is associated with progression to septic shock in severe sepsis patients. *Crit Care Med.* 45: 623–629.

138 Wunderink, R.G., Srinivasan, A., Barie, P.S. et al. (2020). Antibiotic stewardship in the intensive care unit. An official American Thoracic Society workshop report in collaboration with the AACN, CHEST, CDC, and SCCM. *Ann Am Thorac Soc* 17 (5): 531–540. https://doi.org/10.1513/AnnalsATS.202003-188ST.

139 Dingle, K.E., Didelot, X., Quan, T.P. et al. (2017). Modernising medical microbiology informatics group. Effects of control interventions on Clostridium difficile infection in England: an observational study. *Lancet Infect Dis.* 17 (4): 411–421. https://doi.org/10.1016/S1473-3099(16)30514-X.

140 Wicky, P.H., Niedermann, M.S., and Timsit, J.F. (2021). Ventilator-associated pneumonia in the era of COVID-19 pandemic: how common and what is

the impact? *Crit Care.* 25 (1): 153. https://doi.org/10.1186/s13054-021-03571-z.

141 Broadhurst, D., Moureau, N., and Ullman, A.J. (2017). The world congress of vascular access (WoCoVA) skin impairment management advisory panel management of central venous access device-associated skin impairment. *J Wound Ostomy Continence Nurs.* 44 (3): 211–220. https://doi.org/10.1097/WON.0000000000000322.

142 Piazza, G., Campia, U., Hurwitz, S. et al. (2020). Registry of arterial and venous thromboembolic complications in patients with COVID-19. *J Am Coll Cardiol.* 76 (18): 2060–2072. https://doi.org/10.1016/j.jacc.2020.08.070.

143 Al-Samkari, H., Karp Leaf, R.S., Dzik, W.H. et al. (2020). COVID-19 and coagulation: bleeding and thrombotic manifestations of SARS-CoV-2 infection. *Blood* 136 (4): 489–500. https://doi.org/10.1182/BLOOD.2020006520.

144 Moll, M., Zon, R.L., Sylvester, K.W. et al. (2020). VTE in ICU patients with COVID-19. *Chest* 158 (5): 2130–2135. https://doi.org/10.1016/j.chest.2020.07.031.

145 Klok, F.A., Kruip, M.J.H.A., van der Meer, N.J.M. et al. (2020). Incidence of thrombotic complications in critically ill ICU patients with COVID-19. *Thromb Res.* 191: 145–147. https://doi.org/10.1016/j.thromres.2020.04.013.

146 Poissy, J., Goutay, J., Caplan, M. et al. (2020). Pulmonary embolism in patients with COVID-19: awareness of an increased prevalence. *Circulation* 142 (2): 184–186. https://doi.org/10.1161/CIRCULATIONAHA.120.047430.

147 Llitjos, J.F., Leclerc, M., Chochois, C. et al. (2020). High incidence of venous thromboembolic events in anticoagulated severe COVID-19 patients. *J Thromb Haemost.* 18 (7): 1743–1746. https://doi.org/10.1111/jth.14869.

148 Ackermann, M., Verleden, S.E., Kuehnel, M. et al. (2020). Pulmonary vascular endothelialitis, thrombosis, and angiogenesis in Covid-19. *N Engl J Med.* 383: 120–128. https://doi.org/10.1056/nejmoa2015432.

149 Menter, T., Haslbauer, J.D., Nienhold, R. et al. (2020). Postmortem examination of COVID-19 patients reveals diffuse alveolar damage with severe capillary congestion and variegated findings in lungs and other organs suggesting vascular dysfunction. *Histopathology* 77 (2): 198–209. https://doi.org/10.1111/his.14134.

150 Fox, S.E., Akmatbekov, A., Harbert, J.L. et al. (2020). Pulmonary and cardiac pathology in African American patients with COVID-19: an autopsy series from New Orleans. *Lancet Respir Med.* 8 (7): 681–686. https://doi.org/10.1016/S2213-2600(20)30243-5.

151 Wang, J., Hajizadeh, N., Moore, E.E. et al. (2020). Tissue plasminogen activator (tPA) treatment for COVID-19 associated acute respiratory distress syndrome (ARDS): a case series. *J Thromb Haemost.* 18 (7): 1752–1755. https://doi.org/10.1111/jth.14828.

152 Barrett, C.D., Oren-Grinberg, A., Chao, E. et al. (2020). Rescue therapy for severe COVID-19-associated acute respiratory distress syndrome with tissue plasminogen activator: a case series. *J. Trauma Acute Care Surg.* 89 (3): 453–457. https://doi.org/10.1097/TA.0000000000002786.

153 Christie, D.B., Nemec, H.M., Scott, A.M. et al. (2020). Early outcomes with utilization of tissue plasminogen activator in COVID-19–associated respiratory distress: a series of five cases. *J. Trauma Acute Care Surg.* 89 (3): 448–452. https://doi.org/10.1097/TA.0000000000002787.

154 Fraissé, M., Logre, E., Pajot, O. et al. (2020). Thrombotic and hemorrhagic events in critically ill COVID-19 patients: a French monocenter retrospective study. *Crit Care.* 24 (1): 275. https://doi.org/10.1186/s13054-020-03025-y.

155 Herridge, M.S., Tansey, C.M., Matté, A. et al. (2011). Functional disability 5 years after acute respiratory distress syndrome. *N Engl J Med.* 364 (14): 1293–1304.

156 Jackson, J.C., Pandharipande, P.P., Girard, T.D. et al. (2014). Depression, post-traumatic stress disorder, and functional disability in survivors of critical illness in the BRAIN-ICU study: a longitudinal cohort study. *Lancet Respir Med.* 2 (5): 369–379.

157 Desai, S.V., Law, T.J., and Needham, D.M. (2011). Long-term complications of critical care. *Crit Care Med.* 39 (2): 371–379.

158 Chopra, V., Flanders, S.A., O'Malley, M. et al. (2021). Sixty-day outcomes among patients

hospitalized with COVID-19. *Ann Intern Med.* 174: 576–578.

159 Mazza, M.G., De Lorenzo, R., Conte, C. et al. (2020). Anxiety and depression in COVID-19 survivors: role of inflammatory and clinical predictors. *Brain Behav Immun.* 89: 594–600.

160 Ritchie, K., Chan, D., and Watermeyer, T. (2020). The cognitive consequences of the COVID-19 epidemic: collateral damage? *Brain Commun.* 2 (2): fcaa069.

161 Antonio, G.E., Wong, K.T., Hui, D.S. et al. (2003). Thin-section CT in patients with severe acute respiratory syndrome following hospital discharge: preliminary experience. *Radiology* 228 (3): 810–815.

162 Das, K.M., Lee, E.Y., Singh, R. et al. (2017). Follow-up chest radiographic findings in patients with MERS-CoV after recovery. *Indian J Radiol Imaging.* 27 (3): 342–349. doi: 10.4103/ijri. IJRI_469_16.

12

COVID-19 in Pediatrics

Erlinda R. Ulloa[1,2], Kaidi He[3], Erin Chung[4], Delma Nieves[1,2], David E. Michalik[1,5], and Behnoosh Afghani[1,6,7]

[1] *Department of Pediatrics, University of California Irvine School of Medicine, Irvine, CA, USA*
[2] *Division of Pediatric Infectious Diseases, CHOC Children's, Orange, CA, USA*
[3] *Department of Pediatrics, Children's Hospital of Los Angeles, Los Angeles, CA, USA*
[4] *Department of Pediatrics, University of Washington, Seattle Children's Hospital, Seattle, WA, USA*
[5] *Division of Pediatric Infectious Diseases, Miller Children's and Women's Hospital, Long Beach, CA, USA*
[6] *Hospitalist, CHOC Children's, Orange, CA, USA*
[7] *Pediatric Infectious Diseases, University of California Irvine School of Medicine, Irvine, CA, USA*

Abbreviations

AAP	American Academy of Pediatrics
ARDS	acute respiratory distress syndrome
CBC	complete blood count
CDC	Centers for Disease Control and Prevention
CRP	C-reactive protein
CT	computed tomography
CXR	chest radiograph
ECMO	extracorporeal membrane oxygenation
ESR	erythrocyte sedimentation rate
EUA	Emergency Use Authorization
FDA	US Food and Drug Administration
HFNC	high-flow nasal cannula
HOL	hours of life
ICU	intensive care unit
IDSA	Infectious Diseases Society of America
IL-6	interleukin-6
IV	intravenous
IVIG	intravenous immunoglobulin
MIS-C	multisystem inflammatory syndrome in children
NIH	National Institutes of Health
NSAID	nonsteroidal anti-inflammatory drug
PASC	postacute sequelae of SARS-CoV-2
RT-PCR	reverse transcription-polymerase chain reaction
SARS-CoV-2	severe acute respiratory syndrome coronavirus 2
WHO	World Health Organization

Epidemiology

In December 2019, the first cases of coronavirus disease 2019 (COVID-19), the disease caused by severe acute respiratory syndrome coronavirus 2 (SARS-CoV-2), were reported in adults in Wuhan, China. Reports of SARS-CoV-2 infections in children followed, but information remained limited because of the generally mild course and low mortality in pediatric COVID-19. According to early estimates, SARS-CoV-2 infections in children accounted for only 1–5% of all cases [1]. Although proportions were variable by country, a minority of reported COVID-19 cases occurred in children: in June 2020, a review of 29 countries reported percentages ranging from 0.3% in Spain to 13.8% in Argentina [2]. In the United States, SARS-CoV-2 infection rates in children have increased over time but have followed trends in adults [3]. However, the true incidence of SARS-CoV-2 infection in children may be higher than reported because testing in many countries has focused on symptomatic individuals, generally adults. It is unclear why children have less severe illness from COVID-19 compared with adults, but several hypotheses relate it to biological factors, such as decreased angiotensin-converting enzyme 2 expression and viral affinity and/or stronger immune responses as a result of cross-reactivity to human CoV antibodies [4, 5].

SARS-CoV-2 infects children and adolescents of all ages, with a median age of six to seven years [1, 6], but averages may vary because of differences in defining pediatric age ranges. In children younger than five years, as many as half of cases may occur in infants [7]. There may be a slight male predominance in SARS-CoV-2 infection rates [8, 9]. Furthermore, SARS-CoV-2 has disproportionately affected minority children, especially Hispanic and Black (African American, Afro-Caribbean, and African) children [8, 10]. Hispanic and Black children have the highest rates of COVID-19-associated hospitalization [11, 12] and attendant morbidity and mortality [13]. Contributing factors may include low socioeconomic status, larger household size, caregivers working as "essential workers" in high-risk jobs, inequities in healthcare access, and discrimination [10].

The increase in the number of hospitalizations because of COVID-19 has been accompanied by a decline in pediatric hospital admissions for cases unrelated to COVID-19 [14]. That being said, hospitalization rates in children with acute COVID-19 have been significantly lower compared with those in adults [15]. Children with comorbidities have been more likely to be hospitalized [13] and require intensive care, with obesity as the most common risk factor for escalated care [16]. Mortality has been lower in children than in adults. Early studies suggested a 1% mortality rate [9], and a review of fatality rates across 17 developed countries has shown an exponential age-related trend from 0.002% at age 10 years to 0.01% at age 25 years [17]. Persistent symptoms after acute SARS-CoV-2 infection, newly termed post-acute sequelae of SARS-CoV-2 (PASC) in children, but the prevalence of pediatric PASC and duration of symptoms have yet to be fully determined [18].

Multiple variants of SARS-CoV-2 are now circulating globally. The more highly infectious SARS-CoV-2 B.1.1.7 (Alpha) lineage originated in the United Kingdom in the fall of 2020 with subsequent spread to countries worldwide [19]. In 2021, the B.1.617.2 (Delta) variant, a variant of concern due to increased transmissibility, became the predominant variant worldwide. This was accompanied by an increase in hospitalization rates for COVID-19 among children <18 years, particularly in regions with lower COVID-19 vaccination rates [20]. The role of children in SARS-CoV-2 transmission may change with the shifting epidemiology of variants and COVID-19 vaccine uptake. An updated list of SARS-CoV-2 variants can be found on the Centers for Disease Control and Prevention (CDC) website (https://www.cdc.gov/coronavirus/2019-ncov/cases-updates/variant-surveillance/variant-info.html) [21].

Epidemiology of Multisystem Inflammatory Syndrome in Children

In April 2020, reports emerged from the United Kingdom of a severe condition similar to Kawasaki disease or toxic shock syndrome in children exposed to SARS-CoV-2 [22]. This condition, initially named pediatric inflammatory multisystem syndrome temporally associated with SARS-CoV-2, was ultimately designated as multisystem inflammatory syndrome in children (MIS-C) [23]. This rare condition is specific to children, with only a few reports of adults with MIS-C-like symptoms.

Although MIS-C and Kawasaki disease (complete or incomplete) may have many overlapping features (see later MIS-C Clinical Manifestations section), the epidemiology differs from that of classic Kawasaki disease. Children with MIS-C tend to be older, with a median age ranging from seven to nine years [23, 24]. By contrast, in Kawasaki disease, the majority of patients are younger than five years, with a median age of two years [25]. MIS-C has also disproportionately affected Hispanic and Black children [4], as evidenced by higher rates of hospitalization [26]. In contrast, classic Kawasaki disease has a higher incidence in East Asia and in children of Asian descent [27].

Of patients with MIS-C who are hospitalized, roughly 80% require pediatric intensive care unit (ICU) admission, 20% require mechanical ventilation, and up to 50% require vasopressors [23]. Coronary artery aneurysms have been noted in up to 8–13% of patients, and depressed cardiac function in more than half of patients [23, 28–30]. Although children may present in shock, overall prognosis is favorable, and the mortality rate from MIS-C has been low, estimated up to 2% [23, 24, 28, 29].

Transmission in Children

SARS-CoV-2 is transmitted from person to person primarily via respiratory droplets with contribution from aerosolized particles [31, 32]. The ability of the virus to spread in particles highlights the importance of preventative measures like increased ventilation in addition to precautions like masking and distancing.

The average incubation period of SARS-CoV-2 in children is about 5–6 days, with a range of 2–14 days [33], similar to adults. Children may shed viral RNA from the upper respiratory and gastrointestinal tract for two to four weeks [34, 35]. SARS-CoV-2 has been detected longer in stool than in respiratory tract samples [36]. Immunocompromised children can shed for longer than four weeks [37]. Prolonged shedding does not indicate transmissibility of infectious virus.

The role of children in the transmission of SARS-CoV-2 remains a subject of study. Early pediatric cases were noted to be part of family clusters [1], and studies have continued to show significant household transmission risks, likely secondary to the potential for prolonged, close contact between household members [38]. Within households, children one year or younger have been shown to be the most susceptible of all children [2]. These studies have suggested that adults are most often the index cases [39, 40], possibly because adults are more likely to be symptomatic compared with children [41].

In children, estimated proportions of asymptomatic infection range from 15% to 45% [42, 43]. Asymptomatic children may be less likely to transmit SARS-CoV-2, possibly because of more rapid viral clearance, shorter durations of shedding infectious virus, and/or lower viral loads [44]. Children may also be less effective at transmitting droplets and aerosolized virus [45]. Studies of SARS-CoV-2 reverse transcription-polymerase chain reaction (RT-PCR) cycle threshold values or viral loads suggest that asymptomatic children may have less viral RNA or lower viral loads than symptomatic children [34, 46]. However, recent evidence suggests that compared with adults, children likely have similar viral loads in their nasopharynx [47–49], similar secondary infection rates, and can spread the virus to others [50, 51].

In societies with in-person schooling, infection rates in children have been linked to community infection rates [52]. Even when community transmission rates remained high, there have been low transmission rates when mitigation measures (e.g. physical distancing, masking, hand hygiene) were enforced [53, 54]. Adult staff and teachers also appear to play key roles in transmission chains [55], because studies suggest that transmission from students is less likely than from staff [56]. In childcare centers, there has been little evidence of spread from children to childcare providers [57].

Neonatal Transmission

Although neonates can be infected with SARS-CoV-2 antenatally (through the placenta) or perinatally (during the delivery), the greatest risk for infection is thought to be postnatally through environmental exposure, such as infected maternal respiratory secretions [58, 59]. Due to a paucity of data, it is currently not clear whether SARS-CoV-2 can be transmitted vertically from mother to fetus [59]. Antenatal transplacental transmission via maternal viremia appears to be unlikely based on data and prior experience with other respiratory viruses (e.g. influenza, SARS-CoV-1, Middle East respiratory syndrome) [60]. Limited early reports of RT-PCR testing of amniotic fluid, placenta, and maternal vaginal secretions for SARS-CoV-2 did not identify virus in these specimens [61–64]. In neonates born to women who acquired SARS-CoV-2 in the third trimester, no vertical transmission was observed in the 29 neonates tested from the time of delivery to nine days later [60]. Nonetheless, other studies demonstrate early virologic evidence of SARS-CoV-2 in neonates born to infected mothers [65–68]. In one case, placental tissue was positive for SARS-CoV-2 by RT-PCR, as were maternal and neonatal blood samples [69]. In a systematic review of 38 studies of 936 neonates born to SARS-CoV-2-positive mothers, 27 neonates, or 3.2%, tested positive [70]. Although suggestive, these data are not conclusive for in-utero transmission, and more data are needed [59].

Breastfeeding

Currently, there is no clear evidence for SARS-CoV-2 transmission through breast milk, because most studies to date have not detected replication-competent SARS-CoV-2 in breast milk [71, 72]. The CDC [73], the World Health Organization (WHO) [72], and the American Academy of Pediatrics (AAP) [74] encourage mothers with suspected or confirmed COVID-19 to breastfeed (either directly or via expressed breast milk) because the benefits of breast milk outweigh the risks of potential transmission of the virus. Mothers who desire to breastfeed directly should comply with strict preventive precautions, including use of a mask, breast and hand hygiene, and cleaning and sanitizing breast pumps. Expressed breast milk is also an option after similar preventive precautions are taken. In cases where mothers are too ill to breastfeed, caregivers who are not infected or not at increased risk for severe illness from COVID-19 may feed the breast milk to the infant.

Clinical Manifestations

Clinical manifestations of SARS-CoV-2 infection in children continue to evolve since its emergence in late 2019. The course of SARS-CoV-2 infection in children is highly variable and depends on the age and host characteristics. Most children infected with SARS-CoV-2 have no or mild symptoms [75]. US surveillance data highlight that "fever, cough or shortness of breath" account for 60–63% of symptoms in patients aged 0–19 years [76]. The clinical findings in symptomatic children and adolescents are nonspecific (Table 12.1) [77, 78], and many of these symptoms overlap with common pediatric conditions, such as upper and lower respiratory tract infections and gastroenteritis [79]. However, certain symptoms may be more concerning (Table 12.1) and may warrant testing for SARS-CoV-2, particularly in regions with high rates of SARS-CoV-2 community transmission.

Table 12.1   COVID-19 symptoms and definition of suspected cases.

	Concerning symptoms	Nonspecific symptoms
COVID-19 symptoms	Sustained cough Shortness of breath Difficulty breathing Loss of taste or smell	Fever Fatigue Chills/rigors Headache Myalgia Sore throat Congestion/rhinorrhea Nausea Vomiting/diarrhea
COVID-19 suspected	<ul><li>≥1 Concerning symptom(s) **or**</li><li>≥2 Nonspecific symptoms</li><li>Without evidence of another explanatory illness</li></ul>Examples: cellulitis; hand, foot and mouth; group A streptococcal pharyngitis; urinary tract infection Exceptions: bronchiolitis, pneumonia or Severe respiratory illness with at least *one* of the following: ○ Clinical or radiographic evidence of pneumonia ○ Acute respiratory distress syndrome	

Sources: Centers for Disease Control and Prevention [77] and Orscheln et al. [78].

Disease Severity

The clinical spectrum of SARS-CoV-2 infection can be divided into asymptomatic, mild, moderate, severe, or critical disease based on clinical and radiographic criteria (Table 12.2) [80]. Data suggest that up to 45% of pediatric infections are asymptomatic [43]. Disease isolated to the upper respiratory tract is either asymptomatic or mild. In contrast, patients with radiographic evidence of lower respiratory tract involvement can have moderate to critical disease depending on the level of respiratory support required. Careful, regular assessments to determine the severity of infection and risk for progression need to be made, particularly in the setting of a lower respiratory tract infection [81]. Patients with moderate disease have no new or increased oxygen requirement, whereas those with severe disease do. Patients with critical disease are defined as those who require invasive or noninvasive mechanical ventilation (including high-flow nasal cannula [HFNC]). A subset of patients with severe COVID-19 experience development of a hyperinflammatory syndrome, septic shock, and/or acute respiratory distress syndrome (ARDS). This high-risk inflammatory phenotype usually appears during the second week of illness and is characterized by elevated inflammatory markers, escalation of respiratory support to mechanical ventilation, and decreased survival [82]. Although children have lower rates of mechanical ventilation and death than adults, one in three children hospitalized with COVID-19 in the United States (1 March 2020 to 25 July 2020) were admitted to the ICU, a rate similar to that in adults [11].

Mild to Moderate Disease

Many studies have shown that the disease course in the pediatric population is less severe than in adults, and most infected children are asymptomatic or have mild symptoms [75]. Patients with mild disease typically present with upper respiratory tract symptoms, including nasal congestion, sore throat, and cough, along with fever, headache, fatigue, and myalgias. As previously mentioned, these characteristics are not specific enough to differentiate mild infection caused by SARS-CoV-2 from other respiratory viruses. However, gastrointestinal symptoms, such as diarrhea, abdominal pain, and vomiting, may predominate and are seen in up to 20% of patients with SARS-CoV-2 infection [79].

Table 12.2 Spectrum of severe acute respiratory syndrome coronavirus 2 symptom severity.

Asymptomatic	Mild	Moderate	Severe	Critical
Positive SARS-CoV-2 No symptoms	**URI** Fever Fatigue Headache Nasal congestion Sore throat Cough Diarrhea Vomiting Myalgias	**LRTI** Tachypnea Cough Dyspnea WITHOUT hypoxia	**LRTI** Tachypnea Cough Dyspnea WITH hypoxia supplemental O_2 is required	**LRTI** Tachypnea Cough Dyspnea WITH respiratory failure noninvasive or invasive mechanical ventilation (including HFNC) required
		Radiographic pneumonia	Radiographic pneumonia	+/− ARDS +/− Septic shock

ARDS, acute respiratory distress syndrome; HFNC, high-flow nasal cannula; LRTI, lower respiratory tract infection; SARS-CoV-2, severe acute respiratory syndrome coronavirus 2; URI, upper respiratory tract infection.
Source: National Institutes of Health [80].

Patients with moderate illness have radiographic evidence of COVID-19 pneumonia and present with lower respiratory tract symptoms, including dyspnea, tachypnea, and cough without hypoxia.

Severe to Critical Disease

Most pediatric cases do not progress to severe disease and do improve with supportive care alone. Of 277,285 school-aged children with confirmed SARS-CoV-2 laboratory test, 3240 (1.2%) were hospitalized and of those, 404 (0.1%) required ICU admission and 51 (<0.01%) died. At least one underlying condition was noted in 16% of those hospitalized, 27% of those admitted to the ICU, and 28% of those who died [83]. Patients who do develop severe or critical disease often present with shortness of breath, tachypnea, fever and cough, or severe diarrhea, and the disease usually progresses within 7–10 days [84]. In hospitalized patients, the median time from the development of symptoms to admission is typically one to five days for younger children and two to seven days for adolescents [85]. When compared with older children, infants are more likely to present with nonspecific symptoms, such as congestion, fever, and decreased activity [86], and less likely to present with respiratory distress. That being said, a retrospective study of pediatric patients during early stages of the COVID-19 pandemic reported that infants younger than one year were more likely to experience severe or critical illness compared with older children [87].

Pediatric patients hospitalized with COVID-19 illness more frequently suffer from underlying conditions, such as obesity [88], diabetes, asthma, chronic lung disease, sickle cell disease [89], or immunodeficiency [88]. A meta-analysis that analyzed the effect of comorbidities on severity of COVID-19 infection in the pediatric population reported that severe COVID-19 was present in 5.1% of children with comorbidities and in 0.2% without comorbidities. Children with obesity were 2.87 times more likely to have severe disease compared with those without obesity or other comorbidities [90]. Of those patients who were hospitalized, the majority were Hispanic (45%) or Black (24%) [83]. It is not clear why Hispanics and Blacks are at greater risk for acquiring more severe disease with COVID-19. Contributing factors may include genetic factors, living situation, lifestyle conditions, nutritional status, and health disparities, including delayed care because of lack of affordability or uncontrolled chronic illnesses [91].

Infection in Infants (Age <1 Year)

Information on the clinical manifestations of COVID-19 in infants is limited. Infants generally present with difficulty feeding, mild upper respiratory symptoms, and/or fever without an obvious source [86, 92–95]. Infants do not appear to have significant pulmonary disease [93]. When present, respiratory symptoms are similar to those caused by other coronaviruses and influenza [96] and can also manifest as bronchiolitis [97, 98]. In a systematic review of 63 infants (<3 months of age) with laboratory-confirmed SARS-CoV-2, symptoms included fever (73%), cough (38%), rhinitis (36%), respiratory distress (26%), poor feeding (24%), vomiting (14%), and diarrhea (14%) [99]. The majority (92%) of these symptomatic infants were hospitalized [99]. However, most cases were mild to moderate and improved with supportive care alone, while 21% had severe disease and 3% had critical disease requiring mechanical ventilation [99]. In a retrospective study on 46 infants (<12 months of age) hospitalized with SARS-CoV-2, disease was asymptomatic or mild in 4 cases, moderate in 40 cases, and severe in 2 cases [86]. Only four infants had underlying comorbidities [86]. Overall, when compared with older children, infants <1 year of age are more likely to suffer from moderate to severe disease [86, 87, 99].

Cutaneous Manifestations

Many dermatologic manifestations are associated with SARS-CoV-2. In an international registry that included a large representative sample of patients, the most common dermatologic morphologies in 171 COVID-19 laboratory-confirmed cases included morbilliform (22%), pernio-like (18%), urticarial (16%), macular erythema (13%), vesicular (11%), and papulosquamous (9.9%) findings [100]. All of these findings have been described in pediatric patients [101]. The majority of cutaneous findings appear during the acute or postinfectious phase. However, up to 12% have been found to predate the appearance of COVID-19-related symptoms [100]. Pediatric patients with urticarial lesions tend to be asymptomatic, while those with erythema multiforme are either asymptomatic or have mild respiratory or gastrointestinal symptoms [101, 102].

COVID Toes

Acral changes that are pernio-like or chilblains-like have been reported in children with suspected COVID-19 or exposures to COVID-19 [103–107]. These skin findings are usually accompanied by mild or no other symptoms [108]. The feet and toes appear to be more affected than the hands and fingers. They have been described as red or purple patches measuring millimeters to a few centimeters, sometimes with erosions or central graying. Skin biopsy often shows features on histology similar to pernio. The lesions are often associated with coolness of the area, mild pain, and sometimes mild pruritis [108]. The lesions generally resolve within four to eight weeks [108].

Neurologic Symptoms

Neurologic symptoms in the pediatric population as a result of COVID-19 are less common compared with adults, but the number of reports has increased since the start of the pandemic. These patients can present with a variety of symptoms, including acute encephalopathy (altered mental status, lethargy or drowsiness, or agitation), headache, dizziness or light-headedness; ataxia, balance, or coordination problems; and altered sense of smell (anosmia), altered sense of taste (dysgeusia), stroke, Guillain–Barré syndrome, seizure, sympathetic storming, meningitis or encephalitis, and other focal neurologic deficits (such as visual impairment or weakness or numbness) [109]. Overall, the pathophysiology of the neurologic symptoms is not well understood. Some of these symptoms, such as headache, dizziness, and delirium, can occur as a nonspecific consequence of systemic illness. In addition, the lack of unequivocal reports of SARS-CoV-2 being recovered from the cerebrospinal fluid of patients with neurologic involvement strengthens the possibility that some neurologic sequelae are secondary to hypoxia, cytokine involvement, or another indirect mechanism [109].

Atypical Clinical Manifestations

Atypical presentations of SARS-CoV-2 infection may include severe odynophagia, recurrent pneumothorax, and pseudoappendicitis [85]. Whether the atypical manifestations are related to direct viral invasion or immune phenomenon remains to be elucidated.

Imaging Findings

Imaging findings of acute SARS-CoV-2 infection in children are generally nonspecific and milder than those seen in infected adults [110]. The most common lung imaging modalities used in children include chest radiographs (CXRs) and chest computed tomography (CT). By definition, patients with moderate, severe, or critical disease have radiographic evidence of a lower respiratory tract infection [80]. Features typical of viral pneumonia and reactive small airway disease, such as peribronchial thickening and/or opacities, have been observed more frequently in pediatric COVID-19 cases than in adults [111] (Figure 12.1). Other CXR findings commonly reported include pneumonic infiltrates and "white lung" or lung haziness [110] (Figure 12.2). Chest CT findings are similarly nonspecific. The most frequently reported findings include bilateral peripheral and/or subpleural ground-glass and/or consolidative opacities often in the lower lobes of the lungs [110–112] (Figure 12.3). Based on expert opinion from a group of international radiologists with expertise in pediatric thoracic imaging, the "halo" sign is generally observed early in the disease course (early phase) before progressing to ground-glass (progressive phase) and eventually into

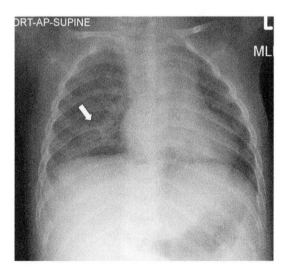

Figure 12.1 Previously healthy 12-month-old boy with positive severe acute respiratory syndrome coronavirus 2 reverse transcription-polymerase chain reaction test who presented with fever and difficulty breathing. Frontal chest radiograph demonstrates patchy right lung opacity (*arrow*). *Source:* Image courtesy of Ali Gholamrezanezhad, MD.

On admission

3 days later

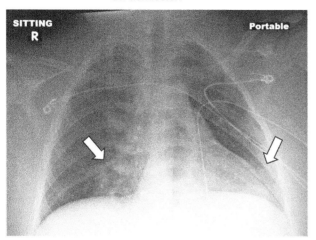
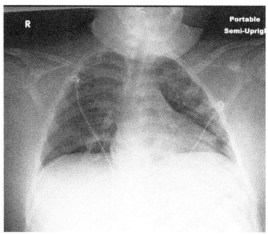

Figure 12.2   A 13-year-old boy with diabetes and positive severe acute respiratory syndrome coronavirus 2 reverse transcription-polymerase chain reaction test presented with tachypnea and oxygen saturation of 93%. Frontal chest radiograph on admission (left) demonstrates right cardiophrenic angle and left lung base air space opacities (*arrows*). Follow-up frontal chest radiograph three days later (right) shows some improvement. *Source:* Image courtesy of Ali Gholamrezanezhad, MD.

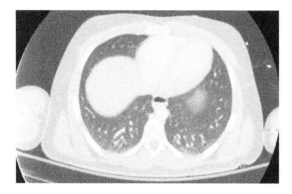

Figure 12.3   Previously healthy 15-year-old boy with positive severe acute respiratory syndrome coronavirus 2 reverse transcription-polymerase chain reaction test who presented with trauma (automobile vs. bike). Axial lung window computed tomography image demonstrates minimal bilateral subpleural ground-glass opacities, which may represent atelectasis or atypical pneumonia. *Source:* Image courtesy of Ali Gholamrezanezhad, MD.

consolidative opacities (developed phase) [111]. Peribronchial thickening and inflammation along the bronchovascular bundle are observed more frequently in the pediatric population compared with the adult population [111]. Findings seen in adults, such as interlobular thickening, air bronchograms, and crazy-paving pattern, are rarer in children [111].

MIS-C Clinical Manifestations

Various reports of a multisystem inflammatory syndrome presenting in children during the COVID-19 pandemic have placed caregivers on high alert for identifying and diagnosing these patients appropriately given that management is different from that of acute COVID-19. Pediatric cases of MIS-C are seen at an increased rate two to six weeks after the acute COVID-19 infection peaks [113–115]. The cause of MIS-C is not clear, but it is postulated that it results from an exaggerated immune response or cytokine storm leading to organ damage triggered by a previous infection with SARS-CoV-2. Multiple health leaders and organizations have created guidelines for identifying and treating these patients [113, 116–119] (Table 12.3). In the United States alone, as of October 2021, 5217 cases of MIS-C were reported that met the CDC case definition and 46 MIS-C deaths [120].

The clinical presentation of MIS-C includes fever ($\geq$38.0 °C) with multisystem ($\geq$2) organ involvement, including cardiac, renal, respiratory, hematologic, gastrointestinal, dermatologic, and/or neurologic manifestations (Table 12.3). Diarrhea and abdominal pain seem to be the most consistent features in reported cases, followed by conjunctivitis, rash, and mucous membrane changes [23]. Shock is also present in a

Table 12.3 Summarized MIS-C case definitions and diagnostic criteria suggested.

	CDC [117]	WHO [118]	RCPCH [119]	ACR [113]
Age	<21 years old	0–19 years old	Child	Child
Fever	**X** ≥ 38.0 °C for ≥24 h Or subjective fever ≥24 h	**X** Fever ≥3 d	**X** Persistent fever >38.5 °C	**X** Unremitting fever >38 °C
Clinical presentation	**X** Clinically severe illness requiring hospitalization **X** (>2) Organ system involvement: • Cardiac • Renal • Respiratory • Hematologic • Gastrointestinal • Dermatologic • Neurologic	**X** 2 of the following: a) Rash or bilateral nonpurulent conjunctivitis or mucocutaneous inflammation signs (oral, hands or feet) b) Hypotension or shock c) Myocardial dysfunction, pericarditis, valvulitis, or coronary abnormalities (including echocardiogram findings or elevated troponin/natriuretic peptide pro-BNP) d) Evidence of coagulopathy (by PT, PTT, elevated D-dimers) e) Acute gastrointestinal problems (diarrhea, vomiting, or abdominal pain)	**X** Evidence of single or multiorgan dysfunction (shock, cardiac, respiratory, renal, gastrointestinal, or neurologic disorder) with additional features *Most common:* Oxygen requirement Hypotension *Sometimes:* • Abdominal pain • Confusion • Conjunctivitis • Cough • Diarrhea • Headache • Lymphadenopathy • Mucous membrane changes • Neck swelling • Rash • Respiratory symptoms • Sore throat • Swollen hands and feet • Syncope • Vomiting	**X** At least 2 of the following: • Rash (polymorphic, maculopapular, or petechial, but not vesicular) • Gastrointestinal symptoms (diarrhea, abdominal pain, or vomiting) • Edema of hands/feet • Oral mucosa changes (red and/or cracked lips, strawberry tongue, or erythema of the oropharyngeal mucosa) • Conjunctivitis (bilateral conjunctival infection without exudate) • Lymphadenopathy • Neurologic symptoms (altered mental status, encephalopathy, focal neurologic deficits, meningismus, or papilledema)

(Continued)

Table 12.3 (Continued)

	CDC [117]	WHO [118]	RCPCH [119]	ACR [113]
Current or recent SARS-CoV-2 infection	**X** By RT-PCR, serology, or antigen test Or COVID-19 exposure within the 4 wk before onset of symptoms	**X** Evidence of COVID-19 (RT-PCR, antigen test or serology positive), or likely contact with patients with COVID-19	SARS-CoV-2 RT-PCR testing may be positive or negative	**X** Epidemiologic link to SARS-CoV-2: • + SARS-CoV-2 by RT-PCR • + SARS-CoV-2 by serology • Preceding illness resembling COVID-19 • Or close contact with an individual with confirmed or suspected COVID-19 in the past 4 wk
Exclusion	**X** No alternate diagnosis	**X** No other obvious microbial cause of inflammation, including bacterial sepsis or staphylococcal or streptococcal shock syndromes	**X** Absence of potential causative organisms (other than SARS-CoV-2) Exclusion of any other microbial cause, including bacterial sepsis, staphylococcal or streptococcal shock syndromes, infections associated with myocarditis such as enterovirus	**X** Rule out other non-MIS-C etiologies
Laboratory workup	**X** Evidence of inflammation including one or more of the following: *Elevated:* • CRP • ESR • Fibrinogen • Procalcitonin • D-dimer • Ferritin • LDH • IL-6 • Neutrophils	**X** Evidence of inflammation, such as: *Elevated* • ESR • CRP • Procalcitonin	**X** Evidence of inflammation: • Neutrophilia • Elevated CRP • Lymphopenia **X All:** • Abnormal fibrinogen • High CRP • High D-dimers • High ferritin • Hypoalbuminemia • Lymphopenia • Neutrophilia in most	**X Tier 1:** check comprehensive metabolic panel, ESR, CRP, and SARS-CoV-2 RT-PCR and/or serologies If CRP >5 or ESR >40 mm/h and at least 1: • Absolute lymphocyte count <1000/μl • Platelet count <150,000/μl • Na <135 mmol/l • Neutrophilia • Hypoalbuminemia

Reduced:
- Lymphocytes
- Albumin

Some:
- Acute kidney injury
- Anemia
- Coagulopathy
- High IL-10
- High IL-6
- Neutrophilia
- Proteinuria
- Raised CK
- Raised LDH
- Raised triglycerides
- Raised troponin
- Thrombocytopenia
- Transaminitis

If the above met, then do Tier 2:
- BNP
- Troponin T
- Procalcitonin
- Ferritin
- PT
- PTT
- D-dimer
- Fibrinogen
- LDH
- UA
- Cytokine panel triglycerides
- SARS-CoV-2 serology
- Blood smear

Imaging

Echocardiogram findings

Echocardiogram and ECG: myocarditis, valvulitis, pericardial effusion, coronary artery dilatation
- CXR: patchy symmetrical infiltrates, pleural effusion
- Abdominal US: colitis, ileitis, lymphadenopathy, ascites, hepatosplenomegaly
- CT chest: as for CXR—may demonstrate coronary artery abnormalities if with contrast

Note: ECG and echocardiogram part of **Tier 2** evaluation

ACR, American College of Rheumatology; BNP, brain natriuretic peptide; CDC, Centers for Disease Control and Prevention; CK, creatinine kinase; CRP, C-reactive protein; CT, computed tomography; CXR, chest X-ray; ECG, electrocardiogram; ESR, erythrocyte sedimentation rate; IL-6, interleukin-6; IL-10, interleukin-10; LDH, lactic acid dehydrogenase; MIS-C, multisystem inflammatory syndrome in children; PT, prothrombin time; PTT, partial thromboplastin time; RCPCH, Royal College of Pediatrics and Child Health; RT-PCR, reverse transcription-polymerase chain reaction; UA, urinalysis; WHO, World Health Organization; X, required as part of case definition/diagnosis.

majority of reported cases and may have components of cardiogenic, distributive, and hypovolemic shock [23]. Infrequently observed is cervical lymphadenopathy (>1.5 cm). Neurologic symptoms are nonspecific and may include headache, irritability, lethargy, altered mental status, neck stiffness, and cranial nerve palsies [23].

MIS-C Mucocutaneous Findings

In contrast with acute COVID-19 infection, MIS-C presents with mucocutaneous findings in the majority of children younger than 5 years [23]. The most common mucocutaneous findings in MIS-C parallel those seen in Kawasaki disease and include bilateral non-purulent conjunctivitis (bulbar or limbic-involving), along with diffuse and nonspecific rash and mucosal changes (e.g. erythema and cracking of lips, strawberry tongue, and/or erythema of oral and pharyngeal mucosa). In the acute phase, extremity changes, including erythema and edema of the hands and feet, can also be seen. As in Kawasaki disease, periungual desquamation has been described as a late finding after acute MIS-C. Other findings described in MIS-C include malar erythema, urticarial eruptions, and periorbital edema. The rash tends to be polymorphic, maculopapular, petechial, but not vesicular. Morbilliform, scarlatiniform, urticarial, and reticulated patterns also have been described [121]. These rashes can be localized, usually to the face or extremities, or widely distributed throughout the body. Mucocutaneous findings generally present after fever starts and last about five days, but they can be present as short as a few hours or persist for longer than a week.

MIS-C Imaging Findings

In MIS-C, imaging generally demonstrates sequalae of systemic hyperinflammation and cardiac decompensation. As a result, MIS-C imaging findings are characteristically distinct from those found in pediatric patients with acute COVID-19, where extrapulmonary abnormalities are rare [122]. Abdominal imaging may show ascites, mesenteric lymphadenopathy, bowel wall thickening, or signs of gallbladder inflammation [122]. Pulmonary imaging typically reveals perihilar interstitial thickening, hilar adenopathy, cardiomegaly, and/or pleural effusions [122]. Chest CT may also show basal consolidation and ground-glass opacities as seen in pediatric patients with acute

COVID-19 [122]. Echocardiogram may be normal or reveal dilation, coronary artery ectasia or aneurysms, or left ventricular systolic dysfunction with depressed ejection fraction [122]. In pediatric patients with MIS-C-related myocarditis, cardiac magnetic resonance imaging may demonstrate edema in the myocardium without fibrosis or focal necrosis [122, 123].

Post-Acute Sequelae of SARS-CoV-2 (PASC) in Children

At the time of this publication, the scientific community is actively working to learn more about the range of short- and long-term health effects associated with COVID-19. Although most people recover and return to normal health after being infected with SARS-CoV-2, some have symptoms that can last for weeks or even months after recovery from acute illness [124]. PASC or "long COVID" has been shown to affect a subset of patients and appears to be more common in women, older individuals, and those with multiple symptoms on initial presentation [125]. It has also been increasingly described in children. Some data suggest that children may have persistent symptoms for a mean of 8.2 months [126]. Most commonly reported pediatric symptoms include fatigue, headache, abdominal pain, muscle and/or joint pain, and changes in energy level, mood, sleep, or concentration [126]. Most children tend to have a period of improvement before symptom recurrence [126]. More research is needed into the underlying pathogenesis and whether risk modification is possible.

Approach to Diagnosis

The following section focuses on SARS-CoV-2 pediatric testing criteria in the United States, which may vary geographically based on community prevalence and test availability. In most regions of the United States, there is an adequate supply of SARS-CoV-2 diagnostic tests and associated supplies to test all patients in whom there is a clinical suspicion of infection. Testing strategies with regard to the type of test (nucleic acid or antigen) and the recommended specimen type are the same for children and adults [75] (see Chapter 3). The following recommendations are based on published guidelines from the CDC, AAP [127], peer-reviewed literature, and expert consensus.

Clinical suspicion of SARS-CoV-2 infection should depend on regional prevalence of SARS-CoV-2. When SARS-CoV-2 transmission is widespread, clinical suspicion of COVID-19 is appropriate in most patients with consistent clinical manifestations, especially fever and lower respiratory tract symptoms [76]. SARS-CoV-2 infection is probable in any patient with a CDC-defined SARS-CoV-2 epidemiologic link in the 14 days before symptom onset [77]. This includes close contact with a confirmed or suspected case of COVID-19, or travel to or residence in regions known to have high rates of community transmission of SARS-CoV-2 [128]. It is difficult to precisely define a "close contact." Per the CDC, a close contact is someone who was within 6 ft of an infected person for a prolonged period ($\geq$15 minutes) or for a cumulative total of $\geq$15 minutes over a 24-hour period within two days of symptom onset or specimen collection of a subsequently positive test [129]. Other examples of "close contact" may include providing care at home to someone who is sick with COVID-19 and/or direct physical contact (e.g. hugging or kissing) or sharing eating or drinking utensils with someone with SARS-CoV-2 [130, 131].

Screening and Diagnosis in Symptomatic Patients

Table 12.1 summarizes the symptom-based criteria that should be used in conjunction with epidemiologic data to raise suspicion for COVID-19 in children and adolescents [77, 78]. The majority of symptoms are nonspecific. However, a subset is deemed concerning because they are either more specific to COVID-19 (anosmia and ageusia), more serious (difficulty breathing and shortness of breath), or more likely to increase transmission (cough). Any one of these concerning symptoms should prompt evaluation by a healthcare provider and/or testing for SARS-CoV-2. COVID-19 severity and presentation can vary (see Table 12.2). Patients with lower respiratory tract symptoms and/or septic shock should also be evaluated for acute SARS-CoV-2 infection.

Evaluating for Coinfections

In children with nonspecific symptoms, it is prudent to rule out other sources of infection, such as cellulitis; classic hand, foot and mouth disease; group A streptococcal pharyngitis; or urinary tract infections [127]. SARS-CoV-2 testing is not recommended routinely if another source of infection that lacks shared symptoms with SARS-CoV-2 (such as cellulitis or urinary tract infection) is identified in the outpatient setting [127]. However, SARS-CoV-2 testing may be required for children being hospitalized to allow for additional isolation precautions, as discussed later [127].

Intercurrent infections may occur with other respiratory pathogens that share overlapping symptoms with SARS-CoV-2 [132–134]. As a result, detection of other respiratory pathogens from nasopharyngeal specimens does not exclude COVID-19 [134]. In a systemic review of SARS-CoV-2, coinfections with respiratory pathogens were observed in 5.6% of children [135]. The most common coinfections included *Mycoplasma pneumoniae* (58%), influenza (11%), and respiratory syncytial virus (9.7%) [135]. It is difficult to distinguish SARS-CoV-2 and influenza based on clinical presentation alone [136]. Therefore, during influenza season, patients should be tested for both [127]. Clinical judgment should be used to rule out other acute illnesses in SARS-CoV-2-positive patients who present with severe or critical illness (such as ARDS and/or septic shock).

COVID Toes

Although the nature of the phenomenon of COVID toes is still being investigated, most children with these acral changes have tested negative for COVID-19 by PCR [100]. That being said, most have high-risk exposures. The typical workup mirrors that for pernio [137], which includes anti-nuclear antibody testing, rheumatoid factor, D-dimer, fibrinogen, complete blood count (CBC) with differential, C3, C4, C-reactive protein (CRP), erythrocyte sedimentation rate (ESR), and antiphospholipid antibodies. It is also appropriate to test for SARS-CoV-2 by RT-PCR and serology, because these symptoms may be caused by a late effect of the virus. These tests are still often negative [100]. Skin biopsy may be recommended in more severe cases.

Screening and Diagnosis in Asymptomatic Patients

Testing of asymptomatic patients is warranted in certain circumstances. Asymptomatic patients who have previously been diagnosed with COVID-19 within the past

90 days (i.e. "COVID-recovered patients") should not be retested because a positive test in this circumstance is unlikely to represent a new, active infection [130].

Ambulatory Testing

There are various indications for testing of the asymptomatic patient in the ambulatory setting. The results may be needed for the purposes of contact tracing of an exposed patient. In which case, exposed patients that are unvaccinated can be tested on or after days 5–7, and they can end quarantine if negative after seven days [130]. Exposed patients that are fully vaccinated do not need to quarantine. As per CDC recommendations, these individuals must wear a mask indoors in public for 14 days following exposure or until a negative test result is obtained 5-7 days after exposure. Testing should also be considered 24–72 hours before any outpatient treatments or procedures requiring anesthesia with high likelihood of aerosol generation, such as those involving the upper respiratory tract. Asymptomatic testing of children may also be required for admission to a hospital or another facility, such as shelters or residential facilities, or for clearance for school, sports, work, or travel [127].

Inpatient and Perioperative Testing

During the pandemic, most pediatric centers have adopted "universal testing" of patients on admission irrespective of clinical symptoms or suspicion for COVID-19. Through such practices, hospitals are able to detect asymptomatic patients who would not have been otherwise detected, as well as presymptomatic patients, to ensure early diagnosis and monitoring. Overall, the goal of this strategy is to allow for the early identification of infected patients to allow for prompt isolation and contact tracing and to prevent hospital-associated transmission.

Perioperative testing should be individualized and guided by regional SARS-CoV-2 prevalence, testing capacity and resources, and local infection prevention and control guidance [138]. The incidence rate of COVID-19 in children undergoing preoperative universal screening has been shown to be <1% [138]. Patients who have planned upcoming procedures or admission should receive molecular-based (i.e. RT-PCR) screening tests only. The optimal timing of preoperative screening is complicated by scheduling logistics and inadequate turnaround times of tests, necessitating testing several days in advance. In a single-site

study carried out when community transmission rates were relatively low, SARS-CoV-2 test results obtained one to three days before surgery were 100% concordant with those on the day of surgery [139]. At times when SARS-CoV-2 community transmission has been high, many pediatric hospitals in the United States have required that anyone with a planned admission, surgical procedure, or aerosol-generating procedure be tested at most 72 hours before admission.

Neonatal Testing

All neonates (≤28 days old) born to mothers with suspected or confirmed COVID-19, regardless of symptoms, should undergo molecular testing for SARS-CoV-2 from a nasopharynx, oropharynx, or nasal swab sample [59]. The sensitivity of a single test specimen in this age group is unknown and continues to be evaluated. Ideally, molecular testing should be obtained from paired nasopharynx and oropharynx samples [140]. However, testing on a single sample is acceptable based on institutional resources, particularly for asymptomatic, term infants [140]. In the case of an initial negative test result, repeat testing should be guided by clinical judgment and institutional testing priorities in discussion with infection prevention and control. For neonates with signs of infection suggestive of COVID-19 (see earlier Infection in Infants (Age <1 Year) section), providers should also consider alternative diagnoses.

The optimal timing of testing after birth is not known. Ideally, neonatal testing may be deferred for asymptomatic neonates until maternal results are available. In symptomatic neonates with a high index of suspicion, testing should be sent even if maternal testing is pending. In general, testing at <24 hours of life (HOL) is not recommended to avoid detecting transient viral nucleic acid [59, 140]. Early testing may also lead to false negative results because viral RNA may not yet be detectable immediately after exposure following birth. In asymptomatic neonates expected to be discharged early (<48 HOL), a single test before discharge (between 24 and 48 HOL) is recommended with plan to follow up pending results by phone [59]. All others should undergo initial testing at 24 HOL and if negative, testing should be repeated at 48 HOL and at 14 days (for admitted infants) [59]. Any neonate requiring admission for postnatal exposure to anyone with suspected or confirmed SARS-CoV-2 should be tested on admission and, if negative, at 7 and 14 days [59]. When testing or test results are not available, all neonates born to mothers with suspected or confirmed infection should be considered as having suspected SARS-CoV-2 infection for the 14-day period of observation [140].

COVID-Recovered Patients

COVID-recovered patients are defined as patients who are at least 10 days status post symptom onset or their first SARS-CoV-2 laboratory-confirmed test from a respiratory source or clinical specimen [141]. For previously symptomatic patients who are severely immunocompromised or those previously admitted for severe to critical illness (see Table 12.2), at least 20 days must have passed since symptoms first appeared [141]. Any patient who was previously symptomatic must also be at least 24 hours out since last fever without the use of fever-reducing medications with improvement in symptoms (e.g. cough, shortness of breath) [141]. Evidence from human studies of immunity after COVID-19 have demonstrated that immunity is present for at least a short duration after recovery from SARS-CoV-2 infection (even when antibody titers in serum are below the level of detection) [142, 143]. Such studies have also shown that reinfection with transmissible virus has not occurred over short time periods after confirmed COVID-19 [142, 143].

Retesting of COVID-Recovered Patients

Cases of reinfection with COVID-19 have been reported but remain rare [144–146]. Retesting for SARS-CoV-2 should be considered in the following instances: (i) new infectious symptoms ≥90 days since first or most recent SARS-CoV-2 infection, (ii) new infectious symptoms without alternate etiology 45–89 days since first or most recent SARS-CoV-2 infection, and (iii) new infectious symptoms with close contact with a person known to have laboratory-confirmed SARS-CoV-2 infection 45–89 days since first SARS-CoV-2 infection [147]. In these cases, a positive result suggests reinfection. If viral specimens from both time points are available, genetic sequencing could be used to further support that reinfection has occurred. Lastly, retesting of an asymptomatic patient with no known exposure to SARS-CoV-2 may be required for transfer to a congregate care setting with testing required as per the protocol for patient

acceptance. In such scenarios, a positive test does not necessarily indicate reinfection.

Testing of COVID-19 Fully Vaccinated Persons

Guidelines about testing of vaccinated persons may change as we learn more about different vaccines and new strains. As of October 2021, fully vaccinated persons with exposure to a suspected or confirmed case of COVID-19 do not need to quarantine or obtain SARS-CoV-2 testing if they (i) are two weeks past their full vaccination series, and (ii) have remained asymptomatic since their COVID-19 exposure [130]. These individuals should still wear a mask in public indoor settings or until they receive a negative test result 5-7 days following the date of their exposure. They should continue to watch for symptoms for 14 days after exposure. SARS-CoV-2 testing is recommended if they become symptomatic [130]. They should isolate if they test positive. Fully vaccinated people who live in a household with someone who is immunosuppressed, at increased risk of severe disease, or unvaccinated (including unvaccinated children) could also consider masking at home for 14 days following a known exposure or until they receive a negative test result. A fully vaccinated person who experiences symptoms consistent with COVID-19 should isolate themselves from others, be clinically evaluated for COVID-19, and tested for SARS-CoV-2 if indicated.

MIS-C Diagnosis

The first step in management of MIS-C is the rapid identification and diagnosis of children at risk. Table 12.3 summarizes the case definition and diagnostic workup recommended by the CDC [117], WHO [118], Royal College of Pediatrics and Child Health (RCPCH) [119], and American College of Rheumatology [113]. The mainstay of MIS-C diagnosis involves evidence or high suspicion based on epidemiologic data of COVID-19 infection in the prior two to six weeks, fever (≥38.0 °C), signs of inflammation with clinical findings (≥2) of rash, conjunctivitis, mucosal erythema, respiratory distress, and gastrointestinal, cardiac, and neurologic involvement. Supportive laboratory evidence includes, but is not limited to, an elevated CRP, ESR, fibrinogen, procalcitonin, D-dimer, ferritin, lactic acid dehydrogenase

(LDH), or interleukin-6 (IL-6), and elevated neutrophils, reduced lymphocytes, low albumin, low sodium, or low platelets. Given the frequent association of MIS-C with cardiac involvement, cardiac testing, including echocardiogram, electrocardiogram, cardiac enzyme or troponin testing, and B-type natriuretic peptide, is suggested to aid in diagnosis and management. The various cardiac manifestations seen in MIS-C include left ventricular dysfunction, coronary artery dilation or coronary artery aneurysm, and electrical conduction abnormalities. Less frequently seen are valvular dysfunction, myocarditis, pericardial effusion and atrioventricular block [113, 148]. The most concerning presentations are those with shock, vital sign instability, and respiratory distress. Various reviews of COVID-19 and MIS-C in children and adolescents have been published from around the world and serve to help guide the clinician in identifying and treating patients with MIS-C [30, 149, 150].

When evaluating a patient with possible MIS-C, it is essential to rule out other acute illnesses, including bacterial sepsis, acute viral myocarditis, toxic shock syndrome, acute appendicitis, and even acute flares of autoimmune conditions such as lupus because notable overlap in presentation exists.

Hyperinflammation in COVID-19 Versus MIS-C

As defined in Table 12.3, MIS-C is characterized by fever, systemic inflammation, and multiorgan dysfunction that occurs in the late phase of SARS-CoV-2 infection. Some patients can develop hyperinflammation in the acute, infectious phase of COVID-19. There may be similarities in the features of some children with MIS-C and COVID-19-associated hyperinflammation because they share features of lymphopenia, coagulopathy, hyperferritinemia, transaminitis, elevated CRP, and elevated LDH. However, patients with hyperinflammation typically present later in the course of acute infection (often during the second week of the respiratory illness) with clinical decline, whereas the time frame of development of MIS-C after COVID-19 exposure is two to six weeks, and affected patients are generally well before onset of symptoms, which tend to appear abruptly. A recent review compared more than 1000 US patients <21 years of age diagnosed with either MIS-C (n = 539) or severe acute COVID-19

(n = 577) [30]. Patients with MIS-C had higher neutrophil/lymphocyte ratio (median, 6.4 vs. 2.7; $P < 0.001$), had higher CRP concentration (median, 152 vs. 33 mg/l; $P < 0.001$), and were more likely to be directly admitted to the ICU (73.8% vs. 43.8%) [30]. Clinical symptoms of gastrointestinal and mucocutaneous involvement and evidence of myocardial dysfunction tend to be more prominent in MIS-C, whereas respiratory involvement is more common in COVID-19 [30]. Antibody testing may help differentiate the two, but this is an area of debate.

Management

It has become challenging for pediatric medical professionals to manage an emerging infection such as SARS-CoV-2 because the existing medical management has been largely studied in adults. There have been trials looking at different treatment modalities in pediatrics, however, the results of some studies have been difficult to interpret because of study design, lack of power, and conflicting reports. Treatment options remain limited to those already being used in adults or those offered largely under the umbrella of a clinical trial. Thus far, the treatment of active SARS-CoV-2 remains supportive, and ongoing clinical trials and research studies hope to shed more light on how to best manage young patients.

Outpatient Management

Most children with a SARS-CoV-2 infection are asymptomatic or have mild symptoms [75]. The mainstay of managing SARS-CoV-2 infections in this population is supportive care and is based on interim guidance provided by a panel of pediatric infectious diseases physicians [81]. Infected children should be isolated as best as is appropriate to minimize transmission to others. These children should also be assessed regularly for signs and symptoms of disease progression.

Supplemental Agents

There are no data to support the use of supplements, such as zinc, vitamin C, or vitamin D, in children infected with or who have been exposed to SARS-CoV-2. Any use of supplemental agents in the setting of outpatient management or postexposure prophylaxis should be done only in the context of a clinical trial. In addition, the CDC has telephone triage guidance for medical practices receiving calls from patients and their family members with COVID-19 infection [151].

The National Institutes of Health (NIH) recommends against the use of zinc supplementation above the recommended dietary allowance for the prevention of COVID-19, except in a clinical trial [152]. With regard to vitamin C or vitamin D, there are insufficient data either for or against their use for the prevention or treatment of COVID-19 [153, 154]. Vitamin C is an antioxidant and free radical scavenger that has anti-inflammatory properties [154]. Vitamin C is also thought to influence cellular immunity and vascular integrity and serves as a cofactor in the generation of endogenous catecholamines [154]. As such, the potential role of high doses of vitamin C in ameliorating inflammation and vascular injury in patients with COVID-19 is being studied, particularly in those with sepsis and ARDS [154]. Vitamin D may have immunomodulatory effects that could potentially protect against COVID-19 infection or decrease the severity of illness [153]. Vitamin D deficiency has been associated with increased risk of pneumonia, and poor outcomes with COVID-19 disease [153]. Therefore, at some centers, vitamin D is part of the standard management of critically ill patients with COVID-19.

Monoclonal Antibodies

The development of monoclonal antibodies for therapy against SARS-CoV-2 has provided some hope of improving outcomes in infected patients. As of October 2021, these monoclonal antibodies include bamlanivimab-etesevimab, casirivimab-imdevimab, as well as sotrovimab. These antibodies work by binding the receptor binding domain of SARS-CoV-2, preventing binding of the virus to host cells [155]. In adults, administration of these agents may lead to more rapid viral clearance and a lower rate of hospitalization when administered early in the course of illness [156]. In children, there are insufficient data to support the use of monoclonal antibodies. Some experts advise against routine administration of monoclonal antibody therapy, with one study citing that in children and adolescents, the usual course of COVID-19 is mild and there is no evidence for safety and efficacy [157].

Bamlanivimab initially obtained Emergency Use Authorization (EUA) under the US Food and Drug Administration (FDA) as monotherapy but is now being deployed in combination with etesevimab following a randomized controlled trial showing that the combination is most effective [158, 159]. In March 2021, the US government stopped distribution of the monotherapy altogether because of a sustained increase in SARS-CoV-2 viral variants in the United States that are resistant to bamlanivimab when administered alone [160]. Data suggest that bamlanivimab with etesevimab retains neutralization activity against the B.1.1.7 (UK) variant but has reduced activity against the Gamma (P.1, Brazil) and Beta (B.1.35, South African) variants [162]. Due to the latter, distribution of bamlanivimab plus etesevimab was paused in the United States. However, distribution of these agents has been reinstated as of October 2021 in states with low rates of these and other resistant variants. Please refer to the FDA website for the latest on banlanivimab plus etesevimab distribution [161]. Casirivimab-imdevimab and sotrovimab have maintained activity against the B.1.1.7 (UK) and B.1.351 (South African) variants [162, 163]. Ongoing evaluation of the efficacy of monoclonal antibodies against new variants remains critical. As of October 2021, efficacy has not been demonstrated in patients already hospitalized with COVID-19.

For high-risk children with mild to moderate SARS-CoV-2 infection who are 12–17 years of age and weigh ≥40 kg, bamlanivimab-etesevimab or casirivimab-imdevimab or sotrovimab can be offered under EUA [156] within 10 days of COVID-19 symptom onset [159, 160, 163]. Only children with certain conditions associated with increased risk for progression to severe disease are eligible. These conditions or comorbidities are defined as chronic respiratory disease, congenital or acquired heart disease, neurodevelopmental disorders, sickle cell disease, a body mass index ≥85th percentile, or a medically related technologic dependence (e.g. tracheostomy, gastrostomy, or positive pressure ventilation) [159, 160, 163]. As of October 2021, these agents should be used only in children younger than 12 years in the setting of a clinical trial, because there is currently no EUA for this age group.

The purpose of monoclonal antibodies is to prevent hospitalization of high-risk patients with SARS-CoV-2 infection. Therefore, use of monoclonal antibodies should be considered only on a case-by-case basis in the outpatient setting. Patients hospitalized for a reason other than COVID-19 or those who do not require new or increased respiratory support as a result of COVID-19 are also eligible [160, 163]. As of October 2021, the use of bamlanivimab-etesevimab and casirivimab-imdevimab have also obtained EUA under the FDA as post-exposure prophylaxis for certain individuals at high risk for acquiring SARS-CoV-2 infection and progression to serious illness if infected [164]. For high-risk patients, post-exposure prophylaxis can be considered for patients who are unvaccinated and either exposed to SARS-COV-2 infected person (having a close contact within 6 feet for at least 15 minutes) or at high risk due to COVID-19 cases in same environment.

Patients hospitalized or requiring supplemental oxygen for COVID-19 should not be given monoclonal antibodies because some data suggest monoclonal antibodies can worsen outcomes in these groups [157]. In some cases, patients may be given monoclonal antibodies under the FDA's compassionate use pathway outside of the EUA [165]. Clinicians considering this treatment for their patients are advised to consult an infectious diseases specialist who can best determine appropriate use, particularly for those patients with high-risk comorbidities.

Inpatient Management

Initial management of pediatric patients hospitalized with SARS-CoV-2 infection consists of clinical stabilization and supportive care for multiple organ systems. Careful monitoring of vital signs and oxygen saturations is important because clinical status can rapidly change. Laboratory workup includes baseline CBC with differential, CRP, D-dimer, ferritin, and LDH. Some hospitals have incorporated IL-6 monitoring. Depending on severity of illness, laboratory monitoring may be daily or two to three times per week. Imaging may be considered on a case-by-case basis.

Respiratory and Cardiac Management

Respiratory management includes supplemental oxygen administration in invasive and noninvasive forms. These include nasal cannula, continuous positive airway pressure, bilevel positive airway pressure, intubation, and ventilator support. When possible, noninvasive ventilation is preferred, and HFNC has been used with success [166]. Infectious diseases consultation is recommended for patients who require supplemental oxygen.

Careful monitoring is required, with assessment for pediatric ICU consultation in patients with rapidly deteriorating clinical status. Careful cardiac monitoring is necessary. Vasopressor support may be necessary in patients with COVID-19 and shock and, in rare cases, extracorporeal membrane oxygenation (ECMO).

Fluid and Electrolytes

Children tend to be become dehydrated faster than adults, so crucial management of dehydration is necessary, especially in neonates, who are at even greater risk. Dynamic parameters, such as skin temperature, capillary refilling time, and/or lactate parameters, can help in assessing fluid response [167].

Hematology

Because COVID-19 has been found to be a hypercoagulable state, venous thromboembolism prophylaxis must be considered in at-risk patients. Hematology consult should be considered in settings of fever, hypoxia, respiratory distress, abnormal CXR, obesity, central venous catheters, and immobilization. Anticoagulation with enoxaparin and heparin has been used [168]. Contraindications for prophylaxis include a gastrointestinal bleed within three months, gastrointestinal ulcers, planned surgery, or bleeding disorders.

Special Populations

Children with acute symptomatic COVID-19 should be admitted if they have preexisting conditions that predispose them to acute worsening of disease. These include, but are not limited to, obesity, asthma, diabetes, immunocompromised, or infants younger than 30 days of age with fever. Clinicians should be aware that existing comorbidities and special patient populations will require individual plans, because disease manifestations in these patients may be more severe than COVID-19 in healthy patients. For example, oncology patients are at increased risk for mortality in comparison with those without underlying disease [169]. In immunocompromised hosts, viral symptoms may also persist for a longer course because of difficulty of clearing the virus. In patients receiving chronic immunosuppressive therapy, COVID-19 manifestation may be different from expected. These patients will need consultation with a specialist regarding reducing immunosuppressive therapy.

Antiviral Therapy

Available evidence, which is of variable quality but evolving rapidly, supports use of remdesivir as the antiviral agent that could be considered as part of COVID-19 management. Remdesivir binds to the SARS-CoV-2 RNA polymerase and leads to premature termination of transcription [155]. Other antivirals, such as lopinavir-ritonavir, have been studied in large randomized clinical trials but are currently not recommended for use in any patient, pediatric or adult [170].

Remdesivir

Data supporting use for remdesivir are conflicting, with multiple clinical trials arriving at discordant conclusions [171–173]. The IDSA and NIH recommend use of remdesivir under specific circumstances, and WHO conditionally recommends against it. A double-blinded randomized controlled trial funded by the NIH, the Adaptive Covid-19 Treatment Trial (ACTT-1), showed that remdesivir significantly reduced the time to recovery compared with placebo [171]. The median time to recovery was 10 days versus 15 days with placebo. Subgroup analysis suggested this was most pronounced for patients who required supplemental oxygen, and suggested a mortality benefit in this group [171]. However, the SIMPLE-Moderate and the SOLIDARITY trials did not show any mortality benefit [172, 173]. The SIMPLE-Moderate was a Gilead-sponsored open-label, randomized trial in patients with moderate COVID-19 that compared (i) standard of care, (ii) 5-day course of remdesivir, and (iii) 10-day course of remdesivir (although this group received a median of 6 days of the drug). There was significant improvement in the 5-day remdesivir group, but not in the 10-day remdesivir group, compared with the standard-of-care group. The authors suggest the effect size was of questionable clinical significance even in the 5-day group, and there was no difference in mortality between groups [172]. The SOLIDARITY trial, an open-label, global multicenter study sponsored by the WHO, randomized patients to one of five treatment options or no study drug with standard of care [171]. There was no significant difference in mortality, length

of hospitalization, or initiation of mechanical ventilation between any of the groups, including remdesivir versus no study drug [171]. All of these trials were done in adult patient populations. A phase 2/3 clinical trial evaluating the pharmacokinetics of remdesivir in children is currently underway; however, those results have not yet been published [174].

Remdesivir is the only drug approved by the FDA for treatment of COVID-19 for hospitalized adults and children aged ≥12 years and weighing ≥40 kg. Remdesivir is additionally FDA authorized via EUA for hospitalized patients with COVID-19 who are 12 years of age and who weigh more than 3.5 kg and children of any age who weigh between 3.5 and 40 kg [175]. As per the Infectious Diseases Society of America (IDSA) and NIH, use of remdesivir is suggested for hospitalized patients who require supplemental oxygen, noninvasive or invasive mechanical ventilation, or ECMO [176]. Remdesivir is most beneficial earlier in the course of illness, so it should be started as soon as possible after a positive test in patients meeting these criteria, particularly in patients who require invasive mechanical ventilation or ECMO.

Remdesivir is dosed with a 5 mg/kg intravenous (IV) loading dose (maximum 200 mg) on day 1, followed by 2.5 mg/kg IV every 24 hours (maximum 100 mg) on days 2–5 [175]. Duration can be extended up to 10 days on a case-by-case basis, usually in consultation with infectious diseases, if not clinically improving and ongoing viral replication is suspected [175]. Remdesivir should be discontinued at time of hospital discharge, even if this occurs before the completion of five days of treatment [175]. Remdesivir carries with it some noteworthy side effects, particularly hepatotoxicity. This agent should not be used in combination with hepatotoxic drugs. Before starting remdesivir, baseline laboratory tests should be obtained, including CBC, prothrombin time/international normalized ratio, comprehensive metabolic panel, and pregnancy test (if applicable). Follow-up laboratory tests should include a comprehensive metabolic panel daily, along with CBC and prothrombin time/international normalized ratio at day 5 if therapy is to be continued (or sooner if concern for toxicity). There is no dose adjustment with renal or hepatic impairment. Remdesivir is not recommended for patients with estimated glomerular filtration rate <30 ml/min because it contains renally cleared metabolites [175, 177]. If used, duration should be limited to five days, and lyophilized powder should be used preferentially to minimize risk for toxicity from cyclodextrin accumulation. Moreover, remdesivir should not be used if alanine aminotransferase is more than 10 times the upper limit of normal [175]. Clinicians should review side effects with families of pediatric patients receiving remdesivir. If an EUA is used, proper consent and documentation should be followed as per FDA and hospital policy. The FDA has created a remdesivir fact sheet for patients and their families [178].

More recently, remdesivir has been used in combination with baricitinib. The FDA has issued an EUA for use of baricitinib in combination with remdesivir for treatment of COVID-19 in hospitalized patients ≥2 years of age who require supplemental oxygen, invasive mechanical ventilation, or ECMO [179].

Glucocorticoids

Glucocorticoids have been shown in randomized control trials to reduce mortality in adults with COVID-19 who required supplemental oxygen or ventilation [180]. SARS-CoV-2 leads to a hyperinflammatory state, and dexamethasone may suppress the immune response, preventing progression to severe disease and further pulmonary injury. Children were not included in the reported data, so it is uncertain whether they experience similar benefit. IDSA recommends corticosteroids in confirmed COVID-19 hospitalized patients with severe COVID-19 requiring supplemental oxygen, ventilation, or ECMO (the same definitions guiding remdesivir use) [176]. The NIH makes similar recommendations and stratifies recommendations by disease severity, determining whether glucocorticoids are to be used alone or in combination with remdesivir [181]. The WHO similarly recommends systemic dexamethasone or other corticosteroids, such as hydrocortisone or prednisone, for patients with severe or critical COVID-19 [182].

In children, corticosteroids should be considered on a case-by-case basis, weighing individual risks and benefits and duration of illness, with children who have been ill for longer durations (e.g. more than 7–10 days) perhaps benefiting more. Moderate-dose corticosteroid therapy is typically used for treatment of pediatric patients who require respiratory support, but caution is advised in those already receiving steroids or with severe immunocompromise. Dexamethasone is the most commonly prescribed at a dose of 0.15 mg/kg orally or IV (maximum dose of 6 mg). Alternatives include equivalent daily doses of methylprednisolone (0.8 mg/kg once daily [maximum dose, 32 mg]) or prednisone (1 mg/kg orally once daily [maximum dose, 40 mg]) [155]. In children being treated for an asthma exacerbation in the setting of COVID-19, higher doses of methylprednisolone are often used (2 mg/kg/day divided twice daily [maximum, 30 mg/dose]). At some pediatric centers, hydrocortisone is used in infants with postmenstrual age <40 weeks: 0.5 mg/kg IV every 12 hours for seven days and then 0.5 mg/kg once daily for three days. The duration of therapy is 10 days or until discharge, whichever is shorter, unless there is another indication for ongoing corticosteroids [176, 183]. Adjunctive corticosteroids may also be considered in patients with ARDS, adrenal dysfunction, or catecholamine refractory septic shock. For patients with adrenal insufficiency, hydrocortisone should be administered in addition to dexamethasone.

When using steroids, clinicians should monitor for hyperglycemia, especially in patients with endocrinopathy such as diabetes. In addition, it is important to keep in mind that prolonged steroids may increase risk for reactivation of latent infection or worsen superimposed bacterial or fungal infections [155]. Dexamethasone is a moderate cytochrome P450 inducer, so careful review of all medications is important [183]. In cases where new oncologic diagnosis is suspected, dexamethasone should be used carefully and in discussion with specialists, because this could mask symptoms and delay the diagnosis.

Nonsteroidal Anti-inflammatory Drugs

No current data connect the use of nonsteroidal anti-inflammatory drugs (NSAIDS), including ibuprofen, to worsening COVID-19-related symptoms and/or death [184]. Currently, the FDA and WHO do not recommend against use of NSAIDS [185]. If patients are chronically taking NSAIDS, they do not necessarily need to be discontinued. However, patients receiving remdesivir therapy should not receive concomitant NSAIDs because of risk for nephrotoxicity [175].

Convalescent Plasma

Convalescent plasma harvested from patients with prior COVID-19 infection has been occasionally used in the setting of adults with COVID-19 pneumonia to hasten recovery. The proposed mechanisms of action include viral neutralization through passive antibodies in patients who have not had time to develop antibodies. In August 2020, the FDA authorized EUA for use of convalescent plasma in hospitalized patients with COVID-19 [186]. This decision was based on descriptive data early in the pandemic in which convalescent plasma showed promise of being a viable agent to treat patients hospitalized with acute COVID-19 [176]. A systematic review and meta-analysis of 10 randomized controlled studies concluded that use of convalescent plasma in patients with COVID-19 does not appear to improve survival or clinical status, shorten hospital stays, or reduce the need for mechanical ventilation [Janiaud-187]. The previous EUA was further revised in February 2021 to authorize only high-titer COVID-19 convalescent plasma use, and only for hospitalized patients with early COVID-19 disease or impaired immunity [188]. For pediatric patients, safety and efficacy of COVID-19 convalescent plasma are inconclusive, with insufficient evidence from the NIH to recommend for against its use for the treatment of COVID-19 in hospitalized children not requiring mechanical ventilation. In pediatric patients who are mechanically ventilated, NIH recommends against its use [181].

Adjunctive Therapy

Hydroxychloroquine

The FDA initially authorized the use of hydroxychloroquine under EUA in March 2020, but this EUA was revoked in June 2020 after further studies showed poor evidence of benefit [189]. In a large controlled trial of adult hospitalized patients in the United Kingdom, hydroxychloroquine did not decrease mortality when compared with standard of care and even resulted in longer median hospital stay. Patients not on ventilators at time of randomization had higher likelihood of intubation and death [190]. Currently, the NIH, WHO, and IDSA recommend against the use of hydroxychloroquine alone and/or with azithromycin [176, 191].

Ivermectin

Ivermectin is an antiparasitic medication [192]. Although ivermectin may inhibit SARS-CoV-2 replication in vitro, the concentration needed to achieve this inhibition in vitro far exceeds the concentrations achieved in human blood or plasma with available dosing strategies. Ivermectin has substantial side effects, including gastrointestinal and neurologic complications such as coma and death; the effective concentration required to treat COVID-19 in humans would be lethal [155]. Neither the IDSA, NIH, nor the FDA recommend using ivermectin outside of a clinical trial [192–194].

IL-6 Inhibitors

IL-6 is a proinflammatory cytokine associated with cytokine storm, systemic inflammation, and multiorgan failure. Therapies targeted against IL-6 include anti-IL6 receptor monoclonal antibodies (mAbs) (e.g. tocilizumab, sarilumab,) or anti-IL6 mAbs (siltuximab). As reflected in the NIH guidelines, data [195, 196, 197] support a role for tocilizumab in severely ill adults early in the course of ICU admission (within 24 hours) who are taking corticosteroids, with rapidly increasing oxygenation needs and systemic inflammation [198]. There is insufficient evidence for the NIH to recommend either for or against the use of tocilizumab in hospitalized children with COVID-19 or MIS-C [195]. FDA has issued EUA for tocilizumab for hospitalized pediatric patients ages 2 years and older with severe COVID-19 [198]. Some pediatric centers use tocilizumab (in addition to steroids) on a case-by-case basis in COVID-19 positive children with evidence of hyperinflammation early in the course of ICU admission (within 24 hours) or in those patients with new onset respiratory failure, rapidly escalating respiratory support and/or hemodynamic instability refractory to fluid resuscitation [195, 198]. Tocilizumab is usually infused over 1 hour and is dosed by total body weight: 12 mg/kg IV for patients < 30 kg and 8 mg/kg for patients > 30 kg (max 800 mg). A second dose may be considered within 12-18 hours of the first dose if there is no clinical improvement [195].

Patients should generally not receive tocilizumab if they received a live, attenuated vaccine within the two weeks prior to therapy due to concern for vaccine strain infection and/or decreased effectiveness of the vaccine. Moreover, tocilizumab should be avoided in a subset of patients who are severely immunocompromised, using other biologic immunomodulators, high ALT, high risk for gastrointestinal perforation, uncontrolled non-SARS-CoV-2 infection, severe neutropenia, severe thrombocytopenia, or known hypersensitivity to tocilizumab [195, 198]. There have been reports of Strongyloides stercoralis in patients with COVID-19 treated with immunomodulators. Therefore, empiric treatment with ivermectin may be considered in patients weighing more than >15 kg from regions where Strongyloides stercoralis is endemic.

Kinase Inhibitors

Kinase inhibitors are divided into two classes, Janus kinase (JAK) inhibitors and Bruton's tyrosine kinase (BTK) inhibitors. JAK inhibitors block phosphorylation and activation of transcription (STAT) proteins, which reduce T-cell activation. In COVID-19, this activity dampens proinflammatory cytokine signaling, including that of IL-2, IL-6, GM-CSF, IFN-gamma, and IL-10. Current JAK inhibitors under investigation include baricitinib and tofacitinib. FDA has issued EUA for a 14-day course of baricitinib in hospitalized patients ages 2 years and older with COVID-19 who require supplemental oxygen, invasive mechanical ventilation, or extracorporeal membrane oxygenation (ECMO). Some pediatric centers use baricitinib (in addition to steroids) on a case-by-case basis in COVID-19 positive children with evidence of hyperinflammation meeting these EUA criteria [179]. Please see EUA fact sheet for dosing, drug monitoring parameters and recommended action [179].

Baricitinib should be used with caution in immunocompromised children given the risk for opportunistic infections and herpesvirus reactivation syndromes. JAK inhibitors should also not be used in patients with known active tuberculosis. Patients should generally not receive baricitinib if they received a live, attenuated vaccine within the two weeks prior to therapy due to concern for vaccine strain infection and/or decreased effectiveness of the vaccine. There have been reports of Strongyloides stercoralis in patients with COVID-19 treated with immunomodulators. Therefore, empiric treatment with ivermectin may be considered in patients weighing more than >15 kg from regions where Strongyloides stercoralis is endemic.

BTK inhibitors act on B-cell antigen receptor and cytokine receptor pathways. Current BTK inhibitors under investigation include acalabrutinib and ibrutinib. The safety and efficacy of BTK inhibitors for pediatric patients has not yet been established [195], and as of October 2021, most experts recommend against the use of these immunomodulators, except in clinical trials.

Superimposed Infections

Bacterial coinfection in the setting of patients with COVID-19 infection is relatively uncommon, occurring in <10% of cases [199, 200]. In a study of adult patients with COVID-19, community-acquired coinfection at diagnosis was uncommon, mainly caused by *Streptococcus pneumoniae* and *Staphylococcus aureus* [201]. Bacterial superinfection should be considered in the presence of laboratory findings of leukocytosis or bandemia or radiographic findings of lobar consolidations [200]. In addition, antibacterial agents may be considered in the setting of persistent fevers, fever relapse, or clinical deterioration.

Fungal coinfection in acute COVID-19 infections are also uncommon. That being said, there has been a noted incidence of *Aspergillus* species complicating COVID-19 pneumonia, now termed coronavirus disease–associated pulmonary aspergillosis. In one small cohort study, coronavirus disease–associated pulmonary aspergillosis was found to occur in up to 20% of critically ill ventilated adult patients [202]. Based on these findings, it seems reasonable to consider adding an antifungal such as voriconazole for pediatric patients with COVID-19 infections who require intensive care, although definitive recommendations for this are lacking.

Management of MIS-C

MIS-C is recognized to be a multiorgan system inflammatory disease that occurs two to six weeks after a patient is infected with SARS-CoV-2. For case definitions, see Table 12.3. Information regarding the management of MIS-C is evolving rapidly for refractory cases. The article by Henderson et al summarizes the most recent updates with the version number included in the title [203]. Readers should consult the most current version of the article. Treatment includes a stepwise approach to reducing the inflammatory burden as quickly as possible with immunomodulatory agents. First-tier treatment regimens include high-dose (2 g/kg) intravenous immunoglobulin (IVIG) with or without glucocorticoids. Glucocorticoids (1–2 mg/kg/day divided twice daily of prednisone, prednisolone, or methylprednisolone) should be used as adjunctive therapy in patients with severe disease (shock or organ-threatening disease) or as intensification therapy in patients with IVIG-refractory disease [113, 203]. Anakinra may also be considered as a steroid-sparing agent in patients with contraindications to long courses of glucocorticoids [113, 203]. As of October, 2021, the American College of Rheumatology recommends intensification treatment with either pulse IV steroids (methylprednisolone 10–30 mg/kg/day IV) or high-dose anakinra (>4 mg/kg/day), or infliximab in certain patients with refractory disease [203]. MIS-C does appear to be a hypercoagulable state, so aspirin and anticoagulants (e.g. enoxaparin) should be considered [113]. The American College of Rheumatology provides guidance with regard to antiplatelet and anticoagulation therapy and duration, which should be tailored to the patient's risk for thrombosis, coronary artery z-scores, and left ventricular function (i.e. ejection fraction) [113]. Low-dose aspirin should be continued at least until ≥4 weeks after diagnosis [113]. Epinephrine, dobutamine, and dopamine are used for patients with septic shock and/or depressed cardiac function [204]. Serial laboratory testing and cardiac assessment should guide decisions to decrease immunomodulatory treatment [203]. Children with MIS-C require a prolonged course of immunomodulatory treatment that may need to extend for two to three weeks, or even longer, to avoid rebound inflammation [203]. Live vaccines should be held for 11 months in patients who receive high-dose IVIG.

Not all patients with MIS-C may require treatment with immunomodulatory agents. In a study by Whittaker et al. [205], 22% of patients with mild MIS-C recovered with supportive care only. The MIS-C Task Force of the American College of Rheumatology noted uncertainty around the empiric use of IVIG in this setting to prevent coronary artery aneurysms [203]. It appears as though some patients with mild symptoms may require only close monitoring by specialists who have expertise in MIS-C, without the use of immunomodulators [203].

Guidance for Return to Sports After SARS-CoV-2 Infection

The following recommendations are based on expert analysis from the American College of Cardiology [206] and review of published guidelines as of March 2021 [207]. Timing with regard to returning to sports is important due to the association of COVID-19 with cardiac damage and myocarditis [208]. Recommendations are subject to change as more information about the cardiac manifestations of COVID-19 in pediatric patients becomes available.

Pediatric patients should refrain from sports for at least 10 days and until asymptomatic for 24 hours without fever-reducing medicines to allow for the full clinical manifestations of COVID-19 to present themselves and to decrease the risk for transmission to others [206]. Pediatric patients may be cleared for sports thereafter if during quarantine they were either asymptomatic or minimally symptomatic without cardiac concerns irrespective of age, or moderately symptomatic with no abnormal cardiac testing for children <12 years of age [206, 207]. Pediatric patients ≥12 years of age with a history of moderate COVID-19 symptoms who want to participate in high-intensity physical activity require an electrocardiogram for clearance [206]. If the electrocardiogram and examination are normal and there are no additional cardiac concerns, the patient may be cleared for participation in sports. If abnormalities are identified, the patient should be referred to pediatric cardiology [206]. For all patients cleared for sports, physical activity should be resumed slowly over a minimum of seven days, and patients should be monitored for symptoms. Any concern for clinical deterioration or cardiac symptoms should prompt further cardiac evaluation and discontinuation of exercise until further notice [207].

All patients with severe acute COVID-19 symptoms should be referred to outpatient cardiology for evaluation at least two weeks after discharge, or sooner if there are cardiac concerns, regardless of age or activity level. Patients should be restricted from exercise and sports until the initial cardiology appointment, with anticipatory guidance that exercise restriction may last up to three to six months [206, 207].

Patients with MIS-C should be followed by pediatric cardiology outpatient. Physical activity in this population may be restricted up to three to six months [206, 207]. However, return to sports is ultimately dictated by pediatric cardiology and/or by a multidisciplinary team.

Vaccines

COVID-19 vaccines are being developed rapidly, and distribution is well underway at the time of this publication. For more information on vaccine platforms and efficacy, please see Chapter on Vaccines in this book. The FDA granted EUA for the Pfizer-BioNTech mRNA COVID-19 vaccine for adolescents ages 12-15 years in May 2021 [209], and for children ages 5-11 years in November 2021 [210].

These vaccines are administered as a two dose series, 21 days apart. An additional dose for immunocompromised children ³12 years is recommended ³28 days after completion of the 2-dose primary series [210]. Available safety and immunogenicity data for Pfizer-BioNTech COVID-19 vaccines in children and adolescents are similar to those seen in young adults [210]. There is no recommendation as of November 2021 in the US for a booster dose in people <18 years to enhance or restore protection that might have waned after the primary vaccination series. Children and adolescents who participated in the Pfizer-BioNTech COVID-19 vaccine clinical trials as well as those vaccinated at large, will be followed to determine the duration of protective effects and the need for booster dosing in this age group. The CDC and AAP recommend COVID-19 vaccination for all children 5 years and older who do not have contraindications to the COVID-19 vaccine, regardless of a history of symptomatic or asymptomatic SARS-CoV-2 infection. These organizations further support the co-administration of routine childhood vaccinations and the Pfizer-BioNTech COVID-19 vaccine. As of November 2021, there are no recommendations for vaccinating children <5 years of age against SARS-CoV-2. However, clinical trials are in progress for children as young as six months of age [211].

Each dose for children ages 5-11 is 10μg, which is one-third the dose approved for those 12 years and older (30mg). Per the CDC, children should receive the age-appropriate vaccine formulation regardless of their size or weight [210]. Therefore, children that will turn 12 years old between their first and second dose, should receive the age-appropriate 30mg Pfizer-BioNTech COVID-19 vaccine [210]. Per the FDA, however, children turning 12 between the two vaccine doses, can receive 10mg or 30mg for both doses [212]. If such dosing occurs, the child is considered fully vaccinated. This is not considered an error and reporting to the Vaccine Adverse Event Reporting System (VAERS) is not indicated.

The most common side effects of the Pfizer-BioNTech COVID-19 vaccine include arm soreness, redness, and swelling at the site of injection, as well as fatigue, headaches and muscle aches that usually last 24-48 hours. Less common side effects are swollen lymph nodes and skin sensitivity. As of October 2021, there have been no cases of transverse myelitis or Guillain-Barré syndrome reported following vaccination among participants of the Pfizer-BioNTech COVID-19 vaccine clinical trials [213]. A history of these conditions is not a contraindication to vaccination with the Pfizer-BioNTech COVID-19 vaccine [213].

Myocarditis has also been reported after vaccination with mRNA COVID-19 vaccines. These cases are very rare and estimated to occur in about 1 in 50,000 people (predominantly males) in their teens and 20s, usually within 4 days of receiving the second dose of an mRNA COVID-19 vaccine [213, 214]. Symptoms may include chest pain, shortness of breath and/or tachycardia or fluttering; and should prompt medical evaluation to ensure proper diagnosis and VAERS reporting. Most people fully recover after a brief hospitalization without any apparent permanent damage to the heart [213, 214]. Infection with SARS-CoV-2 can more frequently cause myocarditis that is often more severe. Therefore, COVID-19 vaccination continues to be recommended by the CDC and AAP. Individuals with a history of myocarditis or pericarditis related to SARS-CoV-2 or other viruses may receive the Pfizer-BioNTech COVID-19 vaccine if i) symptoms have fully resolved; ii) they have no evidence of ongoing heart inflammation; and iii) they have no cardiac sequelae as determined by a medical professional or clinical team [210]. At the time of this publication, it is unclear if people who develop myocarditis related to an mRNA COVID-19 vaccine are at increased risk of further adverse cardiac events following a subsequent dose [210]. Experts currently advise against a subsequent COVID-19 vaccine dose in these individuals unless the theoretical risk of cardiac events is outweighed by the personal risk of severe acute COVID-19 [210].

Data are limited on the safety of COVID-19 vaccines in people with a history of MIS-C. Therefore, case-by-case discussions surrounding post-MIS-C COVID-19 vaccination are important. Most experts recommend deferring COVID-19 vaccination until the patient has recovered clinically from MIS-C, including return to normal cardiac function. Since the risk of reinfection is low in the months after SARS-CoV-2 infection, some experts recommend delaying vaccination for 90 days after diagnosis. Other factors to consider when weighing individual benefits and risks include SARS-CoV-2 community transmission rates and the personal risk of severe acute COVID-19 [210]. MIS-C is exceedingly rare after COVID-19 vaccination. Clinical illnesses compatible with MIS-C in individuals vaccinated against SARS-CoV-2 should be reported to VAERS.

Live vaccines should be delayed for 11 months after receipt of high-dose intravenous immunoglobulin, which is often used in the management of MIS-C. Live vaccines should also be withheld for 3 months in patients who have received immunomodulators for the treatment of COVID-19, such as tocilizumab and baricitinib. Other vaccines, including COVID-19 vaccines, may be administered to children and adolescents without regard to timing of these antibody products or immunomodulators. COVID-19 vaccine should be delayed, however, for 30 days after receipt of anti-SARS-CoV-2 monoclonal antibodies or 90 days after receipt of COVID-19 specific passive antibody products such as COVID-19 convalescent plasma [210]. Vaccines other than COVID-19 vaccines, including inactivated and live vaccines, may be administered without regard to timing of anti-SARS-CoV-2 monoclonal antibodies. Lives vaccines should be delayed at least 7 months after receipt of COVID-19 convalescent plasma [210]. Allergic reactions to mRNA COVID-19 Vaccines are very rare but anaphylactic reactions to the vaccine component, polyethylene glycol has been reported [215]. Therefore, any child with a history of anaphylactic reaction or allergy to polyethylene glycol should not receive the mRNA vaccines.

References

1 Ludvigsson, J.F. (2020). Systematic review of COVID-19 in children shows milder cases and a better prognosis than adults. *Acta Paediatr.* 109: 1088–1095.

2 Li, X., Xu, W., Dozier, M. et al. (2020). The role of children in the transmission of SARS-CoV2: updated rapid review. *J. Glob. Health* 10: 021101.

3 Leidman, E., Duca, L.M., Omura, J.D. et al. (2021). COVID-19 trends among persons aged 0-24 years—United States, march 1 December 12, 2020. *MMWR Morb. Mortal. Wkly Rep.* 70: 88–94.

4 Sinaei, R., Pezeshki, S., Parvaresh, S., and Sinaei, R. (2021). Why COVID-19 is less frequent and severe in children: a narrative review. *World J. Pediatr.* 17: 10–20.

5 Zimmermann, P. and Curtis, N. (2020). Why is COVID-19 less severe in children? A review of the proposed mechanisms underlying the age-related difference in severity of SARS-CoV-2 infections. *Arch. Dis. Child.* 106: 429–429.

6 Lu, X., Zhang, L., Du, H. et al. (2020). SARS-CoV-2 infection in children. *N. Engl. J. Med.* 382: 1663–1665.

7 Bhuiyan, M.U., Stiboy, E., Hassan, M.Z. et al. (2021). Epidemiology of COVID-19 infection in young children under five years: a systematic review and meta-analysis. *Vaccine* 39: 667–677.

8 Baronio, R., Savare, L., Ruggiero, J. et al. (2021). Impact of ethnicity on COVID-19 related hospitalizations in children during the first pandemic wave in northern Italy. *Front. Pediatr.* 9: 625398.

9 Li, B., Zhang, S., Zhang, R. et al. (2020). Epidemiological and clinical characteristics of COVID-19 in children: a systematic review and meta-analysis. *Front. Pediatr.* 8: 591132.

10 Goyal, M.K., Simpson, J.N., Boyle, M.D. et al. (2020). Racial and/or ethnic and socioeconomic disparities of SARS-CoV-2 infection among children. *Pediatrics* 146: e2020009951.

11 Kim, L., Whitaker, M., O'Halloran, A. et al. (2020). Hospitalization rates and characteristics of children aged <18 years hospitalized with laboratory-confirmed COVID-19 - COVID-NET, 14 states, march 1 July 25, 2020. *MMWR Morb. Mortal. Wkly Rep.* 69: 1081–1088.

12 Moore, J.T., Ricaldi, J.N., Rose, C.E. et al. (2020). Disparities in incidence of COVID-19 among underrepresented racial/ethnic groups in counties

identified as hotspots during June 5–18, 2020–22 states, February–June 2020. *MMWR Morb. Mortal. Wkly Rep.* 69: 1122–1126.

13 Moreira, A., Chorath, K., Rajasekaran, K. et al. (2021). Demographic predictors of hospitalization and mortality in US children with COVID-19. *Eur. J. Pediatr.* 180: 1659–1663.

14 Pelletier, J.H., Rakkar, J., Au, A.K. et al. (2021). Trends in US pediatric hospital admissions in 2020 compared with the decade before the COVID-19 pandemic. *JAMA Netw. Open* 4: e2037227.

15 Levin, Z., Choyke, K., Georgiou, A. et al. (2021). Trends in pediatric hospitalizations for coronavirus disease 2019. *JAMA Pediatr.* 175: 415–417.

16 Verma, S., Lumba, R., Dapul, H.M. et al. (2021). Characteristics of hospitalized children with SARS-CoV-2 in the New York City metropolitan area. *Hosp. Pediatr.* 11: 71–78.

17 Levin, A.T., Hanage, W.P., Owusu-Boaitey, N. et al. (2020). Assessing the age specificity of infection fatality rates for COVID-19: systematic review, meta-analysis, and public policy implications. *Eur. J. Epidemiol.* 35: 1123–1138.

18 Ludvigsson, J.F. (2021). Case report and systematic review suggest that children may experience similar long-term effects to adults after clinical COVID-19. *Acta Paediatr.* 110: 914–921.

19 Galloway SE, Paul P, MacCannell DR, et al. Emergence of SARS-CoV-2 B.1.1.7 Lineage — United States, December 29, 2020–January 12, 2021. MMWR Morb Mortal Wkly Rep 2021;70:95–99., DOI: http://dx.doi.org/10.15585/mmwr.mm7003e2. Accessed 22 March 2021.

20 Delahoy MJ, Ujamaa D, Whitaker M, et al. Hospitalizations Associated with COVID-19 Among Children and Adolescents - COVID-NET, 14 States, March 1, 2020-August 14, 2021. MMWR Morb Mortal Wkly Rep. 2021;70(36):1255-1260. Published 2021 Sep 10. doi:10.15585/mmwr.mm7036e2.

21 Centers for Disease Control and Prevention (2021). SARS-CoV-2 variant classifications and definitions. https://www.cdc.gov/coronavirus/2019-ncov/cases-updates/variant-surveillance/variant-info.html (accessed 16 March 2021).

22 Riphagen, S., Gomez, X., Gonzalez-Martinez, C. et al. (2020). Hyperinflammatory shock in children during COVID-19 pandemic. *Lancet* 395: 1607–1608.

23 Feldstein, L.R., Rose, E.B., Horwitz, S.M. et al. (2020). Multisystem inflammatory syndrome in U.S. children and adolescents. *N. Engl. J. Med.* 383: 334–346.

24 Sood, M., Sharma, S., Sood, I. et al. (2021). Emerging evidence on multisystem inflammatory syndrome in children associated with SARS-CoV-2 infection: a systematic review with meta-analysis. *SN Compr. Clin. Med.* 3: 38–47.

25 Centers for Disease Control and Prevention (2020). Kawasaki disease. https://www.cdc.gov/kawasaki/index.html (accessed 4 June 2020).

26 Lee, E.H., Kepler, K.L., Geevarughese, A. et al. (2020). Race/ethnicity among children with COVID-19-associated multisystem inflammatory syndrome. *JAMA Netw. Open* 3: e2030280.

27 Galeotti, C. and Bayry, J. (2020). Autoimmune and inflammatory diseases following COVID-19. *Nat. Rev. Rheumatol.* 16: 413–414.

28 Kaushik, S., Aydin, S.I., Derespina, K.R. et al. (2020). Multisystem inflammatory syndrome in children associated with severe acute respiratory syndrome coronavirus 2 infection (MIS-C): a multi-institutional Study from New York City. *J. Pediatr.* 224: 24–29.

29 Dufort, E.M., Koumans, E.H., Chow, E.J. et al. (2020). Multisystem inflammatory syndrome in children in New York state. *N. Engl. J. Med.* 383: 347–358.

30 Feldstein, L.R., Tenforde, M.W., Friedman, K.G. et al. (2021). Characteristics and outcomes of US children and adolescents with multisystem inflammatory syndrome in children (MIS-C) compared with severe acute COVID-19. *JAMA* 325: 1074–1087.

31 Staudt, A., Saunders, J., Pavlin, J., and Shelton-Davenport, M. (eds.) (2020). *Airborne Transmission of SARS-CoV-2: Proceedings of a Workshop-in Brief*. Washington, DC: National Academies Press.

32 Centers for Disease Control and Prevention (2021). COVID-19 overview and infection prevention and control priorities in non-US healthcare settings. https://www.cdc.gov/coronavirus/2019-ncov/hcp/non-us-settings/overview/index.html (accessed 26 February 2021).

33 Shane, A.L., Sato, A.I., Kao, C. et al. (2020). A pediatric infectious diseases perspective of severe acute respiratory syndrome coronavirus 2 (SARS-CoV-2) and novel coronavirus disease 2019 (COVID-19) in children. *J. Pediatric. Infect. Dis. Soc.* 9: 596–608.

34 Han, M.S., Choi, E.H., Chang, S.H. et al. (2021). Clinical characteristics and viral RNA detection in children with coronavirus disease 2019 in the Republic of Korea. *JAMA Pediatr.* 175: 73–80.

35 DeBiasi, R.L. and Delaney, M. (2021). Symptomatic and asymptomatic viral shedding in pediatric patients infected with severe acute respiratory syndrome coronavirus 2 (SARS-CoV-2): under the surface. *JAMA Pediatr.* 175: 16–18.

36 Peng, D., Zhang, J., Ji, Y., and Pan, D. (2020). Risk factors for redetectable positivity in recovered COVID-19 children. *Pediatr. Pulmonol.* 55: 3602–3609.

37 Pinninti, S.G., Pati, S., Poole, C. et al. (2021). Virological characteristics of hospitalized children with SARS-CoV-2 infection. *Pediatrics* 147: e2020037812.

38 Thompson, H.A., Mousa, A., Dighe, A. et al. (2021). SARS-CoV-2 setting-specific transmission rates: a systematic review and meta-analysis. *Clin. Infect. Dis.* 2021: ciab100.

39 Zhu, Y., Bloxham, C.J., Hulme, K.D. et al. (2020). A meta-analysis on the role of children in severe acute respiratory syndrome coronavirus 2 in household transmission clusters. *Clin. Infect. Dis.* 72: e1146–e1153.

40 Maltezou, H.C., Magaziotou, I., Dedoukou, X. et al. (2020). Children and adolescents with SARS-CoV-2 infection: epidemiology, clinical course and viral loads. *Pediatr. Infect. Dis. J.* 39: e388–e392.

41 O'Leary, S.T. (2021). To spread or not to spread SARS-CoV-2-is that the question? *JAMA Pediatr.* 175: 559–560.

42 Viner, R.M., Ward, J.L., Hudson, L.D. et al. (2020). Systematic review of reviews of symptoms and signs of COVID-19 in children and adolescents. *Arch. Dis. Child.* https://doi.org/10.1136/archdischild-2020-320972.

43 Liguoro, I., Pilotto, C., Bonanni, M. et al. (2020). SARS-COV-2 infection in children and newborns: a systematic review. *Eur. J. Pediatr.* 179: 1029–1046.

44 Hyde, Z. (2021). Difference in SARS-CoV-2 attack rate between children and adults may reflect bias. *Clin. Infect. Dis.* 2021: ciab183.

45 Moschovis, P.P., Yonker, L.M., Shah, J. et al. (2021). Aerosol transmission of SARS-CoV-2 by children and adults during the COVID-19 pandemic. *Pediatr. Pulmonol.*: 56, 1389–94.

46 Kociolek, L.K., Muller, W.J., Yee, R. et al. (2020). Comparison of upper respiratory viral load distributions in asymptomatic and symptomatic children diagnosed with SARS-CoV-2 infection in pediatric hospital testing programs. *J. Clin. Microbiol.* 59: e02593–e02520.

47 Hurst, J.H., Heston, S.M., Chambers, H.N. et al. (2020). SARS-CoV-2 infections among children in the biospecimens from respiratory virus-exposed kids (BRAVE kids) study. *Clin. Infect. Dis.* 2020: ciaa1693.

48 Madera, S., Crawford, E., Langelier, C. et al. (2021). Nasopharyngeal SARS-CoV-2 viral loads in young children do not differ significantly from those in older children and adults. *Sci. Rep.* 11: 3044.

49 Heald-Sargent, T., Muller, W.J., Zheng, X. et al. (2020). Age-related differences in nasopharyngeal severe acute respiratory syndrome coronavirus 2 (SARS-CoV-2) levels in patients with mild to moderate coronavirus disease 2019 (COVID-19). *JAMA Pediatr.* 174: 902–903.

50 Laws, R.L., Chancey, R.J., Rabold, E.M. et al. (2021). Symptoms and transmission of SARS-CoV-2 among children - Utah and Wisconsin, March-May 2020. *Pediatrics* 147: e2020027268.

51 Yonker, L.M., Neilan, A.M., Bartsch, Y. et al. (2020). Pediatric severe acute respiratory syndrome coronavirus 2 (SARS-CoV-2): clinical presentation, infectivity, and immune responses. *J. Pediatr.* 227: 45–52. e5.

52 Mensah, A.A., Sinnathamby, M., Zaidi, A. et al. (2021). SARS-CoV-2 infections in children following the full re-opening of schools and the impact of national lockdown: prospective, national observational cohort surveillance, July–December 2020, England. *J. Infect.* 82: 67–74.

53 Zimmerman, K.O., Akinboyo, I.C., Brookhart, M.A. et al. (2021). Incidence and secondary transmission of SARS-CoV-2 infections in schools. *Pediatrics* 147: e2020048090.

54 Ismail, S.A., Saliba, V., Lopez Bernal, J. et al. (2021). SARS-CoV-2 infection and transmission in educational settings: a prospective, cross-sectional analysis of infection clusters and outbreaks in England. *Lancet Infect. Dis.* 21: 344–353.

55 Gold, J.A.W., Gettings, J.R., Kimball, A. et al. (2021). Clusters of SARS-CoV-2 infection among elementary school educators and students in one School

District - Georgia, December 2020-January 2021. *MMWR Morb. Mortal. Wkly Rep.* 70: 289–292.

56 Xu, W., Li, X., Dozier, M. et al. (2020). What is the evidence for transmission of COVID-19 by children in schools? A living systematic review. *J. Glob. Health* 10: 021104.

57 Gilliam, W.S., Malik, A.A., Shafiq, M. et al. (2021). COVID-19 transmission in US child care programs. *Pediatrics* 147: e2020031971.

58 Raschetti, R., Vivanti, A.J., Vauloup-Fellous, C. et al. (2020). Synthesis and systematic review of reported neonatal SARS-CoV-2 infections. *Nat. Commun.* 11: 5164.

59 Centers for Disease Control and Prevention (2020). Evaluation and management considerations for neonates at risk for COVID-19. https://www.cdc.gov/coronavirus/2019-ncov/hcp/caring-for-newborns.html (accessed 8 December 2020).

60 Schwartz, D.A. (2020). An analysis of 38 pregnant women with COVID-19, their newborn infants, and maternal-fetal transmission of SARS-CoV-2: maternal coronavirus infections and pregnancy outcomes. *Arch. Pathol. Lab. Med.* 144: 799–805.

61 Chen, H., Guo, J., Wang, C. et al. (2020). Clinical characteristics and intrauterine vertical transmission potential of COVID-19 infection in nine pregnant women: a retrospective review of medical records. *Lancet* 395: 809–815.

62 Fan, C., Lei, D., Fang, C. et al. (2021). Perinatal transmission of 2019 coronavirus disease-associated severe acute respiratory syndrome coronavirus 2: should we worry? *Clin. Infect. Dis.* 72: 862–864.

63 Li, Y., Zhao, R., Zheng, S. et al. (2020). Lack of vertical transmission of severe acute respiratory syndrome coronavirus 2, China. *Emerg. Infect. Dis.* 26: 1335–1336.

64 Wang, X., Zhou, Z., Zhang, J. et al. (2020). A case of 2019 novel coronavirus in a pregnant woman with preterm delivery. *Clin. Infect. Dis.* 71: 844–846.

65 Wang, S., Guo, L., Chen, L. et al. (2020). A case report of neonatal 2019 coronavirus disease in China. *Clin. Infect. Dis.* 71: 853–857.

66 Zeng, L., Xia, S., Yuan, W. et al. (2020). Neonatal early-onset infection with SARS-CoV-2 in 33 neonates born to mothers with COVID-19 in Wuhan, China. *JAMA Pediatr.* 174: 722–725.

67 Dong, L., Tian, J., He, S. et al. (2020). Possible vertical transmission of SARS-CoV-2 from an infected mother to her newborn. *JAMA* 323: 1846–1848.

68 Zeng, H., Xu, C., Fan, J. et al. (2020). Antibodies in infants born to mothers with COVID-19 pneumonia. *JAMA* 323: 1848–1849.

69 Vivanti, A.J., Vauloup-Fellous, C., Prevot, S. et al. (2020). Transplacental transmission of SARS-CoV-2 infection. *Nat. Commun.* 11: 3572.

70 Kotlyar, A.M., Grechukhina, O., Chen, A. et al. (2021). Vertical transmission of coronavirus disease 2019: a systematic review and meta-analysis. *Am. J. Obstet. Gynecol.* 224: 35–53.e3.

71 Chambers, C., Krogstad, P., Bertrand, K. et al. (2020). Evaluation for SARS-CoV-2 in breast Milk from 18 infected women. *JAMA* 324: 1347–1348.

72 World Health Organization (2020). Breastfeeding and COVID-19: Scientific Brief. https://www.who.int/news-room/commentaries/detail/breastfeeding-and-covid-19 (accessed 23 June 2020).

73 Centers for Disease Control and Prevention (2020). Care for breastfeeding people: interim guidance on breastfeeding and breast milk feeds in the context of COVID-19. https://www.cdc.gov/coronavirus/2019-ncov/hcp/care-for-breastfeeding-women.html (accessed 3 December 2020).

74 Puopolo KM, Hudak ML, Kimberlin DW, et al. (2020) INITIAL GUIDANCE: management of infants born to mothers with COVID-19. https://www.tn.gov/content/dam/tn/health/documents/cedep/novel-coronavirus/AAP_COVID-19-Initial-Newborn-Guidance.pdf (accessed 2 April 2020).

75 Centers for Disease Control and Prevention (2020). Information for pediatric healthcare providers. https://www.cdc.gov/coronavirus/2019-ncov/hcp/pediatric-hcp.html (accessed 30 December 2020).

76 Stokes, E.K., Zambrano, L.D., Anderson, K.N. et al. (2020). Coronavirus disease 2019 case surveillance - United States, January 22 may 30, 2020. *MMWR Morb. Mortal. Wkly Rep.* 69: 759–765.

77 Centers for Disease Control and Prevention (2020). Coronavirus disease 2019 (COVID-19) 2020 Interim Case Definition. Approved August 5, 2020. https://wwwn.cdc.gov/nndss/conditions/coronavirus-disease-2019-covid-19/case-definition/2020/08/05 (accessed 22 March 2021).

78 Orscheln, R.C., Newland, J.G., and Rosen, D.A. (2021). Practical school algorithms for symptomatic or SARS-CoV-2-exposed students are essential for returning children to in-person learning. *J. Pediatr.* 229: 275–277.

79 Chiappini, E., Licari, A., Motisi, M.A. et al. (2020). Gastrointestinal involvement in children with SARS-COV-2 infection: an overview for the pediatrician. *Pediatr. Allergy Immunol.* 31 ((Suppl 26)): 92–95.

80 National Institutes of Health (2020). Clinical spectrum of SARS-CoV-2 infection. https://www.covid19treatmentguidelines.nih.gov/overview/clinical-spectrum (accessed 17 December 2020).

81 Chiotos, K., Hayes, M., Kimberlin, D.W. et al. (2020). Multicenter initial guidance on use of antivirals for children with coronavirus disease 2019/severe acute respiratory syndrome coronavirus 2. *J. Pediatric. Infect. Dis. Soc.* 9: 701–715.

82 Manson, J.J., Crooks, C., Naja, M. et al. (2020). COVID-19-associated hyperinflammation and escalation of patient care: a retrospective longitudinal cohort study. *Lancet Rheumatol.* 2: e594–e602.

83 Leeb, R.T., Price, S., Sliwa, S. et al. (2020). COVID-19 trends among school-aged children - United States, March 1 September 19, 2020. *MMWR Morb. Mortal. Wkly Rep.* 69: 1410–1415.

84 Ciuca, I.M. (2020). COVID-19 in children: an ample review. *Risk Manag. Healthc. Policy* 13: 661–669.

85 Zachariah, P., Johnson, C.L., Halabi, K.C. et al. (2020). Epidemiology, clinical features, and disease severity in patients with coronavirus disease 2019 (COVID-19) in a Children's Hospital in New York City, New York. *JAMA Pediatr.* 174: e202430.

86 Wei, M., Yuan, J., Liu, Y. et al. (2020). Novel coronavirus infection in hospitalized infants under 1 year of age in China. *JAMA* 323: 1313–1314.

87 Dong, Y., Mo, X., Hu, Y. et al. (2020). Epidemiology of COVID-19 among children in China. *Pediatrics* 145: e20200702.

88 Leon-Abarca, J.A. (2020). Obesity and immunodeficiencies are the main pre-existing conditions associated with mild to moderate COVID-19 in children. *Pediatr. Obes.* 15: e12713.

89 Vilela, T.S., Braga, J.A.P., and Loggetto, S.R. (2021). Hemoglobinopathy and pediatrics in the time of COVID-19. *Hematol. Transfus. Cell Ther.* 43: 87–100.

90 Tsankov, B.K., Allaire, J.M., Irvine, M.A. et al. (2021). Severe COVID-19 infection and pediatric comorbidities: a systematic review and meta-analysis. *Int. J. Infect. Dis.* 103: 246–256.

91 Yancy, C.W. (2020). COVID-19 and African Americans. *JAMA* 323: 1891–1892.

92 Leibowitz, J., Krief, W., Barone, S. et al. (2021). Comparison of clinical and epidemiologic characteristics of Young febrile infants with and without severe acute respiratory syndrome Coronavirus-2 infection. *J. Pediatr.* 229: 41–7.e1.

93 Mithal, L.B., Machut, K.Z., Muller, W.J., and Kociolek, L.K. (2020). SARS-CoV-2 infection in infants less than 90 days old. *J. Pediatr.* 224: 150–152.

94 Meslin, P., Guiomard, C., Chouakria, M. et al. (2020). Coronavirus disease 2019 in newborns and very Young infants: a series of six patients in France. *Pediatr. Infect. Dis. J.* 39: e145–e147.

95 Nathan, N., Prevost, B., and Corvol, H. (2020). Atypical presentation of COVID-19 in young infants. *Lancet* 395: 1481.

96 Vanhems, P., Endtz, H., Dananche, C. et al. (2020). Comparison of the clinical features of SARS-CoV-2, other coronavirus and influenza infections in infants less than 1-year-old. *Pediatr. Infect. Dis. J.* 39: e157–e158.

97 Grimaud, E., Challiol, M., Guilbaud, C. et al. (2020). Delayed acute bronchiolitis in infants hospitalized for COVID-19. *Pediatr. Pulmonol.* 55: 2211–2212.

98 Andre, M.C., Patzug, K., Bielicki, J. et al. (2020). Can SARS-CoV-2 cause life-threatening bronchiolitis in infants? *Pediatr. Pulmonol.* 55: 2842–2843.

99 Mark, E.G., Golden, W.C., Gilmore, M.M. et al. (2021). Community-onset severe acute respiratory syndrome coronavirus 2 infection in Young infants: a systematic review. *J. Pediatr.* 228: 94–100.e3.

100 Freeman, E.E., McMahon, D.E., Lipoff, J.B. et al. (2020). The spectrum of COVID-19-associated dermatologic manifestations: an international registry of 716 patients from 31 countries. *J. Am. Acad. Dermatol.* 83: 1118–1129.

101 Andina, D., Belloni-Fortina, A., Bodemer, C. et al. (2021). Skin manifestations of COVID-19 in children: part 2. *Clin. Exp. Dermatol.* 46: 451–461.

102 Torrelo, A., Andina, D., Santonja, C. et al. (2020). Erythema multiforme-like lesions in children and COVID-19. *Pediatr. Dermatol.* 37: 442–446.

103 Fernandez-Nieto, D., Jimenez-Cauhe, J., Suarez-Valle, A. et al. (2020). Characterization of acute acral skin lesions in nonhospitalized patients: a case series of 132 patients during the COVID-19 outbreak. *J. Am. Acad. Dermatol.* 83: e61–e63.

104 Piccolo, V., Neri, I., Filippeschi, C. et al. (2020). Chilblain-like lesions during COVID-19 epidemic: a preliminary study on 63 patients. *J. Eur. Acad. Dermatol. Venereol.* 34: e291–e293.

105 Recalcati, S., Barbagallo, T., Frasin, L.A. et al. (2020). Acral cutaneous lesions in the time of COVID-19. *J. Eur. Acad. Dermatol. Venereol.* 34: e346–e347.

106 Galvan Casas, C., Catala, A., Carretero Hernandez, G. et al. (2020). Classification of the cutaneous manifestations of COVID-19: a rapid prospective nationwide consensus study in Spain with 375 cases. *Br. J. Dermatol.* 183: 71–77.

107 Freeman, E.E., McMahon, D.E., Lipoff, J.B. et al. (2020). Pernio-like skin lesions associated with COVID-19: a case series of 318 patients from 8 countries. *J. Am. Acad. Dermatol.* 83: 486–492.

108 Landa, N., Mendieta-Eckert, M., Fonda-Pascual, P., and Aguirre, T. (2020). Chilblain-like lesions on feet and hands during the COVID-19 pandemic. *Int. J. Dermatol.* 59: 739–743.

109 Stafstrom, C.E. and Jantzie, L.L. (2020). COVID-19: neurological considerations in neonates and children. *Children (Basel)* 7: 133.

110 Nino, G., Zember, J., Sanchez-Jacob, R. et al. (2021). Pediatric lung imaging features of COVID-19: a systematic review and meta-analysis. *Pediatr. Pulmonol.* 56: 252–263.

111 Foust, A.M., Phillips, G.S., Chu, W.C. et al. (2020). International expert consensus statement on chest imaging in pediatric COVID-19 patient management: imaging findings, imaging study reporting and imaging study recommendations. *Radiol. Cardiothorac. Imaging* 2 (2): e200214.

112 Bayramoglu, Z., Canipek, E., Comert, R.G. et al. (2021). Imaging features of pediatric COVID-19 on chest radiography and chest CT: a retrospective, single-center study. *Acad. Radiol.* 28: 18–27.

113 Henderson, L.A., Canna, S.W., Friedman, K.G. et al. (2020). American College of Rheumatology Clinical Guidance for multisystem inflammatory syndrome in children associated with SARS-CoV-2 and Hyperinflammation in pediatric COVID-19: version 1. *Arthritis Rheumatol.* 72: 1791–1805.

114 Verdoni, L., Mazza, A., Gervasoni, A. et al. (2020). An outbreak of severe Kawasaki-like disease at the Italian epicentre of the SARS-CoV-2 epidemic: an observational cohort study. *Lancet* 395: 1771–1778.

115 Toubiana, J., Poirault, C., Corsia, A. et al. (2020). Kawasaki-like multisystem inflammatory syndrome in children during the covid-19 pandemic in Paris, France: prospective observational study. *BMJ* 369: m2094.

116 Centers for Disease Control and Prevention, Health Alert Network (2020). Multisystem inflammatory syndrome in children (MIS-C) associated with coronavirus disease 2019 (COVID-19). https://emergency.cdc.gov/han/2020/han00432.asp (accessed 14 May 2020).

117 Centers for Disease Control and Prevention (2021). Information for healthcare providers about multisystem inflammatory syndrome in children (MIS-C). https://www.cdc.gov/mis-c/hcp (accessed 17 February 2021).

118 World Health Organization (2020). Multisystem inflammatory syndrome in children and adolescents temporally related to COVID-19. https://www.who.int/news-room/commentaries/detail/multisystem-inflammatory-syndrome-in-children-and-adolescents-with-covid-19 (accessed 15 May 2020).

119 Royal College of Paediatrics and Child Health (2020). Paediatric multisystem inflammatory syndrome temporally associated with COVID-19 (PIMS) - guidance for clinicians. www.rcpch.ac.uk/resources/paediatric-multisystem-inflammatory-syndrome-temporally-associated-covid-19-pims-guidance (accessed 1 May 2020).

120 Centers for Disease Control and Prevention (2021). Health Department-Reported Cases of Multisystem Inflammatory Syndrome in Children (MIS-C) in the United States. https://www.cdc.gov/mis-c/cases/index.html (accessed 20 October 2021).

121 Young, T.K., Shaw, K.S., Shah, J.K. et al. (2021). Mucocutaneous manifestations of multisystem inflammatory syndrome in children during the COVID-19 pandemic. *JAMA Dermatol.* 157: 207–212.

122 Winant, A.J., Blumfield, E., Liszewski, M.C. et al. (2020). Thoracic imaging findings of multisystem inflammatory syndrome in children (MIS-C) associated with COVID-19: what radiologists need to know now. *Radiol. Cardiothorac. Imaging* 2 (4): e200346.

123 Blondiaux, E., Parisot, P., Redheuil, A. et al. (2020). Cardiac MRI in children with multisystem

inflammatory syndrome associated with COVID-19. *Radiology* 297: E283–E288.

124 Centers for Disease Control and Prevention (2020). Long-term effects of COVID-19. https://www.cdc.gov/coronavirus/2019-ncov/long-term-effects.html (accessed 13 November 2020).

125 Sudre, C.H., Murray, B., Varsavsky, T. et al. (2021). Attributes and predictors of long COVID. *Nat. Med.* 27: 626–631.

126 Buonsenso D, Espuny Pujol F, Munblit D, et al. (2021). Clinical characteristics, activity levels and mental health problems in children with long COVID: a survey of 510 children. Preprints. doi:https://doi.org/10.20944/preprints 202103.0271.v1.

127 American Academy of Pediatrics (2021). COVID-19 testing guidance. https://services.aap.org/en/pages/2019-novel-coronavirus-covid-19-infections/clinical-guidance/covid-19-testing-guidance (accessed 5 March 2021).

128 Centers for Disease Control and Prevention (2020). FAQ: COVID-19 data and surveillance. https://www.cdc.gov/coronavirus/2019-ncov/covid-data/faq-surveillance.html (accessed 20 November 2020).

129 Centers for Disease Control and Prevention (2021). Appendices. https://www.cdc.gov/coronavirus/2019-ncov/php/contact-tracing/contact-tracing-plan/appendix.html (accessed 6 March 2021).

130 Centers for Disease Control and Prevention (2021). When to quarantine. https://www.cdc.gov/coronavirus/2019-ncov/if-you-are-sick/quarantine.html (accessed 11 February 2021).

131 Huang, N., Perez, P., Kato, T. et al. (2021). SARS-CoV-2 infection of the oral cavity and saliva. *Nat. Med.* 27: 892–903.

132 Wu, Q., Xing, Y., Shi, L. et al. (2020). Coinfection and other clinical characteristics of COVID-19 in children. *Pediatrics* 146: e20200961.

133 Wu, X., Cai, Y., Huang, X. et al. (2020). Co-infection with SARS-CoV-2 and influenza a virus in patient with pneumonia, China. *Emerg. Infect. Dis.* 26: 1324–1326.

134 Kim, D., Quinn, J., Pinsky, B. et al. (2020). Rates of co-infection between SARS-CoV-2 and other respiratory pathogens. *JAMA* 323: 2085–2086.

135 Hoang, A., Chorath, K., Moreira, A. et al. (2020). COVID-19 in 7780 pediatric patients: a systematic review. *EClinicalMedicine* 24: 100433.

136 Song, X., Delaney, M., Shah, R.K. et al. (2020). Comparison of clinical features of COVID-19 vs seasonal influenza a and B in US children. *JAMA Netw. Open* 3: e2020495.

137 Cappel, J.A. and Wetter, D.A. (2014). Clinical characteristics, etiologic associations, laboratory findings, treatment, and proposal of diagnostic criteria of pernio (chilblains) in a series of 104 patients at Mayo Clinic, 2000 to 2011. *Mayo Clin. Proc.* 89: 207–215.

138 Lin, E.E., Blumberg, T.J., Adler, A.C. et al. (2020). Incidence of COVID-19 in pediatric surgical patients among 3 US Children's hospitals. *JAMA Surg.* 155: 775–777.

139 Lin, E.E., Akaho, E.H., Sobilo, A. et al. (2021). Concordance of Preprocedure testing with time-of-surgery testing for SARS-CoV-2 in children. *Pediatrics* 147: e2020044289.

140 American Academy of Pediatrics (2021). FAQs: management of infants born to mothers with suspected or confirmed COVID-19. https://services.aap.org/en/pages/2019-novel-coronavirus-covid-19-infections/clinical-guidance/faqs-management-of-infants-born-to-covid-19-mothers (accessed 11 February 2021).

141 Centers for Disease Control and Prevention (2021). Interim guidance on duration of isolation and precautions for adults with COVID-19. https://www.cdc.gov/coronavirus/2019-ncov/hcp/duration-isolation.html (accessed 13 February 2021).

142 Ni, L., Ye, F., Cheng, M.L. et al. (2020). Detection of SARS-CoV-2-specific Humoral and cellular immunity in COVID-19 convalescent individuals. *Immunity* 52: 971–977.e3.

143 Robbiani, D.F., Gaebler, C., Muecksch, F. et al. (2020). Convergent antibody responses to SARS-CoV-2 in convalescent individuals. *Nature* 584: 437–442.

144 To, K.K., Hung, I.F., Ip, J.D. et al. (2020). COVID-19 re-infection by a phylogenetically distinct SARS-coronavirus-2 strain confirmed by whole genome sequencing. *Clin. Infect. Dis.* 2020: ciaa1275.

145 Tomassini, S., Kotecha, D., Bird, P.W. et al. (2021). Setting the criteria for SARS-CoV-2 reinfection - six possible cases. *J. Infect.* 82: 282–327.

146 Abu-Raddad, L.J., Chemaitelly, H., Malek, J.A. et al. (2020). Assessment of the risk of SARS-CoV-2 reinfection in an intense re-exposure setting. *Clin. Infect. Dis.* 2020: ciaa1846.

147 Centers for Disease Control and Prevention (2020). Investigative criteria for suspected cases of SARS-CoV-2 reinfection (ICR). https://www.cdc.gov/coronavirus/2019-ncov/php/invest-criteria.html (accessed 27 October 2020).

148 Belhadjer, Z., Meot, M., Bajolle, F. et al. (2020). Acute heart failure in multisystem inflammatory syndrome in children in the context of global SARS-CoV-2 pandemic. *Circulation* 142: 429–436.

149 Jiang, L., Tang, K., Levin, M. et al. (2020). COVID-19 and multisystem inflammatory syndrome in children and adolescents. *Lancet Infect. Dis.* 20: e276–e288.

150 Kaushik, A., Gupta, S., Sood, M. et al. (2020). A systematic review of multisystem inflammatory syndrome in children associated with SARS-CoV-2 infection. *Pediatr. Infect. Dis. J.* 39: e340–e346.

151 Centers for Disease Control and Prevention (2020). Phone advice line tool. https://www.cdc.gov/coronavirus/2019-ncov/hcp/phone-guide/index.html (accessed 18 November 2020).

152 National Institutes of Health (2021). COVID-19 treatment guidelines, zinc. https://www.covid19treatmentguidelines.nih.gov/supplements/zinc (accessed 11 February 2021).

153 National Institutes of Health (2020). COVID-19 treatment guidelines, vitamin D. https://www.covid19treatmentguidelines.nih.gov/supplements/vitamin-d (accessed 17 July 2020).

154 National Institutes of Health (2020). COVID-19 Treatment guidelines, vitamin C. https://www.covid19treatmentguidelines.nih.gov/supplements/vitamin-c (accessed 3 November 2020).

155 Infectious Diseases Society of America (2021). Therapeutics & interventions. https://www.idsociety.org/covid-19-real-time-learning-network/therapeutics-and-interventions (accessed 17 March 2021).

156 Chen, P., Nirula, A., Heller, B. et al. (2021). SARS-CoV-2 neutralizing antibody LY-CoV555 in outpatients with Covid-19. *N. Engl. J. Med.* 384: 229–237.

157 Wolf, J., Abzug, M.J., Wattier, R.L. et al. (2021). Initial guidance on use of monoclonal antibody therapy for treatment of COVID-19 in children and adolescents. *J. Pediatric. Infect. Dis. Soc.* 10: 629–634.

158 Gottlieb, R.L., Nirula, A., Chen, P. et al. (2021). Effect of Bamlanivimab as Monotherapy or in combination with Etesevimab on viral load in patients with mild to moderate COVID-19: a randomized clinical trial. *JAMA* 325: 632–644.

159 Eli Lilly and Company (2021). Fact sheet for health care providers emergency use authorization (EUA). http://pi.lilly.com/eua/bam-and-ete-eua-factsheet-hcp.pdf (accessed 23 March 2021).

160 U.S. Department of Health & Human Services. Bamlanivimab. 2021. https://www.phe.gov/emergency/events/COVID19/investigation-MCM/Bamlanivimab/Pages/default.aspx. Accessed 24 March 2021.

161 Food and Drung Administration. Fact sheet for health care providers emergency use authorization (EUA of Bamlanivimab and Etesevimab Authorized States, Territories, and U.S. Jurisdictions). 2021. <https://www.fda.gov/media/151719/download. Accessed 3 November 2021.

162 Wang P, Nair MS, Liu L, et al. Increased resistance of SARS-CoV-2 variants B.1.351 and B.1.1.7 to antibody neutralization. bioRxiv. 2021. doi:10.1101/2021.01.25.428137

163 Food and Drug Administration. Fact sheet for health care providers emergency use authorization (EUA) of casirivimab and imdevimab. 2021. https://www.fda.gov/media/143892/download. Accessed 16 March 2021.

164 NIH COVID-19 Treatment Guidelines: Anti-SARS-CoV-2 Monoclonal Antibodies. 2021. https://www.covid19treatmentguidelines.nih.gov/therapies/anti-sars-cov-2-antibody-products/anti-sars-cov-2-monoclonal-antibodies/. Accessed October 19, 2021.

165 Rizk, J.G., Forthal, D.N., Kalantar-Zadeh, K. et al. (2021). Expanded access programs, compassionate drug use, and emergency use authorizations during the COVID-19 pandemic. *Drug Discov. Today* 26: 593–603.

166 Raoof, S., Nava, S., Carpati, C., and Hill, N.S. (2020). High-flow, noninvasive ventilation and awake (nonintubation) proning in patients with

coronavirus disease 2019 with respiratory failure. *Chest* 158: 1992–2002.

167 National Institutes of Health (2020). Care of critically ill patients with COVID-19. https://www.covid19treatmentguidelines.nih.gov/critical-care (accessed 17 December 2020).

168 Goldenberg, N.A., Sochet, A., Albisetti, M. et al. (2020). Consensus-based clinical recommendations and research priorities for anticoagulant thromboprophylaxis in children hospitalized for COVID-19-related illness. *J. Thromb. Haemost.* 18: 3099–3105.

169 Giannakoulis, V.G., Papoutsi, E., and Siempos, I.I. (2020). Effect of cancer on clinical outcomes of patients with COVID-19: a meta-analysis of patient data. *JCO Glob. Oncol.* 6: 799–808.

170 National Institutes of Health (2021). COVID-19 treatment guidelines, lopinavir/ritonavir and other hiv protease inhibitors. https://www.covid19treatmentguidelines.nih.gov/antiviral-therapy/lopinavir-ritonavir-and-other-hiv-protease-inhibitors (accessed 11 February 2021).

171 Beigel, J.H., Tomashek, K.M., Dodd, L.E. et al. (2020). Remdesivir for the treatment of Covid-19 - final report. *N. Engl. J. Med.* 383: 1813–1826.

172 Spinner, C.D., Gottlieb, R.L., Criner, G.J. et al. (2020). Effect of Remdesivir vs standard care on clinical status at 11 days in patients with moderate COVID-19: a randomized clinical trial. *JAMA* 324: 1048–1057.

173 Consortium, W.H.O.S.T., Pan, H., Peto, R. et al. (2021). Repurposed antiviral drugs for Covid-19 - interim WHO Solidarity trial results. *N. Engl. J. Med.* 384: 497–511.

174 National Institutes of Health (2021). Study to evaluate the safety, tolerability, pharmacokinetics, and efficacy of remdesivir (GS-5734™) in participants from birth to < 18 years of age with coronavirus disease 2019 (COVID-19) (CARAVAN). https://www.clinicaltrials.gov/ct2/show/NCT04431453 (accessed 17 March 2021).

175 Gilead (2021). Fact sheet for healthcare providers emergency use authorization (EUA) of Veklury® (remdesivir) for hospitalized pediatric patients weighing 3.5 kg to less than 40 kg or hospitalized pediatric patients less than 12 years of age weighing at least 3.5 kg. https://www.gilead.com/-/ media/files/pdfs/remdesivir/eua-fact-sheet-for-hcps.pdf (accessed 16 March 2021).

176 Bhimraj, A., Morgan, R.L., Shumaker, A.H. et al. (2020). Infectious Diseases Society of America guidelines on the treatment and management of patients with COVID-19. *Clin. Infect. Dis.* 2020: ciaa478.

177 Barlow, A., Landolf, K.M., Barlow, B. et al. (2020). Review of emerging pharmacotherapy for the treatment of coronavirus disease 2019. *Pharmacotherapy* 40: 416–437.

178 Gilead (2021). Fact sheet for parents and caregivers Emergency Use Authorization (EUA) of VEKLURY® (remdesivir) for hospitalized children weighing 8 pounds (3.5 kg) to less than 88 pounds (40 kg) or hospitalized children less than 12 years of age weighing at least 8 pounds (3.5 kg) with coronavirus disease 2019 (COVID-19). https://www.gilead.com/-/media/files/pdfs/remdesivir%20/eua-fact-sheet-for-patients-and-caregivers.pdf (accessed 16 March 2021).

179 Eli Lilly and Company (2021). Fact sheet for healthcare providers Emergency Use Authorization (EUA) of baricitinib. http://pi.lilly.com/eua/baricitinib-eua-factsheet-hcp.pdf (accessed 17 March 2021).

180 Group, R.C., Horby, P., Lim, W.S. et al. (2021). Dexamethasone in hospitalized patients with Covid-19. *N. Engl. J. Med.* 384: 693–704.

181 National Institutes of Health (2021). Coronavirus disease 2019 (COVID-19) treatment guidelines. https://www.covid19treatmentguidelines.nih.gov (accessed 20 October 2021).

182 World Health Organization (2020). Corticosteroids for COVID-19. https://www.who.int/publications/i/item/WHO-2019-nCoV-Corticosteroids-2020.1 (accessed 2 September 2020).

183 National Institutes of Health (2020). COVID-19 treatment guidelines, corticosteroids. https://www.covid19treatmentguidelines.nih.gov/immunomodulators/corticosteroids (ccessed 3 November 2020).

184 Wong, A.Y., MacKenna, B., Morton, C.E. et al. (2021). Use of non-steroidal anti-inflammatory drugs and risk of death from COVID-19: an OpenSAFELY cohort analysis based on two cohorts. *Ann. Rheum. Dis.* 80: 943–951.

185 Food and Drug Administration (2020). FDA advises patients on use of non-steroidal anti-inflammatory drugs (NSAIDs) for COVID-19. https://www.fda.gov/drugs/drug-safety-and-availability/fda-advises-patients-use-non-steroidal-anti-inflammatory-drugs-nsaids-covid-19 (accessed 19 March 2020).

186 Food and Drug Administration (2021). Fact sheet for health care providers Emergency Use Authorization (EUA) of COVID-19 convalescent plasma for treatment of hospitalized patients with COVID-19. https://www.fda.gov/media/141478/download (accessed 17 March 2021).

187 Janiaud P, Axfors C, Schmitt AM, et al. Association of convalescent plasma treatment with clinical outcomes in patients with COVID-19: a systematic review and meta-analysis. JAMA 2021;325:1185–95.

188 Food and Drug Administration: FDA Updates Emergency Use Authorization for COVID-19 Convalescent Plasma to Reflect New Data. 2021.

189 Food and Drug Administration (2020). FDA cautions against use of hydroxychloroquine or chloroquine for COVID-19 outside of the hospital setting or a clinical trial due to risk of heart rhythm problems. https://www.fda.gov/drugs/drug-safety-and-availability/fda-cautions-against-use-hydroxychloroquine-or-chloroquine-covid-19-outside-hospital-setting-or (accessed 1 July 2020).

190 RECOVERY Collaborative Group, Horby, P., Mafham, M. et al. (2020). Effect of Hydroxychloroquine in hospitalized patients with Covid-19. *N. Engl. J. Med.* 383: 2030–2040.

191 National Institutes of Health (2020). COVID-19 treatment guidelines, chloroquine or hydroxychloroquine with or without azithromycin. https://www.covid19treatmentguidelines.nih.gov/antiviral-therapy/chloroquine-or-hydroxychloroquine-with-or-without-azithromycin (accessed 9 October 2020).

192 National Institutes of Health (2021). COVID-19 treatment guidelines, ivermectin. https://www.covid19treatmentguidelines.nih.gov/antiviral-therapy/ivermectin (accessed 11 February 2021).

193 Food and Drug Administration (2020). FAQ: COVID-19 and ivermectin intended for animals. https://www.fda.gov/animal-veterinary/product-safety-information/faq-covid-19-and-ivermectin-intended-animals (accessed 16 December 2020).

194 Infectious Diseases Society of America (2021). IDSA guidelines on the treatment and management of patients with COVID-19. https://www.idsociety.org/practice-guideline/covid-19-guideline-treatment-and-management/#toc-14 (accessed 18 March 2021).

195 National Institutes of Health. COVID-19 treatment guidelines. 2020. https://www.covid19treatmentguidelines.nih.gov/therapies/immunomodulators/. Accessed 31 October 2021.

196 RECOVERY Collaborative Group (2021). Tocilizumab in patients admitted to hospital with COVID-19 (RECOVERY): preliminary results of a randomised, controlled, open-label, platform trial. medRxiv. https://www.medrxiv.org/content/10.1101/2021.02.11.21249258v1 (accessed 11 February 2021).

197 REMAP-CAP Investigators, Gordon, A.C., Mouncey, P.R. et al. (2021). Interleukin-6 receptor antagonists in critically ill patients with Covid-19. *N. Engl. J. Med.* 384: 1491–1502.

198 Food and Drug Administration. Fact sheet for healthcare providers. Emergency use authorization for actemra (tocilizumab). https://www.fda.gov/media/150321/download. Accessed on 20 October 2021.

199 Karami, Z., Knoop, B.T., Dofferhoff, A.S.M. et al. (2021). Few bacterial co-infections but frequent empiric antibiotic use in the early phase of hospitalized patients with COVID-19: results from a multicentre retrospective cohort study in the Netherlands. *Infect. Dis. (Lond.)* 53: 102–110.

200 Infectious Diseases Society of America (2021). Co-infection and antimicrobial stewardship. https://www.idsociety.org/covid-19-real-time-learning-network/disease-manifestations--complications/co-infection-and-Antimicrobial-Stewardship (accessed 22 January 2021).

201 Garcia-Vidal, C., Sanjuan, G., Moreno-Garcia, E. et al. (2021). Incidence of co-infections and superinfections in hospitalized patients with COVID-19: a retrospective cohort study. *Clin. Microbiol. Infect.* 27: 83–88.

202 van Arkel, A.L.E., Rijpstra, T.A., Belderbos, H.N.A. et al. (2020). COVID-19-associated pulmonary Aspergillosis. *Am. J. Respir. Crit. Care Med.* 202: 132–135.

203 Henderson, L.A., Canna, S.W., Friedman, K.G. et al. (2020). American College of Rheumatology Clinical Guidance for multisystem inflammatory syndrome in children associated with SARS-CoV-2 and hyperinflammation in pediatric COVID-19: version 2. *Arthritis Rheumatol.* 73: e13–e29.

204 Kwak, J.H., Lee, S.Y., Choi, J.W., and Korean Society of Kawasaki Disease (2021). Clinical features, diagnosis, and outcomes of multisystem inflammatory syndrome in children associated with coronavirus disease 2019. *Clin. Exp. Pediatr.* 64: 68–75.

205 Whittaker, E., Bamford, A., Kenny, J. et al. (2020). Clinical characteristics of 58 children with a pediatric inflammatory multisystem syndrome temporally associated with SARS-CoV-2. *JAMA* 324: 259–269.

206 Dean P.N., Jackson L.B., Paridon S.M. (2020). Returning to play after coronavirus infection: pediatric cardiologists' perspective. https://www.acc.org/latest-in-cardiology/articles/2020/07/13/13/37/returning-to-play-after-coronavirus-infection.

207 American Academy of Pediatrics (2021). COVID-19 interim guidance: return to sports and physical activity. https://services.aap.org/en/pages/2019-novel-coronavirus-covid-19-infections/clinical-guidance/covid-19-interim-guidance-return-to-sports (accessed 1 March 2021).

208 Driggin, E., Madhavan, M.V., Bikdeli, B. et al. (2020). Cardiovascular considerations for patients, health care workers, and health systems during the COVID-19 pandemic. *J. Am. Coll. Cardiol.* 75: 2352–2371.

209 Polack, F.P., Thomas, S.J., Kitchin, N. et al. (2020). Safety and efficacy of the BNT162b2 mRNA Covid-19 vaccine. *N. Engl. J. Med.* 383: 2603–2615.

210 Center for Disease Control Vaccines & Immunizations. https://www.cdc.gov/vaccines/covid-19/planning/children.html#covid19-vax-recommendations. Accessed 31 October 2021.

211 National Institutes of Health. U.S. National Library of Medicine. A study to evaluate safety and effectiveness of mRNA-1273 vaccine in healthy children between 6 months of age and less than 12 years of age. 2021. https://www.clinicaltrials.gov/ct2/show/NCT04796896?term=moderna+6+months&cond=COVID-19&draw=2&rank=1. Accessed 19 March 2021.

212 Food and Drug Administration. Fact Sheet for healthcare providers administering vaccine. Emergency use authorization (EUA) of the Pfizer-Biontech COVID-19 vaccine to prevent coronavirus disease 2019 (COVID-19). Revised 29 October 2021. HYPERLINK "https://urldefense.com/v3/__https:/www.fda.gov/media/153713/download__;!!Hig9073Q!gabigKRkbAQb1JdjCIUa4KlJkGePe56rfAOSW1caZjQg9B5qhz9UwXPyWFXctF-sPw$"https://www.fda.gov/media/153713/download.

213 Infectious Diseases Society of America. Vaccines FAQ. https://www.idsociety.org/covid-19-real-time-learning-network/vaccines/vaccines-information--faq/#safety. Accessed 16 October 2021.

214 Abu Mouch S, Roguin A, Hellou E, Ishai A, Shoshan U, Mahamid L, Zoabi M, Aisman M, Goldschmid N, Berar Yanay N. Myocarditis following COVID-19 mRNA vaccination. Vaccine. 2021 Jun 29;39(29):3790-3793. doi: 10.1016/j.vaccine.2021.05.087.

215 Oliver SE, Gargano JW, Marin M, et al. The Advisory Committee on Immunization Practices' interim recommendation for use of Pfizer-BioNTech COVID-19 vaccine—United States, December 2020. MMWR Morb Mortal Wkly Rep. 2020;69(50):1922-1924. doi:10.15585/mmwr.mm6950e2.

13

Pharmacologic Therapeutics for COVID-19

Amanda M. Burkhardt[1], Angela Lu[2], Isaac Asante[1,3], and Stan Louie[4,5,6]

[1] Clinical Pharmacy Department, School of Pharmacy, University of Southern California, Los Angeles, CA, USA
[2] Department of Pharmacology and Pharmaceutical Sciences, School of Pharmacy, University of Southern California, Los Angeles, CA, USA
[3] Roski Eye Institute, Keck School of Medicine, University of Southern California, Los Angeles, CA, USA
[4] Clinical Pharmacy and Ophthalmology, School of Pharmacy, University of Southern California, Los Angeles, CA, USA
[5] Clinical Experimental Therapeutics Program, School of Pharmacy, University of Southern California, Los Angeles, CA, USA
[6] Ginsburg Institute of Biomedical Technology, Keck School of Medicine, University of Southern California, Los Angeles, CA, USA

Abbreviations

ACE2	angiotensin-converting enzyme 2
AngII	angiotensin II
ARB	angiotensin receptor blocker
ARDS	acute respiratory distress syndrome
AT1R	angiotensin type 1 receptor
AZM	azithromycin
CAR T	chimeric antigen receptor T
CI	confidence interval
CM	camostat
CQ	chloroquine
CRS	cytokine release syndrome
DEX	dexamethasone
EUA	Emergency Use Authorization
FDA	US Food and Drug Administration
GM-CSF	granulocyte-macrophage colony-stimulating factor
HCQ	hydroxychloroquine
IFN-β	interferon-β
IL-6	interleukin-6
IV	intravenous
MERS-CoV	Middle East respiratory syndrome coronavirus
NIH	National Institutes of Health
NK	natural killer
NSP	nonstructural viral protein
NT-proBNP	N-terminal pro-B-type natriuretic peptide
PLpro	papain-like protease
RAAS	renin–angiotensin–aldosterone system
RBD	receptor-binding domain
RBV	ribavirin
RdRp	RNA-dependent RNA polymerase
RDV-TP	remdesivir triphosphate
S	Spike
SARS-CoV-2	severe acute respiratory syndrome coronavirus 2
SOBI	Swedish Orphan Biovitrum AB
TMPRSS2	transmembrane protease serine 2

Virus Life Cycle

Understanding the pathobiology of the novel severe acute respiratory syndrome coronavirus 2 (SARS-CoV-2) is critical to the identification of potential therapeutic targets for drug discovery and development. These insights will further guide scientists in selecting precise targets, which will aid in increasing the margin of safety while exerting maximum antiviral activity. There is a large body of literature detailing the life cycle of SARS-CoV-2 and its associated pathogenesis [1–3].

Current understanding points to the nasal and paranasal cavities as the primary site for viral infection and the source leading to systemic spread. Furthermore, in situ RNA mapping has shown angiotensin-converting enzyme 2 (ACE2) expression to be highest in the nasal cavity, with lower levels of expression descending the respiratory tract [4]. As such, this points to the nasopharyngeal orifice as a predominant route for infection, viral susceptibility, and the entryway for subsequent pulmonary effects.

At the cellular level, SARS-CoV-2 viral entry into host cells is facilitated by viral binding onto ACE2 found on the cell surface. Specifically, the spike (S) protein found on the SARS-CoV-2 viral envelope has a receptor-binding domain (RBD) that interacts with ACE2 found on the host cell surface [5]. These interactions include hydrogen bond and salt bridge formation.

More specifically, the S protein consists of two subunits, S1 and S2. After the attachment of S1 onto cellular ACE2, a conformational change occurs that facilitates S2 virus–host cell membrane fusion. Along with ACE2, cellular transmembrane protease serine 2 (TMPRSS2) acts to cleave the viral S protein to promote viral activation and entry [6, 7]. This process also activates endosomal/lysosomal cysteine proteases, such as cathepsin B and L, which will further facilitate viral uptake into human host cells [8, 9].

Once SARS-CoV-2 has entered the host cell, the viral RNA is released and translated to produce viral proteins while using host cellular machinery. Similar to other viruses, active viral proteins must be liberated via SARS-CoV-2 proteases. The main viral protease is Mpro (3CLpro). This is a viral cysteine protease responsible for viral polyproteins cleavage to release active proteins, such as pp1A, pp1B, and various nonstructural viral proteins (NSP1–16) [10] These events are important in mediating viral replication and transcription of SARS-CoV-2. Because there are no mammalian homologs of Mpro, blockade of this target is less likely to lead to host cytotoxicity and has been prioritized as a high-value drug target for SARS-CoV-2.

SARS-CoV-2 also has a papain-like protease (PLpro) capable of cleaving viral polyproteins. In addition to its metabolic activities, PLpro can inhibit expression of proinflammatory cytokines, such as interferon-β (IFN-β), and chemokines. This is one of many evasion mechanisms that will allow SARS-CoV2 to invade. In this context, CXCL10 and CCL5 are key chemokines that play an important role in suppressing viral replication, where PLpro can inhibit their expression. Thus, the targeting of PLpro has several advantages, where its inhibition not only reduces viral evasion mechanisms and virus replication but also can reduce the death of surrounding uninfected cells while preserving the level of proinflammatory cytokines required for inherent antiviral immune response [11].

An additional virally specific target includes RNA-dependent RNA polymerase (RdRp), which catalyzes viral RNA synthesis. This enzyme is a potential therapeutic target where synthetic nucleoside and nucleotide agents are currently being developed [12]. This is further detailed in the following anti-nucleoside/anti-nucleotide section.

Drug Development for SARS-CoV-2

Because SARS-CoV-2 is a newly identified viral pathogen, there are few virus-specific drug options capable of effectively managing infection and viral proliferation. In general, drug development emerging from benchtop discovery to clinical evaluation may require years to complete. To rapidly address the lack of specific antiviral agents targeting SARS-CoV-2, one strategy is to reposition available agents found to have activity against SARS-CoV-2, including evaluating agents previously proved to be effective in managing SARS-CoV-1 and/or Middle East respiratory syndrome coronavirus (MERS-CoV). Studies have identified 68 drugs with activity against SARS-CoV-1 and MERS-CoV, which were further evaluated for their potential against SARS-CoV-2 [13, 14]. Wide-spectrum antiviral agents, such as ribavirin (RBV), nitazoxanide, chloroquine (CQ), nafamostat, and camostat (CM), have been identified and clinically evaluated for their efficacy and safety in the treatment of SARS-CoV-2. Additional strategies include deploying antiviral agents effective against other viruses, such as remdesivir, oseltamivir, RBV, and favipiravir.

As mentioned earlier, viral targets have been identified to disrupt SARS-CoV-2 interaction with host cells, viral replication, and viral assembly in addition to targeting host immune response to viral infection. Understanding of the protein–protein interactions between SARS-CoV-2 and host cells has led to the design and development of a number of potential compounds [14].

Immune Responses that Contribute to COVID-19 Pathology

After more than a year of intense study in both animal models [15, 16] and human patients [17, 18], we have a better understanding of how SARS-CoV-2 elicits its pathology, which in turn leads to varying degrees of COVID-19-mediated disease severity. As discussed earlier, SARS-CoV-2 requires access to the host replication and processing machinery to complete its life cycle and to produce more viral particles, which it achieves through interaction between viral S protein with ACE2 that is found on the surface of host cells. After the virus enters the host cells, it is eventually detected by components of the host immune response. Paradoxically, the host antiviral response is also responsible for a significant amount of the pathology observed in patients diagnosed with severe COVID-19.

Immune detection of SARS-CoV-2 infection can activate first the innate and subsequently the adaptive branch of the immune system [17–19]. However, we now know that this virus is capable of hijacking this traditional progression of the immune response and exploiting it to cause significant immunopathology [17, 19, 20]. This particularly is the case in patients who experience severe COVID-19. The goal of any immune response is twofold: (1) for the innate immune system to quickly and nonspecifically generate inflammation that will prevent uncontrolled replication of the infectious agent, and (2) for the inflammation generated by the innate immune system to trigger activation of the adaptive immune response that is necessary for full clearance of the infectious agent. This latter process will also generate long-lasting immunologic memory in the form of antibodies, more specifically immunoglobulin G. SARS-CoV-2 turns this paradigm on its head by delaying the normal immune response progression at the innate immune response and generating an uncontrollable and excessive amount of inflammation, which is a hallmark of severe COVID-19. This uncontrolled inflammation is evidenced by the significant elevation of proinflammatory cytokines and chemokines in the serum (e.g. interleukin-6 [IL-6], IL-1ß, IL-2, granulocyte-macrophage colony-stimulating factor [GM-CSF], tumor necrosis factor-α, CXCL8, CCL2). Accompanying cytokine/chemokine response is the appearance of cellular exhaustion markers on the surface of CD8 T cells and natural killer (NK) cells, two adaptive immune cells critical for effective antiviral immune responses. Patients also present with significantly reduced total numbers of lymphocytes (e.g. CD4$^+$, CD8$^+$ T cells, B cells, and NK cells) and an increased neutrophil count [17, 18, 20]. This shift to an innate dominated immune response has been correlated with worse disease outcomes for these patients. We now understand that this inflammation has a significant impact on the natural adaptive immune response to infection by retarding the robustness of antibody responses and limiting the development of immunologic memory, which ultimately has implications for long-term immunity in patients who recover from natural SARS-CoV-2 infections [21, 22].

In addition, this excessive and unchecked inflammation leads to significant damage of healthy bystander cells and tissues locally and systemically, which can lead to the development of pneumonia and eventually acute respiratory distress syndrome (ARDS), septic shock, and/or multiple organ dysfunction in approximately 15–25% of patients hospitalized with severe COVID-19 [17, 19]. ARDS has been previously observed in patients with severe SARS-CoV-1 and MERS-CoV infections. Similar hyperimmune responses have been seen in patients with leukemia who are receiving chimeric antigen receptor T cell (CAR T cell) therapy [23]. In all three of these clinical scenarios, ARDS is induced through the tremendous upregulation of proinflammatory cytokine production by the innate immune system, more commonly referred to as cytokine release syndrome (CRS) – an analogous phenomenon observed in patients with severe COVID-19.

Studies of CRS and CRS-induced ARDS in patients with SARS-CoV, MERS-CoV, and CAR T have identified multiple factors found in these inflammatory pathways that can be targeted by existing therapeutics to mitigate, reduce, and even prevent the immune-mediated pathology. As will be discussed in further detail later, these therapeutics range from broad global immunosuppression to highly specific targeting of individual cytokines to prevent CRS-mediated inflammation, to administration of recombinant cytokines to aid in more productive immune response and resolution of infection.

Challenges to Discover and Deploy Drugs for a New Infectious Agent

In comparison with SARS-CoV-1 and MERS-CoV, SARS-CoV-2 is more highly transmissible, which explains its rapid person-to-person spread leading to the current global pandemic. The spread of this newly discovered virus is aided by the lack of effective treatment modalities. Unfortunately, de novo drug development is a complicated, prolonged, and costly process. As such, the strategy to repurpose or reposition existing compounds can be applied to rapidly accelerate the search for effective antiviral therapies.

Repositioning or repurposing of drugs seeks to develop new applications for preexisting US Food and Drug Administration (FDA)-approved therapeutics. This process leverages existing safety and efficacy data to rapidly advance drug efficacy for new indications. Existing information, such as unexpected side effects or potential interaction with the new target(s), can provide significant insights to repurposing efforts and accelerate the approval process. This strategy reduces the risk and allows preclinical and clinical designs to circumvent potential pitfalls in the drug development process.

Currently, there are 68 drugs with antiviral activity against SARS-CoV-1 and MERS-CoV that were also screened for subsequent activity against SARS-CoV-2 [13, 14]. Compounds such as RBV, nitazoxanide, CQ, nafamostat, and remdesivir were all found to have promise in patients with COVID-19 (summarized in Table 13.1). In addition, screening for anti–SARS-CoV-2 activity with existing antivirals has also identified several potentially active compounds, including penciclovir, a nucleoside analogue with antiherpes properties, which was found to inhibit SARS-CoV-2 [24].

A second approach to drug repositioning was based on existing data detailing the molecular mechanisms of coronavirus interaction with the host cell. Therefore, drugs that presumably could affect human proteins essential for the SARS-CoV-2 life cycle were selected for further analysis. The activity of the anti-inflammatory agent auranofin, which is used to treat rheumatoid arthritis, was assessed. Its proposed mechanism of action involves the inhibition of redox enzymes, induction of endoplasmic reticulum stress, and subsequent activation of the unfolded protein response, which leads to cellular apoptosis.

Therapeutic Classes

Antivirals

Existing antivirals have been investigated for potential efficacy in targeting various stages in the viral life cycle, such as viral attachment, protein processing, replication, and release. In this section, antiviral therapeutics will be classified based on mechanism of action. Figure 13.1 summarizes the SARS-CoV-2 life cycle, where we have highlighted targets and classes of drugs that may be active in suppressing SARS-CoV-2 replication and/or induction of inflammation.

Viral Entry or Attachment Inhibitors

The blockade of viral host cell entry may be effective in preventing viral replication and disease progression. To begin identifying potential agents, we evaluated a database of existing and undeveloped compounds in silico and verified them using in vitro tests to affirm their ability to prevent and/or block SARS-CoV-2 replication.

Because these types of interaction are specific for SARS-CoV-2 binding and cellular penetration, they have been identified as potential targets for COVID-19 therapeutic development. Membrane fusion and cytoplasmic entry of SARS-CoV-2 into ACE2-TMPRSS2–expressing respiratory epithelial cells can provoke inflammatory cytokine production.

The receptor-mediated virus entry is dependent on a serine protease, TMPRSS2 [25–27]. TMPRSS2 primes the S protein found on highly pathogenic human coronaviruses, such as SARS-CoV-1 and MERS-CoV, and facilitates viral entry into the host cell [28].

TMPRSS2 is expressed by airway epithelial cells, cardiac endothelium, microvascular endothelial cells, kidney, and digestive tract, making these systems all potential targets for SARS-CoV-2 infection [25]. Because alveolar type 2 cells express high levels of both ACE2 and TMPRSS2, these cell types are particularly susceptible to SARS-CoV-2 infection [25]. These data have propelled intense investigation and development for blockers of ACE2 and/or TMPRSS2.

Camostat (Foipan)

CM is a serine protease enzyme inhibitor that was initially developed and approved in Japan for the treatment of chronic pancreatitis and postoperative reflux

Table 13.1 Detailed summary of therapeutics investigated for treatment of SARS-CoV2 infections.

Group	Drug(s)	Mechanism of Action	Therapeutic Target	Dosage	Route of Administration	Duration of Therapy	NIH Recommendation
Viral entry or attachment inhibitors	Camostat (CM) Nafamostat (INN)	Serine protease inhibitor	TMPRSS2	200 mg t.i.d. 0.1–0.2 mg/kg/h	PO IV	5 days 7–10 days	Insufficient evidence (under review)
	Upamostat			200 mg or 400 mg q.i.d.	PO	14 days	
	Umifenovir	Inhibits viral cell fusion	Nonspecific: cell membrane	200 mg t.i.d.	PO	7–14 days	
ARBs	Valsartan	1) Block excessive AT1R activation by angiotensin II 2) Upregulate ACE2	AT1R	80 or 160 mg maximum b.i.d.	PO	Up to 14 days	
	Losartan			25 mg daily for three days, 50 mg daily thereafter			
	Telmisartan			40–80 mg daily			
Viral replication inhibitors	Favipiravir	Terminate strand RNA elongation	Viral RNA degradation	1600 mg b.i.d. loading dose, then 800 mg b.i.d.	PO	Up to 7 days	
	Molnupiravir	Inhibits viral RNA replication		200–800 mg b.i.d.	PO	5 days	
	Remdesivir	Inhibits viral RNA-dependent RNA polymerase		200 mg loading dose, then 100 mg daily	IV	10 days	Approved
	Ribavirin	Inhibits guanosine generation		500 mg b.i.d.	PO/IV	14 days	Insufficient evidence
	Oseltamivir	Inhibits neuraminidase enzymes	Viral entry	45–75 b.i.d.	PO	5 days	
Viral protein inhibitors	LPV/r	Protease inhibitor	Viral Proteases	400/100 mg b.i.d.	PO	<2.28 days	Against
	LPV/r + IFN-ß	Protease inhibitor with viral immunomodulator	Viral proteases and viral immunity activation	400/100 mg b.i.d. LPV/r + 0.25 mg injection IFN q.o.d.	PO + SQ	14 days LPV/r, 3 days IFN-ß	
	Disulfiram	Mpro/ATPase inhibitor	Mpro/ATPase	250–500 mg b.i.d.	PO	5 days	Insufficient evidence

Category	Drug	Mechanism	Target	Dose	Route	Duration	Recommendation
Antivirals and antiparasitic agents	Chloroquine HCQ	ACE2 glycosylation inhibitor	Lysosomal and ACE2 modulator	600 mg b.i.d. 800 mg loading dose, then 400 mg b.i.d.	PO	10 days 5 days	Against
	HCQ + AZM	ACE2 inhibitor, immunomodulator	ACE2, IL/IFN	400 mg b.i.d. HCQ, 500 mg daily AZM	PO	5 days	
	AZM	Immunomodulator	IL/IFN	500 mg daily	PO	3 days	Insufficient evidence
	Ivermectin	Inhibits viral entry into nucleus	α/β1 nuclear transport proteins, spike protein	600 or 1200 μg/kg	PO	5 days	
	Nitazoxanide	Protease inhibitor, viral genome synthesis	Mpro, PLpro	500 mg t.i.d.	PO	5 days	Against
Immunotherapy for CRS	PEGASYS/ peginterferon α-2a	Type I IFNs	Activation of viral immunity	180 μg/week for 2 doses	SC	1× per week	Insufficient evidence (under review)
	PEG-intron/ peginterferon α-2a	Type I IFNs	Activation of viral immunity	1 μg/kg	SC	1× per week	
	Recombinant GM-CSF (Sargramostim)	Activation of macrophages	Alveolar wall cells	125 μg/m² b.i.d.	IV or inhaled	5 days	
	Recombinant GM-CSF (Molgramostim)			300 μg	Inhaled	7 days	
	Lenzilumab	Monoclonal antibody	Anti-GM-CSF	600 mg q8h	IV	3 dosages	
	Anakinra	IL-1 receptor antagonism	IL-1 inhibitor	100 mg daily	SQ	10–28 days	
	Sarilumab	IL-6 receptor antagonism	IL-6 receptor	400 mg daily	IV	10 days	
	Tocilizumab			8 mg/kg daily	IV	10–28 days	Approved

(*Continued*)

Table 13.1 (Continued)

Group	Drug(s)	Mechanism of Action	Therapeutic Target	Dosage	Route of Administration	Duration of Therapy	NIH Recommendation
Passive immunity	Casirivimab/ Imdevimab (REGEN-COV)	Recombinant immunoglobulin G1 monoclonal antibody	Spike protein RBD	600/600 mg IV bolus and 300/300 mg maintenance every week	IV/SQ	7 days	Insufficient evidence (under review)
	Bamlanivimab/ Etesevimab			700 mg + 1400 mg, respectively, daily		11 days	
Steroids	DEX	Chemotaxis, vasodilation	GR	6–20 mg daily	IV/PO	5 days	Approved
	Methylprednisolone	Inhibits expression of proinflammatory genes		250–500 mg daily for three days, then 50 mg/day PO	IVP/PO	14 days	Insufficient evidence (under review)
Immunosuppressants	Cyclosporine	Inhibits NF-AT	CypA, calcineurin	Cumulative dose >300 mg	PO	<21 days	
	Cyclosporine + DEX	Anti-inflammatory, immune suppressant	GR, CypA, calcineurin				
	Acalabrutinib	Anti-inflammatory	Bruton's tyrosine kinase	100 mg b.i.d.	PO	10–14 days	
	Baricitinib	Anti-inflammatory	Janus kinase (JAK1 and 2)	4 mg daily	PO	14 days	Approved

ACE2, angiotensin-converting enzyme 2; ARB, angiotensin receptor blocker; AT1R, Angiotensin II type 1 receptor; AZM, azithromycin; CRS, cytokine release syndrome; DEX, dexamethasone; GM-CSF, granulocyte-macrophage colony-stimulating factor; GR, glucocorticoid receptor; HCQ, hydroxychloroquine; IFN, interferon; IL, interleukin; IV, intravenous; IVP, intravenous push; LPV/r, lopinavir/ritonavir; NIH, National Institutes of Health; PO, orally; q.o.d., every other day; RBD, receptor-binding domain; SQ, subcutaneous; TMPRSS2, transmembrane protease serine 2.

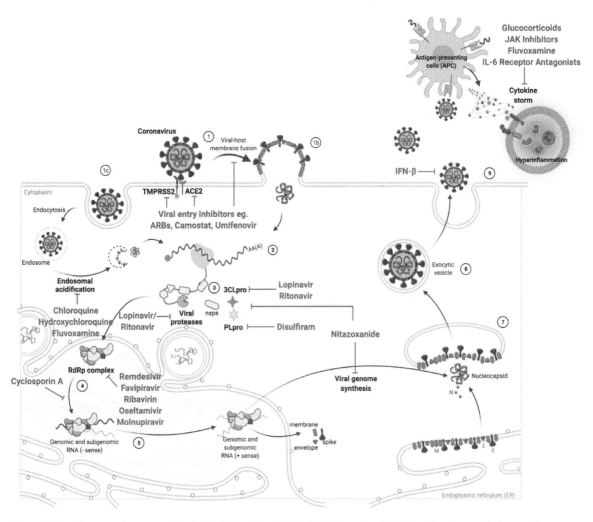

Figure 13.1 Therapeutic entry points in the life cycle of SARS-CoV-2 to reduce infectious burden and inflammation. JAK, Janus kinase.

esophagitis. Interest in CM for SARS-CoV-2 was spurred on by its ability to inhibit TMPRSS2. One in vitro study showed that CM can reduce SARS-CoV-2 infection in Calu-3 lung epithelial cells.

These encouraging in vitro findings led to a phase 2a double-blind, randomized, placebo-controlled, multi-center trial that enrolled adults hospitalized with COVID-19 [29]. Participants were administered 200 mg t.i.d. for five days, compared with placebo. In this small clinical trial, CM was found be ineffective in patients with established COVID-19, where there was no difference in the time to clinical improvements with CM versus placebo [29]. A possible limitation of this trial may be the severity of patient disease at study

entry. In addition, CM may be ineffective once SARS-CoV-2 has entered the cell.

There are continued efforts to determine the role of this potential drug in mitigating SARS-CoV-2 infection and subsequent COVID-19 (ClinicalTrials. gov: NCT04353284, NCT04608266, NCT04625114, NCT04455815, NCT04662073, and NCT04652765). One great advantage of using CM is its low cost (one 100-mg tablet is priced as low as US$0.10–$0.40). This pragmatic treatment strategy has the potential to save the lives of many people, including in lower-income areas. However, to date, there are no clinical data on the use of the drug in blocking or at least reducing viral spread and pathogenesis of any coronaviruses.

Nafamostat

Nafamostat mesylate (INN), a synthetic serine protease inhibitor, has been approved in Japan for the treatment of disseminated intravascular coagulation and pancreatitis. Nafamostat is also a fast-acting proteolytic inhibitor that is used during hemodialysis to prevent the proteolysis of fibrinogen into fibrin [30]. It was shown that nafamostat is a potent antiviral inhibitor capable of blocking viral infections in lung cells [31]. Molecular analyses showed nafamostat exerts anti–SARS-CoV-2 through blocking TMPRSS2 at nanomolar concentrations [28, 32]. Therefore, its antiviral, anti-inflammatory, and anticoagulant properties may be able to attenuate COVID-19 symptoms, disease progression, and complications.

Currently, several clinical trials are ongoing in different countries (ClinicalTrials.gov: NCT04390594, NCT04473053, and NCT04483960) to test its overall efficacy and safety. In these studies, nafamostat is dosed daily between 0.1 and 0.2 mg/kg/h intravenously (IV) for 7–10 days, based on the severity. Although nafamostat is thought to be active alone, it has also been combined with favipiravir, a viral replication inhibitor discussed later in this chapter. This combination is intended to block viral entry and replication. In addition, it is thought that this combination can prevent pathogenic host hypercoagulopathy, which has been reported as a cause of mortality. Although the number of patients in this case series was very small, low mortality rate associated with the combination of favipiravir and nafamostat suggest that this may be a potential treatment for critically ill patients with COVID-19.

Upamostat

Upamostat is a first-in-class orally administered serine protease inhibitor along with urokinase inhibitory properties. More recently, upamostat was found also to inhibit TMPRSS2 activity [33]. It targets human cell factors involved in S protein–mediated viral entry. This approach can potentially minimize development of chemoresistance leading to emergence viral variants. Like other antiviral agents, upamostat exhibits both anti-inflammatory and antiviral activities, making it a strong candidate for evaluation as a potential treatment for COVID-19 infection (ClinicalTrials.gov: NCT04723527).

Currently, it has been granted orphan drug status by the FDA as adjuvant treatment in pancreatic cancer. Its pharmacologic activities target multiple indications, such as COVID-19, cancer, inflammatory lung diseases, and gastrointestinal diseases. The current upamostat dosage is either 200 or 400 mg given daily for 14 days. Its efficacy against SARS-CoV-2 is now under investigation in a phase 2/3 study for treatment in nonhospitalized patients with symptomatic COVID-19 who do not require supplemental oxygen (ClinicalTrials.gov: NCT04723537).

Chloroquine and Hydroxychloroquine

CQ and hydroxychloroquine (HCQ) are tertiary amines used in the treatment of malaria. HCQ is more tolerable and is often also used for the management of autoimmune disorders such as systemic lupus erythematosus. Because HCQ is a less toxic metabolite of CQ and has fewer drug–drug interactions, it is generally preferred over CQ. Both agents have similar molecular pharmacologic mechanisms, where they disrupt host cell lysosomal processing and interfere with cellular autophagy pathways. Specifically, accumulation of CQ and HCQ in the lysosome will increase its pH and thus inhibit lysosomal activity. Downstream effects of lysosomal inhibition include immunomodulatory effects because lysosomes play an important role in antigen processing and major histocompatibility complex class II presentation [34]. Increasing endosomal pH impairs lysosomal and autophagosome maturation.

CQ treatment in patients with COVID-19 has demonstrated an ability to inhibit ACE2 glycosylation, thus potentially interfering with viral binding onto its cognate host receptor [24]. Despite optimistic in vitro data, large clinical trials have produced contradictory findings, in which CQ and HCQ have been found to either lead to unfavorable outcomes or show no significant change as compared with control [35, 36]. Currently, the National Institutes of Health (NIH) does not recommend monotherapy using either CQ or HCQ or in combination with azithromycin (AZM). Prior to being revoked, the FDA had approved Emergency Use Authorization (EUA) of HCQ sulfate taken orally at 800 mg initial dose and 400 mg thereafter in adults and adolescents weighing ≥ 50 kg.

Early in the COVID-19 pandemic, HCQ was also combined with AZM, a macrolide antibiotic with immunomodulatory properties. Because HCQ was found to have some in vitro activity against SARS-CoV-2, studies evaluating this combination were rapidly conducted. Unfortunately, HCQ with or without AZM did not show clinical outcome improvements that included parameters such as admissions into intensive care unit care, need for mechanical ventilation, and overall mortality [37–40]. However, serious safety concerns such as drug-induced cardiac disorders (experienced by 0.3–1.6% of patients), as well as mild to moderate gastrointestinal discomfort, were identified in multiple studies. The most common side effects include headache, dizziness, vomiting, and diarrhea, which affected up to 10% of patients [41].

Modulators of the Renin–Angiotensin–Aldosterone System

Another class of antivirals targeting viral attachment and entry are angiotensin receptor blockers (ARBs). The importance of the renin–angiotensin–aldosterone system (RAAS) has been highlighted in the SARS-CoV-2 pandemic because the virus requires binding to ACE2 to gain access to host cells [1]. Viral targeting of the ACE2 explains some of the sequelae associated with SARS-CoV-1 infection. Therapeutic agents in this class of agents include valsartan, losartan, and telmisartan, which are classified as ARBs. ARBs are traditionally used for the treatment of hypertension and cardiovascular disease. Current understanding is that angiotensin II (AngII) binding to the angiotensin type 1 receptor (AT1R) activates the traditional arm of RAAS pathway, which can promote proinflammatory and vasoconstriction properties. As implied by its name, ARBs completely block AngII binding onto AT1R, which prevents AngII-mediated inflammation and fibrosis. It is thought that blockade of AT1R will enhance AngII binding onto AT2R, which is a proreparative mechanism of RAAS and counters inflammatory activity induced by AngII/AT1R binding [42]. In addition, unbound AngII can also undergo ACE2-mediated metabolism to form Ang(1–7), a ligand for mitochondria assembly protein (Mas), which can also counter the effect of AngII/AT1R activity [43]. Due to the inflammatory modulatory activity, ARBs and other RAAS components have been investigated for their ability to mitigate SARS-CoV-2 morbidities, such as virally induced CRS and ARDS.

Angiotensin Receptor Blockers

Valsartan

Valsartan (Diovan) is an ARB that is currently undergoing clinical evaluation for the prevention of ARDS associated with COVID-19 in hospitalized patients. These double-blinded placebo-controlled studies are still actively recruiting and are evaluating the impact of valsartan on outcomes such as all-cause hospitalization, need for mechanical ventilation, and all-cause mortality. Scientific rationale for using ARBs for SARS-CoV-2 infection is based on the hypothesis that the loss of ACE2 activity may contribute to organ injury [44]. A systematic review and meta-analysis on the effectiveness of angiotensin-converting enzyme inhibitors and ARBs for the treatment of COVID-19 showed no additional risk for mortality for patients receiving either angiotensin-converting enzyme inhibitors or ARBs. The safety of high-dose valsartan for the treatment of hypertension has been assessed previously [45].

Valsartan in combination with sacubitril, a neprilysin inhibitor, is commercially available under the brand name Entresto. Sacubitril/valsartan combination is an FDA-approved combination product for the treatment of chronic heart failure. This combination uses valsartan to block AngII binding onto AT1R and thus reduce profibrotic and hyperproliferative effects. When combined with sacubitril, the fixed combination can also decrease the degradation of natriuretic peptides, thus promoting anti-inflammatory effects [46]. Support for the use of ARBs includes evidence showing significant increases in N-terminal pro-B-type natriuretic peptide (NT-proBNP) in patients with COVID-19 that is thought to be related to cardiac injury in patients with SARS-CoV-2 [47]. Others have supported that elevated NT-proBNP was an independent factor associated with COVID-19 mortality [48]. Moreover, elevated NT-proBNP levels have been shown to induce inflammation in non–SARS-CoV-2 sepsis [49]. Currently, clinical trials are using a valsartan-based dose of 80 or 160 mg up to a maximum dosage of 160 mg b.i.d. (ClinicalTrials.gov: NCT04335786).

Losartan

Like valsartan, losartan (Cozaar) is a nonpeptide ARB that blocks AngII/AT1R engagement. Losartan has also been shown to downregulate transforming growth factor-β expression, which is a key protein in promoting fibrosis [50]. In animal studies, losartan reduced lung fibrosis [51, 52]. In addition, ARBs may improve respiratory failure in patients with COVID-19. A small-scale, single-arm, open-label trial has assessed the safety of losartan with the primary outcome of occurrence of adverse events. Hospitalized patients with respiratory failure were administered oral losartan 25 mg/d for three days, then 50 mg thereafter until day 14 or discharge (ClinicalTrials.gov: NCT04335123) [53]. Compared with control, participants receiving losartan experienced fewer adverse events with an incidence ratio of 0.69 [53]. Further large-scale studies are necessary to determine losartan efficacy in reducing pulmonary complications associated with SARS-CoV-2 infection. Common losartan side effects include headache, dizziness, and fatigue. However, the rates of adverse events associated with ARB usage have been comparable with control, and side effects have not led to study withdrawal [54].

Telmisartan

Compared with other ARBs, telmisartan (Micardis) is 10-fold more potent as compared with losartan and dissociates more slowly from AT1R [55]. Telmisartan is also a partial agonist of peroxisome proliferator-activated receptor γ. Specifically, telmisartan activates peroxisome proliferator-activated receptor γ, which in turn inhibits AT1R gene expression. As such, telmisartan exhibits dual AT1R inhibition properties that can be beneficial for reducing fibrotic effects associated with SARS-CoV-2 infection. One study of telmisartan-treated patients showed shorter time to discharge when compared with control patients. The median discharge day for control patients was 15 days, while with telmisartan it was only nine days. Death by day 30 in the telmisartan-treated groups was 4.29% versus 22.54% among controls ($P = 0.002$) [56]. These exciting results support additional studies using telmisartan to mitigate SARS-CoV-2–related morbidities and mortality.

Comparative studies investigating the safety and efficacy of ARBs, including valsartan and telmisartan, versus placebo have shown all treatments have similar tolerability. Active clinical trials are recruiting patients to further assess drug efficacy for the treatment of COVID-19 (ClinicalTrials.gov: NCT04394117, NCT04364893, and NCT04591210).

These trials assess lung and cardiovascular function with overall survival.

Recombinant ACE2

As has been previously mentioned, ACE2 is the target for SARS-CoV-2 binding. This carboxypeptidase is an important enzyme that metabolizes AngI to form the biologic active peptide, Ang(1–9). In addition, ACE2 can also use AngII as a substrate to form Ang(1–7), which is a natural ligand of mitochondrial assembly (Mas) receptors [57]. Both Ang(1–9) and Ang(1–7) are peptides in the RAAS that are able to counterbalance the effect of AngII/AT1R binding. In addition, ACE2 can also metabolize other peptides found in the RAAS. This includes metabolizing des-Arg bradykinin and neurotensin.

The role of ACE2 expression in relation to SARS-CoV-2 has been demonstrated using ACE2 genetic knockout animal models, where exposure to the virus can activate proinflammatory and fibrotic axes. In addition, age-related reduction of ACE2 expression in lung tissue has correlated with the increased risk for mortality and worsened phenotype in elderly patients with SARS-CoV-2 [58]. Soluble ACE2 was found to bind onto the SARS-CoV-1 S1 domain and was able to block SARS-CoV-1 infectivity in susceptible cells [59]. Thus, soluble ACE2 may act as a decoy for SARS-CoV-2. SARS-CoV-2 infections were suppressed in engineered human tissues by clinical-grade soluble human ACE2 [60], which further supports this hypothesis. The important role of ACE2 is now being realized, where therapeutic approaches using soluble ACE2 (e.g. recombinant human ACE2, APN01, GSK2586881) have been used as potential decoys to neutralize the virus as a result of competitive binding with cellular ACE2.

Ang(1–7)

SARS-CoV-2 attachment onto ACE2 promotes viral penetration [61]. In addition, SARS-CoV-2 binding onto ACE2 can also downregulate the expression of the surface protein. It has been suggested that following SARS-CoV-2/ACE2 internalization will lead to AngII accumulation and reduction in Ang(1–7) [62, 63]. Clinical studies using ACE2 and ARBs showed clinical benefits in SARS-CoV-2–infected patients.

In pulmonary inflammation models such as acute lung injury, lung fibrosis, and ARDS, Ang(1–7) decreased proinflammation cytokine/chemokine biosynthesis and recruitment of inflammatory cells to the lung. These properties correlated with improved pulmonary function.

In addition, SARS-CoV-2–mediated reduction of ACE2 will also increase AngII accumulation, which may partially contribute to vasculopathy, coagulopathy, and inflammation [64]. Because Ang(1–7) binding onto Mas counterbalances AngII/AT1R-mediated proinflammatory and profibrotic effects, reduction of Ang(1–7) may tilt the balance of this homeostasis. Because Ang(1–7) is one of the products of ACE2 metabolism, it stands to reason that exogenous administration of Ang(1–7) may mitigate some of the SARS-CoV-2–mediated vasculopathy, coagulopathy, inflammation, and lung fibrosis. Synthetic Ang(1–7) is currently in clinical evaluation for SARS-CoV-2–mediated adverse events such as lung fibrosis.

There is still controversy over the precise RAAS profile in patients infected with SARS-CoV-2 [64, 65]. What is not controversial are the potential benefits that Ang(1–7) may provide, including anti-inflammatory, antithrombogenic, and antifibrotic activities [66]. Several groups are evaluating the efficacy of Ang(1–7) in phase 1/2 (ClinicalTrials.gov: NCT04633772) and phase 3 clinical trials (ClinicalTrials.gov: NCT04332666). No clinical efficacy data have yet been reported from these studies.

Viral Replication Inhibitors

Favipiravir (Avigan)

Favipiravir (T-705) is an antiviral that was approved in Japan in 2014 to treat pandemic influenza. It is a prodrug that must undergo phosphoribosylation to form favipiravir–ribonucleotide–triphosphate to form the active metabolite. Similar to other nucleobase compounds, the biotransformed metabolite is incorporated into the viral RNA, causing strand RNA elongation blockade. Additional antiviral activity has included the ability to disrupt viral protein synthesis. Finally, favipiravir has been shown to induce lethal viral mutagenesis leading to antiviral activity [67, 68]. Efforts are underway to repurpose favipiravir as an experimental agent against enveloped, positive-sense, single-strand RNA viruses such as SARS-CoV-2,

including mild or asymptomatic infection among outpatients. In the United States, favipiravir is being investigated in a phase 2 randomized, double-blind, placebo-controlled trial to determine whether oral favipiravir decreases the duration of viral shedding better than placebo when given within 72 hours of diagnosis in outpatients with mild or asymptomatic COVID-19.

Another study has shown that COVID-19 patients treated with Favipiravir did not have significantly different recovery rate than that treated with Umifenovir, however, the duration of fever and cough relief time are significantly shorter in Favipiravir group than in Umifenovir group. However, a posthoc analysis showed that COVID-19 patients with moderate severity treated with favipiravir had superior recovery rate than that treated with umifenovir (p=0.0199). The current dosage for trials is 1600 mg by mouth twice daily for one day, followed by 800 mg twice daily (maximum days of therapy is seven days) [69].

Molnupiravir (MK-4482 or EIDD-2801)

Molnupiravir is an orally active experimental antiviral drug developed for the treatment of influenza. Similar to other nucleoside analogues, molnupiravir requires biotransformation to the triphosphate moiety to exert its antiviral activity. Similar to favipiravir, molnupiravir's antiviral activity is to induce lethal viral mutagenesis in animal studies [70]. This promising in vitro anti–SARS-CoV-2 data prompted the initiation of two phase 2/3 trials to determine its ability to reduce mortality and accelerate recovery. In this dosage-finding study, molnupiravir is given at 200, 400, or 800 mg b.i.d. for five days. Among those with a positive viral culture at enrolment, by day five, 24% of placebo participants continued to be COVID-19 culture positive as compared with none treated with molnupiravir ($P = 0.001$). Participants receiving either 400 or 800 mg molnupiravir were virally undetectable as compared with 11.1% for subjects receiving placebo ($P = 0.03$). Time to viral RNA clearance was decreased in participants administered 800 mg molnupiravir versus placebo ($P = 0.01$). These promising results have encouraged further evaluation [71]. In addition, the molecular mechanism of antiviral activity presents safety concerns that need to be investigated thoroughly.

Remdesivir (Veklury)

Remdesivir is a nucleoside analogue with broad-spectrum antiviral activity that was initially developed for Ebola virus infection [72]. Remdesivir, a nucleoside analogue prodrug, has inhibitory effects on pathogenic animal and human coronaviruses such as MERS-CoV, SARS-CoV-1, and SARS-CoV-2. This nucleoside analogue was also found to be active against filoviruses, paramyxoviruses, and pneumoviruses [73, 74]. Like all nucleoside analogues, remdesivir requires biotransformation into the active metabolite, remdesivir triphosphate (RDV-TP). RDV-TP inhibits viral RdRp, which blocks the elongating RNA and has been proposed as the primary mechanism of antiviral action [75]. This antiviral activity can lead to faster recovery and reduced disease severity. Remdesivir has been shown to reduce time to recovery in adults with COVID-19, and it is currently the only antiviral approved by the FDA for the treatment of COVID-19 [76].

As RNA synthesis proceeds, RDV-TP competes with its natural counterpart ATP for chain elongation complementing opposite template U at a random position "i" (stage 2). Steady-state kinetics have shown the efficiency of incorporation of RDV-TP to be three times higher [77, 78], which is unusually efficient for a nucleotide analogue inhibitor. The presence of a 3′-hydroxyl group allows a nucleophilic attack on the next incoming nucleotide, and no significant inhibition is seen at position $i+1$. Three additional nucleotides are incorporated before RNA synthesis is arrested at position $i+3$ (stage 3). Inhibitors of this type are commonly referred to as "delayed chain terminators," in contrast with obligate or classic chain terminators that lack the 3′-hydroxyl group and prevent further nucleotide additions at $i+1$ [79].

Remdesivir is a potent SARS-CoV-2 nucleotide inhibitor that can block viral replication in human nasal and bronchial airway epithelial cells [80]. In addition to its antiviral potency, the safety margin of remdesivir is high where its EC_{50} (effective concentration 50%) = 0.77 μM and selectivity index is >129.87 [24]. On 22 October 2020, the FDA approved remdesivir for use in adults and pediatric patients (≥12 years of age and weighing at least 40 kg) for the treatment of COVID-19 requiring hospitalization. IV administration of remdesivir in the treatment of a patient with COVID-19 resulted in recovery from pneumonia [81]. In subjects receiving remdesivir, nearly 70% of patients had improvement in terms of oxygen requirements, and many patients who were mechanically ventilated were extubated. Patients in the remdesivir group had a shorter time to recovery as compared with the patients receiving placebo group (median, 10 days, as compared with 15 days; rate ratio for recovery, 1.29; 95% confidence interval [CI], 1.12–1.49; $P < 0.001$). Treatment with remdesivir may have ameliorated the progression to more severe respiratory disease, as shown by the lower proportion of serious adverse events caused by respiratory failure among patients in the remdesivir group, as well as a lower incidence of new oxygen use among patients who were not receiving oxygen at enrolment and a lower proportion of patients needing higher levels of respiratory support during the study [82].

In an open-label randomized trial in hospitalized patients (n = 596), two dosage regimens of remdesivir were tested against the standard of care. As a limitation for the study, the standard of care included patients who received HCQ, lopinavir/ritonavir, or AZM. The dosages of remdesivir differed by the duration of 5 versus 10 days. There were no significant differences between the different durations of treatment. However, the five-day remdesivir treatment had significantly higher odds of better clinical status distribution on day 11 than standard of care (odds ratio, 1.65; 95% CI, 1.09–2.48; $P = 0.02$). By day 28, there were more hospital discharges among patients who received remdesivir (89% in the 5-day arm and 90% in the 10-day arm) than those who received standard of care (83%) [83].

The current recommendation for remdesivir, administered IV, is a 200 mg loading dose on day one, followed by 100 mg once-daily maintenance doses for up to nine additional days. This dosage is recommended for adults and children 12 years or older weighing at least 40 kg. For patients not requiring invasive mechanical ventilation and/or extracorporeal membrane oxygenation, the recommended total treatment duration is five days. If a patient does not demonstrate clinical improvement, treatment may be extended for up to five additional days for a total treatment duration of up to 10 days. Clinicians must monitor for signs of hepatotoxicity and reduced renal function. Remdesivir should not be used in combination with other hepatotoxic drugs, and clinicians should monitor hepatic function throughout treatment. Clinicians need to monitor kidney function of all patients receiving remdesivir, particularly those with preexisting renal impairments and those receiving nephrotoxic drugs. Remdesivir use should be avoided in patients with an estimated glomerular filtration rate <30 ml/min or full-term neonates with serum creatinine concentration >1 mg/dl (see FDA EUA Fact Sheet for Heath Providers: https://www.fda.gov/media/137566/download, July 2020).

Ribavirin

RBV is a guanosine analogue with broad-spectrum activity against RNA and DNA viruses [84, 85]. Like other nucleoside analogues, RBV must be biotransformed into the triphosphate moiety and incorporate into the viral nucleic acid elongation strand. Although RBV has significant toxicities, such as anemia, it has been successfully combined with IFNs for the treatment of hepatitis C virus infection. The triphosphate moiety is known to inhibit HCV RNA, while the monophosphate metabolite is an inhibitor of inosine monophosphate dehydrogenase. Other activity attributed to RBV-triphosphate includes inhibition of RNA polymerase as well [86].

In a study evaluating the effect of RBV in COVID-19, the rate of reverse transcriptase-polymerase chain reaction conversion in patients with severe SARS-CoV-2 was compared between RBV recipients and 71 control subjects. Both control and treatment groups had similar baseline laboratory values and clinical characteristics. The negative conversion time for severe SARS-CoV-2 reverse transcriptase-polymerase chain reaction positivity in the RBV group was 12.8 ± 4.1 days, which was lower than in the control group with 14.1 ± 3.5 days ($P = 0.314$). Mortality in the RBV group was 7/41 (17.1%), while the mortality was 17/69 (24.6%) in the control group ($P = 0.475$). Adverse effects were similar between the two treatment groups. Participants with severe COVID-19 who were treated with RBV did not experience more rapid conversion to negative RT-PCR. Further studies are needed to determine the efficacy of RBV in patients with COVID-19 [87].

Oseltamivir

Oseltamivir (Tamiflu) is a drug approved for treatment of influenza A and B. Oseltamivir targets the neuraminidase distributed on the surface of the influenza virus to inhibit the spread of the influenza virus once it enters a cell. This drug has been explored as a potential treatment for SARS-CoV-2 infection; however, one study reported that no positive outcomes were observed with oseltamivir [88]. Oseltamivir is also being evaluated in clinical trials alone (as an adjuvant) or in combination with other agents (ClinicalTrials.gov: NCT04516915 and NCT04558463).

Umifenovir

Umifenovir is an antiviral agent used to treat influenza in China and Russia that is being investigated for the treatment of COVID-19. It is a broad-spectrum antiviral that has activity against various DNA and RNA viruses. Umifenovir exhibits antiviral activity in part through drug interactions with aromatic residues found within glycoproteins involved in viral-cell recognition and fusion [89]. It also has been shown to interfere with the accumulation of clathrin-coated structures intracellularly, which reduces viral uptake through endocytosis [90]. A systematic review and meta-analysis regarding the safety and efficacy of umifenovir across 12 studies has confirmed the safety of umifenovir and indicated that, compared with the control groups, umifenovir was associated with a higher rate of negative PCR test on day 14 [91]. Further large-scale trials are necessary in more diverse patient populations to establish efficacy for COVID-19 progression.

Viral Protein Process Inhibitors

SARS-CoV-2 also has a PLpro capable of cleaving the viral polyproteins. In addition to its metabolic activities, PLpro can inhibit expression of proinflammatory cytokines such as IFN-β and chemokines. Chemokines such as CXCL10 and CCL5 are an important immune response to suppressing viral replication. The targeting of PLpro has several advantages; its inhibition not only suppresses virus replication but also reduces bystander cell toxicity [11]. RdRp catalyzes viral RNA synthesis and is another functional protein that could be used as a therapeutic target to develop synthetic nucleotide drugs [12].

Lopinavir/Ritonavir

Lopinavir/ritonavir (Kaletra or Aluvia) are coformulated HIV-1 protease inhibitors. Ritonavir inhibits cytochrome P450 enzymatic activity and thus prolongs the plasma concentration of lopinavir. This combination has been shown to competitively inhibit viral proteases. These agents are expected to work similarly to inhibit the production of SARS-CoV-2 viral proteins. Lopinavir is thought to provide the bulk of the combination's antiviral effect. Drug interactions with other P450 metabolized drugs are common.

Both proteases of the host cell, which assist the virus during its life cycle, and those of the virus act in a concerted fashion to regulate and coordinate specific steps of the viral propagation, such as (1) the entry and replication of the virus, (2) the maturation of the polyprotein, and (3) the assembly of the secreted virions for further diffusion [92]. Lopinavir is a peptidomimetic molecule that contains a hydroxyethylene scaffold that mimics the peptide linkage typically targeted by the HIV-1 protease enzyme but which by itself cannot be cleaved, thus preventing the activity of the HIV-1 protease [93].

Lopinavir-ritonavir was investigated in an open-label, randomized, controlled trial, where patients with COVID-19 received either lopinavir/ritonavir 400 mg/100 mg orally b.i.d. plus standard of care or standard of care alone. Although no benefit was observed with lopinavir/ritonavir treatment beyond standard care, there was a significant decrease in coronavirus viral load, with no or little coronavirus observed in the follow-up study [94]. Most of the side effects experienced were gastrointestinal.

In a randomized clinical trial, 1616 participants received lopinavir/ritonavir (400/100 mg b.i.d.) compared with 3424 patients receiving standard of care [95]. There were no detectable benefits in terms of reduction in 28-day mortality, duration of hospital stay, or risk of progressing to invasive mechanical ventilation or death. These findings do not support the use of lopinavir/ritonavir for treatment of patients admitted to the hospital with COVID-19 [95]. A 14-day triple combination of lopinavir/ritonavir with eight million international units of recombinant IFN-β (on alternating days) was evaluated in a phase 2 clinical trial (ClinicalTrials.gov: NCT04276688) [96]. This triple-combination therapy was found to be more effective at alleviating COVID-19 symptoms and shortening viral shedding time compared with lopinavir/ritonavir alone [96].

Disulfiram (Antabuse)

One agent with great potential for repurposing is disulfiram (Antabuse), an aldehyde dehydrogenase inhibitor currently used to treat alcohol use disorder. This treatment has more than 60 years of clinical use and an acceptable safety profile. Disulfiram treatment for COVID-19 may be useful because of its ability to reduce hyperinflammation in host cells and inhibition of virus-encoded proteases. Hu et al. [97] showed disulfiram-mediated anti-inflammatory effects. In addition, disulfiram was able to reduce mortality in a sepsis mouse model, suggesting a possible therapeutic effect in patients with severe COVID-19.

The pharmacologic properties ascribed to disulfiram include the ability to inhibit proinflammatory IL-1β release and pyroptosis by blocking the assembly of the homopolymeric gasdermin D pore. In addition, disulfiram was found to be an inhibitor of the SARS-CoV-2 main protease (Mpro) and PLpro in both MERS-CoV and SARS-CoV-1. As aforementioned, both enzymes are needed for viral replication [98–101]. The IC_{50} (inhibitory concentration 50%) values of disulfiram for both proteases are 9.35 and 2–7 μM, respectively, compared with the dosage of disulfiram prescribed for alcohol use disorders (up to 500 mg daily). Lastly, disulfiram can inhibit the ATPase activity of NSP13 and the exoribonuclease activity of NSP14 of SARS-CoV-2 via its Zn^{2+}-ejector function [102].

In a preprint retrospective cohort study among veterans, Fillmore et al. [103] reported that patients treated with disulfiram had a 34% lower risk of SARS-CoV-2 infection compared with those not treated with disulfiram, with a hazard ratio of 0.66 (95% CI: 0.57–0.76; $P < 0.001$).

Additional data are expected from two small ongoing phase 2 clinical trials of disulfiram involving early mild-to-moderate symptomatic (ClinicalTrials.gov: NCT04485130, 60 participants) or hospitalized (ClinicalTrials.gov: NCT04594343, 200 participants) patients with COVID-19.

Antibiotics and Antiparasitic

Azithromycin

AZM is a macrolide antibiotic used for the treatment of bacterial infections that have immunomodulatory activities, including downregulating inflammatory cytokine production, maintaining epithelial cell integrity, and preventing lung fibrosis. In addition, AZM was found to increase Golgi network pH and recycling endosomes, which are used by SARS-CoV-2 for replication [104, 105]. All these properties are potentially important for SARS-CoV-2–mediated pathogenesis, such as acute lung injury and/or fibrosis.

AZM was initially assessed in viral infections for its ability to reduce mortality and requirement for mechanical ventilation days. In a small study conducted early in the COVID-19 pandemic, AZM was combined with HCQ. Participants receiving 600 mg of HCQ with AZM (dosage was not specified) were evaluated for respiratory viral load over time [106]. This study showed a reduction in SARS-CoV-2 PCR positivity.

To further explore these findings, we assessed SARS-CoV-2–positive patients treated with AZM 500 mg daily in a larger study. Patients were randomly assigned to AZM plus standard of care (n = 540) compared with standard of care alone (n = 875) [107]. These participants were also compared with patients receiving other interventions (n = 850). No meaningful benefit was shown for the AZM plus standard of care group (which included HCQ) as compared with standard of care alone (hazard ratio, 1.08; 95% Bayesian credibility interval: 0.95–1.23).

Azithromycin in Combination with HCQ

The results of the COALITION II Clinical Trial corroborate those of COALITION I, which was done by the same study group and evaluated HCQ with or without AZM in patients admitted to the hospital with mild or moderate COVID-19 [108]. In COALITION I, there was no significant difference in outcomes in patients receiving HCQ with or without AZM and no evidence of an increase in adverse events. The results of these trials suggest that AZM might not provide benefit to patients once the disease has progressed, and that patients require hospitalization. Because AZM is a commonly prescribed outpatient therapy for COVID-19, establishing whether it is helpful earlier in the disease course is an important research priority. If

AZM does not have a role in the treatment of COVID-19, avoiding its use would reduce unnecessary antibiotic consumption and AZM's risk for Q-T interval prolongation.

Ivermectin

Ivermectin (Stromectol) is an antiparasitic agent used to treat onchocerciasis, strongyloidiasis, helminthiases, and scabies. Reports have shown that ivermectin can inhibit α/ß-1 nuclear transport proteins. Viruses inhibit these intracellular transport proteins to prevent host antiviral immune response. However, ivermectin was also found to interfere with SARS-CoV-2 S protein onto epithelial cells, which sparked interest in this compound.

Ivermectin is currently being investigated as a treatment for SARS-CoV-2 at 0.2–0.4 mg/kg/d orally for five days (ClinicalTrials.gov: NCT04920942 and NCT04646109). There are research efforts to explore intranasal delivery approaches as well [109]. Ivermectin reduced the amount of cell-associated viral DNA by 99.8% after 24 hours. Further studies are needed to determine the clinical effectiveness of this medicine in humans with COVID-19. Currently, both the FDA and the European Medicines Agency do not recommend the use of ivermectin for patients with COVID-19 because there is yet no clinical evidence of its efficacy in infected patients. A large trial of ivermectin that initially suggested benefit has been withdrawn from the preprint server Research Square (https://www.researchsquare.com/article/rs-100956/v4).

Nitazoxanide

Nitazoxanide (Alinia) is a broad-spectrum antiparasitic agent that was previously found to have antiviral activity against influenza in a phase 2b/3 clinical trial. Initially, nitazoxanide was prescribed for immunocompromised patients with cryptosporidiosis and giardiasis.

Nitazoxanide for COVID-19 was evaluated in a multicenter, randomized, double-blind, placebo-controlled trial, for adult patients presenting up to three days after onset of COVID-19 symptoms with PCR-confirmed illness [110]. Participants were randomized to receive either nitazoxanide (500 mg) or placebo thrice daily for five days. Those receiving nitazoxanide with mild COVID-19 had a more rapid viral load reduction as compared with patients receiving placebo (P = 0.006), but the primary endpoint of time to symptom resolution did not differ between nitazoxanide and placebo groups. The study did affirm the safety of nitazoxanide in patients with COVID-19 [110].

Immunotherapy

Immunotherapy has been gaining popularity as a therapeutic approach to manage a wide range of disease states with an immune component, including cancer, autoimmunity, and infectious disease. Many of the immunotherapeutics that have been used in patients with COVID-19 have already gained FDA approval for use in other immune-mediated diseases, but several of the immunotherapeutics discussed later are new, and their rapid development and deployment in the grips of a global pandemic exemplify that innovation and ingenuity are still very much alive in the field of immunotherapy research and development.

Recombinant Cytokine Therapy

Type I IFNs

IFNs were among the first members of the cytokine family to be described [111]. These cytokines are elicited after immune detection of an invading pathogen and are well-known to evoke antipathogen, especially antiviral, responses after binding their cognate receptors by increasing the lysing activity of NK cells and increasing major histocompatibility complex class I expression by virus-infected cells. Many pathogens have developed mechanisms to downregulate IFN expression to evade detection and potential destruction by immune cells. It has been shown that one mechanism SARS-CoV-2 uses to evade the antiviral effects of type I IFNs is through induction of autoantibody production against endogenous type I IFNs, which prevent these cytokines from binding their cognate receptors and exerting their antiviral effects [112]. As a result, many patients are deficient in their expression of these critical, endogenous antiviral immune mediators during infection.

Three types of IFN have been described: type I, type II, and type III. Expression of type I IFNs, which include IFN-α and IFN-β, has been shown to be downregulated in patients with COVID-19. To combat the SARS-CoV-2–mediated reduction in these essential cytokines, two different recombinant IFN-α therapies

have been given to patients with COVID-19: PEGASYS/ Peginterferon α-2a (180 µg per week for two doses) [113] from Genentech, and 1 µg/kg PEG-Intron/Peginterferon α-2a from Merck (ClinicalTrials.gov: NCT04480138). Each of these drugs has been previously approved to treat chronic hepatitis B and C infection; for hepatitis C, these drugs are typically given with RBV. This recombinant IFN-α therapy in combination with RBV has been evaluated in patients with COVID-19 in clinical trials [114] (ClinicalTrials.gov: NCT04480138) that have demonstrated a reduction in duration of viral shedding and to significantly improve clinical outcomes.

GM-CSF

This granulocyte and macrophage growth factor cytokine underscores the challenge and complexity of treating COVID-19 as it is being analyzed for both therapeutic blockade (see the following section) and recombinant administration [115, 116]. GM-CSF is known to be required for maintenance of pulmonary function and lung-mediated immunity [115, 116]. In lethal influenza-induced lung injury animal models [117, 118], lung-specific overexpression of this cytokine increased survival and protection against secondary infection [115, 119], whereas GM-CSF-deficient animals succumbed to their disease beyond 48 hours after challenge [115, 120]. In patients with ARDS, administration of inhaled GM-CSF has been shown to increase oxygenation. Use of inhaled recombinant GM-CSF (125 µg b.i.d. for five days) in patients with COVID-19 with respiratory failure has been evaluated in a phase 4 clinical trial (SARPAC, ClinicalTrials.gov: NCT04326920) [115], in addition to several other phase 1/2 trials initiated by companies that produce therapeutic GM-CSF [115]. As of the writing of this chapter, the results of this clinical trial have not been posted.

Anticytokine Therapy

IL-1 Receptor Antagonism

IL-1 is a key inflammatory cytokine component involved in cytokine storm, which was also evident in patients with COVID-19. Anakinra (Kineret) is an injectable IL-1 receptor antagonist that was originally developed for the management of rheumatoid arthritis and neonatal-onset multisystem inflammatory disease. Anakinra blocks the activity of the endogenous IL-1 produced in response to inflammatory stimuli via binding to the IL-1 receptor, which prevents binding of IL-1 and the downstream signaling and activating events. Multiple national (Swedish Orphan Biovitrum AB [SOBI], ClinicalTrials.gov: NCT04603742) and international [121, 122] studies have been conducted to determine the potential clinical benefit of anakinra in patients with COVID-19. The dose, dosing schedule, and duration varied between each study, with 100–200 mg of anakinra given to patients multiple times a day for at least 24 hours before switching to once-a-day dosing for several subsequent days [121, 122] (SOBI, ClinicalTrials.gov: NCT04603742). Although anakinra cohort studies used in patients with COVID-19 reduced the need for invasive mechanical ventilation [121], no benefit was observed in patients with mild-to-moderate COVID-19 [122]. These findings need further studies to substantiate their finding. In addition, a phase 2 clinical trial investigating the efficacy of anakinra in prevention of CRS has not yet posted results as of the writing of this chapter (SOBI, ClinicalTrials.gov: NCT04603742).

IL-6 Receptor Antagonism

The inflammatory cytokine IL-6 was quickly confirmed to be a major contributor to host-mediated immunopathology and the cytokine likely to initiate the CRS cytokine storm. As a result, blocking the IL-6 signaling pathway became a priority for the treatment of patients with COVID-19 early in the pandemic. Two IL-6 receptor–blocking monoclonal antibodies had been previously developed for the management of rheumatoid arthritis: sarilumab (Kevzara; Regeneron Pharmaceuticals) and tocilizumab (Actemra; Hoffman-La Roche). Both drugs have been shown to reduce mortality rates in patients with severe COVID-19 and increased survival in the REMAP-CAP clinical trial (ClinicalTrials.gov: NCT02735707) [123]. Interestingly, a phase 2 clinical trial investigating the use of sarilumab alone in patients with COVID-19 did not demonstrate efficacy (ClinicalTrials.gov: NCT04327388) [124], despite both trials analyzing the same concentration and dosing of sarilumab (400 mg

IV, once per day) [123, 124]. This differing conclusion is likely due to the significantly smaller sarilumab group in the REMAP-CAP trial versus the Sanofi and Regeneron trials (48 and 159 patients, respectively). A recent systemic review and meta-analysis concluded that tocilizumab improves outcome compared with patients who do not receive this IL-6 receptor monoclonal antibody [125]. Furthermore, the findings on tocilizumab's efficacy in the REMAP-CAP trial were consistent with the findings of the RECOVERY trial (ClinicalTrials.gov: NCT04381936), suggesting that this is the more effective of the two available therapeutics. On 24 June 2021, the FDA issued an EUA for tocilizumab for the treatment of hospitalized adults and pediatric patients (≥2 years old) who are receiving systemic corticosteroids and require supplemental oxygen or ventilatory support (https://www.fda.gov/media/150321/download).

IL-6 Antagonism

In addition to targeting the IL-6 receptor, it is also possible to directly target secreted IL-6 using the chimeric monoclonal antibody siltuximab (Sylvant). Phase 3 clinical trials began in patients with COVID-19 in December 2020 (SILVAR, ClinicalTrials.gov: NCT04616586) but were terminated in early 2021 after both the REMAP-CAP and RECOVERY trials reported positive results supporting the use of tocilizumab in patients with COVID-19. At this time, the NIH COVID-19 treatment guidelines (https://www.covid19treatmentguidelines.2020.03nih.gov/immunomodulators/interleukin-6-inhibitors) do not recommend the use of siltuximab outside a clinical trial setting.

GM-CSF Antagonism

As discussed in the earlier "Recombinant Cytokine Therapy" section, the field lacks consensus on GM-CSF's role in the immunopathology observed in patients with COVID-19. Although preclinical respiratory tract infection models and non-COVID ARDS patient data suggest an immunoprotective role for GM-CSF in lung tissue [115, 116, 120], other studies recommend targeting of endogenous GM-CSF and postulate that treatment with GM-CSF-boosting therapeutics like sargramostim may actually contribute to ARDS by boosting myeloid cell production and by promoting survival and accumulation of these in the inflammatory lung environment [115, 126, 127].

The humanized GM-CSF targeting monoclonal antibody lenzilumab (Humanigen Inc.) was originally developed to combat CAR T cell–induced CRS [128] and graft-versus-host disease–associated CRS [129], in addition to other inflammatory diseases driven by GM-CSF. Although this monoclonal antibody does not yet have FDA approval for use in CAR T cell recipients, the FDA did approve the initiation of a phase 3 clinical trial to investigate the clinical benefit of this experimental therapeutic for patients with COVID-19-induced ARDS (ClinicalTrials.gov: NCT04351152), although no dosing information has been provided on the clinical trial study page. This trial is still ongoing, and no results were posted at the time this text was written.

Neutralizing Antibody Therapy

Neutralizing antibodies are the cornerstone of immunologic memory. These antibodies are typically produced by the immune system in response to a primary natural infection or vaccination and can persist in the bloodstream at high levels for months, years, or even a lifetime depending on the pathogen or vaccine. However, because of our increased understanding of the immune system coupled with advances in monoclonal antibody technology, exogenous pathogen-specific neutralizing antibodies can now be provided to patients prophylactically, early in the course of illness, or during the height of an infection to mitigate disease severity. In the context of SARS-CoV-2 infection, two different approaches have been used: (1) recombinant monoclonal antibodies specific for viral S protein, and (2) convalescent plasma from patients recovered from COVID-19.

Recombinant Monoclonal Antibodies

Two different recombinant monoclonal antibody regimens have been extensively investigated for their use in patients with COVID-19. The first, casirivimab/imdevimab (REGEN-COV), is a cocktail of two antibodies manufactured by Regeneron Pharmaceuticals that can bind onto nonoverlapping epitopes found on the RBD of S protein. These antibodies are given in combination to prevent mutational escape of the virus

and therapeutic resistance, which has been observed in single-antibody therapies [130]. After showing efficacy in reducing COVID-19-related hospitalizations and intensive care unit visits and overall viral load, the FDA issued an EUA for casirivimab/imdevimab in November 2020 [131]. Phase 3 clinical trial data from April 2021 (ClinicalTrials.gov: NCT04425629) reported that this monoclonal antibody cocktail (1200 mg of both, infused IV) was 81% effective in reducing infection risk for noninfected patients, suggesting it may also have efficacy as a prophylactic therapy alternative to vaccination (ClinicalTrials.gov: NCT04425629). It was also reported that in active infections, casirivimab/imdevimab reduced time to symptom resolution to one week versus three weeks in patients who received placebo (ClinicalTrials.gov: NCT04425629). Although these study results have not yet been officially reviewed and published, this recombinant monoclonal antibody cocktail is currently recommended by the NIH's COVID-19 Treatment Guidelines for high-risk patients with outpatient COVID-19 illness and for close exposures without illness [132].

The second recombinant monoclonal antibody that has been studied in patients with COVID-19 is bamlanivimab (LY-CoV555; AbCellera Biologics and Eli Lilly), which is also specific for epitopes on the S viral protein RBD. In December 2020, bamlanivimab was awarded an EUA from the FDA, but this was revoked in April 2021 after it was found that administration of bamlanivimab alone was not efficacious. Bamlanivimab is currently being investigated in combination with etesevimab (Blaze-1 Trial, ClinicalTrials.gov: NCT04427501) (700 and 1400 mg, respectively) and was awarded an EUA from the FDA in February 2021 for use in patients with COVID-19. This clinical trial is still recruiting patients, and no results have been posted at the time this chapter was compiled.

Convalescent Plasma Therapy

In addition to recombinant monoclonal antibodies, neutralizing antibodies against SARS-CoV-2 S protein can be recovered from the sera of patients recovered from COVID-19. This therapeutic approach, which is also called passive immunotherapy, has been used in past infectious outbreaks [133–135] with limited success. Initial clinical trials evaluating the efficacy of this therapy focused on patients with severe COVID-19 and did not demonstrate good clinical efficacy [136–138], which could be contributed to underpowered studies, limited enrolment, and heterogeneity among the trial participants [136]. Observational studies provided more positive data, and some suggested a clinical benefit for this therapy [139]. Despite receiving an FDA-issued EUA for use of this therapy, the NIH's COVID-19 Treatment Guidelines do not support the use of this therapy above other therapeutics that have better data backing their use [136], and many clinicians and researchers have called for better-organized clinical trials to finally determine the clinical efficacy of this therapy. Additional considerations must be considered for the practical implementation of this therapy, including rolling plasma shortages and inconsistency of neutralizing antibody titers between donors [136].

Other Anti-inflammatory Therapies

Steroids

Steroids are a class of anti-inflammatory therapeutics with pleiotropic activity. These agents, which include prednisone and dexamethasone (DEX), can induce lymphocyte apoptosis, reduce nuclear factor-κB activation, and block leukocyte migration to the site of infection. In addition, steroids decrease cytokine expression.

The use of corticosteroids during a respiratory illness is empirically driven because while mounting an immune response to eliminate a viral infection, the body must not damage native lung tissue. An overactive immune response may result in harm to native lung tissue that is worse than damage from the inciting virus. Using corticosteroids to suppress an immune response may result in an uncontrolled viral infection. Identifying how and when corticosteroids can strike this equilibrium between benefit and harm is a substantial consideration.

DEX is a corticosteroid used in a wide range of conditions for its anti-inflammatory and immunosuppressant effects through T cell inhibition. Clinically, DEX (6 mg IV/PO daily) was evaluated early in the pandemic in a randomized open-label study (ClinicalTrials.gov: NCT04381936). Patients who received DEX had significantly reduced need for mechanical ventilation and oxygen. These findings were further supported by a follow-up study (CoDEX) where 299 adults with suspected

or confirmed COVID-19 with signs and symptoms consistent with moderate to severe ARDS were randomized to receive 20 mg DEX daily for five days and compared with those receiving standard of care (ClinicalTrials.gov: NCT04327401). DEX-treated patients had a statistically significant reduction in mortality and were ventilator free at day 28, as well as having a reduction in Sequential Organ Failure Assessment scores at day seven ($P < 0.004$). In patients hospitalized with COVID-19, the use of DEX resulted in lower 28-day mortality among those who were receiving either invasive mechanical ventilation or oxygen alone at randomization, but notably not among those receiving no respiratory support. NIH guidelines recommend the use of DEX in hospitalized adults requiring oxygen or ventilatory support [140]. Other corticosteroids can be used if DEX is not available.

Cyclosporine

Treatment with cyclosporine leads to a decrease in hyperinflammation and likely decreased viral replication as well [141]. Although cyclosporine is an immunosuppressive drug used in transplant medicine administered to prevent organ rejection, its use for COVID-19 in immunocompetent patients is under investigation (SOLIDARITY study, COQUIMA cohort); these pending investigational phase 1 studies suggest a cumulative dose of at least 300 mg to be administered for a duration of three weeks maximum with trough drug level monitoring.

Several independent studies indicate that cyclosporine inhibits replication of several different coronaviruses in vitro. The cyclosporine-analogue alisporivir has recently been shown to inhibit SARS-CoV-2 in vitro [142]. These findings are promising, although there is no clinical evidence yet for a protective effect to reduce the likelihood of severe COVID-19 or to treat ARDS, which often causes severe morbidity.

Acalabrutinib

Acalabrutinib, sold as Calquence by Acerta Pharma, is a selective inhibitor of Bruton's tyrosine kinase currently approved for the treatment of mantle cell lymphoma, chronic lymphocytic leukemia, or small lymphocytic lymphoma. This small molecule can covalently bind onto Bruton's tyrosine kinase and inhibit its enzymatic activity in B cells, which is important for B cell proliferation, activation, chemotaxis, and adhesion.

The efficacy was initially evaluated in 19 patients hospitalized with severe COVID-19. At study entry, 11 of these patients required supplemental oxygen, while 8 patients received mechanical ventilation. Over a 10- to 14-day treatment course, 100 mg acalabrutinib given enterally for 10 days improved oxygenation in a majority of patients [143] without toxicity. Levels of C-reactive protein and IL-6 normalized in most patients. Normalization of lymphopenia correlated with improved oxygenation. At the end of acalabrutinib treatment, 8 of 11 (72.7%) patients who required supplemental oxygen had been discharged on room air. In addition, four of eight (50%) patients who were on mechanical ventilation were successfully extubated, while two of eight (25%) were discharged on room air. A confirmatory international prospective randomized controlled clinical trial (ClinicalTrials.gov: NCT04346199) among patients who were not ventilator dependent was unable to reach a primary endpoint and was discontinued.

Baricitinib

Baricitinib, sold under the name Olumiant by Eli Lilly, is a selective Janus kinase 1 and 2 inhibitor that has been FDA approved for the treatment of rheumatoid arthritis. This is an orally bioavailable small molecule that inhibits the expression of inflammatory cytokines associated with CRS.

The combination of baricitinib with remdesivir was predicted to have synergy for SARS-CoV-2 when using artificial intelligence algorithms. This combination leverages the ability of Janus kinase inhibitor to inhibit inflammatory cytokines such as IL-1, IL-6, IL-10, and GM-CSF.

These simulations were affirmed in a large clinical study (ClinicalTrials.gov: NCT04401579) where baricitinib was combined with remdesivir and was found to be superior to remdesivir alone in reducing recovery time and accelerating clinical improvements. In this study, patients with COVID-19 received a 200 mg loading dose of remdesivir on day 1 followed by 100 mg daily maintenance doses on days 2–10, or until discharge from hospital or death [144]. Baricitinib was administered as a 4 mg daily dose (via 2-mg tablets or via nasogastric tube) for 14 days, or until discharge from hospital [144]. In addition, this therapeutic combination was associated with fewer serious adverse events [144]. As of this writing, NIH treatment guidelines recommend adding either baricitinib or tocilizumab for individuals with rapidly increasing oxygen needs and systemic inflammation, in addition to corticosteroids [145].

Lenzilumab

Lenzilumab is a humanized monoclonal antibody targeting anti-GM-CSF. Lenzilumab was originally developed to block GM-CSF-mediated signaling, triggering CRS in non-COVID-19 patients. As evidence began to emerge that GM-CSF levels correlated with ARDS and cytokine-mediated lung injury, this therapeutic began to be evaluated in patients with COVID-19. A phase 3 clinical trial reported on the preprint server medRxiv and not yet peer-reviewed, the LIVE-AIR study (ClinicalTrials.gov: NCT04351152), compared lenzilumab with placebo treatment in hypoxic patients with oxygen saturation (SpO$_2$) ≤94% and not on mechanical ventilation. A total of 261 participants were randomized to receive lenzilumab (600 mg in three IV infusions given eight hours apart) and compared with 259 receiving placebo. Lenzilumab recipients showed an improvement in survival without ventilation by 54% when evaluated using a modified intent-to-treat population (hazard ratio, 1.54; 95% CI: 1.02–2.31, $P = 0.041$). This study concluded that lenzilumab was most beneficial for subjects with C-reactive protein (CRP) level <150 mg/L and who were younger than 85 years where lenzilumab treatment can improve survival.

Experimental Therapeutics

PAC-MAN

With the rise of CRISPR technology, scientists are now looking to extend the power of this gene-editing tool in the field of infectious diseases. Investigators at Stanford are using a CRISPR-Cas13 approach, which they call PAC-MAN (Prophylactic Antiviral CRISPR in huMAN cells), to inhibit and destroy viral RNA during an ongoing infection [146]. This approach is still in early in vitro validation, but it has shown significant efficacy in reducing influenza viral load in epithelial cells and has been investigated for its efficacy against SARS-CoV-2 by the same group [147]. Although this technology will likely make little immediate impact for patients with COVID-19, it represents an exciting and new therapeutic modality on the horizon for management of RNA virus–mediated infections.

Single-Domain Antibody

Single-domain antibodies, also called nanobodies, are an antibody fragment containing a single variable domain. Like the more commonly known Y-shaped dual-domain antibodies (known therapeutically as monoclonal antibodies), single-domain antibodies bind selectively to a single antigen. The first single-domain antibodies were engineered from camelid heavy chain antibodies. A significant advantage of single-domain antibodies is their small size that allows for easier production at much higher concentrations, shorter plasma half-life, and better permeability into tissues, all of which are critical considerations for their potential as a therapeutic agent. Single-domain antibodies can also be administered by inhalation, making them an ideal therapeutic candidate for the treatment of respiratory diseases [147, 148]. Furthermore, precedent for use of single-domain antibodies already exists in the FDA-approved blinatumomab (Blincyto, Amgen, Inc.) [149].

Several teams have now identified multiple single-domain antibodies from the serum of RBD-immunized llamas and alpacas that can neutralize the SARS-CoV-2 RBD [147–149]. Although this technology is still at the validation stage, the early findings are promising; this, coupled with the increased flexibility in production, scaling, and administration of single-domain antibodies versus traditional monoclonal antibodies, makes a strong case for this technology to continue to be investigated for its potential in humans.

Exo-CD24

Exosomes are small-membrane vesicles derived from a variety of cell types. Cellular communication has been attributed to the interplay of these. This include dictating cellular proliferation, differentiation, and maturation. Depending on the cell type from which exosomes are derived, they have beneficial or detrimental effects.

CD24 is an extensively glycosylated protein linked to glycosyl-phosphatidylinositol, which is found on cellular surfaces. It was found that exosomes containing CD24 is a negative regulator of inflammation. The rationale is that exosomes overexpressing CD24 isolated and purified from T-REx-293 cells can suppress the CRS. In a phase 1 feasibility and tolerability study, Exo-CD24 was evaluated in 35 patients with moderate to severe COVID-19. In this dosage escalation study, the dosage stratification ranged from 1×10^8 to 100×10^8 exosomal particles given as an aerosolized delivery system for five days (ClinicalTrials.gov: NCT04747574). All 29 participants in this study were discharged after three to five days of treatment. The data from this study are encouraging, and further studies are needed to affirm these critical findings. Currently, Exo-CD24 is in a phase 2 trial in Greece.

Fluvoxamine

Fluvoxamine (brand name Luvox) is a selective serotonin reuptake inhibitor that has been FDA approved for the treatment of obsessive-compulsive disorder and depression. Mechanistically, fluvoxamine is intended to lower inflammatory cytokine production caused by increased activation of the RAAS pathway and may have antiviral effects. A preliminary placebo-controlled trial in 152 patients assessed fluvoxamine efficacy in preventing clinical deterioration. Fluvoxamine 100 mg or placebo was administered three times daily for 15 days, which is higher than conventional dosage used for depression. Despite the high dosages used, this study indicates a decreased likelihood for clinical deterioration in the treatment group as compared with control without notable adverse events noted [150]. Of the 80 participants given fluvoxamine, none experienced deterioration defined by dyspnea or a decrease in oxygen saturation (<92%) as primary outcomes. In contrast, 6/72 (8.3%) patients receiving placebo had notable clinical decline, which was statistically higher than patients receiving fluvoxamine ($P = 0.009$). Large-scale clinical trials are underway to corroborate these findings (ClinicalTrials.gov: NCT04668950).

Clofazimine (Lamprene)

Often used in combination with rifampicin and dapsone to treat multibacillary leprosy, clofazimine inhibits the myeloperoxidase system and exhibits anti-inflammatory effects. Preclinical data have shown clofazimine to be effective in inhibiting the activity of various coronaviruses, including SARS-CoV-2 and MERS-CoV. Its proposed mechanism of action is through inhibition of cell fusion mediated by the S glycoprotein and as an inhibitor of viral helicase. in vivo studies conducted using golden Syrian hamsters demonstrated clofazimine was able to reduce plaque-forming units in the lung tissue by 1–2 $\log_{10}$ compared with untreated control [151]. Currently, the University of Hong Kong is recruiting patients for a controlled phase 2 clinical trial on the effect of short-term (three-day) dual therapy of clofazimine and IFN-ß1b (ClinicalTrials.gov: NCT04465695). Further clinical studies are crucial to elucidating the effect of clofazimine on the alleviation of SARS-CoV-2–induced symptoms.

References

1 V'kovski, P., Kratzel, A., Steiner, S. et al. (2021). Coronavirus biology and replication: implications for SARS-CoV-2. *Nat. Rev. Microbiol.* 19: 155–170.

2 Astuti, I. and Ysrafil (2020). Severe acute respiratory syndrome coronavirus 2 (SARS-CoV-2): an overview of viral structure and host response. *Diabetes Metab. Syndr.* 14: 407–412.

3 Gengler, I., Wang, J.C., Speth, M.M., and Sedaghat, M.M. (2020). Sinonasal pathophysiology of SARS-CoV-2 and COVID-19: a systematic review of the current evidence. *Laryngoscope Investig. Otolaryngol.* 5: 354–359.

4 Hou, Y.J., Okuda, K., Edwards, C.E. et al. (2020). SARS-CoV-2 reverse genetics reveals a variable infection gradient in the respiratory tract. *Cell* 182: 429–446.e414.

5 Lan, J., Ge, J., Yu, J. et al. (2020). Structure of the SARS-CoV-2 spike receptor-binding domain bound to the ACE2 receptor. *Nature* 581: 215–220.

6 Mollica, V., Rizzo, A., and Massari, F. (2020). The pivotal role of TMPRSS2 in coronavirus disease 2019 and prostate cancer. *Future Oncol.* 16: 2029–2033.

7 Gkogkou, E., Barnasas, G., Vougas, K., and Trougakos, I.P. (2020). Expression profiling meta-analysis of ACE2 and TMPRSS2, the putative anti-inflammatory receptor and priming protease of SARS-CoV-2 in human cells, and identification of putative modulators. *Redox. Biol.* 36: 101615.

8 Trougakos, I.P., Stamatelopoulos, K., Terpos, E. et al. (2021). Insights to SARS-CoV-2 life cycle, pathophysiology, and rationalized treatments that target COVID-19 clinical complications. *J. Biomed. Sci.* 28: 9.

9 Liu, T., Luo, S., Libby, P., and Shi, G.P. (2020). Cathepsin L-selective inhibitors: a potentially promising treatment for COVID-19 patients. *Pharmacol. Ther.* 213: 107587.

10 Arya, R., Kumari, S., Pandey, B. et al. (2021). Structural insights into SARS-CoV-2 proteins. *J. Mol. Biol.* 433: 166725.

11 Báez-Santos, Y.M., St John, S.E., and Mesecar, A.D. (2015). The SARS-coronavirus papain-like protease: structure, function and inhibition by designed antiviral compounds. *Antivir. Res.* 115: 21–38.

12 Gao, Y., Yan, L., Huang, Y. et al. (2020). Structure of the RNA-dependent RNA polymerase from COVID-19 virus. *Science* 368: 779–782.

13 Weston, S., Coleman, C.M., Haupt, R. et al. (2020). Broad anti-coronavirus activity of food and drug administration-approved drugs against SARS-CoV-2 *in vitro* and SARS-CoV *in vivo*. *J. Virol.* 94: e01218-20.

14 Jeon, S., Ko, M., Lee, J. et al. (2020). Identification of antiviral drug candidates against SARS-CoV-2 from FDA-approved drugs. *Antimicrob. Agents Chemother.* 64: e00819-20.

15 Rockx, B., Kuiken, T., Herfst, S. et al. (2020). Comparative pathogenesis of COVID-19, MERS, and SARS in a nonhuman primate model. *Science* 368: 1012–1015.

16 Shi, J., Wen, Z., Zhong, G. et al. (2020). Susceptibility of ferrets, cats, dogs, and other domesticated animals to SARS-coronavirus 2. *Science* 368: 1016–1020.

17 Cao, X. (2020, 2020). COVID-19: immunopathology and its implications for therapy. *Nat. Rev. Immunol.* 20: 269–270.

18 Buszko, M., Park, J.H., Verthelyi, D. et al. (2020). The dynamic changes in cytokine responses in COVID-19: a snapshot of the current state of knowledge. *Nat. Immunol.* 21: 1146–1151.

19 Tay, M.Z., Poh, C.M., Rénia, L. et al. (2020). The trinity of COVID-19: immunity, inflammation and intervention. *Nat. Rev. Immunol.* 20: 363–374.

20 Zhang, X., Tan, Y., Ling, Y. et al. (2020). Viral and host factors related to the clinical outcome of COVID-19. *Nature* 583: 437–440.

21 Robbiani, D.F., Gaebler, C., Muecksch, F. et al. (2020). Convergent antibody responses to SARS-CoV-2 in convalescent individuals. *Nature* 584: 437–442.

22 Zohar, T. and Alter, G. (2020). Dissecting antibody-mediated protection against SARS-CoV-2. *Nat. Rev. Immunol.* 20: 392–394.

23 Moore, J.B. and June, C.H. (2020). Cytokine release syndrome in severe COVID-19. *Science* 368: 473–474.

24 Wang, M., Cao, R., Zhang, L. et al. (2020). Remdesivir and chloroquine effectively inhibit the recently emerged novel coronavirus (2019-nCoV) in vitro. *Cell Res.* 30: 269–271.

25 Lisi, L., Lacal, P.M., Barbaccia, M.L., and Graziani, G. (2020). Approaching coronavirus disease 2019: mechanisms of action of repurposed drugs with potential activity against SARS-CoV-2. *Biochem. Pharmacol.* 180: 114169.

26 Morris, G., Bortolasci, C.C., Puri, B.K. et al. (2020). The pathophysiology of SARS-CoV-2: a suggested model and therapeutic approach. *Life. Sci.* 258: 118166.

27 Al-Horani, R.A., Kar, S., and Aliter, K.F. (2020). Potential anti-COVID-19 therapeutics that block the early stage of the viral life cycle: structures, mechanisms, and clinical trials. *Int. J. Mol. Sci.* 21: 5224.

28 Hoffmann, M., Kleine-Weber, H., Schroeder, S. et al. (2020). SARS-CoV-2 cell entry depends on ACE2 and TMPRSS2 and is blocked by a clinically proven protease inhibitor. *Cell* 181: 271–280.e278.

29 Gunst, J.D., Staerke, N.B., Pahus, M.H. et al. (2021). Efficacy of the TMPRSS2 inhibitor camostat mesilate in patients hospitalized with Covid-19-a double-blind randomized controlled trial. *EClinicalMedicine* 35: 100849.

30 Yamamoto, M., Kiso, M., Sakai-Tagawa, Y. et al. (2020). The anticoagulant nafamostat potently inhibits SARS-CoV-2 S protein-mediated fusion in a cell fusion assay system and viral infection in vitro in a cell-type-dependent manner. *Viruses* 12: 629.

31 Ko, M., Jeon, S., Ryu, W.S., and Kim, S. (2021). Comparative analysis of antiviral efficacy of FDA-approved drugs against SARS-CoV-2 in human lung cells. *J. Med. Virol.* 93: 1403–1408.

32 Hoffmann, M., Schroeder, S., Kleine-Weber, H. et al. (2020). Nafamostat mesylate blocks activation of SARS-CoV-2: new treatment option for COVID-19. *Antimicrob. Agents Chemother.* 64: e00754-20.

33 Heinemann, V., Ebert, M.P., Laubender, R.P. et al. (2013). Phase II randomised proof-of-concept study of the urokinase inhibitor upamostat (WX-671) in combination with gemcitabine compared with gemcitabine alone in patients with non-resectable, locally advanced pancreatic cancer. *Br. J. Cancer* 108: 766–770.

34 Schrezenmeier, E. and Dörner, T. (2020). Mechanisms of action of hydroxychloroquine and chloroquine: implications for rheumatology. *Nat. Rev. Rheumatol.* 16: 155–166.

35 Axfors, C., Schmitt, A.M., Janiaud, P. et al. (2021). Mortality outcomes with hydroxychloroquine and chloroquine in COVID-19 from an international collaborative meta-analysis of randomized trials. *Nat. Commun.* 12: 2349.

36 Oren, O., Yang, E.H., Gluckman, T.J. et al. (2020). Use of chloroquine and hydroxychloroquine in COVID-19 and cardiovascular implications: understanding safety discrepancies to improve interpretation and design of clinical trials. *Circ. Arrhythm. Electrophysiol.* 13: e008688.

37 Furtado, R.H.M., Berwanger, O., Fonseca, H.A. et al. (2020). Azithromycin in addition to standard of care versus standard of care alone in the treatment of patients admitted to the hospital with severe COVID-19 in Brazil (COALITION II): a randomised clinical trial. *Lancet* 396: 959–967.

38 Geleris, J., Sun, Y., Platt, J. et al. (2020). Observational study of hydroxychloroquine in hospitalized patients with Covid-19. *N. Engl. J. Med.* 382: 2411–2418.

39 Rosenberg, E.S., Dufort, E.M., Udo, T. et al. (2020). Association of treatment with hydroxychloroquine or azithromycin with in-hospital mortality in patients with COVID-19 in New York state. *JAMA* 323: 2493–2502.

40 Cavalcanti, A.B., Zampieri, F.G., Rosa, R.G. et al. (2020). Hydroxychloroquine with or without azithromycin in mild-to-moderate Covid-19. *N. Engl. J. Med.* 383: 2041–2052.

41 Juurlink, D.N. (2020). Safety considerations with chloroquine, hydroxychloroquine and azithromycin in the management of SARS-CoV-2 infection. *CMAJ* 192: E450–E453.

42 Terenzi, R., Manetti, M., Rosa, I. et al. (2017). Angiotensin II type 2 receptor (AT2R) as a novel modulator of inflammation in rheumatoid arthritis synovium. *Sci. Rep.* 7: 13293.

43 Patel, V.B., Zhong, J.C., Grant, M.B., and Oudit, G.Y. (2016). Role of the ACE2/angiotensin 1-7 axis of the renin-angiotensin system in heart failure. *Circ. Res.* 118: 1313–1326.

44 Vaduganathan, M., Vardeny, O., Michel, T. et al. (2020). Renin-angiotensin-aldosterone system inhibitors in patients with Covid-19. *N. Engl. J. Med.* 382: 1653–1659.

45 Parati, G., Asmar, R., Bilo, G. et al. (2010). Effectiveness and safety of high-dose valsartan monotherapy in hypertension treatment: the ValTop study. *Hypertens. Res.* 33: 986–994.

46 Vitiello, A., La Porta, R., and Ferrara, F. (2021). Scientific hypothesis and rational pharmacological for the use of sacubitril/valsartan in cardiac damage caused by COVID-19. *Med. Hypotheses* 147: 110486.

47 Shi, S., Qin, M., Shen, B. et al. (2020). Association of cardiac injury with mortality in hospitalized patients with COVID-19 in Wuhan, China. *JAMA Cardiol.* 5: 802–810.

48 Gao, L., Jiang, D., Wen, X.S. et al. (2020). Prognostic value of NT-proBNP in patients with severe COVID-19. *Respir. Res.* 21: 83.

49 Li, N., Zhang, Y., Fan, S. et al. (2013). BNP and NT-proBNP levels in patients with sepsis. *Front. Biosci. (Landmark Ed.)* 18: 1237–1243.

50 Choi, J.A., Kim, J.E., Ju, H.H. et al. (2019). The effects of losartan on cytomegalovirus infection in human trabecular meshwork cells. *PLoS One* 14: e0218471.

51 Sellers, S.L., Milad, N., Chan, R. et al. (2018). Inhibition of Marfan syndrome aortic root dilation by losartan: role of angiotensin II receptor type 1-independent activation of endothelial function. *Am. J. Pathol.* 188: 574–585.

52 Guo, F., Sun, Y.B., Su, L. et al. (2015). Losartan attenuates paraquat-induced pulmonary fibrosis in rats. *Hum. Exp. Toxicol.* 34: 497–505.

53 Bengtson, C.D., Montgomery, R.N., Nazir, U. et al. (2021). An open label trial to assess safety of losartan for treating worsening respiratory illness in COVID-19. *Front. Med. (Lausanne)* 8: 630209.

54 Abraham, H.M., White, C.M., and White, W.B. (2015). The comparative efficacy and safety of the angiotensin receptor blockers in the management of hypertension and other cardiovascular diseases. *Drug Saf.* 38: 33–54.

55 Rothlin, R.P., Vetulli, H.M., Duarte, M., and Pelorosso, F.G. (2020). Telmisartan as tentative angiotensin receptor blocker therapeutic for COVID-19. *Drug Dev. Res.* 81: 768–770.

56 Duarte, M., Pelorosso, F., Nicolosi, L.N. et al. (2021). Telmisartan for treatment of Covid-19 patients: an open multicenter randomized clinical trial. *EClinicalMedicine* 37: 100962.

57 Donoghue, M., Hsieh, F., Baronas, E. et al. (2000). A novel angiotensin-converting enzyme-related carboxypeptidase (ACE2) converts angiotensin I to angiotensin 1-9. *Circ. Res.* 87: E1–E9.

58 Xie, X., Xudong, X., Chen, J. et al. (2006). Age- and gender-related difference of ACE2 expression in rat lung. *Life Sci.* 78: 2166–2171.

59 Li, W., Moore, M.J., Vasilieva, N. et al. (2003). Angiotensin-converting enzyme 2 is a functional receptor for the SARS coronavirus. *Nature* 426: 450–454.

60 Monteil, V., Kwon, H., Prado, P. et al. (2020). Inhibition of SARS-CoV-2 infections in engineered human tissues using clinical-grade soluble human ACE2. *Cell* 181: 905–913.e907.

61 Peiró, C. and Moncada, S. (2020). Substituting angiotensin-(1-7) to prevent lung damage in SARS-CoV-2 infection? *Circulation* 141: 1665–1666.

62 Zhang, H., Penninger, J.M., Li, Y. et al. (2020). Angiotensin-converting enzyme 2 (ACE2) as a SARS-CoV-2 receptor: molecular mechanisms and potential therapeutic target. *Intensive Care Med.* 46: 586–590.

63 Liu, Y., Yang, Y., Zhang, C. et al. (2020). Clinical and biochemical indexes from 2019-nCoV infected patients linked to viral loads and lung injury. *Sci. China Life Sci.* 63: 364–374.

64 Miesbach, W. (2020). Pathological role of angiotensin II in severe COVID-19. *TH Open* 4: e138–e144.

65 Kintscher, U., Slagman, A., Domenig, O. et al. (2020). Plasma angiotensin peptide profiling and ACE (angiotensin-converting enzyme)-2 activity in COVID-19 patients treated with pharmacological blockers of the renin-angiotensin system. *Hypertension* 76: e34–e36.

66 Santos, R.A.S., Sampaio, W.O., Alzamora, A.C. et al. (2018). The ACE2/angiotensin-(1-7)/MAS axis of the renin-angiotensin system: focus on angiotensin-(1-7). *Physiol. Rev.* 98: 505–553.

67 Swanstrom, R. and Schinazi, R.F. (2022). Lethal mutagenesis as an antiviral strategy. *Science* 375: 497–498.

68 Arias, A., Thorne, L., and Goodfellow, I. (2014). Favipiravir elicits antiviral mutagenesis during virus replication in vivo. *elife* 3: e03679.

69 Chen, C., Zhang, Y., Huang, J. et al. (2021). Favipiravir versus arbidol for clinical recovery rate in moderate and severe adult COVID-19 patients: a prospective, multicenter, open-label, randomized controlled clinical trial. *Front pharmacol.* 12: 683296.

70 Sheahan, T.P., Sims, A.C., Zhou, S. et al. (2020). An orally bioavailable broad-spectrum antiviral inhibits SARS-CoV-2 in human airway epithelial cell cultures and multiple coronaviruses in mice. *Sci. Transl. Med.* 12: eabb5883.

71 Fischer, W., Eron, J.J., Holman, W. et al. (2021). Molnupiravir, an oral antiviral treatment for COVID-19. *medRxiv* https://doi.org/10.1101/2021.06.17.21258639.

72 Siegel, D., Hui, H.C., Doerffler, E. et al. (2017). Discovery and synthesis of a phosphoramidate prodrug of a pyrrolo[2,1-f][triazin-4-amino] adenine C-nucleoside (GS-5734) for the treatment of Ebola and emerging viruses. *J. Med. Chem.* 60: 1648–1661.

73 Lo, M.K., Jordan, R., Arvey, A. et al. (2017). GS-5734 and its parent nucleoside analog inhibit Filo-, Pneumo-, and Paramyxoviruses. *Sci. Rep.* 7: 43395.

74 Sheahan, T.P., Sims, A.C., Graham, R.L. et al. (2017). Broad-spectrum antiviral GS-5734 inhibits both epidemic and zoonotic coronaviruses. *Sci. Transl. Med.* 9: eaal3653.

75 Tchesnokov, E.P., Gordon, C.J., Woolner, E. et al. (2020). Template-dependent inhibition of coronavirus RNA-dependent RNA polymerase by remdesivir reveals a second mechanism of action. *J. Biol. Chem.* 295: 16156–16165.

76 Boutzoukas, A.E., Benjamin, D.K., and Zimmerman, K.O. (2021). Remdesivir: preliminary data and clinical use versus recommended use. *Pediatrics* 147: e2021050212.

77 Gordon, C.J., Tchesnokov, E.P., Feng, J.Y. et al. (2020). The antiviral compound remdesivir potently inhibits RNA-dependent RNA polymerase from Middle East respiratory syndrome coronavirus. *J. Biol. Chem.* 295: 4773–4779.

78 Gordon, C.J., Tchesnokov, E.P., Woolner, E. et al. (2020). Remdesivir is a direct-acting antiviral that inhibits RNA-dependent RNA polymerase from severe acute respiratory syndrome coronavirus 2 with high potency. *J. Biol. Chem.* 295: 6785–6797.

79 Tchesnokov, E.P., Obikhod, A., Schinazi, R.F., and Götte, M. (2008). Delayed chain termination protects the anti-hepatitis B virus drug entecavir from excision by HIV-1 reverse transcriptase. *J. Biol. Chem.* 283: 34218–34228.

80 Pizzorno, A., Padey, B., Julien, T. et al. (2020). Characterization and treatment of SARS-CoV-2 in nasal and bronchial human airway epithelia. *Cell Rep. Med.* 1: 100059.

81 Holshue, M.L., DeBolt, C., Lindquist, S. et al. (2020). First case of 2019 novel coronavirus in the United States. *N. Engl. J. Med.* 382: 929–936.

82 Beigel, J.H., Tomashek, K.M., Dodd, L.E. et al. (2020). Remdesivir for the treatment of Covid-19 – final report. *N. Engl. J. Med.* 383: 1813–1826.

83 Spinner, C.D., Gottlieb, R.L., Criner, G.J. et al. (2020). Effect of Remdesivir vs standard care on clinical status at 11 days in patients with moderate COVID-19: a randomized clinical trial. *JAMA* 324: 1048–1057.

84 Sidwell, R.W., Huffman, J.H., Khare, G.P. et al. (1972). Broad-spectrum antiviral activity of Virazole: 1-beta-D-ribofuranosyl-1,2,4-triazole-3-carboxamide. *Science* 177: 705–706.

85 Te, H.S., Randall, G., and Jensen, D.M. (2007). Mechanism of action of ribavirin in the treatment of chronic hepatitis C. *Gastroenterol Hepatol. (N Y).* 3: 218–225.

86 Maag, D., Castro, C., Hong, Z., and Cameron, C.E. (2001). Hepatitis C virus RNA-dependent RNA polymerase (NS5B) as a mediator of the antiviral activity of ribavirin. *J. Biol. Chem.* 276: 46094–46098.

87 Tong, S., Su, Y., Yu, Y. et al. (2020). Ribavirin therapy for severe COVID-19: a retrospective cohort study. *Int. J. Antimicrob. Agents* 56: 106114.

88 Wang, D., Hu, B., Hu, C. et al. (2020). Clinical characteristics of 138 hospitalized patients with 2019 novel coronavirus-infected pneumonia in Wuhan, China. *JAMA* 323: 1061–1069.

89 Kadam, R.U. and Wilson, I.A. (2017). Structural basis of influenza virus fusion inhibition by the

antiviral drug Arbidol. *Proc. Natl Acad. Sci. U S A.* 114: 206–214.

90 Blaising, J., Lévy, P.L., Polyak, S.J. et al. (2013). Arbidol inhibits viral entry by interfering with clathrin-dependent trafficking. *Antivir. Res.* 100: 215–219.

91 Huang, D., Yu, H., Wang, T. et al. (2021). Efficacy and safety of umifenovir for coronavirus disease 2019 (COVID-19): a systematic review and meta-analysis. *J. Med. Virol.* 93: 481–490.

92 Simmons, G., Zmora, P., Gierer, S. et al. (2013). Proteolytic activation of the SARS-coronavirus spike protein: cutting enzymes at the cutting edge of antiviral research. *Antivir. Res.* 100: 605–614.

93 De Clercq, E. (2009). Anti-HIV drugs: 25 compounds approved within 25 years after the discovery of HIV. *Int. J. Antimicrob. Agents.* 33: 307–320.

94 Lim, J., Jeon, S., Shin, H.Y. et al. (2020). Case of the index patient who caused tertiary transmission of COVID-19 infection in Korea: the application of Lopinavir/Ritonavir for the treatment of COVID-19 infected pneumonia monitored by quantitative RT-PCR. *J. Korean Med. Sci.* 35: e79.

95 RECOVERY Collaborative Group (2020). Lopinavir-ritonavir in patients admitted to hospital with COVID-19 (RECOVERY): a randomised, controlled, open-label, platform trial. *Lancet* 396: 1345–1352.

96 Hung, I.F., Lung, K.C., Tso, E.Y. et al. (2020). Triple combination of interferon beta-1b, lopinavir-ritonavir, and ribavirin in the treatment of patients admitted to hospital with COVID-19: an open-label, randomised, phase 2 trial. *Lancet* 395: 1695–1704.

97 Hu, J.J., Liu, X., Xia, S. et al. (2020). FDA-approved disulfiram inhibits pyroptosis by blocking gasdermin D pore formation. *Nat. Immunol.* 21: 736–745.

98 Jin, Z., Du, X., Xu, Y. et al. (2020). Structure of M^{pro} from SARS-CoV-2 and discovery of its inhibitors. *Nature* 582: 289–293.

99 Ma, C., Hu, Y., Townsend, J.A. et al. (2020). Ebselen, disulfiram, Carmofur, PX-12, Tideglusib, and Shikonin are nonspecific promiscuous SARS-CoV-2 main protease inhibitors. *ACS Pharmacol. Transl. Sci.* 3: 1265–1277.

100 Smith, E., Davis-Gardner, M.E., Garcia-Ordonez, R.D. et al. (2020). High-throughput screening for drugs that inhibit papain-like protease in SARS-CoV-2. *SLAS Discov.* 25: 1152–1161.

101 Sargsyan, K., Lin, C.C., Chen, T. et al. (2021). Correction: multi-targeting of functional cysteines in multiple conserved SARS-CoV-2 domains by clinically safe Zn-ejectors. *Chem. Sci.* 12: 6210.

102 Chen, T., Fei, C.Y., Chen, Y.P. et al. (2021). Synergistic inhibition of SARS-CoV-2 replication using disulfiram/Ebselen and Remdesivir. *ACS Pharmacol Transl Sci.* 4: 898–907.

103 Fillmore, N., Bell, S., Shen, C. et al. (2021). Disulfiram use is associated with lower risk of COVID-19: a retrospective cohort study. *PLoS One* 16: e0259061.

104 Touret, F., Gilles, M., Barral, K. et al. (2020). in vitro screening of a FDA approved chemical library reveals potential inhibitors of SARS-CoV-2 replication. *Sci. Rep.* 10: 13093.

105 Poschet, J.F., Perkett, E.A., Timmins, G.S., and Deretic, V. (2020). Azithromycin and ciprofloxacin have a chloroquine-like effect on respiratory epithelial cells. *bioRxiv* https://doi.org/10.1101/2020.03.29.008631.

106 Gautret, P., Lagier, J.C., Parola, P. et al. (2020). Hydroxychloroquine and azithromycin as a treatment of COVID-19: results of an open-label non-randomized clinical trial. *Int. J. Antimicrob. Agents* 56: 105949.

107 PRINCIPLE Trial Collaborative Group (2021). Azithromycin for community treatment of suspected COVID-19 in people at increased risk of an adverse clinical course in the UK (PRINCIPLE): a randomised, controlled, open-label, adaptive platform trial. *Lancet* 397: 1063–1074.

107 Oldenburg, C.E. and Doan, T. (2020). Azithromycin for severe COVID-19. *Lancet* 396: 936–937.

108 Errecalde, J., Lifschitz, A., Vecchioli, G. et al. (2021). Safety and pharmacokinetic assessments of a novel Ivermectin nasal spray formulation in a pig model. *J. Pharm. Sci.* 110: 2501–2507.

110 Rocco, P.R.M., Silva, P.L., Cruz, F.F. et al. (2021). Early use of nitazoxanide in mild COVID-19 disease: randomised, placebo-controlled trial. *Eur. Respir. J.* 58: 2003725.

111 Dinarello, C.A. (2007). Historical insights into cytokines. *Eur. J. Immunol.* 37 (Suppl 1): S34–S45.

112 Bastard, P., Michailidis, E., Hoffmann, H.H. et al. (2021). Auto-antibodies to type I IFNs can underlie adverse reactions to yellow fever live attenuated vaccine. *J. Exp. Med.* 218: e20202486.

113 El-Lababidi, R.M., Mooty, M., Bonilla, M.F., and Salem, N.M. (2020). Treatment of severe pneumonia due to COVID-19 with peginterferon alfa 2a. *IDCases* 21: e00837.

114 Pandit, A., Bhalani, N., Bhushan, B.L.S. et al. (2021). Efficacy and safety of pegylated interferon alfa-2b in moderate COVID-19: a phase II, randomized, controlled, open-label study. *Int. J. Infect. Dis.* 105: 516–521.

115 Lang, F.M., Lee, K.M., Teijaro, J.R. et al. (2020). GM-CSF-based treatments in COVID-19: reconciling opposing therapeutic approaches. *Nat. Rev. Immunol.* 20: 507–514.

116 Mehta, P., Chambers, R.C., and Dagna, L. (2021). Granulocyte-macrophage colony stimulating factor in COVID-19: friend or foe? *Lancet Rheumatol.* 3: e394–e395.

117 Subramaniam, R., Hillberry, Z., Chen, H. et al. (2015). Delivery of GM-CSF to protect against influenza pneumonia. *PLoS One* 10: e0124593.

118 Huang, H., Li, H., Zhou, P., and Ju, D. (2010). Protective effects of recombinant human granulocyte macrophage colony stimulating factor on H1N1 influenza virus-induced pneumonia in mice. *Cytokine* 51: 151–157.

119 Halstead, E.S., Umstead, T.M., Davies, M.L. et al. (2018). GM-CSF overexpression after influenza a virus infection prevents mortality and moderates M1-like airway monocyte/macrophage polarization. *Respir. Res.* 19: 3.

120 Ballinger, M.N., Paine, R., Serezani, C.H. et al. (2006). Role of granulocyte macrophage colony-stimulating factor during gram-negative lung infection with Pseudomonas aeruginosa. *Am. J. Respir. Cell Mol. Biol.* 34: 766–774.

121 Huet, T., Beaussier, H., Voisin, O. et al. (2020). Anakinra for severe forms of COVID-19: a cohort study. *Lancet Rheumatol.* 2: e393–e400.

122 CORIMUNO-19 Collaborative Group (2021). Effect of anakinra versus usual care in adults in hospital with COVID-19 and mild-to-moderate pneumonia (CORIMUNO-ANA-1): a randomised controlled trial. *Lancet. Respir. Med.* 9: 295–304.

123 REMAP-CAP Investigators, Gordon, A.C., Mouncey, P.R. et al. (2021). Interleukin-6 receptor antagonists in critically ill patients with Covid-19. *N. Engl. J. Med.* 384: 1491–1502.

124 Lescure, F.X., Honda, H., Fowler, R.A. et al. (2021). Sarilumab in patients admitted to hospital with severe or critical COVID-19: a randomised, double-blind, placebo-controlled, phase 3 trial. *Lancet Respir. Med.* 9: 522–532.

125 Petrelli, F., Cherri, S., Ghidini, M. et al. (2021). Tocilizumab as treatment for COVID-19: a systematic review and meta-analysis. *World J Methodol.* 11: 95–109.

126 Potey, P.M., Rossi, A.G., Lucas, C.D., and Dorward, D.A. (2019). Neutrophils in the initiation and resolution of acute pulmonary inflammation: understanding biological function and therapeutic potential. *J. Pathol.* 247: 672–685.

127 Sanofi-Aventis (2017). Leukine (sargramostim) package insert. US Food and Drug Administration. https://www.accessdata.fda.gov/drugsatfda_docs/label/2017/103362s5237lbl.pdf

128 Sterner, R.M., Sakemura, R., Cox, M.J. et al. (2019). GM-CSF inhibition reduces cytokine release syndrome and neuroinflammation but enhances CAR-T cell function in xenografts. *Blood* 133: 697–709.

129 Tugues, S., Amorim, A., Spath, S. et al. (2018). Graft-versus-host disease, but not graft-versus-leukemia immunity, is mediated by GM-CSF-licensed myeloid cells. *Sci. Transl. Med.* 10: eaat8410.

130 Baum, A., Fulton, B.O., Wloga, E. et al. (2020). Antibody cocktail to SARS-CoV-2 spike protein prevents rapid mutational escape seen with individual antibodies. *Science* 369: 1014–1018.

131 Coronavirus (COVID-19) update: FDA authorizes monoclonal antibodies for treatment of COVID-19. US Food and Drug Administration. 2020. https://www.fda.gov/news-events/press-announcements/coronavirus-covid-19-update-fda-authorizes-monoclonal-antibodies-treatment-covid-19

132 COVID-19 Treatment Guidelines Panel. Coronavirus disease 2019 (COVID-19) treatment guidelines: anti-SARS-CoV-2 monoclonal antibodies. National Institutes of Health. 2021. https://www.covid19treatmentguidelines.nih.gov/therapies/statement-on-casirivimab-plus-imdevimab-as-pep

133 Beigel, J.H., Aga, E., Elie-Turenne, M.C. et al. (2019). Anti-influenza immune plasma for the treatment of patients with severe influenza A: a randomised, double-blind, phase 3 trial. *Lancet Respir. Med.* 7: 941–950.

134 van Griensven, J., Edwards, T., de Lamballerie, X. et al. (2016). Evaluation of convalescent plasma for Ebola virus disease in Guinea. *N. Engl. J. Med.* 374: 33–42.

135 Winkler, A.M. and Koepsell, S.A. (2015). The use of convalescent plasma to treat emerging infectious diseases: focus on Ebola virus disease. *Curr. Opin. Hematol.* 22: 521–526.

136 Katz, L.M. (2021). (A little) clarity on convalescent plasma for Covid-19. *N. Engl. J. Med.* 384: 666–668.

137 Li, L., Zhang, W., Hu, Y. et al. (2020). Effect of convalescent plasma therapy on time to clinical improvement in patients with severe and life-threatening COVID-19: a randomized clinical trial. *JAMA* 324: 460–470.

138 Simonovich, V.A., Burgos Pratx, L.D., Scibona, P. et al. (2021). A randomized trial of convalescent plasma in Covid-19 severe pneumonia. *N. Engl. J. Med.* 384: 619–629.

139 Joyner, M.J., Carter, R.E., Senefeld, J.W. et al. (2021). Convalescent plasma antibody levels and the risk of death from Covid-19. *N. Engl. J. Med.* 384: 1015–1027.

140 Hage, R., Steinack, C., and Schuurmans, M.M. (2020). Calcineurin inhibitors revisited: a new paradigm for COVID-19? *Braz. J. Infect. Dis.* 24: 365–367.

141 COVID-19 Treatment Guidelines Panel. Coronavirus disease 2019 (COVID-19) treatment guidelines: corticosteroids. National Institutes of Health. 2021. https://www.covid19 treatmentguidelines.nih.gov/therapies/ immunomodulators/corticosteroids

142 Softic, L., Brillet, R., Berry, F. et al. (2020). Inhibition of SARS-CoV-2 infection by the Cyclophilin inhibitor Alisporivir (Debio 025). *Antimicrob. Agents Chemother.* 64: e00876-20.

143 Roschewski, M., Lionakis, M.S., Sharman, J.P. et al. (2020). Inhibition of Bruton tyrosine kinase in patients with severe COVID-19. *Sci Immunol.* 5: eabd0110.

144 Kalil, A.C., Patterson, T.F., Mehta, A.K. et al. (2021). Baricitinib plus Remdesivir for hospitalized adults with Covid-19. *N. Engl. J. Med.* 384: 795–807.

145 COVID-19 Treatment Guidelines Panel. Coronavirus disease 2019 (COVID-19) treatment guidelines: therapeutic management of hospitalized adults with COVID-19. National Institutes of Health. 2021. https://www. covid19treatmentguidelines.nih.gov/management/ clinical-management/hospitalized-adults-- therapeutic-management/

146 Abbott, T.R., Dhamdhere, G., Liu, Y. et al. (2020). Development of CRISPR as an antiviral strategy to combat SARS-CoV-2 and influenza. *Cell* 181: 865–876.e812.

147 Koenig, P.A., Das, H., Liu, H. et al. (2021). Structure-guided multivalent nanobodies block SARS-CoV-2 infection and suppress mutational escape. *Science* 371: eabe6230.

148 Xiang, Y., Nambulli, S., Xiao, Z. et al. (2020). Versatile and multivalent nanobodies efficiently neutralize SARS-CoV-2. *Science* 370: 1479–1484.

149 Sasisekharan, R. (2021). Preparing for the future – nanobodies for Covid-19? *N. Engl. J. Med.* 384: 1568–1571.

150 Lenze, E.J., Mattar, C., Zorumski, C.F. et al. (2020). Fluvoxamine vs placebo and clinical deterioration in outpatients with symptomatic COVID-19: a randomized clinical trial. *JAMA* 324: 2292–2300.

151 Yuan, S., Yin, X., Meng, X. et al. (2021). Clofazimine broadly inhibits coronaviruses including SARS-CoV-2. *Nature* 593, 418–423.

14

Co-infections and Secondary Infections in COVID-19 Pneumonia

Sanaz Katal[1*], Liesl S. Eibschutz[2*], Amit Gupta[3], Sean K. Johnston[2], Lucia Flors[2], and Ali Gholamrezanezhad[2]

[1] St Vincent's Hospital Medical Imaging Department, Melbourne, Victoria, Australia
[2] Department of Radiology, Keck School of Medicine, University of Southern California, Los Angeles, CA, USA
[3] Department of Radiology, University Hospitals Cleveland Medical Center, Cleveland, OH, USA
* Sanaz Katal and Liesl S. Eibschutz are co-first authors.

Abbreviations

ARDS	acute respiratory distress syndrome
CT	computed tomography
CXR	chest x-ray
GGO	ground-glass opacity
IAV	influenza A virus
IBV	influenza B virus
ICU	intensive care unit
IFD	invasive fungal disease
IgM	immunoglobulin M
IPA	invasive pulmonary aspergillosis
MRI	magnetic resonance imaging
PCP	*Pneumocystis jirovecii* pneumonia
RSV	respiratory syncytial virus
RT-PCR	reverse transcriptase-polymerase chain reaction
SARS-CoV-2	severe acute respiratory syndrome coronavirus 2
Th	T helper (cell)

Over the past two years, the coronavirus disease 2019 (COVID-19) pandemic has affected millions globally. The novel coronavirus, severe acute respiratory syndrome coronavirus 2 (SARS-CoV-2), primarily affects the respiratory tract. Although in many patients a clinical and radiologic reversal begins and lung lesions regress, some patients can develop secondary infections with bacterial, fungal, viral, and parasitic pathogens. Because previous coronaviruses, such as SARS-CoV and Middle East respiratory syndrome coronavirus, and respiratory viruses, such as influenza, are associated with co-infection, a high index of suspicion for super-imposed infection is vital in patients with COVID-19 [1]. The prevalence rate of co-infection has been reported to vary from 4% [2] to 42% [3].

Although typical imaging presentations of COVID-19 have been widely reported, there are limited data regarding the imaging features of secondary infections or co-infections. In addition, many COVID-19 radiologic findings are atypical or nonspecific. Therefore, any acute change in the clinical picture or radiologic findings of patients with COVID-19 should prompt a rapid and expert clinical assessment to exclude superimposed infections.

Bacterial Co-infections

A recent meta-analysis demonstrated that 3.5% and 14.3% of patients with COVID-19 had bacterial co-infection and bacterial secondary infection, respectively [4]. The most common organisms reported were *Streptococcus pneumoniae, Staphylococcus aureus, Klebsiella pneumoniae, Mycoplasma pneumoniae, Chlamydia pneumoniae, Legionella pneumophila,* and *Acinetobacter baumannii.* Ultimately, these COVID-19-associated infections contribute to high morbidity and mortality because one large retrospective multicenter study noted bacterial co-infection in half of hospitalized patients who died of COVID-19 [5].

Coronavirus Disease 2019 (COVID-19): A Clinical Guide, First Edition. Edited by Ali Gholamrezanezhad and Michael P. Dube.

Streptococcus pneumoniae

S. pneumoniae is the primary bacterial cause of community-acquired pneumonia and may co-infect patients with COVID-19. Given the high mortality rate of pneumococcal infection (which can range from 10% to 36%), it is imperative to quickly identify the microorganism, particularly in vulnerable populations, such as the elderly and immunocompromised patients [6]. However, diagnosis can be obscured because of the similar radiologic appearance of pneumococcal pneumonia and COVID-19. The most common radiologic appearance of pneumococcal pneumonia is that of a unilateral lobar consolidation, but it can sometimes present as bilateral or interstitial infiltrates [7–9].

Zhou et al. [7] compared the computed tomography (CT) features of COVID-19 with pneumococcal pneumonia. Ground-glass opacities (GGOs) and interlobular septal thickening (crazy paving pattern) on chest CT were significantly more common in COVID-19 than *S. pneumoniae* pneumonia. Although these radiologic findings are not diagnostic, they may suggest an additional diagnosis. Co-infection with *S. pneumoniae* should be suspected in patients with COVID-19 who have sudden worsening of symptoms or new radiologic findings. Suspected pneumococcal infection can then be confirmed by bacterial isolation in sputum, blood cultures, or detection of pneumococcal antigen in urine.

Klebsiella

K. pneumoniae has also been found to complicate COVID-19 pneumonia. A case report in Japan [8] described a fatal case of superimposed, hypervirulent *K. pneumoniae* in an 87-year-old patient with confirmed SARS-CoV-2 infection. Although the initial chest x-ray (CXR) was unremarkable, as the patient's condition worsened, a repeat CXR demonstrated new infiltrates in the left lung and pleural effusion. Subsequent microbial investigation yielded *K. pneumoniae*.

At our center, a 54-year-old woman with proven COVID-19 infection presented with an admission CT noting multifocal patchy GGOs and unilateral consolidations consistent with COVID-19 pneumonia. She was treated with antiviral agents and corticosteroids, and her condition quickly improved. Eleven days later, however, this patient underwent a second CT scan because of persistent low oxygen saturation, without cough or fever. Radiologic findings demonstrated new parenchymal opacities, coarse reticular pattern, a bulging fissure sign, and new air space consolidations. Bronchoalveolar lavage subsequently confirmed superimposed *Klebsiella* infection (Figure 14.1).

In another case of concurrent COVID-19 and *Klebsiella* pneumonia, chest CT revealed a large cavitation, emerging consolidation on top of previously seen GGOs and interlobular septal thickening (resulting in a crazy paving pattern), cystic changes, and traction bronchiectasis [9]. Uncommon imaging features in COVID-19 pneumonia, such as new consolidation or cavitation (Figure 14.2), should raise suspicion for possible co-infections.

Mycoplasma pneumoniae

M. pneumoniae is another important bacterial copathogen found in patients with COVID-19, with rates of co-infection ranging from 1% to 40% [10]. In a case report by Huang et al. [11], a patient with concomitant *M. pneumoniae* and SARS-CoV-2 recovered well after combination therapy. The CXR showed patchy bilateral consolidative opacities, and high-resolution CT showed patchy GGOs with septal thickening (crazy paving pattern) and peribronchovascular consolidation. Imaging findings of *M. pneumoniae* alone include peribronchovascular reticular opacities, air space consolidation, and nodular opacities on CXR and GGOs (86%) and air space consolidation (79%) on high-resolution CT, making it difficult to distinguish between COVID-19 and *M. pneumoniae* based on clinical and radiologic patterns alone [12]. This highlights the value of complementary serologic investigations of suspected cases. After administering azithromycin, the patient's clinical condition and imaging findings improved, and elevated mycoplasma IgM and IgG levels returned to normal [11].

Many authors report a high prevalence of superimposed *M. pneumoniae* infection in pediatric patients with COVID-19, particularly with the delta variant. In a study of 81 children admitted to the hospital for COVID-19, 33% of children had co-infection, with *M. pneumoniae* being the most common pathogen [13]. Surprisingly, there were no significant differences in symptomatology in these children compared with those without co-infection. On CT, air space consolidation

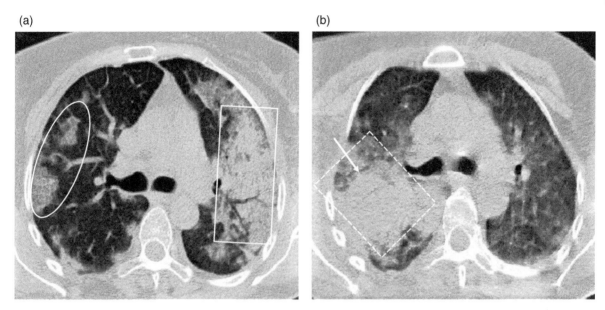

Figure 14.1 *Klebsiella* superinfection on COVID-19. RT-PCR-positive COVID-19 pneumonia in a 54-year-old woman. (a) CT scan on admission (day 1) shows multifocal patchy GGOs (*circle*) and air space consolidations (*box*). She received an antiviral agent and corticosteroids, and her condition improved significantly. (b) On day 11, she underwent a second CT scan because of persistent low O_2 saturation without fever or cough, which displayed new air space consolidations in right upper lobe and right lower lobe (*dotted box*) with a decrease in some of the previously seen GGOs. Culture of bronchoalveolar lavage confirmed superimposed *Klebsiella* infection.

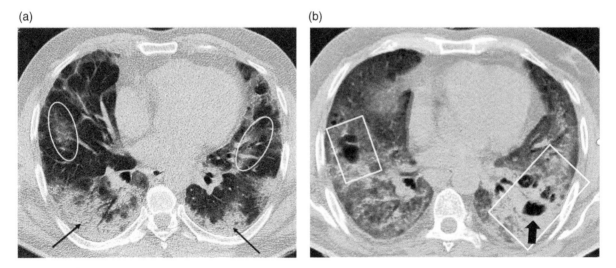

Figure 14.2 Mixed fungal superinfection on COVID-19. RT-PCR-positive COVID-19 pneumonia in a 56-year-old man. (a) CT scan on the first day of admission displays multifocal patchy GGOs (*circles*) and air space consolidations (*arrows*) with predominantly peripheral distribution. After standard treatment with remdesivir and corticosteroid and partial improvement, he developed a fever, dyspnea, and low O_2 saturation. (b) Follow-up CT scan on day 14 shows worsened air space consolidations with internal areas of cavitation (*boxes*), some of them with air–fluid levels (*thick arrow*). He underwent bronchoscopy, and culture of bronchoalveolar lavage showed mixed fungal (aspergillosis) and gram-negative (*Klebsiella*) infection.

was more common in the children with superimposed infection compared with those without. However, this radiologic correlation may be biased because lung consolidation is the most common CT finding in children with *M. pneumoniae* infection [14].

Pseudomonas aeruginosa

Qu et al. [14] recently reported a *Pseudomonas* co-infection in a patient hospitalized for COVID-19. Admission CT indicated basilar and peripheral pre-dominant GGOs and early consolidations. After one week of hospitalization, the patient had worsening respiratory failure. Repeat CT at this time point demonstrated confluent consolidations bilaterally along with new pleural effusions. *P. aeruginosa* was isolated from bronchoalveolar lavage. Although some authors call for prophylactic antibiotic therapy on admission in hospitalized patients with severe COVID-19, many do not support widespread use of empiric antibiotics because it can promote resistance [15]. Despite a relatively low incidence of proven bacterial co-infections in patients with COVID-19, more than 70% of patients received

antibiotics in one study (mostly broad-spectrum agents) [4]. Judicious prescription of antibiotics should be encouraged to preserve their future effectiveness and avoid unnecessary adverse effects.

In another case of *Pseudomonas* co-infection, a 62-year-old man presented to the hospital with acute hypoxemia and proven COVID-19. CXR on admission indicated multifocal peripheral patchy and hazy opacities (Figure 14.3a). CT showed basilar and peripheral predominant GGOs and early consolidations, typical of COVID-19 pneumonia (Figure 14.3b,c). He was given supplemental oxygen and hydroxychloroquine. The next day, he was transferred to the intensive care unit (ICU) because of severe acute chest pain, hypotension, and worsening respiratory failure requiring intubation and mechanical ventilation. He received empiric therapy for bacterial pneumonia. Workup revealed myocardial infarction requiring emergent coronary artery stenting. Repeat CT one week later demonstrated more confluent consolidations bilaterally along with new pleural effusions (Figure 14.3d,e). Subsequently, a bronchoalveolar lavage showed *P. aeruginosa*, and antibiotic therapy was switched to meropenem, with improvement.

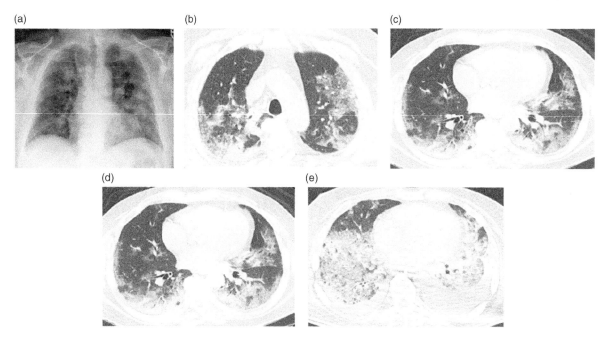

(a) (b) (c)
(d) (e)

Figure 14.3 *Pseudomonas* superinfection with COVID-19. A 62-year-old man presented with acute hypoxemia and positive PCR for COVID-19. Initial frontal radiograph (a) shows multifocal peripheral patchy air space opacities (*arrows*), confirmed on axial CT images (b, c), which show basilar and peripheral predominant GGOs and consolidative opacities, typical for COVID-19 pneumonia. Over the next week, his oxygen demands increased and follow-up CT (d, e) demonstrated more confluent consolidations bilaterally along with new pleural effusions. Subsequent bronchial lavage/pleural cultures returned with *Pseudomonas aeruginosa*.

Legionella

Other atypical bacteria have been shown to infect patients with COVID-19 at surprisingly high rates. Xing et al. [16] described a rate of *Legionella* co-infection in Chinese patients with COVID-19 of 20% (n = 68). Notably, environmental factors may have played a role in these results. The pandemic forced many buildings to temporarily shut down, and decreased water usage increased the levels of stagnant or standing water in plumbing systems, thus creating conditions favorable for *Legionella* [17]. Superimposed Legionnaires' disease in patients with COVID-19 has severe and potentially fatal outcomes.

Verhasselt et al. [18] noted a 41-year-old man with no recent travel history who initially presented with cough, fever, and dyspnea. Before admission, he was empirically treated with azithromycin and ceftriaxone for four days. After a *Legionella* antigen result returned positive, intravenous levofloxacin was substituted. After weeks of hospitalization, the patient remained critically ill, receiving mechanical ventilation.

Another case study from early 2020 reported an 80-year-old man with diarrhea, cough, and malaise seven days after returning from a Nile cruise [19]. The strong correlation between cruise ships and Legionnaires' disease prompted *Legionella* testing, and both urinary antigen for *Legionella* and reverse transcriptase-polymerase chain reaction (RT-PCR) for COVID-19 were positive. Although CXR was not clinically significant, chest CT demonstrated patchy, peripheral GGOs bilaterally (Figure 14.4). Unfortunately, this co-infection proved fatal.

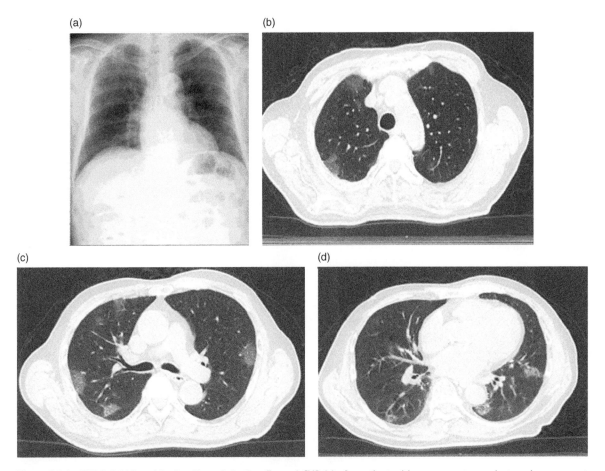

Figure 14.4 SARS-CoV-2 and *Legionella* co-infection. Frontal CXR (a) of a patient with severe acute respiratory derangement and confirmed SARS-CoV-2 and *Legionella* co-infection reveals no definite significant abnormality. However, on axial CT scan images (b–d) obtained on day 7 of illness, there are bilateral subpleural predominant patchy GGOs. *Source:* Arashiro et al. [19].

These studies highlight the importance of considering bacterial co-infection in patients infected with SARS-CoV-2. Although clinical and local epidemiologic data should guide the diagnosis of the precise copathogen, considering radiologic findings, previous travel history, and environmental factors can promote early detection of co-infection and help avoid fatal outcomes.

Fungal Superinfection

Certain authors note that severe SARS-CoV-2 infection can increase the risk for invasive fungal disease (IFD), such as invasive pulmonary aspergillosis (IPA), invasive candidiasis, mucormycosis, or *Pneumocystis jirovecii* pneumonia (PCP) [20]. It is speculated that certain pathophysiologic characteristics of COVID-19 facilitate secondary fungal infections, because the systemic immune dysregulation associated with COVID-19 concurrent with decreased T lymphocytes may alter innate immunity [21]. Because SARS-CoV-2 can yield extensive pulmonary disease and subsequent alveolo-interstitial lesions, patients are at higher risk for invasive fungal infections. In addition, the extensive use of steroids and broad-spectrum antibiotics may result in the development or exacerbation of superimposed fungal diseases.

Pulmonary Aspergillosis

Aspergillus superinfection in critically ill patients with COVID-19 is associated with poorer outcomes and a longer duration of hospitalization and supportive therapies [22]. Given its high mortality, tremendous vigilance is needed, particularly when treating patients with comorbidities and/or on immunosuppressive therapies. It is well documented that influenza complicated by acute respiratory distress syndrome (ARDS) increases risk for IPA even in the absence of predisposing immunocompromise [23]. Thus, clinicians should consider IPA in the differential diagnosis of critically ill patients with COVID-19 with ARDS who are experiencing an acute change in status.

In a large case series by Zhu et al. [24], 23.3% (60/243) of patients with COVID-19 had co-infection with *Aspergillus*. Additional studies from Belgium and the Netherlands reported the incidence of IPA in patients with COVID-19 requiring ICU admission to be 20.6% (7/34) and 19.6% (6/31), respectively. Clinical characteristics and predisposing risk factors in these patients included hypertension, diabetes mellitus, obesity, chronic obstructive pulmonary disease, hypercholesterolemia, and ischemic heart disease, which were also the most common comorbidities in COVID-19-associated IPA. However, 14.7% of patients did not have any comorbidities [25]. Other risk factors for IPA in critically ill patients with COVID-19 include mechanical ventilation, prolonged duration of ventilation, corticosteroid use, immunosuppressive treatments, central venous catheters, prolonged hospital stay, and surgical procedures [26]. A review by Wang et al. [27] noted ARDS followed by liver damage and acute kidney injury as the most likely complications. Lai et al. [25] estimated the overall fatality rate of IPA in COVID-19 to be 64.7% (20/34). These findings indicate the importance of early detection and treatment.

Wang et al. [27] showed that in the early phase of COVID-19 complicated by IPA, typical features of aggressive pneumoconiosis were seen, including dendritic signs and nodules with cavities. However, in the late phase of the co-infection, the imaging findings of IPA were atypical, and some lesions were difficult to identify because of pulmonary consolidations or interstitial changes. Other findings have also been reported, such as peripheral nodules, reverse halo sign, the air crescent sign, GGOs, nodular consolidations, crazy paving pattern, pleural effusion, and pulmonary cysts [28, 29].

Recently, the consensus definitions of IFD from the European Organization for Research and Treatment of Cancer and the Mycoses Study Group Education and Research Consortium defined three diagnostic groups as "proven," "probable," and "possible" IFD [30]. According to these criteria, probable IFD requires the presence of at least one host factor, a clinical feature, and mycologic evidence in immunocompromised patients. For clinical criteria, specific imaging findings have also been included. For example, the presence of one of the four following patterns on a CT scan will categorize a patient as probable IPA: dense, well-circumscribed lesions with or without a halo sign; air crescent sign; cavity, wedge-shaped; and segmental or lobar consolidations. However, these guidelines have not been validated for diagnosing IFD in critically ill patients in the absence of a predisposing risk factor. Thus, other authors recently proposed that the presence of multiple pulmonary nodules or lung cavitation in critically ill patients with COVID-19 should prompt a comprehensive evaluation for IPA, because these imaging features are rarely reported in SARS-CoV-2 alone [31].

Radiologic findings of IPA can vary based on type and level of immunosuppression. For example, infiltrates or nodules with a halo sign are common CT findings in neutropenic patients but are nonspecific for IPA in other groups [32]. In nonneutropenic patients with IPA, bronchopneumonia, segmental/subsegmental and patchy consolidation, cavitation, pleural effusions, GGOs, tree-in-bud opacities, and atelectasis are frequently seen on CT. In addition, the air crescent sign is a late and nonspecific sign in this patient population [33].

The diagnosis of IPA requires a high level of suspicion, careful respiratory sampling, processing of respiratory cultures, and attention to radiologic features. In a case report from Australia [34], initial CXR showed poorly defined pulmonary opacities bilaterally, located principally in the lower lungs and right midlung. Testing for COVID-19 was positive. On day 16, the patient's condition deteriorated rapidly, CXR showed significant progression of bilateral consolidative opacities (worse in the lower zones), and *Aspergillus fumigatus* complex was isolated from endotracheal aspirate. On day 45, the patient's condition continued to worsen, and chest CT at this time point demonstrated bilateral air space consolidations and fibrosis, along with a probable small segmental pulmonary embolism in the left upper lobe, known sequelae of COVID-19 pneumonia. This case report again suggests that radiographic findings cannot definitively determine the causative pathogen. Due to the remarkable overlap in CT findings between IFD and COVID-19 alone, imaging may help distinguish only typical COVID pneumonia and typical IPA. However, atypical or indeterminate radiographical features of COVID-19 may create a diagnostic dilemma. Therefore, the importance of combining radiologic, clinical, and laboratory assessments cannot be overemphasized. Figure 14.5 demonstrates another case of IPA in a patient with COVID-19.

(a)

(b)

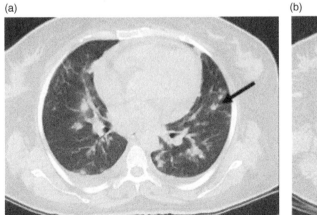
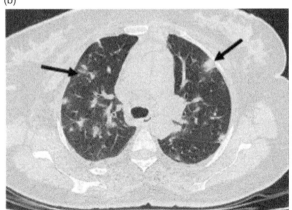

Figure 14.5 Aspergillosis superinfection in COVID-19. A 42-year-old female patient with newly diagnosed acute myeloid leukemia who recently underwent standard combination chemotherapy. (a, b) Axial chest CT images on day 8 showed multiple vessel-related nodular opacities with ground-glass halo with central and peripheral distribution (*arrows*) with small bilateral pleural effusion. The imaging findings are more typical for an invasive fungal infection and atypical for COVID-19. She tested positive for SARS-CoV-2 and *Aspergillus fumigatus*. *Source:* Nasri et al. [35].

Mucormycosis

Mucormycosis is an uncommon opportunistic fungal infection characterized by necrosis and tissue infarction resulting from angioinvasion by fungal hyphae. The infection is a rapidly progressive highly fatal disease that typically affects immunocompromised patients. It can be classified into different clinical forms based on anatomic location, including pulmonary, rhinocerebral, cutaneous, gastrointestinal, and disseminated disease. Although the morbidity and mortality of invasive aspergillosis have declined over the past few years, the prognosis of mucormycosis has not significantly improved because of the lack of specific diagnostic biomarkers, difficulty culturing the causative fungi, and the limited efficacy of antifungal agents against Mucorales [36]. Thus, early diagnosis and a high index of suspicion are critical to beginning appropriate antifungal therapy.

COVID-19-associated pulmonary mucormycosis in hospitalized patients often has fatal outcomes. A case report by Garg et al. [37] noted a probable IFD in a patient with COVID-19 with end-stage renal disease and diabetes. CXR on admission indicated common COVID-19 findings, including diffuse interstitial opacities bilaterally, and subsequent RT-PCR returned positive for SARS-CoV-2. After 14 days of remdesivir, dexamethasone, and supportive therapies, the patient improved, with radiologic resolution. However, three days later, the patient developed a new cough with expectoration. A CXR on day 21 showed a right upper lobe pulmonary cavity with intracavitary contents and a minor right-sided pleural effusion. Sputum culture grew *Rhizopus*, and after treatment with liposomal amphotericin B for probable pulmonary mucormycosis, the patient was discharged 54 days later.

Certain authors have recognized specific chest CT findings that favor the diagnosis of pulmonary mucormycosis over pulmonary aspergillosis. These include pleural effusion, reverse halo sign, and ≥10 pulmonary nodules [38–40]. Reverse halo sign in particular was much more common in patients with mucormycosis than in those with invasive aspergillosis (54% vs. 6%, respectively), whereas some airway-invasive features, such as peribronchial consolidations, clusters of centrilobular nodules, and bronchial wall thickening, were more frequently seen in patients with aspergillosis. In immunocompromised hosts, the CT reverse halo sign is one of the strongest indicators of pulmonary mucormycosis [41]. Although these radiologic features cannot yield exact diagnoses, awareness of these radiologic trends may guide physicians in reaching the correct diagnosis sooner and promptly initiate empiric therapeutic interventions.

Rhinocerebral mucormycosis can spread from the paranasal sinus across bony barriers, including into the orbit, and these patients typically present with acute localized pain or pain radiating to the eye, orbital swelling, nasal ulcer with black eschar, orbital cellulitis, visual defects, headache, and proptosis (Figure 14.6).

Early imaging aids in evaluating the extent of involvement of this highly fatal condition, which requires prompt aggressive treatment. Because the CT findings of rhinocerebral mucormycosis include evidence of simple sinusitis or intracranial abscess, a negative CT cannot exclude the diagnosis. Thus, cranial magnetic resonance imaging (MRI) is generally preferred given its superior assessment of cerebral and orbital involvement. Suggestive features on MRI include sinusitis, soft tissue swelling, intracranial disease progression, intracranial abscess, involvement of the cavernous sinus with thrombophlebitis, multifocal infarction, and orbital involvement [37, 42]. In addition, contrast-enhanced MRI can be used to track the spread of perineural infection, which presents as postcontrast enhancement along the nerve and/or high T2 signal. Another key MRI finding is the black turbinate sign, which indicates devitalized mucosa, thus generating a hypointense mucosal appearance [43].

In a case report [44], an 82-year-old man with diabetes with confirmed SARS-CoV-2 infection developed orbital mucormycosis during hospitalization (under treatment with meropenem, oral oseltamivir, and parenteral methylprednisolone). MRI of the brain, paranasal sinuses, and orbits displayed soft tissue swelling in the right preseptal, premaxillary, malar, and retrobulbar areas, as evidenced by T2 and fluid-attenuated inversion recovery hyperintensity. In addition, mild right proptosis was noted, as well as enlarged right extraocular muscles. Sinusitis evidenced by increased mucosal thickening was evident in the right frontal, maxillary, and ethmoid sinus. The patient underwent nasal biopsy showing broad aseptate filamentous fungal hyphae suggestive of mucormycosis. Despite antifungal measures, his condition deteriorated, and he died six days later.

Werthman-Ehrenreich [45] also reported a 33-year-old woman with diabetic ketoacidosis who presented with altered mental status and proptosis

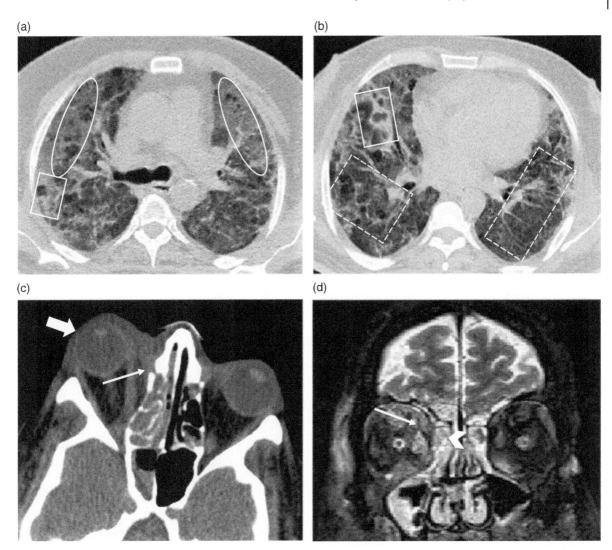

Figure 14.6 Rhino-orbital mucormycosis and COVID-19 co-infection. RT-PCR-positive COVID-19 pneumonia in a 55-year-old male patient with poorly controlled diabetes mellitus. (a, b) Lung CT scan at the second week of infection on ICU admission shows extensive bilateral confluent consolidations (*box*), GGOs (*circles*), and coarse reticular pattern (*dotted boxes*) associated with interstitial septal thickening. He underwent standard of care treatment with remdesivir and corticosteroid. On day 4 of admission, he developed right-sided proptosis and chemosis. (c, d) Orbital CT scan (c) and MRI (d) in coronal T2-weighted sequence display opacification of right ethmoidal, frontal, and maxillary sinuses showing relative T2-weighted hypointense appearance (*chevrons*). An ill-defined lesion is seen in medial right orbit (*thin arrows*) involving extraconal space leading to proptosis of globe (*thick arrow*). Paranasal sinus culture confirmed rhino-orbital mucormycosis. He eventually died during admission after intracranial spread of fungal infection.

and was ultimately diagnosed with COVID-19 and concomitant mucormycosis orbital compartment syndrome.

Pneumocystis jirovecii Pneumonia

There has been increasing recognition of PCP occurring with or succeeding severe COVID-19 (Figure 14.7),

primarily in immunocompromised subjects. A recent study of 108 critically ill patients with COVID-19 found that 9% also tested positive for *P. jirovecii* on bronchial alveolar lavage [46]. Established risk factors for this superimposed infection in patients with COVID-19 include lymphocytopenia, ARDS requiring adjunctive steroids, and multiple immunosuppressive therapies [47].

(a)

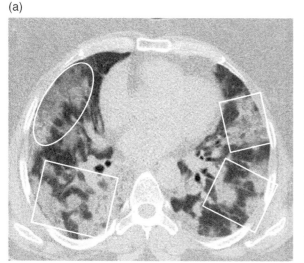

(b)

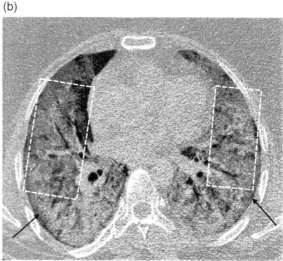

Figure 14.7   PCP in COVID-19. RT-PCR-positive COVID-19 pneumonia in a 57-year-old woman. (a) Chest CT image on day 1 shows bilateral multifocal consolidations (*boxes*) and patchy GGOs (*circle*) with dominant peripheral distribution. The patient did not respond well to routine standard of care treatment, and corticosteroid was continued. Due to persistent hypoxemia and respiratory distress, a second CT was obtained on day 18 of admission in the ICU (b), which showed extensive bilateral confluent GGOs and associated septal thickening (*dotted boxes*). Relative subpleural sparing is also noted in lower lobes (*arrows*). Diagnostic bronchoscopy was not performed because of respiratory distress. Considering the new imaging findings, she underwent a treatment trial for PCP, her condition dramatically improved, and she was discharged.

Radiologic diagnosis of PCP in patients with SARS-CoV-2 infection can be extremely challenging because of overlap in imaging characteristics. To differentiate these two infections, Bhat et al. [48] reported key radiologic findings present in PCP infection, such as cystic changes, pneumothorax, and fine reticular patterns. Some reported chest CT findings with PCP and COVID-19 co-infection include apical cystic changes, diffuse GGOs, dense consolidation, and pneumothorax [48]. Diffuse bilateral GGOs and small nodular foci of consolidation [49] and extensive subpleural and paramediastinal cystic changes with subpleural ground-glass changes bilaterally [50] have also been reported.

In a case report by Rubiano et al. [51], a 36-year-old critically ill patient with COVID-19 was found to have AIDS and PCP. On admission, his CXR showed diffuse hazy pulmonary opacifications. CT pulmonary angiography showed diffuse upper and lower lobe GGOs without pulmonary embolism. The patient was started on vancomycin and cefepime for possible bacterial pneumonia. However, his condition worsened, and repeat CXR showed heterogeneous bilateral alveolar opacities with scattered air bronchograms. Because the opacities were somehow less dense than expected for COVID-19 and for the patient's level of hypoxemia,

he received empiric trimethoprim-sulfamethoxazole and prednisone. Bronchoscopy with bronchoalveolar lavage was positive for PCP, and RT-PCR was positive for SARS-CoV-2. Despite specific therapies, he died on day 26 of hospital admission.

Physicians should retain a broad differential diagnosis in patients with COVID-19 who are immunocompromised or demonstrate atypical clinical presentations. In addition, COVID-19 and *Pneumocystis* co-infection should be seriously considered in critically ill patients, even in the absence of traditional risk factors for PCP.

Trichosporon asahii Fungemia

A recent study noted co-infection with *Trichosporon asahii* fungemia in five critically ill COVID-19 patients in Brazil [52]. All were previously exposed to risk factors that increased their risk for fungal co-infection, such as prior broad-spectrum antibiotics and echinocandin therapy, prolonged corticosteroid use, and a central venous catheter. Fully 60% of patients with superimposed *Trichosporon* infection died within two weeks of diagnosis.

Segrelles-Calvo et al. [53] reported on a 58-year-old man with a history of malignancy and 12 days of nonproductive cough, dyspnea, and fever. Lymphopenia was noted. RT-PCR for COVID-19 was positive, and CXR on admission demonstrated left lobe air space consolidation. Azithromycin, hydroxychloroquine, lopinavir/ritonavir, methylprednisolone, and tocilizumab were given. After 12 days of hospitalization, the patient's status worsened, and he required intubation and mechanical ventilation. On day 19 of hospital admission, he had persistent fever and respiratory failure. Sputum culture indicated drug-resistant *P. aeruginosa* and *Stenotrophomonas maltophilia*. Chest CT at this time showed a moderate pleural effusion, bilateral consolidations, and findings suggesting a pleuropulmonary fistula. The patient was given appropriate antibiotics. After not improving, bronchoalveolar lavage on day 28 was positive for *Trichosporon asahii*. On day 38, the patient passed away as a result of septic shock.

Histoplasmosis

Other authors have recently identified cases of histoplasmosis concurrent with COVID-19 infection primarily in endemic regions. Stasiak et al. [54] described a 37-year-old Brazilian woman who presented with a 12-day history of fever, chest pain, and night sweats. Initial CT scan showed small pleural effusion and two irregular pulmonary opacities with central necrosis in the left lung. Molecular testing for histoplasmosis returned positive. She began itraconazole and was discharged. Six weeks later, this patient returned with the same symptoms and underwent a fluorodeoxyglucose-positron emission tomography/CT to distinguish between active and resolved infection. This noted significant fluorodeoxyglucose uptake (maximum standardized uptake value [SUVmax] = 6) in the original pulmonary opacities and positive lymph nodes in the cervical region, left lung and hepatic hilum, and mediastinum, thus indicating active infection. However, pulmonary opacities in a ground-glass pattern were now visible in the right lower lobe, highly suggestive of COVID-19 infection. RT-PCR testing returned positive. Interestingly, the patient's symptoms stayed mild, and she was discharged without hospitalization. Six weeks later, repeat positron emission tomography/CT indicated resolution of the right lower lobe pulmonary opacities in a ground-glass pattern and further decrease in size of the left lobe opacities. This case describes the importance of having a low threshold for COVID-19 in patients with recurring fever and exacerbation of otherwise well-controlled fungal disease.

In southern Brazil, a 43-year-old woman with a 21-year history of HIV with poor adherence to antiretroviral treatment presented to the hospital with fever, disorientation, cough, and dyspnea [55]. Initial RT-PCR for COVID-19 was negative. Chest CT on admission demonstrated multiple centrilobular nodules, bilateral GGOs, and diffuse bronchial wall thickening (Figure 14.8a). An abdominal CT

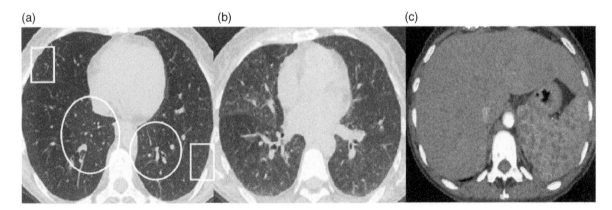

(a) (b) (c)

Figure 14.8 Superimposed histoplasmosis infection on COVID-19. A 43-year-old woman with a 21-year history of HIV infection and poor adherence to antiretroviral treatment recently tested positive for COVID-19. Initial chest CT axial image (a) shows subtle patchy bilateral GGOs (*circle*), diffuse bronchial wall thickening, and subtle centrilobular nodules (*box*). Abdominal CT showed hepatosplenomegaly (images not shown). Eight days later, chest (b) and abdominal CT scans (c) were repeated because of worsening symptoms, which show worsening of ground-glass opacities and centrilobular nodules and numerous splenic hypodense nodules concerning for disseminated granulomatous infection. The patient tested positive for urinary *H. capsulatum* antigen. *Source:* Basso et al. [55].

showed hepatosplenomegaly. The patient was empirically treated for neurotoxoplasmosis and discharged. However, she returned eight days later with worsening symptoms, and RT-PCR for COVID-19 was now positive. Chest and abdominal CT scans were repeated with the former indicating worsening of GGOs and micronodules, and the latter demonstrating hepatosplenomegaly with numerous splenic hypodense nodules and retroperitoneal lymphadenopathy (Figure 14.8b,c). At this point, urine *Histoplasma capsulatum* antigen returned positive, and she started oral itraconazole and was discharged.

Superimposed miliary histoplasmosis can also sometimes occur in patients with COVID-19. In an Argentinian patient with COVID-19 with prior history of HIV [56], initial chest CT showed a bilateral diffuse micronodular interstitial pattern, suggestive of superimposed miliary histoplasmosis. Bertolini et al. [57] noted both miliary-pattern infiltrates and bilateral peripheral multifocal GGOs in a person with HIV with both histoplasmosis and COVID-19 co-infection.

Parasitic

Strongyloidiasis

Superimposed parasitic infection in patients with COVID-19 is rare. Specifically, superimposed strongyloidiasis in immunocompromised patients with COVID-19 has been described, even after a short course of low-dose glucocorticoids or a single high dose of dexamethasone [56]. Although strongyloidiasis is often asymptomatic in immunocompetent patients, it can present with mild gastrointestinal or respiratory symptoms and a linear pruritic rash known as larva currens [58]. In immunocompromised patients, a disseminated infection or "hyperinfection" can occur and potentially cause meningitis or bacterial sepsis [56].

Both COVID-19 and strongyloidiasis share many of the same clinical and radiologic findings, such as dyspnea, fever, and gastrointestinal symptoms and bilateral lung infiltrates. Given their overlapping presentations, it can be exceedingly difficult to distinguish such co-infections; thus, high clinical suspicion and a thorough diagnostic workup are vital for an accurate diagnosis, particularly in patients with prior travel history to endemic areas or those with poor sanitation.

In a case report by Lier et al. [59], a 68-year-old patient presented to the hospital after eight days of myalgia, chills, dyspnea, and nausea. This patient had emigrated from Ecuador to the United States 20 years prior. RT-PCR was positive for COVID-19, and CXR indicated patchy air space opacities bilaterally in the mid to lower lung zones. One day after admission, the patient developed respiratory failure requiring intubation along with three courses of methylprednisolone (40 mg intravenously every eight hours) and one dose of tocilizumab (intravenously at 8 mg/kg). On day 18, this patient developed fever, eosinophilia, and confusion, and serpiginous tracks on chocolate agar raised suspicion for strongyloidiasis, but *Strongyloides* serology was negative. Repeat CXR on day 21 revealed unchanged multifocal pulmonary opacities bilaterally. The patient progressively worsened and was diagnosed with probable meningitis associated with disseminated strongyloidiasis after immunosuppressive treatment for COVID-19. On day 30, chest CT scan was notable for diffuse peripheral GGOs and peribronchial consolidation in the right lower lobe. Repeat *Strongyloides* serology on day 38 returned positive. After extensive treatment and more than 40 days of hospitalization, this patient was discharged.

Recent research has suggested that parasitic co-infection in patients with COVID-19 can have a favorable impact on the severity of COVID-19 infection. Certain authors have noted that patients with COVID-19 who reside in developing countries such as Africa have less severe COVID-19 symptoms than that of the industrialized world [60]. In a study of 751 patients with COVID-19 in Ethiopia, Wolday et al. [60] reported a significant inverse correlation between the presence of parasitic co-infection and COVID-19 severity. Gebrecherkos et al. [61] found similar findings and noted that patients with COVID-19 with parasitic, protozoa, or helminth co-infection had a lower probability of developing severe COVID-19. Although a normal viral immune response involves T helper (Th) 1 cell–based responses, a parasitic infestation may shift to a Th2 cell response and decrease the level of Th1 cell–associated inflammation. Thus, co-infection with parasites may promote immune tolerance, possibly muting COVID-19-induced hyperinflammation.

Viral

Influenza

Many authors have reported influenza superinfection in patients with COVID-19. In a study by Ozaras et al. [62], six patients with COVID-19 were diagnosed with influenza co-infection by RT-PCR. Of those six, five patients demonstrated classic COVID-19 radiographic findings, such as nonspecific peripheral lesions in both lobes, patchy GGOs and consolidation opacities, shrinking lesion contour, and bronchial wall thickening. One patient, however, showcased classic influenza findings on chest CT, which consisted of central lesions that favor inferior lobes, cluster-like GGOs, nonshrinking lesion contour, and an absence of bronchial wall thickening. Yue et al. [63] in Wuhan identified three groups of patients: those infected with COVID-19 alone, co-infection with influenza A virus (IAV), and co-infection with influenza B virus (IBV). Between January 2020 and February 2021, 176 patients (n = 307) had either IAV or IBV co-infection. Patients with IBV co-infection had more severe disease indicated by more extensive CT abnormalities and lymphopenia, while patients with IAV co-infection had fewer abnormalities. However, this study is limited by failing to account for prognostic factors such as age or comorbidities.

To further characterize radiographic findings in IAV (H1N1) and COVID-19, Yin et al. [64] compared the common CT findings. Linear opacification, crazy paving pattern, pleural thickening, and vascular enlargement were more common in COVID-19 pneumonia, while bronchiectasis and pleural effusion were more frequently seen in influenza A (H1N1) pneumonia. Although these findings are not pathognomonic, new-onset bronchiectasis or pleural effusion in a patient with COVID-19 may be indicative of superimposed IAV infection and prompt further workup.

Because IAV replicates in type 2 pneumocytes, cells that SARS-CoV-2 preferentially infects, there may be some synergy between the viruses [65]. Interestingly, Bai et al. [66] noted that in IAV-infected type 2 pneumocytes, mRNA levels of the ACE2 receptor were threefold higher than baseline; thus, influenza infection may exacerbate and/or increase susceptibility to COVID-19 infection. In addition, these authors conducted mouse studies on SARS-CoV-2 and IAV co-infection and described that infection with IAV before COVID-19 can enhance SARS-CoV-2 infectivity and viral entry. Mice co-infected with SARS-CoV-2 and IAV were shown to have more severe lung damage, evident by histopathologic changes reminiscent of alveolar necrosis and increased SARS-CoV-2 viral load. Further research is necessary to determine the exact correlations between influenza co-infection and COVID-19 severity.

Dengue

Although the rates of many seasonal illnesses plummeted because of mask mandates and strict social distancing guidelines, rates of dengue fever in 2020 surpassed case counts from the last decade combined in some areas [67]. Other authors noted dengue cases reaching or outnumbering COVID-19 cases in endemic areas [68]. However, other studies found the opposite, with COVID-19 cases skyrocketing and few reported cases of dengue fever [69]. Lustig et al. [70] recently argued that this disagreement in rates could be attributed to serologic cross-reactivity between dengue and COVID-19, thus generating false-positive antibody test results.

In addition to serologic cross-reactivity, overlapping clinical and radiologic similarities between the two diseases have made accurate diagnosis of dengue co-infection in patients with COVID-19 a challenging task [71]. COVID-19 often presents as an acute undifferentiated febrile illness, and in many endemic countries, dengue virus is considered the most likely cause, making them hard to distinguish on clinical grounds [72]. The symptoms of both dengue and COVID-19 include myalgia, fever, malaise, gastrointestinal symptoms, and headache. Leukopenia with lymphopenia can also be present in both early dengue and early COVID-19 infection. However, the presence or absence of viral exanthem may guide clinicians to the correct diagnosis, because this finding is frequently seen with dengue fever and is uncommon in COVID-19 infection.

The radiologic findings of superimposed dengue infection in patients with COVID-19 mimics that of a typical viral pneumonia. In a systematic review analyzing dengue and COVID-19 co-infection, the authors noted GGOs in five patients, bilateral lung opacities in four patients, splenomegaly and pleural effusion in one patient, and normal CXR or CT in the remaining patients [73]. Thus, chest imaging findings do not play an active role in distinguishing COVID-19 and dengue fever co-infection because of their similarities. However, imaging can be helpful in elucidating extrapulmonary manifestations (i.e. splenomegaly, hepatomegaly, and ascites) in the absence of serologic results. Tiwari et al. [74] recently reported a pediatric case of COVID-19 encephalitis with superimposed dengue shock syndrome. RT-PCR for COVID-19 and serum dengue antigen test returned positive, and the patient's CXR demonstrated reticulonodular opacities bilaterally without any evidence of pleural effusion. Contrast-enhanced brain CT showed ill-defined hypodensities in the bilateral frontal lobes, bilateral temporal lobe, basal ganglia, right parietal lobe, corpus callosum, midbrain, and pons, consistent with viral encephalitis (Figure 14.9). These imaging findings were suggestive of COVID-19-associated encephalitis with superimposed dengue shock syndrome. This case emphasizes the importance of testing for prevalent pathogens in endemic regions because of the possibility of detrimental viral synergy.

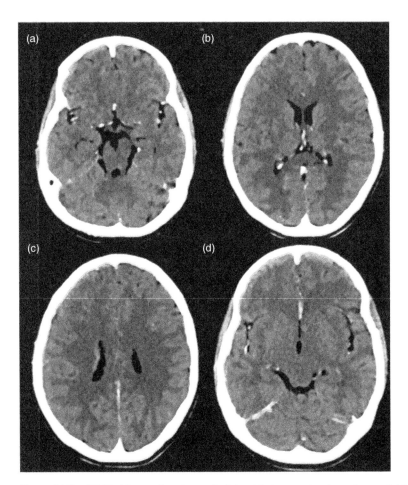

Figure 14.9 COVID-19-associated encephalitis with dengue shock syndrome. A 14-year-old girl presented with high-grade fever, headache, vomiting, respiratory distress, and hypotensive shock. Nasopharyngeal PCR tests for SARS-CoV-2 and serum dengue NS1 antigen were positive. Contrast-enhanced axial CT images showing ill-defined marked hypodensities in midbrain (a), thalamus (b), corpus callosum and bilateral periventricular area (c), and basal ganglia and bilateral frontal lobes (d). Given the clinical context, laboratory testing results, and patient's demographics (resident of an area endemic for dengue fever), the image findings are suggestive of viral encephalitis. *Source:* Tiwari et al. [74], reproduced with permission from BMJ Publishing Group Ltd.

Certain studies report varying levels of severity and outcome of superimposed dengue infection in patients with COVID-19. Saddique et al. [75] noted high morbidity and mortality in patients with superimposed dengue infection. Estofolete et al. [76] reported a 60-year-old obese woman who presented with headache, fever, myalgia, and retro-orbital pain. She was diagnosed with dengue and discharged with symptomatic treatment. However, she returned eight days later with respiratory failure requiring mechanical ventilation. RT-PCR for both COVID-19 and dengue antigen returned positive. A chest CT showed extensive bilateral consolidative opacities and GGOs (Figure 14.10). She was admitted to the ICU, underwent hemodialysis, and received antibiotics and heparin. Four days later, the patient developed anisocoria, and a CT brain showed extensive hypodense injury in the left cerebellar and cerebral hemispheres representative of subacute ischemic injury. Midline shift and ventricle compression were also suggested because of parenchymal edema. The patient died soon after.

Bicudo et al. [77] described a 56-year-old woman with a mild course of dengue and COVID-19 co-infection. The patient presented to the hospital after 12 days of sore throat, anosmia, mild dyspnea, headache, and fever. RT-PCR for COVID-19 was subsequently positive, but immunoglobulin M (IgM) and IgG antibody tests for dengue were negative. A chest CT showed peripheral GGOs bilaterally, representative of COVID-19 infection. Three days later, the patient developed diarrhea/nausea, as well as a pruritic, erythematous maculopapular rash, in addition to her previous symptoms. At this time point, repeat RT-PCR for both dengue and COVID-19 returned positive, and IgM and IgG antibody tests for dengue converted to positive. Due to mild symptoms, she was discharged after supportive treatment.

Respiratory Syncytial Virus

With the recent emergence of the COVID-19 delta variant, reports of COVID-19 and respiratory syncytial virus (RSV) co-infection have been observed [78]. RSV

(a) (b)

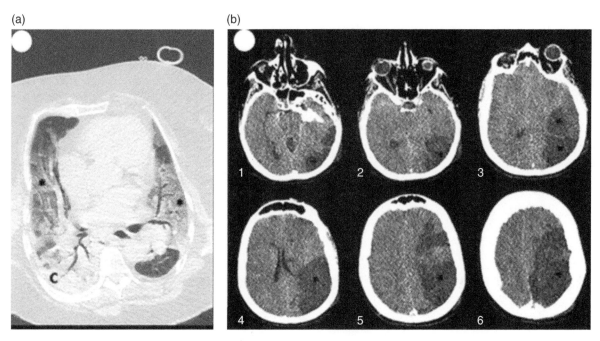

Figure 14.10 Fatal stroke caused by dengue virus co-infection in COVID-19. A 60-year-old obese woman who presented to the emergency department with headache, fever, myalgia, and retroorbital pain. (a) Chest CT images on day 8 show extensive bilateral consolidative opacities (*C*) and GGOs (*asterisks*). (b) Brain CT images on day 12 show an extensive hypodense injury (*asterisks*) involving the left cerebral and cerebellar hemispheres (*1–6*), inferring an area of subacute ischemic vascular injury, and edema in the left cerebral hemisphere, with a compressive effect and midline deviation. *Source:* Estofolete et al. [76].

is a common respiratory viral infection that has traditionally been an important cause of hospitalization in patients younger than 12 months [79]. However, distinguishing COVID-19 and RSV infection can be a difficult task because of the similarities between both their clinical and radiologic findings. Clinically, both COVID-19 and RSV present with rhinorrhea, cough, and fatigue. As far as radiologic findings, both viral infections are associated with bilateral GGOs and consolidations. In a case report by Jiang et al. [80], the authors noted a six-year-old girl with both RSV and human metapneumovirus superimposed on COVID-19. Chest CT showed GGOs, and after two weeks of treatment, she was discharged without residual symptoms.

Interestingly, it appears that children infected with two or more pathogens have a mild disease course, thus suggesting these organisms may be colonizers rather than pathogens. Wu et al. [81] reported that 51% (n = 74) of children demonstrated superimposed infection, with 42% of the children noted to have two or more pathogens other than SARS-CoV-2. The most common offenders were *M. pneumoniae* alone (11/34), *M. pneumoniae* with RSV (2/34), *M. pneumoniae* with Epstein–Barr virus (2/34), cytomegalovirus alone (2/34), cytomegalovirus and Epstein–Barr virus (1/34), and one child with *M. pneumoniae*, influenza A and B, and RSV. Unfortunately, no clinical associations were determined between the children with co-infections and the presence or absence of CT findings. However, of the 74 children, only 50% had abnormal CT findings that resembled a mild viral pneumonia. Most of the children had very mild symptoms and/or were asymptomatic. Further research is necessary to determine the exact correlation between severity, symptomatology, and radiologic findings in children with superimposed infections.

Summary

Although many patients with COVID-19 present with mild or moderate disease, patients with preexisting conditions may require hospitalization with intensive care and mechanical ventilation, increasing their risk for secondary infection. These bacterial, fungal, viral, and parasitic co-infections have not only increased the morbidity and mortality of COVID-19 but also created a challenging diagnostic dilemma for clinicians. Thus, any acute change in status or imaging findings of patients with COVID-19, such as the presence of new cavitation or worsened consolidations, should prompt thorough workup to exclude superimposed opportunistic infection. Because co-infection can worsen the prognosis in many high-risk COVID-19 patients, such as the immunocompromised, physicians should have a greater index of suspicion for superimposed infection in this population. In addition, antibiotics, corticosteroids, and antifungal therapy should be prescribed judiciously to preserve their future effectiveness and avoid colonization by multidrug-resistant pathogens with high mortality. Ultimately, combining imaging and laboratory findings, epidemiologic data, and detailed clinical history can help clinicians identify opportunistic infections earlier and greatly improve patient outcomes.

References

1 Joseph, C., Togawa, Y., and Shindo, N. (2013). Bacterial and viral infections associated with influenza. *Influenza Other Respir. Viruses* 7 (Suppl 2): 105–113.

2 Cao, B., Wang, Y., Wen, D. et al. (2020). A trial of lopinavir-ritonavir in adults hospitalized with severe Covid-19. *N. Engl. J. Med.* 382 (19): 1787–1799.

3 Wang, L., He, W., Yu, X. et al. (2020). Coronavirus disease 2019 in elderly patients: characteristics and prognostic factors based on 4-week follow-up. *J. Infect.* 80 (6): 639–645.

4 Langford, B.J., So, M., Raybardhan, S. et al. (2020). Bacterial co-infection and secondary infection in patients with COVID-19: a living rapid review and meta-analysis. *Clin. Microbiol. Infect.* 26 (12): 1622–1629.

5 Zhou, F., Yu, T., Du, R. et al. (2020). Clinical course and risk factors for mortality of adult inpatients with COVID-19 in Wuhan, China: a retrospective cohort study. *Lancet* 395: 1054–1062.

6 Martens, P., Worm, S.W., Lundgren, B. et al. (2004). Serotype-specific mortality from invasive Streptococcus

pneumoniae disease revisited. *BMC Infect. Dis.* 4: 21. https://doi.org/10.1186/1471-2334-4-21.

7 Zhou, J., Liao, X., Cao, J. et al. (2021). Differential diagnosis between the coronavirus disease 2019 and Streptococcus pneumoniae pneumonia by thin-slice CT features. *Clin. Imaging* 69: 318–323.

8 Hosoda, T., Harada, S., Okamoto, K. et al. (2021). COVID-19 and fatal sepsis caused by Hypervirulent Klebsiella pneumoniae, Japan, 2020. *Emerg. Infect. Dis.* 27 (2): 556–559.

9 Ammar, A., Drapé, J.L., and Revel, M.P. (2021). Lung cavitation in COVID-19 pneumonia. *Diagn. Interv. Imaging* 102 (2): 117–118.

10 Akbari, H. (2020). Prevalence of Mycoplasma pneumonia coinfection among patients with COVID-19: a systematic review. *Arch. Med. Lab. Sci.* 6 (1): 1–6. (e3).

11 Huang, A.C., Huang, C.G., Yang, C.T., and Hu, H.C. (2020). Concomitant infection with COVID-19 and mycoplasma pneumoniae. *Biomed. J.* 43 (5): 458–461.

12 Reittner, P., Müller, N.L., Heyneman, L. et al. (2000). Mycoplasma pneumoniae pneumonia: radiographic and high-resolution CT features in 28 patients. *AJR Am. J. Roentgenol.* 174: 37–41.

13 Li, Y., Wang, H., Wang, F. et al. (2021). Co-infections of SARS-CoV-2 with multiple common respiratory pathogens in infected children: a retrospective study. *Medicine* 100 (11): e24315. https://doi.org/10.1097/MD.0000000000024315.

14 Qu, J., Cai, Z., Liu, Y. et al. (2021). Persistent bacterial coinfection of a COVID-19 patient caused by a genetically adapted Pseudomonas aeruginosa chronic colonizer. *Front. Cell. Infect. Microbiol.* 11: 641920.

15 Contou, D., Claudinon, A., Pajot, O. et al. (2020). Bacterial and viral co-infections in patients with severe SARS-CoV-2 pneumonia admitted to a French ICU. *Ann. Intensive Care* 10: 119. https://doi.org/10.1186/s13613-020-00736-x.

16 Xing, Q., Li, G., Xing, Y., et al. (2020). Precautions Are Needed For COVID-19 Patients With Coinfection Of Common Respiratory Pathogens. medRxiv. https://doi.org/10.1101/2020.02.29.20027698. Accessed 12 Sep 2021.

17 Pattinson, M. (2021). ESGLI guidance for managing legionella in building water systems during the COVID-19 pandemic. PWTAG, The Pool Water Treatment Advisory Group. https://www.pwtag.org/

esgli-guidance-managing-legionella-building-water-systems-covid-19-pandemic.

18 Verhasselt, H.L., Buer, J., Dedy, J. et al. (2021). COVID-19 co-infection with legionella pneumophila in 2 tertiary-care hospitals, Germany. *Emerg. Infect. Dis.* 27 (5): 1535–1537. https://doi.org/10.3201/eid2705.203388.

19 Arashiro, T., Nakamura, S., Asami, T. et al. (2020). SARS-CoV-2 and legionella co-infection in a person returning from a Nile cruise. *J. Travel Med.* 27 (3): taaa053.

20 Pemán, J., Ruiz-Gaitán, A., García-Vidal, C. et al. (2020). Fungal co-infection in COVID-19 patients: should we be concerned? *Rev. Iberoam. Micol.* 37 (2): 41–46.

21 Gangneux, J.P., Bougnoux, M.E., Dannaoui, E. et al. (2020). Invasive fungal diseases during COVID-19: we should be prepared. *J. Mycol. Med.* 30 (2): 100971. https://doi.org/10.1016/j.mycmed.2020.100971.

22 Chong, W.H. and Neu, K.P. (2021). Incidence, diagnosis and outcomes of COVID-19-associated pulmonary aspergillosis (CAPA): a systematic review. *J. Hosp. Infect.* 113: 115–129. https://doi.org/10.1016/j.jhin.2021.04.012.

23 Waldeck, F., Boroli, F., Suh, N. et al. (2020). Influenza-associated aspergillosis in critically-ill patients: a retrospective bicentric cohort study. *Eur. J. Clin. Microbiol. Infect. Dis.* 39 (10): 1915–1923.

24 Zhu, X., Ge, Y., Wu, T. et al. (2020). Co-infection with respiratory pathogens among COVID-2019 cases. *Virus Res.* 285: 198005.

25 Lai, C.C. and Yu, W.L. (2021). COVID-19 associated with pulmonary aspergillosis: a literature review. *J. Microbiol. Immunol. Infect.* 54 (1): 46–53. https://doi.org/10.1016/j.jmii.2020.09.004.

26 Ezeokoli, O.T., Gcilitshana, O., and Pohl, C.H. (2021). Risk factors for fungal co-infections in critically ill COVID-19 patients, with a focus on Immunosuppressants. *J. Fungi (Basel, Switzerland)* 7 (7): 545. https://doi.org/10.3390/jof7070545.

27 Wang, J., Yang, Q., Zhang, P. et al. (2020). Clinical characteristics of invasive pulmonary aspergillosis in patients with COVID-19 in Zhejiang, China: a retrospective case series. *Crit. Care* 24 (1): 299.

28 Lescure, F.X., Bouadma, L., Nguyen, D. et al. (2020). Clinical and virological data of the first cases of COVID-19 in Europe: a case series. *Lancet Infect. Dis.* 20 (6): 697–706. https://doi.org/10.1016/S1473-3099(20)30200-0.

29 Prattes, J., Valentin, T., Hoenigl, M. et al. (2021). Invasive pulmonary aspergillosis complicating COVID-19 in the ICU – a case report. *Med. Mycol. Case Rep.* 31: 2–5. https://doi.org/10.1016/j.mmcr. 2020.05.001.

30 Donnelly, J.P., Chen, S.C., Kauffman, C.A. et al. (2019). Revision and update of the consensus definitions of invasive fungal disease from the European Organization for Research and Treatment of cancer and the mycoses study group education and research consortium. *Clin. Infect. Dis.* 71 (6): 1367–1376. https://doi.org/10.1093/cid/ciz1008.

31 Koehler, P., Bassetti, M., Chakrabarti, A. et al.; European Confederation of Medical Mycology; International Society for Human Animal Mycology; Asia Fungal Working Group; INFOCUS LATAM/ ISHAM Working Group; ISHAM Pan Africa Mycology Working Group; European Society for Clinical Microbiology; Infectious Diseases Fungal Infection Study Group; ESCMID Study Group for Infections in Critically Ill Patients; Interregional Association of Clinical Microbiology and Antimicrobial Chemotherapy; Medical Mycology Society of Nigeria; Medical Mycology Society of China Medicine Education Association; Infectious Diseases Working Party of the German Society for Haematology and Medical Oncology; Association of Medical Microbiology; Infectious Disease Canada(2021). Defining and managing COVID-19-associated pulmonary aspergillosis: the 2020 ECMM/ ISHAM consensus criteria for research and clinical guidance. *Lancet Infect. Dis.* 21 (6): e149–e162.

32 Lim, C., Seo, J.B., Park, S.Y. et al. (2012). Analysis of initial and follow-up CT findings in patients with invasive pulmonary aspergillosis after solid organ transplantation. *Clin. Radiol.* 67 (12): 1179–1186.

33 Donnelly, J.P., Chen, S.C., Kauffman, C.A. et al. (2020). Revision and update of the consensus definitions of invasive fungal disease from the European Organization for Research and Treatment of cancer and the mycoses study group education and research consortium. *Clin. Infect. Dis.* 71 (6): 1367–1376.

34 Sharma, A., Hofmeyr, A., Bansal, A. et al. (2021). COVID-19 associated pulmonary aspergillosis (CAPA): an Australian case report. *Med. Mycol. Case Rep.* 31: 6–10.

35 Nasri, E., Shoaei, P., Vakili, B. et al. (2020). Fatal invasive pulmonary aspergillosis in COVID-19 patient with acute myeloid leukemia in Iran. *Mycopathologia* 185 (6): 1077–1084.

36 Petrikkos, G., Skiada, A., Lortholary, O. et al. (2012). Epidemiology and clinical manifestations of mucormycosis. *Clin. Infect. Dis.* 54 (Suppl 1): S23–S34.

37 Garg, D., Muthu, V., Sehgal, I.S. et al. (2021). Coronavirus disease (Covid-19) associated mucormycosis (CAM): case report and systematic review of literature. *Mycopathologia* 186 (2): 289–298.

38 Chamilos, G., Marom, E.M., Lewis, R.E. et al. (2005). Predictors of pulmonary zygomycosis versus invasive pulmonary aspergillosis in patients with cancer. *Clin. Infect. Dis.* 41 (1): 60–66.

39 Legouge, C., Caillot, D., Chrétien, M.L. et al. (2014). The reversed halo sign: pathognomonic pattern of pulmonary mucormycosis in leukemic patients with neutropenia? *Clin. Infect. Dis.* 58 (5): 672–678.

40 Jung, J., Kim, M.Y., Lee, H.J. et al. (2015). Comparison of computed tomographic findings in pulmonary mucormycosis and invasive pulmonary aspergillosis. *Clin. Microbiol. Infect.* 21 (7): 684. e11-8.

41 Georgiadou, S.P., Sipsas, N.V., Marom, E.M., and Kontoyiannis, D.P. (2011). The diagnostic value of halo and reversed halo signs for invasive mold infections in compromised hosts. *Clin. Infect. Dis.* 52 (9): 1144–1155.

42 Alekseyev, K., Didenko, L., and Chaudhry, B. (2021). Rhinocerebral mucormycosis and COVID-19 pneumonia. *J. Med. Cases* 12 (3): 85–89. https://doi. org/10.14740/jmc3637.

43 Chen, I.W. and Lin, C.W. (2019). Rhino-orbital-cerebral mucormycosis. *CMAJ* 191 (16): E450.

44 Mehta, S. and Pandey, A. (2020). Rhino-orbital mucormycosis associated with COVID-19. *Cureus* 12 (9): e10726. https://doi.org/10.7759/cureus.10726.

45 Werthman-Ehrenreich, A. (2021). Mucormycosis with orbital compartment syndrome in a patient with COVID-19. *Am. J. Emerg. Med.* 42: 264.e5–264.e8.

46 Alanio, A., Dellière, S., Voicu, S. et al. (2021). The presence of Pneumocystis jirovecii in critically ill patients with COVID-19. *J. Infect.* 82 (4): 84–123. https://doi.org/10.1016/j.jinf.2020.10.034.

47 Beumer, M.C., Koch, R.M., van Beuningen, D. et al. (2019). Influenza virus and factors that are associated with ICU admission, pulmonary co-infections and ICU mortality. *J. Crit. Care* 50: 59–65.

48 Bhat, P., Noval, M., Doub, J.B., and Heil, E. (2020). Concurrent COVID-19 and Pneumocystis jirovecii pneumonia in a severely immunocompromised 25-year-old patient. *Int. J. Infect. Dis.* 99: 119–121.

49 Menon, A.A., Berg, D.D., Brea, E.J. et al. (2020). A case of COVID-19 and *Pneumocystis jirovecii* coinfection. *Am. J. Respir. Crit. Care Med* 202 (1): 136–138.

50 Coleman, H., Snell, L.B., Simons, R. et al. (2020). Coronavirus disease 2019 and *Pneumocystis jirovecii* pneumonia: a diagnostic dilemma in HIV. *AIDS* 34 (8): 1258–1260.

51 Rubiano, C., Tompkins, K., Sellers, S.A. et al. (2020). Pneumocystis and severe acute respiratory syndrome coronavirus 2 co-infection: a case report and review of an emerging diagnostic dilemma. *Open Forum Infect. Dis.* 8 (1): ofaa633.

52 Nobrega de Almeida, J. Jr., Moreno, L., Francisco, E.C. et al. (2021). Trichosporon asahii superinfections in critically ill COVID-19 patients overexposed to antimicrobials and corticosteroids. *Mycoses* 64 (8): 817–822. https://doi.org/10.1111/myc.13333.

53 Segrelles-Calvo, G., Araújo, G., Llopis-Pastor, E., and Frasés, S. (2021). Trichosporon asahii as cause of nosocomial pneumonia in patient with COVID-19: a triple co-infection. *Arch. Bronconeumol.* 57 (Suppl 2): 46–48. https://doi.org/10.1016/j.arbres.2020.11.007.

54 Stasiak, C., Nigri, D., Cardoso, F. et al. (2021). Case report: incidental finding of COVID-19 infection after positron emission tomography/CT imaging in a patient with a diagnosis of histoplasmosis and recurring fever. *Am. J. Trop. Med. Hyg.* 104 (5): 1651–1654. https://doi.org/10.4269/ajtmh.20-0952.

55 Basso, R.P., Poester, V.R., Benelli, J.L. et al. (2021). COVID-19-associated histoplasmosis in an AIDS patient. *Mycopathologia* 186 (1): 109–112.

56 Verweij, P.E., Chiller, T.M., and Santiso, G. (2020). Coronavirus disease 2019 (COVID-19) in a patient with disseminated histoplasmosis and HIV-A case report from Argentina and literature review. *J. Fungi (Basel)* 6 (4): 275.

57 Bertolini, M., Mutti, M.F., Barletta, J.A. et al. (2020). COVID-19 associated with AIDS-related disseminated histoplasmosis: a case report. *Int. J. STD AIDS* 31 (12): 1222–1224.

58 De Wilton, A., Nabarro, L.E., Godbole, G.S. et al. (2021). Risk of *Strongyloides* hyperinfection syndrome when prescribing dexamethasone in severe COVID-19. *Travel Med. Infect. Dis.* 40: 101981.

59 Lier, A.J., Tuan, J.J., Davis, M.W. et al. (2020). Case report: disseminated Strongyloidiasis in a patient with COVID-19. *Am. J. Trop. Med. Hyg.* 103 (4): 1590–1592.

60 Wolday, D., Gebrecherkos, T., Arefaine, Z. et al. (2021). Effect of co-infection with intestinal parasites on COVID-19 severity: a prospective observational cohort study. *Eclinicalmedicine* 39: 101054. https://doi.org/10.1016/j.eclinm.2021.101054.

61 Gebrecherkos, T., Gessesse, Z., Kebede, Y. et al. (2021). Effect of co-infection with parasites on severity of COVID-19. *medRxiv* 2021.2002.2002.21250995. https://doi.org/10.1101/2021.02.02.21250995.

62 Ozaras, R., Cirpin, R., Duran, A. et al. (2020). Influenza and COVID-19 coinfection: report of six cases and review of the literature. *J. Med. Virol.* 92: 2657–2665. https://doi.org/10.1002/jmv.26125.

63 Yue, H., Zhang, M., Xing, L. et al. (2020). The epidemiology and clinical characteristics of co-infection of SARS-CoV-2 and influenza viruses in patients during COVID-19 outbreak. *J. Med. Virol.* 92 (11): 2870–2873. https://doi.org/10.1002/jmv.26163.

64 Yin, Z., Kang, Z., Yang, D. et al. (2020). A comparison of clinical and chest CT findings in patients with influenza A (H1N1) virus infection and coronavirus disease (COVID-19). *Am. J. Roentgenol.* 215 (5): 1065–1071. https://doi.org/10.2214/ajr.20.23214.

65 Dadashi, M., Khaleghnejad, S., Abedi Elkhichi, P. et al. (2021). COVID-19 and influenza co-infection: a systematic review and meta-analysis. *Front. Med. (Lausanne)* 8: 681469. https://doi.org/10.3389/fmed.2021.681469.

66 Bai, L., Zhao, Y., Dong, J. et al. (2021). Coinfection with influenza A virus enhances SARS-CoV-2 infectivity. *Cell Res.* 31: 395–403. https://doi.org/10.1038/s41422-021-00473-1.

67 Carosella, L.M., Pryluka, D., Maranzana, A. et al.; COVIDENGUE study Group(2021). Characteristics of patients co-infected with severe acute respiratory syndrome coronavirus 2 and dengue virus, Buenos Aires, Argentina, march-June 2020. *Emerg. Infect. Dis.* 27 (2): 348–351. https://doi.org/10.3201/eid2702.203439.

68 Cardona-Ospina, J.A., Arteaga-Livias, K., Villamil-Gómez, W.E. et al. (2021). Dengue and COVID-19,

overlapping epidemics? An analysis from Colombia. *J. Med. Virol.* 93: 522–527.

69 Phadke, R., Mohan, A., Çavdaroğlu, S. et al. (2021). Dengue amidst COVID-19 in India: the mystery of plummeting cases. *J. Med. Virol.* 93 (7): 4120–4121. https://doi.org/10.1002/jmv.26987.

70 Lustig, Y., Keler, S., Kolodny, R. et al. (2021). Potential antigenic cross-reactivity between severe acute respiratory syndrome coronavirus 2 (SARS-CoV-2) and dengue viruses. *Clin. Infect. Dis.* 73 (7): e2444–e2449.

71 Luhulima, D., Soetowo, T., and Amelia, R. (2021). Cross-reaction antibody test between SARS-CoV-2 and dengue hemorrhagic fever in Indonesia. *Indones. J. Clin. Pathol. Med. Lab.* 27 (2): 224. https://doi.org/10.24293/ijcpml.v27i2.1681.

72 Nasomsong, W., Luvira, V., and Phiboonbanakit, D. (2020). Case report: dengue and COVID-19 co-infection in Thailand. *Am. J. Trop. Med. Hyg.* 104 (2): 487–489.

73 Tsheten, T., Clements, A.C.A., Gray, D.J. et al. (2021). Clinical features and outcomes of COVID-19 and dengue co-infection: a systematic review. *BMC Infect. Dis.* 21: 729. https://doi.org/10.1186/s12879-021-06409-9.

74 Tiwari, L., Shekhar, S., Bansal, A., and Kumar, P. (2020). COVID-19 with dengue shock syndrome in a child: co-infection or cross-reactivity? *BMJ Case Rep.* 13 (12): e239315.

75 Saddique, A., Rana, M.S., Alam, M.M. et al. (2020). Emergence of co-infection of COVID-19 and dengue: a serious public health threat. *J. Infect.* 81 (6): e16–e18. https://doi.org/10.1016/j.jinf.2020.08.009.

76 Estofolete, C.F., Machado, L.F., Zini, N. et al. (2021). Presentation of fatal stroke due to SARS-CoV-2 and dengue virus coinfection. *J. Med. Virol.* 93: 1770–1775. https://doi.org/10.1002/jmv.26476.

77 Bicudo, N., Bicudo, E., Costa, J.D. et al. (2020). Co-infection of SARS-CoV-2 and dengue virus: a clinical challenge. *Braz. J. Infect. Dis.* 24 (5): 452–454.

78 Giannattasio, A., Maglione, M., D'Anna, C. et al. (2021). Silent RSV in infants with SARS-CoV-2 infection: a case series. *Pediatr. Pulmonol.* 56 (9): 3044–3046. https://doi.org/10.1002/ppul.25465.

79 Walsh, E.E. and Hall, C.B. (2015). Respiratory syncytial virus (RSV). In: *Mandell, Douglas, and Bennett's Principles and Practice of Infectious Diseases*, 1948–1960. New York: Elsevier.e3. https://doi.org/10.1016/B978-1-4557-4801-3.00160-0.

80 Jiang, S., Liu, P., Xiong, G. et al. (2020). Coinfection of SARS-CoV-2 and multiple respiratory pathogens in children. *Clin. Chem. Lab. Med.* 58: 1160–1161.

81 Wu, Q., Xing, Y., Shi, L. et al. (2020). Coinfection and other clinical characteristics of COVID-19 in children. *Pediatrics* 146 (1): e20200961. https://doi.org/10.1542/peds.2020-0961.

15

COVID-19: Neurology Perspective

Kiandokht Keyhanian[1], Raffaella Pizzolato Umeton[1,2], Babak Mohit[3], Brooke McNeilly[1], and Mehdi Ghasemi[1]

[1] Department of Neurology, University of Massachusetts Medical School, Worcester, MA, USA
[2] Department of Neurology, Massachusetts General Hospital, Harvard Medical School, Boston, MA, USA
[3] Sleep Disorders Center, Division of Pulmonary and Critical Care Medicine, Department of Medicine, University of Maryland School of Medicine, Baltimore, MD, USA

Abbreviations

ACE2	angiotensin-converting enzyme 2
ADEM	acute disseminated encephalomyelitis
AED	antiepileptic drug
ARDS	acute respiratory distress syndrome
BBB	blood–brain barrier
CNS	central nervous system
CRP	C-reactive protein
CRS	cytokine release syndrome
CSF	cerebrospinal fluid
CT	computed tomography
EEG	electroencephalography
EMG/NCS	electromyography/nerve conduction study
FLAIR	fluid-attenuated inversion recovery
GBS	Guillain–Barré syndrome
HEV	hemagglutinating encephalomyelitis virus
ICD-10	International Classification of Disease, 10th Revision
ICU	intensive care unit
IgG	immunoglobulin G
IL-6	interleukin-6
IVIG	intravenous immunoglobulin
MAL	macrophage activation-like syndrome
MERS	Middle East respiratory syndrome
MOG	myelin oligodendrocyte glycoprotein
NRP-1	neuropilin-1
RT-PCR	reverse transcription-polymerase chain reaction
SARS-CoV-2	severe acute respiratory syndrome coronavirus 2
WBC	white blood cell

The earliest reports of an atypical pneumonia epidemic in Wuhan, China, in December 2019 were associated with a novel strain of coronavirus, first retrieved from lower respiratory tract samples of four cases on 7 January 2020 [1]. The virus was later named severe acute respiratory syndrome coronavirus 2 (SARS-CoV-2) [2]; the disease was classified as coronavirus disease 2019 (COVID-19) and assigned the International Classification of Disease, 10th Revision (ICD-10) Code of U07-U012 [3]. Although the primary mode of attack of the SARS-CoV-2 is reported to be through respiratory pathways, early in the pandemic, reports from Wuhan, China, showed that some patients with COVID-19 also showed neurologic signs, such as headache, nausea, and vomiting [4]. The objective of this chapter is to review the neurologic signs and conditions associated with SARS-CoV-2 infection and COVID-19.

Coronavirus Disease 2019 (COVID-19): A Clinical Guide, First Edition. Edited by Ali Gholamrezanezhad and Michael P. Dube.
© 2023 John Wiley & Sons Ltd. Published 2023 by John Wiley & Sons Ltd.

Epidemiology and Transmission Mode

On 11 March 2020, the World Health Organization declared COVID-19 as a pandemic. As of the first anniversary of the declaration of a pandemic, by mid-March 2021, there have been more than 125 million cases with 2.5 million deaths reported from 192 countries [5], as well as the effects on billions of livelihoods with widespread social and economic ramifications in every continent around the globe. Clinical manifestations were initially reported to range from asymptomatic to severe symptomatic disease and a case fatality rate of 2.3% [6]. COVID-19 commonly manifests with dry cough, fever, fatigue, and dyspnea [7]. Symptoms of anosmia [7, 8] and ageusia [7] were later added as distinguishing symptoms. Although the majority of cases of COVID-19 have mild symptoms, some cases led to a cytokine storm followed by acute respiratory distress syndrome (ARDS) [9], thromboembolic events, septic shock, multiorgan failure, and ultimately death [10–12]. The time from exposure to onset of symptoms averages at 5 days but may vary between 2 and 14 days [7].

Early in the pandemic, SARS-CoV-2 was thought to be spread through droplets and contaminated surfaces, while evidence of aerosolized spread was limited [13]. Later evidence emerged, suggesting that the pathogen may also be spread through aerosols [14]. SARS-CoV-2 is primarily spread between people during close contact, most often through small droplets produced during coughing, sneezing, or talking [7]. Infection through touching a contaminated surface and then touching the face is now known to be less common [7]. Droplets are known to fall to the ground or surfaces, and do not travel through air over long distances [7]. SARS-CoV-2 is most contagious during the first three days after the onset of symptoms, although spread is possible before symptoms appear and from people who do not show symptoms [7].

The standard method of diagnosis of COVID-19 is by detecting the SARS-CoV-2 RNA through a real-time reverse transcription-polymerase chain reaction (RT-PCR) test collected via a nasopharyngeal swab [15]. Imaging through computed tomography (CT) of the chest also has been a reliable source for diagnosis in individuals where there is a high suspicion of infection based on symptoms and risk factors [16].

Route to the Nervous System

So far, there are three suggested pathways for coronaviruses to enter the central nervous system (CNS): (i) retrograde through neurons, (ii) angiotensin-converting enzyme 2 (ACE-2) expression in neurons, and (iii) hematogenous dissemination [17, 18]. In addition, damage to the CNS is mediated by an indirect effect of the virus causing a cytokine storm [19, 20].

Retrograde Pathway Through Neurons

Olfactory Pathway

The olfactory nerve contains bipolar neurons, which tie the nasal epithelium to the CNS via brain stem, specifically midbrain, hypothalamus, basal ganglia, and finally, cortex [21, 22]. Some viral families, such as Herpesviridae, Coronaviridae, Flaviviridae, Togaviridae, and Rhabdoviridae families, can affect the olfactory nerve through the nasal epithelium bridge, so the olfactory nerve is considered a unique direct gate from periphery to CNS [23]. There are evidences showing the presence of prior coronavirus family members in the CNS and using the olfactory tract as their mean in early stages of infection [24, 25]. The presence of hyposmia in a large number of patients with COVID-19 implies the existence of SARS-CoV-2 in the olfactory system [20]. In a multicentric cohort in Europe, there were symptoms of olfactory dysfunction in 85.6% of the patients with mild to moderate COVID-19 infection and, interestingly, in 11.8% of these patients, olfactory symptoms preceded other symptoms [26]. Coolen et al. [27] could show the presence of SARS-CoV-2 only in olfactory bulbs. However, a contrasting research study suggested that SARS-CoV-2 is more likely to target human olfactory epithelium via Bowman's cells, sustentacular cells, mucosal cells, and olfactory stem cells and might not directly enter olfactory sensory neurons [28]. Another controversy involves the presence or absence of ACE-2 receptors in the olfactory system. Although single-cell transcriptional analysis demonstrated absence of ACE-2 receptors in glial cells and olfactory sensory neurons and some other olfactory cells pathway [12, 29], there is evidence for the presence of the ACE-2 receptor on the surface of cilia cells in the olfactory system [20]. Another proposed mechanism for viral entry is through the anterograde vesicular axonal pathway and affecting olfactory receptor neurons and olfactory endothelia [12, 29]. Dendrites of olfactory sensory neurons have an unprotected exposure to inspirational air in the nose [30]. Lastly, SARS-CoV-2 triggers a cytokine storm both systemically and locally from accessory cells in the olfactory system, which might contribute to the damage in the olfactory system [22, 29]. Interestingly, magnetic resonance imaging (MRI) has shown hyperintensity in olfactory bulb and posterior gyrus rectus, which is assumed as olfactory cortex in a patient with anosmia [31].

Other Cranial Nerves

Other points in the body that are plausible ways of viral entry and access to the nervous system are lung, gastrointestinal tract, and conjunctiva. These locations bring our attention to the trigeminal and the vagal nerves. Previously, influenza virus and hemagglutinating encephalomyelitis virus (HEV) were demonstrated to be able to enter nerve endings and travel retrogradely [32, 33]. SARS-CoV-2 is very well known to involve the lung and gastrointestinal tract. Therefore, vagal nerve afferents can be a potential point of viral entry and transport virus retrograde to CNS [4, 34]. Other local peripheral nerves that reside in the gastrointestinal system are also potential gateways for virus through their exposure to other cells [35–37]. Moreover, there is evidence of the presence of SARS-CoV-2 RNA in conjunctiva in patients with conjunctivitis. Thus, the trigeminal nerve, which has sensory fibers in conjunctiva, as well as interaction with nociceptive cells in nasal cavity, can be considered as a potential gateway for viral entry to the CNS [36, 38].

Direct Infection Through ACE-2 Expression

SARS-CoV-2 expresses spike-like proteins on its surface, which has affinity to ACE-2 receptors. ACE-2 is expressed in respiratory and gastrointestinal systems, as well as the nervous system, and is very crucial for cardiac function, blood pressure control, oxygen exchange at the level of alveoli, and the rennin–angiotensin system [39, 40]. One way for neuronal infection is ACE-2 expression that is further discussed in mechanisms of CNS complications.

Hematogenous Pathway

When the blood–brain barrier (BBB) is disrupted, this may provide a potential source of infection spread to the CNS. CNS invasion can be through direct attack or through migration of infected leukocytes to the CNS [35]. Using infected leukocytes to attack the CNS through a mechanism called "Trojan Horse" is thought to be the mechanism HIV and Zika virus use for reaching the CNS [18, 41, 42]. Previously influenza and other viruses in the coronavirus family demonstrated their potential to cross a damaged BBB [23, 24, 43]. Mouse hepatitis virus is a coronavirus that can enter the CNS through disruption of the BBB [44–46]. SARS-CoV was found in human cerebrum during its pandemic [47], and also SARS-CoV-2 was found within brain endothelial capillary pericytes during human postmortem studies that strongly support hematogenous spread of SARS-CoV-2 to the CNS [48].

Several mechanisms have been proposed for disrupting the BBB by coronaviruses, including interaction with ACE-2, disrupting tight junctions, and neuroinflammation. Endothelial cells in the BBB express ACE-2, which is a target for SARS-CoV, and attacking this target encourages more penetration of virus to the CNS [18, 49]. Mouse hepatitis virus also seems to be capable of disrupting tight junctions of endothelial cells in the microvascular system and lead to increased permeability [50]. In addition, an increased inflammatory state and cytokine storm as a result of coronavirus infection might cause increased permeability of the BBB, making the CNS more vulnerable to infection [18, 51].

Mechanisms for CNS Complications

Neuronal Infection

For any viral infection and entry to the host cell, the most critical determinant of affinity and infectivity to the host is receptor recognition. When there is the strongest binding affinity between host receptor and viral antigen, there is the greatest chance of infection. If a new virus in a family builds a sturdier and stronger bond with the host receptor, natural selection would most likely choose this strain over prior ones. The affinity of host receptor and viral antigen is determined by the combination of amino residues in the binding domain and their hydrophilic versus hydrophobic propensities. Among viruses, RNA viruses have the highest rate of mutation, which makes them much more adaptable to the host while giving them the best chance of reaching the most favorable of combination of amino acid residues in their host binding domain [52].

The Coronaviridae family is a group of RNA viruses with oval shape covered by an envelope of spike (S) glycoproteins. Having a spike as envelope and being oval gives them a crown figure under electron microscopy. *Corona* means "crown" and is originating from this figure [20, 53]. Although SARS-CoV and SARS-CoV-2 have an analogous 3D structure and homology in terms of trimeric S proteins combination, their receptor binding affinity toward ACE-2 is different due to new series of mutations [54–56]. One of these mutation series involves ACE-2 hotspot 31, which includes a hydrophobic location for a salt bridge between Lys31 in host receptor and its counterpart in coronavirus. In the earlier civet-SARS-CoV, lysine interacted with lysine on the other side, leading to steric and electrostatic interference between host and virus salt bridge [57]. Subsequently, after a mutation caused substitution of lysine with asparagine in the viral domain to interact with lysine-31 in the ACE-2 host domain, affinity toward human ACE-2 and SARS-COV increased and facilitated interspecies viral transmission. Several similar mutations have taken place during coronaviruses evolution; some were more favorable and some were unfavorable for viral transmission. We still observe the variable affinities of SARS-CoV versus SARS-CoV-2 toward human ACE-2 receptor [57]. As discussed previously, ACE-2 receptor, which is a target for SARS-CoV-2, is expressed in multiple tissues, including glial cells and neurons in the CNS [49]. If the virus can penetrate the CNS via prior discussed mechanisms, then its main targets are neurons and glial cells [58, 59]. Cells with ACE-2 receptor are also particularly abundant in brain stem and are involved in regulating the cardiovascular system via the reticular activating system [60]. Despite a large amount of evidence for affinity of coronaviruses to ACE-2, ACE-2 is not the sole mechanism of viral entry to the cells. Some liver cells, despite very low or nonexpression of ACE-2 receptor, could become infected with coronaviruses [61, 62]. Another proposed receptor for SARS-CoV-2 is human protein neuropilin-1 (NRP-1). Mouse models showed that NRP-1 allows viral entry to the CNS, and antibodies against NRP-1

can block human cells infection by SARS-CoV [63]. Also, retrograde infection of neurons through synaptic routes is another infection pathway as discussed earlier [32, 64]. HEV is one of the coronavirus models that favors the retrograde pathway. Because HEV infects human cells, endoplasmic reticulum–Golgi intermediate compartments start producing viral particles and assemble them into virions that would be eventually secreted from the nerve cells into the adjacent matrix [64–66]. Delayed involvement of brain after inoculation of SARS-COV and HCoV-OC43 intranasally is a support for retrograde transmission of virus [22, 67].

Eventually, after cell infection with coronaviruses, cell death will follow. Several pathways are involved in cell death, including apoptosis, pyroptosis, autophagy, or phagocytosis by innate immune cells [68, 69]. After massive cell death in critical brain pathways, life-threatening consequences, such as cardiac or respiratory arrest, might occur. Cells that contain viral antigens have been found in brain stem regions, including nucleus ambiguus and solitarius [4, 66, 70].

Neuroinflammation

Immune response toward SARS-CoV-2 follows two phases, innate and adaptive immune responses. The main components of innate immune response are neutrophils, macrophages, and natural killer cells, while lymphocytes, whether T cells as cytotoxic CD8[+] or CD4[+] T helper cells, as well as B cells, play the most important parts in the adaptive immune response [66]. In studies that determined the total amount of different cell types in patients infected by SARS-CoV-2, there was an enhanced response of neutrophils compensated by a decrease in total number of lymphocytes, monocytes, eosinophilic cells, and basophilic cells. Although the absolute number of lymphocytes is reduced after SARS-CoV-2 infection, the main affected cell types are regulatory and memory T helper cells, while the total number of naive T cells and proinflammatory T helper CD4[+] IL-17[+] cells might increase [71–74]. Increase in proinflammatory cell lines results in a boost of inflammatory cytokine production or cytokine storm. The main proinflammatory cytokines that are released seem to be interleukin-6 (IL-6), tumor necrosis factor-α (TNF-α), IL-2, IL-7, and granulocyte colony-stimulating factor. This heavy cytokine release can be called "cytokine release syndrome (CRS)" or can be the result of "secondary hemophagocytic lymphohistiocytosis," also called "macrophage activation-like syndrome (MAL)" [75, 76]. CRS is a catastrophic phenomenon followed sometimes by sepsis after organ transplantation, CAR T cell therapy, and some viral infections. Common clinical features of CRS are fever, hypotension, and encephalopathy, as well as bone marrow suppression and eventually multiorgan failure [76, 77]. MAL generally complicates hematologic malignancies and infections and also shares most of these clinical features [71]. Moderate to severe cases of SARS-CoV-2 infection demonstrated an increase in IL-6, which occurs in both CRS and MAL [19]. Increased IL-6 and tumor necrosis factor-α assists disruption of BBB [78, 79], eventually leading to CNS involvement and complications, such as encephalitis, demyelination, and necrotizing events in the CNS and Guillain–Barré syndrome (GBS) in the peripheral nervous system [80–85]. The monoclonal antibody against IL-6 receptor tocilizumab demonstrated some benefit in treating severe cases of SARS-CoV-2 infection presumably by reducing the damage an IL-6 storm could make [77, 86, 87]. However, as of yet, there is not sufficient evidence to clarify the exact role of systemic inflammation versus local inflammation as a result of the direct viral infection or hypoxia, which is a common complication of SARS-CoV-2 infection.

Other Mechanisms

Generally, a disease process involving lung might cause CNS complications, and CNS diseases can cause respiratory distress as well while they contain centers for respiration and cardiovascular regulation [88]. As previously described, brain stem infection with SARS-CoV-2 has been previously demonstrated, and it can cause damage to respiratory and cardiovascular centers in the brain stem when causing massive cell death in these centers leading to respiratory/cardiovascular arrest [4, 66, 70]. In some patients with SARS-CoV-2 lung infection complicated by ARDS, the pathophysiology of ARDS seems to be atypical, because despite severity of hypoxemia, they show relatively preserved lung mechanics. It is possible that this type of ARDS is a result of dysregulated lung perfusion and hypoxic vasoconstriction due to damage in brain stem centers for the respiratory/cardiovascular system and not exclusively in lung [89]. Also, when lungs are involved severely by infection, an interruption in alveolar gas exchange might lead to anaerobic metabolism in

brain cells and cause "infectious toxic encephalopathy," which is a sort of CNS hypoxia. In turn, CNS hypoxia would result in cell swelling and interstitial edema, and eventually increased intracranial hypertension and its complications [20, 88]. Hypoxic brain damage may also trigger the loop of local microglial activation and systemic inflammation [20, 90].

An additional complication of SARS-CoV-2 infection similar to other coronaviruses, including SARS and Middle East respiratory syndrome (MERS) [91, 92], is activating the hypercoagulable state. There is evidence of hypercoagulability in patients with SARS-CoV-2 infection that is measurable by thrombocytopenia, increased D-dimer level, and prolongation of prothrombin time and activated partial thromboplastin time [93]. As expected, potential complications of increased hypercoagulability, such as ischemic strokes and cerebral venous sinus thrombosis, are seen, along with myocardial infarction or pulmonary embolism [94, 95]. Despite this thrombotic tendency, there have been reports of cerebral hemorrhage [96] in patients with SARS-CoV-2 infection. The exact mechanism for thrombophilic or hemorrhagic tendencies during SARS-CoV-2 infection is not well understood yet. However, one of the proposed mechanisms is overactivation of nicotinamide adenine dinucleotide phosphate oxidase 2 (NOX-2) in serum of SARS-CoV-2-infected patients causing excessive production of reactive oxygen species [97]. NOX-2 overactivation was demonstrated in both severe SARS-CoV-2 infection and in milder cases with thrombotic complications [97]. Also, coagulopathy is an end result of thrombocytopenia, which is a common finding in SARS-CoV-2 infection [98]. To explain hemorrhagic cerebral events, there are theories implicating ACE-2 disruption by SARS-CoV-2 infection causing dysregulation of cerebral blood flow, hypertension, and arterial wall rupture, rendering the CNS to hemorrhagic events [99].

Neurologic Manifestations

Patients with SARS-CoV-2 infection may also experience neurologic symptoms and complications (Table 15.1) [54, 73, 100–121]. Early investigation in Wuhan, China, revealed that ~36% of patients with COVID-19 had neurologic presentations that included dizziness (16.8%), headache (13.1%), skeletal muscle injury (myalgia combined with elevated serum creatinine kinase [CK] level [hyper-CKemia], 10.7%), decreased level of consciousness (7.5%),

Table 15.1   COVID-19-related neurologic clinical presentation.

Region	Patients	Age (yr)	Female (%)	Neurologic symptoms (%)	References
China (799)	113 deaths	68 (median)	30 (27)	Myalgia (19), headache (10), dizziness (9), ↓ consciousness (22)	[54]
	161 recovered	51 (median)	73 (45)	Myalgia (24), headache (12), dizziness (7), ↓ consciousness (1)	
China	214	52.7 (mean)	127 (59.3)	Dizziness (16.8), headache (13.1), skeletal muscle injury (10.7), ↓ consciousness (7.5), ageusia (5.6), anosmia (5.1), stroke (2.8, ischemic [66.3], hemorrhagic [16.7]), nerve pain (2.3), visual change (1.4), ataxia (0.5), seizure (0.5)	[100]
China	41	49 (median)	11 (29)	Headache (8), myalgia or fatigue (44)	[101]
China (710)	52 critically ill	59.7 (mean)	17 (33)	Headache (6), myalgia (11.5), malaise (35)	[102]
China	138	56 (median)	63 (45.7)	Fatigue (69.6), myalgia (34.8), dizziness (9.4), headache (6.5)	[103]
China	99	55.5 (mean)	32 (32)	Myalgia (11), confusion (9), headache (8)	[104]
China	452	58 (mean)	217 (48)	Myalgia (21.4), confusion (0.7), headache (11.4), dizziness (8.1), fatigue (46.4)	[73]
China	140	57 (median)	69 (49.3)	Fatigue (75)	[105]
China	85 fatal cases	65.8 (mean)	23 (27.1)	Fatigue (58.8), myalgia (16.5), headache (4.7)	[106]
China	221	55 (median)	113 (51.1)	Fatigue (70.6), headache (7.7)	[107]
China	917	48.7 (mean)	417 (44.8)	↓ Consciousness (2.7), stroke (1.1), muscle cramp (0.2), headache (0.2), occipital neuralgia (0.1), tremor/tic (0.2)	[108]
China	645	Not reported	317 (49.1)	Myalgia (11), fatigue (18.3), headache (10.4)	[109]
China	91	50 (median)	54 (59.34)	Fatigue (44), headache (7.7), myalgia (5.5), back discomfort (3.3)	[110]
China	62	41 (median)	27 (43.5)	Headache (34), myalgia or fatigue (52)	[111]
China	90	50 (mean)	51 (56.7)	Fatigue/weakness (21), myalgia (28), headache (4)	[112]
China	149	45.11 (mean)	68 (45.6)	Headache (8.7), myalgia (3.4)	[113]
China	137	57 (median)	76 (55.5)	Myalgia or fatigue (32.1%), headache (9.5)	[114]
China	13	34 (median)	3 (23.1)	Myalgia 3 (23.1), headache (23.1)	[115]
China	262	47.5 (median)	216 (82.4)	Fatigue (26.3), headache (6.5)	[116]
China	1099	47 (median)	459 (41.9)	Headache (13.6), fatigue (38.1), myalgia/arthralgia (14.9)	[117]
China	50	43.9 (mean)	21 (42)	Headache (10), myalgia (16), fatigue (16)	[118]
South Korea	28	42.6 (mean)	13 (46.1)	Myalgia (14.3), fatigue (10.7)	[119]
India	21	40.3 (mean)	7 (33.3)	Headache (14.3)	[120]
South Iran	113	53.75 (mean)	42 (37.2)	Fatigue (66.4), myalgia or arthralgia (61.1), headache (53.1), dizziness or vertigo (39.8)	[121]

ageusia (5.6%), anosmia (5.1%), stroke (2.8%), nerve pain (2.3%), visual impairment (1.4%), seizure (0.5%), and ataxia (0.5%) [100]. Patients with severe COVID-19 infection were found to have more neurologic manifestations, primarily impaired consciousness, stroke, and skeletal muscle injury [100]. Patients older than 60 years had higher rates of neurologic manifestations and mortality [108]. In addition, new onset of neurologic critical events (e.g. impaired consciousness and stroke) increased mortality risk by six times in patients with COVID-19 [108]. In general, the most common reported neurologic symptoms in patients with COVID-19 include fatigue/malaise, myalgia, headache, impaired consciousness, dizziness, ageusia, and anosmia; less common manifestations are visual acuity change, nerve pain, occipital neuralgia, ataxia, tremor, and tic. An increasing number of case reports and series also demonstrate that various neurologic conditions and autoimmune complications occur in relation with SARS-CoV-2 infection, which mainly include GBSs, myopathy and rhabdomyolysis, encephalopathy, meningoencephalitis, encephalomyelitis, myelitis, and acute cerebrovascular events.

Guillain–Barré Syndromes

Classic GBS typically presents with acute (less than four weeks) ascending muscle weakness, decreased deep tendon reflexes, occasional sensation changes in the form of sensory loss or radicular pain, and less frequently cranial nerve involvement [122]. Treatment of GBS is based on symptoms with the utmost emphasis on respiratory monitoring because respiratory failure is the most feared complication. Supportive care and immunotherapy, including intravenous immunoglobulin (IVIG) and plasmapheresis, are the effective treatments, with intravenous steroids proving to be ineffective [123].

GBS cases are thought in large part to result from the development of postinfectious autoimmunity. Approximately two-thirds of cases may have had a viral illness one to three weeks before the neurologic manifestations [124]. Thus, unsurprisingly, GBS outbreaks have been observed alongside viral epidemics, including those with coronaviruses (i.e. MERS-CoV and SARS-CoV) [124, 125], with the first SARS-CoV-2 (COVID-19) case reported in January 2020 [126].

Abu-Rumeileh et al. [127] performed an extensive systematic review compiling 73 documented cases of GBS and variants worldwide in patients with known SARS-CoV-2 [127]. A predominant portion of the patients had the classic COVID-19 symptoms, such as cough (72%), fever (74%), diarrhea (18%), dyspnea (64%), ageusia (22%), and anosmia (21%). Most of these patients presented with classic clinical GBS findings of rapidly progressive ascending paralysis, areflexia, varying degrees of sensory changes, and cranial nerve involvement. Sixty-two cases had documented electromyography/nerve conduction study (EMG/NCS) results, with demyelinating features seen in 48 of the cases, axonal damage features in only 9 cases, and 5 cases showing a mix of demyelinating and axonal features. Overall, 82% of the patients met criteria for acute inflammatory demyelinating polyneuropathy, 13% for acute motor and sensory axonal neuropathy, and 5% for acute motor axonal neuropathy. About 71% of the patients who underwent CSF analysis had the classic albuminocytologic dissociation [127]. Significant is that every CSF sample tested for COVID-19 with the real-time RT-PCR, 31 in total, tested negative, thus leading to the assumption of no active intrathecal SARS-CoV-2 replication or root infection. This finding, along with favorable outcomes post-IVIG, may suggest an underlying autoimmune process. Overall, IVIG led to a favorable improvement, if not complete resolution of symptoms, in the 60 patients who received it. Anti-GD1b and anti-GM1 were positive in two cases, strengthening the assumption of an autoimmune etiology; however, negative antibodies were found on 33 other occurrences. Thus, there is no solid evidence at this time of an underlying autoimmune process, but this is something that warrants further future investigation [127].

Molecular mimicry induces antibodies against different gangliosides (GM1, GD1a, GT1a, and GQ1b) in some of the axonal-type GBS variants, and the targets of these antibodies are known to be expressed in the peripheral nerves [124]. There is evidence that SARS-CoV-2 S protein binds to sialic acid–containing glycoprotein and gangliosides on the cell surfaces leading to increased viral transmissibility [128]. Thus, there is potential for cross reaction to occur if the epitopes from the SARS-CoV-2 antigens are able to react with the peripheral nerve glycolipids and trigger the formation of cellular autoimmunity. Therefore, checking anti-ganglioside antibodies could lead to further insight into the disease pathophysiology and this proposed mechanism in the future.

Skeletal Muscle Injury

An early clinical study from Wuhan [100] reported that skeletal muscle injury, defined as myalgia plus hyper-CKemia, was present in about 11% of patients with COVID-19. Although case reports of rhabdomyolysis with CK levels as high as >11,000 U/l have been reported in patients with COVID-19 [129–131], an association of SARS-CoV-2 with either viral or necrotizing autoimmune myositis is still elusive. Two reported cases may indirectly suggest a SARS-CoV-2-triggered necrotizing autoimmune myositis [130, 131]. The first case is a man, aged 88 years, from New York, presenting with acute, painful bilateral proximal lower-limb weakness and hyperCKemia (13,581 U/l) [131] who was found to be COVID positive and started on hydroxychloroquine; his weakness and CK levels improved one week later. The second case is a man, aged 60 years, from Wuhan, with six-day COVID-positive pneumonia and fever who seven days later, despite improvement in his clinical condition, developed painful proximal muscle weakness with hyperCKemia (11,842 U/l) and elevated C-reactive protein (CRP) and benefited from IVIG therapy [130]. A more recent study also reported six intensive care unit (ICU)-admitted cases (age between 51 and 72 years) with COVID-19 who had acute flaccid quadriplegia [132]. EMG/NCS showed myopathic features in all of these patients, and CK levels were normal to mildly elevated (highest level of 1274 U/l), suggesting the presence of critical illness myopathy [132]. Overall, these observations may necessitate pursuing more investigations, such as muscle biopsy and antibody screening in some patients with COVID-19 with signs of skeletal muscle injury, because treatment with IVIG may potentially improve functional outcomes in these patients. Notably, ACE-2 is shown to be expressed in skeletal muscles [133]; thus, evaluation of direct SARS-CoV-2 infection of skeletal muscle fibers should be studied.

Encephalopathy

The potential neurotropism and neuroinvasive capability of human coronavirus infections have been described in the literature. These viruses are able to reach the brain mainly through the olfactory bulb or hematogenous route, causing inflammation and demyelination, probably related to abnormal host immune responses with autoimmunity and/or direct CNS damage as a result of viral replication and infiltration [24]. With regard to SARS-CoV-2, ACE-2 and transmembrane protease, serine 2 (TMPRSS2) expressed in the oligodendrocytes are documented co-receptors for its entry; therefore, a direct involvement of white matter in the case of encephalitis related to COVID-19 infection is possible [134, 135], although a postinfectious immune-mediated process is also a possible etiology (Figure 15.1) [136]. A retrospective study [137] of 235 ICU COVID-19-positive patients showed that 21% experienced neurologic symptoms. MRI data from 27 of 50 (37) patients showed cortical FLAIR (fluid-attenuated inversion recovery) abnormalities with cortical diffusion restriction, leptomeningeal enhancement, or cortical blooming artifact in a nonspecific pattern, as well as subcortical and deep white matter FLAIR lesions in only 3 patients. Interestingly, there was no correlation between the MRI findings and patients' symptomatology. Half of the patients with cortical FLAIR abnormalities also underwent a lumbar puncture, and cerebrospinal fluid (CSF) findings included elevated proteins (mean, 80 mg/dl; range, 60–110 mg/dl), normal cell count, glucose level, immunoglobulin G (IgG) index, oligoclonal bands, and albumin, as well as negative real-time RT-PCR for SARS-CoV-2 [137]. A case report from the United Kingdom described a case of rhombencephalitis with involvement of the right inferior cerebellar peduncle who presented with fever and respiratory symptoms, progressive unsteady gait, diplopia, limb ataxia, altered sensation in the right arm, hiccups, and dribbling when eating. CSF test results showed normal protein, normal white blood cell (WBC) counts, and negative bacterial culture [138]. Neuropathology reports of 18 brain specimens from encephalopathic patients showed foci of perivascular lymphocytes and focal leptomeningeal inflammation, confirming the presence of brain inflammatory changes related to COVID-19, although these findings were reported as rare and did not support an underlying diagnosis of encephalitis. Immunohistochemical analyses to detect SARS-CoV-2 by real-time RT-PCR were negative, and the virus was

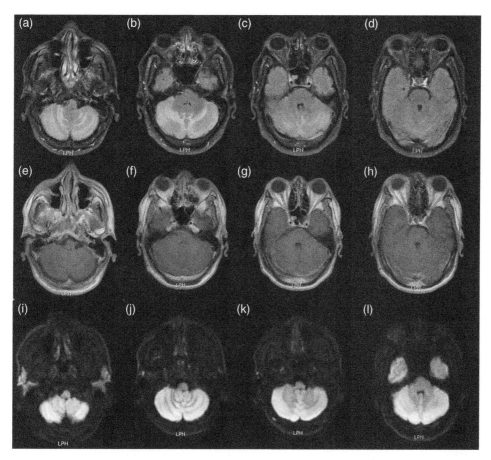

Figure 15.1 Axial T2 fluid-attenuated inversion recovery (a–d), T1 with contrast (e–h), and diffusion-weighted imaging (i–l) brain magnetic resonance imaging (MRI) sequences of a 39-year-old man who, five weeks after his self-recovered nasopharyngeal reverse transcription-polymerase chain reaction–proved COVID-19 infection, presented to the emergency department with three-day worsening vomiting, tiredness, elevated blood pressure, acute confusion, and gait ataxia. The brain MRI demonstrated bilateral cerebellar edema with effacement of cisterns and crowding of the foramen magnum, without restricted diffusion or gross abnormal enhancement, consistent with post-COVID-19 inflammatory cerebellitis. The other infectious and metabolic workup was unremarkable, and the serum severe acute respiratory syndrome coronavirus 2 immunoglobulin G was positive at the time. The patient's condition improved with supportive care, including intravenous fluid and blood pressure management, with no residual neurologic symptoms at eight weeks of outpatient follow-up. Imaging was performed on a 1.5-Tesla system. LPH, left posterior head axis.

detected at low levels in only five patients, which could be secondary to direct infiltration in the brain or hematogenous spread of viral RNA [139]. On the basis of available studies, virus is not usually detected in CSF by RT-PCR except in rare cases, and pleocytosis is usually absent. Interestingly, there is the report of a 39-year-old man with delirium that progressed to somnolence, coma, and death and in which postmortem neuropathology of brain specimens detected SARS-CoV-2 antigen by immunohistochemistry and viral RNA by in situ hybridization [140].

The number of cases of encephalopathy as one of the presenting symptoms or complications of COVID-19 is rapidly accumulating. Encephalitis is secondary to an inflammatory process of the brain and surrounding tissues with a broad spectrum of symptoms that include altered mental status, headache, behavioral changes, and psychiatric disturbances in association with focal neurologic signs (e.g. paresthesia, weakness) (Figure 15.1). Meningitis instead is an inflammatory process involving the meninges and spinal cord and manifests usually as neck stiffness, fever, headache, photophobia, or phonophobia. Seizures could also be part of the encephalitis and meningitis presentation [141, 142]. Encephalitis and meningitis can present with symptoms of diverse severity, which makes the proper diagnosis in patients with mild manifestations difficult. In addition, the inability to distinguish the underlying process (infectious or toxic-metabolic) based only on the symptoms causes further complexity in the diagnosis and management of encephalopathies, in which there is no evidence of direct invasion by the virus. Many patients with a severe form of COVID-19 infection may present with altered mental status from the toxic-metabolic processes as a result of hypoxia, electrolyte derangements, metabolic disturbances, and multiorgan failure, without necessarily presenting involvement of the CNS. Also, a few patients with COVID-19 presented with a rare form of acute necrotizing encephalopathy without CSF PCR for SARS-CoV-2 data [83, 143, 144]. Acute necrotizing encephalopathy is characterized by neuroinflammation secondary to cytokine storm with multifocal symmetric lesions in the gray and white matter without direct viral damage. In addition, there are also reports of demyelinating lesions. A case report of a 54-year-old woman admitted initially for respiratory distress caused by COVID-19 infection with only a history of mild elevated blood pressure under treatment showed lesions in the white matter and globus pallidus. Her Glasgow Coma Scale score was 14 with altered sensorium, but her neurologic examination was nonfocal on admission, then rapidly deteriorated and required endotracheal intubation. She was treated with hydroxychloroquine, azithromycin, and amoxicillin-clavulanic acid and kept sedated for two days. After discontinuation of sedation, the patient remained obtunded for a long period, and this prompted neuroimaging and further investigations. Brain MRI showed bilateral asymmetric restricted diffusion lesions without hemorrhage or enhancement in the supratentorial periventricular white matter and globus pallidus, without involvement of the thalamus, striatum, and posterior fossa. Two days later, she had a repeated MRI brain that showed homogeneous contrast enhancement of the lesions with negative vascular images. CSF studies, performed twice (on admission and nine days after), were reportedly unremarkable, including real-time RT-PCR for SARS-CoV-2. The patient received steroids for suspected demyelination

12 days later after her hospitalization upon a negative nasopharyngeal PCR with subsequent slight improvement of her mental status and residual right-sided hemiplegia [145]. There is also a case of myelin oligodendrocyte glycoprotein (MOG)-associated encephalitis reported in a 23-year-old man admitted for cognitive slowing and personality changes, left-sided headache, and dysesthesias who was found to be COVID-19 positive. MRI brain showed diffuse left-hemispheric cortical FLAIR hyperintensity in association with left-hemispheric leptomeningeal enhancement. A lumbar puncture showed elevated opening pressure (33 cm H_2O), 0 RBCs, 57 WBCs with lymphocytic predominance, and normal glucose and protein levels, as well as negative oligoclonal bands. Viral testing was negative. Serum MOG antibody results were positive, while the CSF autoimmune encephalopathy panel was negative. On treatment with a five-day course of intravenous methylprednisolone, he improved clinically and radiographically [146]. Demyelination has been described to be associated with coronavirus, both in murine animal models [147] and in a pediatric patient with acute disseminated encephalomyelitis (ADEM) [148].

In a retrospective observational case series from Wuhan [100] of 214 patients with laboratory-confirmed diagnosis, 24.8% had CNS manifestation and 7.5% presented with encephalopathy. Neurologic manifestation appeared to be more commonly associated with severe COVID-19 infection compared with nonsevere infection, with encephalopathy present in 14.8% of cases versus 2.4% ($P < 0.001$), respectively. The severe cases have in common older age and more comorbidities (hypertension, diabetes, malignancies, vascular diseases of kidney issues), with only a small proportion presenting with typical symptoms such as fever or cough. The severe cases also showed marked inflammatory response with higher levels of WBC counts, neutrophil counts, blood urea nitrogen, D-dimer, and CRP, and reduced lymphocyte and platelet counts. The neurologic complications usually tended to appear a few days after the admission, with associated higher mortality rate. Other case reports described encephalopathic patients who presented with new onset of seizure as a manifestation of COVID-19 meningoencephalitis [82, 141, 142].

Given the complexity of patients with COVID-19 with encephalopathies, recognition of underlying encephalitis/meningitis is not easy with lack of CSF or serologic biomarkers [137, 149]. Therefore, detailed neurologic examination, as well the use of electrophysiologic studies (i.e. electroencephalography [EEG]), CSF analysis, and brain imaging, can help in early diagnosis and treatment of these conditions with possible better outcomes [150–152]. Seizures should also be suspected in patients with COVID-19 with unclear or prolonged altered sensorium given the fact that cases of clinical or subclinical seizures or status epilepticus have been reported [142]. Seizure could be direct brain viral damage or related to toxic-metabolic derangements [141]. Antiepileptic drugs (AEDs) are usually recommended after the initial diagnosis of seizure to prevent further episodes for a period of six weeks with subsequent taper in one to two weeks [141]. Many patients with COVID-19 who manifest seizures are often critically ill; therefore, the use of intravenous AEDs is recommended with reduced side effects on respiratory and cardiac status (i.e. levetiracetam and/or brivaracetam). Phenytoin and valproic acid should be avoided in patients treated with extracorporeal membrane oxygenation because this interferes with the pharmacokinetics of highly protein-bound AEDs [141].

Meningoencephalitis

The lack of evidence of direct viral damage in the brain represented by the inability to detect the virus in the CSF suggests that SARS-CoV-2 only rarely causes encephalitis via this mechanism [153]. It is not possible to exclude meningoencephalitis as a consequence of immune-mediated inflammation or induction of an autoimmune response via molecular mimicry [136]. The first case of COVID-19 encephalitis with associated laboratory confirmation was reported in Beijing in a patient with altered mental status, seizures, slow pupillary response, persistent hiccups, hyperreflexia, and meningeal irritation. CSF studies were normal with the exception of increased opening pressure and positive PCR for SARS-CoV-2 [38, 152]. This case report was published in Chinese, and it lacked further data to support the diagnosis. Several other cases were then reported with clinical presentation consistent with meningoencephalitis without positive CSF studies [82, 154]. These cases had in common the presence of CSF pleocytosis, mildly elevated proteins with normal MRI, and again negative SARS-CoV-2 CSF PCR [57, 155, 156]. Other case reports of meningoencephalitis with

positive nasopharyngeal swab but negative CSF PCR for SARS-CoV-2 had elevated CSF protein levels with sometimes associated lymphocytosis. Some of the cases had MRI findings with white matter and cortical abnormalities and contrast enhancement compatible with meningoencephalitis. An underlying autoimmune etiology was suspected for both MRI positive and negative patients, and these patients underwent treatment with plasmapheresis. Improvements of the clinical status were observed in five of six patients, and MRI findings were reversible in all patients with positive MRI [157, 158]. Improvement with immunotherapy was also seen in another similar case in Italy [156]. Another case of COVID-19 meningoencephalitis [82] was reported in a young patient with headache, fatigue, fever with worsening mental status and new onset of seizure, and clear meningeal signs on examination. Blood work showed pleocytosis, CT scan of the head was negative, and interestingly, SARS-CoV-2 was detected only in the CSF and not in the nasopharyngeal swab. CSF showed elevated opening pressure and 12 WBCs mainly mononuclear; MRI showed diffusion-weighted imaging hyperintensity at the level of the wall of the inferior horn of the right ventricle and FLAIR abnormalities in the right mesial temporal lobe and hippocampus. It is noteworthy to mention that false RT-PCR positivity could be the result of sample contamination from shed airborne virus [134]. A French study on brain 2-desoxy-2-fluoro-D-glucose-positron-emission tomography/CT imaging in four patients with COVID-19 encephalopathy showed frontal hypometabolism and cerebellar hypermetabolism in all of them [159]. All patients responded to immunotherapy, reflecting an underlying immune process that targets possibly the prefrontal and orbitofrontal cortices. This pattern is different from the global cortical hypometabolism seen in a patient with delirium [160]. Interestingly, cerebellar hypermetabolism is usually seen in paraneoplastic cerebellar degeneration, pointing toward an autoimmune process targeting this region. This imaging modality could be helpful in differentiating patients with delirium as part of their COVID-19 manifestation [161].

The exact pathogenetic mechanism of autoimmune encephalitis in the setting of COVID-19 is unclear, and it has been hypothesized that cytokine storm with direct damage to the BBB and increased leukocyte migration to the brain [142], as well as dysregulation of viral immunity mediated by molecular mimicry, could be implicated [156]. The latter hypothesis is supported by the presence of positive CSF autoantibodies in encephalopathic patients found to have SARS-CoV-2. Franke et al. [162] analyzed the CSF of 11 patients with COVID-19 admitted to the ICU in different German hospitals. SARS-CoV-2 PCR in CSF was negative in all patients, while 3 of 11 patients had mild pleocytosis, 4 of 11 had elevated protein, and a few of them also had positive oligoclonal bands. All patients had an increased level of neurofilament light chain, one patient showed Yo antibodies in serum and CSF, two patients had positive myelin antibodies in serum, and one patient had positive IgG *N*-methyl-D-aspartate receptor antibodies. Interestingly, it was noted that IgG staining patterns in vessel endothelium, perinuclear antigens, astrocytic proteins, and neuropil of basal ganglia, hippocampus, and olfactory bulb indicate the presence of antigenic epitopes not currently known [162]. Another case report from Italy showed a case of *N*-methyl-D-aspartate receptor autoimmune encephalitis in an Ecuadorian man with COVID-19 positivity who presented with psychomotor agitation, anxiety, delusions, and hallucinations and responded to IVIG treatment [163].

Indeed, a trial with immunomodulatory therapies can be crucial to diagnose, as well as to confirm, autoimmune encephalitis. Further case reports of patients with suspected viral or autoimmune meningoencephalitis with detailed description of their presentation, workup, and response to treatment are also needed. As said, CSF PCR may be not reliable for the diagnosis because SARS-CoV-2 dissemination in the brain and its positivity may be transient with extremely low titer [164]. Furthermore, the test is not widely available. Therefore, a detailed and accurate neurologic examination and standard diagnostic studies such as EEG, CSF analyses, and brain imaging are crucial for the diagnosis of COVID-19-associated meningoencephalitis without delaying appropriate treatment.

Metabolic Encephalopathy

Many cases of severe COVID-19 encephalopathy are related to underlying toxic-metabolic derangements. A retrospective study of 799 patients with COVID-19 [54] showed that 22% of those who died had encephalopathy on admission, whereas only 1% of patients who recovered from infection had encephalopathy. This could point toward a possible negative prognostic factor of encephalopathy as the initial presentation. Headache without neurologic symptoms or signs was reported in 10% of the deceased patients versus 12% of the recovered patients. Metabolic derangements were more common in deceased patients than those who recovered, and 20% of the deceased patients suffered from hypoxic encephalopathy secondary to pulmonary inflammation. In this study, no laboratory studies were conducted to rule out viral encephalitis/meningitis, underlying seizures, and nonconvulsive status epilepticus, making it difficult to completely exclude an underlying viral encephalitis as the cause of encephalopathy and death. A study from France [165] showed that 84% of patients with ARDS and COVID-19 presented with neurologic signs, such as agitation (69%), corticospinal tract signs (67%), and dysexecutive syndrome with inattention, disorientation, or poorly organized movements in response to command (36%). MRI of the brain was performed in 13 of the 54 patients reported in the study. Notably, these patients did not have any focal signs suggestive of stroke, although 23% had an underlying ischemic stroke, 62% had leptomeningeal enhancement, and all the patients who underwent perfusion imaging showed bilateral frontotemporal hypoperfusion. A small proportion of the patients (8/54) had an EEG that showed nonspecific changes or bilateral frontal slowing, and a smaller proportion (7/54) had CSF studies showing no cells or other signs of infection with negative RT-PCR assays for SARS-CoV-2 in all samples. Usually, encephalopathies related to toxic metabolic causes resolve with improvement of the infection with supportive treatment.

Acute Myelitis

Acute myelitis is a known complication of viral infections as direct involvement of the spinal cord or via a secondary autoimmune mechanism such as what is seen in ADEM. Myelitis could also be an early manifestation of other neuroimmunologic disorders such as multiple sclerosis and neuromyelitis optica spectrum disorders or MOG-associated disease. Little is known about the association between SARS-CoV-2 and acute myelitis. A report of seven cases of acute myelitis, with only spinal cord (four cases) or with associated with brain involvement (three cases), has been published in relation to COVID-19 [84, 138, 166–170]. Six patients had upper respiratory symptoms related to COVID-19 2–25 days before the onset of neurologic symptoms of myelitis. SARS-CoV-2 RT-PCR was negative in the CSF of five patients. Overall, the functional outcome was favorable in six patients after treatment with either steroids or plasmapheresis. A case from Spain [171], a 68-year-old woman with acute necrotizing myelitis in association with COVID-19 who experienced seven-day radicular neck pain, right facial numbness, left hand numbness and weakness, gait instability, and general hyperreflexia preceded by fever and cough, was found to have transverse myelitis from the medulla oblongata to C7 with negative blood testing for anti–aquaporin-4, MOG, and anti-phospholipid antibodies. CSF studies showed elevated protein level and pleocytosis with no oligoclonal band, normal IgG index, no anti-neuronal surface antibody, and negative SARS-CoV-2 PCR. After 5-day course of methylprednisolone, she had worsening symptoms, and repeated spinal MRI showed a new area of central necrosis at the T1 level with peripheral enhancement that prompted further treatment with plasmapheresis and another course of five-day methylprednisolone followed by slow tapering oral prednisone with clinical improvement. The exact pathophysiology mechanism in acute necrotizing myelitis is unknown, probably related to a postviral autoimmune cytokine storm [172]. Two cases of ADEM were also reported in the literature with typical MRI findings of FLAIR and T2 hyperintensity in the subcortical and deep white matter [173, 174]. One case of suspected COVID-19-ADEM also had a brain biopsy that showed features of both acute hemorrhagic leukoencephalitis and ADEM [175]. One case of COVID-19-related acute flaccid myelitis has been described with suggestive clinical findings and supportive imaging data [176].

Acute Cerebrovascular Events

Acute cerebrovascular events also can occur in the setting of SARS-CoV-2 infection [150, 177]. Several pathophysiologic mechanisms have been suggested that may underlie such neurologic complications, which include: (i) direct vascular endothelial injury by SARS-CoV-2 after CNS invasion [149], (ii) development of coagulopathy and thromboembolism via endothelial damage or inflammatory cytokines [95, 178, 179], and (iii) cardioemboli from direct damage of the myocardium by SARS-CoV-2 [180]. Early investigation also showed that ~6% of patients with confirmed COVID-19 presented with acute cerebrovascular events (mainly ischemic strokes). It was found that these patients had an overall more severe course as evidenced by higher levels of inflammatory markers and D-dimer levels, older age, and more comorbidities (particularly hypertension) [100]. A study on 1419 patients with COVID-19 in Spain reported 8 patients (0.6%) presented with cerebrovascular events (6 with acute ischemic stroke and 2 with transient ischemic attack) [96]. A similar incidence was found in another large retrospective study of 3556 patients with COVID-19, of which 32 (0.9%) presented with ischemic stroke (65.6% cryptogenic and 34.4% embolic stroke of undetermined source) [181]. Stroke patients with COVID-19 are usually older than 50 years and present with higher National Institutes of Health Stroke Scale score on admission [181], severe disease course, immunocompromise, and different comorbidities and cardiovascular risk factors [96, 100]. However, it is noteworthy that a case report from New York City showed five patients with COVID-19 younger than 50 years who had large-vessel ischemic stroke [152]. Although data on the prognosis of SARS-CoV-2-associated stroke are scarce, the overall outcome appears to be poor, which could be a result of older age, more comorbidities, and more severe COVID-19 course in these patients [96, 98, 182–184]. Cerebral venous thrombosis is also reported in both adults and pediatric patients with COVID-19, which could be fatal in these cases [94, 185–188]. Headache was found to be the presenting symptom in the majority of these cases that was accompanied by various focal neurologic deficits, confusion, and decreased level of consciousness [94, 186–188]. Elevated acute-phase reactants (CRP and ferritin), hypercoagulability factors (D-dimer and activated partial thromboplastin time), and abnormal platelet counts are reported in patients with COVID-19 with cerebral venous thrombosis [94, 186–188], indicating that a hypercoagulability state related to SARS-CoV-2 infection may underlie such neurologic complications. Central venous thrombosis with thrombocytopenia also has been associated with the AstraZeneca chimpanzee adenovirus vector vaccine ChAdOx1-S [189]. Clearly more clinical studies are needed to delineate the best therapeutic approaches for patients with COVID-19 who experience acute cerebrovascular events.

Therapeutic Strategies

As previously described, various therapeutic approaches have been considered for treatment of neurologic complications related to SARS-CoV-2 infection, which include IVIG or plasma exchange for GBS and skeletal muscle injury; intravenous or oral steroids, as well as plasmapheresis, for acute myelitis and autoimmune encephalitis; and antiseizure drugs for seizures. Antimalarial drugs, such as dexamethasone, RNA-dependent RNA polymerase inhibitors, such as remdesivir, and biologic agents, such as tocilizumab, interferons, and convalescent plasma, have demonstrated some benefits for these conditions [190]. The US Food and Drug Administration has approved remdesivir for severely ill hospitalized patients [191]. This drug is a broad-spectrum antiviral that can inhibit SARS-CoV-2 replication and thereby improve clinical symptoms, recovery, and mortality rate [192]. The Randomized Evaluation of COVID-19 Therapy (RECOVERY) trial has also found that dexamethasone caused a lower 28-day mortality rate in patients with COVID-19 receiving either invasive mechanical ventilation or oxygen alone at randomization, but not in those receiving no respiratory support [193]. Although data on dexamethasone and remdesivir look promising for COVID-19 in general, whether this therapeutic approach is effective on the neurologic manifestations of COVID-19 needs further investigation.

Promising data on preventive methods using COVID-19 vaccination [194–196] and initiation of vaccination worldwide will undoubtedly be effective in reducing the incidence rate, as well as the number of severe cases, of COVID-19. Thus, we may expect to have fewer neurologic manifestations or complications via global vaccination. This assumption needs to be pursued in vaccinated populations in the future.

Conclusion

Various neurologic manifestations and complications of SARS-CoV-2 infection can occur before, during, and after the onset of general COVID-19 manifestations. The most common neurologic presentations related to COVID-19 include headache, dizziness, muscular or radicular/neuropathic pain, impaired consciousness, confusion, fatigue, ageusia, anosmia, seizure, and ataxia. Important neurologic conditions related to SARS-CoV-2 also include GBSs, myopathy/rhabdomyolysis, encephalopathy, meningoencephalitis, encephalomyelitis, acute myelitis, and acute cerebrovascular events. The exact etiology of these complications is still elusive. Direct viral infection to both central and peripheral nervous systems, neuroinflammation, postviral-triggered autoimmune response, hypercoagulability, vasculopathy, and metabolic or hypoxic injury are among suggested mechanisms. Therapeutic approaches to overcome or prevent COVID-19 include three main considerations: (i) targeting the infection with antiviral medications, monoclonal antibodies, or convalescent plasma therapy; (ii) targeting inflammatory hyperactivation with immunomodulatory agents and cytokine inhibitors; and (iii) COVID-19 vaccines [197]. Especially with the consideration of vaccination worldwide, hopefully the pandemic will end soon.

References

1 Zhu, N., Zhang, D., Wang, W. et al. (2020). A novel coronavirus from patients with pneumonia in China, 2019. *N. Engl. J. Med.* 382 (8): 727–733.

2 Gorbalenya, A.E., Baker, S.C., Baric, R.S. et al. (2020). Severe acute respiratory syndrome-related coronavirus: the species and its viruses – a statement of the coronavirus study group. *bioRxiv*. doi:2020.02.07.937862.

3 World Health Organization (WHO) (2019). International Classification of Disease (ICD-10) Version 2019. Chapter XXII. Codes for special purposes (U00-U85). https://icd.who.int/browse10/2019/en#/U07.

4 Li, Y.C., Bai, W.Z., and Hashikawa, T. (2020). The neuroinvasive potential of SARS-CoV2 may play a role in the respiratory failure of COVID-19 patients. *J. Med. Virol.* 92 (6): 552–555.

5 Dong, E., Du, H., and Gardner, L. (2020). An interactive web-based dashboard to track COVID-19 in real time. *Lancet Infect. Dis.* 20 (5): 533–534.

6 Novel Coronavirus Pneumonia Emergency Response Epidemiology Team (2020). The epidemiological characteristics of an outbreak of 2019 novel coronavirus diseases (COVID-19) in China. *Zhonghua Liu Xing Bing Xue Za Zhi* 41 (2): 145–151.

7 Centers for Disease Control and Prevention (CDC) (2020). Coronavirus disease 2019 (COVID-19). https://www.cdc.gov/coronavirus/2019-ncov/ symptoms-testing/symptoms.html.

8 Moein, S.T., Hashemian, S.M.R., Mansourafshar, B. et al. (2020). Smell dysfunction: a biomarker for COVID-19. *Int. Forum Allergy Rhinol.* 10 (8): 944–950.

9 Ye, Q., Wang, B., and Mao, J. (2020). The pathogenesis and treatment of the 'cytokine Storm' in COVID-19. *J. Infect.* 80 (6): 607–613.

10 Bikdeli, B., Madhavan, M.V., Jimenez, D. et al. (2020). COVID-19 and thrombotic or thromboembolic disease: implications for prevention, antithrombotic therapy, and follow-up: JACC state-of-the-art review. *J. Am. Coll. Cardiol.* 75 (23): 2950–2973.

11 Cascella, M., Rajnik, M., Cuomo, A. et al. (2020). *Features, evaluation and treatment coronavirus (COVID-19). StatPearls.* Treasure Island, FL: StatPearls Publishing.

12 Murthy, S., Gomersall, C.D., and Fowler, R.A. (2020). Care for critically ill patients with COVID-19. *JAMA* 323 (15): 1499–1500.

13 Pyankov, O.V., Bodnev, S.A., Pyankova, O.G., and Agranovski, I.E. (2018). Survival of aerosolized coronavirus in the ambient air. *J. Aerosol Sci.* 115: 158–163.

14 van Doremalen, N., Bushmaker, T., Morris, D.H. et al. (2020). Aerosol and surface stability of SARS-CoV-2 as compared with SARS-CoV-1. *N. Engl. J. Med.* 382 (16): 1564–1567.

15 World Health Organization (WHO). Laboratory testing for coronavirus disease (COVID-19) in suspected human cases. https://www.who.int/ publications-detail/ laboratory-testing-for-2019-novel-coronavirus-in-suspected-human-cases-20200117.

16 Salehi, S., Abedi, A., Balakrishnan, S., and Gholamrezanezhad, A. (2020). Coronavirus disease 2019 (COVID-19): a systematic review of imaging findings in 919 patients. *AJR Am. J. Roentgenol.* 215: 87–93.

17 Dodding, M.P. and Way, M. (2011). Coupling viruses to dynein and kinesin-1. *EMBO J.* 30 (17): 3527–3539.

18 Nagu, P., Parashar, A., Behl, T., and Mehta, V. (2021). CNS implications of COVID-19: a comprehensive review. *Rev. Neurosci.* 32 (2): 219–234.

19 Wan, S., Yi, Q., Fan, S. et al. (2020). Characteristics of lymphocyte subsets and cytokines in peripheral blood of 123 hospitalized patients with 2019 novel coronavirus pneumonia (NCP). *medRxiv*: 10.1101/2020.02.10.20021832.

20 Wu, Y., Xu, X., Chen, Z. et al. (2020). Nervous system involvement after infection with COVID-19 and other coronaviruses. *Brain Behav. Immun.* 87: 18–22.

21 Mussa, B.M., Srivastava, A., and Verberne, A.J. (2021). COVID-19 and neurological impairment: hypothalamic circuits and beyond. *Viruses* 13 (3): 498.

22 Netland, J., Meyerholz, D.K., Moore, S. et al. (2008). Severe acute respiratory syndrome coronavirus infection causes neuronal death in the absence of encephalitis in mice transgenic for human ACE2. *J. Virol.* 82 (15): 7264–7275.

23 Koyuncu, O.O., Hogue, I.B., and Enquist, L.W. (2013). Virus infections in the nervous system. *Cell Host Microbe* 13 (4): 379–393.

24 Desforges, M., Le Coupanec, A., Dubeau, P. et al. (2019). Human coronaviruses and other respiratory viruses: underestimated opportunistic pathogens of the central nervous system? *Viruses* 12 (1): 14.

25 Mori, I. (2015). Transolfactory neuroinvasion by viruses threatens the human brain. *Acta Virol.* 59 (4): 338–349.

26 Lechien, J.R., Chiesa-Estomba, C.M., De Siati, D.R. et al. (2020). Olfactory and gustatory dysfunctions as a clinical presentation of mild-to-moderate forms of the coronavirus disease (COVID-19): a multicenter European study. *Eur. Arch. Otorhinolaryngol.* 277: 2251–2261.

27 Coolen, T., Lolli, V., Sadeghi, N. et al. (2020). Early postmortem brain MRI findings in COVID-19 non-survivors. *Neurology* 95: e2016–e2027. https://doi. org/10.1212/WNL.0000000000010116.

28 Brann, D., Tsukahara, T., Weinreb, C. et al. (2020). Non-neural expression of SARS-CoV-2 entry genes in the olfactory epithelium suggests mechanisms underlying anosmia in COVID-19 patients. *bioRxiv* https://doi.org/10.1101/2020.03.25.009084.

29 Jakhmola, S., Indari, O., Chatterjee, S., and Jha, H.C. (2020). SARS-CoV-2, an underestimated pathogen of the nervous system. *SN Compr. Clin. Med.* 2: 2137–2146.

30 Mori, I., Nishiyama, Y., Yokochi, T., and Kimura, Y. (2005). Olfactory transmission of neurotropic viruses. *J. Neurovirol.* 11 (2): 129–137.

31 Politi, L.S., Salsano, E., and Grimaldi, M. (2020). Magnetic resonance imaging alteration of the brain in a patient with coronavirus disease 2019 (COVID-19) and anosmia. *JAMA Neurol.* 77 (8): 1028–1029.

32 Andries, K. and Pensaert, M.B. (1980). Immunofluorescence studies on the pathogenesis of hemagglutinating encephalomyelitis virus infection in pigs after oronasal inoculation. *Am. J. Vet. Res.* 41 (9): 1372–1378.

33 Matsuda, K., Park, C., Sunden, Y. et al. (2004). The vagus nerve is one route of transneural invasion for intranasally inoculated influenza a virus in mice. *Vet. Pathol.* 41 (2): 101–107.

34 Toljan, K. (2020). Letter to the editor regarding the viewpoint "evidence of the COVID-19 virus targeting the CNS: tissue distribution, host-virus interaction, and proposed neurotropic mechanism". *ACS Chem. Neurosci.* 11 (8): 1192–1194.

35 Bostancıklıoğlu, M. (2020). Temporal correlation between neurological and gastrointestinal symptoms of SARS-CoV-2. *Inflamm. Bowel Dis.* 26: e89–e91.

36 Lima, M., Siokas, V., Aloizou, A.-M. et al. (2020). Unraveling the possible routes of SARS-COV-2 invasion into the central nervous system. *Curr. Treat. Options Neurol.* 22 (11): 1–15.

37 Wong, S.H., Lui, R.N., and Sung, J.J. (2020). Covid-19 and the digestive system. *J. Gastroenterol. Hepatol.* 35 (5): 744–748.

38 Sun, T. and Guan, J. (2020). Novel coronavirus and the central nervous system. *Eur. J. Neurol.* 27: e52.

39 Vaduganathan, M., Vardeny, O., Michel, T. et al. (2020). Renin–angiotensin–aldosterone system inhibitors in patients with Covid-19. *N. Engl. J. Med.* 382 (17): 1653–1659.

40 Xu, J. and Lazartigues, E. (2020). Expression of ACE2 in human neurons supports the neuro-invasive potential of COVID-19 virus. *Cell. Mol. Neurobiol.* https://doi.org/10.1007/s10571-020-00915-1.

41 Ayala-Nunez, N.V., Follain, G., Delalande, F. et al. (2019). Zika virus enhances monocyte adhesion and transmigration favoring viral dissemination to neural cells. *Nat. Commun.* 10 (1): 1–16.

42 Kaul, M., Garden, G.A., and Lipton, S.A. (2001). Pathways to neuronal injury and apoptosis in HIV-associated dementia. *Nature* 410 (6831): 988–994.

43 Wang, S., Le, T.Q., Kurihara, N. et al. (2010). Influenza virus-cytokine-protease cycle in the pathogenesis of vascular hyperpermeability in severe influenza. *J. Infect. Dis.* 202 (7): 991–1001.

44 Bleau, C., Filliol, A., Samson, M., and Lamontagne, L. (2015). Brain invasion by mouse hepatitis virus depends on impairment of tight junctions and Beta interferon production in brain microvascular endothelial cells. *J. Virol.* 89 (19): 9896–9908.

45 Cabirac, G.F., Soike, K.F., Butunoi, C. et al. (1993). Coronavirus JHM OMP1 pathogenesis in owl monkey CNS and coronavirus infection of owl monkey CNS via peripheral routes. *Adv. Exp. Med. Biol.*: 347–352.

46 Cowley, T.J. and Weiss, S.R. (2010). Murine coronavirus neuropathogenesis: determinants of virulence. *J. Neurovirol.* 16 (6): 427–434.

47 Ding, Y., He, L., Zhang, Q. et al. (2004). Organ distribution of severe acute respiratory syndrome (SARS) associated coronavirus (SARS-CoV) in SARS patients: implications for pathogenesis and virus transmission pathways. *J. Pathol.* 203 (2): 622–630.

48 Paniz-Mondolfi, A., Bryce, C., Grimes, Z. et al. (2020). Central nervous system involvement by severe acute respiratory syndrome coronavirus-2 (SARS-CoV-2). *J. Med. Virol.* 92 (7): 699–702.

49 Hamming, I., Timens, W., Bulthuis, M.L. et al. (2004). Tissue distribution of ACE2 protein, the functional receptor for SARS coronavirus. A first step in understanding SARS pathogenesis. *J. Pathol.* 203 (2): 631–637.

50 Mecha, M., Carrillo-Salinas, F.J., Mestre, L. et al. (2013). Viral models of multiple sclerosis: neurodegeneration and demyelination in mice infected with Theiler's virus. *Prog. Neurobiol.* 101–102: 46–64.

51 Erickson, M.A., Dohi, K., and Banks, W.A. (2012). Neuroinflammation: a common pathway in CNS diseases as mediated at the blood-brain barrier. *Neuroimmunomodulation* 19 (2): 121–130.

52 Wu, K., Peng, G., Wilken, M. et al. (2012). Mechanisms of host receptor adaptation by severe acute respiratory syndrome coronavirus. *J. Biol. Chem.* 287 (12): 8904–8911.

53 Schoeman, D. and Fielding, B.C. (2019). Coronavirus envelope protein: current knowledge. *Virol. J.* 16 (1): 69.

54 Chen, T., Wu, D., Chen, H. et al. (2020). Clinical characteristics of 113 deceased patients with coronavirus disease 2019: retrospective study. *BMJ* 368: m1091.

55 Li, F., Li, W., Farzan, M., and Harrison, S.C. (2005). Structure of SARS coronavirus spike receptor-binding domain complexed with receptor. *Science* 309 (5742): 1864–1868.

56 Ziegler, C.G.K., Allon, S.J., Nyquist, S.K. et al. (2020). SARS-CoV-2 receptor ACE2 is an interferon-stimulated gene in human airway epithelial cells and is detected in specific cell subsets across tissues. *Cell* 181 (5): 1016–1035.e19.

57 Yin, R., Feng, W., Wang, T. et al. (2020). Concomitant neurological symptoms observed in a patient diagnosed with coronavirus disease 2019. *J. Med. Virol.* 92: 1782–1784.

58 Baig, A.M., Khaleeq, A., Ali, U., and Syeda, H. (2020). Evidence of the COVID-19 virus targeting the CNS: tissue distribution, host–virus interaction, and proposed neurotropic mechanisms. *ACS Chem. Neurosci.* 11 (7): 995–998.

59 Palasca, O., Santos, A., Stolte, C. et al. (2018). TISSUES 2.0: an integrative web resource on mammalian tissue expression. *Database (Oxford)* 2018: bay028.

60 Xia, H. and Lazartigues, E. (2008). Angiotensin-converting enzyme 2 in the brain: properties and future directions. *J. Neurochem.* 107 (6): 1482–1494.

61 Prabakaran, P., Xiao, X., and Dimitrov, D.S. (2004). A model of the ACE2 structure and function as a SARS-CoV receptor. *Biochem. Biophys. Res. Commun.* 314 (1): 235–241.

62 To, K. and Lo, A.W. (2004). Exploring the pathogenesis of severe acute respiratory syndrome (SARS): the tissue distribution of the coronavirus (SARS-CoV) and its putative receptor, angiotensin-converting enzyme 2 (ACE2). *J. Pathol. Soc. Great Br. Ir.* 203 (3): 740–743.

63 Daly, J.L., Simonetti, B., Klein, K. et al. (2020). Neuropilin-1 is a host factor for SARS-CoV-2 infection. *Science* 370 (6518): 861–865.

64 Hara, Y., Hasebe, R., Sunden, Y. et al. (2009). Propagation of swine hemagglutinating encephalomyelitis virus and pseudorabies virus in dorsal root ganglia cells. *J. Vet. Med. Sci.* 71 (5): 595–601.

65 Li, Y.-C., Bai, W.-Z., Hirano, N. et al. (2012). Coronavirus infection of rat dorsal root ganglia: ultrastructural characterization of viral replication, transfer, and the early response of satellite cells. *Virus Res.* 163 (2): 628–635.

66 Steardo, L., Steardo, L. Jr., Zorec, R., and Verkhratsky, A. (2020). Neuroinfection may contribute to pathophysiology and clinical manifestations of COVID-19. *Acta Physiol (Oxf.)* 229: e13473.

67 Dube, M., Le Coupanec, A., Wong, A.H.M. et al. (2018). Axonal transport enables neuron-to-neuron propagation of human coronavirus OC43. *J. Virol.* 92 (17): e00404–e00418.

68 Varga, Z., Flammer, A.J., Steiger, P. et al. (2020). Endothelial cell infection and endotheliitis in COVID-19. *Lancet* 395 (10234): 1417–1418.

69 Yang, N. and Shen, H.-M. (2020). Targeting the endocytic pathway and autophagy process as a novel therapeutic strategy in covid-19. *Int. J. Biol. Sci.* 16 (10): 1724.

70 Xia, H. and Lazartigues, E. (2010). Angiotensin-converting enzyme 2: central regulator for cardiovascular function. *Curr. Hypertens. Rep.* 12 (3): 170–175.

71 Karakike, E. and Giamarellos-Bourboulis, E.J. (2019). Macrophage activation-like syndrome: a distinct entity leading to early death in sepsis. *Front. Immunol.* 10: 55.

72 Lagunas-Rangel, F.A. (2020). Neutrophil-to-lymphocyte ratio and lymphocyte-to-C-reactive protein ratio in patients with severe coronavirus disease 2019 (COVID-19): a meta-analysis. *J. Med. Virol.* 92: 1733–1734.

73 Qin, C., Zhou, L., Hu, Z. et al. (2020). Dysregulation of immune response in patients with COVID-19 in Wuhan, China. *Clin. Infect. Dis.*: 71, 762–78.

74 Xu, Z., Shi, L., Wang, Y. et al. (2020). Pathological findings of COVID-19 associated with acute respiratory distress syndrome. *Lancet Respir. Med.* 8 (4): 420–422.

75 Mehta, P., McAuley, D.F., Brown, M. et al. (2020). COVID-19: consider cytokine storm syndromes and immunosuppression. *Lancet* 395 (10229): 1033–1034.

76 Zhang, H., Penninger, J.M., Li, Y. et al. (2020). Angiotensin-converting enzyme 2 (ACE2) as a SARS-CoV-2 receptor: molecular mechanisms and potential therapeutic target. *Intensive Care Med.* 46: 586–590.

77 Le, R.Q., Li, L., Yuan, W. et al. (2018). FDA approval summary: tocilizumab for treatment of chimeric antigen receptor T cell-induced severe or life-threatening cytokine release syndrome. *Oncologist* 23 (8): 943.

78 Ichiyama, T., Shoji, H., Kato, M. et al. (2002). Cerebrospinal fluid levels of cytokines and soluble tumour necrosis factor receptor in acute disseminated encephalomyelitis. *Eur. J. Pediatr.* 161 (3): 133–137.

79 Linker, R.A., Lühder, F., Kallen, K.-J. et al. (2008). IL-6 transsignalling modulates the early effector phase of EAE and targets the blood-brain barrier. *J. Neuroimmunol.* 205 (1–2): 64–72.

80 Alberti, P., Beretta, S., Piatti, M. et al. (2020). Guillain-Barré syndrome related to COVID-19 infection. *Neurol. Neuroimmunol. Neuroinflamm.*: 7(4), e741.

81 McAbee, G.N., Brosgol, Y., Pavlakis, S. et al. (2020). Encephalitis associated with COVID-19 infection in an 11 year-old child. *Pediatr. Neurol.* 109: 94.

82 Moriguchi, T., Harii, N., Goto, J. et al. (2020). A first case of meningitis/encephalitis associated with SARS-Coronavirus-2. *Int. J. Infect. Dis.* 94: 55–58.

83 Poyiadji, N., Shahin, G., Noujaim, D. et al. (2020). COVID-19–associated acute hemorrhagic necrotizing encephalopathy: imaging features. *Radiology* 296: e119–e120.

84 Zanin, L., Saraceno, G., Panciani, P.P. et al. (2021). SARS-CoV-2 can induce brain and spine demyelinating lesions. *Acta Neurochir. (Wein)* 163: 331–334.

85 Zhang, T., Rodricks, M.B., and Hirsh, E. (2020). COVID-19-associated acute disseminated encephalomyelitis: a case report. *medRxiv* https://doi.org/10.1101/2020.04.16.20068148.

86 Gordon, A.C., Mouncey, P.R., Al-Beidh, F. et al. (2021). Interleukin-6 receptor antagonists in critically ill patients with Covid-19 – preliminary report. *medRxiv* doi:2021.01.07.21249390.

87 Xu, X., Han, M., Li, T. et al. (2020). Effective treatment of severe COVID-19 patients with tocilizumab. *Proc. Natl Acad. Sci. USA* 117: 10970–10975.

88 Abdennour, L., Zeghal, C., Deme, M., and Puybasset, L. (2012). Interaction brain-lungs. *Ann. Fr. Anesth. Reanim.* 31: e101–e107.

89 Gattinoni, L., Coppola, S., Cressoni, M. et al. (2020). Covid-19 does not lead to a "typical" acute respiratory distress syndrome. *Am. J. Respir. Crit. Care Med.* 201: 1299–1300.

90 Liu, F. and Mccullough, L.D. (2013). Inflammatory responses in hypoxic ischemic encephalopathy. *Acta Pharmacol. Sin.* 34 (9): 1121–1130.

91 Giannis, D., Ziogas, I.A., and Gianni, P. (2020). Coagulation disorders in coronavirus infected patients: COVID-19, SARS-CoV-1, MERS-CoV and lessons from the past. *J. Clin. Virol.* 127: 104362.

92 Merad, M. and Martin, J.C. (2020). Pathological inflammation in patients with COVID-19: a key role for monocytes and macrophages. *Nat. Rev. Immunol.* 20: 355–362.

93 Violi, F., Pastori, D., Cangemi, R. et al. (2020). Hypercoagulation and antithrombotic treatment in coronavirus 2019: a new challenge. *Thromb. Haemost.* 120 (6): 949–956.

94 Hughes, C., Nichols, T., Pike, M. et al. (2020). Cerebral venous sinus thrombosis as a presentation of COVID-19. *Eur. J. Case Rep. Intern. Med.* 7 (5): 001691.

95 Klok, F.A., Kruip, M.J.H.A., van der Meer, N.J.M. et al. (2020). Confirmation of the high cumulative incidence of thrombotic complications in critically ill ICU patients with COVID-19: an updated analysis. *Thromb. Res.* 191: 148–150.

96 Cantador, E., Nunez, A., Sobrino, P. et al. (2020). Incidence and consequences of systemic arterial thrombotic events in COVID-19 patients. *J. Thromb. Thrombolysis* 50: 543–547.

97 Violi, F., Oliva, A., Cangemi, R. et al. (2020). Nox2 activation in Covid-19. *Redox Biol.* 36: 101655.

98 Wang, H.Y., Li, X.L., Yan, Z.R. et al. (2020). Potential neurological symptoms of COVID-19. *Ther. Adv. Neurol. Disord.* 13:1756286420917830.

99 Sharifi-Razavi, A., Karimi, N., and Rouhani, N. (2020). COVID-19 and intracerebral haemorrhage: causative or coincidental? *New Microbes New Infect.* 35: 100669.

100 Mao, L., Jin, H., Wang, M. et al. (2020). Neurologic manifestations of hospitalized patients with coronavirus disease 2019 in Wuhan, China. *JAMA Neurol.* 77: 683–690.

101 Huang, C., Wang, Y., Li, X. et al. (2020). Clinical features of patients infected with 2019 novel coronavirus in Wuhan, China. *Lancet* 395 (10223): 497–506.

102 Yang, X., Yu, Y., Xu, J. et al. (2020). Clinical course and outcomes of critically ill patients with SARS-CoV-2 pneumonia in Wuhan, China: a single-centered, retrospective, observational study. *Lancet Respir. Med.* 8 (5): 475–481.

103 Wang, D., Hu, B., Hu, C. et al. (2020). Clinical characteristics of 138 hospitalized patients with 2019 novel coronavirus–infected pneumonia in Wuhan, China. *JAMA* 323 (11): 1061–1069.

104 Chen, N., Zhou, M., Dong, X. et al. (2020). Epidemiological and clinical characteristics of 99 cases of 2019 novel coronavirus pneumonia in Wuhan, China: a descriptive study. *Lancet* 395 (10223): 507–513.

105 Zhang, J.J., Dong, X., Cao, Y.Y. et al. (2020). Clinical characteristics of 140 patients infected with SARS-CoV-2 in Wuhan, China. *Allergy* 75: 1730–1741.

106 Du, Y., Tu, L., Zhu, P. et al. (2020). Clinical features of 85 fatal cases of COVID-19 from Wuhan: a retrospective observational study. *Am. J. Respir. Crit. Care Med.* 201: 1372–1379.

107 Zhang, G., Hu, C., Luo, L. et al. (2020). Clinical features and short-term outcomes of 221 patients with COVID-19 in Wuhan, China. *J. Clin. Virol.* 127: 104364.

108 Xiong, W., Mu, J., Guo, J. et al. (2020). New onset neurologic events in people with COVID-19 infection in 3 regions in China. *Neurology* 95: e1479–e1487. https://doi.org/10.1212/WNL.0000000000010034.

109 Zhang, X., Cai, H., Hu, J. et al. (2020). Epidemiological, clinical characteristics of cases of SARS-CoV-2 infection with abnormal imaging findings. *Int. J. Infect. Dis.* 94: 81–87.

110 Qian, G.-Q., Yang, N.-B., Ding, F. et al. (2020). Epidemiologic and clinical characteristics of 91 hospitalized patients with COVID-19 in Zhejiang, China: a retrospective, multi-Centre case series. *QJM* 113: 474–481.

111 Xu, X.W., Wu, X.X., Jiang, X.G. et al. (2020). Clinical findings in a group of patients infected with the 2019 novel coronavirus (SARS-Cov-2) outside of Wuhan, China: retrospective case series. *BMJ* 368: m606.

112 Xu, X., Yu, C., Qu, J. et al. (2020). Imaging and clinical features of patients with 2019 novel coronavirus SARS-CoV-2. *Eur. J. Nucl. Med. Mol. Imaging* 47 (5): 1275–1280.

113 Yang, W., Cao, Q., Qin, L. et al. (2020). Clinical characteristics and imaging manifestations of the 2019 novel coronavirus disease (COVID-19): a multi-center study in Wenzhou city, Zhejiang, China. *J. Infect.* 80 (4): 388–393.

114 Liu, K., Fang, Y.Y., Deng, Y. et al. (2020). Clinical characteristics of novel coronavirus cases in tertiary hospitals in Hubei Province. *Chin. Med. J.* 133 (9): 1025–1031.

115 Chang, D., Lin, M., Wei, L. et al. (2020). Epidemiologic and clinical characteristics of novel coronavirus infections involving 13 patients outside Wuhan, China. *JAMA* 323 (11): 1092–1093.

116 Tian, S., Hu, N., Lou, J. et al. (2020). Characteristics of COVID-19 infection in Beijing. *J. Infect.* 80 (4): 401–406.

117 Guan, W.-j., Ni, Z.-y., Hu, Y. et al. (2020). Clinical characteristics of coronavirus disease 2019 in China. *N. Engl. J. Med.* 382 (18): 1708–1720.

118 Xu, Y.-H., Dong, J.-H., An, W.-M. et al. (2020). Clinical and computed tomographic imaging features of novel coronavirus pneumonia caused by SARS-CoV-2. *J. Infect.* 80 (4): 394–400.

119 Bigaut, K., Mallaret, M., Baloglu, S. et al. (2020). Guillain-Barré syndrome related to SARS-CoV-2 infection. *Neurol. Neuroimmunol. Neuroinflamm.* 7 (5): e785.

120 Gupta, N., Agrawal, S., Ish, P. et al. (2020). Clinical and epidemiologic profile of the initial COVID-19 patients at a tertiary care Centre in India. *Monaldi Arch. Chest Dis.* 90 (1) https://doi.org/10.4081/monaldi.2020.1294.

121 Shahriarirad, R., Khodamoradi, Z., Erfani, A. et al. (2020). Epidemiological and clinical features of 2019 novel coronavirus diseases (COVID-19) in the south of Iran. *BMC Infect. Dis.* 20 (1): 427.

122 Shahrizaila, N., Lehmann, H.C., and Kuwabara, S. (2021). Guillain-Barré syndrome. *Lancet* 397 (10280): 1214–1228.

123 Rocha Cabrero, F. and Morrison, E.H. (2020). *Miller Fisher Syndrome. StatPearls*. Treasure Island, FL: StatPearls Publishing.

124 Wakerley, B.R. and Yuki, N. (2013). Infectious and noninfectious triggers in Guillain-Barré syndrome. *Expert. Rev. Clin. Immunol.* 9 (7): 627–639.

125 Kim, J.E., Heo, J.H., Kim, H.O. et al. (2017). Neurological complications during treatment of Middle East respiratory syndrome. *J. Clin. Neurol.* 13 (3): 227–233.

126 Zhao, H., Shen, D., Zhou, H. et al. (2020). Guillain-Barré syndrome associated with SARS-CoV-2 infection: causality or coincidence? *Lancet Neurol.* 19 (5): 383–384.

127 Abu-Rumeileh, S., Abdelhak, A., Foschi, M. et al. (2021). Guillain-Barré syndrome spectrum associated with COVID-19: an up-to-date systematic review of 73 cases. *J. Neurol.* 268: 1133–1170.

128 Fantini, J., Di Scala, C., Chahinian, H., and Yahi, N. (2020). Structural and molecular modelling studies reveal a new mechanism of action of chloroquine and hydroxychloroquine against SARS-CoV-2 infection. *Int. J. Antimicrob. Agents* 55 (5): 105960.

129 Gefen, A.M., Palumbo, N., Nathan, S.K. et al. (2020). Pediatric COVID-19-associated rhabdomyolysis: a case report. *Pediatr. Nephrol.* 35: 1517–1520.

130 Jin, M. and Tong, Q. (2020). Rhabdomyolysis as potential late complication associated with COVID-19. *Emerg. Infect. Dis.* 26 (7): 1618–1620.

131 Suwanwongse, K. and Shabarek, N. (2020). Rhabdomyolysis as a presentation of 2019 novel coronavirus disease. *Cureus* 12 (4): e7561.

132 Madia, F., Merico, B., Primiano, G. et al. (2020). Acute myopathic quadriplegia in patients with COVID-19 in the intensive care unit. *Neurology* 95: 492–494. https://doi.org/10.1212/WNL.0000000000010280.

133 Cabello-Verrugio, C., Morales, M.G., Rivera, J.C. et al. (2015). Renin-angiotensin system: an old

player with novel functions in skeletal muscle. *Med. Res. Rev.* 35 (3): 437–463.

134 Needham, E.J., Chou, S.H., Coles, A.J., and Menon, D.K. (2020). Neurological implications of COVID-19 infections. *Neurocrit. Care.* 32: 667–671.

135 Sellner, J., Taba, P., Öztürk, S., and Helbok, R. (2020). The need for neurologists in the care of COVID-19 patients. *Eur. J. Neurol.* 27: e31–e32.

136 Koralnik, I.J. and Tyler, K.L. (2020). COVID-19: a global threat to the nervous system. *Ann. Neurol.* 88 (1): 1–11.

137 Kandemirli, S.G., Dogan, L., Sarikaya, Z.T. et al. (2020). Brain MRI findings in patients in the intensive care unit with COVID-19 infection. *Radiology* (1): 297, E232–295.

138. Wong, P.F., Craik, S., Newman, P. et al. (2020). Lessons of the month 1: a case of rhombencephalitis as a rare complication of acute COVID-19 infection. *Clin. Med. (Lond.)* 20: 293–294.

139 Solomon, I.H., Normandin, E., Bhattacharyya, S. et al. (2020). Neuropathological features of Covid-19. *N. Engl. J. Med.* 383: 989–992.

140 Xu, J., Zhong, S., Liu, J. et al. (2005). Detection of severe acute respiratory syndrome coronavirus in the brain: potential role of the chemokine mig in pathogenesis. *Clin. Infect. Dis.* 41 (8): 1089–1096.

141 Asadi-Pooya, A.A. (2020). Seizures associated with coronavirus infections. *Seizure* 79: 49–52.

142 Sohal, S. and Mossammat, M. (2020). COVID-19 presenting with seizures. *IDCases* 20: e00782.

143 Radmanesh, F., Rodriguez-Pla, A., Pincus, M.D., and Burns, J.D. (2020). Severe cerebral involvement in adult-onset hemophagocytic lymphohistiocytosis. *J. Clin. Neurosci.* 76: 236–237.

144 Dixon, L., Varley, J., Gontsarova, A. et al. (2020). COVID-19-related acute necrotizing encephalopathy with brain stem involvement in a patient with aplastic anemia. *Neurol. Neuroimmunol. Neuroinflamm.* 7 (5): e789.

145 Brun, G., Hak, J.F., Coze, S. et al. (2020). COVID-19-white matter and globus pallidus lesions: demyelination or small-vessel vasculitis? *Neurol. Neuroimmunol. Neuroinflamm.* 7 (4): e777.

146 Peters, J., Alhasan, S., Vogels, C.B.F. et al. (2021). MOG-associated encephalitis following SARS-COV-2 infection. *Mult. Scler. Relat. Disord.* 50: 102857.

147 Wu, G.F., Dandekar, A.A., Pewe, L., and Perlman, S. (2000). CD4 and CD8 T cells have redundant but not identical roles in virus-induced demyelination. *J. Immunol.* 165 (4): 2278–2286.

148 Yeh, E.A., Collins, A., Cohen, M.E. et al. (2004). Detection of coronavirus in the central nervous system of a child with acute disseminated encephalomyelitis. *Pediatrics* 113 (1 Pt 1): e73–e76.

149 Baig, A.M. (2020). Neurological manifestations in COVID-19 caused by SARS-CoV-2. *CNS Neurosci. Ther.* 26 (5): 499–501.

150 Asadi-Pooya, A.A. and Simani, L. (2020). Central nervous system manifestations of COVID-19: a systematic review. *J. Neurol. Sci.* 413: 116832.

151 Liu, K., Pan, M., Xiao, Z., and Xu, X. (2020). Neurological manifestations of the coronavirus (SARS-CoV-2) pandemic 2019-2020. *J. Neurol. Neurosurg. Psychiatry* 91: 669–670.

152 Oxley, T.J., Mocco, J., Majidi, S. et al. (2020). Large-vessel stroke as a presenting feature of Covid-19 in the young. *N. Engl. J. Med.* 382 (20): e60.

153 Iadecola, C., Anrather, J., and Kamel, H. (2020). Effects of COVID-19 on the nervous system. *Cell* 183: 16–27.e1.

154 Huang, Y.H., Jiang, D., and Huang, J.T. (2020). SARS-CoV-2 detected in cerebrospinal fluid by PCR in a case of COVID-19 encephalitis. *Brain Behav. Immun.* 87: 149.

155 Bernard-Valnet, R., Pizzarotti, B., Anichini, A. et al. (2020). Two patients with acute meningoencephalitis concomitant with SARS-CoV-2 infection. *Eur. J. Neurol.* 27 (9): e43–e44.

156 Pilotto, A., Odolini, S., Masciocchi, S. et al. (2020). Steroid-responsive encephalitis in coronavirus disease 2019. *Ann. Neurol.* 88 (2): 423–427.

157. Bernard-Valnet, R., Pizzarotti, B., Anichini, A. et al. (2020). Two patients with acute meningoencephalitis concomitant to SARS-CoV-2 infection. *Eur. J. Neurol.* 27: e43–e44.

158 Dogan, L., Kaya, D., Sarikaya, T. et al. (2020). Plasmapheresis treatment in COVID-19-related autoimmune meningoencephalitis: case series. *Brain Behav. Immun.* 87: 155–158.

159 Delorme, C., Paccoud, O., Kas, A. et al. (2020). COVID-19-related encephalopathy: a case series with brain FDG-positron-emission tomography/computed tomography findings. *Eur. J. Neurol.* 27 (12): 2651–2657.

160 Haggstrom, L.R., Nelson, J.A., Wegner, E.A., and Caplan, G.A. (2017). 2-(18)F-fluoro-2-deoxyglucose positron emission tomography in delirium. *J. Cereb. Blood Flow Metab.* 37 (11): 3556–3567.

161 Hosseini, A.A., Shetty, A.K., Sprigg, N. et al. (2020). Delirium as a presenting feature in COVID-19: Neuroinvasive infection or autoimmune encephalopathy? *Brain Behav. Immun.* 88: 68–70.

162 Franke, C., Ferse, C., Kreye, J. et al. (2021). High frequency of cerebrospinal fluid autoantibodies in COVID-19 patients with neurological symptoms. *Brain Behav. Immun.* 93: 415–419.

163 Panariello, A., Bassetti, R., Radice, A. et al. (2020). Anti-NMDA receptor encephalitis in a psychiatric Covid-19 patient: a case report. *Brain Behav. Immun.* 87: 179–181.

164 Ye, M., Ren, Y., and Lv, T. (2020). Encephalitis as a clinical manifestation of COVID-19. *Brain Behav. Immun.* 88: 945–946.

165 Helms, J., Kremer, S., Merdji, H. et al. (2020). Neurologic features in severe SARS-CoV-2 infection. *N. Engl. J. Med.* 382: 2268–2270.

166 AlKetbi, R., AlNuaimi, D., AlMulla, M. et al. (2020). Acute myelitis as a neurological complication of Covid-19: a case report and MRI findings. *Radiol. Case Rep.* 15 (9): 1591–1595.

167 Munz, M., Wessendorf, S., Koretsis, G. et al. (2020). Acute transverse myelitis after COVID-19 pneumonia. *J. Neurol.* 267: 2196–2197.

168 Novi, G., Rossi, T., Pedemonte, E. et al. (2020). Acute disseminated encephalomyelitis after SARS-CoV-2 infection. *Neurol. Neuroimmunol. Neuroinflamm.* 7 (5): e797.

169 Sarma, D. and Bilello, L.A. (2020). A case report of acute transverse myelitis following novel coronavirus infection. *Clin. Pract. Cases Emerg. Med.* 4 (3): 321–323.

170 Valiuddin, H., Skwirsk, B., and Paz-Arabo, P. (2020). Acute transverse myelitis associated with SARS-CoV-2: a case-report. *Brain Behav. Immun. Health* 5: 100091.

171 Sotoca, J. and Rodríguez-Álvarez, Y. (2020). COVID-19-associated acute necrotizing myelitis. *Neurol. Neuroimmunol. Neuroinflamm.* 7 (5): e803.

172 Kansagra, S.M. and Gallentine, W.B. (2011). Cytokine storm of acute necrotizing encephalopathy. *Pediatr. Neurol.* 45 (6): 400–402.

173 Zanin, L., Saraceno, G., Panciani, P.P. et al. (2020). SARS-CoV-2 can induce brain and spine

demyelinating lesions. *Acta Neurochir.* 162 (7): 1491–1494.

174 Zhang, T., Hirsh, E., Zandeieh, S., and Rodricks, M.B. (2021). COVID-19-associated acute multi-infarct encephalopathy in an asymptomatic CADASIL patient. *Neurocrit. Care.* 34 (3): 1099–1102.

175 Reichard, R.R., Kashani, K.B., Boire, N.A. et al. (2020). Neuropathology of COVID-19: a spectrum of vascular and acute disseminated encephalomyelitis (ADEM)-like pathology. *Acta Neuropathol.* 140 (1): 1–6.

176 Abdelhady, M., Elsotouhy, A., and Vattoth, S. (2020). Acute flaccid myelitis in COVID-19. *BJR Case Rep.* 6 (3): 20200098.

177 Benussi, A., Pilotto, A., Premi, E. et al. (2020). Clinical characteristics and outcomes of inpatients with neurologic disease and COVID-19 in Brescia, Lombardy, Italy. *Neurology* 95: e910–e920.

178 Lodigiani, C., Iapichino, G., Carenzo, L. et al. (2020). Venous and arterial thromboembolic complications in COVID-19 patients admitted to an academic hospital in Milan, Italy. *Thromb. Res.* 191: 9–14.

179 Zhang, Y., Xiao, M., Zhang, S. et al. (2020). Coagulopathy and Antiphospholipid antibodies in patients with Covid-19. *N. Engl. J. Med.* 382 (17): e38.

180 Guo, T., Fan, Y., Chen, M. et al. (2020). Cardiovascular implications of fatal outcomes of patients with coronavirus disease 2019 (COVID-19). *JAMA Cardiol.* 5: 811–818.

181 Yaghi, S., Ishida, K., Torres, J. et al. (2020, 2020). SARS2-CoV-2 and stroke in a New York Healthcare System. *Stroke* 51: e179.

182 Dafer, R.M., Osteraas, N.D., and Biller, J. (2020). Acute stroke care in the coronavirus disease 2019 pandemic. *J. Stroke Cerebrovasc. Dis.* 29: 104881.

183 Lahiri, D. and Ardila, A. (2020). COVID-19 pandemic: a neurological perspective. *Cureus* 12: e7889.

184 Siniscalchi, A. and Gallelli, L. (2020). Could COVID-19 represent a negative prognostic factor in patients with stroke? *Infect. Control Hosp. Epidemiol.* 41: 1115–1116.

185 Bastidas, H.I., Márquez-Pérez, T., García-Salido, A. et al. (2021). Cerebral venous sinus thrombosis in a pediatric patient with COVID-19. *Neurol. Clin. Pract.* 11 (2): e208–e210. https://doi.org/10.1212/CPJ.0000000000000899.

186 Cavalcanti, D.D., Raz, E., Shapiro, M. et al. (2021). Cerebral venous thrombosis associated with COVID-19. *AJNR Am. J. Neuroradiol.* 48: 121–124.

187 Garaci, F., Di Giuliano, F., Picchi, E. et al. (2020). Venous cerebral thrombosis in COVID-19 patient. *J. Neurol. Sci.* 414: 116871.

188 Poillon, G., Obadia, M., Perrin, M. et al. (2021). Cerebral venous thrombosis associated with COVID-19 infection: causality or coincidence? *J. Neuroradiol.* 48: 121–124.

189 Pharmacovigilance Risk Assessment Committee (PRAC) (2021). Signal assessment report on embolic and thrombotic events (SMQ) with COVID-19 Vaccine (ChAdOx1-S [recombinant]) – COVID-19 Vaccine AstraZeneca (Other viral vaccines). https://www.ema.europa.eu/en/documents/prac-recommendation/signal-assessment-report-embolic-thrombotic-events-smq-covid-19-vaccine-chadox1-s-recombinant-covid_en.pdf (accessed July 8, 2021).

190 Chibber, P., Haq, S.A., Ahmed, I. et al. (2020). Advances in the possible treatment of COVID-19: a review. *Eur. J. Pharmacol.* 883: 173372.

191 Lamb, Y.N. (2020). Remdesivir: first approval. *Drugs* 80 (13): 1355–1363.

192 Frediansyah, A., Nainu, F., Dhama, K. et al. (2021). Remdesivir and its antiviral activity against COVID-19: a systematic review. *Clin. Epidemiol. Global Health* 9: 123–127.

193 Horby, P., Lim, W.S., Emberson, J.R. et al. (2021). Dexamethasone in hospitalized patients with Covid-19 - preliminary report. *N. Engl. J. Med.* 384: 693–704.

194 Baden, L.R., El Sahly, H.M., Essink, B. et al. (2021). Efficacy and safety of the mRNA-1273 SARS-CoV-2 vaccine. *N. Engl. J. Med.* 384 (5): 403–416.

195 Logunov, D.Y., Dolzhikova, I.V., Shcheblyakov, D.V. et al. (2021). Safety and efficacy of an rAd26 and rAd5 vector-based heterologous prime-boost COVID-19 vaccine: an interim analysis of a randomised controlled phase 3 trial in Russia. *Lancet* 397 (10275): 671–681.

196 Polack, F.P., Thomas, S.J., Kitchin, N. et al. (2020). Safety and efficacy of the BNT162b2 mRNA Covid-19 vaccine. *N. Engl. J. Med.* 383 (27): 2603–2615.

197 Vabret, N., Britton, G.J., Gruber, C. et al. (2020). Immunology of COVID-19: current state of the science. *Immunity* 52 (6): 910–941.

16

COVID-19: Cardiology Perspective

Michael DiVita[1], Meshe Chonde[1], Megan Kamath[1], Darko Vucicevic[1], Ashley M. Fan[2], Arnold S. Baas[1], and Jeffrey J. Hsu[1,3]

[1]Division of Cardiology, Department of Medicine, UCLA Health, Los Angeles, CA, USA
[2]Department of Pharmaceutical Services, UCLA Health, Los Angeles, CA, USA
[3]Division of Cardiology, Department of Medicine, Veterans Affairs Greater Los Angeles Healthcare System, Los Angeles, CA, USA

Abbreviations

ACC	American College of Cardiology
ACE-2	angiotensin-converting enzyme 2
ACEi	angiotensin-converting enzyme inhibitor
ACoCS	acute COVID-19 cardiovascular syndrome
ACS	acute coronary syndrome
AHA	American Heart Association
ARB	angiotensin receptor blocker
BNP	B-type natriuretic peptide
CCL	cardiac catheterization laboratory
CFR	case fatality rate
CMR	cardiac magnetic resonance imaging
CRP	C-reactive protein
CT	computed tomography
DVT	deep vein thrombosis
ECG	electrocardiogram
ICU	intensive care unit
IL-6	interleukin-6
IVIG	intravenous immunoglobulin
LMWH	low-molecular-weight heparin
LVEF	left ventricular ejection fraction
MI	myocardial infarction
MIS-A	multisystem inflammatory syndrome in adults
MIS-C	multisystem inflammatory syndrome in children
NIH	National Institutes of Health
PASC	postacute sequelae of SARS-CoV-2
PCI	percutaneous coronary intervention
PE	pulmonary embolism
PIMS	pediatric inflammatory multisystem syndrome
POTS	postural orthostatic tachycardia syndrome
PPE	personal protective equipment
SARS-CoV-2	severe acute respiratory syndrome coronavirus 2
STEMI	ST-segment elevation myocardial infarction
VTE	venous thromboembolism

Coronavirus disease 2019 (COVID-19), caused by infection with the novel severe acute respiratory syndrome coronavirus 2 (SARS-CoV-2), has become a worldwide pandemic since its outbreak from Wuhan, China in December 2019. Although clinically this disease manifests primarily with respiratory symptoms such as shortness of breath, cough, fever, and fatigue, there have been several cardiac manifestations observed as well. Often, it is difficult to distinguish between cardiac and respiratory manifestations because both present with dyspnea. Sometimes, symptoms more typical of cardiac disease, such as chest pain or palpitations, may be present. This chapter will review the epidemiology, mechanisms of action, manifestations, and management of cardiovascular diseases associated with COVID-19.

Coronavirus Disease 2019 (COVID-19): A Clinical Guide, First Edition. Edited by Ali Gholamrezanezhad and Michael P. Dube.
© 2023 John Wiley & Sons Ltd. Published 2023 by John Wiley & Sons Ltd.

Epidemiology

Older age is widely recognized as the strongest risk factor for mortality in COVID-19. Cardiovascular comorbidities have also consistently shown to be associated with greater risk for adverse clinical outcomes and more severe disease. Hypertension, diabetes mellitus, and cardiovascular disease (i.e. coronary artery disease, congestive heart failure) have been most strongly associated with worse outcomes and death. Hypertension has the strongest association, present in 15–30% of patients with severe disease and as much as 48% in nonsurvivors. Diabetes has been observed in 10–20% of patients with severe disease (31% of nonsurvivors) and cardiovascular disease in 8–16% with severe disease (13% of nonsurvivors) [1, 2]. Notably, however, these comorbidities are more frequent in people with advanced age. It is possible that the poor outcomes observed in these populations are a reflection of age rather than comorbidities.

The rate of cardiac injury observed in COVID-19 is variable (mostly based on definition) but appears to be more prevalent in patients with known cardiovascular comorbidities and hospitalized patients. Studies have observed cardiac injury in 7–28% of hospitalized patients and 22% of those who require intensive care unit (ICU) care [3–5]. Cardiac injury is associated with worse outcomes, including ICU admission and death [3, 4]. One study identified the mortality rate of individuals hospitalized with subsequent evidence of cardiac injury (i.e. elevated troponin) to be as high as 51.2%, compared with 4.5% in those without evidence of cardiac injury [4].

The case fatality rate (CFR) has also been shown to be significantly increased in patients with cardiovascular comorbidities compared with those without comorbidities. One study suggested a CFR of 0.9% in patients without comorbidities compared with a CFR of 6% with hypertension, 7.3% with diabetes, and 10.5% with cardiovascular disease [6].

Potential Mechanisms of Cardiovascular System Involvement in COVID-19

The effects of SARS-CoV-2 on the cardiovascular system and subsequent cardiac injury are not completely understood. Multiple mechanisms have been proposed, and the effects are likely multifactorial (Figure 16.1).

Direct Viral Myocardial Injury

To gain entry into a cell, SARS-CoV-2 binds to the cell surface receptor angiotensin-converting enzyme 2 (ACE-2). The virus membrane then fuses with the host cell membrane, and the viral genome is deposited in the host cell cytoplasm for translation and replication. Although the main target for SARS-CoV-2 appears to be respiratory epithelial cells, ACE-2 also exists on myocardium and vascular endothelial cells (Figure 16.2) [8], providing a theoretical mechanism for direct viral infection of the heart and blood vessels, with resultant myocarditis and vasculitis, respectively. In addition, infection-mediated vasculitis may result in monocyte and lymphocyte infiltration of the arterial and venous walls, which causes vascular endothelial injury and subsequent myocardial injury [7].

An early case report demonstrated the presence of viral particles in an endomyocardial biopsy sample from a patient with COVID-19 and fulminant cardiogenic shock, although it remained unclear if this occurred via direct viral invasion of cardiomyocytes [9]. A subsequent autopsy study performed on 277 hearts from patients with COVID-19, however, found SARS-CoV-2-related myocarditis to be rare, present in less than 2% of the specimens analyzed [10]. Thus, although direct viral myocardial injury may be possible, it is overall considered to be a rare occurrence.

Microvascular Injury

A prominent finding in COVID-19 has been thrombosis, both in the microvascular circulation and in larger vessels [11]. Likely, this hypercoagulable state is the result of an overwhelming imbalance between the coagulation and fibrinolytic systems from an infection-mediated cause, such as disseminated intravascular coagulopathy. Platelet activation is also known to be enhanced in sepsis and inflammation, which may contribute to the formation of thrombus. It has been hypothesized that myocardial injury may be the result of thrombus formation in the myocardial vasculature and resultant microvascular dysfunction.

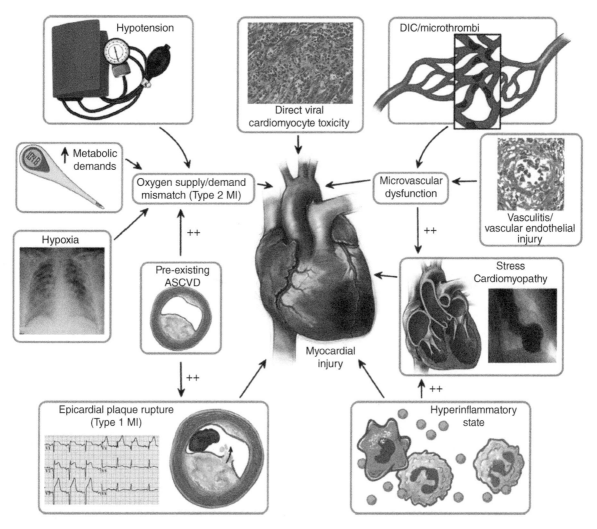

Figure 16.1 Multiple mechanisms for severe acute respiratory syndrome coronavirus 2 interaction with the cardiovascular system. *Source:* Reproduced with permission from Atri et al. [7].

Acute Coronary Syndrome

There are multiple mechanisms by which a systemic viral infection may lead to a greater risk for coronary plaque destabilization and subsequent acute coronary syndrome (ACS). The immune response to an acute viral infection of an arterial wall will cause a surge of cytokines and inflammatory mediators leading to localized vessel inflammation [12]. This inflammatory response may be more pronounced within segments containing coronary plaques and cause subsequent plaque rupture and ACS. In addition, viral products in the systemic circulation can generate an innate immune receptor activation that results in activation of immune

cells residing in preexisting atheroma. Activation of these cells may trigger destabilization of the plaque and subsequent plaque rupture, causing ACS.

Oxygen Supply and Demand Mismatch

Mismatch between oxygen supply and demand without significant coronary artery occlusion, known as a type 2 myocardial infarction (MI), has been hypothesized as another mechanism for myocardial injury. Severe physiologic stress and demand for oxygen by the myocardium during COVID-19-induced sepsis may lead to inadequate oxygen supply and subsequent

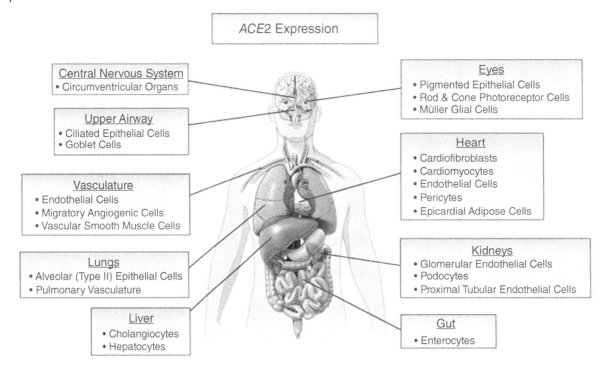

ACE2 Expression

Central Nervous System
• Circumventricular Organs

Upper Airway
• Ciliated Epithelial Cells
• Goblet Cells

Vasculature
• Endothelial Cells
• Migratory Angiogenic Cells
• Vascular Smooth Muscle Cells

Lungs
• Alveolar (Type II) Epithelial Cells
• Pulmonary Vasculature

Liver
• Cholangiocytes
• Hepatocytes

Eyes
• Pigmented Epithelial Cells
• Rod & Cone Photoreceptor Cells
• Müller Glial Cells

Heart
• Cardiofibroblasts
• Cardiomyocytes
• Endothelial Cells
• Pericytes
• Epicardial Adipose Cells

Kidneys
• Glomerular Endothelial Cells
• Podocytes
• Proximal Tubular Endothelial Cells

Gut
• Enterocytes

Figure 16.2 Angiotensin-converting enzyme 2 (ACE2) is found on myocardial, vascular endothelial cells and a variety of other cells within the body. *Source:* Reproduced with permission from Gheblawi et al. [8].

myocardial injury. This oxygen supply and demand mismatch may be further exacerbated by coinciding hypoxemia as a result of respiratory failure, further inducing or perpetuating myocardial injury.

Systemic Hyperinflammatory Response

Previous studies have demonstrated that cardiomyopathy in sepsis is partially mediated by inflammatory cytokines such as tumor necrosis factor-α, interleukin-6 (IL-6), IL-1β, interferon gamma, and IL-2. Significant elevations in levels of inflammatory biomarkers and cytokines, such as IL-6, C-reactive protein (CRP), tumor necrosis factor-α, IL-2 receptor, and ferritin, have also been observed in COVID-19 [13], thus suggesting another mechanism for myocardial injury.

Myocardial Injury in Acute COVID-19

Acute Coronary Syndrome

Although COVID-19 is associated with many cardiovascular complications, there has been a decline observed in the number of catheterization lab activations for acute ST-segment elevation myocardial infarctions (STEMIs) and hospitalizations for ACS during the pandemic [14]. This is speculated to be due to reluctance of patients to seek medical attention or potential misdiagnosis given the focus on evaluation for respiratory symptoms, and not necessarily a decline in acute coronary events. Regardless, STEMI and ACS remain important conditions that require immediate therapy, whether because of a direct effect of SARS-CoV-2 or coincidental occurrence during the pandemic.

Clinical Presentation

The clinical manifestations of ACS during the COVID-19 pandemic, regardless of whether occurring in conjunction with active SARS-CoV-2 infection, are similar to symptoms experienced during typical myocardial ischemia. The typical symptom will be chest pain, usually described as a pressure-like sensation, or anginal equivalent. Chest pain may be associated with radiation to the left arm or jaw, shortness of breath, and/or diaphoresis. It is important to note that chest pain is a relatively less common presenting manifestation of COVID-19 [13, 15], and report of such symptoms should raise suspicion for an acute coronary event.

Diagnosis

The definition of an acute MI caused by atherothrombotic coronary artery occlusion, also known as a type 1 MI, is unchanged from the standard definition provided by the 4th Universal Definition of MI [16]. As such, the diagnosis of ACS during the COVID-19 pandemic remains unchanged as well. For any patient with suspected ACS, a history and physical examination, electrocardiogram (ECG), and troponin should be obtained as rapidly as possible (usually within 10 minutes of presentation). The physical examination should include assessment of vital signs, auscultation of the heart and lungs, and assessment for signs of congestive heart failure. In a STEMI, the ECG will show ST-segment elevation in two or more contiguous leads with reciprocal changes, and cardiac biomarkers (i.e. troponin) will be elevated. In the case of non-STEMI, elevated biomarkers without ST-segment elevation on ECG will be observed.

Given the prevalence of myocardial injury without coronary artery occlusion (referred to as type 2 MI) [16] seen in COVID-19, a high index of suspicion should be maintained for the possibility of noncoronary myocardial injury, such as myocarditis, when elevated biomarkers are observed without ECG changes in COVID-positive or probable patients. If a type 2 MI is suspected, noninvasive testing with coronary computed tomography (CT) angiography or myocardial perfusion imaging should be performed to confirm the absence of significant coronary artery disease. In addition, the presence of ST-segment elevation on ECG, especially in the setting of atypical symptoms, may signal an alternative diagnosis such as stress cardiomyopathy (also known as Takotsubo cardiomyopathy) or myocarditis. In these situations, additional imaging, such as transthoracic echocardiogram or point-of-care ultrasound, to identify wall motion abnormalities may be helpful.

During the pandemic, the emergency department (ED) evaluation should become an even more vital part of the evaluation of patients with ACS. ED assessments should be focused on making the proper diagnosis of ACS while also assessing COVID-19 status and the potential need for additional interventions, such as intubation for respiratory failure. As point-of-care COVID-19 tests become available, all patients presenting with STEMI should be routinely screened before transfer to the cardiac catheterization laboratory (CCL) to better characterize the patient's infectious status and allow for optimized care.

Management

STEMI

As per American College of Cardiology (ACC)/American Heart Association (AHA)/Society for Cardiovascular Angiography and Interventions guidelines (Table 16.1), for any patient with a true STEMI, irrespective of COVID-19 status, primary percutaneous coronary intervention (PCI) should remain the standard of care. One caveat to this recommendation being for patients who present with severe respiratory failure as a result of COVID-19 or other extremist condition where mortality rate is believed to be excessively high, then pursual of comfort care may be more appropriate. Any high-grade stenosis found in a non-culprit vessel should be treated during the index procedure to minimize potential exposure of staff during a staged procedure. Patients who are hemodynamically stable after primary PCI should be admitted to a step-down or telemetry unit with plans for an early discharge (<48 hours), in an effort to preserve availability of critical care beds [17].

Anytime a patient is required to be brought to the CCL for intervention, emphasis should be placed on maintaining safety of all healthcare workers and staff throughout the procedure. This includes ensuring appropriate personal protective equipment (PPE) is provided for and worn by all staff throughout the duration of the case. Given the high risk of aerosolizing-generating procedures (i.e. endotracheal intubation, noninvasive positive pressure ventilation, or cardiopulmonary resuscitation) occurring during a catheterization, it is recommended that all personnel wear N95 masks. In the event that endotracheal intubation is required, a powered air-purifying respirator (PAPR) should be worn. Utilization of a negative pressure procedure room is preferred for all cases if available.

There has been evidence to suggest higher thrombogenicity in patients with STEMI and concomitant COVID-19. In a study by Choudry et al. [18], higher rates of multivessel thrombosis, stent thrombosis, glycoprotein IIb/IIIa use, and thrombectomy use in patients

Table 16.1 American College of Cardiology/American Heart Association guidelines for the care of patients with acute myocardial infarction during the COVID-19 pandemic.

All patients with STEMI should initially undergo evaluation in the ED.

- Patients should be evaluated in the ED before CCL activation to ensure appropriate risks are assessed.
- All patients require the placement of a face mask to prevent droplet contamination of the CCL and environment before transport.

CCL staff and physicians should have appropriate PPE for safe performance of the procedure, including gowns, gloves, full face mask, and an N95 respiratory mask. If N95 masks are to be reused between cases by a single HCW, then an additional surgical mask should be worn on top of this mask. The number of HCWs present during the procedure should be limited to only those essential for patient care and procedure support.

Patients with respiratory compromise should be intubated before arrival in the CCL if possible.

- If intubation is required in the CCL, all personnel should have complete PPE and exposures should be minimized to essential team members only.
- For all procedures at high risk for aerosolization, PAPRs should be considered.

Proper PPE training should be provided and practiced by physicians and CCL staff involved in all cases, and extra consideration should be given to the protection of trainees with high-risk patients and procedures.

Primary PCI should remain the default strategy in patients with clear evidence of a STEMI; if a primary PCI approach is not feasible, a pharmacoinvasive approach may be considered.

During the COVID-19 period, there may be delays in door-to-balloon times that result from evaluation and/or management of patients with COVID-19. This can be documented in the medical record and coded in the NCDR CathPCI version 5 as follows:

- If primary PCI for STEMI, code "Yes" for Seq. #7850 (patient-centered reason for delay in PCI) and select "Other" in Seq. #7851 (delay reason).
- If primary thrombolytic therapy for STEMI, code "Yes" for Seq. #14208 (patient reason for delay in thrombolytic).

Within the CCL, a single negative pressure procedure room with essential supplies only is preferable for the care of known COVID-19-positive or -probable patients with a terminal clean after the procedure.

To preserve ICU beds, all hemodynamically stable patients with STEMI after PCI should be admitted to an intermediate care telemetry unit with plan for early (<48 h) discharge.

CCL, cardiac catheterization laboratory; COVID-19, coronavirus disease 2019; ED, emergency department; HCW, healthcare worker; ICU, intensive care unit; NCDR, National Cardiovascular Data Registry; PAPR, powered air-purifying respirator; PCI, percutaneous coronary intervention; PPE, personal protective equipment; STEMI, ST-elevation myocardial infarction.
Source: Adapted with permission from Mahmud et al. [17].

with STEMI was observed in COVID-19-positive patients compared to those who were COVID-19 negative. This also translated into longer hospital length of stays and greater need for intensive care services.

For patients with STEMI presenting to a non-PCI-capable center, primary PCI should remain the standard of care if rapid transfer to a PCI-capable center is possible (<120 minutes from first medical contact to PCI-capable center). If rapid transfer is not possible, an initial pharmacologic strategy with fibrinolysis should be implemented with subsequent transfer to a PCI-capable center. However, patients found to be COVID-19 positive should be discussed in additional detail with the referral center to ensure no unnecessary exposure to staff during the transfer process.

It is important to note that in the United States where regional systems for primary PCI are in place, a strategy of fibrinolysis in all COVID-19-positive patients with STEMI is not recommended. Fibrinolysis should be reserved for non-PCI-capable centers when transfer to a PCI-capable center cannot be achieved within 120 minutes from first medical contact. Close monitoring of regional STEMI systems and transfer processes should be performed, and adjustments to protocols should be made as needed.

Non-STEMI

Patients with NSTE-ACS (non-STEMI or unstable angina) without high-risk features, regardless of COVID-19 status, should be treated initially with standard medical therapy including dual antiplatelet therapy and therapeutic anticoagulation.

For COVID-19-positive or -probable patients, urgent coronary angiography and possible PCI should be pursued only in the presence of high-risk clinical features (i.e. Global Registry of Acute Coronary Events [GRACE] score > 140, thrombolysis in myocardial infarction score [TIMI] ≥ 3) or hemodynamic instability. In the absence of high-risk features, coronary angiography should be deferred until a future date when resolution of the infection has occurred.

In COVID-19-negative patients, an early invasive approach should be pursued as clinically indicated.

Out-of-Hospital Cardiac Arrest

Patients with resuscitated out-of-hospital cardiac arrest caused by acute MI represent a high-risk subgroup of patients with ACS. Emergent coronary angiography and PCI should remain a priority in the presence of persistent ST elevations suggestive of a true coronary artery occlusion. In patients without ST elevations after resuscitation, an early invasive approach should be deferred unless hemodynamic instability ensues or acute coronary occlusion remains high on the differential diagnosis.

Thrombosis and Pulmonary Embolism

Thrombosis and thrombotic disease, both of the arterial and venous circulations, have been a well-described component of COVID-19 [11]. The occurrence of thrombotic disease is likely multifactorial, including direct effects of the virus, such as direct endothelial injury, and indirect effects of the infection, such as the development of a severe inflammatory response or disseminated intravascular coagulopathy. In addition, traditional underlying risk factors, such as genetic procoagulant abnormalities or immobility as a result of critical disease, may be contributing.

These hypercoagulable states manifest as derangements in hemostatic parameters, including mild thrombocytopenia and elevated D-dimer levels. Prolongation of prothrombin time and international normalized ratio have also been observed. Elevated levels of inflammatory markers, such as CRP, ferritin, and IL-6, have been observed and may suggest a correlation between the inflammatory response observed and a procoagulant state.

Venous thromboembolism (VTE), including deep vein thrombosis (DVT) and pulmonary embolism (PE), is very common in acutely ill patients with COVID-19, seen in as many as one-third of patients in the ICU despite prophylactic anticoagulation [19]. However, randomized clinical trials testing therapeutic doses of anticoagulation in patients with COVID-19 admitted to the ICU did not improve outcomes compared with routine prophylactic anticoagulation doses [20, 21]. Conversely, another large trial found that there may be benefit to therapeutic anticoagulation in hospitalized patients with COVID-19 not admitted to the ICU, although these results have yet to be published at the time of this writing [22].

Clinical Presentation

VTE in COVID-19-positive or -probable patients mimics the typical VTE presentation in prepandemic times. Acute DVT presents with unilateral (occasionally bilateral) extremity swelling, warmth, and tenderness. In extreme cases with extensive thrombosis, patients may present with signs of phlegmasia, including severe pain, swelling, cyanosis, edema, and venous gangrene of the extremity. PE presents with chest pain, shortness of breath, hypoxemia (often disproportionate to known respiratory pathologies), and signs of right ventricular failure, including tachycardia, elevated jugular venous pressure, and potentially hypotension. In extreme cases, patients may present with syncope or cardiac arrest.

Diagnosis

Evaluation and diagnosis of VTE in patients with COVID-19 should be based on clinical features. Although laboratory values may be helpful in prognosticating disease severity and outcomes, evaluation for VTE should not be based off these abnormal findings alone. However, given the high prevalence of VTE in patients with COVID-19, clinicians should maintain a high level of suspicion in the presence of appropriate clinical features.

In individuals with a suspected DVT, venous compression ultrasonography should be performed if possible. Prone positioning in severely ill patients may pose difficulty in performing ultrasonography or alternative imaging studies.

If PE is suspected, a normal D-dimer in patients with low to intermediate pretest probability for PE should be sufficient to exclude the diagnosis of PE. If pretest probability remains high despite a normal D-dimer value, or the patient has an elevated D-dimer value with intermediate or greater pretest probability, then further imaging should be pursued. Computed tomography with pulmonary angiography is the preferred test for the diagnosis of PE. A ventilation/perfusion scan also can be considered, but results may be inconclusive in patients with significant respiratory involvement from COVID-19. In addition, the ventilation component of the ventilation/perfusion scan may unnecessarily expose healthcare workers to COVID-19 and may be deferred during this examination.

When performing imaging studies, the risk for exposure to healthcare workers and other individuals should be appropriately weighed against the benefits of obtaining the study. If patients are critically ill with high risk for mortality, deferral of imaging may be appropriate.

Management

Therapeutic anticoagulation is the mainstay of VTE treatment. Selection of anticoagulant agent should take into consideration clinical situations and other comorbidities, such as renal or hepatic dysfunction. In critically ill patients, parenteral anticoagulation (i.e. unfractionated heparin, low-molecular-weight heparin [LMWH]) may be preferred. Downsides to using unfractionated heparin include longer time to achieve therapeutic effect and increased exposure of healthcare workers when performing frequent activated partial thromboplastin time blood draws. For these reasons, LMWH may be preferred when appropriate. In noncritical patients and outpatients, oral anticoagulation with direct oral anticoagulants or parenteral therapy with LMWH may be preferred to facilitate early hospital discharge, minimize the need for therapeutic monitoring, and reduce utilization of healthcare resources compared with oral vitamin K antagonists.

With regard to reperfusion strategies for acute PE, patients with hemodynamically stable intermediate-risk PE, also known as submassive PE (defined as biomarker or echocardiographic evidence of right ventricular strain without hypotension), should be treated with therapeutic anticoagulation and monitored closely. If further deterioration is observed, systemic fibrinolysis or catheter-based interventions can be considered. In patients with hemodynamically unstable high-risk PE, also known as massive PE (defined as the presence of hypotension), systemic fibrinolysis is indicated as first-line therapy assuming no absolute contraindications.

In general, interventional-based therapies for VTE have not demonstrated significant benefit over traditional medical therapy. As such, these therapies should be saved for patients with severe disease, such as venous thrombosis with phlegmasia or disease refractory to traditional therapy [23].

Acute Myocarditis and Cardiogenic Shock

Acute myocarditis with resultant cardiogenic shock and circulatory collapse is one of the acute cardiovascular effects of COVID-19 that has been reported. Before the COVID-19 pandemic, the annual incidence of myocarditis from all causes was about 22 cases per 100,000 people [24], with the most common etiology in the United States being viral [25]. As of the time of this publication, however, there remains limited information on the presentation, diagnosis, and management of COVID-19-associated myocarditis, because this disease process is still relatively novel [26]. Currently, there is no established definition of COVID-19-associated myocarditis. We define it as acute myocardial injury that occurs in acute COVID-19 illness, which commonly results in acute left ventricular or biventricular dysfunction in the absence of obstructive epicardial disease [27].

As mentioned earlier in this chapter, the mechanism of myocardial injury is not completely understood and likely multifactorial. It is clear, however, that myocardial injury is associated with more severe complications and increased mortality [28]. Driggin and colleagues [23] estimated that 7% of COVID-19 deaths result from myocarditis. Meanwhile, others have estimated that 32% of COVID-19 reported deaths are accompanied by heart failure, with acute myocardial injury with heart failure being listed as a contributing factor [29]. However, the overall incidence is difficult to assess due to the limited sample size of the aforementioned studies. Although an early CMR study raised concern for a high prevalence of myocarditis among patients recovering from COVID-19 [30], subsequent studies have revealed that this may have been an overestimate. Evaluation of young and professional athletes recovering from COVID-19 has found an overall low prevalence of clinical myocarditis in this relatively low-risk group [31, 32].

Clinical Presentation

The clinical presentation of acute myocarditis is characterized by symptoms such as chest pain and dyspnea [33, 34]. Signs include ST-segment deviation (either elevation or depression) on 12-lead ECG, elevations in cardiac biomarkers (i.e. troponin and B-type natriuretic peptide [BNP]), and the presence of left ventricular and/or right ventricular hypokinesis on echocardiography. Commonly preceding this presentation is a viral prodrome of fever, dry cough, myalgias, headache, and other influenza-like symptoms [35]. The constellation of myocardial dysfunction in the absence of epicardial coronary disease following this viral prodrome is suggestive of acute myocarditis; however, diagnosing the cause is challenging because the majority of cases of myocarditis in the United States are presumed to be viral in etiology [25].

Diagnosis

Diagnosis may be improved by imaging, such as cardiac magnetic resonance imaging (CMR) or CT scan. CMR can be beneficial by following the Lake Louise Consensus Criteria for the diagnosis of myocarditis, which requires the presence of at least two of the following findings to meet diagnostic criteria: (i) myocardial edema; (ii) irreversible cell injury as indicated by the presence of delayed gadolinium enhancement; and (iii) hyperemia or capillary leak [36]. CMR findings from reports of SARS-CoV-2 myocarditis have included biventricular dysfunction [37], diffuse myocardial edema, pseudohypertrophy [34], and late gadolinium enhancement [37]. Contrast-enhanced CT with ECG gating is an effective alternative [26].

Endomyocardial biopsy is generally not recommended given potential exposure risk to staff and lack of evidence to support change in management based on findings. If performed, findings demonstrate an acute inflammatory process with diffuse T-lymphocytic infiltrates with interstitial edema and limited necrosis without fibrosis. Thus far, however, molecular analysis of tissue specimens has not consistently demonstrated the presence of SARS-CoV-2 within cardiomyocytes themselves [9, 26].

Management

Currently, there is a lack of treatment for SARS-CoV-2 viral myocarditis. Previously studied therapies for myocarditis include cyclosporine and azathioprine [38], intravenous immunoglobulin (IVIG) [39], and corticosteroids [40], although their routine use for myocarditis management has not been recommended. Use of IVIG has been suggested by some small case series [41, 42] as a potential for further study and may be used as salvage therapy in presumed viral myocarditis [43]. In the absence of a definitive medical therapy, management should focus on providing hemodynamic support with vasopressor and inotropic agents as needed, and the addition of mechanical circulatory support if necessary. Expert consultation with an advanced heart failure team or multidisciplinary shock team should be considered, with potential transfer of patients to specialized centers when these teams are not available at the treating facility. Mechanical ventilation is also sometimes necessary given the acute respiratory failure, which can ensue secondary to cardiac failure in patients afflicted by SARS-CoV-2-induced myocarditis.

For those individuals who achieve clinical improvement, persistence of reduced ventricular systolic function necessitates initiation of guideline-directed medical therapy as per ACC/AHA guidelines for heart failure. Usually the initiation of this therapy occurs later in the hospital course, such as nearing discharge [27]. In addition, standard post-myocarditis recommendations should be followed, including abstinence from competitive sports or aerobic activity for three to six months [27].

Pericarditis

Pericarditis is inflammation localized to the pericardium. Its association with COVID-19 infection has not been well described, although a study of healthy college athletes recovering from COVID-19 found that nearly 40% had delayed enhancement of their pericardial tissue on CMR [44]. Generally, the most common etiology in the United States is viral [45]. The incidence of pericarditis has been reported to be between

3.3 and 27.7 cases per 100,000 people [46, 47]. At the time of this publication however, there remains limited information on the presentation, diagnosis, and management of SARS-CoV-2-associated pericarditis [26].

The pathogenesis for COVID-19-associated pericarditis is not well described, although there are several proposed mechanisms. Similar to the purported pathophysiology of myocarditis, the pericardial cells may suffer direct toxicity from infection via ACE-2 receptor-mediated entry in pericardial mesothelial cells [27] followed by viral replication and damage via the impairment of stress granule formation [26], which may occur in the initial presentation. The activation of the inflammatory cascade and release of proinflammatory cytokines may lead to infiltration of the pericardium by inflammatory cells resulting in further cell injury and either a local (pericarditis) or diffuse (myopericarditis) process [27, 48].

Clinical Presentation

The clinical presentation of acute pericarditis is characterized by symptoms of chest pain and dyspnea [49], which are worse when lying flat and alleviated when leaning forward [50]. Commonly preceding pericarditis is a viral prodrome of fever, dry cough, myalgias, headache, and other influenza-like symptoms [35], which may make it difficult to discern and diagnose.

Patients with pericarditis commonly have vital signs within normal limits [50], and the presence of an abnormality such as hypotension or tachycardia may suggest an alternative diagnosis or the presence of a complication such as cardiac tamponade [51, 52].

Diagnosis

Twelve-lead ECG may show diffuse ST-segment elevation and PR depression with reciprocal changes in lead aVR, although findings may be focal as well [50, 53]. Laboratory studies may reveal leukocytosis [49, 53], elevated inflammatory markers such as CRP [49, 53], and elevated BNP [51]. Troponin levels should not be elevated unless there is associated myocardial injury, such as in myopericarditis. Transthoracic echocardiography will demonstrate preserved ventricular function [49–51], bright and echogenic pericardium [50], and usually an associated pericardial effusion [49]. The presence of ventricular systolic dysfunction is not

typical of isolated pericarditis, and this finding should raise suspicion for myocardial involvement and possibly a myopericarditis [37, 51].

CT imaging or CMR also can be helpful in the diagnosis of pericarditis. CT imaging allows for assessment of pericardial thickening and the identification of a pericardial effusion [53]. CT may also allow for better imaging when echocardiography is challenging [54]. CMR can be beneficial in the diagnosis of pericarditis, and its use has increased because of its ability to gather additional information, such as better definition of the pericardium, assessment of pericardial thickening, identification of inflammation/scar with late gadolinium enhancement, and evaluation for associated myocardial involvement [44, 50]. In addition, although CT imaging is a relatively rapid test and can be used in pre-procedure planning such as pericardiocentesis or pericardiectomy to provide anatomic information, CMR can assess hemodynamic information, such as evaluation for constrictive pericarditis [55].

Management

Thus far, there have been only case reports illustrating acute pericarditis in the setting of acute COVID-19 [49–51], and data remain incomplete on the optimal management. Generally, treatment of acute pericarditis is focused on reduction of pericardial inflammation. Nonsteroidal anti-inflammatory drugs (NSAIDs) are the mainstay of treatment, along with colchicine [49, 56]. In patients in whom NSAIDs may be contraindicated, corticosteroids can be used as an alternative, although there remains concern of an increased risk for recurrent pericarditis with this treatment modality [56]. Currently, the use of these medications in treating COVID-19 pericarditis has not been well studied, but their usage has not been linked to any worse cardiovascular or pulmonary adverse effects [56, 57].

NSAIDs and colchicine have relatively tolerable side effect profiles with the exception of nephrotoxicity [58]. At this time, corticosteroids, specifically dexamethasone, are commonly used in patients who develop acute respiratory failure with COVID-19, and their use may potentially provide treatment for COVID-19-associated pericarditis, leading to possible underdiagnosis [37]. To date, there has been no large trial examining the efficacy of these therapies in the treatment of acute pericarditis associated with

SARS-CoV-2 infection; however, several small case reports have illustrated the safety and efficacy of colchicine [49, 50, 53] and NSAIDs [49, 56] in patients with COVID-19.

Kawasaki Disease, Multisystem Inflammatory Syndrome in Children, Pediatric Multisystem Syndrome, Multisystem Inflammatory Syndrome in Adults, and Acute COVID-19 Cardiovascular Syndrome: Overlapping Post-COVID-19 Inflammatory Cardiac Syndromes

Kawasaki disease (mucocutaneous lymph node syndrome) is a rare but potentially severe systematic inflammatory syndrome first described in 1967 as affecting children, adolescents, and rarely adults [59]. This disease is characterized by fever (>39 °C for >5 days) and diffuse inflammation involving multiple systems, including skin (diffuse rash often involving trunk, genital area, palms and soles of feet leading to desquamation), eyes (conjunctivitis, uveitis, papilledema), mouth (cracked lips, swollen tongue), neurologic (sensorineural hearing loss, ataxia, aseptic meningitis, facial nerve palsy), lymph nodes (adenopathy in the neck, typically >1.5 cm), gastrointestinal (diarrhea, abdominal pain, emesis), musculoskeletal (arthralgia and arthritis), kidneys (proteinuria, acute kidney injury, tubulointerstitial nephritis, hemolytic uremic syndrome, immune complex–mediated nephropathy), genitourinary (urethritis/meatitis, hydrocele), pulmonary (cough, respiratory distress, infiltrates, or nodules), and cardiac (coronary artery aneurysm, myocarditis, valvulitis, arrhythmias) [60].

Early in the COVID-19 pandemic, children, adolescents, and some younger adults were characterized as having milder or even no symptoms compared with adults with COVID-19, especially those adults with significant comorbidities. However, several investigators in the United Kingdom [61, 62], Italy [63], Spain [64], and the United States [65] described case series of children and adolescents with a post-COVID-19 multisystem hyperinflammatory syndrome

termed multisystem inflammatory syndrome in children (MIS-C) or pediatric inflammatory multisystem syndrome (PIMS), typically greater than four weeks after COVID-19 exposure. In a study of 184 patients with MIS-C in New York City, MIS-C had a higher incidence among Black and Hispanic children when compared with White children [66]. These clinical findings shared many of the clinical and laboratory features of Kawasaki disease and toxic shock syndrome, such as persistent fever, rash, mucocutaneous manifestations, adenopathy, abdominal pain, diarrhea, lethargy-irritability-confusion, and cardiac involvement, with up to 20% of patients demonstrating coronary artery aneurysms as typically observed in Kawasaki disease. In the Italian series, this post-COVID-19 Kawasaki disease incidence was 30-fold greater than typically observed in the general population before the COVID-19 pandemic. In addition, patients with MIS-C or PIMS were on average older (8–10 years) than typical patients with Kawasaki disease (<5 years); more often presented with shock, myocarditis, and left ventricular dysfunction (>50%); and had significantly greater elevations in markers of systemic inflammation (erythrocyte sedimentation rate, CRP, ferritin) and cardiac involvement (elevated troponin and BNP). Furthermore, more than half of patients with MIS-C or PIMS required ICU level of care, with greater than 50% requiring vasopressors and inotropes, and some even requiring temporary mechanical circulatory support with left ventricular assist device or extracorporeal membrane oxygenation [64, 67, 68].

Reflecting the severity of the systemic inflammatory syndrome and multisystem involvement, mortality in these series ranged from 1% to 3%. A recent systems immunologic approach to analyzing cytokine storm differences in patients with COVID-19, Kawasaki disease, or MIS-C demonstrates that the hyperinflammation of MIS-C differs from that in acute COVID-19. Furthermore, T-cell subsets discriminate MIS-C from Kawasaki disease, and IL-17 drives Kawasaki disease, but not the MIS-C inflammatory state [69].

Recently, the Centers for Disease Control and Prevention reported a case series of 16 post-COVID-19 adult patients, aged 20–50 years, with similar multisystem inflammatory findings to MIS-C and PIMS, including cardiac involvement. This process was termed multisystem inflammatory syndrome in adults

(MIS-A), indicating that this syndrome is no longer isolated to the pediatric or adolescent population [70]. To add to the list and confusion of post-COVID-19 inflammatory syndromes affecting the cardiovascular syndrome, MIS-A also is very similar to another post-COVID-19 inflammatory syndrome termed acute COVID-19 cardiovascular syndrome (ACoCS) [27]. In the rapidly evolving science of COVID-19, it is likely that there is significant clinical overlap in the inflammatory cardiovascular conditions of Kawasaki disease, MIS-C/PIMS, MIS-A, and ACoCS as illustrated in Figure 16.3 [71].

Clinical Presentation

In general, patients with MIS-C or PIMS tended to demonstrate three presentation phenotypes: (i) neurologic with confusion, ataxia, headache, seizures, and focal neurologic deficits; (ii) gastrointestinal with diarrhea and severe abdominal pain mimicking an acute abdomen; and (iii) cardiac with a Kawasaki disease-like presentation.

Diagnosis

Classic Kawasaki disease is diagnosed clinically with the AHA criteria of fever for >5 days and four of five of the following: (i) erythema of oral and pharyngeal mucosa; (ii) bilateral bulbar conjunctival injection without exudate; (iii) rash (maculopapular, diffuse erythroderma, or erythema multiforme-like); (iv) erythema and edema of the hands and feet in the acute phase and/or periungual desquamation in the subacute phase; and (v) cervical lymphadenopathy (≥1.5 cm in diameter), usually unilateral [60]. Recently, the Centers for Disease Control and

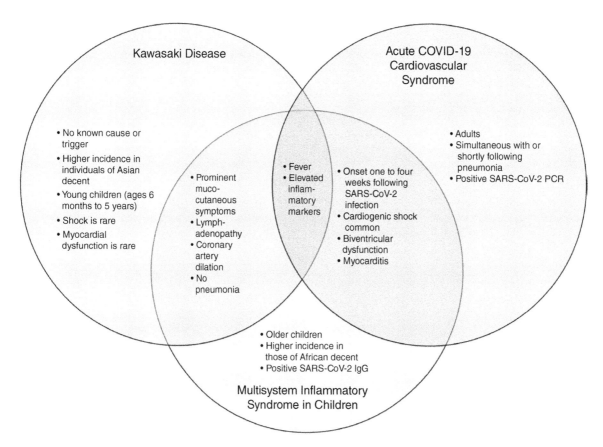

Figure 16.3 Venn diagram comparing the characteristics of Kawasaki disease, multisystem inflammatory syndrome in children, and acute COVID-19 cardiovascular syndrome. *Source:* Reproduced with permission from Most et al. [71].

Prevention has established clinical diagnostic criteria for MIS-C: individual aged <21 years with fever, laboratory evidence of inflammation, and evidence of clinically severe illness requiring hospitalization, with multisystem (≥2) organ involvement (cardiac, renal, respiratory, hematologic, gastrointestinal, dermatologic, or neurologic); and/or alternative plausible diagnoses; and positive for current or recent SARS-CoV-2 infection by RT-PCR, serology, or antigen test; or exposure to a suspected or confirmed COVID-19 case within the four weeks before the onset of symptoms [72]. Notably, in the initial case series of patients with MIS-C, PIMS, and MIS-A, who are typically presenting four weeks after initial COVID-19 infection, up to 50% of individuals at that time are RT-PCR negative for COVID-19, but prior infection was confirmed by antibody or antigen testing.

Laboratory confirmation of inflammation includes elevations in CRP, ESR, ferritin, procalcitonin, D-dimer, LDH, IL-6, and neutrophil count with reduced lymphocyte count. Biologic markers of cardiac involvement include elevations in troponin and BNP. In general, as compared with patients with Kawasaki disease, individuals with MIS-C, PIMS, MIS-A, and ACoCS tend to demonstrate significantly greater elevations in laboratory evidence of inflammation and cardiac markers. Cardiac testing should include ECG to assess for myocardial injury, ischemia, perimyocarditis, conduction abnormalities, and arrhythmias. Echocardiography is essential to evaluate not only left and right ventricular systolic function but also to assess for diastolic dysfunction, abnormal global longitudinal strain, valvular dysfunction, pericardial effusion, and coronary artery ectasia or aneurysmal development in the pediatric and adolescent population (using coronary z-scores >2.0) [73]. Other cardiac imaging modalities that may be indicated include CMR to assess for myocardial scar and/or coronary CT angiography to noninvasively assess the coronary arteries [74] and invasive coronary angiography in the setting of an ACS.

Management

A multidisciplinary treatment approach including consultants from infectious disease, cardiology, critical care, and rheumatology is warranted to manage these complex patients. Active COVID-19 illness is managed per guidelines and may include, as indicated by the latest guidelines, remdesivir and dexamethasone. For Kawasaki disease, MIS-C, PIMS, MIS-A, and ACoCS, IVIG and corticosteroids are essential to reduce the intensive inflammatory response and to prevent development of coronary artery aneurysms. Second-line anti-inflammatory therapies that have been used include anakinra, infliximab, and tocilizumab. Addition of aspirin to prevent arterial thrombosis and heparin for DVT prophylaxis may also be beneficial. ICU care, including arrhythmia monitoring, broad-spectrum antibiotics, vasopressor and inotrope therapy, mechanical ventilation, and circulatory support, may be utilized as clinically dictated [67, 68]. Once patients have clinically recovered from the initial illness, careful follow-up of cardiac function, including serial echocardiography to follow left ventricular and right ventricular systolic function recovery and to monitor coronary artery aneurysms, is recommended.

Arrhythmias in Acute COVID-19

Patients with severe COVID-19 illness frequently experience hypoxemia, a hyperinflammatory state, and possibly myocardial injury, which are all associated with an increased risk for cardiac arrhythmias. Indeed, early in the pandemic, Wang et al. [1] reported the incidence of arrhythmias in patients with COVID-19 admitted to the ICU in Wuhan, China, to be as high as 44.4%. Arrhythmias were less common in the non-ICU patient cohort (6.9%). In a similar retrospective analysis of 393 patients in New York, the incidence of arrhythmias was 18.5% in patients on mechanical ventilation versus 1.9% in patients who did not require ventilatory support [75]. More severe COVID-19 infection characterized by admission to the ICU and the need for ventilatory support has been shown to be a risk factor for development of both atrial and ventricular tachyarrhythmias [76, 77]. Interestingly, no such association was found for bradyarrhythmias in multivariate analysis [76]. Arrhythmias seem to be less prevalent in clinically stable patients with COVID-19 as reported in a single-day snapshot study from Italy, in which only 9% of patients had arrhythmic events [78]. The incidence rate of malignant ventricular arrhythmias was as high as 11% in patients who died of COVID-19 infection in the New York area, with an incidence rate of atrioventricular block of 6% in the same patient population [79].

In addition, significant hypokalemia and hypomagnesaemia can be present in patients with COVID-19 [80], because of binding and degradation of ACE-2 by SARS-CoV-2 [81], leading to increased renin–angiotensin–aldosterone system activity and urinary potassium excretion [82]. These electrolyte disturbances can predispose to the development of significant ventricular arrhythmias, including torsades de pointes [83].

Management

Treatment of arrhythmias in patients diagnosed with COVID-19 infection should follow the same principles used in the general population, because there are currently no available data to suggest the benefits of any COVID-19-specific therapy. Advanced Cardiac Life Support Guidelines should be followed in all patients with unstable arrhythmias. Special precautions should be undertaken to minimize the exposure of staff to infected patients [84]. In addition, secondary causes of arrhythmias, such as electrolyte imbalance, hypoxemia, myocardial ischemia, or drug interactions, should be recognized and addressed [85].

High-grade atrioventricular nodal blocks and symptomatic bradycardia refractory to medical therapy should be acutely treated with insertion of a temporary pacemaker. Permanent pacemaker placement should be postponed until patients recover from COVID-19, because bradyarrhythmias might be transient in the setting of critical illness, and implantation during acute infection may lead to higher risk for device infection [86].

In patients with COVID-19 who experience atrial tachyarrhythmias requiring anticoagulation (i.e. atrial fibrillation or atrial flutter), the risks and benefits should be carefully considered. Although COVID-19 can be associated with a hypercoagulable state [12], there are no data to suggest the need to deviate from standard anticoagulation protocols in these patients. Parenteral anticoagulants such as heparin are preferable in hospitalized patients, because both oral vitamin K antagonists and direct oral anticoagulants can interact with antiviral and experimental medications used for treatment of COVID-19 infection (remdesivir, lopinavir/ritonavir, tocilizumab, hydroxychloroquine) and potentially increase the risk for bleeding [87].

Beta blockers and calcium channel blockers, with careful monitoring, can be used for a rate control strategy of tachyarrhythmias. Antiarrhythmics such as flecainide, propafenone, amiodarone, and dofetilide should be used with caution, especially if they are concomitantly used with experimental COVID-19 treatments such as hydroxychloroquine, azithromycin, and/or lopinavir/ritonavir. QT interval and electrolyte levels need to be carefully monitored to minimize the risk for life-threatening ventricular tachyarrhythmias [84, 86, 87].

Postural Orthostatic Tachycardia Syndrome

Although the autonomic nervous system was previously defined as the parasympathetic, sympathetic, and enteric nervous systems [88], more recently it has been proposed that the extended autonomic nervous system is responsible for maintaining the fine balance of crucial interactions between the nervous system and the immune system [89]. Sympathetic activation and pro-inflammatory cytokine release have now been well described in COVID-19 illness [90], while vagal stimulation likely contributes to the anti-inflammatory response and may represent a potential target for neuroimmune modulation in the treatment of COVID-19 [91].

Autonomic dysfunction has been implicated as an important causal factor in the severity of acute illness and the long-term sequelae of neurologic manifestations associated with COVID-19 [92]. Infection is a known trigger for the development of postural orthostatic tachycardia syndrome (POTS) [93, 94]. Chronic fatigue, malaise, and changes in heart rate variability associated with autonomic dysfunction were also noted in patients with a history of COVID-19 [95].

Clinical Presentation

Orthostatic intolerance syndromes include orthostatic hypotension, vasovagal syncope, and POTS [93]. Clinical characteristics include a sustained heart rate increase of >30 beats/min within 10 minutes of standing up and may also encompass symptoms such as light-headedness, palpitations, tremulousness, generalized weakness, blurred vision, and fatigue [96]. It is also postulated that these symptoms may be exacerbated not only by the patients' underlying chronic comorbidities that affect other organ systems but also by the prolonged inactivity and deconditioning that may accompany the inciting infection [97].

Diagnosis

The diagnosis of orthostatic intolerance in a patient with COVID-19 requires attention to detail, beginning with a comprehensive history and physical examination. General examination should include vital signs such as temperature, orthostatic blood pressures and heart rate measurements, and pulse oximetry. If feasible, orthostatic blood pressures should be taken with blood pressure measured five minutes after lying supine and then three minutes after active standing. Further diagnostic testing may include head-up tilt testing, which is considered the gold standard for diagnosis of POTS [98].

Additional cardiac testing is largely dependent on the clinical setting and the severity of the illness. This may include external extended ECG monitoring or implantable loop recorders, 24-hour ambulatory blood pressure monitoring, exercise ECG, echocardiography, and Valsalva maneuver. Initial laboratory evaluation to look for anemia, electrolyte disorders, thyroid disease, adrenal hormone abnormalities, and elevated catecholamines is prudent. Noncardiac testing for autonomic dysfunction in other organ systems should be considered on a case-by-case basis [96]. The American Autonomic Society published a position statement recommending the continuation of necessary autonomic function testing during the COVID-19 pandemic with specific attention to infection prevention measures while maintaining accuracy of testing [99].

Management

The management of autonomic dysfunction in patients with COVID-19 is predicated primarily on education about the condition and reassurance. Implementation of fluid and salt repletion, counter-pressure maneuvers, compression garments, and isometric exercises can be helpful in controlling symptoms. Avoidance of exacerbating factors is also crucial in symptom control. Pharmacotherapy for autonomic dysfunction can be considered if initial measures fail [96]. Interestingly, the use of ivabradine in patients with POTS was associated with an improvement in heart rate and some measures of quality of life compared with placebo [100]. Notably, this study was not performed on patients with COVID-19-related POTS, and at this time, there are currently no data to suggest that POTS in this population should be approached differently. The initial data on effects of autonomic dysfunction in patients who have survived COVID-19 suggests that the pathophysiologic mechanisms behind patient symptoms need to be further elucidated [93], given the complex intersections of immunity, infection, and preexisting comorbidities.

Postacute Sequelae of SARS-COV-2 Infection

Months into the COVID-19 pandemic, the medical community gained an increasing awareness that a substantial portion of patients recovering from COVID-19 continued to exhibit lingering, sometimes debilitating symptoms several weeks to months after the initial infection. Recognition of this syndrome of continued symptoms was largely spurred by patients themselves [101], and the phenomenon was initially termed "long COVID" [102], with the afflicted collectively called "long haulers." More recently, these sequelae of symptoms have been renamed postacute sequelae of SARS-CoV-2 (PASC) infection. A precise definition has not yet been established, although it generally describes either the persistence or development of new symptoms related to COVID-19 weeks to months after the acute illness.

The true prevalence of PASC remains to be determined. An early study conducted in Rome, Italy, found that 87% of hospitalized patients continued to have at least one symptom approximately two months after their discharge [103], while another study from Wuhan, China, described 76% of patients reporting at least one symptom six months after their initial infection [104]. Fatigue was the most commonly reported symptom in both studies, and in the study from Wuhan, women were more likely than men to experience symptoms of fatigue/muscle weakness and anxiety/depression. In addition, a slightly higher percentage of female patients (81%) experienced at least one symptom six months after diagnosis compared with male patients (73%) [104].

The etiology of PASC remains unknown at this time, but its features resemble those of chronic disease syndromes, such as chronic fatigue syndrome and mast cell degranulation syndrome.

Whether cardiovascular system involvement is present in PASC remains unclear. Some of the reported symptoms include chest pain, palpitations/tachycardia, and dyspnea. In an editorial written by physicians in the United Kingdom who had personally contracted COVID-19, the authors described experiencing cardiac conditions such as myocarditis or pericarditis, microvascular angina, cardiac arrhythmias (atrial flutter and atrial fibrillation), and dysautonomia (including POTS) [101]. The prevalence of these cardiovascular issues in the recovered population remains to be determined, and the etiology has not been well established at this time.

Long-Term Management of COVID-19 Cardiovascular Disease

Due to the novelty of the COVID-19 pandemic, data on the long-term risks and sequelae of the disease remain limited [105], particularly for those patients who have experienced cardiovascular disease [2, 3, 106]. As described earlier in this chapter, acute cardiovascular manifestations include acute MI, myocarditis and heart failure, pericarditis, arrhythmias, and thromboembolic disease [105]. Although the initial myocardial injury may recover, there is a theoretical concern that affected tissue may continue to undergo damage, including fibrosis, and in turn lead to the development of ongoing cardiomyopathies, heart failure, and arrhythmias [107]. It is unclear how long this process may take, which risk factors may hasten development, which therapeutic interventions may attenuate it, or which patients will be most at risk. A recent study of patients who recovered from COVID-19 demonstrated elevated troponin levels, lower left ventricular ejection fraction (LVEF), elevated T1/T2 signaling, and late gadolinium enhancement on CMR at a median of 71 days after infection [30].

Of these potential sequelae, myocarditis during the recovery period remains the area of greatest interest and debate. The diagnosis of myocarditis in patients who have recovered from COVID-19 should be reserved for those who have a clinical syndrome of myocarditis, including symptoms (e.g. chest pain, dyspnea, exercise intolerance) and objective evidence of myocardial injury (e.g. serum troponin elevation, new arrhythmias or conduction abnormalities, left ventricular wall motion abnormalities on echocardiography, characteristic inflammatory findings on CMR). Although inflammatory features on CMR may help to support the diagnosis of myocarditis, they should not be used alone to make the diagnosis in the absence of a clinical syndrome [108, 109]. An endomyocardial biopsy is not usually needed in this setting, although it is the gold standard to confirm the diagnosis of myocarditis [108]. In addition, significant epicardial coronary artery disease should be ruled out with coronary angiography (via CT or cardiac catheterization).

For patients who have recovered from COVID-19 in the ambulatory setting with a diagnosis of myocarditis, an assessment of LVEF should be performed by transthoracic echocardiography or CMR, and guideline-directed medical therapy for heart failure initiated accordingly [110]. There is insufficient evidence at this time to support the use of immunosuppressive or antiviral agents for the treatment of myocarditis in patients who have recovered from COVID-19. Biomarkers of myocardial injury (e.g. troponin, brain natriuretic peptide) and inflammation (e.g. CRP, erythrocyte sedimentation rate) may be helpful in the initial assessment and for monitoring trajectory during treatment and recovery, although no data at this time show that such monitoring impacts outcomes in this population.

Due to concerns for myocarditis-related ventricular arrhythmias that may occur in the setting of ongoing inflammation, it is recommended that athletic patients avoid competition for three to six months after the initial diagnosis [108, 109]. Return to competition can be considered after that time if LVEF and cardiac/inflammatory biomarkers have normalized and no concerning findings are seen on maximal exercise treadmill testing and ambulatory ECG monitoring. Similarly, nonathlete patients should refrain from strenuous exercise, with a similar workup performed before increasing the intensity of their exercise regimen. Consideration for device therapy should follow the AHA/ACC guidelines for heart failure and arrhythmia management [110, 111].

Meanwhile, as we continue to learn more about the long-term cardiovascular sequelae of COVID-19, patients with related myocarditis should continue to be followed closely by a cardiologist, with implementation of newly recommended therapies and management strategies as they arise in clinical studies. At this time, there are no clear guidelines on the outpatient follow-up and continued long-term treatment of patients with cardiovascular manifestations of SARS-CoV-2. Some have advocated that in addition to routine postdischarge management, screening for residual cardiac disease should be undertaken, which can be challenging, especially when some manifestations can be subclinical [105]. Routine testing includes clinical evaluation, laboratory testing with CBC, chemistries D-dimer, anticardiolipin, CRP, von Willebrand factor, cardiac monitoring with ECG, and echocardiography within two to six months [105, 112]. In addition, given the concern for myocarditis, cardiomyopathy, and subsequent arrhythmias, advanced imaging with CMR or CT/PET is also usually performed. This has led to some institutions developing dedicated clinics to care for these COVID cardiology patients [105, 112].

Cardiovascular Effects of COVID-19 Treatments

As the knowledge and experience with COVID-19 treatment options continues to evolve and grow, clinicians must consider the potential for cardiovascular complications from several treatment options and must select optimal treatment strategies for patients with preexisting cardiovascular disease.

At this time, several options trialed for the treatment of COVID-19 have known adverse cardiovascular effects. Hydroxychloroquine and chloroquine were early suggested treatment options during the COVID-19 pandemic. Hydroxychloroquine and chloroquine are 4-amionoquinolones, which are structurally different by just one hydroxyl group. Because of this, they share a similar mechanism, pharmacokinetic profile, and adverse effects, although hydroxychloroquine has a lower incidence of and less severe toxicities compared with chloroquine [113, 114]. Although in vitro studies of these agents demonstrated positive effects of viral inhibition, several randomized controlled trials and observational studies have not shown beneficial effects of these agents for the prevention or treatment of COVID-19 [113, 115–117]. Importantly, hydroxychloroquine and chloroquine have several known cardiotoxic effects. Both drugs are known to prolong the QT interval by blocking the inward rectifier potassium ion channel, which impairs ventricular repolarization, broadens the cardiac action potential, and therefore prolongs the QT interval [113]. Because prolonged QTc can lead to torsades de pointes, a potentially lethal ventricular tachyarrhythmia, this toxicity must be considered, particularly in the setting of additional agents that also have the potential to prolong the QT interval. The National Institutes of Health (NIH) COVID-19 Treatment Guidelines Panel and the Infectious Diseases Society of America currently recommend against the use of hydroxychloroquine, with or without azithromycin, for the treatment of COVID-19 in patients who are hospitalized. For nonhospitalized patients, the panel also recommends against the use of hydroxychloroquine, with or without azithromycin, for the treatment of COVID-19, except in a clinical trial. The panel further states that hydroxychloroquine or chloroquine should be used only if necessary in combination with other medications that pose a moderate to high risk for QT prolongation [114, 118]. It is important for clinicians to be aware of these recommendations and the potential for ongoing cardiovascular risks if patients have received hydroxychloroquine and additional QTc-prolonging agents, particularly because of the long half-life of hydroxychloroquine, which is about 40 days [119].

Another agent that has been studied for the management of COVID-19 that has cardiovascular considerations is azithromycin. Azithromycin is a macrolide antibiotic, which also possesses anti-inflammatory and immunomodulatory effects [120]. Azithromycin has been used as adjunctive treatment for respiratory infections and conditions, such as acute respiratory distress syndrome, to provide antibacterial coverage and for the potential benefit of decreasing the inflammatory response and providing immunomodulation [120, 121]. Several studies have evaluated the use of azithromycin, particularly in combination with hydroxychloroquine, for the treatment of patients with COVID-19, but to date, these studies have not demonstrated beneficial effects [122, 123]. Because macrolide antibiotics have been shown to prolong the QT interval, clinicians must consider this risk in treatment, particularly if additional agents that also prolong the QT interval are used. Numerous studies have demonstrated increased cardiac risk, particularly when azithromycin and hydroxychloroquine are used concomitantly [124, 125]. The current Infectious Diseases Society of America and NIH COVID-19 Treatment Guidelines Panel recommend against the use of azithromycin in combination with hydroxychloroquine for the management of hospitalized or nonhospitalized patients with COVID-19 [114, 118]. However, for patients with confirmed COVID-19, if additional bacterial pneumonia or sepsis is suspected, empiric antibiotics should be administered [114, 126]. Although data are limited at this time, it is suspected that similar pathogens, which would cause community-acquired pneumonia, would also affect patients with COVID-19 [126]. Therefore, azithromycin may be used in these scenarios. It is recommended that antibiotics are guided by the antimicrobial stewardship policies and discontinued if a bacterial infection is not confirmed [126].

Remdesivir is a nucleoside analogue prodrug that inhibits viral RNA polymerases. At this time, remdesivir is the only direct-acting antiviral approved by the US Food and Drug Administration for treatment of COVID-19 in certain populations. Despite the widespread use of remdesivir, there is still limited knowledge regarding its adverse effects, particularly the potential cardiovascular side effects [127]. There are published case reports describing cardiovascular adverse effects associated with the use of remdesivir, including marked sinus bradycardia and QT prolongation with T-wave abnormalities. These patients experienced resolution of symptoms with the discontinuation of remdesivir [127, 128]. Data from the remdesivir manufacturer's compassionate use program for adult patients with severe COVID-19 showed that of 53 patients, 8% experienced hypotension and 6% had atrial fibrillation [129]. Notably, there was a very low incidence of cardiac adverse effects noted in the Adaptive Covid-19 Treatment Trial (ACTT-1), with only 1.9% versus 1.4% of patients experiencing cardiac arrest in the remdesivir versus placebo groups, and only 0.9% versus 0.2% of patients experiencing atrial fibrillation, respectively [130]. At this time, additional surveillance and research are necessary to determine causality and mechanism for any potential cardiotoxicity with remdesivir. Healthcare providers should ensure appropriate monitoring and caution are used, particularly for patients with preexisting cardiovascular disease.

There are additional medication-related considerations for clinicians managing patients with preexisting cardiovascular disease, particularly because of the increased risk for severe COVID-19 in this patient population.

There has been much interest in the impact of angiotensin-converting enzyme inhibitors (ACEis) and angiotensin receptor blockers (ARBs) in COVID-19 severity. SARS-CoV-2 binds to the ACE-2 receptor to gain entry into host cells [131]. ACE-2 is expressed on the surface of epithelial cells in the lungs, intestines, kidneys, and blood vessels [132]. Some previous literature has demonstrated that the use of ACEis or ARBs can lead to an upregulation of the ACE-2 receptor [133]. Additional agents, including sodium glucose cotransporter 2 inhibitors, thiazolidinediones, and ibuprofen, can also increase expression of ACE-2 [133, 134]. This potential upregulation of the ACE-2 receptor has raised concern for whether ACEis and ARBs increase the infectivity of COVID-19 and therefore should be discontinued or avoided. Conversely, experimental studies have shown that ACEis and ARBs reduce severe lung injury in certain viral pneumonias, and therefore have been speculated to be beneficial in COVID-19 [135]. To date, several studies have assessed the impact of ACEis and ARBs on COVID-19 infectivity and disease severity and found no significant associations [136–138]. Additional clinical trials are continuing to evaluate the impact of either continuing or discontinuing ACEi or ARB therapies. At this time, the AHA, ACC, Heart Failure Society of America, European Society of Cardiology, and the NIH COVID-19 Treatment Guidelines Panel recommend that patients who are currently prescribed ACEi or ARB therapies continue therapy, because there are not enough data to support beneficial or adverse outcomes among patients with COVID-19 who are receiving these therapies [114, 135, 139]. This is an important counseling point for providers to educate patients on due to the known risks of abrupt withdrawal of renin–angiotensin–aldosterone system inhibitors in high-risk patients, such as patients with heart failure or history of a previous MI [140].

In addition, for providers managing patients with COVID-19 and known cardiovascular disease, they should also consider the use of 3-hydroxy-3-methyl-glu taryl-coenzyme A reductase inhibitors, or "statin" medications. Interest in statin therapy for patients with COVID-19 has grown because of statin's anti-inflammatory, antithrombotic, and immunomodulatory effects [141]. Similarly to ACEis and ARBs, statins also have been shown to experimentally upregulate ACE-2 expression [142]. After cell entry via ACE-2, SARS-CoV-2 downregulates ACE-2 expression. ACE-2 is a counterregulatory enzyme of the renin–angiotensin system, which catalyzes the conversion of angiotensin II to angiotensin-(1–7). Angiotensin-(1–7) opposes the damaging effects of angiotensin II, including increased oxidative stress, inflammation, and fibrosis. These effects are thought to be responsible for the severe lung injury seen in many patients with COVID-19 [141]. Therefore, the effects of statins, ACEis, and ARBs upregulating ACE-2 are theoretically beneficial in the management of COVID-19. To date, there is insufficient evidence from randomized controlled trials examining the use of statins in patients with COVID-19. Several studies have demonstrated conflicting results regarding the benefit of statins in reducing COVID-19 disease severity, mortality, or recovery [143–145]. Currently, the NIH COVID-19 Treatment Guidelines Panel recommends that patients who are receiving statin therapy for the treatment or prevention of cardiovascular disease are continued on statin therapy, but statins should not be used for the treatment of COVID-19 except in clinical trials [114]. When continuing statin therapy, clinicians must weigh the potential benefit with safety risks of statins. Conditions such as liver injury, myotoxicity, and rhabdomyolysis-related kidney injury may occur more frequently in severe COVID-19 infections; therefore, statin therapy may need to be at least temporarily held [141]. Furthermore, providers should be aware of potential drug interactions, because most statins undergo metabolism via the hepatic isoenzyme cytochrome P450 3A4, and other COVID-19 treatments may impact this.

Patients with preexisting cardiovascular disease are at a greater risk for acquiring more severe COVID-19 infections [146]. Although the knowledge and experience will continue to grow with treatments for COVID-19, healthcare providers must consider the safety and effectiveness of the current management strategies for this vulnerable patient population.

COVID-19 in Special Populations

The COVID-19 pandemic has had a devastating impact on patients with underlying cardiovascular conditions. Two specific populations of cardiovascular patients who warrant particular attention are those with chronic heart failure and those who have undergone heart transplantation.

Chronic Heart Failure

In patients with chronic heart failure, SARS-CoV-2 infection has been shown to increase the risk for mortality approximately twofold compared with similar patients without heart failure [147]. Interestingly, though, patients with chronic heart failure and systolic dysfunction did not have increased risk when compared with those with preserved function [147]. In addition, viral infections such as influenza and other respiratory pathogens can be triggers for acute heart failure exacerbations, leading to increased hospitalizations and mortality [148].

With regard to specialized management of patients with chronic heart failure and COVID-19, currently, no robust data are available to support specific therapies for this population. Although there was initial ambiguity on the safety of guideline-directed heart failure therapies such as ACEi and ARBs, these have since been shown to be safe to continue, as discussed in the previous section [147]. Importantly, special attention should be paid to this population, even those without COVID-19, to ensure that they continue to seek routine care for their heart failure from their medical providers. During the initial phase of the pandemic, there was an increase in deaths caused by cardiovascular disease in certain regions of the United States, and the concern is that this was an indirect effect of pandemic-related aspects, such as delayed cardiovascular care [149].

Heart Transplant Recipients

SARS-CoV-2 infection has also raised special concerns in heart transplant recipients. Solid organ transplant recipients have mortality rates up to 18% [150], with heart transplant recipients found to have mortality rates as high as 25–30% with COVID-19 [151, 152]. Infected heart transplant recipients generally present with similar symptoms as those in the general population, including dyspnea, fever, and cough, but they may also have atypical presenting symptoms such as diarrhea [150], potentially leading to late presentation or even missed diagnosis. Mortality in this population appears to be primarily due to respiratory failure [151], similar to nontransplant recipients [153]. In addition, prior coronary intervention, presence of allograft vasculopathy, and higher New York Heart Association class were also associated with higher mortality [151]. Although some had biomarker elevations indicative of myocardial injury [150, 154], most patients had normal-appearing left ventricular function [151, 152, 154], although some developed right ventricular dysfunction and elevated pulmonary artery pressures [154].

In addition, there are special considerations with regard to the management of immunosuppression regimens in transplant recipients with COVID-19. In the case of moderate to severe infection, it is recommended to withhold mycophenolate mofetil, mammalian target of rapamycin inhibitors, or azathioprine [155]. Thus far, there have not been any well-studied COVID-19 therapies specifically used in heart transplant recipients. The use of dexamethasone has been shown to reduce mortality in patients with COVID-19 who require mechanical ventilation or supplemental oxygen, and it has low potential of clinically significant interaction with immunosuppression [156]. Remdesivir has been shown to decrease the time to recovery in patients with COVID-19 pneumonia [130], but given

its potential to interact with tacrolimus, sirolimus, and cyclosporine metabolism, levels of these medications should be closely monitored. Other therapies, such as IL-6 inhibitors, are currently being evaluated as potential therapies, and because certain IL-6 inhibitors may increase cytochrome P450 metabolism, levels of common immunosuppressive agents (tacrolimus, sirolimus, and cyclosporine) should again be monitored closely [157].

The early studies conducted in vaccine development excluded transplant recipients; thus, robust safety data in this population are not yet available. However, a small study of transplant recipients performed after the public release of the first two mRNA vaccines (Pfizer-BioNTech and Moderna) have shown them to be relatively safe and well tolerated, with adverse reaction profiles similar to those seen in the general population [158]. Data on the durability of vaccination is still being investigated, but results thus far suggest persistence of neutralizing antibodies at least up to four months [159]. However, these findings may be different in transplant recipients because of their immunosuppressed state. Commonly, transplant recipients undergo initial B- or T-cell ablative therapy around the time of their transplant, which will reduce their ability to mount an appropriate response to the vaccine; as such, most professional societies have recommended administering the vaccine at least one month posttransplant or at least three months after if B- or T-cell ablative therapy was used [155, 157, 160]. The potential use of SARS-CoV-2 monoclonal antibodies for prophylaxis in solid organ transplant recipients is promising but needs further study.

Conclusion

As the COVID-19 pandemic continues to evolve, so too will our knowledge on the cardiovascular implications of this disease. There is an ongoing need to better understand both the acute and long-term cardiovascular effects of COVID-19, as well as optimal management strategies. Continued research and collaboration will be vital to our ability to better diagnose and treat the cardiovascular manifestations associated with this disease, and thus allow for optimal outcomes of patients afflicted by this unprecedented virus.

References

1 Wang, D., Hu, B., Hu, C. et al. (2020). Clinical characteristics of 138 hospitalized patients with 2019 novel coronavirus-infected pneumonia in Wuhan, China. *JAMA* 323: 1061–1069.

2 Zheng, Y.-Y., Ma, Y.-T., Zhang, J.-Y., and Xie, X. (2020). COVID-19 and the cardiovascular system. *Nat. Rev. Cardiol.* 17: 259–260.

3 Zhou, F., Yu, T., Du, R. et al. (2020). Clinical course and risk factors for mortality of adult inpatients with COVID-19 in Wuhan, China: a retrospective cohort study. *Lancet* 395: 1054–1062.

4 Shi, S., Qin, M., Shen, B. et al. (2020). Association of cardiac injury with mortality in hospitalized patients with COVID-19 in Wuhan, China. *JAMA Cardiol.* 5: 802–810.

5 Guo, T., Fan, Y., Chen, M. et al. (2020). Cardiovascular implications of fatal outcomes of patients with coronavirus disease 2019 (COVID-19). *JAMA Cardiol.* 5: 811–818.

6 Clerkin, K.J., Fried, J.A., Raikhelkar, J. et al. (2020). COVID-19 and cardiovascular disease. *Circulation* 141: 1648–1655.

7 Atri, D., Siddiqi, H.K., Lang, J.P. et al. (2020). COVID-19 for the cardiologist: basic virology, epidemiology, cardiac manifestations, and potential therapeutic strategies. *JACC Basic Transl. Sci.* 5: 518–516.

8 Gheblawi, M., Wang, K., Viveiros, A. et al. (2020). Angiotensin-converting enzyme 2: SARS-CoV-2 receptor and regulator of the renin-angiotensin system: celebrating the 20th anniversary of the discovery of ACE2. *Circ. Res.* 126: 1456–1474.

9 Tavazzi, G., Pellegrini, C., Maurelli, M. et al. (2020). Myocardial localization of coronavirus in COVID-19 cardiogenic shock. *Eur. J. Heart Fail.* 22: 911–915.

10 Halushka, M.K. and Vander Heide, R.S. (2021). Myocarditis is rare in COVID-19 autopsies: cardiovascular findings across 277 postmortem examinations. *Cardiovasc. Pathol.* 50: 107300.

11 Bikdeli, B., Madhavan, M.V., Jimenez, D. et al. (2020). Global COVID-19 thrombosis collaborative group, endorsed by the ISTH, NATF, ESVM, and the IUA, supported by the ESC working group on pulmonary circulation and right ventricular function. COVID-19 and thrombotic or thromboembolic disease: implications for prevention, antithrombotic therapy, and follow-up: JACC state-of-the-art review. *J. Am. Coll. Cardiol.* 75: 2950–2973.

12 Connors, J.M. and Levy, J.H. (2020). COVID-19 and its implications for thrombosis and anticoagulation. *Blood* 135: 2033–2040.

13 Chen, G., Wu, D., Guo, W. et al. (2020). Clinical and immunological features of severe and moderate coronavirus disease 2019. *J. Clin. Invest.* 130: 2620–2629.

14 Pericàs, J.M., Hernandez-Meneses, M., Sheahan, T.P. et al. (2020). Hospital Clínic cardiovascular infections study group. COVID-19: from epidemiology to treatment. *Eur. Heart J.* 41: 2092–2112.

15 Chen, N., Zhou, M., Dong, X. et al. (2020). Epidemiological and clinical characteristics of 99 cases of 2019 novel coronavirus pneumonia in Wuhan, China: a descriptive study. *Lancet* 395: 507–513.

16 Thygesen, K., Alpert, J.S., Jaffe, A.S. et al. (2018). Fourth universal definition of myocardial infarction. *Circulation* 138: e618–e651. https://doi.org/10.1161/CIR.0000000000000617.

17 Mahmud, E., Dauerman, H.L., Welt, F.G.P. et al. (2020). Management of Acute Myocardial Infarction during the COVID-19 pandemic: a position statement from the Society for Cardiovascular Angiography and Interventions (SCAI), the American College of Cardiology (ACC), and the American College of Emergency Physicians (ACEP). *J. Am. Coll. Cardiol.* 76: 1375–1384.

18 Choudry, F.A., Hamshere, S.M., Rathod, K.S. et al. (2020). High thrombus burden in patients with COVID-19 presenting with ST-segment elevation myocardial infarction. *J. Am. Coll. Cardiol.* 76: 1168–1176.

19 Klok, F.A., Kruip, M.J.H.A., van der Meer, N.J.M. et al. (2020). Incidence of thrombotic complications in critically ill ICU patients with COVID-19. *Thromb. Res.* 191: 145–147.

20 The REMAP-CAP, ACTIV-4a, ATTACC Investigators and Zarychanski, R. (2021). Therapeutic anticoagulation in critically Ill patients with

Covid-19 – preliminary Report. *medRxiv* https://doi.org/10.1101/2021.03.10.21252749.

21 INSPIRATION Investigators, Sadeghipour, P., Talasaz, A.H. et al. (2021). Effect of intermediate-dose vs standard-dose prophylactic anticoagulation on thrombotic events, extracorporeal membrane oxygenation treatment, or mortality among patients with COVID-19 admitted to the intensive care unit: the INSPIRATION randomized clinical trial. *JAMA* 325: 1620.

22 National Institutes of Health (2021). Full-dose blood thinners decreased need for life support and improved outcome in hospitalized COVID-19 patients. https://www.nih.gov/news-events/news-releases/full-dose-blood-thinners-decreased-need-life-support-improved-outcome-hospitalized-covid-19-patients (accessed 4 May 2021).

23 Driggin, E., Madhavan, M.V., Bikdeli, B. et al. (2020). Cardiovascular considerations for patients, health care workers, and health systems during the COVID-19 pandemic. *J. Am. Coll. Cardiol.* 75: 2352–2371.

24 Kariyanna, P.T., Sutarjono, B., Grewal, E. et al. (2020). A systematic review of COVID-19 and myocarditis. *Am. J. Med. Case Rep.* 8: 299–305.

25 Kociol, R.D., Cooper, L.T., Fang, J.C. et al. (2020). Recognition and initial management of fulminant myocarditis: a scientific statement from the American Heart Association. *Circulation* 141: e69–e92.

26 Siripanthong, B., Nazarian, S., Muser, D. et al. (2020). Recognizing COVID-19-related myocarditis: the possible pathophysiology and proposed guideline for diagnosis and management. *Heart Rhythm* 17: 1463–1471.

27 Hendren, N.S., Drazner, M.H., Bozkurt, B., and Cooper, L.T. (2020). Description and proposed management of the acute COVID-19 cardiovascular syndrome. *Circulation* 141: 1903–1914.

28 Lippi, G., Lavie, C.J., and Sanchis-Gomar, F. (2020). Cardiac troponin I in patients with coronavirus disease 2019 (COVID-19): evidence from a meta-analysis. *Prog. Cardiovasc. Dis.* 63: 390–391.

29 Ruan, Q., Yang, K., Wang, W. et al. (2020). Clinical predictors of mortality due to COVID-19 based on an analysis of data of 150 patients from Wuhan, China. *Intensive Care Med.* 46: 846–848.

30 Puntmann, V.O., Carerj, M.L., Wieters, I. et al. (2020). Outcomes of cardiovascular magnetic resonance imaging in patients recently recovered from coronavirus disease 2019 (COVID-19). *JAMA Cardiol.* 5: 1265–1273.

31 Martinez, M.W., Tucker, A.M., Bloom, O.J. et al. (2021). Prevalence of inflammatory heart disease among professional athletes with prior COVID-19 infection who received systematic return-to-play cardiac screening. *JAMA Cardiol.* 2021: e210565.

32 Moulson, N., Petek, B.J., Drezner, J.A. et al. (2021). SARS-CoV-2 cardiac involvement in young competitive athletes. *Circulation* 144 https://doi.org/10.1161/CIRCULATIONAHA.121.054824.

33 Hu, H., Ma, F., Wei, X., and Fang, Y. (2021). Coronavirus fulminant myocarditis treated with glucocorticoid and human immunoglobulin. *Eur. Heart J.* 42: 206.

34 Sala, S., Peretto, G., Gramegna, M. et al. (2020). Acute myocarditis presenting as a reverse Tako-Tsubo syndrome in a patient with SARS-CoV-2 respiratory infection. *Eur. Heart J.* 41: 1861–1862.

35 Guan, W.-J., Ni, Z.-Y., Hu, Y. et al. (2020). Clinical characteristics of coronavirus disease 2019 in China. *N. Engl. J. Med.* 382: 1708–1720.

36 Friedrich, M.G., Sechtem, U., Schulz-Menger, J. et al. (2009). International consensus group on cardiovascular magnetic resonance in myocarditis. Cardiovascular magnetic resonance in myocarditis: a JACC white paper. *J. Am. Coll. Cardiol.* 53: 1475–1487.

37 Inciardi, R.M., Lupi, L., Zaccone, G. et al. (2020). Cardiac involvement in a patient with coronavirus disease 2019 (COVID-19). *JAMA Cardiol.* 5: 819.

38 Mason, J.W., O'Connell, J.B., Herskowitz, A. et al. (1995). A clinical trial of immunosuppressive therapy for myocarditis. The myocarditis treatment trial Investigators. *N. Engl. J. Med.* 333: 269–275.

39 McNamara, D.M., Holubkov, R., Starling, R.C. et al. (2001). Controlled trial of intravenous immune globulin in recent-onset dilated cardiomyopathy. *Circulation* 103: 2254–2259.

40 Chen, H.S., Wang, W., Wu, S.N., and Liu, J.P. (2013). Corticosteroids for viral myocarditis. *Cochrane Database Syst. Rev.* 2013: CD004471.

41 Cao, W., Liu, X., Bai, T. et al. (2020). High-dose intravenous immunoglobulin as a therapeutic option

for deteriorating patients with coronavirus disease 2019. *Open Forum Infect. Dis.* 7: ofaa102.

42 Li, A., Garcia-Bengochea, Y., Stechel, R., and Azari, B.M. (2020). Management of COVID-19 myopericarditis with reversal of cardiac dysfunction after blunting of cytokine storm: a case report. *Eur. Heart. J. Case Rep.* 4: 1–6.

43 Magnani, J.W. and Dec, G.W. (2006). Myocarditis: current trends in diagnosis and treatment. *Circulation* 113: 876–890.

44 Brito, D., Meester, S., Yanamala, N. et al. (2021). High prevalence of pericardial involvement in college student athletes recovering from COVID-19. *JACC Cardiovasc. Imaging* 14: 541–555.

45 Imazio, M., Gaita, F., and LeWinter, M. (2015). Evaluation and treatment of pericarditis: a systematic review. *JAMA* 314: 1498–1506.

46 Imazio, M., Cecchi, E., Demichelis, B. et al. (2008). Myopericarditis versus viral or idiopathic acute pericarditis. *Heart* 94: 498–501.

47 Kytö, V., Sipilä, J., and Rautava, P. (2014). Clinical profile and influences on outcomes in patients hospitalized for acute pericarditis. *Circulation* 130: 1601–1606.

48 Cooper, L.T. (2009). Myocarditis. *N. Engl. J. Med.* 360: 1526–1538.

49 Faraj, R., Belkhayat, C., Bouchlarhem, A. et al. (2021). Acute pericarditis revealing COVID-19 infection: case report. *Ann. Med. Surg. (Lond.)* 62: 225–227.

50 Kumar, R., Kumar, J., Daly, C., and Edroos, S.A. (2020). Acute pericarditis as a primary presentation of COVID-19. *BMJ Case Rep.* 13: e237617.

51 Hua, A., O'Gallagher, K., Sado, D., and Byrne, J. (2020). Life-threatening cardiac tamponade complicating myo-pericarditis in COVID-19. *Eur. Heart J.* 41: 2130–2120.

52 Dabbagh, M.F., Aurora, L., D'Souza, P. et al. (2020). Cardiac tamponade secondary to COVID-19. *JACC Case Rep.* 2: 1326–1330.

53 Sauer, F., Dagrenat, C., Couppie, P. et al. (2020). Pericardial effusion in patients with COVID-19: case series. *Eur. Heart J. Case Rep.* 4: 1–7.

54 Cremer, P.C., Kumar, A., Kontzias, A. et al. (2016). Complicated pericarditis: understanding risk factors and pathophysiology to inform imaging and treatment. *J. Am. Coll. Cardiol.* 68: 2311–2328.

55 Klein, A.L., Abbara, S., Agler, D.A. et al. (2013). American Society of Echocardiography clinical recommendations for multimodality cardiovascular imaging of patients with pericardial disease: endorsed by the Society for Cardiovascular Magnetic Resonance and Society of cardiovascular computed tomography. *J. Am. Soc. Echocardiogr.* 26: 965–1012. e15.

56 Imazio, M., Brucato, A., Lazaros, G. et al. (2020). Anti-inflammatory therapies for pericardial diseases in the COVID-19 pandemic: safety and potentiality. *J. Cardiovasc. Med. (Hagerstown)* 21: 625–629.

57 Little, P. (2020). Non-steroidal anti-inflammatory drugs and covid-19. *BMJ* 368: m1185.

58 Imazio, M. and Adler, Y. (2013). Treatment with aspirin, NSAID, corticosteroids, and colchicine in acute and recurrent pericarditis. *Heart Fail. Rev.* 18: 355–360.

59 Kawasaki, T., Kosaki, F., Okawa, S. et al. (1974). A new infantile acute febrile mucocutaneous lymph node syndrome (MLNS) prevailing in Japan. *Pediatrics* 54: 271–276.

60 McCrindle, B.W., Rowley, A.H., Newburger, J.W. et al. (2017). Diagnosis, treatment, and long-term Management of Kawasaki Disease: a scientific statement for health professionals from the American Heart Association. *Circulation* 135: e927–e999.

61 Riphagen, S., Gomez, X., Gonzalez-Martinez, C. et al. (2020). Hyperinflammatory shock in children during COVID-19 pandemic. *Lancet* 395: 1607–1608.

62 Whittaker, E., Bamford, A., Kenny, J. et al. (2020). Clinical characteristics of 58 children with a pediatric inflammatory multisystem syndrome temporally associated with SARS-CoV-2. *JAMA* 324: 259–269.

63 Verdoni, L., Mazza, A., Gervasoni, A. et al. (2020). An outbreak of severe Kawasaki-like disease at the Italian epicentre of the SARS-CoV-2 epidemic: an observational cohort study. *Lancet* 395: 1771–1778.

64 Moraleda, C., Serna-Pascual, M., Soriano-Arandes, A. et al. (2021). Multi-inflammatory syndrome in children related to severe acute respiratory syndrome coronavirus 2 (SARS-CoV-2) in Spain. *Clin. Infect. Dis.* 72: e397–e401.

65 Cheung, E.W., Zachariah, P., Gorelik, M. et al. (2020). Multisystem inflammatory syndrome related

to COVID-19 in previously healthy children and adolescents in New York City. *JAMA* 324: 294–296.

66 Lee, E.H., Kepler, K.L., Geevarughese, A. et al. (2020). Race/ethnicity among children with COVID-19–associated multisystem inflammatory syndrome. *JAMA Netw. Open* 3: e2030280.

67 Feldstein, L.R., Rose, E.B., Horwitz, S.M. et al. (2020). Multisystem inflammatory syndrome in U.S. children and adolescents. *N. Engl. J. Med.* 383: 34–346.

68 Kaushik, A., Gupta, S., Sood, M. et al. (2020). A systematic review of multisystem inflammatory syndrome in children associated with SARS-CoV-2 infection. *Pediatr. Infect. Dis. J.* 39: e340–e346.

69 Consiglio, C.R., Cotugno, N., Sardh, F. et al. (2020). The immunology of multisystem inflammatory syndrome in children with COVID-19. *Cell* 183: 968–81.e7.

70 Morris, S.B., Schwartz, N.G., Patel, P. et al. (2020). Case series of multisystem inflammatory syndrome in adults associated with SARS-CoV-2 infection - United Kingdom and United States, march-august 2020. *MMWR Morb. Mortal. Wkly Rep.* 69: 1450–1456.

71 Most, Z.M., Hendren, N., Drazner, M.H., and Perl, T.M. (2021). Striking similarities of multisystem inflammatory syndrome in children and a myocarditis-like syndrome in adults: overlapping manifestations of COVID-19. *Circulation* 143: 4–6.

72 Centers for Disease Control and Prevention (2020). Multisystem inflammatory syndrome in children (MIS-C) associated with coronavirus disease 2019 (COVID-19). https://emergency.cdc.gov/han/2020/han00432.asp.

73 Matsubara, D., Kauffman, H.L., Wang, Y. et al. (2020). Echocardiographic findings in pediatric multisystem inflammatory syndrome associated with COVID-19 in the United States. *J. Am. Coll. Cardiol.* 76: 1947–1961.

74 van Stijn-Bringas, D.D., Planken, R.N., Groenink, M. et al. (2020). Coronary artery assessment in Kawasaki disease with dual-source CT angiography to uncover vascular pathology. *Eur. Radiol.* 30: 432–441.

75 Goyal, P., Choi, J.J., Pinheiro, L.C. et al. (2020). Clinical characteristics of Covid-19 in New York City. *N. Engl. J. Med.* 382: 2372–2374.

76 Bhatla, A., Mayer, M.M., Adusumalli, S. et al. (2020). COVID-19 and cardiac arrhythmias. *Heart Rhythm* 17: 1439–1444.

77 Colon, C.M., Barrios, J.G., Chiles, J.W. et al. (2020). Atrial arrhythmias in COVID-19 patients. *JACC Clin Electrophysiol.* 6: 1189–1190.

78 Sala, S., Peretto, G., De Luca, G. et al. (2020). Low prevalence of arrhythmias in clinically stable COVID-19 patients. *Pacing Clin. Electrophysiol.* 43: 891–893.

79 Turagam, M.K., Musikantow, D., Goldman, M.E. et al. (2020). Malignant arrhythmias in patients with covid-19: incidence, mechanisms, and outcomes. *Circulation: Arrhythmia Electrophysiol. 2020* 13: e008920. https://doi.org/10.1161/CIRCEP.120.008920.

80 Chen, D., Li, X., Song, Q. et al. (2020). Assessment of hypokalemia and clinical characteristics in patients with coronavirus disease 2019 in Wenzhou, China. *JAMA Netw. Open* 3: e2011122.

81 Moreno-P, O., Leon-Ramirez, J.-M., Fuertes-Kenneally, L. et al. (2020). COVID19-ALC research group. Hypokalemia as a sensitive biomarker of disease severity and the requirement for invasive mechanical ventilation requirement in COVID-19 pneumonia: a case series of 306 Mediterranean patients. *Int. J. Infect. Dis.* 100: 449–454.

82 Bielecka-Dabrowa, A., Mikhailidis, D.P., Jones, L. et al. (2012). The meaning of hypokalemia in heart failure. *Int. J. Cardiol.* 158: 12–17.

83 Digby, G.C., Pérez Riera, A.R., Barbosa Barros, R. et al. (2011). Acquired long QT interval: a case series of multifactorial QT prolongation. *Clin. Cardiol.* 34: 577–582.

84 Lakkireddy, D.R., Chung, M.K., Gopinathannair, R. et al. (2020). Guidance for cardiac electrophysiology during the COVID-19 pandemic from the Heart Rhythm Society COVID-19 task force; electrophysiology section of the American College of Cardiology; and the electrocardiography and arrhythmias Committee of the Council on clinical cardiology, American Heart Association. *Heart Rhythm* 17: e233–e241.

85 Dherange, P., Lang, J., Qian, P. et al. (2020). Arrhythmias and COVID-19: a review. *JACC Clin Electrophysiol.* 6: 1193–1204.

86 Saenz, L.C., Miranda, A., Speranza, R. et al. (2020). Recommendations for the organization of

electrophysiology and cardiac pacing services during the COVID-19 pandemic: Latin American Heart Rhythm Society (LAHRS) in collaboration with: Colombian College of Electrophysiology, Argentinian Society of Cardiac Electrophysiology (SADEC), Brazilian Society of Cardiac Arrhythmias (SOBRAC), Mexican Society of Cardiac Electrophysiology (SOMEEC). *J. Interv. Card. Electrophysiol.* 59: 307–313.

87 Russo, V., Rago, A., Carbone, A. et al. (2020). Atrial fibrillation in COVID-19: from epidemiological association to pharmacological implications. *J. Cardiovasc. Pharmacol.* 76: 138–145.

88 Kenney, M.J. and Ganta, C.K. (2014). Autonomic nervous system and immune system interactions. *Compr. Physiol.* 4: 1177–1200.

89 Goldstein, D.S. (2020). The extended autonomic system, dyshomeostasis, and COVID-19. *Clin. Auton. Res.* 30: 299–315.

90 Fudim, M., Qadri, Y.J., Ghadimi, K. et al. (2020). Implications for Neuromodulation therapy to control inflammation and related organ dysfunction in COVID-19. *J. Cardiovasc. Transl. Res.* 13: 894–899.

91 Díaz, H.S., Toledo, C., Andrade, D.C. et al. (2020). Neuroinflammation in heart failure: new insights for an old disease. *J. Physiol.* 598: 33–59.

92 Verstrepen, K., Baisier, L., and De Cauwer, H. (2020). Neurological manifestations of COVID-19, SARS and MERS. *Acta Neurol. Belg.* 120: 1051–1060.

93 Miglis, M.G., Prieto, T., Shaik, R. et al. (2020). A case report of postural tachycardia syndrome after COVID-19. *Clin. Auton. Res.* 30: 449–451.

94 Thieben, M.J., Sandroni, P., Sletten, D.M. et al. (2007). Postural orthostatic tachycardia syndrome: the Mayo clinic experience. *Mayo Clin. Proc.* 82: 308–313.

95 Lo, Y.L., Leong, H.N., Hsu, L.Y. et al. (2005). Autonomic dysfunction in recovered severe acute respiratory syndrome patients. *Can. J. Neurol. Sci.* 32: 264.

96 Fedorowski, A. (2019). Postural orthostatic tachycardia syndrome: clinical presentation, aetiology and management. *J. Intern. Med.* 285: 352–366.

97 Dani, M., Dirksen, A., Taraborrelli, P. et al. (2021). Autonomic dysfunction in 'long COVID': rationale, physiology and management strategies. *Clin. Med.* 21: e63–e67.

98 Brignole, M., Moya, A., de Lange, F.J. et al. (2018). ESC scientific document group. Practical instructions for the 2018 ESC guidelines for the diagnosis and management of syncope. *Eur. Heart J.* 39: e43–e80.

99 The American Autonomic Society, Figueroa, J.J., Cheshire, W.P. et al. (2020). Autonomic function testing in the COVID-19 pandemic: an American autonomic society position statement. *Clin. Auton. Res.* 30: 295–297.

100 Taub, P.R., Zadourian, A., Lo, H.C. et al. (2021). Randomized trial of Ivabradine in patients with hyperadrenergic postural orthostatic tachycardia syndrome. *J. Am. Coll. Cardiol.* 77: 861–871.

101 Gorna, R., MacDermott, N., Rayner, C. et al. (2021). Long COVID guidelines need to reflect lived experience. *Lancet* 397: 455–457.

102 Mahase, E. (2020). Covid-19: what do we know about "long covid"? *BMJ* 370: m2815.

103 Carfì, A., Bernabei, R., and Landi, F. (2020). Gemelli against COVID-19 post-acute care study group. Persistent symptoms in patients after acute COVID-19. *JAMA* 324: 603–605.

104 Huang, C., Huang, L., Wang, Y. et al. (2021). 6-month consequences of COVID-19 in patients discharged from hospital: a cohort study. *Lancet* 397: 220–232.

105 Mitrani, R.D., Dabas, N., and Goldberger, J.J. (2020). COVID-19 cardiac injury: implications for long-term surveillance and outcomes in survivors. *Heart Rhythm* 17: 1984–1990.

106 Bhatraju, P.K., Ghassemieh, B.J., Nichols, M. et al. (2020). Covid-19 in critically ill patients in the Seattle region - case series. *N. Engl. J. Med.* 382: 2012–2022.

107 Suthahar, N., Meijers, W.C., Silljé, H.H.W., and de Boer, R.A. (2017). From inflammation to fibrosis- molecular and cellular mechanisms of myocardial tissue Remodelling and perspectives on differential treatment opportunities. *Curr. Heart Fail. Rep.* 14: 235–250.

108 Maron, B.J., Udelson, J.E., Bonow, R.O. et al. (2015). Eligibility and disqualification recommendations for competitive athletes with cardiovascular abnormalities: task force 3: hypertrophic cardiomyopathy, arrhythmogenic right ventricular cardiomyopathy and other cardiomyopathies, and myocarditis: a scientific statement from the American Heart Association and American College of Cardiology. *Circulation* 132: e273–e280.

109 Kim, J.H., Levine, B.D., Phelan, D. et al. (2021). Coronavirus disease 2019 and the athletic heart: emerging perspectives on pathology, risks, and return to play. *JAMA Cardiol.* 6: 219–227.

110 Yancy, C.W., Jessup, M., Bozkurt, B. et al. (2017). 2017 ACC/AHA/HFSA focused update of the 2013 ACCF/AHA guideline for the Management of Heart Failure: a report of the American College of Cardiology/American Heart Association task force on clinical practice guidelines and the Heart Failure Society of America. *Circulation*;136 ;e137–61. doi: https://doi.org/10.1161/CIR.0000000000000509.

111 Al-Khatib, S.M., Stevenson, W.G., Ackerman, M.J. et al. (2018). 2017 AHA/ACC/HRS guideline for management of patients with ventricular arrhythmias and the prevention of sudden cardiac death: a report of the American College of Cardiology/American Heart Association task force on clinical practice guidelines and the Heart Rhythm Society. *Circulation* 138: e272–e391. https://doi.org/10.1161/CIR.0000000000000549.

112 Becker, R.C. (2020). Anticipating the long-term cardiovascular effects of COVID-19. *J. Thromb. Thrombolysis* 50: 512–524.

113 Khuroo, M.S. (2020). Chloroquine and hydroxychloroquine in coronavirus disease 2019 (COVID-19). Facts, fiction and the hype: a critical appraisal. *Int. J. Antimicrob. Agents* 56: 106101.

114 Centers for Disease Control and Prevention (2021). COVID-19 treatment guidelines panel. https://www.covid19treatmentguidelines.nih.gov.

115 RECOVERY Collaborative Group, Horby, P., Mafham, M. et al. (2020). Effect of hydroxychloroquine in hospitalized patients with Covid-19. *N. Engl. J. Med.* 383: 2030–2040.

116 Geleris, J., Sun, Y., Platt, J. et al. (2020). Observational study of hydroxychloroquine in hospitalized patients with Covid-19. *N. Engl. J. Med.* 382: 2411–2418.

117 Cavalcanti, A.B., Zampieri, F.G., Rosa, R.G. et al. (2020). Coalition Covid-19 Brazil I Investigators. Hydroxychloroquine with or without azithromycin in mild-to-moderate Covid-19. *N. Engl. J. Med.* 383: 2041–2052.

118 Bhimraj, A., Morgan, R.L., Shumaker, A.H. et al. (2020). Infectious diseases society of America guidelines on the treatment and Management of Patients with COVID-19. *Clin. Infect. Dis.* 2020: ciaa478.

119 Tett, S.E. (1993). Clinical pharmacokinetics of slow-acting antirheumatic drugs. *Clin. Pharmacokinet.* 25: 392–407.

120 Kanoh, S. and Rubin, B.K. (2010). Mechanisms of action and clinical application of macrolides as immunomodulatory medications. *Clin. Microbiol. Rev.* 23: 590–615.

121 Kawamura, K., Ichikado, K., Takaki, M. et al. (2018). Adjunctive therapy with azithromycin for moderate and severe acute respiratory distress syndrome: a retrospective, propensity score-matching analysis of prospectively collected data at a single center. *Int. J. Antimicrob. Agents* 51: 918–924.

122 Rosenberg, E.S., Dufort, E.M., Udo, T. et al. (2020). Association of treatment with hydroxychloroquine or azithromycin with in-hospital mortality in patients with COVID-19 in New York state. *JAMA* 323: 2493–2502.

123 Furtado, R.H.M., Berwanger, O., Fonseca, H.A. et al. (2020). Azithromycin in addition to standard of care versus standard of care alone in the treatment of patients admitted to the hospital with severe COVID-19 in Brazil (COALITION II): a randomised clinical trial. *Lancet* 396: 959–967.

124 Ramireddy, A., Chugh, H., Reinier, K. et al. (2020). Experience with Hydroxychloroquine and azithromycin in the coronavirus disease 2019 pandemic: implications for QT interval monitoring. *J. Am. Heart Assoc.* 9: e017144.

125 Bessière, F., Roccia, H., Delinière, A. et al. (2020). Assessment of QT intervals in a case series of patients with coronavirus disease 2019 (COVID-19) infection treated with Hydroxychloroquine alone or in combination with azithromycin in an intensive care unit. *JAMA Cardiol.* 5: 1067–1069.

126 Metlay, J.P. and Waterer, G.W. (2020). Treatment of community-acquired pneumonia during the coronavirus disease 2019 (COVID-19) pandemic. *Ann. Intern. Med.* 173: 304–305.

127 Gubitosa, J.C., Kakar, P., Gerula, C. et al. (2020). Marked sinus Bradycardia associated with Remdesivir in COVID-19: a case and literature review. *JACC Case Rep.* 2: 2260–2264.

128 Gupta, A.K., Parker, B.M., Priyadarshi, V., and Parker, J. (2020). Cardiac adverse events with Remdesivir in COVID-19 infection. *Cureus* 12: e11132.

129 Grein, J., Ohmagari, N., Shin, D. et al. (2020). Compassionate use of Remdesivir for patients with severe Covid-19. *N. Engl. J. Med.* 382: 2327–2336.

130 Beigel, J.H., Tomashek, K.M., Dodd, L.E. et al. (2020). Remdesivir for the treatment of Covid-19-final report. *N. Engl. J. Med.* 383: 1813–1826.

131 Zhang, P., Zhu, L., Cai, J. et al. (2020). Association of Inpatient use of angiotensin-converting enzyme inhibitors and angiotensin II receptor blockers with mortality among patients with hypertension hospitalized with COVID-19. *Circ. Res.* 126: 1671–1681.

132 Wan, Y., Shang, J., Graham, R. et al. (2020). Receptor recognition by the novel coronavirus from Wuhan: an analysis based on decade-long structural studies of SARS coronavirus. *J. Virol.* 94: e00127-20.

133 Solaru, K.W. and Wright Jr. J.T. 2020. COVID-19 and use of drugs targeting the renin-angiotensin-system. American College of Cardiology. https://www.acc.org/latest-in-cardiology/articles/2020/07/15/13/12/covid-19-and-use-of-drugs-targeting-the-renin-angiotensin-system.

134 Fang, L., Karakiulakis, G., and Roth, M. (2020). Are patients with hypertension and diabetes mellitus at increased risk for COVID-19 infection? *Lancet Respir. Med.* 8: e21.

135 Bozkurt, B., Kovacs, R., and Harrington, B. (2020). Joint HFSA/ACC/AHA statement addresses concerns re: using RAAS antagonists in COVID-19. *J. Card. Fail.* 26: 370.

136 Reynolds, H.R., Adhikari, S., Pulgarin, C. et al. (2020). Renin-angiotensin-aldosterone system inhibitors and risk of Covid-19. *N. Engl. J. Med.* 382: 2441–2448.

137 Mancia, G., Rea, F., Ludergnani, M. et al. (2020). Renin-angiotensin-aldosterone system blockers and the risk of Covid-19. *N. Engl. J. Med.* 382: 2431–2440.

138 Hakeam, H.A., Alsemari, M., Duhailib, Z.A. et al. (2021). Association of angiotensin-converting enzyme inhibitors and angiotensin II blockers with severity of COVID-19: a multicenter, prospective study. *J. Cardiovasc. Pharmacol. Ther.* 26: 244–252.

139 European Society of Cardiology 2020. Position statement of the ESC council on hypertension on ACE-inhibitors and angiotensin receptor blockers. https://www.escardio.org/Councils/Council-on-Hypertension-(CHT)/News/position-statement-of-the-esc-council-on-hypertension-on-ace-inhibitors-and-ang.

140 Vaduganathan, M., Vardeny, O., Michel, T. et al. (2020). Renin-angiotensin-aldosterone system inhibitors in patients with Covid-19. *N. Engl. J. Med.* 382: 1653–1659.

141 Lee, K.C.H., Sewa, D.W., and Phua, G.C. (2020). Potential role of statins in COVID-19. *Int. J. Infect. Dis.* 96: 615–617.

142 Castiglione, V., Chiriacò, M., Emdin, M. et al. (2020). Statin therapy in COVID-19 infection. *Eur. Heart J. Cardiovasc. Pharmacother.* 6: 258–259.

143 Scheen, A.J. (2020). Statins and clinical outcomes with COVID-19: meta-analyses of observational studies. *Diabetes Metab.* 47: 101220.

144 Butt, J.H., Gerds, T.A., Schou, M. et al. (2020). Association between statin use and outcomes in patients with coronavirus disease 2019 (COVID-19): a nationwide cohort study. *BMJ Open* 10: e044421.

145 Fan, Y., Guo, T., Yan, F. et al. (2020). Association of Statin use with the in-hospital outcomes of 2019-coronavirus disease patients: a retrospective study. *Front. Med. (Lausanne)* 7: 584870.

146 Matsushita, K., Ding, N., Kou, M. et al. (2020). The relationship of COVID-19 severity with cardiovascular disease and its traditional risk factors: a systematic review and meta-analysis. *Glob. Heart* 15: 64.

147 Alvarez-Garcia, J., Lee, S., Gupta, A. et al. (2020). Prognostic impact of prior heart failure in patients hospitalized with COVID-19. *J. Am. Coll. Cardiol.* 76: 2334–2348.

148 Kytömaa, S., Hegde, S., Claggett, B. et al. (2019). Association of influenza-like illness activity with hospitalizations for heart failure: the atherosclerosis risk in communities study. *JAMA Cardiol.* 4: 363–369.

149 Wadhera, R.K., Shen, C., Gondi, S. et al. (2021). Cardiovascular deaths during the COVID-19 pandemic in the United States. *J. Am. Coll. Cardiol.* 77: 159–169.

150 Pereira, M.R., Mohan, S., Cohen, D.J. et al. (2020). COVID-19 in solid organ transplant recipients: initial report from the US epicenter. *Am. J. Transplant.* 20: 1800–1808.

151 Bottio, T., Bagozzi, L., Fiocco, A. et al. (2021). COVID-19 in heart transplant recipients: a multicenter analysis of the northern Italian outbreak. *JACC Heart Fail.* 9: 52–61.

152 Latif, F., Farr, M.A., Clerkin, K.J. et al. (2020). Characteristics and outcomes of recipients of heart transplant with coronavirus disease 2019. *JAMA Cardiol.* 5: 1165–1169.

153 Zheng, Z., Peng, F., Xu, B. et al. (2020). Risk factors of critical & mortal COVID-19 cases: a systematic literature review and meta-analysis. *J. Infect.* 81: e16–e25.

154 Rivinius, R., Kaya, Z., Schramm, R. et al. (2020). COVID-19 among heart transplant recipients in Germany: a multicenter survey. *Clin. Res. Cardiol.* 109: 1531–1539.

155 International Society for Heart and Lung Transplantation 2021. Guidance from the ISHLT regarding the SARS CoV-2 pandemic. https:// ishlt.org/covid-19-information (accessed 14 April 2021).

156 RECOVERY Collaborative Group, Horby, P., Lim, W.S. et al. (2021). Dexamethasone in hospitalized patients with Covid-19. *N. Engl. J. Med.* 384: 693–704.

157 National Institutes of Health 2020. Special considerations in solid organ transplant, hematopoietic stem cell transplant, and cellular therapy candidates, donors, and recipients. https:// www.covid19treatmentguidelines.nih.gov/ special-populations/transplant (accessed 14 April 2021).

158 Boyarsky, B.J., Ou, M.T., Greenberg, R.S. et al. (2021). Safety of the first dose of SARS-CoV-2 vaccination in solid organ transplant recipients. *Transplantation* 105: e56–e57.

159 Widge, A.T., Rouphael, N.G., Jackson, L.A. et al. (2021). Durability of responses after SARS-CoV-2 mRNA-1273 vaccination. *N. Engl. J. Med.* 384: 80–82.

160 American Society of Transplantation 2021. COVID-19 vaccine FAQ sheet. https://www.myast. org/sites/default/files/Education/2021%2003%20 02%20COVID19%20VACCINE%20FAQS_ update%20v4%20FINAL%20%281%29.pdf (accessed 3 March 2021).

17

COVID-19: Oncologic and Hematologic Considerations

Diana L. Hanna[1,2], Caroline I. Piatek[3], Binh T. Ngo[4], and Heinz-Josef Lenz[1]

[1] Division of Medical Oncology, Norris Comprehensive Cancer Center, University of Southern California, Los Angeles, CA, USA
[2] Hoag Cancer Center, Newport Beach, CA, USA
[3] Jane Anne Nohl Division of Hematology, Keck School of Medicine, University of Southern California, Los Angeles, CA, USA
[4] Department of Dermatology, Keck School of Medicine, University of Southern California, Los Angeles, CA, USA

Abbreviations

ASCO	American Society of Clinical Oncology
CDC	Centers for Disease Control and Prevention
FDA	US Food and Drug Administration
G-CSF	granulocyte colony-stimulating factor
ICU	intensive care unit
ITP	immune thrombocytopenia
mRNA	messenger RNA
NCCN	National Comprehensive Cancer Network
RT-PCR	reverse transcription-polymerase chain reaction
SARS-CoV-2	severe acute respiratory syndrome coronavirus 2
SCT	stem cell transplantation
TKI	tyrosine kinase inhibitor

The Natural History of COVID-19 in Patients with Cancer

Worldwide estimates of prevalence of coronavirus disease 2019 (COVID-19) infections vary considerably from 1% to 10% among patients with malignancy [1, 2]. Among patients with cancer, subgroups with more prevalent COVID-19 infection include men, patients older than 65 years, African Americans, Hispanics, and those with lung or hematologic malignancies [3]. Conversely, estimates of cancer incidence among patients with COVID-19 differ across countries and within the United States and range from 1% to 20% [4–6]. Multiple factors may influence this variability in estimates, including testing and reporting practices and accuracy, presence of viral variants, immunocompromised host status, and other comorbidities.

Similarly, data are conflicting regarding the impact of recent cancer diagnosis, type of cancer, and active or recent therapy on the incidence, morbidity, and mortality from COVID-19. In a population-based survey, patients with cancer had a 60% increased risk of having a positive COVID-19 test [2]. Indeed, those receiving chemotherapy or immunotherapy had a more than twofold increased risk of a positive test compared with patients with cancer not receiving treatment [2]. A meta-analysis of 15 studies of patients with COVID-19 (N = 3019) concluded that those with cancer have a much higher mortality than those without cancer, with an overall case fatality rate of 22.4%, including a significantly increased rate seen in men and patients older than 65 years of age [7]. Although several studies have demonstrated increased risk for morbidity and mortality from COVID-19 in patients with cancer, particularly those with lung or hematologic malignancies, others have shown comparable outcomes [8]. Certain analyses may be limited by lack of propensity score adjustment, selection bias, recall bias, and evolving disease or practice patterns [9]. Due to the heterogeneity of populations, there are limitations to these data, and additional studies are warranted.

Diagnosing COVID-19 in Patients with Cancer: Clinical, Serologic, and Imaging Considerations

Severe acute respiratory syndrome coronavirus 2 (SARS-CoV-2) is a betacoronavirus, and the initial presentation of COVID-19 is that of an ordinary upper respiratory viral illness. Patients commonly present with fever, chills, sore throat, rhinorrhea, malaise, chest pain, dyspnea, headache, nausea/vomiting, diarrhea, ageusia, and anosmia, and these presenting symptoms are similar in patients with cancer. As with any patient, a thorough history identifying potential exposures, vaccination status, and physical examination should be conducted. What distinguishes COVID-19 is an inflammatory phase of hyperimmunity and coagulopathy. This inflammatory phase supervenes in up to 20% of patients, most commonly manifesting as an organizing multilobar pneumonia with hypoxia [10]. Although COVID-19 must be considered in patients with suggestive symptoms, the differential should not be prematurely narrowed and other etiologies should be explored, including other viral syndromes and bacterial pneumonia. Moreover, therapy-related adverse events, particularly immune-mediated effects and progression of cancer, must also be considered. Dermatologic manifestations may include morbilliform rash, urticaria, vesicular lesions, necrotic vascular lesions, or pernio-like acral lesions (also known as "COVID toes") and should be distinguished from cancer therapy-related rashes or other skin toxicities.

Molecular-based reverse transcription-polymerase chain reaction (RT-PCR) is the gold standard and most used diagnostic test for detection of SARS-CoV-2 RNA. Antigen-based rapid testing, including home tests, varies in sensitivity from 58% to 79% but is useful for confirmation of typical COVID-19 symptoms when positive and allow prompt treatment [11]. Acutely symptomatic patients should have a confirmatory RT-PCR performed. A combination multiplex PCR is recommended when considering other respiratory pathogens, such as influenza and respiratory syncytial virus, in addition to SARS-CoV-2. In symptomatic patients, a negative RT-PCR usually excludes a COVID-19 diagnosis. However, a negative test in the setting of suspicious symptoms for COVID-19 should prompt repeat testing. Nasopharyngeal or nasal turbinate swabs are the most accessible and appropriate diagnostic samples. Bronchoalveolar lavage or aerosol-generating procedures, such as induced sputum, should be limited and reserved for situations when testing from deep sampling is required to clarify a suspicious diagnosis or test for other potential pathogens.

On clinical recovery from COVID-19, patients may have prolonged viral shedding that correlates with severity of the illness. In a comprehensive meta-analysis, the mean duration of SARS-CoV-2 RNA shedding was 17.0 days in the upper respiratory tract, 14.6 days in the lower respiratory tract, and 17.2 days in stool [12]. Patients with cancer who are infected with SARS-CoV-2 may have more prolonged viral shedding. In a series of patients with hematologic malignancies undergoing hematopoietic stem cell transplantation (SCT) or chimeric antigen receptor T cell therapies who were infected with COVID-19, shedding of viable virus RNA was detected for up to 78 days after the onset of symptoms [13]. However, viral shedding and active infection must be distinguished from each other, and infectivity appears lower than implied by positive PCR samples [14]. A balance must be achieved between delaying cancer-directed therapy and ensuring adequate COVID-19 resolution, as well as mitigating the risk for spread to other patients in the cancer center. To this end, practice patterns vary with respect to requiring negative COVID-19 testing after infection before returning to a cancer center and/or resuming systemic therapy or radiation.

Serologic tests measure antibodies to SARS-CoV-2 in the blood to find evidence of prior infection or exposure. Timing and type of exposure to an infected individual, as well as type of malignancy and proximity of cancer therapy, should be considered when interpreting results. These tests are only moderately useful in patients with cancer who may have depressed immunity because of their inherent illness or cancer treatment.

On imaging, a particularly difficult diagnostic challenge may be distinguishing evolving COVID-19 infection with organizing pneumonia from progression of primary lung cancer or pulmonary metastases, including the presence of lymphangitic spread or carcinomatosis, as well as chemotherapy- or radiation-induced pneumonitis [15, 16]. Although certain therapies, such as steroids, may address multiple etiologies concurrently, the decision to modify cancer-directed therapy is more nuanced and must be made with caution in accordance with the patient's overall prognosis and wishes regarding goals of care (see also the following two sections).

COVID-19 Therapeutics in Patients with Cancer

For patients with cancer who test positive for COVID-19 and have mild or no symptoms, isolation at home with supportive care may be appropriate. Proactive remote monitoring; early identification of moderate, severe, or worsening disease; and aggressive symptom control are critical and may reduce the need for hospitalization [17]. Patients who present with dyspnea, hypoxemia (O_2 saturation <94% on room air), or signs or symptoms to suggest hypoxia, including altered mentation, will warrant urgent hospital evaluation. Barrier methods of protection, including masks and face shields, blocking respiratory transmission are very useful but not easy to follow in households.

Following are recommendations derived from the Centers for Disease Control and Prevention (CDC) and National Comprehensive Cancer Network (NCCN) regarding the outpatient and inpatient therapeutics for patients with cancer who are infected with COVID-19.

Monoclonal Antibodies (Casirivimab/Imdevimab, Sotrovimab, and Bamlanivimab/Etesevimab)

Based on an Emergency Use Authorization issued by the US Food and Drug Administration (FDA), outpatients with mild to moderate COVID-19 at high risk for severe COVID-19, including patients with cancer who are immunosuppressed, are eligible to receive one of the following monoclonal antibodies directed against SARS-CoV-2. These treatments should be given as soon as possible after diagnosis and within 7–10 days of symptom onset. They are not authorized for use in asymptomatic or hospitalized patients. Following is a summary of currently used agents:

- Casirivimab/imdevimab 600 mg/600 mg IV (or subcutaneous if IV not available)
- Bamlanivimab/etesevimab 700 mg/1400 mg IV
- Sotrovimab 500 mg IV

Casirivimab/imdevimab and bamlanivimab/etesevimab are also authorized for use as postexposure prophylaxis in patients with mild to moderate COVID-19 who are at risk for severe disease and are not fully vaccinated or not expected to mount an adequate immune response to vaccination. Sotrovimab is a very interesting antibody that targets an evolutionarily conserved epitope of sarbecoviruses, and thus may have a broader spectrum of activity against viruses other than SARS-CoV-2. In fact, the origin of the antibody was isolation from a patient with SARS-CoV-1 [18].

Remdesivir

Remdesivir, an intravenous nucleotide analogue, may lead to more rapid clinical improvement and is recommended for inpatients hospitalized for COVID-19 pneumonia with hypoxia, but who not yet require mechanical ventilation or extracorporeal membrane oxygenation. Liver function tests should be monitored daily. The risks and benefits of therapy should be weighed in patients with renal insufficiency. Remdesivir may be considered in hospitalized patients without hypoxemia and in those at higher risk for infection progression at the following dosing:

- Remdesivir 200 mg IV × 1 day, then 100 mg/day for 5–10 days

In an observational study of 2186 patients with cancer, remdesivir significantly reduced 30-day mortality compared with other therapies (including hydroxychloroquine, azithromycin, steroids, and tocilizumab in various combinations), but not compared with control subjects who received no treatment [19].

Glucocorticoids

Glucocorticoid therapy is recommended for patients with active malignancy hospitalized for COVID-19 pneumonia with hypoxemia who are on supplemental oxygen or receiving ventilatory support. There is unclear benefit of corticosteroids if patients are neutropenic or otherwise immunosuppressed (e.g. in bone marrow transplant patients on immune suppression). Following is a summary of currently used agents:

- Dexamethasone 6 mg/day for 10 days or shorter if discharged from hospital sooner
- Alternatives: hydrocortisone 150 mg/day, methylprednisolone 32 mg/day, prednisone 40 mg/day

Baricitinib and Other Janus Kinase Inhibitors

An Emergency Use Authorization was issued for the Janus kinase inhibitor baricitinib, in combination with remdesivir, in patients hospitalized for COVID-19 requiring supplemental oxygen or ventilation support. Baricitinib may also be used in patients receiving low-flow oxygen but with increasing oxygen requirements despite use of steroids. Tofacitinib has also shown clinical benefit and may be considered. Following is a summary of currently used agents:

- Baricitinib 4 mg orally daily for 14 days or shorter if discharged from the hospital sooner
- Tofacitinib 10 mg orally b.i.d. for 14 days or shorter if discharged from the hospital sooner

Tocilizumab and Other Interleukin-6 Inhibitors

Tocilizumab should be considered in patients hospitalized with COVID-19 who require at least high-flow oxygen or mechanical ventilation and are receiving glucocorticoids. This is ideally administered within 96 hours of hospital admission and within 24–48 hours of initiating intensive care unit (ICU) level of care. Following is the recommended regimen:

- Tocilizumab 8 mg/kg IV single dose

Convalescent Plasma

Convalescent plasma has not demonstrated a consistent survival benefit in studies of the general population hospitalized for COVID-19 [20–23]. However, convalescent plasma was shown to reduce 30-day all-cause mortality in patients with hematologic malignancies in whom humoral immunity is particularly compromised [24]. In this multi-institutional retrospective cohort study, 30-day mortality was significantly improved in patients admitted to the ICU and who required mechanical ventilation [24]. This survival benefit remained significant after adjusting for age, sex, ethnicity, performance status, timing of last cancer therapy, obesity, hypertension, renal or pulmonary disease, and receipt of chemotherapy within three months of COVID-19 diagnosis [24].

Therefore, in patients with hematologic malignancies, the use of convalescent plasma is recommended in conjunction with other approved therapeutics. A dose of one or more high-titer units is recommended. The best outcomes are likely to occur in those who receive high-titer units within a few days of COVID-19 diagnosis or admission to hospital early in the course of infection.

Molnupiravir

Molnupiravir is an oral ribonucleoside analogue that inhibits SARS-CoV-2 replication and is active against different variants, including the Delta variant. It is investigational at the time of this publication [25, 26], although preliminary reported results are encouraging. Among outpatients with mild to moderate COVID-19 at risk for severe disease, those who received molnupiravir within five days of symptom onset had a significantly reduced risk for hospitalization or death by approximately 50% (7.3% vs. 14.1% with placebo) as reported in a press release from the sponsor [27].

Other drugs not mentioned earlier should not be prescribed outside the context of a clinical trial or based on updated approvals and guidelines.

Interactions between COVID-19 therapeutics and anticancer drugs have been identified, and the French Society for Oncology Pharmacy has published a review addressing known interactions to guide clinicians in decision making regarding COVID-19 and antineoplastic therapy [28].

Patients with COVID-19 may have secondary infections with fungal, bacterial, and/or other viral pathogens. The clinical implication of such co-infections is not entirely clear, but they might contribute significantly to morbidity or mortality, especially among those who required admission to the ICU.

Practical Considerations in the Management of Patients with Cancer

Patients with cancer require frequent evaluation and follow-up, and they often must receive chemotherapy at infusion centers. Telemedicine is useful to permit surveillance of patients at home, but the practicality of caring for cancer patients often requires in-person evaluation and treatment at medical facilities. Certainly, air handling, decontamination, and barrier methods of protection to block respiratory transmission, including masks and face shields, are very useful. However, the transportation of patients, often requiring assistance from relatives, introduces many opportunities for infection.

Offering in-person versus remote visits has been a swinging pendulum following the phases of the pandemic. In general, in-person consultations are ideal for delivering information regarding initial cancer diagnosis, new treatment plan, disease relapse or progression, and goals of care transitions [29]. During sensitive discussions, allowing one person in the room with the patient can allow for a more supportive and empathic in-person visit.

The following recommendations have been issued by the American Society of Clinical Oncology (ASCO) [30] and are in accordance with CDC guidelines:

- When scheduling appointments, inform patients that appointments will need to be rescheduled for any of following reasons:
  - If the patient develops symptoms of a respiratory infection (e.g. cough, shortness of breath, fever, chills, myalgias, sore throat, new loss of taste or smell, or other flu-like symptoms) on the day they are scheduled to be seen, instruct patients to call the office before departing for their appointment (or sooner)
  - If they have symptoms of COVID-19 within the 10 days before their appointment
  - If they have been diagnosed with COVID-19 infection within 10 days before their appointment

  - If they have had contact with someone with suspected or confirmed COVID-19 infection within 14 days before their scheduled appointment

Advise patients that they are required to put on a face mask or other face covering, regardless of symptoms, before entering the facility and throughout their visit.

Contact the patient 48–72 hours before the appointment to screen for symptoms of cough, shortness of breath, fever, chills, myalgias, sore throat, new loss of taste or smell, or other flu-like symptoms. If symptoms are present, triage protocols should be used to determine whether an appointment is necessary or if the patient can be managed from home. If the patient can be managed from home, the patient should be instructed to contact their primary care physician if symptoms worsen or do not resolve within 14 days. The patient appointment should be rescheduled when he or she is determined to be no longer infectious.

Limit access to the facility through one point of entry, if possible. If there are multiple points of entry, screening must occur at all entrances. Facility access should exclude nonessential vendors and allow only essential ancillary services.

Implement face masks for everyone entering the facility, regardless of symptoms, to help prevent transmission from infected individuals who may not have symptoms of COVID-19.

Include signage with COVID-19 screening questions and visualization of symptoms for all patients/visitors, as well as patient education materials and illustrations of proper hygiene for infection prevention and symptoms to report. Provide signage and patient education materials in language(s) appropriate for your patient population.

Patient screening status and COVID-positive status should be documented prior to the patient entering the facility (e.g. electronic medical record, patient identification wristband with date of screening). However, the value of routine prescreening with RT-PCR for COVID-19 in outpatients with cancer pending start of therapy has been called into question [31] and is not recommended.

Patients receiving myelosuppressive cancer-directed therapy who become infected with COVID-19 may be at an increased risk for serious complications, hospitalization, and death [7, 32, 33]. Multiple meta-analyses addressing this issue have shown no definitive, significant interaction between targeted therapy, immunotherapy, or surgery and outcomes in patients with cancer and COVID-19. However, there have been mixed findings, notably with respect to the effects of chemotherapy and radiation. The decision to delay cancer screening and diagnostic procedures and specific cancer-directed therapies must be individualized between the patient and oncologist and should take into account the following:

- Curative versus palliative intent of the intervention
- Performance status, comorbidities (including baseline cognitive and/or sensory impairment, underlying nonmalignant immunocompromise, or cardiopulmonary disease), and vaccination status
- Natural history of the cancer, including the risk for recurrence or progression with interruption of therapy
- Risks or adverse effects of the intervention (e.g. degree and duration of myelosuppression, perioperative morbidity/mortality)
- Psychosocial support system, proximity to a healthcare facility, access to telehealth and to remote nursing/monitoring capabilities

ASCO has issued guidelines for clinicians and patients faced with these decisions, along with links to resources from other respective medical societies depending on the nature of the intervention [34].

Cancer Screening and Diagnosis

COVID-19 caused a 60–99% reduction in screening procedures for breast, colorectal, cervical, and prostate cancers between January and June 2020 [35–38]. Importantly, rates of diagnostic mammography were reduced by approximately 80% during this period as well compared with prepandemic rates [36]. In July 2020, there was a notable lag in the rebound of screening mammography in Hispanic and Asian women, where the volumes had reached only 72.7% and 51.3% of prepandemic rates, respectively [36, 39]. In addition, the rebound in screening for colorectal cancer remained about 15% less than prepandemic levels across all individuals [36]. Delayed screening eventually leads to increased rates of later-stage diagnoses and cancer-related mortality and may contribute to racial disparities in outcomes [36, 40, 41].

Ultimately, the decision to resume screening will follow the rates of infection and available resources in a particular community, as well as the risk of the individual patient. Patients with symptoms concerning for cancer requiring diagnostic evaluation, imaging, and procedures should be prioritized, followed by screening examinations for individuals deemed high risk (i.e. based on germline predisposition or other factors), and then examinations for people at average risk. Such a stratified approach where missed screening examinations are caught up in a delayed (rather than immediate) fashion may strike the optimal balance between available resources and an increase in required capacity, while not compromising the outcomes of cancer incidence and mortality [42–46].

Post-COVID-19 messenger RNA (mRNA) vaccine ipsilateral axillary adenopathy has emerged as a confounder in the interpretation of radiologic imaging and screening studies, especially mammograms, with the incidence varying between 2% and 20% across studies, depending on type, first versus second dose, and timing of the vaccine [47, 48]. According to published guidelines from the Radiology Scientific Expert Panel and others, if clinically safe, routine screening and other imaging should be completed before an mRNA COVID-19 vaccination or four to six weeks after the second vaccine dose [49, 50]. Importantly, clinically indicated imaging for evaluating symptoms or for treatment planning, assessing response, and complications should not be delayed because of prior vaccination [49]. If vaccination is occurring concurrently with urgently needed cancer imaging, vaccination in the contralateral arm or thigh may be appropriate [50]. Information, including type of vaccine, date administered, and injection site, should be collected in preimaging questionnaires or made otherwise readily available in the medical record to guide imaging interpretation by radiologists and clinicians [49].

With respect to mammograms, unilateral axillary adenopathy warrants a Breast Imaging Reporting and Data System (BI-RADS) 0 designation (incomplete examination, need additional imaging evaluation and/or prior mammograms for comparison) for future assessment [51]. In addition to diagnostic workup for alternative causes of the axillary adenopathy, short-term follow-up mammography is recommended in 4–12 weeks after the second vaccination [51]. If ipsilateral axillary lymphadenopathy persists beyond six weeks after the final vaccine dose, then further clinical evaluation, including ultrasound, should be pursued [50].

Specific recommendations regarding the timing of radiologic imaging and the adenoviral As26.COV2.S (Janssen COVID-19) vaccine are not as clear, but similar principles as earlier may be applied.

Cancer Therapy: Cytotoxic Chemotherapy

Studies have yielded mixed findings regarding the impact of cytotoxic therapy on mortality from COVID-19. In a report from the National COVID Cohort Collaborative representing 50 US medical centers (N = 398 579; 15% COVID-19-positive), all-cause mortality was found to be higher in patients with cancer who had received cytotoxic chemotherapy within the last 30 days [52]. Additional factors associated with increased mortality among COVID-19-positive patients included age ≥65 years, male sex, Southern or Western US residence, hematologic malignancy, multiple tumor sites, and adjusted Charlson Comorbidity Index ≥4 [52]. Similarly, a multicenter COVID-19 analysis from Wuhan, China (N = 13 077; 1.8% with cancer) reported that patients with cancer, particularly those with advanced malignancy or who had received chemotherapy within the last two weeks, were more likely to progress to severe COVID-19 [53]. In contrast, researchers from the UK Coronavirus Cancer Monitoring Project Team suggest that the impact of cancer therapy on mortality depends on tumor type and found receipt of chemotherapy not to be associated with outcomes among those who develop COVID-19 [54]. Another smaller study (N = 306) also demonstrated a lack of association between receiving chemotherapy within 35 days and severe COVID-19 (as defined earlier) or a critical COVID-19 event defined as respiratory failure, septic shock, and/or multiple organ dysfunction or failure [55].

Importantly, the form of chemotherapy must be considered, and multiple studies have illustrated only certain or more myelosuppressive regimens to impact severity of COVID-19. In a British population study, receipt of cancer regimens with a 10–50% risk of grade 3 or 4 neutropenia or lymphopenia within the last 12 months was more likely to have severe COVID-19 and associated mortality than lower-risk regimens [56]. In another study from the COVID-19 and Cancer

Consortium (N = 4966), receipt of chemotherapy within 3 months of COVID-19 diagnosis predicted significantly increased COVID-19 severity and worse 30-day all-cause mortality, with platinum-etoposide, R-CHOP-like regimens, and DNA methyltransferase inhibitors being associated with the highest mortality [57]. Although the broad, prolonged myelosuppression expected with these regimens likely impacts outcomes, multiple complex factors are at play, including the impact on T cell and B cell lymphodepletion, presence of pulmonary tumor involvement, use and dose of steroids, and resulting impact on the inflammatory response. Relatedly, the presence of lymphopenia, neutropenia, and thrombocytopenia have all been shown to be negative prognosticators in hospitalized patients with cancer and COVID-19, although these laboratory findings are almost always multifactorial in etiology [55].

Ultimately, the decision to administer chemotherapy must be individualized, with the most difficult decisions being made in patients receiving highly myelosuppressive regimens with curative intent.

Among noninfected patients with cancer, routinely holding or delaying chemotherapy is not recommended. However, in cancer centers heavily affected by active COVID-19, where chemotherapy must be prioritized, or where the risks of COVID-19 outweigh the risk of interrupting chemotherapy, alternative treatment strategies may be necessary and pursued. Alternate treatment approaches may include a treatment holiday for patients in deep, durable remission, using oral chemotherapy or noncytotoxic regimens, adjusting the schedule to allow for fewer in-person visits, or at least temporary transfer of care to another center [58].

Among patients who test positive for SARS-CoV-2, chemotherapy should be held until a patient assessment is completed and a discussion is had regarding next steps in management. In accordance with CDC and ASCO guidelines, chemotherapy may be resumed once transmission-based precautions are discontinued. Institutions will vary with respect to using time since initial symptoms or first positive test (i.e. non-test-based, time and/or symptom-based) versus test-based protocols to discontinue infection-control precautions and resume cancer therapy. Certain institutions will use a hybrid approach that combines both test-based and non-test-based strategies.

In patients who remain asymptomatic, the time-based approach mandates at least 10 days have passed since the first positive viral diagnostic test, or at least 20 days in severely immunocompromised patients, including patients with hereditary and acquired immune deficiencies (e.g. common variable immunodeficiency, receiving highly myelosuppressive regimens or more than ≥20 mg prednisone daily equivalent for ≥2 weeks, begin within 1 year of receiving solid organ transplant) before discontinuation of infection-control precautions.

In symptomatic patients with a positive SARS-CoV-2 test, the time-based approach requires at least 10–20 days have elapsed since the first positive test (up to 20 days for those with severe or critical COVID-19), 24 hours have passed since resolution of fever without the use of antipyretics, and there is overall clinical improvement before discontinuation of infection-control precautions. Resolution of symptoms for at least 72 hours is another commonly adapted approach.

As alluded to earlier, the requirement for a subsequent negative PCR test within 48–72 hours of resuming therapy may be useful and preferable in certain circumstances, including in patients who develop severe or critical COVID-19, who are severely immunocompromised, or who are pending start of highly myelosuppressive or prolonged duration of chemotherapy. However, this should be weighed against the possibility of persistent viral shedding and unnecessary risk for delaying cancer-directed therapy in patients who are asymptomatic and may not be infectious. Complex decisions such as these should be made in conjunction with infectious disease and infection prevention specialists. If the patient is deemed clinically stable and safe to resume chemotherapy, the patient should be placed in isolation from other patients in the cancer center with dedicated staff and standard distancing precautions.

Cancer Therapy: Immunotherapy, Targeted Agents, and Biologics

As with cytotoxic chemotherapy, analyses have demonstrated varying conclusions regarding the impact of immunotherapy on outcomes in patients with COVID-19 and cancer. Researchers from Memorial Sloan Kettering found recent use of immune checkpoint inhibitors to predict hospitalization and severe COVID-19, a finding that was independent of cancer type (lung vs. non-lung cancer) and in the absence of concomitant immune-mediated pneumonitis [54]. However, these findings should be interpreted with caution given the retrospective nature of the study and other potential confounders. Even the authors of this study concluded that their findings were not sufficient to alter treatment decisions. Furthermore, most available studies to date suggest no significant impact of immune checkpoint inhibitors on clinical outcomes from COVID-19 in patients with lung or other cancers [1, 59–62]. In a meta-analysis, for example, receipt of immunotherapy within 30 days was not associated with COVID-19 severity or death in patients with cancer [32]. In summary, checkpoint inhibitor therapy is likely safe to be continued in most patients, especially those with asymptomatic COVID-19.

With respect to targeted drugs and biologics that are not checkpoint inhibitors or B cell depleting, including tyrosine kinase inhibitors (TKIs), endocrine or hormonal therapies (e.g. androgen, estrogen blockade), and monoclonal antibodies (e.g. antiangiogenics, anti–epidermal growth factor receptor agents), available studies are in agreement and suggest these do not impact outcomes in patients with cancer infected with COVID-19. One class of TKIs, Burton tyrosine kinase inhibitors used for hematologic malignancies (e.g. ibrutinib for chronic lymphocytic leukemia), have been associated with improved outcomes and less severe COVID-19 infection [63–65], although randomized/controlled studies are needed for more definitive conclusions. In summary, administration of targeted and biologic therapies may be given without interruption or delay alongside standard distancing and other precautions to minimize COVID-19 exposure and transmission. In cancer centers heavily impacted by active COVID-19, home administration of intramuscular or subcutaneous injections may be considered to reduce the number of in-person visits and minimize patient exposure [58].

Cancer Therapy: Radiation Therapy

The nature of external beam radiotherapy requiring on-site daily treatments has posed unique challenges to radiation oncologists caring for patients with cancer.

To this end, the American Society for Radiation Oncology along with the National Institute for Health and Care Excellence have issued guidance on how to prioritize radiotherapy according to cancer type, intent of therapy, dose already administered, planned schedule or fractionation, and evolving goals of care [66, 67].

Patients undergoing radiotherapy or chemoradiotherapy with curative intent for a rapidly proliferating cancer should proceed without interruption, particularly if treatment has already started and/or there is considerable risk for clinical deterioration that cannot be compensated for with a treatment gap [67]. Importantly, patients requiring urgent palliative radiation, such as those with malignant spinal cord compression or other emergent situations (malignant tumor bleeding, superior vena cava syndrome) should proceed with therapy without interruption [66, 67]. Among patients receiving adjuvant radiation, treatment should proceed as planned, minimizing delays as much as possible, especially for cancers with higher rates of recurrence. Among patients with non-life-threatening conditions in whom treatment delays are unlikely to impact outcomes, such as patients with low-risk prostate cancer or ductal carcinoma in situ, treatment delays or interruptions may be considered on an individual basis and depending on the status of COVID-19 rates and resources at the cancer center.

For noninfected patients or those with asymptomatic or mildly symptomatic COVID-19, the earlier guidelines should be followed as deemed feasible, using standard distancing and isolation precautions. For patients with moderate or severe COVID-19, radiotherapy should be interrupted until the patient is deemed clinically stable and safe to resume therapy and as infection precautions are discontinued per CDC guidelines. A designated linear accelerator may be considered for COVID-19-positive patients, and treatment visits can be performed in the linear accelerator vault or via telemedicine [30]. COVID-19-positive patients should have the last appointments of the day on the machine and should remain in these time slots for at least 10 days and/or until improvement in symptoms and at least 24 hours have passed since resolution of fever without the use of fever-reducing medications. If there are multiple patients under investigation for COVID-19 and COVID-19-positive patients on treatment, they should be treated in consecutive slots at the end of the day. Facilities should conduct a thorough wipe-down of all surfaces between each patient under investigation or COVID-19-positive patient [30].

Cancer Therapy: Cellular Therapy and Hematopoietic Transplantation

Patients who have undergone hematopoietic cell transplantation (HCT) are at increased risk for complications and death from COVID-19, with approximately 15% of affected patients with severe disease requiring mechanical ventilation and more than 30% 30-day mortality [68]. Development of COVID-19 within one year of transplantation, age ≥50 years, and having a disease indication of lymphoma as compared with plasma cell disorder/myeloma have been associated with a higher risk for mortality [68]. Accordingly, special precautions should be taken regarding the management of patients with HCT and donors.

The American Society for Transplantation and Cellular Therapy has issued guidelines for HCT recipients presenting with respiratory symptoms, as well as considerations for HCT candidates and donors around the time of planned HCT or cellular therapies [69]. For HCT or cellular therapy recipients who test positive for COVID-19, refer to the earlier Monoclonal Antibodies (Casirivimab/Imdevimab, Sotrovimab, and Bamlanivimab/Etesevimab) section for management considerations.

All HCT and cellular therapy candidates should undergo screening for SARS-CoV-2 by PCR in respiratory specimens no more than two to three days before planned procedures, including peripheral blood stem cell mobilization, bone marrow harvest, T cell collection, and conditioning/lymphodepletion [69]. In candidates who test positive for SARS-CoV-2 or who have household SARS-CoV-2 exposure, all such procedures should be deferred for at least 14 days, until the patient is asymptomatic and has two consecutive negative PCR tests ≥24 hours apart independent of symptoms [69]. In patients who are clinically recovered but with persistent RNA detection, the decision to wait for PCR clearance must be weighed against the urgency of proceeding with HCT because prolonged shedding may persist beyond the presence of replication-competent virus [69]. When feasible and appropriate, bridge therapy should be considered in patients with multiple myeloma or germ cell tumors. Multidisciplinary management involving the infectious disease, cardiology, and pulmonary consultants is prudent in patients pending HCT or cellular therapy, and follow-up CT imaging and pulmonary function tests are recommended for patients recovering from COVID-19 [69].

With respect to HCT donors, individuals who test positive for SARS-CoV-2 in a respiratory sample are typically considered ineligible to donate. However, if there is no severe disease and the donor has been asymptomatic for at least 28 days, they may be considered for donation on a case-by-case basis [69]. Similarly, those who had a close contact with a person diagnosed with COVID-19 should be excluded from donation for at least 28 days, although asymptomatic individuals may be considered for earlier donation on a case-by-case basis with a negative SARS-CoV-2 by PCR [69].

Candidates and donors should avoid nonessential travel, practice social distancing, wear masks in public, and avoid crowds and large gatherings during the 28 days before planned procedures [69].

Bone marrow transplant units must take strict infection-prevention precautions to protect HCT recipients and donors. All admitted patients and visitors should be screened for symptoms or contact with a known COVID-19-positive individual at a single entry point, and healthcare workers should be screened daily. Patients with COVID-19 symptoms should be isolated, with testing conducted at designated locations outside of the transplant unit/clinic. Healthcare workers should wear face masks, as well as eye protection, on patient care units. Healthcare workers should use respirators in addition to airborne and droplet/contact precautions (gloves, gown, N95, eye protection) for care of COVID-19-positive patients. Hospitals may follow different policies of when to remove droplet/contact precautions, including time based, test based, or a combination of both (see earlier Cancer Therapy: Cytotoxic Chemotherapy section). The time-based strategy requires that at least 20 days have passed since symptom onset, as well as 24 hours since the last fever and symptoms have resolved. Alternatively, the test-based strategy requires two documented negative SARS-CoV-2 respiratory PCR tests at least 24 hours apart from each other.

Patients should adhere to universal masking in all clinical spaces and inpatient areas. There should be a limit on allowed hospital visitors. Outpatient in-person appointments should be limited to essential visits, and telemedicine should be used when appropriate.

Oncologic Surgery

Primary resection is essential to the curative management of localized solid tumors. At the height of the pandemic, surgical oncology societies issued guidelines on the timing of tumor resection, which weighed the risk for disease progression against that of COVID-19 infection in the perioperative setting, while considering available hospital resources. Indeed, the COVIDSurg Collaborative, an international multicenter cohort, examined the rate of pulmonary complications and mortality among patients with SARS-CoV-2 undergoing elective and emergent surgery [70]. Pulmonary complications occurred in more than 50% of patients, and 30-day mortality was 38% in this group, with increased morality among patients with cancer (odds ratio, 1.55) [70]. Restrictions have lessened as infections have declined and with increased vaccination. Nonetheless, there are still regions in the United States and abroad that are confronted with high transmission rates and strained resources.

Among patients residing in areas with persistent high rates of COVID-19 infection, one approach may be to proceed with neoadjuvant therapy as a bridge to definitive surgery. This is perhaps particularly relevant in patients with indolent malignancies who may receive neoadjuvant hormone therapy, such as ER$^+$/PR$^+$ breast cancer or low-risk prostate cancer. However, most cancer-related surgeries are deemed urgent and cannot be delayed. As such, all patients are recommended to have COVID-19 testing before any planned procedure or surgery, regardless of vaccination status, with surgery delayed in patients who test positive.

On an institutional level, the decision to resume elective procedures requires a stepwise, flexible, multidisciplinary approach in the setting of a steady decline in COVID-19 infections and hospitalizations. At Columbia University, operations have been assigned a resource intensity score that classifies the procedure based on personnel/space, devices, expendables, and postoperative/recovery resources, as well as the urgency of the operation [71]. Hospital divisions then assign operations according to the resources available on a given day [71], with shorter cases being prioritized over longer ones of similar urgency [71]. Another framework termed the "medically necessary, time-sensitive procedure" score and endorsed by the American College of Surgeons uses patient-, procedure-, and disease-related factors to triage procedures, with higher scores associated with poorer perioperative outcomes, increased risk for COVID-19 transmission to the healthcare team, and/or increased hospital resource use, and lower scores corresponding to lower risk and higher priority procedures [72]. Furthermore, the implementation of COVID-19-free surgical pathways, which includes complete segregation of the operating theater, critical care areas, and inpatient ward areas, has been associated with significantly decreased rates of 30-day postoperative pulmonary complications (pneumonia, acute respiratory distress syndrome, unexpected ventilation) in individuals undergoing elective cancer surgery [72].

Guidance from the Society of Surgical Oncology, American College of Surgeons, European Society of Medical Oncology, NCCN, among others, is continually updated to offer decision-making support on surgery for specific cancers, and a summary of international recommendations in 23 languages is available for patients [73].

Thromboembolism in Patients with Cancer and COVID-19

Cancer and COVID-19 are established hypercoagulable states, yet the risk for arterial and venous thrombosis and bleeding in patients with cancer infected with COVID-19 is similar to those without cancer [74, 75]. Patients admitted to the hospital with COVID-19 should undergo baseline laboratory testing, including complete blood cell count, activated partial thromboplastin time, international normalized ratio, fibrinogen, and D-dimer, and receive prophylactic dosing of anticoagulation, preferably with low-molecular-weight heparin. For patients with confirmed deep vein thrombosis or pulmonary embolism, therapeutic anticoagulation with low-molecular-weight heparin or unfractionated hepa-

rin is recommended. Full-dose anticoagulation may also be considered in patients with clinical respiratory deterioration and no alternative explanation. Therapeutic anticoagulation should be continued for a minimum of three months, until the patient is fully recovered from COVID-19 and has no remaining risk factors for recurrent venous thromboembolism, including no evidence of malignancy and completion of any planned cancer-directed therapy.

Clinical Trials

Clinical trials are a cornerstone of cancer care, and as with cancer-directed therapies, patients with COVID-19 are encouraged to enroll in studies as feasible and appropriate. Importantly, data regarding the immunogenicity of COVID-19 vaccines in patients with cancer are lacking, and many trials are ongoing to address this question. Other studies are examining the impact of specific COVID-19 therapeutics in patients with cancer, the role of remote monitoring on adverse events and hospitalizations, and supportive care measures to prevent long-term consequences of infection.

Enrollment in oncology clinical trials inevitably decreased during the pandemic. For many patients with cancer, especially those with rare tumor types or actionable genetic alterations, clinical trials afford access to otherwise unavailable therapies that may prolong life with quality. As restrictions lessened, regulatory authorities, including the FDA, recognized that protocol deviations would be unavoidable, and that protocol modifications would be necessary to permit resumption of clinical trial enrollment [76, 77].

COVID-19 and Other Vaccinations

The mainstay of prevention of COVID-19 is vaccination. The currently authorized vaccines in the United States include: (1) the inoculations of spike protein mRNA (Pfizer-BioNTech and Moderna) which inserts the spike protein mRNA sequence into cells; and (2) adenoviral vaccine (Johnson & Johnson/Janssen), a replication-incompetent virus. In the rest of the world, other adenoviral (Astra Zeneca AZD1222, Sputnik V) and inactivated virus vaccines (Sinopharm and

Sinovac) have been approved for use. The mRNA products are the most commonly used in the United States. The spike protein mRNA inoculation triggers cellular production of spike protein outside the lungs, resulting in an immune reaction that is protective against SARS-CoV-2 infection and the typical pulmonary clinical deterioration of infected patients [78]. The degree of protection against infection appears to diminish with time, and a third, or booster, shot has been recommended six to eight months after the initial vaccination [79, 80].

The benefits of receiving one of the FDA-authorized mRNA and adenoviral COVID-19 vaccines (Pfizer-BioNTech, Moderna, and Johnson & Johnson/Janssen) outweigh the known risks in patients with cancer. The NCCN has issued guidelines regarding the timing and selection of patients with cancer for COVID-19 vaccination [81]. In patients with cancer, diminished immune response, along with various chemotherapeutic agents, may limit the protective immunity conferred by COVID vaccines [82], and the use of booster shots is highly recommended.

For patients enrolled in oncology clinical trials, sponsors have specific criteria on timing of vaccination with respect to investigational therapy. In general, the COVID-19 vaccine should be administered as soon as available. In the absence of specific protocol instructions, the COVID-19 and Cancer Clinical Trials Working Group outlined recommendations for patients enrolled in trials based on form of therapy [76]:

- For patients in screening studies, vaccines should be administered once available. One exception is those undergoing breast cancer screening, in which screening examinations should be conducted before the first dose of a COVID-19 vaccine or four to six weeks after the second dose of a COVID-19 vaccine.
- For patients enrolled in phase 1 trials, the start of most anticancer agents (especially first-in-human agents with an unknown adverse effect profile) should be deferred until after all vaccine adverse effects have improved to grade ≤1 and ≥72 hours after vaccination. Vaccination should be avoided on the day of drug infusion and anytime during the dose-limiting toxicity period. For agents associated with a potential risk for cytokine-release syndrome, defer vaccination until after the dose-limiting toxicity window or delay administration of the investigational agent for two weeks after vaccine administration.
- For patients enrolled in phase 2 or 3 trials, timing of vaccination should be guided by the mechanism of action of the investigational drug.
- For patients receiving cytotoxic chemotherapy, vaccines should be administered approximately one to two weeks before or after the dose to increase the potential for the immune system to mount a response. For those undergoing intensive induction regimens for hematologic malignancies, vaccines should be delayed until absolute neutrophil recovery.
- For patients receiving targeted therapy (e.g. TKIs), immunotherapy (e.g. checkpoint inhibitors, anti-CD20 antibodies), hormone therapy, and epigenetic therapy, vaccines should be administered once available.
- For patients undergoing hematopoietic SCT or adoptive cell therapies, vaccines should be administered at least three months after completion of therapy [81].
- For patients undergoing radiation, vaccines should be administered once available, unless significant myelosuppression is anticipated (e.g. total body radiation), in which case vaccines should be administered on immune reconstitution.
- For patients undergoing surgical procedures, vaccines should be administered on full recovery from postoperative complications or at least one week before surgery.

An additional, third dose or booster vaccination is advised in the following patients and should be at least 28 days after completing the Pfizer or Moderna mRNA 2-dose series:

- Received cancer therapy within one year of the initial vaccine administration
- Have a newly diagnosed or recurrent cancer and who will be receiving cancer therapy
- Have active hematologic malignancies regardless of receiving current cancer therapy
- SCT recipients and those who received engineered cellular therapy (e.g. chimeric antigen receptor T cells), prioritizing those who are ≤2 years postprocedure
- Allogeneic SCT recipients who are actively receiving immunosuppressive therapy or with a history of graft-versus-host disease regardless of the time posttransplant

In individuals who have had prior COVID-19-directed monoclonal antibodies or convalescent plasma, the CDC recommends vaccination at least 90 days after receipt of treatment [83].

Another special population is patients with preexisting immune thrombocytopenia (ITP). Cases of de novo ITP have been reported in SARS-CoV-2 vaccine recipients. Among 109 patients with known ITP who received SARS-CoV-2 vaccine, 19 experienced an ITP exacerbation defined as $\geq$50% decline in platelet count, nadir platelet count of <30 000/mm^3 with >20% decrease from baseline, and/or use of rescue therapy. Patients with history of splenectomy and those who received at least five lines of prior therapy were at highest risk for ITP exacerbation [84]. Among de novo cases and exacerbations, most patients responded to ITP-directed treatment [84]. The presence of ITP is not a strict contraindication to SARS-CoV-2 vaccination, but diligent monitoring is warranted.

Thromboembolic events, including thrombosis with thrombocytopenia syndrome (or vaccine-induced immune thrombotic thrombocytopenia), have been reported in predominantly young women receiving an adenoviral vector vaccine (Johnson & Johnson or AstraZeneca). This is thought be mediated through antiplatelet autoantibodies that activate platelets. To date, there have been no associations between thrombosis with thrombocytopenia syndrome and cancer patients, but patients who have a history of heparin-induced thrombocytopenia and/or thrombosis should be counseled to receive another vaccine [81].

Other vaccinations, including seasonal influenza, should be administered and not delayed per standard practice. At least a 72-hour period between vaccinations or until the resolution of any vaccine-associated side effects may be advised to allow for recovery and adequate immune response for subsequent inoculations.

See Cancer Screening and Diagnosis section regarding the timing and interpretation of radiologic imaging around COVID-19 vaccination.

Supportive Care

In accordance with ASCO, American Society of Hematology, NCCN, European Society for Medical Oncology, and others, the following recommendations regarding supportive care medications and procedures may guide the care of patients with cancer.

For patients living far from the cancer center or in communities with high infection rates, telemedicine may be used to remotely monitor and manage intracycle therapy-related adverse events in between required in-person appointments for treatment and may be crucial in reducing the rate of emergency department visits and inpatient hospitalizations. To this end, home health nursing agencies may assist with remote symptom and vital sign checks, laboratory monitoring, and providing supportive care, including intravenous hydration, antibiotics, among others.

The routine use of steroids for preventive and active antiemetic therapy, pain management, central nervous system metastases, infusion-related reactions, cytokine release syndrome, and immune-mediated and therapy-related adverse events should continue per standard of care.

In light of studies suggesting higher mortality in patients with cancer and COVID-19 receiving more myelosuppressive regimens, as well as the negative prognostic impact of neutropenia and leukopenia, many oncologists have liberalized the use of myeloid growth factor support (e.g. short- and long-acting granulocyte colony-stimulating factor [G-CSF]). Indeed, NCCN and European Society for Medical Oncology lowered the threshold for prophylactic use for regimens from >20% to >10% risk for febrile neutropenia [29, 85]. Short-acting G-CSF may be favored over long-acting, pegylated formulations because of reports of acute respiratory distress syndrome associated with neutrophil recovery [86–89], although there is no strict contraindication to use of long-acting G-CSF, especially in the outpatient setting. For patients with febrile neutropenia, testing for COVID-19 should be incorporated into the diagnostic algorithm, and standard institutional guidelines should be followed for management.

With respect to disease- or therapy-related anemia, the use of erythropoietin-stimulating agents may be used per standard of care, with no evidence that this compromises outcomes from COVID-19 infection. Transfusion of red blood cells should follow previously established guidance from the American Society of Hematology, using the minimum number of units needed to ensure symptom relief or hemodynamic stability.

A common question posed by patients with active or prior cancer is the utility of prophylactic medications, including antiviral therapy, steroids, antibacterials, or other antimicrobials or monoclonal antibodies for the prevention of COVID-19. At this time, there is no definitive evidence to support the use of such prophylactic medications for patients or household members, and COVID-19 vaccination and standard precautions, including distancing and wearing face masks, should continue to be encouraged.

For patients with central venous catheters, it is standard to flush ports every four to six weeks. However, the frequency may be extended to up to every 12 weeks without compromising safety [90], and this may be considered in areas with high infection rates.

Use and Impact of Telemedicine on Caring for Patients with Cancer

The routine use of telemedicine has distanced oncologists from established patients but also connected those who could otherwise not travel far for subspecialized consultations and facilitated remote symptom monitoring and clinical trial consideration. This practice will undoubtedly continue beyond the pandemic and is anticipated to improve clinical trial accrual in the future.

Based on a systematic literature review, an ASCO Expert Panel issued standards and practice recommendations on when to implement telehealth oncology visits [91]. In many situations, telemedicine visits may be appropriate in areas with high infection rates or transmission and may lead to patient satisfaction when circumstances otherwise limit interactions between providers and patients to telephone triage [91]. Nevertheless, in-person visits remain the standard approach and according to the ASCO Expert Panel are especially preferred in the following clinical settings: initial consultations; initial delivery of antineoplastic treatment; delivery of key information, including new cancer diagnosis or treatment plan, disease relapse or progression, and no further cancer treatment decisions; complex cancer needs as identified by the healthcare provider; physical examination for diagnosis or follow-up; patients with hearing, vision, or cognition limitations; and patients with

inadequate or limited technologic capacity, or lower levels of health literacy [91].

Survivorship and Surveillance After Cancer Therapy

Cancer survivors are at an intermediate risk for COVID-19-related complications, compared with individuals with no cancer history and patients with active cancer [92–94]. This risk is further shaped by type of malignancy, timing of cancer diagnosis, and presence of comorbidities, including residual adverse effects of cancer-directed therapy. Expectedly, cancer diagnosis within the last one to two years, hematologic (vs. nonhematologic) malignancy, and preexisting cardiopulmonary disease have been associated with increased risk for hospitalization and death among cancer survivors who are infected with COVID-19 [92–94].

Similar to screening examinations, the decision to resume surveillance in-person visits, imaging, and procedures will be guided by infection rates and available resources in a particular community, as well as the risk to the individual patient. The safety and appropriateness of delaying routine surveillance for patients who have completed cancer therapy or who are on active surveillance will depend on the risk for disease recurrence or progression. In areas with high infection rates, remote monitoring with telemedicine visits and home laboratory assessments may be used to triage patients accordingly for further warranted imaging and procedures.

An important facet of surveillance is monitoring for cardiac sequalae of prior cancer therapy because patients with cardiovascular disease are at increased risk for complications and death from COVID-19, independent of a history of malignancy. Accordingly, the International Cardio-Oncology Society and the American College of Cardiology Cardio-Oncology and Imaging Councils have issued expert consensus statements on a more focused imaging surveillance strategy and utility of cardiac biomarkers [95, 96].

Cancer survivors, especially adolescents/young adults and the elderly, have been uniquely affected by the pandemic, particularly those with a more recent cancer diagnosis. Issues related to anxiety, psychological distress posed by the pandemic, and the cancer diagnosis, as well as any underlying cognitive impairment, should be considered in each patient when planning survivorship care [97–100].

Palliative Care and Advance Care Planning

Palliative and best supportive care remain critical in the management of patients with advanced, incurable cancer. Among the most painful and difficult aspects of the pandemic has been the separation of families while patients with cancer are hospitalized. Moreover, having discussions about end of life or change in goals of care with progressive cancer with or without COVID-19 is especially difficult when done remotely rather than in person. Therefore, proactive conversations about prognosis and goals of care, including Physician Orders for Life-Sustaining Treatment, are essential, because patients with progressive malignancy and severe COVID-19 have a guarded prognosis [101–103].

After COVID-19: The Natural History of Cancer in the Postpandemic Era

As the peak of the pandemic has passed worldwide, the immediate impact of COVID-19 on cancer care has included reduced screening procedures with potentially increased mortality expected to manifest in the coming years. In addition to reduced screening procedures, the more immediate and unfortunate impact of the pandemic has been delayed initial cancer diagnoses among symptomatic patients. Amidst the tragedy of the pandemic, the world also witnessed unprecedented interdisciplinary collaborations and efforts within the medical profession within and across institutions.

"Empathy" or "compassion fatigue," a precursor to or subtype of burnout that is marked by hyperarousal (hypervigilance, irritability), avoidance of stressful situations, and reexperiencing difficult events, has been brought to the forefront during the COVID-19 pandemic [104, 105]. Compassion fatigue is relevant in all healthcare professionals, including nurses, therapists, ancillary staff, medical trainees undergoing unprecedented forms of clinical education to seasoned oncologists, all faced with even more heightened daily exposure to suffering and death in addition to personal strife, moral distress, and responding to challenges to evidenced-based medicine [105]. Strategies to mitigate compassion fatigue and burnout are aimed at protecting an individual's psychological, cognitive, social, and spiritual health [104]. These include stress reduction strategies, monitoring by peers and supervisors, and taking regular (even if brief) breaks [104]. Hopefully, the emphasis on mental health within the healthcare community will remain once the pandemic is finally behind us and will lead to implementation of programmatic interventions to continually assess and address oncology team needs and improve emotional well-being [105].

The long-term sequalae of COVID-19 infection are beginning to be realized, and outcomes and challenges unique to patients with cancer remain to be seen. Controversies will remain in the management of patients with cancer in the era of COVID-19 as the natural history of Delta and other variants evolves and data emerge regarding the impact of cancer-directed therapies and other comorbidities. Oncologists and other healthcare providers must adapt accordingly and have informed conversations with patients who are facing cancer to optimize clinical outcomes.

References

1 Fillmore, N.R., La, J., Szalat, R.E. et al. (2021). Prevalence and outcome of COVID-19 infection in cancer patients: a national Veterans Affairs study. *J. Natl. Cancer Inst.* 113 (6): 691–698.

2 Lee, K.A., Ma, W., Sikavi, D.R. et al. (2021). Cancer and risk of COVID-19 through a general community survey. *Oncologist* 26 (1): e182–e185.

3 Wang, Q., Berger, N.A., and Xu, R. (2021). Analyses of risk, racial disparity, and outcomes among US patients with cancer and COVID-19 infection. *JAMA Oncol* 7 (2): 220–227.

4 Desai, A., Sachdeva, S., Parekh, T., and Desai, R. (2020). COVID-19 and cancer: lessons from a pooled meta-analysis. *J. Glob. Oncol.* 6: 557–559.

5 Onder, G., Rezza, G., and Brusaferro, S. (2020). Case-fatality rate and characteristics of patients dying in relation to COVID-19 in Italy. *JAMA* 323 (18): 1775–1776.

6 Richardson, S. et al. (2020). Presenting characteristics, comorbidities, and outcomes among 5700 patients hospitalized with COVID-19 in the New York City area. *JAMA* 323 (20): 2052–2059.

7 Zhang, H. et al. (2021). Clinical characteristics and outcomes of COVID-19-infected cancer patients: a systematic review and meta-analysis. *J. Natl. Cancer Inst.* 113 (4): 371–380.

8 Brar, G. et al. (2020). COVID-19 severity and outcomes in patients with cancer: a matched cohort study. *J. Clin. Oncol.* 38 (33): 3914–3924.

9 Curigliano, G. (2020). Cancer patients and risk of mortality for COVID-19. *Cancer Cell* 38 (2): 161–163.

10 Griffin, D.O. et al. (2021). The importance of understanding the stages of COVID-19 in treatment and trials. *AIDS Rev.* 23 (1): 40–47.

11 Dinnes, J. et al. (2021). Rapid, point-of-care antigen and molecular-based tests for diagnosis of SARS-CoV-2 infection. *Cochrane Database Syst. Rev.* 3: CD013705.

12 Cevik, M. et al. (2021). SARS-CoV-2, SARS-CoV, and MERS-CoV viral load dynamics, duration of viral shedding, and infectiousness: a systematic review and meta-analysis. *Lancet Microbe* 2 (1): e13–e22.

13 Aydillo, T. et al. (2020). Shedding of viable SARS-CoV-2 after immunosuppressive therapy for cancer. *N. Engl. J. Med.* 383 (26): 2586–2588.

14 Widders, A., Broom, A., and Broom, J. (2020). SARS-CoV-2: the viral shedding vs infectivity dilemma. *Infect. Dis. Health* 25 (3): 210–215.

15 Ippolito, E. et al. (2020). COVID-19 and radiation induced pneumonitis: overlapping clinical features of different diseases. *Radiother. Oncol.* 148: 201–202.

16 Katal, S., Aghaghazvini, L., and Gholamrezanezhad, A. (2020). Chest-CT findings of COVID-19 in patients with pre-existing malignancies; a pictorial review. *Clin. Imaging* 67: 121–129.

17 Pritchett, J.C. et al. (2021). Association of a Remote Patient Monitoring (RPM) program with reduced hospitalizations in cancer patients with COVID-19. *J. Oncol. Pract.* 17 (9): e1293–e1302.

18 Gupta, A., Gonzalez-Rojas, Y., Juarez, E. et al. (2021). Early treatment for Covid-19 with SARS-CoV-2 neutralizing antibody Sotrovimab. *N. Engl. J. Med.* 385 (21): 1941–1950.

19 Rivera, D.R. et al. (2020). Utilization of COVID-19 treatments and clinical outcomes among patients with cancer: a COVID-19 and cancer consortium (CCC19) cohort study. *Cancer Discov.* 10 (10): 1514–1527.

20 Piechotta, V. et al. (2021). Convalescent plasma or hyperimmune immunoglobulin for people with COVID-19: a living systematic review. *Cochrane Database Syst. Rev.* 5: CD013600.

21 Li, L. et al. (2020). Effect of convalescent plasma therapy on time to clinical improvement in patients with severe and life-threatening COVID-19: a randomized clinical trial. *JAMA* 324 (5): 460–470.

22 Simonovich, V.A. et al. (2021). A randomized trial of convalescent plasma in Covid-19 severe pneumonia. *N. Engl. J. Med.* 384 (7): 619–629.

23 RECOVERY Collaborative Group (2021). Convalescent plasma in patients admitted to hospital with COVID-19 (RECOVERY): a randomised controlled, open-label, platform trial. *Lancet* 397 (10289): 2049–2059.

24 Thompson, M.A., Henderson, J.P., Shah, P.K. et al. (2021). Association of convalescent plasma therapy with survival in patients with hematologic cancers and COVID-19. *JAMA Oncol.* 7 (8): 1167–1175.

25 Bakowski, M.A. et al. (2021). Drug repurposing screens identify chemical entities for the development of COVID-19 interventions. *Nat. Commun.* 12 (1): 3309.

26 Sheahan, T.P., Sims, A.C., Zhou, S. et al. (2020). An orally bioavailable broad-spectrum antiviral inhibits SARS-CoV-2 in human airway epithelial cell cultures and multiple coronaviruses in mice. *Sci. Transl. Med.* 12 (541): eabb5883.

27 Merck & Co., Inc. (2021). Merck and Ridgeback's Investigational Oral Antiviral Molnupiravir Reduced the Risk of Hospitalization or Death by Approximately 50 Percent Compared to Placebo for Patients with Mild or Moderate COVID-19 in Positive Interim Analysis of Phase 3 Study. https://www.merck.com/news/merck-and-ridgebacks-investigational-oral-antiviral-molnupiravir-reduced-the-risk-of-hospitalization-or-death-by-approximately-50-percent-compared-to-placebo-for-patients-with-mild-or-moderat.

28 Slimano, F. et al. (2020). Cancer, immune suppression and coronavirus disease-19 (COVID-19): need to manage drug safety (French Society for Oncology Pharmacy [SFPO] guidelines). *Cancer Treat. Rev.* 88: 102063.

29 Curigliano, G. et al. (2020). Managing cancer patients during the COVID-19 pandemic: an ESMO multidisciplinary expert consensus. *Ann. Oncol.* 31 (10): 1320–1335.

30 American Society of Clinical Oncology (2021). ASCO special report: a guide to cancer care delivery during the COVID-19 pandemic. https://www.asco.org/sites/new-www.asco.org/files/content-files/2020-ASCO-Guide-Cancer-COVID19.pdf.

31 Xie, Z., Saliba, A.N., Abeykoon, J. et al. (2021). Outcomes of COVID-19 in patients with cancer: a closer look at pre-emptive routine screening strategies. *J. Oncol. Pract.* 17 (9): e1382–e1393.

32 Yekeduz, E., Utkan, G., and Urun, Y. (2020). A systematic review and meta-analysis: the effect of active cancer treatment on severity of COVID-19. *Eur. J. Cancer* 141: 92–104.

33 Liu, H. et al. (2021). The effect of anticancer treatment on cancer patients with COVID-19: a systematic review and meta-analysis. *Cancer Med.* 10 (3): 1043–1056.

34 American Society of Clinical Oncology (2021). Anti-cancer therapy for patients with COVID-19 infection: should cancer therapy be delayed in patients who are infected with COVID-19? https://www.asco.org/covid-resources/patient-care-info/cancer-treatment-supportive-care.

35 McBain, R.K. et al. (2021). Decline and rebound in routine cancer screening rates during the COVID-19 pandemic. *J. Gen. Intern. Med.* 36 (6): 1829–1831.

36 Sprague, B.L. et al. (2021). Changes in mammography use by Women's characteristics during the first 5 months of the COVID-19 pandemic. *J. Natl. Cancer Inst.* 113 (9): 1161–1167.

37 Bakouny, Z. et al. (2021). Cancer screening tests and cancer diagnoses during the COVID-19 pandemic. *JAMA Oncol.* 7 (3): 458–460.

38 Chen, R.C. et al. (2021). Association of cancer screening deficit in the United States with the COVID-19 pandemic. *JAMA Oncol.* 7 (6): 878–884.

39 Velazquez, A.I. et al. (2021). Trends in breast cancer screening in a safety-net hospital during the COVID-19 pandemic. *JAMA Netw. Open* 4 (8): e2119929.

40 Alagoz, O., Lowry, K.P., Kurian, A.W. et al. (2021). Impact of the COVID-19 pandemic on breast cancer mortality in the US: estimates from collaborative simulation modeling. *J. Natl. Cancer Inst.* 113 (11): 1484–1494.

41 Toss, A. et al. (2021). Two-month stop in mammographic screening significantly impacts on breast cancer stage at diagnosis and upfront treatment in the COVID era. *ESMO Open* 6 (2): 100055.

42 Kregting, L.M. et al. (2021). Effects of cancer screening restart strategies after COVID-19 disruption. *Br. J. Cancer* 124 (9): 1516–1523.

43 Castanon, A. et al. (2021). Recovery strategies following COVID-19 disruption to cervical cancer screening and their impact on excess diagnoses. *Br. J. Cancer* 124 (8): 1361–1365.

44 Helsper, C.W., Campbell, C., Emery, J. et al. (2020). Cancer has not gone away: a primary care perspective to support a balanced approach for timely cancer diagnosis during COVID-19. *Eur. J. Cancer Care (Engl.)* 29 (5): e13290.

45 Maida, M. (2020). Screening of gastrointestinal cancers during COVID-19: a new emergency. *Lancet Oncol.* 21 (7): e338.

46 Neal, R.D. et al. (2020). Cancer care during and after the pandemic. *BMJ* 370: m2622.

47 Adin, M.E. et al. (2021). Association of COVID-19 mRNA vaccine with ipsilateral axillary lymph node reactivity on imaging. *JAMA Oncol.* 7 (8): 1241–1242.

48 Robinson, K.A. et al. (2021). Incidence of axillary adenopathy in breast imaging after COVID-19 vaccination. *JAMA Oncol.* 7 (9): 1395–1397.

49 Becker, A.S. et al. (2021). Multidisciplinary recommendations regarding post-vaccine adenopathy and radiologic imaging: radiology scientific expert panel. *Radiology* 300 (2): E323–E327.

50 Lehman, C.D. et al. (2021). Unilateral lymphadenopathy after COVID-19 vaccination: a practical management plan for radiologists across specialties. *J. Am. Coll. Radiol.* 18 (6): 843–852.

51 Society of Breast Imaging (2021). SBI recommendations for the management of axillary adenopathy in patinets with recent COVID-19 vaccination. https://www.sbi-online.org/Portals/0/Position%20Statements/2021/SBI-recommendations-for-managing-axillary-adenopathy-post-COVID-vaccination.pdf.

52 Sharafeldin, N. et al. (2021). Outcomes of COVID-19 in patients with cancer: report from the national COVID cohort collaborative (N3C). *J. Clin. Oncol.* 39 (20): 2232–2246.

53 Tian, J. et al. (2020). Clinical characteristics and risk factors associated with COVID-19 disease severity in patients with cancer in Wuhan, China: a multicentre, retrospective, cohort study. *Lancet Oncol.* 21 (7): 893–903.

54 Robilotti, E.V. et al. (2020). Determinants of COVID-19 disease severity in patients with cancer. *Nat. Med.* 26 (8): 1218–1223.

55 Jee, J. et al. (2020). Chemotherapy and COVID-19 outcomes in patients with cancer. *J. Clin. Oncol.* 38 (30): 3538–3546.

56 Clift, A.K. et al. (2020). Living risk prediction algorithm (QCOVID) for risk of hospital admission and mortality from coronavirus 19 in adults: national derivation and validation cohort study. *BMJ* 371: m3731.

57 Grivas, P. et al. (2021). Association of clinical factors and recent anticancer therapy with COVID-19 severity among patients with cancer: a report from the COVID-19 and cancer consortium. *Ann. Oncol.* 32 (6): 787–800.

58 Mulvey, T.M. and Jacobson, J.O. (2020). COVID-19 and cancer care: ensuring safety while transforming care delivery. *J. Clin. Oncol.* 38 (28): 3248–3251.

59 Lee, L.Y. et al. (2020). COVID-19 mortality in patients with cancer on chemotherapy or other anticancer treatments: a prospective cohort study. *Lancet* 395 (10241): 1919–1926.

60 Luo, J. et al. (2020). Impact of PD-1 blockade on severity of COVID-19 in patients with lung cancers. *Cancer Discov.* 10 (8): 1121–1128.

61 Garassino, M.C. et al. (2020). COVID-19 in patients with thoracic malignancies (TERAVOLT): first results of an international, registry-based, cohort study. *Lancet Oncol.* 21 (7): 914–922.

62 Trojaniello, C., Vitale, M.G., and Ascierto, P.A. (2021). Checkpoint inhibitor therapy for skin cancer may be safe in patients with asymptomatic COVID-19. *Ann. Oncol.* 32 (5): 674–676.

63 Treon, S.P. et al. (2020). The BTK inhibitor ibrutinib may protect against pulmonary injury in COVID-19-infected patients. *Blood* 135 (21): 1912–1915.

64 Chong, E.A. et al. (2020). BTK inhibitors in cancer patients with COVID-19: "The Winner Will be the One Who Controls That Chaos" (Napoleon Bonaparte). *Clin. Cancer Res.* 26 (14): 3514–3516.

65 Roschewski, M., Lionakis, M.S., Sharman, J.P. et al. (2020). Inhibition of Bruton tyrosine kinase in patients with severe COVID-19. *Sci. Immunol.* 5 (48): –eabd0110.

66 American Society for Radiation Oncology (ASTRO) (2021). COVID-19 clinical guidance. https://www.astro.org/Daily-Practice/COVID-19-Recommendations-and-Information/Clinical-Guidance.

67 National Institute for Health and Care Excellence (NICE). (2021). COVID-19 rapid guideline: delivery of systemic anticancer treatments. NICE. www.nice.org.uk/guidance/ng161.

68 Sharma, A. et al. (2021). Clinical characteristics and outcomes of COVID-19 in haematopoietic stem-cell transplantation recipients: an observational cohort study. *Lancet Haematol.* 8 (3): e185–e193.

69 Waghmare, A. et al. (2020). Guidelines for COVID-19 management in hematopoietic cell transplantation and cellular therapy recipients. *Biol. Blood Marrow Transplant.* 26 (11): 1983–1994.

70 COVIDSurg Collaborative (2020). Mortality and pulmonary complications in patients undergoing surgery with perioperative SARS-CoV-2 infection: an international cohort study. *Lancet* 396 (10243): 27–38.

71 Coleman, N.L., Argenziano, M., and Fischkoff, K.N. (2020). Developing an algorithm to guide resumption of operative activity in the COVID-19 pandemic and beyond. *Ann. Surg.* 272 (3): e236–e239.

72 Prachand, V.N. et al. (2020). Medically necessary, time-sensitive procedures: scoring system to ethically and efficiently manage resource scarcity and provider risk during the COVID-19 pandemic. *J. Am. Coll. Surg.* 231 (2): 281–288.

73 Mauri, D. et al. (2020). Summary of international recommendations in 23 languages for patients with cancer during the COVID-19 pandemic. *Lancet Oncol.* 21 (6): 759–760.

74 Moll, M. et al. (2020). VTE in ICU patients with COVID-19. *Chest* 158 (5): 2130–2135.

75 Patell, R. et al. (2020). Incidence of thrombosis and hemorrhage in hospitalized cancer patients with COVID-19. *J. Thromb. Haemost.* 18 (9): 2349–2357.

76 Desai, A. et al. (2021). COVID-19 vaccine guidance for patients with cancer participating in oncology clinical trials. *Nat. Rev. Clin. Oncol.* 18 (5): 313–319.

77 U.S. Department of Health and Human Services, Food and Drug Administration, Center for Drug Evaluation and Research (CDER), Center for Biologics Evaluation and Research (CBER), Center for Devices and Radiological Health (CDRH), Oncology Center of Excellence (OCE) Office of Good Clinical Practice (OGCP). (2021). Conduct of clinical trials of medical products during the COVID-19 public health emergency. Food and Drug Administration (FDA). https://www.fda.gov/media/136238/download.

78 Thomas, S.J. et al. (2021). Safety and efficacy of the BNT162b2 mRNA Covid-19 vaccine through 6 months. *N. Engl. J. Med.* 385 (19): 1761–1773.

79 Goldberg, Y., Mandel, M., Bar-On, Y.M. et al. (2021). Waning immunity after the BNT162b2 vaccine in Israel. *N. Engl. J. Med.* 385 (24): e85.

80 Levin, E.G., Lustig, Y., Cohen, C. et al. (2021). Waning immune humoral response to BNT162b2 Covid-19 vaccine over 6 months. *N. Engl. J. Med.* 385 (24): e84.

81 National Comprehensive Cancer Network. Recommendations of the National Comprehensive Cancer Network® (NCCN®) COVID-19 Vaccination Advisory Committee. COVID-19, version 8.2021. https://bit.ly/2Y4IFO5 (accessed 6 November 202)1.

82 Rajan, S. et al. (2021). COVID-19 vaccination for cancer patients: evidence, priority, and practice. *Vaccine* 39 (36): 5075–5077.

83 Centers for Disease Control and Prevention (2022). Interim clinical considerations for use of COVID-19 vaccines currently authorized in the United States. CDC. https://www.cdc.gov/vaccines/covid-19/clinical-considerations/covid-19-vaccines-us.html.

84 Lee, E.J., Beltrami-Moreira, M., Hanny Al-Samkari, H. et al. (2022). SARS-CoV-2 vaccination and ITP in patients with de novo and preexisting ITP. *Blood* 139 (10): 1564–1574.

85 Griffiths, E.A., Alwan, L.M., Bachiashvili, K. et al. (2020). Considerations for use of hematopoietic growth factors in patients with cancer related to the COVID-19 pandemic. *J. Natl. Compr. Cancer Netw.* https://doi.org/10.6004/jnccn.2020.7610.

86 Ergun, Y. et al. (2021). Is it safe to use long-acting G-CSF for febrile neutropenia prophylaxis in COVID-19 pandemic? *J. Oncol. Pract.* 17 (7): 455–456.

87 Lasagna, A. et al. (2020). How to use prophylactic G-CSF in the time of COVID-19. *J. Oncol. Pract.* 16 (11): 771–772.

88 Nawar, T. et al. (2020). Granulocyte-colony stimulating factor in COVID-19: is it stimulating more than just the bone marrow? *Am. J. Hematol.* 95 (8): E210–E213.

89 Taha, M., Sharma, A., and Soubani, A. (2020). Clinical deterioration during neutropenia recovery after G-CSF therapy in patient with COVID-19. *Respir. Med. Case Rep.* 31: 101231.

90 Diaz, J.A. et al. (2017). Phase II trial on extending the maintenance flushing interval of implanted ports. *J. Oncol. Pract.* 13 (1): e22–e28.

91 Zon, R.T. et al. (2021). Telehealth in oncology: ASCO standards and practice recommendations. *J. Oncol. Pract.* 17 (9): 546–564.

92 Kuderer, N.M. et al. (2020). Clinical impact of COVID-19 on patients with cancer (CCC19): a cohort study. *Lancet* 395 (10241): 1907–1918.

93 Mangone, L., Gioia, F., Mancuso, P. et al. (2021). Cumulative COVID-19 incidence, mortality and prognosis in cancer survivors: a population-based study in Reggio Emilia, northern Italy. *Int. J. Cancer* 149: 820–826.

94 Williamson, E.J. et al. (2020). Factors associated with COVID-19-related death using OpenSAFELY. *Nature* 584 (7821): 430–436.

95 Baldassarre, L.A. et al. (2021). Cardiovascular care of the oncology patient during COVID-19: an expert consensus document from the ACC cardio-oncology and imaging councils. *J. Natl. Cancer Inst.* 113 (5): 513–522.

96 Lenihan, D. et al. (2020). Cardio-oncology care in the era of the coronavirus disease 2019 (COVID-19) pandemic: an international cardio-oncology society (ICOS) statement. *CA Cancer J. Clin.* 70 (6): 480–504.

97 Kosir, U. et al. (2020). The impact of COVID-19 on the cancer care of adolescents and young adults and their well-being: results from an online survey conducted in the early stages of the pandemic. *Cancer* 126 (19): 4414–4422.

98 Nekhlyudov, L. et al. (2020). Addressing the needs of cancer survivors during the COVID-19 pandemic. *J. Cancer Surviv.* 14 (5): 601–606.

99 Jones, J.M. et al. (2021). Readdressing the needs of cancer survivors during COVID-19: a path forward. *J. Natl. Cancer Inst.* 113 (8): 955–961.

100 Leach, C.R. et al. (2021). Cancer survivor worries about treatment disruption and detrimental health outcomes due to the COVID-19 pandemic. *J. Psychosoc. Oncol.* 39 (3): 347–365.

101 Curtis, J.R., Kross, E.K., and Stapleton, R.D. (2020). The importance of addressing advance care planning and decisions about do-not-resuscitate orders during novel coronavirus 2019 (COVID-19). *JAMA* 323 (18): 1771–1772.

102 Ueda, M., Martins, R., Hendrie, P.C. et al. (2020). Managing cancer care during the COVID-19 pandemic: agility and collaboration toward a common goal. *J. Natl. Compr. Cancer Netw.* 18 (4): 366–369.

103 Friedman, D.N. et al. (2021). COVID-19-related ethics consultations at a cancer center in New York City: a content review of ethics consultations during the early stages of the pandemic. *J. Oncol. Pract.* 17 (3): e369–e376.

104 Back, A.L., Deignan, P.F., and Potter, P.A. (2014). Compassion, compassion fatigue, and burnout: key insights for oncology professionals. *Am. Soc. Clin. Oncol. Educ. Book* 34: e454–e459.

105 Hlubocky, F.J. et al. (2021). Impact of the COVID-19 pandemic on oncologist burnout, emotional well-being, and moral distress: considerations for the cancer organization's response for readiness, mitigation, and resilience. *J. Oncol. Pract.* 17 (7): 365–374.

18

COVID-19: Dermatology Perspective

Sabha Mushtaq[1], Fabrizio Fantini[2], and Sebastiano Recalcati[2]

[1] *Department of Dermatology, Venereology and Leprology, Government Medical College and associated hospitals, University of Jammu, Jammu, India*
[2] *Department of Dermatology, ASST Lecco, Alessandro Manzoni Hospital, Lecco, Italy*

Abbreviations

CLL	chilblain-like lesion
PM	protective measure
SARS-CoV-2	severe acute respiratory syndrome coronavirus 2

The main clinical feature of coronavirus disease 2019 (COVID-19) infection is interstitial pneumonia, which may progress to acute respiratory distress syndrome. Reports of skin involvement associated with severe acute respiratory syndrome coronavirus 2 (SARS-CoV-2) infection emerged from different parts of the world as the pandemic progressed, but their exact incidence and pathophysiology still remain largely unknown. The COVID-19 pandemic is also indirectly impacting the care and management of other dermatological diseases. Another issue has been the cutaneous adverse reactions caused by the unprecedented use of personal protective measures (PMs) by healthcare professionals and other frontline workers. This can not only affect the compliance to the PMs but can also be a route for acquiring SARS-CoV-2 infection as a result of the impaired skin barrier. In this chapter, we aim to present the various aspects of the COVID-19 pandemic.

Cutaneous Manifestations of COVID-19

The occurrence of skin lesions as a part of the clinical presentation of COVID-19 has been supported by many case reports, case series, and systematic reviews [1–6]. The cutaneous manifestations may precede the respiratory symptoms, occur simultaneously, or appear late in the course of illness. They may sometimes be the only clinical sign in otherwise asymptomatic SARS-CoV-2 carriers. Timely recognition of these cutaneous signs and symptoms associated with SARS-CoV-2 infection helps in early identification of cases, which is important in slowing down the virus transmission and hence the disease burden and prognosis. Dermatologists therefore should keep a high index of suspicion when their consultation is sought for such skin findings. Skin lesions associated with SARS-CoV-2 infection have been reported to occur with a frequency ranging from 0.2% to 24% in different studies [6, 7]. Various classifications and algorithms have been proposed (Table 18.1) [8–13]. A simplified classification was proposed by one of the authors of this chapter based on a retrospective cohort study of 345

Table 18.1 Proposed classifications/categorization of COVID-19-associated cutaneous manifestations.

Authors	Year (country)	Classification

Marzano et al. [8]	May 2020 (Italy)	Two groups and six patterns:
		a) Inflammatory group:
		  i) Urticarial rash
		  ii) Confluent erythematous–maculopapular–morbilliform rash
		  iii) Papulovesicular exanthem
		b) Vasculopathic and vasculitic group:
		  i) Chilblain-like acral pattern
		  ii) Livedo reticularis–livedo racemosa-like pattern
		  iii) Purpuric "vasculitic" pattern

Gisondi et al. [9]	June 2020 (Italy)	Four patterns:
		  i) Exanthema (varicella-like, papulovesicular, morbilliform rash)
		  ii) Vascular (chilblain-like, purpuric/petechial, livedoid lesions)
		  iii) Urticarial eruption
		  iv) Acropapular eruption

Galván et al. [10]	July 2020 (Spain)	Five patterns:
		  i) Pseudochilblain
		  ii) Other vesicular eruptions
		  iii) Urticarial lesions
		  iv) Maculopapular eruptions
		  v) Livedo or necrosis

Potekaev et al. [11]	July 2020 (Russia)	Six patterns:
		  i) Cutaneous vasculitides
		  ii) Papulosquamous rashes and pityriasis rosea
		  iii) Measles-like rashes
		  iv) Papulovesicular rashes
		  v) Urticarial rash
		  vi) Cutaneous adverse drug reactions

Ortega-Quijano et al. [12]	August 2020 (Spain)	Three groups and six patterns:
		a) Nonblanching rash
		  i) Generalized (rash with petechiae)
		  ii) Acral violaceous (acral ischemia)
		  iii) Reticulated vascular pattern (livedo reticularis)
		b) Blanching rash
		  i) Wheals, dermographism (urticarial rash)
		  ii) No wheals or dermographism (erythematous rash)
		c) Vesicular rash (vesicles or secondary crusts/erosions)

Recalcati et al. [13]	December 2020 (Italy)	Three groups and seven patterns:
		a) Exanthems
		  i) Maculopapular
		  ii) Urticarial
		  iii) Vesicular
		  iv) Erythema multiforme
		b) Vascular lesions
		  i) Vasculitic lesions
		  ii) Chilblain-like lesions
		c) Other cutaneous manifestations
		  i) Alopecia
		  ii) Indirect cutaneous manifestations (reactivation of other skin diseases, aggravation of preexisting skin conditions, cutaneous manifestations after therapies or hospitalization, adverse effects as a result of personal protective measures)

Sources: Marzano et al. [8]; Gisondi et al. [9]; Galván Casas et al. [10]; Potekaev et al. [11]; Ortega-Quijano et al. [12]; Recalcati et al. [13].

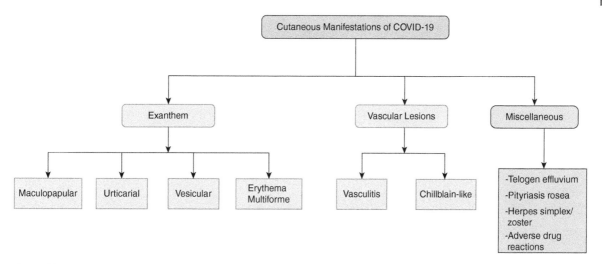

Figure 18.1 A simplified classification of cutaneous manifestations of COVID-19.

patients [13]. Six patterns of cutaneous lesions have been proposed that fall into two broad groups: exanthem group and a group of vascular lesions. A miscellaneous group is also included in the classification (Figure 18.1).

Exanthem Group

The exanthem group comprises cutaneous lesions characteristic of an early viremic phase, similar to eruptions occurring in the course of other common viral infections. Purpura, observed in a few cases, could represent a secondary phenomenon during the natural evolution of the exanthem, perhaps enhanced by the altered coagulated state linked to SARS-CoV-2.

Maculopapular Pattern

Maculopapular rash is one of the most commonly documented cutaneous manifestations in SARS-CoV-2 infection, reported with a frequency of 44–70% [2, 8, 12]. It has been reported in all age groups, although more frequently in middle-aged and older adult patients (mean age, 58.3 years). The eruption can be asymptomatic or associated with pruritus of variable intensity. The rash starts on the trunk and spreads centrifugally (Figure 18.2). The erythematous

maculopapular lesions are confluent, symmetric, and may have a purpuric component. Lesions frequently appear early on and last for a mean of 6.7 days. In our experience, this presentation is associated with a more severe course of COVID-19, often necessitating hospitalization and intensive care. The possibility of adverse drug reaction in these patients cannot be easily ruled out [6, 8].

Urticarial Rash

The frequency of urticarial rash has ranged between 7% and 26% in different cohorts of patients with COVID-19 [1, 2, 6–8]. Urticarial lesions appeared in adults (mean age, 51.8 years), typically presenting at the beginning of a SARS-CoV-2 infection. The hives mostly affected the trunk and lasted a mean of 7.8 days, with itchiness in many places (Figure 18.3). Angioedema has also been reported in a few cases [13, 14]. Urticarial lesions are usually associated with a less severe disease course and good prognosis.

Vesicular Pattern

A vesicular pattern is less commonly reported and may include small monomorphic vesicles, bullous eruption, and chickenpox-like lesions. The eruption mainly affects the trunk and can be localized or disseminated

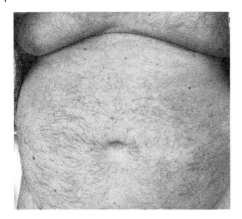

Figure 18.2   Maculopapular rash on the trunk.

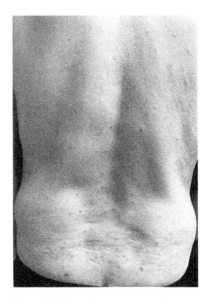

Figure 18.4   Vesicular rash on the trunk.

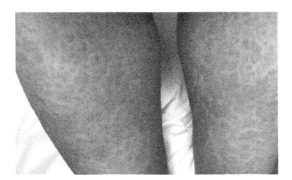

Figure 18.3   Urticarial rash on the lower limbs.

(Figure 18.4) [6, 15]. In our cohort of patients, middle-aged patients were more commonly affected (mean age, 50.6 years). The rash often appeared early in the course of the disease and lasted for a mean duration of 8.8 days. Pruritus was present in up to 50% of our patients. Patients with a vesicular pattern showed variable disease severity and often required hospitalization. It is important to rule out other viral infections.

Erythema Multiforme

In our cohort of patients with COVID-19, erythema multiforme-like lesions were observed in a few patients (mean age, 59.25 years). The lesions consisted of erythematous infiltrated papules with targetoid morphology and central vesiculation in some cases (Figure 18.5). The onset of rash occurred at a mean of six days after the COVID-19 infection and lasted for about 10 days. Pruritus was a significant symptom in many patients. In some instances, erythema multiforme-like lesions can be present simultaneously with chilblain-like

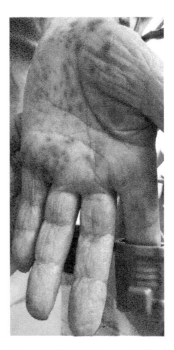

Figure 18.5   Erythema multiforme lesions on the hands.

lesions (CLLs). The disease severity in these patients varied from mild to moderate.

Vascular Lesions

In the group of vascular lesions, likely caused by a delayed vasculopathic mechanism, a distinction was made between vasculitic lesions and CLL subset, because the latter was related to a well-defined setting of young patients, with reproducible lesions and an always good prognosis. Vascular lesions are probably due to an unbalanced coagulation state and might represent a COVID-19-specific complication. SARS-CoV-2 may induce a prothrombotic state, leading in some cases to the formation of microthrombi in the dermal vessels as a result of inflammation, platelet activation, and endothelial dysfunction [13]. It is unknown so far if the cutaneous vascular lesions might signal vessel damage to other organs.

Vasculitic Lesions

In our experience, vasculitic skin signs usually have a delayed onset, appearing on average 16.7 days after the onset of COVID-19 systemic symptoms. In addition to classic cutaneous small vessel vasculitis, we also documented livedo reticularis, thrombosis, and acro-ischemia. Elderly patients (mean age, 68.14 years) were more frequently affected, and this occurrence heralded a poor prognosis, requiring hospitalization and intensive care. Although livedo reticularis was transitory and resolved completely without any specific therapy, thrombosis and acro-ischemia lasted longer, necessitating treatment with low-molecular-weight heparin.

Chilblain-like Lesions

A presentation of CLLs has been labeled with various other names, such as "COVID toes," "acral cutaneous lesions," "pseudochilblain," and "pernio-like lesions." The occurrence of CLLs in association with COVID-19 is still a matter of debate. We have seen about 32 patients with CLLs unrelated to cold exposure or comorbidities, but only 4 of them showed evidence of SARS-CoV-2 infection demonstrated via polymerase chain reaction and serologic testing. Other investigators reported similar percentages of laboratory findings [16]. CLLs typically affect young patients (mean age, 16.3 years), predominantly involving the feet and hands. CLLs appeared late over the disease course and typically affected children and young adults. Typically, erythematous-violaceous macules and papules, which may turn bullous, are associated with swelling of the affected digits (Figure 18.6). The acral eruption may have a purpuric component or a targetoid morphology

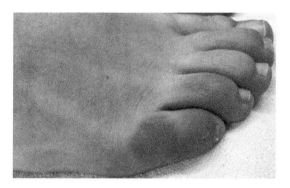

Figure 18.6 Chilblain-like lesions on the right foot.

and is occasionally painful. The occurrence of CLLs portended a good prognosis, with spontaneous resolution within a month in most cases [5, 6]. Relapses were observed [17]. The lesions might result from a delayed immunologic reaction against viral particles, probably mediated by type I interferon [13]. Frequent serologic nonreactivity could be caused by the limitation of available commercial serologic tests. Alternatively, a vigorous innate immune response against the virus, able to control the infection without effectively generating neutralizing antibodies through the adaptive response, may be implicated. As a result, affected patients might not be protected from COVID-19 reinfection.

Miscellaneous Cutaneous Manifestations

Other skin manifestations may be indirectly produced by SARS-CoV-2 infection. Telogen effluvium may occur, after a mean of three months, in patients previously hospitalized for COVID-19 [18]. Occurrence of herpes simplex, herpes zoster, and pityriasis rosea in the course of COVID-19 infection may be explained with the reactivation of latent viruses. Cutaneous adverse reactions to drugs and pressure sores as a result of prolonged pronation can also be observed in affected patients.

Treatment

The majority of the cutaneous manifestations are self-resolving. Symptomatic treatment with antihistamines, topical corticosteroids, and short courses of systemic corticosteroids in some cases has been used. Patients who experience development of thromboses required proper low-molecular-weight heparin therapy, whereas patients with livedo reticularis and CLLs underwent complete resolution without systemic therapy.

Cutaneous Adverse Effects Caused by Use of Personal PMs against SARS-CoV-2

Use of PMs against the SARS-CoV-2 infection may lead to cutaneous adverse effects, either directly related to the use of PMs or through an aggravation of preexisting skin diseases, such as acne, rosacea, atopic dermatitis, and seborrheic dermatitis. The PMs included wearing of masks, gloves, full-body personal protective equipment, and hand hygiene measures, such as use of soap and water and sanitizers. Contact dermatitis, acne, and related disorders such as rosacea and perioral dermatitis, different types of eczema, and urticaria were observed in decreasing order of frequency. Increased washing frequency was the most common culprit. Wearing the personal protective equipment for longer duration increased the severity of symptoms. Most of the patients were managed symptomatically and counseled for adhering to a good skin care routine [19].

Challenges Posed by the COVID-19 Pandemic for Dermatology: Impact on Dermatological Diseases, Dermatology Services, and Dermatology Practice

Corticosteroids and immunosuppressants are central to the treatment of many dermatological diseases and are often lifesaving in some serious dermatoses. In this respect, risk for increased susceptibility to SARS-CoV-2 infection appears to influence treatment decisions. Recommendations and vade mecum have been proposed by various dermatology societies, but the decision should be made on a case-by-case basis, weighing the benefit/risk ratio [20]. Safety of biologic treatment of psoriasis has been evaluated from various centers, and neither an increased susceptibility to SARS-CoV-2 infection nor an increased severity in treated patients when compared with the general population

has so far been reported [21–23]. COVID-19 has had a tremendous impact on the delivery of dermatology services partly because of lockdowns and partly because of diversion of healthcare resources and manpower toward handling of the COVID-19 pandemic. Access to dermatologic services was greatly reduced during the pandemic, particularly for the lower socioeconomic classes. Although accessibility to health care was already a problem for the poor in developing nations, the COVID-19 pandemic brought to fore the nonuniformity and disparity in their healthcare systems. For example, the periodic visits of patients to leprosy clinics were hindered by a variety of factors, such as restrictions on public transport, lack of money, fear of acquiring COVID-19, among others. In addition, leprosy prevention activities came to a halt, such as active case finding in endemic areas, awareness programs, chemoprophylaxis of contacts, and other community-based campaigns. The reduced access to dermatologic facilities can translate into delayed diagnoses and a spur of severe cases in the near future [24]. Dermatology practice has also seen considerable transformation as a result of the COVID-19 pandemic [25, 26]. A web-based global survey conducted in April 2020, including 733 respondents, showed a decrease in the percentage of dermatologists providing in-person consultations, as well as of hospital services and conducting procedures. A significant increase in the use of teledermatology (up to threefold) was noted. WhatsApp was the most common platform used for consultation, and video conferencing was the most common mode opted. Teledermatology proved to be a boon for patients at the peak of the pandemic amidst the total lockdowns, and it holds promise for the future for providing easily accessible dermatology care [25].

Dermatology Registries in Response to COVID-19

In response to the unprecedented challenges posed by the COVID-19 pandemic, dermatology societies across the globe have developed patient registries with the goal of increasing knowledge of the dermatologic manifestations and impact of COVID-19 on dermatologic patients [27–31].

Conclusion

Cutaneous involvement during SARS-CoV-2 infection is well documented, and the spectrum of skin manifestations is heterogeneous. Being aware of these cutaneous manifestations and keeping a high index of suspicion are crucial. The recognition of cutaneous manifestations in asymptomatic patients could be helpful for epidemiologic control, especially in areas where diagnostic tests are scarce. In response to the COVID-19 pandemic, we have seen great collaborations across medical specialties and tremendous cooperation among international healthcare communities and policymakers to tackle the health crises brought by the novel coronavirus SAR-CoV-2.

References

1 Recalcati, S. (2020). Cutaneous manifestations in COVID-19: a first perspective. *J Eur Acad Dermatol Venereol.* 34: e212–e213.

2 De Giorgi, V., Recalcati, S., Jia, Z. et al. (2020). Cutaneous manifestations related to coronavirus disease 2019 (COVID-19): a prospective study from China and Italy. *J Am Acad Dermatol.* 83: 674–675.

3 Recalcati, S., Barbagallo, T., Frasin, L.A. et al. (2020). Acral cutaneous lesions in the time of COVID-19. *J Eur Acad Dermatol Venereol.* https://doi.org/10.1111/jdv.16533.

4 Recalcati, S., Piconi, S., Franzetti, M. et al. (2020). Colchicine treatment of Covid-19 presenting with cutaneous rash and myopericarditis. *Dermatol Ther.* https://doi.org/10.1111/dth.13891.

5 Recalcati, S. and Fantini, F. (2020). Chilblain-like lesions during the COVID-19 pandemic: early or late sign? *Int J Dermatol.* 59: e268–e269. https://doi.org/10.1111/ijd.14975.

6 Singh, H., Kaur, H., Singh, K., and Sen, C.K. (2021). Cutaneous manifestations of COVID-19: a systematic review. *Adv Wound Care* (New Rochelle) 10 (2): 51–80. https://doi.org/10.1089/wound.2020.1309.

7 Askin, O., Altunkalem, R.N., Altinisik, D.D. et al. (2020). Cutaneous manifestations in hospitalized patients diagnosed as COVID-19. *Dermatol Ther.* 33 (6): e13896.

8 Marzano, A.V., Cassano, N., Genovese, G. et al. (2020). Cutaneous manifestations in patients with COVID-19: a preliminary review of an emerging issue. *Br J Dermatol.* 183 (3): 431–442.

9 Gisondi, P., PIaserico, S., Bordin, C. et al. (2020). Cutaneous manifestations of SARS-CoV-2 infection: a clinical update. *J Eur Acad Dermatol Venereol.* 34 (11): 2499–2504.

10 Galván Casas, C., Catala, A.C., Carretero Hernández, G. et al. (2020). Classification of the cutaneous manifestations of COVID-19: a rapid prospective nationwide consensus study in Spain with 375 cases. *Br J Dermatol.* 183 (1): 71–77.

11 Potekaev, N.N., Zhukova, O.V., Protsenko, D.N. et al. (2020). Clinical characteristics of dermatologic manifestations of COVID-19 infection: case series of 15 patients, review of literature, and proposed etiological classification. *Int J Dermatol.* 59 (8): 1000.

12 Ortega-Quijano, D., Jimenez-Cauhe, J., Selda-Enriquez, G. et al. (2020). Algorithm for the classification of COVID-19 rashes. *J Am Acad Dermatol.* 83 (2): e103–e104.

13 Recalcati, S., Gianotti, R., and Fantini, F. (2021). COVID-19: the experience from Italy. *Clin Dermatol.* 39 (1): 12–22. https://doi.org/10.1016/j.clindermatol.2020.12.008.

14 Najafzadeh, M., Shahzad, F., Ghaderi, N. et al. (2020). Urticaria (angioedema) and COVID-19 infection. *J Eur Acad Dermatol Venereol.* 34 (10): e568–e570.

15 Genovese, G., Moltrasio, C., Berti, E., and Marzano, A.V. (2021). Skin manifestations associated with COVID-19: current knowledge and future perspectives. *Dermatology.* 237: 1–12.

16 Baeck, M. and Herman, A. (2021). COVID toes: where do we stand with the current evidence? *Int J Infect Dis.* 102: 53–55. https://doi.org/10.1016/j.ijid.2020.10.021.

17 Recalcati, S., Barbagallo, T., Tonolo, S. et al. (2021). Relapse of chilblain-like lesions during the second wave of COVID-19. *J Eur Acad Dermatol Venereol.* 35: e315–e316. https://doi.org/10.1111/jdv.17168. Online ahead of print.

18 Mieczkowska, K., Deutsch, A., Borok, J. et al. (2021). Telogen effluvium: a sequela of COVID-19. *Int J Dermatol.* 60 (1): 122–124.

19 Mushtaq, S., Terzi, E., Recalcati, S. et al. (2021). Cutaneous adverse effects due to personal protective measures during COVID-19 pandemic: a study of 101 patients. *Int. J. Dermatol.* 60: 327–331. https://doi.org/10.1111/ijd.15354.

20 Niaki, O.Z., Anadkat, M.J., Chen, S.T. et al. (2020). Navigating immunosuppression in a pandemic: a guide for the dermatologist from the COVID task force of the medical dermatology society and Society of Dermatology Hospitalists. *J Am Acad Dermatol.* 83 (4): 1150–1159.

21 Carugno, A., Gambini, D.M., Raponi, F. et al. (2020). COVID-19 and biologics for psoriasis: a high-epidemic area experience – Bergamo, Lombardy, Italy. *J Am Acad Dermatol.* 83 (1): 292–294.

22 Camela, E., Fabbrocini, G., Cinelli, E. et al. (2021). Biologic therapies, psoriasis, and COVID-19: our experience at the psoriasis unit of the University of Naples Federico II. *Dermatology* 237: 13–14.

23 Piaserico, S., Gisondi, P., Cazzaniga, S., and Naldi, L. (2020). Lack of evidence for an increased risk of severe COVID-19 in psoriasis patients on biologics: a cohort study from Northeast Italy. *Am J Clin Dermatol.* 21 (5): 749–751.

24 Mahato, S., Bhattarai, S., and Singh, R. (2020). Inequities towards leprosy-affected people: a challenge during COVID-19 pandemic. *PLoS Negl Trop Dis.* 14 (7): e0008537.

25 Bhargava, S., McKeever, C., and Kroumpouzos, G. (2021). Impact of COVID-19 pandemic on dermatology practices: results of a web-based, global survey. *Int J Women's Dermatol.* 7: 217–213.

26 Litchman, G.H., Marson, J.W., and Rigel, D.S. (2021). The continuing impact of COVID-19 on dermatology practice: office workflow, economics, and future implications. *J. Am Acad Dermatol.* 84 (2): 576–579.

27 Freeman, E.E., McMahon, D.E., Lipoff, J.B. et al. (2020). The spectrum of COVID-19-associated dermatologic manifestations: an international registry of 716 patients from 31 countries. *J Am Acad Dermatol.* 83 (4): 1118–1129.

28 Guelimi, R., Salle, R., and Dousset, L. (2020). Manifestations cutanées au cours l'épidémie de COVID-19: étude COVID-Skin de la Société française de dermatologie. *Ann Dermatol Venereol.* 147 (12): A135.

29 Mahil, S.K., Yiu, Z.Z.N., Mason, K.J. et al. (2020). Global reporting of cases of COVID-19 in psoriasis and atopic dermatitis: an opportunity to inform care during a pandemic. *Br J Dermatol.* 183 (2): 404–406.

30 Naik, H.B., Alhusayen, R., Frew, J. et al. (2020). Global hidradenitis Suppurativa COVID-19 registry: a registry to inform data-driven management practices. *Br J Dermatol.* 183 (4): 780–781. https://doi.org/10.1111/bjd.19345.

31 Balogh, E.A., Heron, C., Feldman, S.R., and Huang, W.W. (2020). SECURE-psoriasis: a de-identified registry of psoriasis patients diagnosed with COVID-19. *J Dermatol Treat.* 31 (4): 327. https://doi.org/10.1080/09546634.2020.1753996.

19

COVID-19: Ophthalmology Perspective

Hashem Al-Marzouki[1], Benjamin P. Hammond[2], Wendy W. Huang[3], and Angela N. Buffenn[4]

[1] Department of Ophthalmology, College of Medicine, King Saud bin Abdulaziz University for Health Sciences, King Abdulaziz Medical Center, Jeddah, Saudi Arabia
[2] Flaum Eye Institute, University of Rochester Medical Center, Rochester, NY, USA
[3] Phoenix Children's Hospital, Ophthalmology, Phoenix, AZ, USA
[4] The Vision Center, Children's Hospital Los Angeles, Roski Eye Institute, Keck School of Medicine, University of Southern California, Los Angeles, CA, USA

Abbreviations

CRAO	central retinal artery occlusion
CRVO	central retinal vein occlusion
IV	intravenous
MIS	multisystem inflammatory syndrome
MIS-C	multisystem inflammatory syndrome in children
RVO	retinal vein occlusion
SARS-CoV-2	severe acute respiratory syndrome coronavirus 2

The viruses within the *Coronaviridae* family are a heterogeneous group known to infect humans and other animals [1, 2]. Although the most typical infections manifest with respiratory tract and gastrointestinal symptoms, they can cause a spectrum of other clinical findings [3]. The most common ocular manifestation in patients with coronavirus disease 2019 (COVID-19) is conjunctivitis, and the prevalence of all ocular manifestations is variable, ranging from 3% to 23% [4]. The novel severe acute respiratory syndrome coronavirus 2 (SARS-CoV-2) has been detected in human tears and a host of ocular structures, including the aqueous humor, vitreous, and retina [5–8]. Orbital and periorbital involvement are rare. However, there have been reports of COVID-19 orbital cellulitis and inflammation, such as dacryoadenitis and myositis. In addition, eyelid dermatitis and emphysema have been described. Although a full clinical picture is still emerging, intraocular effects from SARS-CoV-2 to date have been relatively uncommon. We describe ophthalmologic clinical perspectives for clinicians to consider in patients with COVID-19.

Conjunctiva and Sclera

Conjunctivitis

Clinical Findings and Evaluation

One of the most commonly reported ocular symptoms related to COVID-19 is a follicular conjunctivitis, which is typical in viral conjunctivitis. This form of conjunctivitis is characterized by hyperemia, copious tearing, redness or injection, swelling, and, rarely, pseudomembranes [9]. It can be bilateral or unilateral and may be more prevalent in the pediatric population but with a milder course [10]. In the setting of COVID-19, conjunctivitis can be accompanied by corneal involvement presenting with corneal staining with fluorescein in a pattern similar to herpes simplex virus keratitis [11]. In most cases, conjunctivitis was accompanied with systemic symptoms, including cough, fever, fatigue, diarrhea, and myalgia. However, conjunctivitis as the only sign and symptom of COVID-19 has occurred [12].

Management and Prognosis

Detection of SARS-CoV-2 with real-time reverse transcriptase-polymerase chain reaction in conjunctival samples is relatively low yield with low sensitivity [13]. However, conjunctival swabs while the patient is symptomatic, in addition to nasopharyngeal swabs, are still encouraged [14]. Although no formal treatment protocol has been established and in most cases treatment is supportive, there have been reports of treatment with topical ganciclovir (Zirgan), oral valacyclovir or acyclovir, fluoroquinolones, and artificial tears [15]. The benefit of topical steroids is yet to be established and is best started by an ophthalmologist. Patients with isolated conjunctivitis maintained normal vision after infection and returned to their previous baseline. To date, there have been no reports of long-term vision loss from keratoconjunctivitis in patients with COVID-19.

Episcleritis

Clinical Findings and Evaluation

Episcleritis associated with COVID-19 has been characterized by sectoral epibulbar hyperemia free of staining with fluorescein. Symptoms include foreign body sensation, light sensitivity, redness, and epiphora. Ocular symptoms were accompanied by cough, fever, headache, anosmia, and shortness of breath. Ophthalmic findings may precede systemic symptoms [16, 17].

Management and Prognosis

Episcleritis is differentiated from conjunctivitis and scleritis by slit-lamp examination. Treatment involves topical steroids. Symptoms resolved after treatment in each case. Episcleritis has a known association with other conditions involving vasculitis. Given what we know now about the effect of COVID-19 on the vascular system, it is posited that this finding may be an indicator of underlying systemic vasculitis. It is unknown whether episcleritis is a prognostic indicator in patients with COVID-19 [16, 17].

Anterior Segment

Uveitis

Uveitis has been reported mainly in children and adults with postinfectious multisystem inflammatory syndrome (MIS) after COVID-19 infection [18–21]. MIS (MIS-C in children and MIS-A in adults) is an inflammatory condition that can affect multiple body parts, including the eye, and has been shown to occur after COVID-19 infection (Figure 19.1) [18–21]. MIS-C has been shown to share multiple clinical features in

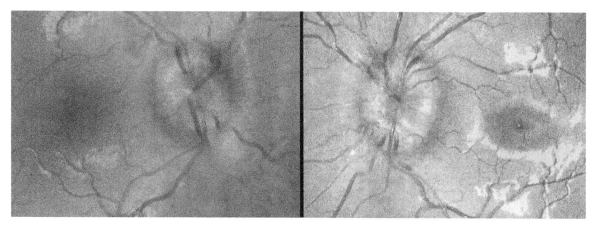

Figure 19.1 Bilateral optic disc edema in a child with fever of unknown origin and presumed MIS-C. The child had positive COVID-19 antibodies after COVID-19 infection. Vision was initially 20/20 but decreased after the onset of anterior uveitis in one eye. Given that the optic nerve edema was bilateral, there was no afferent pupillary defect. Later, the child was diagnosed with tubulointerstitial nephritis secondary to dehydration and nonsteroidal anti-inflammatory drugs in the setting of tubular injury from COVID-19. The optic disc edema resolved after treatment, and vision improved to 20/40 bilaterally.

common with Kawasaki disease [22], and the identification of uveitis in MIS-C further supports a clinical link between these two conditions.

Clinical Findings and Evaluation

Clinical symptoms and signs of uveitis include photophobia, eye pain, blurred vision, conjunctival injection, and occasionally floaters. Pediatric patients are more likely to be asymptomatic than adults. Diagnosis is confirmed by identifying evidence of intraocular inflammation by slit-lamp examination, including inflammatory cells in the anterior or posterior chamber, keratic precipitates, and iris adhesions to the cornea or lens. Uveitis can cause intraocular hypertension and glaucoma. One report noted a case of glaucoma that was not responsive to medical management and required surgical intervention [21].

Causes of uveitis are multitudinal, including a variety of autoimmune, infectious, and idiopathic causative factors. Appropriate workup is determined by the clinical presentation but is generally broad when clinically indicated. Some infectious causes are diagnosed with polymerase chain reaction testing of aqueous or vitreous samples, but the utility of this in suspected COVID-19-related uveitis has not been established.

Management and Prognosis

Uveitis is typically treated by an ophthalmologist with topical steroid and cycloplegic medication. Rheumatology is often involved in cases involving systemic inflammatory conditions. Vision-threatening complications can occur in severe cases that are challenging to control or in chronic cases that are inadequately treated. These complications can include cataract, glaucoma, and phthisis bulbi. In challenging or recalcitrant cases, systemic immunosuppression can be used. Many cases related to a postinfectious or infectious cause respond well to topical treatment, and vision is often preserved with prompt treatment.

Corneal Graft Rejection

Multiple reports have detailed corneal transplant rejection after COVID-19 infection and immunization [23–27]. Corneal graft rejection is an uncommon phenomenon, in part because the eye is a site of immune privilege. Although meta-analysis has shown that graft rejection after vaccination is uncommon after any solid organ transplantation [28], there have been concerns in the past about vaccinations triggering corneal graft rejection [29–31]. The etiology by which a vaccination or nonocular infection would trigger graft rejection is not clearly understood.

Clinical Findings and Evaluation

Patients with corneal graft failure can present with decreased vision, eye redness, eye pain, and photophobia. Diagnosis is made on slit-lamp examination with findings that include corneal edema, Descemet folds, keratic precipitates, anterior chamber cells, corneal neovascularization, and infiltrates or inflammation seen at various levels of the cornea. Corneal graft failure after transplant for an infectious keratitis, such as herpes simplex virus, may represent reactivation of the infection, and workup, if appropriate, is based on the suspected organism.

Management and Prognosis

Steroids are the mainstay in managing acute corneal graft rejection. This can be delivered topically, through periocular injection, or orally. Cycloplegics can be added if photophobia is severe. If caught early, most graft rejections are halted with relative preservation of vision. Complete graft failure can occur, necessitating repeat corneal graft.

Neuro-ophthalmic Complications

Clinical Findings and Evaluation

Several neuro-ophthalmic manifestations of COVID-19 infection have been reported since the start of the pandemic. Examples include cranial nerve palsy, pseudotumor cerebri or intracranial hypertension, encephalopathy, occipital stroke, Miller Fisher syndrome, myasthenia gravis, and Adie tonic pupil [32–34]. Cranial nerve palsies were most commonly reported and presented as new-onset esotropia secondary to sixth nerve palsy and exotropia with ptosis from third nerve palsy [32]. Systemic symptoms were typically severe; however, there was one reported third nerve palsy in an asymptomatic child [33]. It is believed these may be a result of viral neurotropism, triggered autoimmunity, and vasculitis with coagulopathy.

Management and Prognosis

Workup and testing varied based on presentation. Serologic studies, lumbar puncture, magnetic resonance imaging, strabismus evaluation, visual field test, and optical coherence tomography were the main testing modalities implemented [32–34]. Treatments varied and included intravenous (IV) immunoglobulin in the cases of myasthenia gravis and Miller Fisher syndrome, IV steroids, and observation in cases of isolated cranial nerve palsies [32–34]. In observed cranial nerve palsy cases, recovery ranged from complete resolution of secondary strabismus to persistent diplopia and rectus muscle atrophy [33].

Optic Nerve

Active COVID-19 Infection

Clinical Findings and Evaluation

Optic neuritis is a reported manifestation of active COVID-19 infection. This is characterized by unilateral or bilateral acute vision loss, pain, and an afferent pupillary defect. On ophthalmic examination, an edematous elevated optic nerve head (Figure 19.2) can sometimes be seen, but not always. Patients with retrobulbar optic neuritis present with a normal-appearing optic nerve on fundus examination. Optic neuritis with COVID-19 has been reported in both adult and pediatric populations [35–37]. One patient reported findings consistent with acute disseminated encephalomyelitis and anti-myelin oligodendrocyte glycoprotein antibody–associated disease [38].

Optic neuritis is known to be an immune-mediated demyelination process. The association with viral illnesses is well known. The ability of SARS-CoV-2 to induce a complex multisystem immune response is now becoming more established and supports the concept that infection may lead to triggering optic neuritis.

Management and Prognosis

Initial workup for optic neuritis included magnetic resonance imaging, lumbar puncture, and tests for anti-myelin oligodendrocyte glycoprotein antibody, aquaporin-4 antibodies, neuromyelitis optica antibodies (IgG), and pertinent inflammatory markers based on systemic findings. Patients were treated with standard pulse dose IV methylprednisolone and oral prednisolone taper [35–38].

Patients regained vision after treatment [35–37]. The long-term prognosis is unknown. Optic neuritis can have a relapsing and remitting disease course. Whether that is the case with COVID-19-related optic neuritis is not known. It is now known that the timing

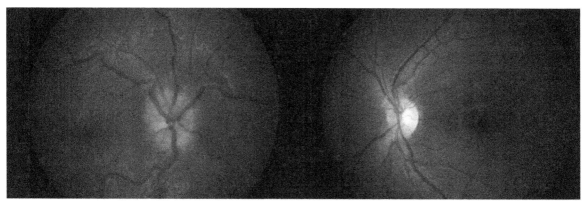

Right Eye   Left Eye

Figure 19.2 Example of optic nerve edema (right eye) caused by optic neuritis. Vision was hand motion in the affected eye at the time of diagnosis, and the examination showed an afferent pupillary defect in the right eye. After treatment with IV and oral steroids, the vision began to slowly improve. At the time of this publication, vision remained low but had improved to 6/200.

of steroid treatment can play a role in the systemic disease course of COVID-19 infections. However, it is uncertain whether treatment for optic neuritis with IV steroids should be modified depending on the phase of the disease.

Optic Nerve and Retinal Changes After COVID-19 Infection

A recent study has indicated that the optic nerve may be affected in patients with COVID-19 even without reported visual symptoms [39]. The study compared optical coherence tomography findings of the optic nerve and macula between COVID-19-recovered individuals and matched control subjects and found that there are significant increases in thickness in certain cell layers of the retina and optic nerve head [39]. These findings suggest that the optic nerve is affected in asymptomatic cases with secondary retina changes. These layers were also significantly thicker in patients with neurologic symptoms [39]. What this means regarding long-term prognosis is not known.

Retina

Retinal Microangiopathy

Retinal microangiopathy is damage to small precapillary vessels and is demonstrated by small hemorrhages within the retina and cotton wool spots (swelling of the retina caused by ischemia). Multiple authors have reported cases series that document retinal microangiopathy seen in association with SARS-CoV-2 infection [40–43]. This is not surprising given other reports have detailed thrombotic complications, including thrombotic microangiopathy, in a variety of organ systems [44–46].

Clinical Findings and Evaluation

Fundoscopic examination is needed to identify hemorrhages and cotton wool spots, which are typically asymptomatic and common in other conditions, such as diabetes and hypertension. A dilated fundoscopic examination will be most sensitive in identifying these changes.

Management and Prognosis

No treatment is needed, and vision is typically preserved. It is possible that retinal microangiopathy may be a marker for microvascular disease within other organ systems, although an association has not been established [43]. In the absence of other risk factors for microangiopathy, such as diabetes or hypertension, the condition is not expected to progress.

Central Retinal Vein Occlusion

Retinal vein occlusions (RVOs) occur because of thrombosis of large retinal veins, most commonly in patients who are hypertensive. A hypercoagulable state can also lead to vein occlusions and is the suspected cause of the multiple reports of central retinal vein occlusion (CRVO) in association with SARS-CoV-2 infection [47–50]. Most of the patients in these reports required hospital admission because of the severity of COVID-19 symptoms, and a majority had SARS-CoV-2 pneumonia. Concurrent deep vein thrombosis was also identified [49].

RVO has been reported after COVID vaccination and is likely associated with vaccine-induced immune thrombotic thrombocytopenia [51, 52]. Vaccine-induced immune thrombotic thrombocytopenia is caused by anti-platelet factor 4 antibodies activating platelets through their FcγRIIa receptors [52]. As a result, it would be reasonable to screen for anti-platelet factor 4 antibodies in a patient with RVO after COVID-19 vaccination.

Clinical Findings and Evaluation

RVO can produce blurred vision or be asymptomatic depending on the degree of occlusion. In the reported cases, all patients showed mild-to-severe decreased visual acuity (20/40 to 20/200). Fundoscopic examination may demonstrate venular dilation with or without tortuosity, retinal hemorrhages, optic disc edema, macular edema, and areas of retinal whitening. A fluorescein angiogram may be helpful in confirming the diagnosis and severity of the occlusion.

Workup should include assessment of blood pressure and laboratory evaluation. The laboratory workup should be done to assess for a hypercoagulable state, systemic inflammatory markers, complete blood cell count, renal function, blood sugars, and lipids.

Management and Prognosis

Two of the case reports were treated with systemic steroids. Steroids were given in the first case to treat suspected optic neuritis before a diagnosis of CRVO was made, and the second case received methylprednisolone to treat vasculitis. Improvement in symptoms and blood markers for inflammation and coagulopathy were noted in both cases [47, 50]. The role of systemic steroids in RVO treatment in the setting of COVID-19 infection is unclear but may be beneficial when vasculitis is suspected. Intravitreal injection of anti-vascular endothelial growth factor medications may be appropriate in some clinical settings. Systemic anticoagulation should be considered given the underlying hypercoagulable state, and clinicians should be vigilant in looking for signs of thrombosis affecting other organ systems.

Many cases of RVO will show improvement in vision following treatment, although vision loss can be severe. These patients need to be managed for chronic complications resulting from retinal ischemia, including neovascular glaucoma and chronic macular edema.

Central Retinal Artery Occlusion

Central retinal artery occlusions (CRAOs) occur as a result of either thrombosis or embolus occluding a major ophthalmic artery, and they may have arteritic and nonarteritic causes. CRAO is treated as a stroke equivalent and is an ophthalmic emergency. CRAO in association with SARS-CoV-2 infection has been reported [53–55]. All reported patients had been severely ill with pneumonia, and concurrent deep venous thrombosis was reported in one case [53]. Vision loss, as is typical with CRAO, was profound. Workup did not identify an embolic source, and hypercoagulopathy leading to retinal artery thrombosis was the suspected cause.

Clinical Findings and Evaluation

Patients will typically describe painless and acute loss of vision, although a critically ill patient may be less likely to recognize the timing or severity of vision changes. Retinal examination may show attenuation of the retinal arteries, diffuse retinal whitening as a result of ischemia, and a cherry-red spot at the fovea.

A thrombus or embolus in the artery may be visible, and a fluorescein angiogram may be used to confirm the diagnosis.

Workup should include neuroimaging to evaluate for other signs of acute cerebrovascular injury. Evaluation of the carotid arteries for clinically significant stenosis and the heart for thrombus or vegetation is important to rule out an embolic source. Telemetry should be considered to evaluate for atrial fibrillation. Additional workup should include laboratory tests to evaluate for arteritis risk (including giant cell arteritis), coagulopathy, other inflammatory markers, complete blood cell count, and other risk factors for chronic vascular disease. The majority of cases of CRAO and CRVO in the setting of SARS-CoV-2 showed hypercoagulability, and the risk for other systemic thrombotic events should be carefully considered and evaluated when appropriate.

Management and Prognosis

CRAO typically carries a poor visual prognosis. Proposed treatments have included thrombolytics, intraocular pressure lowering with medication or anterior chamber paracentesis, and ocular massage. These interventions have failed to show a conclusive benefit. Careful attention should be paid to the risk for extraocular events. Appropriate interventions should be taken to limit the risk for another cerebrovascular accident, especially if an embolic source is likely. If thrombosis is suspected, interventions to limit the risk for other thrombotic events should be considered. The optimal regimen to limit and treat thrombotic events related to SARS-CoV-2 is still being determined.

Orbit

Orbital Cellulitis

Orbital cellulitis and sinusitis have been reported in patients with COVID-19 in the absence of any history of chronic sinusitis. It has been proposed that upper respiratory tract infection, secondary to COVID-19, affects the process of mucociliary clearance in the sinuses, leading to bacterial sinusitis and secondary orbital cellulitis [4].

Clinical Findings and Evaluation

Clinically, patients with COVID-19 can present with eyelid swelling, redness, pain, and discomfort in addition to upper respiratory tract infection. Ocular signs are similar to typical orbital cellulitis and include chemosis, conjunctivitis, limited motility, afferent pupillary defect, and proptosis. The radiologic findings include opacification of the sinuses, consistent with sinusitis. The radiologic features of some patients with COVID-19 can mimic invasive fungal-related sinusitis, such as periantral fat infiltration, despite negative fungal cultures. This can occur in patients who are immunocompetent and have no previous history of chronic sinusitis. Complications reported in orbital cellulitis in the setting of COVID-19 include subperiosteal fluid collection, cavernous sinus thrombosis, and intracranial extension [4].

Management and Prognosis

Broad-spectrum antibiotics are suggested to cover gram-positive and anaerobic bacteria, with a good prognosis. In addition, surgical drainage of the infected sinus and orbital abscess may be required [4].

Orbital Inflammation

Orbital inflammation, specifically myositis and dacryoadenitis, has been reported in patients with COVID-19, with no infectious or autoimmune cause identified [56].

Clinical Findings and Evaluation

Clinically, patients with COVID-19 can present with eyelid swelling, pain, and discomfort in the absence of significant COVID-related symptoms. Ocular signs include redness, eyelid swelling, proptosis, and limited motility. Radiologic findings reveal muscle enlargement with tendon involvement and/or lacrimal gland swelling, in addition to proptosis and intraorbital fat stranding [56].

Management and Prognosis

It is unclear whether the orbital inflammation that occurs in patients with COVID-19 is secondary to COVID-19 infection or represents an autoimmune response to the virus. However, other underlying infectious or autoimmune diseases must be ruled out. The response of myositis and dacryoadenitis to steroids, with or without azithromycin, is complete recovery [57]. In the setting of orbital inflammation, azithromycin is not used routinely but may reduce the viral load in patients with COVID-19 [56, 57]. When the clinical diagnosis is uncertain, broad-spectrum antibiotic coverage should be considered [56, 58].

Rhino-orbital Mucormycosis

Orbital mucormycosis has been reported among patients with COVID-19, especially those with type 2 diabetes, which has been identified as an independent risk factor for both COVID-19 and mucormycosis. It is postulated that COVID-19 increases the risk for mucormycosis for the following reasons [59]:

1) COVID-19 can lead to endothelialitis, thrombosis, and reduced CD4 and CD8 T cell levels, which predispose the patient to mucormycosis.
2) If a steroid is required in the presence of diabetes, it can cause hyperglycemia and phagocytosis impairment, thereby increasing vulnerability to mucormycosis.
3) COVID-19 increases cytokine (IL-6) levels and intracellular free iron, while also predisposing the patient to fungal infection.

Clinical Findings and Evaluation

Clinically, patients with COVID-19 present with eyelid swelling, redness, chemosis, and limited motility. In addition, the involvement of the optic nerve and secondary cavernous sinus thrombosis can lead to reduced vision and ophthalmoplegia, respectively. Mucormycosis should be highly suspected in any patient with underlying uncontrolled diabetes or who is immunocompromised, especially in the presence of black nasal crusts. A nasal, orbital, or sinus biopsy of the necrotic tissue is often required to confirm the diagnosis. The radiologic findings include sinusitis and orbital infiltration. In addition, imaging may show cavernous sinus and thrombotic involvement of the internal carotid artery, as well as a defective nasal septum and osteonecrosis of the orbital bone in invasive fungal disease [59, 60].

Management and Prognosis

Patients usually require hospital admission for systemic antifungal treatment, surgical drainage, debridement, and control of underlying comorbidity and diabetes [59, 60]. The prognosis is usually poor despite aggressive treatment.

Orbital Emphysema

Cutaneous emphysema with orbital involvement has been reported in patients with COVID-19 who are seriously ill and require intubation and ventilation. Clinically, they present with facial and eyelid involvement, as well as subconjunctival emphysema. Usually the patient will have normal visual and optic nerve function, with no sign of compartment syndrome or vascular occlusion. Cutaneous and orbital emphysema is believed to occur as a secondary condition to positive end-expiratory pressure and prone positioning of the patient. The condition resolves spontaneously once the underlying cause is controlled [61, 62].

Conclusions

Coronaviruses that infect humans can affect all layers of the eye, orbit, and periorbital space. Intraocular effects from SARS-CoV-2 have been uncommon. Likewise, orbital and periorbital involvement are rare. Infrequently, ophthalmic findings may precede systemic symptoms. The full clinical picture continues to emerge regarding the impact COVID-19 has on vision, the eye, and surrounding ocular structures. It is important for physicians and other healthcare providers to be aware of the impact COVID-19 can have on the eye and vision so that ophthalmologists can be appropriately consulted. Management of patients infected with COVID-19 often requires a team approach.

References

1 Hartenian, E., Nandakumar, D., Lari, A. et al. (2020). The molecular virology of coronaviruses. *J. Biol. Chem.* 295 (37): 12910–12934. https://doi.org/10.1074/jbc.REV120.013930.

2 Seah, I. and Agrawal, R. (2020). Can the coronavirus disease 2019 (COVID-19) affect the eyes? A review of coronaviruses and ocular implications in humans and animals. *Ocul. Immunol. Inflamm.* 28 (3): 391–395. https://doi.org/10.1080/09273948.2020.1738501.

3 Wiersinga, W.J., Rhodes, A., Cheng, A.C. et al. (2020). Pathophysiology, transmission, diagnosis, and treatment of coronavirus disease 2019 (COVID-19): a review. *JAMA* 324 (8): 782–793. https://doi.org/10.1001/jama.2020.12839.

4 Turbin, R.E., Wawrzusin, P.J., Sakla, N.M. et al. (2020). Orbital cellulitis, sinusitis and intracranial abnormalities in two adolescents with COVID-19. *Orbit* 39 (4): 305–310. https://doi.org/10.1080/01676830.2020.1768560.

5 Yan, Y., Diao, B., Liu, Y. et al. (2020). Severe acute respiratory syndrome coronavirus 2 Nucleocapsid protein in the ocular tissues of a patient previously infected with coronavirus disease 2019. *JAMA Ophthalmol.* 138 (11): 1201–1204. https://doi.org/10.1001/jamaophthalmol.2020.3962.

6 Sawant, O.B., Singh, S., Wright, R.E. 3rd et al. (2021). Prevalence of SARS-CoV-2 in human post-mortem ocular tissues. *Ocul. Surf.* 19: 322–329. https://doi.org/10.1016/j.jtos.2020.11.002.

7 Koo, E.H., Eghrari, A.O., Dzhaber, D. et al. (2021). Presence of SARS-CoV-2 viral RNA in aqueous humor of asymptomatic individuals. *Am J. Ophthalmol.* 230: 151–155. https://doi.org/10.1016/j.ajo.2021.05.008.

8 Casagrande, M., Fitzek, A., Püschel, K. et al. (2020). Detection of SARS-CoV-2 in human retinal biopsies of deceased COVID-19 patients. *Ocul. Immunol. Inflamm.* 28 (5): 721–725. https://doi.org/10.1080/09273948.2020.1770301.

9 Navel, V., Chiambaretta, F., and Dutheil, F. (2020). Haemorrhagic conjunctivitis with pseudomembranous related to SARS-CoV-2. *Am. J. Ophthalmol. Case Rep.* 19: 100735. https://doi.org/10.1016/j.ajoc.2020.100735.

10 Valente, P., Iarossi, G., Federici, M. et al. (2020). Ocular manifestations and viral shedding in tears of pediatric patients with coronavirus disease 2019: a preliminary report. *J. AAPOS* 24 (4): 212–215.

11 Cheema, M., Aghazadeh, H., Nazarali, S. et al. (2020). Keratoconjunctivitis as the initial medical

presentation of the novel coronavirus disease 2019 (COVID-19). *Can. J. Ophthalmol.* 55 (4): e125–e129. https://doi.org/10.1016/j.jcjo.2020.03.003.

12 Scalinci, S.Z. and Trovato, B.E. (2020). Conjunctivitis can be the only presenting sign and symptom of COVID-19. *IDCases* 20: e00774. https://doi.org/10.1016/j.idcr.2020.e00774.

13 Rokohl, A.C., Grajewski, R.S., Wawer Matos, P.A. et al. (2021). No secret hiding place? Absence of SARS-CoV-2 on the ocular surface of 1145 hospitalized patients in a pandemic area. *Graefes Arch. Clin. Exp. Ophthalmol.* 259 (6): 1605–1608. https://doi.org/10.1007/s00417-021-05086-3.

14 Sirakaya, E., Sahiner, M., and Aslan Sirakaya, H. (2021). A patient with bilateral conjunctivitis positive for SARS-CoV-2 RNA in a conjunctival sample. *Cornea* 40 (3): 383–386. https://doi.org/10.1097/ICO.0000000000002485.

15 Chen, L., Deng, C., Chen, X. et al. (2020). Ocular manifestations and clinical characteristics of 535 cases of COVID-19 in Wuhan, China: a cross-sectional study. *Acta Ophthalmol.* 98 (8): e951–e959. https://doi.org/10.1111/aos.14472.

16 Méndez Mangana, C., Barraquer Kargacin, A., and Barraquer, R.I. (2020). Episcleritis as an ocular manifestation in a patient with COVID-19. *Acta Ophthalmol.* 98 (8): e1056–e1057. https://doi.org/10.1111/aos.14484.

17 Otaif, W., Al Somali, A.I., and Al, H.A. (2020). Episcleritis as a possible presenting sign of the novel coronavirus disease: a case report. *Am. J. Ophthalmol. Case Rep.* 20: 100917. https://doi.org/10.1016/j.ajoc.2020.100917.

18 Bettach, E., Zadok, D., Weill, Y. et al. (2021). Bilateral anterior uveitis as a part of a multisystem inflammatory syndrome secondary to COVID-19 infection. *J. Med. Virol.* 93 (1): 139–140. https://doi.org/10.1002/jmv.26229.

19 Wong Chung, J.E.R.E., Engin, Ö., Wolfs, T.F.W. et al. (2021). Anterior uveitis in paediatric inflammatory multisystem syndrome temporally associated with SARS-CoV-2. *Lancet* 397 (10281): e10. https://doi.org/10.1016/S0140-6736(21)00579-1.

20 Karthika, I.K., Gulla, K.M., John, J. et al. (2021). COVID-19 related multi-inflammatory syndrome presenting with uveitis – a case report. *Indian J. Ophthalmol.* 69 (5): 1319–1321. https://doi.org/10.4103/ijo.IJO_52_21.

21 Alonso, R.S., Alonso, F.O.M., Fernandes, B.F. et al. (2021). COVID-19-related ocular hypertension secondary to anterior uveitis as part of a multisystemic inflammatory syndrome. *J. Glaucoma* 30 (5): e256–e258. https://doi.org/10.1097/IJG.0000000000001835.

22 Consiglio, C.R., Cotugno, N., Sardh, F. et al. (2020). The immunology of multisystem inflammatory syndrome in children with COVID-19. *Cell* 183 (4): 968–981.e7. doi:https://doi.org/10.1016/j.cell.2020.09.016.

23 Bitton, K., Dubois, M., Courtin, R. et al. (2021). Descemet's membrane endothelial keratoplasty (DMEK) rejection following COVID-19 infection: a case report. *Am. J. Ophthalmol. Case Rep.* 23: 101138. https://doi.org/10.1016/j.ajoc.2021.101138.

24 Jin, S.X. and Juthani, V.V. (2021). Acute corneal endothelial graft rejection with coinciding COVID-19 infection. *Cornea* 40 (1): 123–124. https://doi.org/10.1097/ICO.0000000000002556.

25 Singh, G. and Mathur, U. (2021). Acute graft rejection in a COVID-19 patient: co-incidence or causal association? *Indian J. Ophthalmol.* 69 (4): 985–986. https://doi.org/10.4103/ijo.IJO_3701_20.

26 Wasser, L.M., Roditi, E., Zadok, D. et al. (2021). Keratoplasty rejection after the BNT162b2 messenger RNA vaccine. *Cornea* 40 (8): 1070–1072. https://doi.org/10.1097/ICO.0000000000002761.

27 Phylactou, M., Li, J.O., and Larkin, D.F.P. (2021). Characteristics of endothelial corneal transplant rejection following immunisation with SARS-CoV-2 messenger RNA vaccine. *Br. J. Ophthalmol.* 105 (7): 893–896. https://doi.org/10.1136/bjophthalmol-2021-319338.

28 Mulley, W.R., Dendle, C., Ling, J.E.H., and Knight, S.R. (2018). Does vaccination in solid-organ transplant recipients result in adverse immunologic sequelae? A systematic review and meta-analysis. *J. Heart Lung Transplant.* 37 (7): 844–852. https://doi.org/10.1016/j.healun.2018.03.001.

29 Lockington, D. (2021). Keratoplasty rejection risk associated with recent vaccination-the pragmatic approach. *Cornea* 40: 1374–1376. https://doi.org/10.1097/ICO.0000000000002818.

30 Matoba, A. (2021). Corneal allograft rejection associated with herpes zoster recombinant adjuvanted vaccine. *Cornea* https://doi.org/10.1097/ICO.0000000000002787.

31 Wertheim, M.S., Keel, M., Cook, S.D., and Tole, D.M. (2006). Corneal transplant rejection following influenza vaccination. *Br. J. Ophthalmol.* 90 (7): 925. https://doi.org/10.1136/bjo.2006.093187.

32 Tisdale, A.K., Dinkin, M., and Chwalisz, B.K. (2021). Afferent and efferent neuro-ophthalmic complications of coronavirus disease 19. *J. Neuroophthalmol.* 41 (2): 154–165. https://doi.org/10.1097/WNO.0000000000001276.

33 de Oliveira, M.R., Lucena, A.R.V.P., Higino, T.M.M., and Ventura, C.V. (2021). Oculomotor nerve palsy in an asymptomatic child with COVID-19. *J. AAPOS* 25: 169–170. https://doi.org/10.1016/j.jaapos.2021.02.001.

34 Ortiz-Seller, A., Martínez Costa, L., Hernández-Pons, A. et al. (2020). Ophthalmic and neuro-ophthalmic manifestations of coronavirus disease 2019 (COVID-19). *Ocul. Immunol. Inflamm.* 28 (8): 1285–1289. https://doi.org/10.1080/09273948.2020.1817497.

35 Gold, D.M. and Galetta, S.L. (2021). Neuro-ophthalmologic complications of coronavirus disease 2019 (COVID-19). *Neurosci. Lett.* 742: 135531. https://doi.org/10.1016/j.neulet.2020.135531.

36 Parvez, Y., AlZarooni, F., and Khan, F. (2021). Optic neuritis in a child with COVID-19: a rare association. *Cureus* 13 (3): e14094. https://doi.org/10.7759/cureus.14094.

37 Sawalha, K., Adeodokun, S., and Kamoga, G.R. (2020). COVID-19-induced acute bilateral optic neuritis. *J. Investig. Med. High Impact Case Rep.* 8:2324709620976018. doi:https://doi.org/10.1177/2324709620976018.

38 Zhou, S., Jones-Lopez, E.C., Soneji, D.J. et al. (2020). Myelin oligodendrocyte glycoprotein antibody-associated optic neuritis and myelitis in COVID-19. *J. Neuroophthalmol.* 40 (3): 398–402. https://doi.org/10.1097/WNO.0000000000001049.

39 Burgos-Blasco, B., Güemes-Villahoz, N., Vidal-Villegas, B. et al. (2021). Optic nerve and macular optical coherence tomography in recovered COVID-19 patients. *Eur. J. Ophthalmol.* https://doi.org/10.1177/11206721211001019.

40 Pereira, L.A., Soares, L.C.M., Nascimento, P.A. et al. (2020). Retinal findings in hospitalised patients with severe COVID-19. *Br. J. Ophthalmol.* https://doi.org/10.1136/bjophthalmol-2020-317576.

41 Invernizzi, A., Torre, A., Parrulli, S. et al. (2020). Retinal findings in patients with COVID-19: results from the SERPICO-19 study. *EClinicalMedicine* 27: 100550. https://doi.org/10.1016/j.eclinm.2020.100550.

42 Bansal, R., Markan, A., Gautam, N. et al. (2021). Retinal involvement in COVID-19: results from a prospective retina screening program in the acute and convalescent phase. *Front. Med. (Lausanne)* 8: 681942. https://doi.org/10.3389/fmed.2021.681942.

43 Landecho, M.F., Yuste, J.R., Gándara, E. et al. (2021). COVID-19 retinal microangiopathy as an in vivo biomarker of systemic vascular disease? *J. Intern. Med.* 289 (1): 116–120. https://doi.org/10.1111/joim.13156.

44 Boudhabhay, I., Rabant, M., Roumenina, L.T. et al. (2021). Case report: adult post-COVID-19 multisystem inflammatory syndrome and thrombotic microangiopathy. *Front. Immunol.* 12: 680567. https://doi.org/10.3389/fimmu.2021.680567.

45 Tiwari, N.R., Phatak, S., Sharma, V.R., and Agarwal, S.K. (2021). COVID-19 and thrombotic microangiopathies. *Thromb. Res.* 202: 191–198. https://doi.org/10.1016/j.thromres.2021.04.012.

46 Jhaveri, K.D., Meir, L.R., Flores Chang, B.S. et al. (2020). Thrombotic microangiopathy in a patient with COVID-19. *Kidney Int.* 98 (2): 509–512. https://doi.org/10.1016/j.kint.2020.05.025.

47 Invernizzi, A., Pellegrini, M., Messenio, D. et al. (2020). Impending central retinal vein occlusion in a patient with coronavirus disease 2019 (COVID-19). *Ocul. Immunol. Inflamm.* 28 (8): 1290–1292. https://doi.org/10.1080/09273948.2020.1807023.

48 Walinjkar, J.A., Makhija, S.C., Sharma, H.R. et al. (2020). Central retinal vein occlusion with COVID-19 infection as the presumptive etiology. *Indian J. Ophthalmol.* 68 (11): 2572–2574. https://doi.org/10.4103/ijo.IJO_2575_20.

49 Gaba, W.H., Ahmed, D., Al Nuaimi, R.K. et al. (2020). Bilateral central retinal vein occlusion in a 40-year-old man with severe coronavirus disease 2019 (COVID-19) pneumonia. *Am. J. Case Rep.* 21: e927691. https://doi.org/10.12659/AJCR.927691.

50 Sheth, J.U., Narayanan, R., Goyal, J., and Goyal, V. (2020). Retinal vein occlusion in COVID-19: a novel entity. *Indian J. Ophthalmol.* 68 (10): 2291–2293. https://doi.org/10.4103/ijo.IJO_2380_20.

51 The Royal College of Ophthalmologists (2021). Safety alert: retinal vein occlusions post COVID vaccination https://www.rcophth.ac.uk/2021/05/retinal-vein-occlusions-post-covid-vaccination/.

52 Greinacher, A., Selleng, K., Mayerle, J. et al. (2021). Anti-platelet factor 4 antibodies causing VITT do not cross-react with SARS-CoV-2 spike protein. *Blood* 138: 1269–1277. https://doi.org/10.1182/blood.2021012938.

53 Dumitrascu, O.M., Volod, O., Bose, S. et al. (2020). Acute ophthalmic artery occlusion in a COVID-19 patient on apixaban. *J. Stroke Cerebrovasc. Dis.* 29 (8): 104982. https://doi.org/10.1016/j.jstrokecerebrovasdis.2020.104982.

54 Acharya, S., Diamond, M., Anwar, S. et al. (2020). Unique case of central retinal artery occlusion secondary to COVID-19 disease. *IDCases* 21: e00867. https://doi.org/10.1016/j.idcr.2020.e00867.

55 Montesel, A., Bucolo, C., Mouvet, V. et al. (2020). Case report: central retinal artery occlusion in a COVID-19 patient. *Front. Pharmacol.* 11: 588384. https://doi.org/10.3389/fphar.2020.588384.

56 Eleiwa, T., Abdelrahman, S.N., ElSheikh, R.H., and Elhusseiny, A.M. (2021). Orbital inflammatory disease associated with COVID-19 infection. *J. AAPOS* 25: 232–234. https://doi.org/10.1016/j.jaapos.2021.04.002.

57 Gautret, P., Lagier, J.C., Parola, P. et al. (2020). Clinical and microbiological effect of a combination of hydroxychloroquine and azithromycin in 80 COVID-19 patients with at least a six-day follow up: a pilot observational study. *Travel Med. Infect. Dis.* 34: 101663. https://doi.org/10.1016/j.tmaid.2020.101663.

58 Martínez Díaz, M., Copete Piqueras, S., Blanco Marchite, C., and Vahdani, K. (2021). Acute dacryoadenitis in a patient with SARS-CoV-2 infection. *Orbit* https://doi.org/10.1080/01676830.2020.1867193.

59 Singh, A.K., Singh, R., Joshi, S.R., and Misra, A. (2021). Mucormycosis in COVID-19: a systematic review of cases reported worldwide and in India. *Diabetes Metab. Syndr.* 15 (4): 102146. https://doi.org/10.1016/j.dsx.2021.05.019.

60 Ashour, M.M., Abdelaziz, T.T., Ashour, D.M. et al. (2021). Imaging spectrum of acute invasive fungal rhino-orbital-cerebral sinusitis in COVID-19 patients: a case series and a review of literature. *J. Neuroradiol.* 48: 319–324. https://doi.org/10.1016/j.neurad.2021.05.007.

61 Das, D., Anwer, Z., Kumari, N., and Gupta, S. (2020). Unilateral orbital emphysema in a COVID-19 patient. *Indian J. Ophthalmol.* 68 (11): 2535. https://doi.org/10.4103/ijo.IJO_2385_20.

62 Stevens, D.V., Tran, A.Q., and Kim, E. (2020). Complications of orbital emphysema in a COVID-19 patient. *Ophthalmology* 127 (7): 990. https://doi.org/10.1016/j.ophtha.2020.05.011.

20

COVID-19: Nutrition Perspectives

Emma J. Ridley[1,2], Lee-anne S. Chapple[3,4,5], Aidan Burrell[1,6], Kate Fetterplace[7,8], Amy Freeman-Sanderson[9,10,11], Andrea P. Marshall[12,13], and Ary Serpa Neto[1]

[1] Australian and New Zealand Intensive Care Research Centre, School of Public Health and Preventative Medicine, Monash University, Melbourne, VIC, Australia
[2] Nutrition Department, The Alfred Hospital, Melbourne, VIC, Australia
[3] Adelaide Medicine School, University of Adelaide, Adelaide, SA, Australia
[4] Intensive Care Unit, Royal Adelaide Hospital, Adelaide, SA, Australia
[5] Centre for Research Excellence in Nutritional Physiology, Adelaide, SA, Australia
[6] Intensive Care Unit, The Alfred Hospital, Melbourne, VIC, Australia
[7] Allied Health Department (Clinical Nutrition), Royal Melbourne Hospital, Melbourne, VIC, Australia
[8] Department of Critical Care, Melbourne Medical School, The University of Melbourne, Melbourne, VIC, Australia
[9] Graduate School of Health, University of Technology Sydney, Sydney, NSW, Australia
[10] Speech Pathology Department & Intensive Care Unit, Royal Prince Alfred Hospital, Sydney, NSW, Australia
[11] Critical Care Division, The George Institute for Global Health, Sydney, NSW, Australia
[12] Gold Coast Health, Southport, QLD, Australia
[13] School of Nursing and Midwifery, Griffith University, Southport, QLD, Australia

Abbreviations

ASPEN/SCCM	American Society of Parenteral and Enteral Nutrition/Society of Critical Care Medicine
BMI	body mass index
CI	confidence interval
CPAP	continuous positive airway pressure
ECMO	extracorporeal membrane oxygenation
EN	enteral nutrition
ESPEN	European Society for Clinical Nutrition and Metabolism
GI	gastrointestinal
GRV	gastric residual volume
HFNC	high-flow nasal cannulae
ICU	intensive care unit
IMV	invasive mechanical ventilation
NMB	neuromuscular blockade
NIV	noninvasive ventilation
OR	odds ratio
PN	parenteral nutrition
PPE	personal protective equipment

Nutrition across hospitalization is likely to play an integral role through the COVID-19 process; comorbid diseases and premorbid nutrition status predict the need for hospitalization and admission to the intensive care unit (ICU); nutrition-impacting symptoms and medical management may impair nutrition adequacy; and reestablishing adequate nutrition intake is integral for recovery from long COVID-19. This chapter will provide a comprehensive look at the unique aspects of providing nutrition therapy for hospitalized patients with coronavirus disease 2019 (COVID-19), including those who are critically ill, from admission to recovery, covering nutrition-impacting symptoms, medical management, nutrition screening and assessment, and nutrition practices of delivery and monitoring of nutrition support. It will also provide perspective on the implications of a global pandemic on caseload, resourcing, stock shortages, and the logistics of managing the nutrition care of highly infectious patients.

Patients with COVID-19 may be at nutrition risk before hospital admission because they often present with at least one comorbidity, such as obesity, diabetes, cardiovascular disease, or chronic lung disease [1, 2]. The presence of these comorbidities, particularly obesity, also increases the likelihood of patients requiring an ICU admission.

A range of unique physiological symptoms occur in patients with COVID-19 that are likely to impact nutrition intake. Data to date describe a loss of taste (dysgeusia) and smell (dysnomia) (34–59%) [3, 4], reduced appetite (78%) [5], and gastrointestinal (GI) symptoms, including diarrhea, nausea, and vomiting (10%) [6–8]. Sustained nutrition deficits may also occur before ICU admission, as a result of these symptoms [1, 7, 9].

COVID-19 causes significant metabolic disturbance with hypermetabolism up to 200% of predicted values reported [10]. Persistent fevers are a contributing factor observed in ~95–98% of patients [6, 7, 11] (associated with a ~10–15% increase in energy requirements for every 1 °C increase in body temperature [12]). An aggressive proinflammatory immune response is also expected, causing increased glucocorticoid and catecholamine production with increased insulin sensitivity, and poor glycemic control [13]. In addition, medical therapy processes required for critically ill patients with COVID-19, including organ support, sedation, and need for ventilation, will further dictate nutrition management.

General considerations for nutrition care of patients with COVID-19 admitted to the hospital and ICU will be discussed in this chapter. Insufficient supplies of nutrition formula and associated consumables have been reported, along with low staffing levels impeding the ability to deliver nutrition therapy. The need for remote assessment and less frequent reviews as a result of staffing levels are also likely to impact the quality of nutrition care. For patients eating orally, intake may be limited by physiologic barriers and restrictions on food service management systems and visitors, affecting meal delivery, menu choice, and feeding assistance.

Inadequate nutrition during and after ICU admission is likely to impact nutrition status and impede recovery. Weight loss of >10% body weight has been reported in both noncritically ill and critically ill patients with COVID-19 [14]. Weight loss at ICU discharge in a small cohort of patients with COVID-19 has been shown to correlate with longer ICU stay [14], while having a greater muscle mass predicted successful extubation (odds ratio [OR], 1.02; 95% confidence interval [CI]: 1.00–1.03; $P = 0.017$), shorter ICU stay (OR, 0.97; 95% CI: 0.95–0.99; $P = 0.03$), and decreased hospital mortality (hazard ratio, 0.98; 95% CI: 0.96–0.99; $P = 0.02$) [15].

The speed at which COVID-19 has progressed globally means there is an absence of high-quality COVID-19-specific nutrition data. Given this, the concepts discussed throughout this chapter are based on the available data, an understanding of how the clinical characteristics of COVID-19 may affect nutrition practices, and implementation of relevant principles from international clinical practice guidelines for the nutrition care of the general ICU and hospitalized patient.

Safety Considerations for Nutrition Processes and Practice When Caring for Patients with COVID-19

Staff safety should be considered the top priority for all staff involved across all aspects of the nutrition care process for patients with COVID-19, including formal training on the use of personal protective equipment (PPE) and mask fit testing [16]. Familiarization of those involved in nutrition care with the hierarchy of hazard control and donning and doffing PPE with the assistance of a PPE spotter may also help to protect staff [17].

Measures to protect the workforce include limiting the number of staff attending "hot zones" and locating them separately or in small groups to prevent exposure of the whole workforce [18]. Where possible, nutrition consultations could be completed remotely, with the use of telemedicine, electronic medical records, and by using family members; however, it is important to ensure that appropriate and safe nutrition care is maintained, recognizing that a completely remote model of care may increase the risk for nutrition failure [19]. Bundling face-to-face care for multiple patients within a hot zone should be considered or using one staff member to attend the hot zone while others remain remote is an appropriate hybrid model. Nutrition or ward-based assistants can also undertake several components of nutrition screening and management on the ward, limiting the number of face-to-face staff. Tasks may include assistance with monitoring of oral intake, quantification of oral nutrition supplement compliance, liaison with bedside staff regarding menu preferences, assistance with food service tasks, assistance with facilitating ICU transfers, and obtaining weight histories [16].

Nutrition in the Noncritically Ill Hospitalized Patient with COVID-19

This section focuses on the clinical management and associated nutrition implications for patients with severe or nonsevere COVID-19 who are located within the hospital setting but outside of the ICU.

Treatment for COVID-19 and Associated Nutrition Impacts

Research into clinical interventions for the treatment of COVID-19 has been prolific since the start of the pandemic. While severe COVID-19 can be defined by the presence of $SpO_2 <90\%$ on room air and/or signs of severe respiratory distress, nonsevere COVID-19 is defined as an absence of any signs of severe COVID-19 [20].

Steroids

Systemic corticosteroids are among the most studied drugs for patients with COVID-19. Polled evidence suggests that daily treatment with intravenous corticosteroids for 7–10 days is associated with reduced mortality in hospitalized patients with severe COVID-19 [21]. Steroids should not be used in patients with nonsevere

COVID-19. Hyperglycemia and insulin resistance are already features of COVID-19, and the use of steroids compounds this impact, resulting in greater hyperglycemia that is sometimes resistant to insulin therapy, requiring both short- and long-acting insulin in some circumstances. Blood glucose levels should continue to be monitored when steroids are administered.

Other Treatments

Other potential treatments for patients with COVID-19 include the use of neutralizing monoclonal antibodies (casirivimab and imdevimab or sotrovimab), interleukin-6 receptor blockers (tocilizumab or sarilumab), Janus kinase inhibitors (baricitinib or tofacitinib), and antivirals (remdesivir). These drugs may be associated with nutrition-impacting symptoms such as stomach pain (interleukin-6 receptor blockers and baricitinib), diarrhea (sarilumab, Janus kinase inhibitors), nausea (Janus kinase inhibitors and remdesivir), and loss of appetite (tofacitinib).

Other interventions that may be applied on the ward and in the ICU are covered in the following section, including noninvasive ventilation (NIV).

Nutrition Screening and Assessment in Noncritically Ill Patients

Malnutrition in noncritically ill patients with COVID-19 is common, with a prevalence rate of 15–80%, and is an independent predictor for all-cause mortality [4, 22–25]. Therefore, screening for malnutrition using a validated screening tool is recommended in major international guidelines [7, 26, 27]. Screening can facilitate timely assessment and prioritization of resources when the hospital system is under strain. The most appropriate nutrition risk screening tool to use is dependent on the clinical setting and preexisting institutional processes. Where possible, existing processes should be maintained but may be adapted to manage the challenges that COVID-19 presents. Malnutrition screening should be undertaken by appropriately trained health professionals on hospital admission. Patients identified at high risk on screening should undergo a formal evaluation for malnutrition to allow implementation of targeted nutrition interventions.

Clinicians have used modified techniques to assess patients via phone interview or with assistance from family members [19]. Validated nutrition screening and malnutrition assessment tools for use in the hospital setting are presented in Table 20.1 [29, 32, 33].

Nutrition Interventions and Monitoring of Nutrition Progress

The timing of assessment and appropriate nutrition intervention should be informed by baseline malnutrition risk or those with complex medical histories. A suggested algorithm is provided in Figure 20.1 [16]. Nutrition deficits before hospital admission, during hospitalization, and the possible trajectory of recovery should also be considered.

In patients at low and moderate risk for malnutrition, a standard protocol of a "high energy and high protein diet order" with or without nutrition supplements is an appropriate first-line management [16]. This is especially true when staff resources may limit timely individual assessment. Patients at high nutrition risk or diagnosed with malnutrition, and those who have received limited to no nutrition for ≥3 days should be provided with an individualized nutrition care plan [31, 34]. Given that restrictions on staff contact time with patients are likely to impair appropriate monitoring of dietary intake and weight changes, repeat screening for malnutrition and close monitoring is recommended because the risk for malnutrition developing during hospitalization is high, even in those who were considered low risk on previous screening.

On the hospital ward, oral nutrition will be the most common mode of nutrition; however, it should be acknowledged that it will likely be inadequate [16, 35]. Monitoring of nutrition throughout hospitalization is crucial, including intake and weight (where possible). High-risk patients should be reviewed at least twice weekly and lower-risk patients at least weekly [16, 19, 36]. If patients are not receiving adequate oral nutrition (<50% of energy and protein targets), nutrition support should be escalated to enteral nutrition (EN) within five to seven days [16, 34]. Parenteral nutrition (PN) should be considered only if EN is not feasible or is inadequate [34].

Nutrition in the Critically Ill Patient with COVID-19

This section will focus on the nutrition needs, treatments, and practices specific to the critically ill patient with COVID-19.

Nutrition Screening and Assessment in Critically Ill Patients

As with patients on the hospital ward, critically ill patients with COVID-19 are anticipated to be at a similar or even greater risk for malnutrition and declining nutrition status given the numerous risk factors experienced by these patients. Consequently, nutrition risk screening within 48 hours of admission is recommended for critically ill patients with COVID-19. It is important to note that nutrition risk will vary depending on the tool used, and that these tools have many limitations (summarized in Table 20.1).

Guidelines

Evidence-based guidelines to support nutrition care of the critically ill patient have been available for many years and the methodologic quality, recommendations, and comprehensiveness differ. Differences likely exist owing to question formulation, search terms and databases used, inclusion and exclusion criteria, review criteria, and low methodological quality or lack of evidence that results in expert opinion being used to formulate recommendations. Despite evidence-based recommendations to inform nutrition care practices for critically ill patients, delivery of nutrition can often be less than that prescribed [37]. Table 20.2 summarizes two of the main evidence-based guidelines for nutrition care of the general critically ill patient [27, 38].

A number of COVID-19-specific nutrition guidelines for critically ill patients have been rapidly developed early in the pandemic that included recommendations largely similar to previously published guidelines for critical care nutrition [16, 28, 30, 39–46]. Ten of the COVID-19-specific guidelines recommend early EN for patients in the prone position and high-energy, high-protein diets with nutrition supplements

Table 20.1 Nutrition risk screening and assessment tools for use in the hospital setting and their limitations.

Tool	Tool Measures	Setting	Recommended in COVID-19 Nutrition Guideline	Limitations
Nutrition Risk Screening Tools				
Malnutrition Universal Screening Tool (MUST)	• BMI • Recent weight loss • Acute disease effect score	ICU and ward	INDI guidelines [28] ESPEN Nutrition screening guidelines [29]	Does not include recent dietary intake so may be less sensitive to detecting future risk
Malnutrition Screening Tool (MST)	• Recent weight loss • Appetite	Ward	INDI guidelines	Simplicity limits sensitivity
Nutrition Risk Screening 2002 (NRS-2002)	• BMI • Recent weight loss • Recent intake • Disease severity • Age	ICU	ESPEN ICU guidelines [29]	More complex to complete than other screening tools
Nutrition Risk in Critically ill (NUTRIC) score	• Age • Injury severity • Comorbidities • Days in hospital before ICU admission +/− interleukin-6	ICU	ATID guidelines [30]	Injury severity scores also incorporate age and comorbidities
Nutrition Assessment Tools				
Mini Nutritional Assessment—Short Form (MNA-SF)	• BMI • Recent weight loss • Recent intake • Mobility • Psychological well-being	Ward- elderly	Nil	Low completion rates shown in practice Content validity not reported
Subjective Global Assessment (SGA)	• Recent weight loss • Recent intake • Nutrition impact symptoms • Disease severity • Age • Physical signs, fat/muscle loss	Ward	Nil	Requires significant training to conduct Time consuming
Global Leadership Initiative on Malnutrition (GLIM)	• BMI • Recent weight loss • Reduced muscle mass • Recent intake • Inflammation	Ward	ESPEN-endorsed consensus statement [31]	

ATID, Israeli Dietetic Association; BMI, body mass index; ESPEN, European Society for Clinical Nutrition and Metabolism; ICU, intensive care unit; INDI, Irish Nutrition and Dietetic Institute.
Sources: Anthony [32], Kondrup et al. [29], and Reber et al. [33].

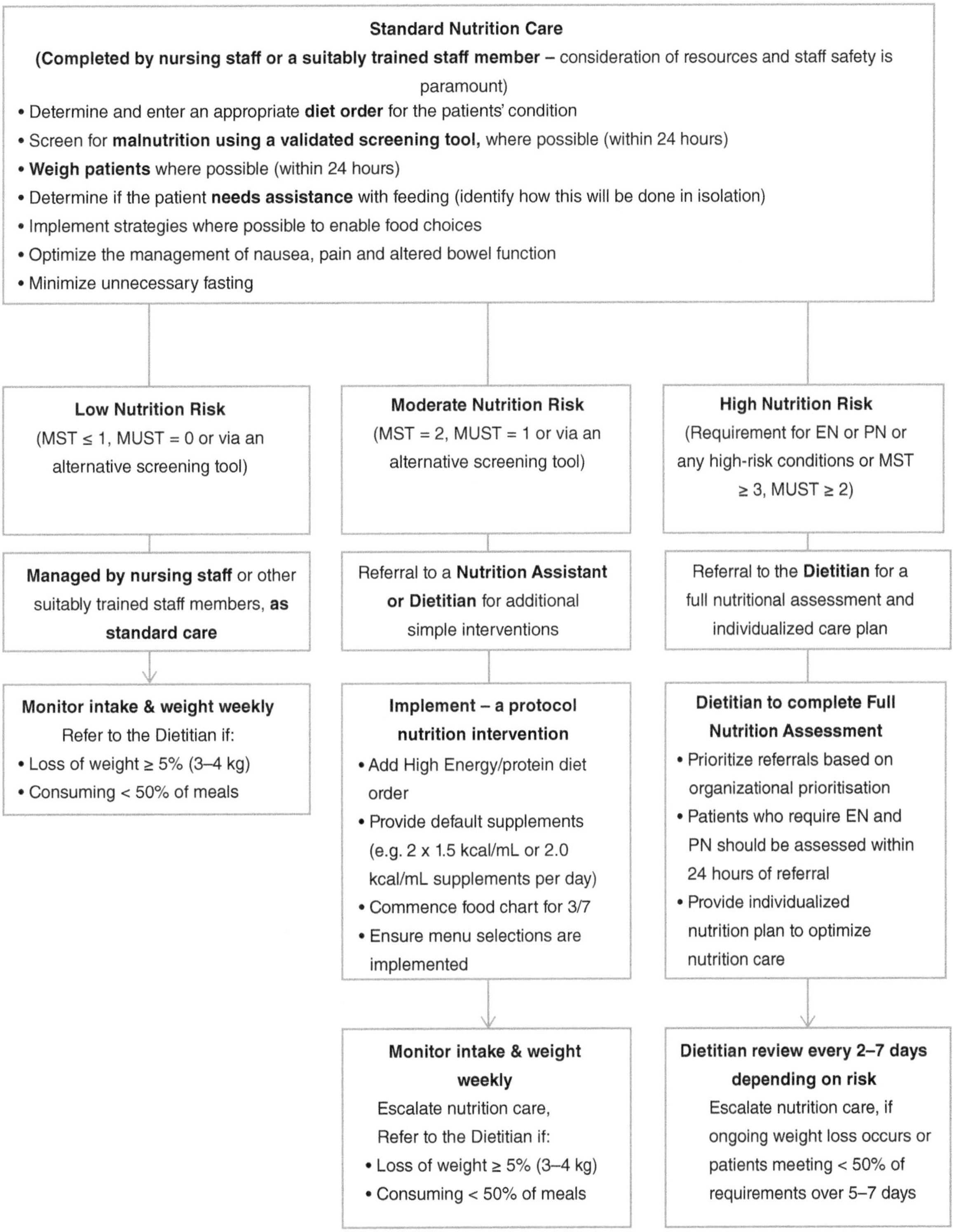

Standard Nutrition Care

(Completed by nursing staff or a suitably trained staff member – consideration of resources and staff safety is paramount)

• Determine and enter an appropriate **diet order** for the patients' condition
• Screen for **malnutrition using a validated screening tool,** where possible (within 24 hours)
• **Weigh patients** where possible (within 24 hours)
• Determine if the patient **needs assistance** with feeding (identify how this will be done in isolation)
• Implement strategies where possible to enable food choices
• Optimize the management of nausea, pain and altered bowel function
• Minimize unnecessary fasting

Low Nutrition Risk	**Moderate Nutrition Risk**	**High Nutrition Risk**
(MST ≤ 1, MUST = 0 or via an alternative screening tool)	(MST = 2, MUST = 1 or via an alternative screening tool)	(Requirement for EN or PN or any high-risk conditions or MST ≥ 3, MUST ≥ 2)

Managed by nursing staff or other suitably trained staff members, **as standard care**	Referral to a **Nutrition Assistant or Dietitian** for additional simple interventions	Referral to the **Dietitian** for a full nutritional assessment and individualized care plan

Monitor intake & weight weekly	**Implement – a protocol nutrition intervention**	**Dietitian to complete Full Nutrition Assessment**
Refer to the Dietitian if: • Loss of weight ≥ 5% (3–4 kg) • Consuming < 50% of meals	• Add High Energy/protein diet order • Provide default supplements (e.g. 2 x 1.5 kcal/mL or 2.0 kcal/mL supplements per day) • Commence food chart for 3/7 • Ensure menu selections are implemented	• Prioritize referrals based on organizational prioritisation • Patients who require EN and PN should be assessed within 24 hours of referral • Provide individualized nutrition plan to optimize nutrition care

Monitor intake & weight weekly	**Dietitian review every 2–7 days depending on risk**
Escalate nutrition care, Refer to the Dietitian if: • Loss of weight ≥ 5% (3–4 kg) • Consuming < 50% of meals	Escalate nutrition care, if ongoing weight loss occurs or patients meeting < 50% of requirements over 5–7 days

Figure 20.1 Acute ward nutrition algorithm for management of patients with COVID-19. EN, enteral nutrition; MST, Malnutrition Screening Tool; MUST, Malnutrition Universal Screening Tool; PN, parenteral nutrition. *Source:* Adapted from Chapple et al. [16].

Table 20.2 Key recommendations in two main clinical practice guidelines for the critically ill (not COVID-19 specific).

Guideline	ASPEN/SCCM (2016) [26]	ESPEN (2019) [27]
Basis of recommendation	Observational studies, RCTs, and consensus opinion from topic experts	Observational studies, RCTs, and consensus opinion from topic experts
General Recommendations		
Energy requirements	• Use IC *(Quality: very low)* • In the absence of IC, use 25–30 kcal/kg/day *(EC)*	• Use IC *(Grade: B^a)* • In the absence of IC, use VO_2 or VCO_2 predictive equations *(Grade: 0^a)*
Protein requirements	1.2–2 g/kg/day *(Quality: very low)*	1.3 g/kg/day delivered progressively *(Grade: 0^a)*
Commencement of EN^b	• Early EN (24–48 hours) for patients who cannot maintain volitional intake *(Quality: very low)* • Patients at low nutrition risk, well-nourished, and/or with low disease severity do not require specialized nutrition therapy over the first week in ICU *(EC)* • For patients at high nutrition risk or severely malnourished, EN should advance to goal as quickly as tolerated over 24–48 hours (while monitoring for refeeding) *(Quality: very low)*	• Early EN (within 48 hours) *(Grade: A^a)* • Hypocaloric nutrition (<70% of EE) in the early acute phase (ICU days 1–3) *(Grade: B^a)* • If using IC, isocaloric nutrition (80–100% EE) can be progressively implemented after day 3 *(Grade: 0^a)* • If using predictive equations, hypocaloric nutrition (<70% of EE) for the first week *(Grade: B^a)*
Commencement of PN	• Exclusive PN (when oral intake or EN contraindicated): for patients at low nutrition risk, withhold for the first 7 days *(Quality: very low)* • For patients at high nutrition risk or severely malnourished, start as soon as possible *(EC)* • Supplemental PN^c: for all patients, it should be considered after 7–10 days if unable to meet >60% of energy and protein requirements by EN *(Quality: moderate)*	• Start exclusive PN (when oral intake or EN contraindicated) within 3–7 days *(Grade: B^a)* • Early and progressive PN (when oral or EN contraindicated) for severely malnourished *(Grade: 0^a)* • Consider supplemental PN^c on a case-by-case basis *(Grade: 0^a)*
Recommendations for Obese Patients		
Energy	• Indirect calorimetry preferred over predictive equation *(EC)* • If IC used, target 65–70% of a measured requirement (for all classes of obesity) *(EC)* • If IC unavailable *(EC)*; BMI 30–50 kg/m²: 11–14 kcal/kg ABW; BMI > 50: 22–25 kcal/kg/IBW	• Isocaloric high-protein diet (Grade 0) • IC preferred over predictive equation (Grade 0) General recommendation for all ICU patients • In the early acute phase of illness, aim for <70% (before day 3) (Grade B) • After day 3, increase to 80–100% of measured or estimated REE
Protein	• BMI 30–40; 2 kg IBW/day *(EC)* • BMI ≥ 40; 2.5 g/kg IBW/day *(EC)*	• Guided by urinary nitrogen loss or lean body mass determination (GPP) • If the above not possible, 1.3 g/kg ABW (GPP)

Table 20.2 (Continued)

Guideline	ASPEN/SCCM (2016) [26]	ESPEN (2019) [27]
Weight adjustment method	No specific statement regarding weight adjustment	Three methods proposed for BMI > 25 (not graded): • IBW: $0.9 \times$ height (in cm) $- 100$ (male) (or 106 [female]) • For energy requirement calculation, add 20–25% of the excess body weight (actual body weight $-$ ideal body weight) to the IBW as above • For protein "ABW"; IBW + 1/3 actual body weight

[a] ESPEN Grade of recommendation: A = at least one high-quality meta-analysis, systematic review, or RCT; B = based on a body of evidence from well-conducted observational studies; 0 = case studies, expert opinion, or evidence extrapolated from high-quality systematic reviews or observational studies (recommendation refers to "can be aimed for" rather than best practice).
[b] Commencement of EN in hemodynamically stable patients who are unable to maintain oral intake.
[c] Supplemental PN: when all nutritional requirements are unable to be met by EN (i.e. due to intolerance, fasting, etc.).
ABW, adjusted body weight; ASPEN/SCCM, American Society of Parenteral and Enteral Nutrition/Society of Critical Care Medicine; EC, expert consensus; EE, energy expenditure; EN, enteral nutrition; ESPEN, European Society for Clinical Nutrition and Metabolism; GPP, good practice point; IC, indirect calorimetry; IBW, ideal body weight; PN, parenteral nutrition; RCT, randomized controlled trial; REE, resting energy expenditure; VCO_2, carbon dioxide production; VO_2, oxygen consumption.
Sources: McClave et al. [26] and Singer et al. [27].

for nonintubated patients identified as being at high nutrition risk. Notably, many guidelines were developed before availability of specific COVID-19 data, and hence recommendations may change as care and evidence evolves. Considerations of the local context, patient populations, resources, and staff experience and training are important when tailoring recommendations for inclusion in local guidelines. Table 20.3 summarizes a selection of consensus and evidence-based guidelines for nutrition care specific to the critically ill patient with COVID-19. Table 20.4 provides an overview of topics covered in all 10 of the COVID-19-specific nutrition guidelines.

Therapies for COVID-19 and Associated Nutrition Impacts

Patients with severe or critical COVID-19 are typically cared for in the ICU. Although this group is relatively small compared with the total population of COVID-19 cases, they have a high mortality rate (20–40%) [47], and survivors often have a prolonged hospital stay requiring significant healthcare resources. Management of COVID-19 within the ICU predominately focuses on treating respiratory failure, but treatment of other organ failures, including renal, cardiovascular, and GI, may be required. Figure 20.2 summarizes medical management for patients with COVID-19 as recommended in current clinical practice guidelines.

Noninvasive Oxygen Therapy

A number of therapies to manage hypoxia and respiratory failure in patients with COVID-19 exist. Conventional oxygen therapy (nasal prongs/venturi mask) are commonly used because they allow a higher fraction of inspired oxygen and can be titrated to the patient's oxygen saturations. High-flow nasal cannulae (HFNC) are commonly used in more severe disease, because they enable compression, humidification, and warming of inspired air. Although there is little direct evidence in COVID-19, HFNC has been shown to reduce the need for intubation in patients without COVID-19 and has been recommended as first-line treatment in international guidelines in patients with hypoxic respiratory failure [48].

Continuous positive airway pressure (CPAP) enables the noninvasive application of positive end-expiratory pressure throughout the respiratory cycle to aid alveolar recruitment and optimize oxygen delivery. Although COVID-19 guidelines recommend CPAP be

Table 20.3 Selected COVID-19-specific nutrition guidelines and key recommendations.

Guidelines	Energy Requirements	Protein Requirements	Route of Feeding	Formula Prescription	Initiation and Considerations	Monitoring (GRVs)
ASPEN [44]	First week: 15–20 kcal/kg/day[a]	1.2–2.0 g/kg/day[a]	EN is preferred to PN EN contraindication: *High nutrition risk:* commence PN as early as possible *Low nutrition risk:* may delay PN for 5–7 days	Standard high-protein (≥20% protein) polymeric isosmotic EN in acute phase	24–36 h of ICU admission (or within 12 h of intubation) Low-dose EN (hypocaloric or trophic), advancing to full-dose EN over the first week	Do not routinely monitor GRVs
AuSPEN [16]	Days 1–5: Standard feed rate 50 mL/h, 1.25 kcal/mL Day 6+: 25 kcal/kg/day (up to 30 kcal/kg/day for severely unwell patients + prolonged admission)[b]	≥1.2 g/kg/day[b]	No recommendation for commencement of EN Supplemental PN: consider where postpyloric EN is not possible and intake is consistently <50% of targets over 5–7 days	Use energy-dense EN formula (1.25–1.5 kcal/mL)	Low nutrition risk: within 24 h of ICU admission High nutrition risk: assess before EN commencement	300 mL cutoff (8 hourly). Stop monitoring in nonprone patients if GRVs are <300 mL for >48 h
BDA [41]	N/A	N/A	Consider an NGT on admission, postpyloric tube if persistently high GRVs PN: consider if postpyloric feeding is not available	Avoid large volumes/high rates of EN. Consider 1.3/1.5 kcal/mL EN	N/A	Use local cutoff for nonprone patients and 300-mL cutoff (4 hourly) for prone patients
ESPEN [40]	Use IC where safe, if so: days 1–3: <70% of measured REE Days >3–7: progression to 80–100% measured REE If using predictive equation: <70% estimated target for first week	1.3 g/kg/day[c] delivered progressively	Oral + ONS preferred, followed by EN EN contraindication: PN to be considered Supplemental PN: case-by-case basis if not tolerating full-dose EN during the first week in ICU	N/A	24–48 h during hospitalization	500-mL cutoff

[a] Adjusted targets recommended in obesity.

[b] Adjusted body weight should be used for overweight and obese patients as per usual site method.

[c] 1.3 g/kg "adjusted body weight" (ABW) protein equivalents per day is recommended. ABW is calculated as ideal body weight + (ABW – ideal body weight) × 0.33.

[d] Different targets recommended in obesity using an ABW.

ASPEN, American Society for Parenteral and Enteral Nutrition; AuSPEN, Australasian Society for Parenteral and Enteral Nutrition; BDA, British Dietetic Association; ESPEN, European Society for Parenteral and Enteral Nutrition; EN, enteral nutrition; GRV, gastric residual volume; NGT, nasogastric tube; ONS, oral nutrition supplementation; PN, parenteral nutrition.

Table 20.4 Summary of content presented in each nutrition guideline for critically ill patients admitted with COVID-19.

Guideline or Practice Recommendation Society	Nutrition Risk Screening	Nutrition Requirements/ Prescription	Timing of Initiation	Route of Feeding	Mode of Feeding	Formula Prescription	Monitoring	Specific Patient Populations/ Conditions	Equipment Considerations	Workforce Recommendations
ANSISA [43]	√	√	X	√	√	√	X	X	X	X
ASPEN [44]	√	√	√	√	√	√	√	√	X	X
AuSPEN [16]	√	√	√	√	√	√	√	√	√	√
BDA [41]	X	X	X	√	√	√	√	√	√	√
BRASPEN [42]	√	√	√	√	X	√	√	X	X	X
ESPEN [40]	√	√	√	√	X	X	√	√	X	√
IDA [39]	X	√	√	√	√	√	X	√	X	√
INDI [28]	√	X	√	√	√	√	√	√	X	X
ATID [30]	√	√	√	√	X	√	√	√	X	√
TDA [46]	√	√	X	√	X	√	X	X	X	X

ANSISA, Italian Association of Medical Specialists in Dietetics and Clinical Nutrition; ASPEN, American Society for Parenteral and Enteral Nutrition; ATID: Israeli Dietetic Association; AuSPEN, Australasian Society for Parenteral and Enteral Nutrition; BDA, British Dietetic Association; BRASPEN: Brazilian Society of Parenteral and Enteral Nutrition; ESPEN, European Society for Clinical Nutrition and Metabolism; INDI: Irish Nutrition and Dietetic Institute; TDA: Turkish Dietetic Association.

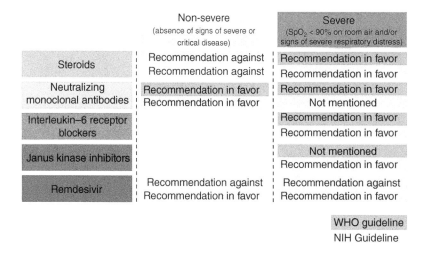

Figure 20.2 Summary of medical management for patients with COVID-19 as recommended in current clinical practice guidelines. NIH, National Institutes of Health; WHO, World Health Organization.

considered in patients with persistent hypoxia ($FiO_2 \geq 0.4$) who are able to tolerate it, the exact impact is unclear. NIV, also known as bilevel positive pressure, is a form of noninvasive positive pressure ventilation. CPAP and NIV may be delivered via traditional face mask or helmet.

The type of oxygen support provided can pose varying challenges for the provision of nutrition, with nutrition deficits reported in patients without COVID-19 receiving oxygen therapy in ICU [16]. HFNC can impact nutrition through drying of the mucous membrane, causing a dry mouth that may impact mastication ability, swallow effort, and laryngeal function [49]. Patients who require CPAP or NIV have considerable fatigue and increased metabolic requirements as a result of work of breathing. Moreover, there is often a concern regarding the need to escalate quickly to mechanical ventilation, meaning patients often fast for long periods. Patients are often unable to tolerate adequate periods without CPAP or NIV to allow nutrition intake, and if they can, they are often exhausted. Patients with increased respiratory rate and altered oxygen levels are at increased risk for dysphagia and tracheal aspiration [50]. Appropriate screening and assessment of swallow practices should be adopted to optimize swallowing safety and efficiency with oral intake [51]. Premorbid nutrition status, as well as the anticipated duration of CPAP/NIV, should be used as a guide for managing nutrition in

these patients (as previously discussed). For some patients, a short period with little to no nutrition may be tolerated. However, for patients at high nutrition risk or requiring prolonged oxygen support, a fine-bore nasogastric tube for EN with or without oral diet should be considered. Where this is not possible, PN may be appropriate.

Invasive Ventilation

Invasive mechanical ventilation (IMV) is required in up to 70% of patients admitted to the ICU when patients fail to respond to HFNC, CPAP, or NIV, and it is strongly associated with worse outcomes (predominantly as a marker of illness severity) [52].

For patients receiving IMV, volitional nutrition intake is not possible, and hence EN is recommended (detailed in "Nutrition Provision, Choice of Nutrition Mode, and Monitoring" section). Considerable guidance exists regarding nutrition provision in patients receiving MV, both with and without COVID-19 (detailed in the following sections and Table 20.2).

Neuromuscular Blockade

COVID-19 guidelines suggest a cautious approach for the use of neuromuscular blockade (NMB) in patients with moderate to severe respiratory failure with a preference of intermittent bolus dosing over continuous infusions [21, 53, 54]. NMB combined with the use of opioids, other sedation agents, and the impact of critical illness itself can lead to GI stasis and intolerance [55]. Research has suggested that metabolic rate is reduced in patients with COVID-19 who are paralyzed (in both obese and nonobese patients energy expenditure was measured as 17.9 kcal/kg actual body weight nonobese versus 19.5 kcal/kg in obese; $P = 0.027$) [56].

Prone Positioning

In non-COVID-19 disease, prone position has been shown to reduce 90-day mortality when used early in illness and for prolonged sessions (>12 hours) [57]; subsequently, it is recommended in all major COVID-19 guidelines for IMV patients. Awake proning may also be considered in patients with mild to moderate disease. Awake proning is associated with a reduction in need for intubation and is generally safe, although it may be difficult to tolerate in some patients, may increase aspiration risk because of positioning, and is required for >8 hours per day to provide benefit [58].

In patients receiving IMV in the prone position, maintenance of gastric feeding is encouraged. EN should be turned off and the nasogastric tube aspirated before any position change, with EN recommenced once the patient is settled and ventilating well. In the setting of impaired GI motility, postpyloric feeding or supplemental PN may be indicated. For awake non-IMV patients, oral intake may be possible while prone; however, it is likely to be practically difficult, and the duration of proning required restricts the opportunity for adequate intake. In situations of prolonged proning where adequate nutrition cannot be maintained orally, enteral feeding should be considered.

Extracorporeal Membrane Oxygenation

Extracorporeal membrane oxygenation (ECMO) is a form of life support that removes blood via large cannulae and oxygenates, and removes carbon dioxide and then returns it to the body. Despite early reports of poor outcomes, ECMO has been adopted widely as a treatment approach in patients with COVID-19, based on its use in non-COVID severe respiratory failure [59]. However, ECMO is resource intense, and many patients suffer significant complications, including prolonged hospital stay; hence this treatment should be applied in experienced centers and carefully selected patients only.

Provision of nutrition to patients receiving ECMO should follow recommendations for general critically ill patients [60]. GI intolerance is a common concern due to the requirement for sedation and sometimes paralysis, reduced movement, reduction in perfusion to the GI tract in some circumstances, and higher illness acuity in general. Moreover, significant cumulative nutrition deficits can occur because of prolonged length of stay if not appropriately managed.

Nutrition Provision, Choice of Nutrition Mode, and Monitoring

It is accepted practice in critically ill patients that EN should be commenced early (within 24–48 hours of admission to ICU) at a relatively low dose, increasing to target slowly over the first three days [26, 27]. The use of early EN has been associated with reduced mortality and a reduced risk for infection in meta-analyses, as well as maintenance of the integrity of the GI tract [61]. The use of PN is more conflicting, with guidelines suggesting PN be started between days 3 and 7 of ICU stay, or perhaps earlier in those at significant nutrition risk [26, 27, 62]. Despite guideline recommendations, it has been consistently documented that in usual care, energy and protein delivery is only approximately half that prescribed [37, 63]. Given the challenges associated with service delivery and the pressure on healthcare systems during a pandemic, nutrition delivery could be even lower in patients with COVID-19.

Oral nutrition intake has not been well investigated in critical illness. Recent data suggest that energy and protein intake is around 30% of prescription when no additional nutrition supplements are provided, both within the ICU and after ICU discharge [64, 65]. This is an important consideration in patients with COVID-19 who may have nutrition compromise before hospital admission, may be on NIV for extended periods, and may struggle to return to usual eating habits (barriers discussed later in "Organization and System Considerations for Nutrition Management" section).

In nonventilated patients, oral intake should be encouraged with close attention paid to adequacy. In patients who are IMV or in whom oral intake is inadequate, EN, provided by a gastric tube, should be the first line of nutrition considered. However, it should be acknowledged that in patients who are sedated, paralyzed, and may have GI tract edema, poor gastric motility is likely. Where GI intolerance occurs, postpyloric feeding may be considered, particularly where it is usual practice at that site to maintain safe practice. In centers where access to postpyloric feeding is infrequent or delayed, use of PN to supplement EN may be more appropriate to bridge the nutrition gap. Finally, where all other attempts fail, provision of total PN is appropriate. Due to the prolonged hospital duration for patients with severe COVID-19, close attention to nutrition is important to prevent cumulative deficits. Figure 20.3 provides a flowchart for decision making regarding modes of nutrition in the ICU, and Table 20.2 summarizes general nutrition guideline recommendations for critically ill patients.

Energy and Protein Requirements

A feature of critical illness is a significant metabolic response due to deranged hormonal and inflammatory responses [66]. Early in illness, a decrease in energy expenditure occurs (the ebb phase); the duration of which is directly proportional to the degree of injury/illness (more severe illness/injury/illness leads to longer shutdown). Although there is no defined "turning point" or biomarker that signals change in metabolic rate, approximately 48–72 hours after injury or illness metabolism changes to the "flow phase," characterized by significant increases in metabolic rate and breakdown of tissue (including muscle) to provide fuel for recovery [66]. The final phase more recently discussed is known as the "recovery phase." The recent European Society for Clinical Nutrition and Metabolism (ESPEN) guidelines have defined the early acute phase as days 1–2, the late acute phase as days 3–7, and the recovery phase as after day 7 [27]. Longer duration of illness, degree of inflammation, severity of COVID-19, and presence of fever, obesity, and high muscle mass are all associated with a higher metabolic rate. These factors should be considered when deciding what energy targets to deliver. The impact of disease phase, organ dysfunction, and inflammation on metabolism is summarized in Table 20.5 [67].

Estimation of Energy Expenditure

Energy expenditure is most commonly estimated using a predictive equation in critical illness due to their ease of application and availability. However, equations are known to be inaccurate when compared with a measured estimate because of individual body composition variation and extrapolation of the equation from the population in which they were developed compared with the population used [66, 68].

Predictive equations have greater inaccuracies at the extremes of weight, which is a significant issue given the high prevalence of obesity in patients with COVID-19. Clinical Practice Guidelines vary in their recommendations for energy delivery for obese critically ill patients, from hypocaloric, high-protein feeding (American Society of Parenteral and Enteral Nutrition/Society of Critical Care Medicine [ASPEN/SCCM]) to provision at the same level as patients within the healthy weight range, all informed by low-level evidence and without data as to the impact on functional recovery [69]. A study in 20 obese critically ill patients with a mean (standard deviation) body mass index (BMI) of 40.1 (8.6) kg/m^2 compared the ASPEN SCCM guideline recommendations for hypocaloric feeding to a measured expenditure and found that the median [interquartile range] guideline recommendation was 950 [595–1254] kcal lower than the measured expenditure at baseline [70]. It is common for obese patients to have a higher metabolic rate than lean counterparts because of their higher overall muscle mass (which is the greatest driver of metabolic rate), increasing the risk for underfeeding.

Indirect calorimetry is known to be the gold standard for assessing energy expenditure in critical illness by measuring oxygen consumption and carbon dioxide production via connection to a patient's mechanical ventilator, providing a direct assessment of the individual metabolic response [66] and an approximation of the resting metabolic rate. The technology is not widely used internationally, and some safety concerns have been raised with COVID-19 because of the risk for aerosol generation during setup and testing [16]. However, safe testing procedures have been proposed, and several studies have demonstrated it can be practically performed in this population within an ICU that has prior experience [27]. In 22 critically

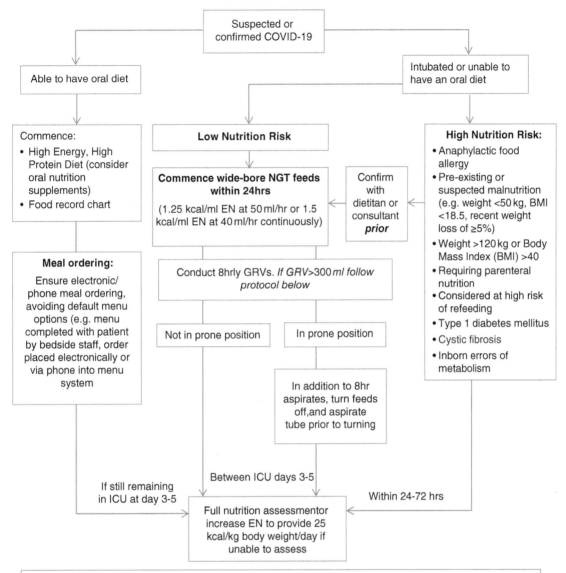

Figure 20.3 ICU nutrition algorithm for management of patients with COVID-19. *Source:* Adapted from Chapple et al. [16].

- Please use in conjunction with local nutrition policy and procedures.
- **The dietitian or treating consultant may elect to commence the standard algorithm in high nutrition risk patients**
- Medical and nursing teams to please contact the dietitian if a nutritional assessment is necessary earlier than stated in the algorithm.
- For first GRV >300ml commence prokinetics as per usual site practices (e.g. metoclopramide IV 10mg 6-hourly ***together with*** erythromycin IV 200mg bd) for 24 –72 hrs where possible and no contraindications exist.
- If GRV remains >300ml, despite prokinetics, consider post-pyloric feeding or supplemental PN.
- Nutrition support should be escalated if energy and protein delivery are <50% of prescribed targets for ≥5-7 days.

Table 20.5 Definition of disease phase in the course of critical illness.

Disease Phase	Organ Dysfunction	Inflammation	Metabolic State	Approximate Duration
Acute Phase				
Early acute phase	Severe or increasing (multiple) organ dysfunction	Progressive inflammation	Catabolic	• 1–3 days • In severe COVID-19, this phase may last >3 days. Inflammation and organ dysfunction should be used as an indicator
Late acute phase	Stable or improving organ dysfunction	Regressive inflammation	Catabolic-anabolic	• 2–4 days • In patients with severe COVID-19, this phase may occur after day 7
Postacute phase				
Convalescence/ rehabilitation	Largely restored function	Resolution of inflammation	Anabolic	• >7 days
Chronic phase	Persistent organ dysfunction	Persistent immune suppression	Catabolic	• >7 days • In severe COVID-19, this phase may last for weeks to months

Source: Adapted from Elke et al. [67].

ill patients with COVID-19 (mean BMI of 30.7 kg/m^2, 55% obese, and approximately 14% receiving NMB), the median [interquartile range] measured resting metabolic rate in obese individuals was 17.5 [12–19] kcal/kg actual body weight, 21 (20–23.5) kcal/kg, and 31.5 (24.8–36) kcal/kg on days 0–7, 7–14, and 14–21, respectively ($P < 0.05$). In nonobese individuals, it was 19.2 (16.9–20.7) kcal/kg actual body weight, 26 (24.5–35.5) kcal/kg, and 29 (23–34.5) kcal/kg on days 0–7, 7–14, and 14–21, respectively ($P < 0.05$) [10]. This increase in energy expenditure from day 3 of ICU stay was supported by a second study, indicating the change to the flow state of metabolism as illness progresses [56]. The duration of hypermetabolism is likely to be extended in severe COVID-19 and will be proportional to the severity of illness (with sicker patients being hypermetabolic for longer) [10, 71].

In summary, early in illness and regardless of patient BMI, a conservative energy estimate should be used at around 20 kcal/kg, increasing to 25 kcal/kg by days 3–5 [27]. From day 7, metabolic rate can increase in patients with COVID-19 to around 30 kcal/kg. There is no consensus as to which predictive equation is more accurate for use in patients with COVID-19; hence

close attention should be paid to factors that impact metabolism, and nutrition delivery should be quantified to avoid long-term nutrition consequences of overprovision or underprovision.

In obese critically ill patients, an adjusted body weight should be used to prevent overfeeding, with careful attention as to the phase and severity of illness. The modified Penn State Equation has shown to be the most accurate predictive equation in critically ill patients aged >60 years with a BMI > 30 [72]. Table 20.2 summarizes guideline recommendations for energy and protein needs, as well as the methods to adjust body weight in patients with obesity.

Nonnutritional Energy

Energy provided from nonnutritive sources should be monitored (including 25 and 50% dextrose [providing 4 kcal/g carbohydrate] and 1 and 2% propofol [provides 1.1 and 0.5 kcal/mL, respectively]). Lipid infusion rates should not exceed 0.11 g/kg/h or a maximum of 2 g/kg/day [73]; when PN is being provided with propofol, maximum infusion rates for lipid should be carefully monitored. Energy contribution from nonnutritional sources can be significant and can lead to overfeeding of energy; energy delivery from medical nutrition therapy may need to be modified to account for this, which may lead to protein deficit. Supplementation with an enteral protein supplement or an intravenous amino acid may be required to meet a basic recommendation of 1.2 g/kg protein delivery.

Protein

Limited definitive evidence exists as to the amount of protein that critically ill patients require, and the impact on outcomes is lacking. It is generally accepted that because of the degree of inflammation and catabolism associated with severe COVID-19, a minimum of 1.2 g/kg should be targeted. This is supported by clinical practice recommendations (Tables 20.2 and 20.3) [16, 26, 27].

Micronutrients and Trace Elements

Although there has been much interest in the role of micronutrients in the immune response to COVID-19, no definitive evidence exists as to a benefit above that recommended for normal health. It should be considered that with prolonged underprovision of energy and protein, micronutrients will also be suboptimal. Supplementation of micronutrients and trace elements to the normal recommended amounts for health may be necessary in patients with a long length of stay and in whom nutrition provision is inadequate or in those premorbidly malnourished. Micronutrients and trace elements should be provided as standard in PN to prevent deficiency.

Management of Complications

Hyperglycemia

Stress-induced hyperglycemia is common in critical illness (occurring in up to 50% of patients often without prior history of diabetes) and is a feature of severe COVID-19 due to increased inflammation and stress hormones such as cortisol related to glycemic control [74]. A blood glucose target of 6–10 mmol/L (106–180 mg/dl) is acceptable depending on region, with tighter targets associated with increased mortality [75]. A continuous insulin infusion directed via a guideline should be used to maintain the appropriate blood glucose target. The impact of nutrition on hyperglycemia is variable but is not often a significant contributing factor unless overfeeding with PN is occurring. Attention should be paid to overall glucose infusion rates, with an aim not to exceed the maximum glucose oxidation rate of 4–7 g/min/kg (5–10 g/kg/day), especially when PN is being provided [73]. Modifications to EN can be made by reducing the overall carbohydrate load while maintaining adequate energy delivery.

GI Intolerance

Patients with COVID-19 can present with GI symptoms such as nausea, vomiting, and diarrhea. This, along with the addition of multiple sedative and paralyzing agents for ventilation, can lead to intolerance in the form of raised gastric residual volumes (GRVs) and/or regurgitation/vomiting. In an analysis of 323 adult mechanically ventilated patients who received EN, 56% had an occurrence of raised GRVs, vomiting, or abdominal distention [76]. Feeding intolerance in ICU was independently associated with increased risk for death (hazard ratio, 3.32; 95% CI: 1.97–5.6), while presentation with one or more GI symptoms and obesity (BMI > 40) were both protective. GI intolerance has also been associated with higher 28-day mortality in patients without COVID-19 [77]. Hence GI intolerance should be managed but also observed as an indicator of potential negative outcome.

Monitoring of GI intolerance following normal site practices (using a GRV cutoff of 250–500 mL) is appropriate, and it is generally accepted that dual prokinetics of metoclopramide at 10 mg q.i.d. and erythromycin at 200 mg b.i.d. are the most effective in the absence of contraindications [78]. Although there are limited document reports, it appears that the risk for COVID-19 transmission from gastric contents appears to be low (and a question as to whether the virus would survive the low-pH environment of the GI tract); moreover, the PPE required in the hospital setting to prevent airborne transmission should be adequate to reduce any possible risk of transmission with exposure to gastric contents.

Constipation is common in critical illness [79] and likely to occur with significant and prolonged use of sedation, analgesia, and paralysis [80]. Constipation can cause abdominal distention, nausea, and vomiting [81] and may reduce EN delivery [80]. Although prophylactic laxative bowel regimens may be used in some clinical areas, there are limited data evaluating this treatment; consequently, a recommendation for their use is not supported [81].

Post-ICU Acute Care Management, Including Dysphagia and Multidisciplinary Care

In ICU survivors, nutrition deficits (particularly in patients consuming intake orally) are greater post-ICU than in the ICU, and for patients with COVID-19, a number of nutrition-impacting symptoms have been shown to persist after ICU discharge [35, 64]. These nutrition-impacting symptoms and their effect on nutrition intake and outcomes are presented in Figure 20.4 and discussed in further detail later [55, 82–93].

Dysphagia: Features and Recovery

In patients with COVID-19, iatrogenic causes and key body systems have been attributed to dysphagia onset and severity, in particular, injury to the respiratory and neurological systems [94]. A large proportion of patients admitted to the ICU require prolonged mechanical ventilation, known to contribute to subsequent dysphagia [95, 96], and two-thirds of ICU patients experiencing dysphagia present with at least one neurological symptom [97, 98].

From the evidence to date, up to 50% of patients admitted to the ICU for COVID-19 require swallow assessment [99], of which >90% are diagnosed with oropharyngeal dysphagia on initial assessment [94, 99–101]. Ongoing assessment and management of swallow function are key, because although the majority of patients return to their baseline diet, the rate of complete recovery at hospital discharge varies between 44% [100] and 70% [94, 99, 101]. In a group of 41 patients who required tracheostomy placement during their admission, at posthospital discharge follow-up (average 54 days), 17.1% still required some degree of food modification or limitations (e.g. avoiding hard textured foods or specific food preparation), and 4.9% of these patients were nil orally, thereby requiring EN [102]. Rehabilitation of swallow function should commence as early as possible [103] using principles of neuroplasticity to promote timely and meaningful recovery [104].

Multidisciplinary Care

Management and rehabilitation of nutrition, including swallowing function, after ICU admission requires a multidisciplinary approach [105]. Instrumental multidisciplinary assessments such as fiberoptic endoscopic evaluation can be incorporated into a rehabilitation framework to inform swallow function, inform oral intake recommendations, and optimize nutrition outcomes [106].

To provide adequate nutrition therapy in survivors of critical illness, ongoing monitoring of nutrition adequacy and potential barriers to intake are required. In general survivors of critical illness, nutrition deficits are greatest in patients receiving oral nutrition alone [35, 64], and hence the provision of EN until oral intake is established is recommended [16]. Close monitoring for patients receiving both oral and EN/PN is recommended with use of ward-based and nutrition assistants where staff pressures are present [16].

To optimize recovery, care should always be patient centered, empowering people to engage in care that is meaningful to them [107, 108]. Participation in treatment decisions and goal planning may require personal communication supports, because communication function is reduced for people admitted to the ICU during the COVID-19 pandemic [109]. Patient engagement in food choices and meal planning with considerations of personal and cultural beliefs can optimize intake.

Organization and System Considerations for Nutrition Management

Workforce and Stock/Supply Considerations

Quality care for critically ill patients requires a multidisciplinary approach [110]. This is particularly important in the context of a COVID-19 surge when usual human and physical resources might be stretched. In most settings, workforce expansion will be required.

Nutrition-Impacting Symptoms

Altered respiratory function
- Airway and respiratory function are impacted [93,95]
- Dyspnoea (shortness of breath) common [93,95]
- Alteration of breath-swallow synchrony impacting swallow efficiency and safety, can lead to reduced volume and textures of oral intake
- Frequency and extended duration of artificial ventilation delays recommencement of oral intake [102]

Cognitive & executive function
- Delirium prevalence up to 84% of patients in ICU [78]
- Persistent and protracted delirium beyond ICU, exacerbated by reduced reorientation practices due to visitor and staff restrictions [81]
- Mood disturbances including anxiety and depression reported in 1/3 general ICU patients 6 months after hospital discharge [82]
- Implications on swallow function, food refusal, appetite, and ability to self feed [79,90]

Dysphagia
- Difficulty or disordered swallow function
- Impacts across sensory and motor functions during the eating and swallowing process
- Efficiency of swallow (such as chewing) reduced [89,94]
- Safety during oral intake compromised (e.g. airway protection) [95, 96, 97]

Sensory loss
- Sensory loss may occur due to inflammation or direct injury of the neural pathways [83,84]
- Dampened or complete loss of taste (dysgeusia) [94]
- Dysnomia (loss of smell) commonly reported as initial symptom and can persist beyond hospital admission [85]
- Reduced enjoyment and hence volume of oral intake

Fatigue
- Most common symptom reported post discharge [86]
- 68% of survivors experienced persistent fatigue 4-6 weeks following discharge [87]
- Patients requiring hospitalisation for COVID-19 report protracted fatigue at 7 months [88]
- Implications on the ability to self-feed, chewing fatigue, and engagement in appetite-stimulating physical therapy [51]

Body function
- Volume of consumed calories and protein
- Ability to eat variety of food and fluid textures
- Ability to taste/smell food
- Sensation of satiety

Activities
- Self-feeding and manipulation of equipment
- Active engagement in rehabilitation activities
- Awareness of eating, and ability to consume a meal

Participation
- Social engagement at mealtimes
- Ability to eat in varied environments
- Enjoyment of oral intake

images: Flaticon.com

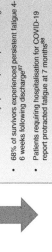
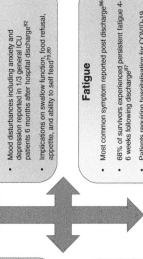

Figure 20.4 Nutrition-impacting symptoms. *Sources:* Helms et al. [82], Pandharipande et al. [83], and Merriweather et al. [84].

Identifying staff with skills transferrable to the acute care setting and who have previous hospital or ICU experience may be helpful [17]. A dedicated training package and education support are required to maintain high-quality and safe patient care. Skill sets should be considered when identifying those who can assist, ensuring a mix of senior and less experienced staff. Dietitians may also be well placed to assist with undertaking nutrition-related patient care more typically undertaken by nursing staff (e.g. assisting with changing EN formulae or giving sets). This is especially true if nursing staff from outside of the acute care environment are assisting and are unfamiliar with usual processes.

During a COVID-19 surge, it is likely that an increased number of nutritionally at-risk patients might be admitted to hospitals and the ICU. The use of protocolized nutrition orders may be helpful in ensuring timely initiation of EN for patients where volitional intake is not possible and for adjustment of EN targets throughout the patient's ICU stay [16]. These strategies may help ensure initiation and progression of EN when a dietitian is unable to review patients as regularly as might occur during usual practice. A balance between minimizing patient contact but also providing the best quality care needs to be found. An increased scope of practice for dietitians with tasks such as nasogastric or postpyloric feeding tube insertion may assist in alleviating nursing and medical workload; however, practice changes such as these should be planned before implementation. When additional staff are being used to assist with workload, the most experienced staff should see the sickest patients and oversee the work of more inexperienced staff.

Consideration should also be given to availability of equipment and formula, which can be disrupted by supply and logistic factors, as well as increased demands. Early engagement of local government, health agencies, and networks to secure additional stock is recommended. Forecasting of patients requiring nutrition supplements, medical nutrition therapy products, and hardware such as feeding pumps, nasogastric tubes, and giving sets should be done early, and strategies to manage shortage in any areas planned. This might include ensuring the availability of gravity feeding sets with a protocol ready to be implemented to ensure patients are able to receive EN, even when enteral feeding pumps are unavailable.

Food Service Considerations

The patient's ability to select their own food greatly impacts nutrition intake [111]. A challenge that has presented itself during the COVID-19 pandemic is that food service staff have been deemed nonessential for clinical care, and therefore in many organizations they are unable to enter "hot zones." Depending on the hospital's food service system, this may present a challenge for food ordering and delivery. Strategies such as electronic applications or phone ordering should be implemented to ensure patients receive meal choices [16]. The development of a default COVID-19 diet protocol may also be beneficial to provide high-energy and high-protein foods, including supplements, for patients awaiting nutrition assessment by a dietitian or to manage low-risk patients, as per the earlier recommendations [16].

Organization-wide food service contingency planning should be undertaken to plan for events where food service staff or the facilities are impacted and/or furloughed because of a COVID-19 outbreak. This may include backup food supplies in storage, such as frozen meals, and additional staff who could provide assistance in the event of staff shortages [16].

Considerations in an Overwhelmed Hospital System

The overall goal should be to maintain as close as possible to usual care, but when changes are required, to ensure care is safe. Preplanning is critical to ensure strategies are in place to respond to periods of staff shortages, and education and support are available to allow inexperienced staff to work safely in complex conditions and the likely possibility of stock and equipment shortages.

Follow-up for COVID-19-Related Nutrition Issues After Hospital Discharge

As the COVID-19 pandemic becomes endemic, considerations for long-term follow-up need to be developed [17]. At least 50% of ICU survivors report a new mild disability six months after hospital discharge, with reduced rates of self-reported quality of life compared with their preadmission function [112]. A portion of patients who have had COVID-19 will also develop long-COVID, with risk factors including preexisting frailty and functional impairment, a prolonged ICU stay, delirium, and sepsis.

Developed by the Intensive Care Society in conjunction with other multidisciplinary organizations, the Post-ICU Presentation Screen tool identifies nutrition and swallow function as key items requiring ongoing assessment and management [113]. Persistent symptoms in survivors of COVID-19 may impact nutrition and return to normal eating, including fatigue, reduced function, and pain one year after diagnosis. Specific multidisciplinary guidance exists for ICU follow-up after COVID-19, which needs to extend beyond hospital discharge, with follow-up screening recommended at a minimum of 2–6 weeks after discharge and again at 12 weeks and beyond [17]. Items to discuss with survivors should include weight check at each appointment, ongoing or new nutrition-impacting symptoms, and functional issues that may impact access to food or shopping and cooking. Figure 20.5 provides a summary of 12 items that should be considered at and after hospital discharge in relation to nutrition.

Conclusion

Attention to nutrition provision and care processes should be paid for all patients hospitalized with COVID-19. At a minimum, patients should be screened on admission to hospital to determine the level of nutrition intervention required. In patients with severe COVID-19, the development of malnutrition and significant nutrition deficits are likely if nutrition is not prioritized as an important element of care. Patients with severe COVID-19 are likely to have challenges with nutrition provision due to the disease process itself, but also other treatments provided to them (including resulting in GI intolerance, prolonged hypermetabolism, delayed and interrupted nutrition provision). Workforce and models of care should be arranged to provide the best quality, safe care that the available resources allow. This may include using staff with external skills who can assist, support staff, and train new staff to assist. All patients who have been hospitalized for COVID-19 should be considered for nutrition-impacting symptoms during recovery and at hospital discharge, and particular focus should be given to those who have had severe disease and/or a long hospital stay. Support and attention should be paid to addressing factors likely to impact nutrition after discharge, including the ability to prepare food, shop and cook, the degree of weakness, and the existing presence of long COVID.

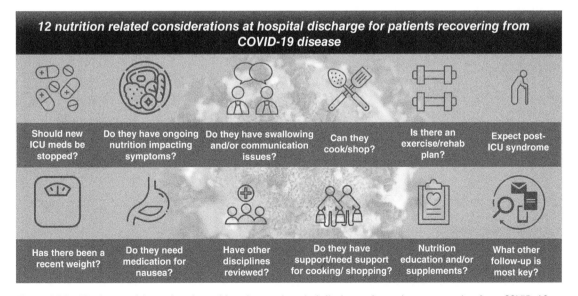

Figure 20.5 Twelve nutrition-related considerations at hospital discharge for patients recovering from COVID-19. *Source:* Adapted from Iwashyna et al. [114].

References

1 Minnelli, N., Gibbs, L., Larrivee, J. et al. (2020). Challenges of maintaining optimal nutrition status in COVID-19 patients in intensive care settings. *J. Parenter. Enteral Nutr.* 44 (8): 1439–1446.

2 Liu, D., Cui, P., Zeng, S. et al. (2020). Risk factors for developing into critical COVID-19 patients in Wuhan, China: a multicenter, retrospective, cohort study. *EClinicalMedicine* 25: 100471.

3 Giacomelli, A., Pezzati, L., Conti, F. et al. (2020). Self-reported olfactory and taste disorders in patients with severe acute respiratory coronavirus 2 infection: a cross-sectional study. *Clin. Infect. Dis.* 71 (15): 889–890.

4 Di Filippo, L., De Lorenzo, R., D'Amico, M. et al. (2021). COVID-19 is associated with clinically significant weight loss and risk of malnutrition, independent of hospitalisation: a post-hoc analysis of a prospective cohort study. *Clin. Nutr.* 40 (4): 2420–2426.

5 Pan, L., Mu, M., Yang, P. et al. (2020). Clinical characteristics of COVID-19 patients with digestive symptoms in Hubei, China: a descriptive, cross-sectional, multicenter study. *Am. J. Gastroenterol.* 115: 766–773.

6 Guan, W.-j., Ni, Z.-y., Hu, Y. et al. (2020). Clinical characteristics of coronavirus disease 2019 in China. *N. Engl. J. Med.* 382 (18): 1708–1720.

7 Huang, B.Y., Tsai, M.R., Hsu, J.K. et al. (2020). Longitudinal change of metabolite profile and its relation to multiple risk factors for the risk of developing hepatitis B-related hepatocellular carcinoma. *Mol. Carcinog.* 59 (11): 1269–1279.

8 Wang, D., Hu, B., Hu, C. et al. (2020). Clinical characteristics of 138 hospitalized patients with 2019 novel coronavirus–infected pneumonia in Wuhan, China. *JAMA* 323 (11): 1061–1069.

9 Richardson, S., Hirsch, J.S., Narasimhan, M. et al. (2020). Presenting characteristics, comorbidities, and outcomes among 5700 patients hospitalized with COVID-19 in the New York City area. *JAMA* 323 (20): 2052–2059.

10 Whittle, J., Molinger, J., MacLeod, D. et al. (2020). Persistent hypermetabolism and longitudinal energy expenditure in critically ill patients with COVID-19. *Crit. Care* 24 (1): 581.

11 Zhou, F., Yu, T., Du, R. et al. (2020). Clinical course and risk factors for mortality of adult inpatients with COVID-19 in Wuhan, China: a retrospective cohort study. *Lancet* 395 (10229): 1054–1062.

12 Del Bene, V.E. (1990). Temperature. In: *Clinical Methods: The History, Physical, and Laboratory Examinations*, 3e. Boston: Butterworths.

13 Prompetchara, E., Ketloy, C., and Palaga, T. (2020). Immune responses in COVID-19 and potential vaccines: lessons learned from SARS and MERS epidemic. *Asian Pac. J. Allergy Immunol.* 38 (1): 1–9.

14 Haraj, N.E., El Aziz, S., Chadli, A. et al. (2021). Nutritional status assessment in patients with Covid-19 after discharge from the intensive care unit. *Clin. Nutr. ESPEN* 41: 423–428.

15 Damanti, S., Cristel, G., Ramirez, G.A. et al. (2021). Influence of reduced muscle mass and quality on ventilator weaning and complications during intensive care unit stay in COVID-19 patients. *Clin. Nutr.* https://doi.org/10.1016/j.clnu.2021.08.004.

16 Chapple, L.S., Fetterplace, K., Asrani, V. et al. (2020). Nutrition management for critically and acutely unwell hospitalised patients with coronavirus disease 2019 (COVID-19) in Australia and New Zealand. *Aust. Crit. Care* 33 (5): 399–406.

17 Australian and New Zealand Intensive Care Society (ANZICS) (2020). ANZICS COVID-19 Guidelines Version 4. Melbourne, Australia; ANZICS; https://www.anzics.com.au/wp-content/uploads/2021/09/ANZICS-COVID-19-Guidelines-Version-4.pdf.

18 Marshall, A.P., Austin, D.E., Chamberlain, D. et al. (2021). A critical care pandemic staffing framework in Australia. *Aust. Crit. Care* 34 (2): 123–131.

19 Mulherin, D.W., Walker, R., Holcombe, B. et al. (2020). ASPEN report on nutrition support practice processes with COVID-19: the first response. *Nutr. Clin. Pract.* 35 (5): 783–791.

20 World Health Organization (2020). Clinical management of COVID-19: interim guidance, Geneva: World Health Organization.

21 Rochwerg, B., Siemieniuk, R.A., Agoritsas, T. et al. (2020). A living WHO guideline on drugs for covid-19. *BMJ* 370: m3379.

22 Wei, C., Liu, Y., Li, Y. et al. (2020). Evaluation of the nutritional status in patients with COVID-19. *J. Clin. Biochem.* 67 (2): 116–121.

23 Rives-Lange, C., Zimmer, A., Merazka, A. et al. (2021). Evolution of the nutritional status of

COVID-19 critically-ill patients: a prospective observational study from ICU admission to three months after ICU discharge. *Clin. Nutr.* https://doi.org/10.1016/j.clnu.2021.05.007.

24 Mendes, A., Serratrice, C., Herrmann, F.R. et al. (2021). Nutritional risk at hospital admission is associated with prolonged length of hospital stay in old patients with COVID-19. *Clin. Nutr.* https://doi.org/10.1016/j.clnu.2021.03.017.

25 Bedock, D., Lassen, P.B., Mathian, A. et al. (2020). Prevalence and severity of malnutrition in hospitalized COVID-19 patients. *Clin. Nutr. ESPEN* 40: 214–219.

26 McClave, S.A., Taylor, B.E., Martindale, R.G. et al. (2016). Guidelines for the provision and assessment of nutrition support therapy in the adult critically ill patient: Society of Critical Care Medicine (SCCM) and American Society for Parenteral and Enteral Nutrition (ASPEN). *JPEN J. Parenter. Enteral Nutr.* 40 (2): 159–211.

27 Singer, P., Blaser, A.R., Berger, M.M. et al. (2019). ESPEN guideline on clinical nutrition in the intensive care unit. *Clin. Nutr.* 38 (1): 48–79.

28 Irish Nutrition and Dietetic Institute (2020). COVID-19 Dietetic care pathway Version 1 and guides to commencing enteral and parenteral nutrition in adult patients in intensive care with suspected or confirmed COVID-19 Version 2. https://learning.indi.ie/course/view.php?id=47

29 Kondrup, J., Allison, S.P., Elia, M. et al. (2003). ESPEN guidelines for nutrition screening 2002. *Clin. Nutr.* 22 (4): 415–421.

30 Anbar, R, Poulin, D, Dolgich-Maza, M, et al. (2020). Feeding the critically Ill mechanically ventilated patient during the COVID-19 epidemic. https://www.atid-eatright.org.il/prdFiles/Feeding%20the%20Critically%20Ill%20Mechanically%20Ventilated%20Patient%20during%20the%20Covid%20%D7%A1%D7%95%D7%A4%D7%99.pdf.

31 Jensen, G.L., Cederholm, T., Correia, M. et al. (2019). GLIM criteria for the diagnosis of malnutrition: a consensus report from the global clinical nutrition community. *JPEN J. Parenter. Enteral Nutr.* 43 (1): 32–40.

32 Anthony, P.S. (2008). Nutrition screening tools for hospitalized patients. *Nutr. Clin. Pract.* 23 (4): 373–382.

33 Reber, E., Gomes, F., Vasiloglou, M.F. et al. (2019). Nutritional risk screening and assessment. *J. Clin. Med.* 8 (7): 1065.

34 Barazzoni, R., Bischoff, S.C., Breda, J. et al. (2020). ESPEN expert statements and practical guidance for nutritional management of individuals with SARS-CoV-2 infection. *Lijec. Vjesn* 142 (3-4): 75–84.

35 Chapple, L.S., Deane, A.M., Heyland, D.K. et al. (2016). Energy and protein deficits throughout hospitalization in patients admitted with a traumatic brain injury. *Clin. Nutr.* 35 (6): 1315–1322.

36 Pironi, L., Sasdelli, A.S., Ravaioli, F. et al. (2021). Malnutrition and nutritional therapy in patients with SARS-CoV-2 disease. *Clin. Nutr.* 40 (3): 1330–1337.

37 Ridley, E.J., Peake, S.L., Jarvis, M. et al. (2018). Nutrition therapy in Australia and New Zealand intensive care units: an international comparison study. *JPEN J. Parenter. Enteral Nutr.* 42 (8): 1349–1357.

38 Reintam Blaser, A., Starkopf, J., Alhazzani, W. et al. (2017). Early enteral nutrition in critically ill patients: ESICM clinical practice guidelines. *Intensive Care Med.* 43 (3): 380–398.

39 Indian Dietetic Association. MNT guidelines for COVID-19. Indian guidance for COVID-19 patients. (2020). http://idaindia.com/mnt-guirdelines-for-covid-19.

40 Barazzoni, R., Bischoff, S.C., Breda, J. et al. (2020). ESPEN expert statements and practical guidance for nutritional management of individuals with SARS-CoV-2 infection. *Clin. Nutr.* 39 (6): 1631–1638.

41 Bear, D and Terblanche, E. (2020). Critical Care Specialist Group Guidance on management of nutrition and dietetic services during the COVID-19 pandemic, Version 2.1. https://www.bda.uk.com/resource/critical-care-dietetics-guidance-covid-19.html (accessed 11 May 2020).

42 Campos, L.F., Barreto, P.A., Duprat, G., et al. BRASPEN's nutritional statement for coping with COVID-19 in hospitalized patients. https://www.cfn.org.br/wp-content/uploads/2020/03/Parecer-BRASPEN-COVID-19.pdf.pdf (accessed 23 Mar 2020).

43 Cena, H., Maffoni, S., Braschi, V. et al. (2020). Position paper of the Italian association of medical specialists in dietetics and clinical nutrition (ANSISA) on nutritional management of patients with COVID-19 disease. *Med. J. Nutrition Metab.* 13 (2): 113–117.

44 Martindale, R., Patel, J.J., Taylor, B. et al. (2020). Nutrition therapy in critically ill patients with coronavirus disease 2019. *JPEN J. Parenter. Enteral Nutr.* 44 (7): 1174–1184.

45 Singer, P., Pichard, C., and De Waele, E. (2020). Practical guidance for the use of indirect calorimetry during COVID 19 pandemic. *Clin. Nutr. Exp.* 33: 18–23.

46 Turkish Dietetic Association (2020). Turkish dietetic association's recommendations on nutrition and COVID-19. EFAD. https://www.efad.org/wp-content/uploads/2022/04/turkish-dietetic-association-nutrition-recommendations-about-coronavirus-covid-19-1.pdf.

47 Armstrong, R.A., Kane, A.D., Kursumovic, E. et al. (2021). Mortality in patients admitted to intensive care with COVID-19: an updated systematic review and meta-analysis of observational studies. *Anaesthesia* 76 (4): 537–548.

48 Frat, J.P., Thille, A.W., Mercat, A. et al. (2015). High-flow oxygen through nasal cannula in acute hypoxemic respiratory failure. *N. Engl. J. Med.* 372 (23): 2185–2196.

49 Arizono, S., Oomagari, M., Tawara, Y. et al. (2021). Effects of different high-flow nasal cannula flow rates on swallowing function. *Clin. Biomech. (Bristol, Avon)* 89: 105477.

50 Steele, C.M. and Cichero, J.A. (2014). Physiological factors related to aspiration risk: a systematic review. *Dysphagia* 29 (3): 295–304.

51 Brodsky, M.B., Suiter, D.M., Gonzalez-Fernandez, M. et al. (2016). Screening accuracy for aspiration using bedside water swallow tests: a systematic review and meta-analysis. *Chest* 150 (1): 148–163.

52 Burrell, A.J., Broadley, T., and Udy, A.A. (2021). Outcomes for patients with COVID-19 admitted to Australian intensive care units during the first four months of the pandemic. *Med. J. Aust.* 214: 23–30.

53 National Institutes of Health. COVID-19 Treatment Guidelines Panel. Coronavirus disease 2019 (COVID-19) treatment guidelines. 2021. https://www.covid19treatmentguidelines.nih.gov. Accessed 5 Nov 2021.

54 Alhazzani, W., Evans, L., Alshamsi, F. et al. (2021). Surviving sepsis campaign guidelines on the management of adults with coronavirus disease 2019 (COVID-19) in the ICU: first update. *Crit. Care Med.* 49 (3): e219–e234.

55 Chapple, L., Weinel, L., Abdelhamid, Y. et al. (2018). Observed appetite and nutrient intake three months after ICU discharge. *Clin. Nutr.* 38 (3): 1215–1220.

56 Karayiannis, D., Maragkouti, A., Mikropoulos, T. et al. (2021). Neuromuscular blockade administration is associated with altered energy expenditure in critically ill intubated patients with COVID-19. *Clin. Nutr.* https://doi.org/10.1016/j.clnu.2021.05.009.

57 Guerin, C., Reignier, J., Richard, J.C. et al. (2013). Prone positioning in severe acute respiratory distress syndrome. *N. Engl. J. Med.* 368 (23): 2159–2168.

58 Ehrmann, S., Li, J., Ibarra-Estrada, M. et al. (2021). Awake prone positioning for COVID-19 acute hypoxaemic respiratory failure: a randomised, controlled, multinational, open-label meta-trial. *Lancet Respir. Med.* 9: 1387–1395.

59 Barbaro, R.P., MacLaren, G., Boonstra, P.S. et al. (2020). Extracorporeal membrane oxygenation support in COVID-19: an international cohort study of the extracorporeal life support organization registry. *Lancet* 396 (10257): 1071–1078.

60 Alfred ECMO Guideline. Nutrition. 2021. https://ecmo.icu/daily-care-organ-support-in-ecmo-nutrition/?parent=menuautoanchor-44&def=true. Accessed 5 Nov 2021.

61 Doig, G.S., Heighes, P.T., Simpson, F. et al. (2009). Early enteral nutrition, provided within 24 h of injury or intensive care unit admission, significantly reduces mortality in critically ill patients: a meta-analysis of randomised controlled trials. *Intensive Care Med.* 35 (12): 2018–2027.

62 Ridley, E.J. (2021). Parenteral nutrition in critical illness: total, supplemental or never? *Curr. Opin. Clin. Nutr. Metab. Care* 24 (2): 176–182.

63 Cahill, N.E., Dhaliwal, R., Day, A.G. et al. (2010). Nutrition therapy in the critical care setting: what is "best achievable" practice? An international multicenter observational study. *Crit. Care Med.* 38 (2): 395–401.

64 Ridley, E.J., Parke, R.L., Davies, A.R. et al. (2019). What happens to nutrition intake in the post–intensive care unit hospitalization period? An observational cohort study in critically ill adults. *JPEN J. Parenter. Enteral Nutr.* 43 (1): 88–95.

65 Moisey, L.L., Pikul, J., Keller, H. et al. (2021). Adequacy of protein and energy intake in critically ill adults following liberation from mechanical ventilation is dependent on route of nutrition delivery. *Nutr. Clin. Pract.* 36 (1): 201–212.

66 Lambell, K.J., Tatucu-Babet, O.A., Chapple, L.A. et al. (2020). Nutrition therapy in critical illness: a review of the literature for clinicians. *Crit. Care* 24 (1): 35.

67 Elke, G., Hartl, W.H., Kreymann, K.G. et al. (2019). Clinical nutrition in critical care medicine – guideline of the German Society for Nutritional Medicine (DGEM). *Clin. Nutr. ESPEN* 33: 220–275.

68 Tatucu-Babet, O.A., Ridley, E.J., and Tierney, A.C. (2016). Prevalence of underprescription or overprescription of energy needs in critically ill mechanically ventilated adults as determined by indirect calorimetry: a systematic literature review. *JPEN J. Parenter. Enteral Nutr.* 40 (2): 212–225.

69 Ridley, E.J., Lambell, K., and Peake, S. (2019). Obesity and nutrition in critical illness. *ICU Manag. Pract.* 19 (3): 162–166.

70 Ridley, E.J., Tierney, A., King, S. et al. (2020). Measured energy expenditure compared with best-practice recommendations for obese, critically ill patients – a prospective observational study. *JPEN J. Parenter. Enteral Nutr.* 44 (6): 1144–1149.

71 Niederer, L.E., Miller, H., Haines, K.L. et al. (2021). Prolonged progressive hypermetabolism during COVID-19 hospitalization undetected by common predictive energy equations. *Clin. Nutr. ESPEN* 45: 341–350.

72 Frankenfield, D. (2011). Validation of an equation for resting metabolic rate in older obese, critically ill patients. *JPEN J. Parenter. Enteral Nutr.* 35 (2): 264–269.

73 Sobotka, L. (ed.) (2011). *Basics in Clinical Nutrition*, 4e. Czech Republic: Publishing House Galen.

74 Nickson, C. (2020). Stress induced hyperglycaemia. Life in the Fastlane. https://litfl.com/stress-induced-hyperglycaemia. Accessed 5 Nov 2021.

75 Investigators, N.-S.S., Finfer, S., Chittock, D.R. et al. (2009). Intensive versus conventional glucose control in critically ill patients. *N. Engl. J. Med.* 360 (13): 1283–1297.

76 Liu, R., Paz, M., Siraj, L. et al. (2021). Feeding intolerance in critically ill patients with COVID-19. *Clin. Nutr.* https://doi.org/10.1016/j.clnu.2021.03.033.

77 Reintam Blaser, A., Poeze, M., Malbrain, M.L. et al. (2013). Gastrointestinal symptoms during the first week of intensive care are associated with poor outcome: a prospective multicentre study. *Intensive Care Med.* 39 (5): 899–909.

78 Nguyen, N.Q., Chapman, M., Fraser, R.J. et al. (2007). Prokinetic therapy for feed intolerance in critical illness: one drug or two? *Crit. Care Med.* 35 (11): 2561–2567.

79 Chapman, M.J., Nguyen, N.Q., and Deane, A.M. (2013). Gastrointestinal dysmotility: evidence and clinical management. *Curr. Opin. Clin. Nutr. Metab. Care* 16 (2): 209–216.

80 Patel, P.B., Brett, S.J., O'Callaghan, D. et al. (2020). Methylnaltrexone for the treatment of opioid-induced constipation and gastrointestinal stasis in intensive care patients. Results from the MOTION trial. *Intensive Care Med.* 46 (4): 747–755.

81 Hay, T., Bellomo, R., Rechnitzer, T. et al. (2019). Constipation, diarrhea, and prophylactic laxative bowel regimens in the critically ill: a systematic review and meta-analysis. *J. Crit. Care* 52: 242–250.

82 Helms, J., Kremer, S., Merdji, H. et al. (2020). Delirium and encephalopathy in severe COVID-19: a cohort analysis of ICU patients. *Crit. Care* 24 (1): 491.

83 Pandharipande, P.P., Ely, E.W., Arora, R.C. et al. (2017). The intensive care delirium research agenda: a multinational, interprofessional perspective. *Intensive Care Med.* 43 (9): 1329–1339.

84 Merriweather, J.L., Salisbury, L.G., Walsh, T.S. et al. (2016). Nutritional care after critical illness: a qualitative study of patients' experiences. *J. Hum. Nutr. Diet.* 29 (2): 127–136.

85 Hosey, M.M. and Needham, D.M. (2020). Survivorship after COVID-19 ICU stay. *Nat. Rev. Dis. Primers.* 6 (1): 60.

86 Ahmed, H., Patel, K., Greenwood, D.C. et al. (2020). Long-term clinical outcomes in survivors of severe acute respiratory syndrome and Middle East respiratory syndrome coronavirus outbreaks after hospitalisation or ICU admission: a systematic review and meta-analysis. *J. Rehabil. Med.* 52 (5): jrm00063.

87 Vergara, J., Lirani-Silva, C., Brodsky, M.B. et al. (2021). Potential influence of olfactory, gustatory, and pharyngolaryngeal sensory dysfunctions on swallowing physiology in COVID-19. *Otolaryngol. Head Neck Surg.* 164 (6): 1134–1135.

88 Najjar, S., Najjar, A., Chong, D.J. et al. (2020). Central nervous system complications associated with SARS-CoV-2 infection: integrative concepts of pathophysiology and case reports. *J. Neuroinflammation* 17 (1): 231.

89 Hopkins, C., Surda, P., Whitehead, E. et al. (2020). Early recovery following new onset anosmia during the COVID-19 pandemic – an observational cohort study. *J. Otolaryngol. Head Neck Surg.* 49: 26.

90 Cares-Marambio, K., Montenegro-Jimenez, Y., Torres-Castro, R. et al. (2021). Prevalence of potential respiratory symptoms in survivors of hospital admission after coronavirus disease 2019 (COVID-19): a systematic review and meta-analysis. *Chron. Respir. Dis.* 18: 14799731211002240.

91 D'Cruz, RA-O, Waller, MA-O, Perrin, F, et al. (2021). Chest radiography is a poor predictor of respiratory symptoms and functional impairment in survivors of severe COVID-19 pneumonia. *ERJ Open Res.* 10.1183/23120541.00655-2020.

92 Fernández-de-las-Peñas, C., Palacios-Ceña, D., Gómez-Mayordomo, V. et al. (2022). Fatigue and dyspnoea as main persistent post-COVID-19 symptoms in previously hospitalized patients: related functional limitations and disability. *Respiration* 101 (2): 132–141.

93 Dziewas, R., Warnecke, T., Zürcher, P. et al. (2020). Dysphagia in COVID-19 – multilevel damage to the swallowing network? *Eur. J. Neurol.* 27: e46–e47.

94 Archer, S.K., Iezzi, C.M., and Gilpin, L. (2021). Swallowing and voice outcomes in patients hospitalized with COVID-19: an observational cohort study. *Arch. Phys. Med. Rehabil.* 102 (6): 1084–1090.

95 Brodsky, M.B., Levy, M.J., Jedlanek, E. et al. (2018). Laryngeal injury and upper airway symptoms after oral endotracheal intubation with mechanical ventilation during critical care: a systematic review. *Crit. Care Med.* 46 (12): 2010, 2017.

96 Brodsky, M.B., Nollet, J.L., Spronk, P.E. et al. (2020). Prevalence, pathophysiology, diagnostic modalities, and treatment options for dysphagia in critically ill patients. *Am. J. Phys. Med. Rehabil.* 99 (12): 1164–1170.

97 Lima, M.S., Sassi, F.C., Medeiros, G.C. et al. (2020). Preliminary results of a clinical study to evaluate the performance and safety of swallowing in critical patients with COVID-19. *Clinics* 75: e2021.

98 Martin-Martinez, A., Ortega, O., Viñas, P. et al. (2021). COVID-19 is associated with oropharyngeal dysphagia and malnutrition in hospitalized patients during the spring 2020 wave of the pandemic. *Clin. Nutr.* https://doi.org/10.1016/j.clnu.2021.06.010.

99 Dawson, C., Capewell, R., Ellis, S. et al. (2020). Dysphagia presentation and management following coronavirus disease 2019: an acute care tertiary Centre experience. *J. Laryngol.* 134 (11): 981–986.

100 Osbeck Sandblom, H., Dotevall, H., Svennerholm, K. et al. (2021). Characterization of dysphagia and laryngeal findings in COVID-19 patients treated in the ICU – an observational clinical study. *PLoS One* 16 (6): e0252347.

101 Regan, J., Walshe, M., Lavan, S. et al. (2021). Post-extubation dysphagia and dysphonia amongst adults with COVID-19 in the Republic of Ireland: a prospective multi-site observational cohort study. *Clin. Otolaryngol.* 46 (6): 1290–1299.

102 Rouhani, M.J., Clunie, G., Thong, G. et al. (2021). A prospective study of voice, swallow, and airway outcomes following tracheostomy for COVID-19. *Laryngoscope* 131 (6): E1918–E1925.

103 Freeman-Sanderson, A., Ward, E.C., Miles, A. et al. (2021). A consensus statement for the management and rehabilitation of communication and swallowing function in the ICU: a global response to COVID-19. *Arch. Phys. Med. Rehabil.* 102 (5): 835–842.

104 Langton-Frost, N. and Brodsky, M. (2022). Speech-language pathology approaches to neurorehabilitation in acute care during COVID-19: capitalizing on neuroplasticity. *PM R* 14 (2): 217–226.

105 Brodsky, M.B., Pandian, V., and Needham, D.M. (2020). Post-extubation dysphagia: a problem needing multidisciplinary efforts. *Intensive Care Med.* 46 (1): 93–96.

106 Boggiano, S., Williams, T., Gill, S.E. et al. (2021). Multidisciplinary management of laryngeal pathology identified in patients with COVID-19 following trans-laryngeal intubation and tracheostomy. *J. Intensive Care Soc.* https://doi.org/10.1177/17511437211034699.

107 Tobiano, G., Jerofke-Owen, T., and Marshall, A.P. (2021). Promoting patient engagement: a scoping review of actions that align with the interactive care model. *Scand. J. Caring Sci.* 35 (3): 722–741.

108 Haines, K.J., Hibbert, E., Leggett, N. et al. (2021). Transitions of care after critical illness – challenges to recovery and adaptive problem solving. *Crit. Care Med.* 49 (11): 1923–1931.

109 Freeman-Sanderson, A., Rose, L., and Brodsky, M.B. (2020). Coronavirus disease 2019 (COVID-19) cuts ties with patients' outside world. *Aust. Crit. Care* 33 (5): 397–398.

110 Parker, A.M., Brigham, E., Connolly, B. et al. (2021). Addressing the post-acute sequelae of SARS-CoV-2 infection: a multidisciplinary model of care. *Lancet Respir. Med.* 9: 1328–1341.

111 Dijxhoorn, D.N., Mortier, M., van den Berg, M.G.A. et al. (2019). The currently available literature on inpatient foodservices: systematic review and critical appraisal. *J. Acad. Nutr. Diet.* 119 (7): 1118–41.e36.

112 Hodgson, C.L., Udy, A.A., Bailey, M. et al. (2017). The impact of disability in survivors of critical illness. *Intensive Care Med.* 43 (7): 992–1001.

113 UKROC Rehabilitation Collaborative, Kings College London; Turner-Stokes L; members of the Intensive Care Society working group 2021. The Post-ICU Presentation Screen (PICUPS). Kings College London and Intensive Care Society UK. https://www.rcslt.org/wp-content/uploads/media/docs/Covid/202006--ICSPICUPSTool.pdf. (accessed 5 Nov 2021).

114 Iwashyna, J. et al. (2022). The dirty dozen: common errors on discharging patients recovering from critical illness. Life in the Fast Lane.https://litfl.com/the-dirty-dozen-common-errors-on-discharging-patients-recovering-from-critical-illness.

21

COVID-19: Nursing Perspective

Michelle Zappas[1], Dalia Copti[1], Cynthia Sanchez[1], Janett A. Hildebrand[1], and Sharon O'Neill[2]

[1] *Department of Nursing, Suzanne Dworak-Peck School of Social Work, University of Southern California, Los Angeles, CA, USA*
[2] *New York University Rory Meyers College of Nursing, New York, NY, USA*

Abbreviations

ARDS	acute respiratory distress syndrome
BiPAP	bilevel positive airway pressure
CDC	Centers for Disease Control and Prevention
HFNC	high-flow nasal cannula
ICT	interdisciplinary care team
ICU	intensive care unit
IL-6	interleukin-6
NIV	noninvasive ventilation
PPE	personal protective equipment
POC	people of color

On 11 March 2020, the World Health Organization declared a coronavirus disease 2019 (COVID-19) pandemic. Ironically, during 2020, nurses celebrated the year of the nurse and midwife. Nurses understand the irony that this unprecedented global pandemic hit during this year. As most Americans sheltered in place, nurses and other healthcare professionals continued to go to work and deliver quality care to their patients. Nurses have been at the forefront of all aspects of patient care – from systems planning, surge response, education of the public, triage, treating patients, discharging patients, and more recently in vaccination efforts. In the inpatient setting, nurses monitored and provided empathic care to critically ill patients who were facing intense isolation and fear.

Crisis care, the care provided during much of the COVID-19 pandemic, impacts patients, families, communities, and healthcare providers [1]. Clinicians have faced moral and ethical conflicts during this time. Stress, fatigue, lack of time, increased patient volume, and workload with an unprecedented demand for expertise and experience have impacted our healthcare system. Nurses respond to surges in patients and workloads and accommodate new procedures, protocols, and forming a new normal.

Care of the Patient in the Inpatient Setting

Resources

Personal Protective Equipment

In prepandemic times, intensive care units (ICUs) averaged 90% full, with limited capacity and resources for the surges of critically ill patients as seen during the COVID-19 pandemic [2]. Adequate personal protective equipment (PPE) has been an issue since early on in the pandemic. As the United States realized that PPE demand far exceeded its supply, the Centers for Disease Control and Prevention (CDC) restructured its guidelines to allow hospitals to amend their PPE policies. Healthcare workers were permitted and even encouraged to reuse PPE, moving from patient to patient without changing their masks or gowns [3]. Although this seems unique and outside standard practices, it is a response that aligns with guidelines

Coronavirus Disease 2019 (COVID-19): A Clinical Guide, First Edition. Edited by Ali Gholamrezanezhad and Michael P. Dube.
© 2023 John Wiley & Sons Ltd. Published 2023 by John Wiley & Sons Ltd.

during disasters and emergencies when the focus is on saving as many lives as possible. When resources are scarce, the focus changes from the individual patient to improving outcomes for larger groups of people [4–6]. This change in focus is consistent with the crisis capacity as defined by the Institute of Medicine in 2010 [7]: "Crisis capacity is defined as adapting spaces, staff, and resources so that . . . you're doing the best you can with what you have. Staff may be asked to practice outside of the scope of their usual expertise. Supplies may have to be reused and recycled. In some circumstances, resources may become completely exhausted."

The CDC created a PPE burn rate calculator, which can help healthcare facilities calculate, plan, and optimize PPE use. The facility enters the number of boxes in stock – gowns, gloves, surgical masks, respiratory equipment, face shields – and then enters the number of patients at their facility [8]. The spreadsheet-based model, in turn, calculates the facility's burn rate for each type of PPE entered. Calculating this rate enables users to project how long the PPE supply will last.

Healthcare entities use general strategies based on the capacity of the facility's PPE. The CDC recommends a three-tiered approach; their levels are conventional, contingency, and crisis capacity [3]. Conventional capacity is the engineering and administrative measures already incorporated into daily practices to optimize PPE [3]. Proper training on the use of PPE includes donning and doffing strategies to prolong the use of PPE. Contingency capacity strategies include temporarily suspending annual fit testing and using equipment beyond their shelf date or prioritizing them for higher-risk activities [3]. At crisis capacity, alternatives to PPE extend the use of disposable PPE when possible [3].

Limiting Hospital Visits

Limiting the number of patients entering hospital settings can also help bolster supplies. Nurse advice lines and telemedicine allow for access to care and the ability to triage patients accordingly. Screening patients with COVID-19 symptoms or those who have been in direct contact with someone with severe acute respiratory syndrome coronavirus 2 infection before healthcare visits reduce the flow of patients and preserve PPE supplies [9]. Limiting the healthcare providers involved in patient care and limiting the number of face-to-face encounters with the patient and visitors to

the facility also decrease the influx of people [9]. Without visitors at the bedside, nurses have assumed the responsibility of calling or scheduling specific times to call and keep families informed of the status of their loved ones. These measures keep family members reassured and updated on the patient's condition, and they decrease transmission risk.

Adjusting Nursing Practices

The world adapted during this time of the pandemic, becoming innovative and improving our new normal, even in these most extreme circumstances. Nurses are no exception. They have managed PPE and staffing shortages in creative ways. Aggregating nursing-related activities to cut down on the number of times the nurse must enter the room and don and doff PPE is one way that conserves resources and allows patients to rest [10]. Positioning as much equipment outside of the patient's room helps reduce the number of times the nurse needs to enter the room [10]. Control panels for ventilators and intravenous pumps with extension tubing allow nurses to adjust settings, bags, medication, and rate changes from outside [10]. Video conferencing with a camera in the room allows multiple team members to assess the patient without a physical presence [10].

Nursing Staffing Issues

Before the pandemic, there was a shortage of nurses, which experts expect to grow to more than half a million registered nurses by 2030 [11]. These prepandemic trends result from an aging population, a retiring population of nurses, and barriers in nursing education. Compounded with the burnout and fatigue faced by nurses during this pandemic, this number will likely grow. There has been an increase in demand for emergency departments and ICU nurses since COVID-19 began. This shortage and increased nursing needs resulted in a redeployment of staff, float, and travel nurses cross-trained to care for patients with COVID-19. Nurses working in other hospital areas, such as psychiatry, pediatrics, obstetrics, and outpatient settings, have routinely been assigned to the ICU and COVID-19 floors. Nurses report a lack of preparation for the crisis. The shortage of nurses and lack of preparedness impact patient care.

When nurses are understaffed, there is a reduction in patient satisfaction, increased patient mortality, and increased readmissions [12]. Due to increased patient volumes and a nursing shortage, patient care fell below the standard. Intubated and sedated patients need to be turned every two hours to prevent pressure ulcers that were often left for longer-to-perform interventions and treatments on other patients with higher acuity. Hospitals bypassed laws protecting the safety of patients and nurses to account for the nursing shortages [13]. The typical ratio in the ICU went from one to two patients per nurse to up to five or six [13].

Reducing Nonessential Visits

Hospitals should cancel all nonessential procedures and visits during surges, providing other nurses and healthcare personnel to support patient care activities. These nurses should receive orientation and training in acute care and COVID-19. Nurses should be identified to work in the facility; state-specific emergency licensure waivers and requirements can help temporarily increase the number of nursing personnel [9]. The use of float nurses is not an ideal solution. Nurses should stay in one location because it builds their skill set and decreases the risk for disease transmission. Facilities may pause personal or elective time off but need to consider nurses' mental health. The benefits of time off for burnout prevention and handling stress should be weighed [9].

On a more hopeful note, there is an increase in applications to all healthcare providers because of the media attention, including medical and nursing schools. "How to become a nurse" is one of the most searched terms in 2021 [14]. Applications to nursing and medical schools have increased [14]. National Public Radio has labeled this the "Fauci effect" [14]. With the emergence of a more hardworking and altruistic generation of healthcare professionals motivated by the racial injustices and other unique challenges we have faced this year, the positive side of this pandemic is that we have an energized nursing workforce [14].

Nursing Interventions

Prone Positioning Spontaneously Breathing Patients

In a 2015 study of nonintubated, spontaneously breathing patients with hypoxemic acute respiratory failure, Scaravilli et al. [15] found that the prone position improves patient oxygenation and outcomes. Prone therapy is encouraged in COVID-19 lung-injured patients who are not intubated and on supplemental oxygen. It enhances secretion clearance, recruits the posterior lung regions that often become atelectatic, and improves ventilation/perfusion matching overall, reducing the need for supplemental oxygen and helping to heal the injured lung.

Patient self-directed prone therapy should be considered in alert and awake nonintubated patients requiring nasal cannula oxygen who can follow instructions. Self-proning is contraindicated in patients with neck, facial, or abdominal conditions or chest wall devices that prevent a safe prone position. Equipment necessary for this intervention includes a comfortable bed, pillows, towels, and telemetry with pulse oximetry with an oxygen titration protocol. A suction canister, Ambu bag, and bite block should be set up and positioned in the room.

The nurse should educate the patient about the potential benefit of self-directed prone position therapy and make sure that other healthcare providers have been instructed on the benefits and risks of self-directed prone position therapy. The nurse should ensure that the patient's oxygen source is secure and that the call light is within the patient's reach. For the first couple of sessions, the nurse should instruct the patient on the method of proning and determine which items (pillows, towels, sheets) will help with comfort. Nurses teach the patient the best times of the day or night for the self-prone position; a specific schedule helps with compliance and encouragement or positional aid from staff.

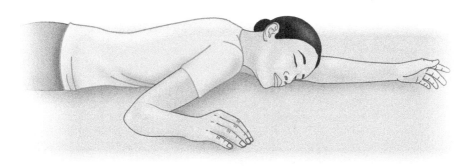

Patients should be encouraged to remain in the prone position for a minimum of three and a maximum of eight hours at one time. Current recommendations include putting the patient prone two to three times a day for a total time of 16 hours every 24 hours. When a patient requires greater than 6 L of oxygen per minute or develops excess work of breathing, the nurse should notify the respiratory specialist. The patient may reduce the frequency or total duration of the prone position therapy when the patient's oxygen requirements improve and remain consistent for at least 48 hours.

Prone Positioning Intubated Patients

Nursing care of the patient in a prone position presents unique challenges, particularly if the need arises for intubation. As such, the management of patients who are intubated and placed in either supine or prone positioning requires a multidisciplinary approach and advanced level of knowledge from the nursing staff, particularly concerning medication administration, side effects, adverse effects, hemodynamic monitoring, and potential complications. As mentioned earlier, not all patients may be candidates for prone therapy, because the process of proning and the position itself has a risk for complications [16]. Hemodynamic instability, massive facial edema, malfunction of renal replacement therapy (continuous or hemodialysis), and potential dislodgement of invasive equipment, such as an endotracheal tube, chest tube, or central lines, represent several possible risks associated with prone therapy [17].

Prone positioning can significantly improve oxygenation in patients, particularly those with moderate to severe acute respiratory distress syndrome (ARDS), and is a viable option for intubated patients with refractory hypoxemia despite mechanical ventilatory support. As such, the decision to prone an intubated patient requires careful consideration and involves multidisciplinary training to safely and successfully perform. Administration of neuromuscular blockade as a pharmacologic nursing intervention requires advanced training and critical thinking. When effectively used, it may reduce the risk of additional ventilator-associated lung injury and allow lung-protective ventilation, subsequently improving the patient's respiratory system compliance. In addition, management of ventilator settings must be coordinated

with the physician staff and respiratory therapy to implement further recruitment maneuvers that promote gas exchange and the reopening of stiff, atelectatic lungs resulting from ARDS [16]. Furthermore, physically placing the intubated patient in a prone position requires a team of healthcare providers to achieve successfully, including, but not limited to, nursing, respiratory, physician, and ancillary staff. Controlled proning therapy ensures calculated movements to maintain hemodynamic stability and adequate oxygenation and prevent accidental dislodging of lines and tubes.

Modes of Oxygen Delivery: High-Flow Nasal Cannula, Bilevel Positive Airway Pressure, and Mechanical Ventilation

Limiting the spread of COVID-19 infection to healthcare workers has been, and continues to be, a significant concern across hospitals worldwide. In the ICU setting in particular, nurses are among the most exposed to the virus due to the amount of time spent in rooms providing direct patient care. Because respiratory droplets and aerosolized particles are the predominant modes of COVID-19 transmission, initial concerns centered on the avoidance of aerosol-generating procedures and interventions that could potentially disperse viral particles, including awake (nonintubated) proning and the use of a high-flow nasal cannula (HFNC) and noninvasive ventilation (NIV) modes. However, mitigating these risks by avoiding NIV has been shown to adversely affect patient outcomes, demonstrating the high mortality associated with patients requiring invasive ventilation and the subsequent difficulty in successfully extubating these patients. With time and experience, the management of patients with COVID-19-induced pneumonia and ARDS has evolved to include the use of awake proning, HFNC, and NIV to avoid mechanical intubation and subsequent barotrauma and healthcare-acquired pneumonia [18].

HFNC uses heated and humidified oxygen that is delivered via nasal cannula. As such, it is often more comfortable and better tolerated when compared with bilevel positive airway pressure (BiPAP)/continuous positive airway pressure, which typically requires a mask to ensure an effective seal. HFNC delivers pressure-related and pH-appropriate oxygen flow, usually ranging from 40 to 80 l/min. This generation of oxygen flow physiologically reduces dead space and subsequently improves ventilatory efficiency, more so than standard oxygen therapy (i.e. nasal cannula, simple mask, nonrebreather). HFNC is also advantageous from a nursing and multidisciplinary standpoint. The nasal interface makes it easy and safe to apply, allows for increased mobility compared with BiPAP or invasive ventilation, and does not impede speech or eating during its use, further contributing to its increased tolerability among patients [18].

Although HFNC provides better oxygenation to patients than standard therapy, it ultimately is not as good an oxygenator as NIV, which provides more significant mean airway pressure by physiologically balancing intrinsic and external positive end-expiratory pressure. NIV includes modalities such as BiPAP and, similarly, continuous positive airway pressure. NIV is a pressure-targeted oxygen delivery modality that provides pressure support to augment inhalation and increases functional residual capacity, both of which improve overall oxygenation and lung compliance. Although superior in oxygenating, when compared with HFNC, NIV may not be as well tolerated among patients, requiring increased precautions and monitoring while in use. For example, it is often not well accepted among claustrophobic patients due to its typical oxygen delivery via orofacial mask and may even lead to facial abrasions or pressure injuries.

In addition, the forced inspiratory pressure in NIV can make communication with patients difficult, because it muffles their speech under the face mask and, more critically, can increase their risk for aspiration. Decreased compliance and tolerability are more likely with NIV, because removing the device is required for eating and specific multidisciplinary therapy interventions [18]. Patients may also try to remove their masks because of feelings of claustrophobia or to facilitate communication better. For these reasons, the use of NIV requires closer observation and monitoring by nursing staff, including redirection and interventions to reduce anxiety while the oxygen delivery device is in place.

Patients with mild to moderate acute respiratory failure from COVID-19 can experience a rapid deterioration in respiratory status, subsequently requiring intubation and mechanical ventilation. One of the most severe complications from viral pneumonia, such as COVID-19, is the development of ARDS, a severe acute inflammatory lung injury associated with a significant mortality rate, often as high as 40–50%. The ARDS Network Trial provides a prominent clinical resource for these patients and is the most extensive and most used study in clinical practice. The Trial Network reduced mortality by 22% and increased the number of ventilator-free days among patients with acute lung injury and ARDS [19]. As recommended by the ARDS Network trial, intubated patients with ARDS should be placed on ventilator settings that provide the low tidal volume and adequate positive end-expiratory pressure lung-protective strategy [19]. This strategic use of lower tidal volumes during ventilation in patients with acute lung injury and ARDS may reduce further lung injury and the release of inflammatory mediators. Nurses must coordinate with respiratory therapy and medical staff to obtain and monitor arterial blood gas results, because this approach may cause respiratory acidosis and decrease arterial oxygenation. As discussed previously, the spontaneous modes of ventilation used with NIV enhance synchrony and comfort with the oxygen delivery device, eliminating the need for deep sedation. However, patients who require intubation often cannot tolerate invasive ventilation without sedation and may even require paralytics to facilitate oxygenation and ventilator synchrony [18]. One of the essential nursing considerations of intubated patients is sedation to enhance ventilator synchrony and comfort, because nurses are responsible for administering sedation and monitoring its desired effects.

As was seen early in the pandemic, discouraging the use of NIV in patients with COVID-19 may prematurely increase the need for intubation, subsequently increasing the morbidity and mortality associated with invasive ventilation and decrease ventilator availability. Some hospitals and providers do not favor noninvasive approaches. They prefer early intubation, while others use NIV more commonly, which present different nursing considerations for implementing interventions, administering medications, and tailoring therapies appropriately [18]. In an observational study of 459 ICU patients across 50 countries, Bellani et al. [20] discussed that NIV was associated with higher ICU mortality in patients with ARDS. Although NIV may stabilize a patient's clinical course in the short term, it should not delay intubation when most appropriate. Although controversial data exist to support the advantages and disadvantages of HFNC and NIV related to intubation/reintubation rates and overall mortality, they remain effective modalities for oxygen delivery that are safe and often better tolerated in patients with COVID-19 pneumonia who are mild to moderately hypoxemic [18].

Pressure-Related Injuries and Other Nursing Interventions

Pressure-related injuries have grown as a result of increased endotracheal tube placements and holders, and patients being too unstable to move. When preventative measures such as repositioning patients and redistribution of pressure cannot be performed, essential interventions include keeping the skin clean and dry with a pH-appropriate skin cleanser and protected from excess moisture. The care of healthy skin includes water-based skin emollients and barrier creams to maintain skin hydration. Other nursing-related interventions consist of packing axilla with ice or using a cooling blanket to promote fever reduction in patients who have exceeded their dosing of acetaminophen.

Medications

The pandemic has made the general public and the medical community question the capricious nature of evidence-based medicine. A study consists of data promoting effective treatment for COVID-19, and then a subsequent study contains points that denounce the same information. Early in the pandemic, the COVID-19 "cocktail" consisted of hydroxychloroquine and azithromycin at many centers. Now our therapeutics are more aimed at antiviral drugs and anti-inflammatory agents, including corticosteroids. Even seasoned ICU nurses have had difficulty navigating new medications and protocols. With nursing shortages and the deployment of nurses into critical care situations with little training, it can be even more difficult. These critically ill patients may need

ventilation; many become septic and require medications to support circulation or renal replacement therapy.

The pathogenesis of COVID-19 virtually affects all organ systems, making a specific, targeted approach to treatment difficult. The virus gains entry into the host via angiotensin-converting enzyme 2 and primarily replicates in the mucosal epithelium of the respiratory tract and, in some individuals, the gastrointestinal mucosa as well. The overactivation of T cells leads to immune dysfunction, which can result in a cytokine storm, and in combination with pulmonary edema, leads to the development of ARDS [21]. Over the last year, pharmacologic therapies that target this overwhelming inflammatory response have emerged as "first-line" treatment for hospitalized patients with COVID-19. However, their safety and effectiveness remain a significant concern.

Hydroxychloroquine/chloroquine was one of the first drugs given to patients early on in the pandemic, primarily for its immunosuppressive properties, along with azithromycin. However, this combination produced an increased incidence of QT prolongation of greater than 500 ms, predisposing patients to lethal arrhythmias and requiring close cardiac monitoring [21]. Remdesivir, an antiviral, has shown inhibitory activity against severe acute respiratory syndrome coronavirus 1, the cause of severe acute respiratory syndrome and Middle East respiratory syndrome coronavirus, the Middle East respiratory syndrome by reducing lung virus levels and subsequent lung damage, making the drug a potentially successful candidate for the treatment of severe acute respiratory syndrome coronavirus 2 (COVID-19) as well. Results of a double-blind, randomized control trial by Beigel et al. [22] demonstrated a shortened recovery time of 11 days versus 15 days in patients who received a 10-day course of remdesivir compared with placebo, as well as a 3–5% reduction in mortality rate within the first 15–29 days. However, known adverse effects of remdesivir include decreased hemoglobin level and lymphocyte count and increased serum creatinine, hepatic transaminases, and glucose levels. Because remdesivir is eliminated by the renal route, patients with severe renal dysfunction are typically not candidates for receiving remdesivir therapy.

Anti-inflammatory agents, including ruxolitinib and tocilizumab, are used in combination with corticosteroids (dexamethasone, methylprednisolone) to reduce the overwhelming inflammatory response caused by COVID-19 and to help mitigate further multiorgan dysfunction. Ruxolitinib, a Janus-associated kinase 1/2 inhibitor, is hypothesized to be effective against elevated cytokine levels but may also cause mild to moderate anemia [21]. Levels of interleukin-6 (IL-6) correlate with COVID-19 severity, suggesting its role in overall immune dysfunction and development of ARDS. The inflammatory cytokine IL-6 promotes multiple proinflammatory effects, suggesting potential benefit from pharmacologic IL-6 antagonism. Tocilizumab, a monoclonal antibody that works against IL-6, is used to treat several inflammatory diseases and has been shown to yield better outcomes in patients with severe COVID-19 pneumonia. Given that this drug is a potent immunosuppressant, patients who receive tocilizumab require ongoing monitoring for adverse effects, such as serious infection (particularly opportunistic), worsening pneumonia, hypersensitivity, liver dysfunction, and bleeding [23]. However, no increase in infections has been reported from large clinical trials of tocilizumab.

Other anti-inflammatory agents such as dexamethasone, a powerful corticosteroid, have also been highly studied and used in the inpatient management of COVID-19 for patients requiring supplemental oxygen. Dexamethasone is typically administered to patients once daily for up to 10 days, benefits those with a longer duration of symptoms, reduces mortality, and decreases hospital stay length. As with all corticosteroids, immunosuppression and subsequent or worsening infection are a risk and require ongoing monitoring of laboratory tests, mainly white blood cell count and blood sugar levels, because there can be significant increases in these values [21].

Finally, vaccines and immune therapy are among the more recent strategies to combat the virus and mitigate the spread. Several large pharmaceutical companies within the United States have developed COVID-19 vaccines that have since become available to the general adult population. One such example is the development of a new mRNA vaccine that has been a topic of both interest and speculation because it is a new approach to vaccination. In contrast to a live or inactivated vaccine, which puts a weakened or inactive form of a virus into the host, the mRNA vaccine teaches the host's cells how to make a protein that subsequently triggers an immune response. These novel vaccines are considered safe and effective and are held to the same rigorous safety and effectiveness standards as all other vaccines approved by the Food and Drug Administration within the United States. Nurses can use widely available resources, such as the CDC's website, to safely educate patients on the possible symptoms after receiving a COVID-19 vaccine [24]. Side effects may occur within a few days after receiving the vaccine and most commonly include pain, redness, and swelling of the injection site, as well as fatigue, headache, muscle pain, chills, fever, and nausea, with a rare chance of anaphylaxis [24]. Nurses also can encourage patients to register and report their side effects using smartphone-based tools or report adverse effects to the Vaccine Adverse Event Reporting System [25].

The CDC's website offers extensive information and resources for healthcare workers and the general population regarding the available COVID-19 vaccine options, their development process, studied efficacy, and possible side effects after immunization. As smartphone-based tools and applications (apps) become widely used and, increasingly, a preferred method to access and exchange information, one such app that can be recommended to vaccinated individuals is the CDC's V-safe After Vaccination Health Checker. The app uses text messaging and web surveys that provide personalized health check-ins after receiving the vaccine. Patients can tell the CDC any side effects they may be experiencing. The app sends questionnaires to follow up either daily, weekly, or monthly, depending on when the individual was vaccinated. Patients should know that the V-safe app does not provide medical advice, cannot schedule COVID-19 vaccination appointments, and does not serve as an official record of having received the vaccine. The app, however, can remind patients of when their second vaccine dose may be due and ultimately provides vital feedback to the CDC about the recipient's postvaccination experience [25].

The pharmacologic management of intubated patients relies heavily on the nurse. It directly affects a patient's tolerability to mechanical ventilation and may even lead to clinical improvements in their condition. Adequate sedation of intubated patients is imperative, because any accidental line or tube dislodgement can result in life-threatening complications. The use of sedation, analgesia, and more critically, the role of neuromuscular blockade in ARDS improve oxygenation by preventing ventilator dyssynchrony from breath stacking [16]. However, nurses sedating an intubated patient require advanced training, critical thinking, and knowledge of various medications, analgesics, sedatives, and paralytic agents, including their desired and adverse effects. Intubated patients in the prone position require close monitoring. They often experience more hemodynamic instability, muscle paralysis, device displacement, and increased sedation than intubated patients in the supine position [17]. Intubated patients may also benefit from inhaled pulmonary vasodilators, such as nitric oxide and epoprostenol. When inhaled, they work directly in the functional lung units by vasodilating pulmonary vasculature and improving ventilation/perfusion matching, subsequently improving oxygenation. The dilatory effects of these drugs also decrease right ventricle afterload and thus warrant close hemodynamic monitoring. The role of pulmonary vasodilators may not improve mortality, but they can be beneficial in the short-term treatment of patients with hypoxemia refractory to traditional therapies that are used [16].

Nutritional Management

The catabolic state associated with critical illness requires an increase in nutrition to meet the patient's needs and prevent further cell injury because of an overwhelming proinflammatory state. Providing nutrition to the intubated and prone patient requires a multidisciplinary approach that includes, but is not limited to, the primary nurse, physician, registered dietician, and pharmacist. Guidelines recommend beginning enteral feeding within the first 24–48 hours for critically ill patients, provided they can tolerate it and are hemodynamically stable. For patients who cannot maintain enteral routes of feeding, parenteral nutrition offers an alternative, posing a higher risk for infectious morbidity. Up to 50–60% of critically ill patients experience delayed gastric emptying, resulting from multiple factors, such as medications (sedation,

paralytics, vasopressors) and immobility. For example, vasopressors, especially in high doses, affect motor function in the gastrointestinal tract and may contribute to delayed gastric emptying. In addition, sedative and analgesic agents, particularly opiates, are known to cause constipation. Nursing care strategies that aim to increase a patient's tolerance to enteral nutrition include head of bed elevation and use of prokinetic agents, such as metoclopramide or erythromycin [26].

The evidence and guidelines for COVID-19 are constantly evolving. Posted guidelines accessible for nurses can help. Nurses sharing best practices between coworkers, colleagues, and peers within and outside one's institution can also be helpful. Nurses should keep up to date with reliable, peer-reviewed resources, such as the CDC, National Institutes of Health, World Health Organization, or hospitals and university websites.

Advance Care Planning

Advance care planning provides the patient a voice of self-determination and allows thoughtful discussion among the individual, their supportive persons, and the healthcare provider. The COVID-19 pandemic exposed systemic injustice as patients and their support persons confronted the ethical dilemma of end-of-life care. As mechanical ventilation became imminent, there was limited time to make informed decisions. Due to the required isolation, there was a sense of helplessness as communication was via video or telephone call. Disenfranchised minority populations were more likely to elect full code status because "do not resuscitate" was associated with allowing providers to give up on them [27].

Often the prognosis for patients with severe COVID-19 is poor. Hospitalized patients with COVID-19 have a 26–32% chance of admission to the ICU [28]. Hospitalized patients were more likely to have ARDS, developing in 20–42% of hospitalized patients overall and 67–85% of patients in the ICU [28]. The mortality rate ranged from 39% to 72% in the ICU and a median length of hospital stay of 10–13 days [28]. Many patients who were intubated did not get extubated. Many providers compare hospital treatment of COVID-19 to battlefield conditions with patients requiring triage. Preferably, the initiation of conversations regarding life-prolonging interventions should occur well before the illness infects us. This fast-moving infectious disease has left families and healthcare providers with little time to discuss general life-prolonging interventions. Clinicians historically have been reluctant to start these conversations. Still, with the realization of our mortality with COVID-19 affecting younger and healthier populations, there is a need to expand advance care directive conversations. Discussing advance directives with all patients admitted to the hospital for COVID-19, or any acute illness, needs to occur early in the admission. Each state's attorney general website provides advance directive forms that meet the individual legal requirements governing their use. This discussion should include the education of the patients and their families about life-saving procedures and potential prognosis. When the prognosis is poor, providers should relay the patient's status to the family and advocate an end to the patient's suffering. Unsuccessful attempts of cardiopulmonary resuscitation can put providers at additional risk for COVID-19 exposure because the aerosolized particles spread widely.

Interdisciplinary Care

The interdisciplinary care team (ICT) consists of professionals from various disciplines working together to improve the patient's physical, psychological, and spiritual needs. Each practitioner is knowledgeable of their responsibility and must provide the intervention or service based on the patient's progression through the hospital stay. A well-functioning team member's autonomy includes making recommendations to the care plan based on the patient's health status. The team corresponds to where the patient receives care (i.e. ICU, general medical wards, or rehabilitation) and the patient's needs (i.e. RN, hospitalist, physician specialist, respiratory therapist, or physical therapist). Although the literature is replete with various successful ICT models, a systematic review by Pannick et al. [29] provides some evidence that collaboration between team members coupled with collective interventions may decrease care complications. Some studies have shown that ICTs may prolong hospital stays to meet the patient's identified medical and social needs [29]. Before the COVID pandemic, team members had access to each other but, more importantly, could speak directly to the patient and their support persons on a scheduled basis. Social distancing and COVID lockdowns erected communication barriers.

Innovative ICT models arose to address the multiorgan complications of COVID-19 coupled with underlying chronic disease. Standardization of an ICT model may be difficult because of the geographical region, type of facility (rural, safety net, or academic hospital), and diversity of the patient population. Current literature does not define the best combination of disciplines required to care for patients with COVID-19 infection. As a result, external ICT teams can be convened to provide COVID guidelines and recommendations based on the limited patient data, insufficient hospital resources, and physician subspecialty limitations [30–32].

When the patient transfers out of the ICU, they require rehabilitation and support to progress in their recovery. Based on the sequelae of both the disease and treatments (i.e. ventilator intubation), the rehabilitation team consists of a physician or hospitalist, registered nurse, and respiratory, physical, occupational, or speech therapist. Other ancillary services that provide consultation to the team include social workers, pharmacists, nutritionists, and spiritual services. Leadership in the group is fluid and interchangeable as the patient progresses. Unfortunately, many patients may not receive sufficient rehabilitation services because of a lack of available personnel and isolation precautions.

It is well established that interprofessional teams improve patient outcomes. For an interprofessional team to function well, trust, role clarity, expertise, and communication are needed. The interprofessional team is integral to critical or intensive care delivery. There are organizational constraints with shift changes, and multiple providers/teams caring for the patient throughout the day and night can be a barrier to interprofessional collaboration. Attention to team dynamics is helpful; familiarity within the team and the innate sense of trust and respect for fellow team members and knowledge of practice styles can be beneficial. With the guidelines and choices constantly evolving, clear guidelines and explicit communication of leadership changes can improve the efficiency of the ICT.

Discharge Planning: Transition to Outpatient/Specialty Care

The aims of hospital discharge planning for the patient are multifold: determine the appropriate discharge destination if they cannot return to the setting they lived in before admission, identify the requirements for a smooth and safe transition, and begin meeting identified postdischarge needs. This process requires seamless communication and coordination between the discharge planner, healthcare providers, key contact(s) at the discharge destination, available community resources, and the patient and their support persons. The discharge planner may be a nurse, social worker, or other trained individual who modifies and updates the care plan based on the patient's progression in their hospital stay or changes at the discharge destination. Properly executed discharge planning enhances the patient's ability to progress toward the goals of their after-discharge care plan and helps prevent readmission to the hospital [33].

There is no nationally accepted standard to identify which patient requires discharge planning. The process is initiated at the time of admission or at least 48 hours before discharge. The care plan involves assessing the patient's functional status, cognitive ability, self-care capability, and the availability and capacity of family or friends to provide support and care. Other factors that drive discharge planning are postdischarge facility admission processes (if the patient does not return to their home), required services from skilled professionals, access to timely outpatient follow-up visits, and prescribed medication accessibility. In a Cochrane Review by Gonçalves-Bradley et al. [34], discharge planning provided a slight reduction in hospital length of stay and decreased readmission rates in the older population. Due to the heterogeneity of the interventions and outcomes across the studies, the interpretation of the data was limited. Thus, discharge planning is a fluid process that requires individualization based on the needs of the patient.

Conversely, numerous factors influence a smooth discharge transition process. Limitations imposed by either the payor or total lack of funding delay planning, complicate recovery, lead to readmission, or increase morbidity and mortality. Social risk factors or social determinants of health beget fragmentation in care and may account for 25–60% of deaths in the United States [35]. Unstable housing, food deserts, isolation, low health literacy, and language barriers directly impact the individual's understanding of their diagnosis, discharge destination, lifestyle choices, medication adherence, and post-hospital follow-up requirements [35]. Discharge planners faced these social circumstances before the COVID-19 pandemic; the process became more challenging as hospitals steadily filled up with patients infected with COVID-19 presenting with a mosaic of symptoms compounded with a new onset of mental health issues. There was a disproportionate effect of the COVID-19 pandemic in the minority population, mostly Black, Latinx, and Native Americans [36]. Hypertension, diabetes mellitus, and obesity are most associated with severe COVID-19 symptoms and are highly prevalent in these minority populations. COVID-19 revealed structural racism as discharge planners faced barriers in developing high-quality patient care plans.

The COVID-19 pandemic further fragmented the discharge planning process as hospitals expedited discharges to manage the constant influx of admissions. Some patients transitioned from the ICU or mechanical ventilation to discharge without adequate physical and occupational therapy because of a lack of hospital personnel or concerns of viral spread [37]. COVID-19 survivors experienced higher functional loss, frailty, and mental health disorders without adequate community resources to improve health outcomes. Support persons lacked a thorough understanding of the posthospitalization sequelae that required continued care, the interventions necessary to improve functional ability, the medication regimens, the healthcare provider follow-up, and the list goes on. Aside from the items on a discharge plan, the support person's age and digital divide directly impacted goal accomplishment.

Once discharged from the hospital, the patient or their support persons could not access hospital personnel for clarification or assistance with the discharge care plan. The ease of scheduling one-week follow-up office visits with primary care providers and specialists was fleeting. Many ambulatory clinics closed or scheduled telehealth office visits only. Rehabilitation services or durable medical equipment was inaccessible because of lack of coverage or funding, or the business was closed as a result of the COVID-19 pandemic. As restrictions ease, access remains problematic.

Home Services and Transition to Home

Discharge planning ideally begins at admission [38], with nursing staff working with families, discussing possible care needs, and handling common symptoms and discomforts associated with the diagnosis. The planners discuss warning signs that the patient's relapse needs immediate attention and reassurance of expected standard progress. Infection-control measures for COVID-19 make in-person conversations unfeasible, with no family at the bedside to teach, and nurses converse with families on the phone.

A lack of communication between the family and nursing can lead to poor outcomes at home and increase readmission risk [38]. Further complicating care is a new circumstance referred to as family clustering. Multiple family unit members or household members contract COVID-19 either concurrently or subsequently to the first person bringing it to the family unit. Family clustering underscores the health inequities affecting people of color (POC). The COVID-19 pandemic has disproportionately affected POC with a higher prevalence of disease, increased mortality, and more severe complications [39]. The risk for family clustering is most significant for POC, who are more than two times as likely to live in a multigenerational household [39]. According to Garg et al. [40], persons with significant chronic conditions and the elderly should avoid exposure to COVID-19. Family clustering affects not only the discharge plan for the patient because of the lack of healthy family members to receive discharge education and instructions but also the availability of qualified family members to support decision making for the end-of-life, palliative care or discharge to long-term facilities [39].

PPE, home oxygen, and assistive devices, such as walkers, bedside commodes, beds, lifts, and wheelchairs, may need to be ordered and coordinated with discharge planning to ensure a smooth transition for in-home care. In-home care also may require physical therapy, occupational therapy, home health nurses, caregivers, and social workers. During the pandemic, the usual home health agency initiation of care within 24–48 hours can stretch to over 3–4 days [41]. According to Garg et al. [40], the highest rate of COVID-19 admissions was among older adults, with almost 90% of those persons having at least one or more comorbidities. Tenner-Hooban [41] recommends creating a telehealth-based transitional team for patients returning to home care until the home health agency can formally assume the patient's care at home. This team can support the patient and their family by monitoring vital signs, answering questions about medications or equipment, and triaging status changes to support caregivers' decision-making process. This telehealth team would be especially beneficial to vulnerable families who experience a lag time because of overburdened hospital resources before initiating formal home health care.

With little known about the long-term sequelae of COVID-19 infection, the need for infection-control measures and supplies at home makes discharge planning for the COVID-19 patient even more critical. Chopra et al. [42] found that at 60 days after hospital discharge, one in five patients' primary care providers had not seen them, with 15% requiring hospital readmission. Symptoms in this group included respiratory problems, emotional distress, and the inability to return to normal activities of daily living. Atalla et al. [43] found higher readmission rates for persons with comorbidities with increased respiratory distress, because the most common reason for readmission was increased respiratory distress. Readmissions tended to be longer than the initial admission. Readmissions can add further burden to hospitals whose resources are already thinly stretched in this pandemic.

Infection-control measures at home with COVID-19 and the need to limit the number of persons exposed to infected individuals exacerbate caregiver fatigue, in addition to the need to limit the number of persons who expose themselves to contagious individuals and prevent family clustering. The social disparities that underpin the increased risk for comorbidities also disproportionately affect POC and the socioeconomically disadvantaged. The burden of COVID-19 could result in the further marginalization of these populations [44]. Many of the resources needed to care for postdischarge COVID-19 patients at home (e.g. PPE, isolating contagious persons to a separate room, hiring outside caretakers, and medical equipment) are often not accessible to families with limited financial resources. Family caregivers can be supported by being provided PPE (at least enough for a few days) and instructed on its proper use, the use of homemade masks, and other PPE at the hospital before discharge. Assessing the capacity for caring for seriously ill families in the home, including caregivers in tele-health visits, and encouraging caregivers to use their other family members for other home tasks should be done where possible. Encourage families, where possible, to use online resources, such as the National Alliance of Caregivers (https://www.caregiving.org), which has COVID-19 resources for families and links to government websites [45].

Humanization of Care

Critical care nursing during COVID-19 has meant caring for intubated patients sedated in a bed for weeks at a time. Family members have been unable to say goodbye. The clergy have failed to perform last rites due to limitations in visitors and nonessential staff. The absence of visitors by the bedside to tell stories and give character can lead to patients becoming just a body in a bed. Nurses and other caregivers need to consider the humanization of care during these stressful times.

An association between social isolation and loneliness exists, resulting in physical and mental deterioration [46]. Self-isolation, quarantine, shelter-in-place orders, and social distancing have negatively impacted people's mental health with COVID-19. A patient's average length of stay with COVID-19 is nearly two weeks. Nurses are often the only personal contact and contact to the outside that a COVID-19 patient has. Nurses have had to communicate with relatives and keep relatives updated during each of their patient's stay. Television, radios, and the coordination of Facetime or chatting by iPads and mobile phones can help patients stay connected with the outside world during their prolonged stays. It may be beneficial to install a video camera with secure access in the room to allow the family to check in on the patient and to see and talk to the patient [10].

Head-to-toe PPE has created communication barriers in and of itself. It is difficult to see faces, let alone name badges, under the face masks, shields, and gowns. The noisy equipment and background can impede communication, particularly for hearing-impaired patients who cannot read lips or view facial expressions. Writing the staff's name and profession on the back of suits or caps can help orient patients to who is in the room. The use of the whiteboard for communication may also help.

The COVID-19 pandemic has raised our awareness of mortality and uncertainty, enhanced by our 24 hours a day, 7 days a week media coverage with continuous reports regarding new cases and the increasing death toll. Nurses have had to provide end-of-life care to severely ill patients whose conditions are rapidly deteriorating. In addition, healthcare workers who have avoided COVID-19 are now covering for sick people or have left the workforce. Encountering death on an unprecedented scale and caring for our ill, dying coworkers and even family members have impacted the health and well-being of nurses and other health professionals. The increasing workload, fatigue, and pressure, as well as the moral damage that comes from losing patients, adds to a decline in empathy and depersonalization – in turn, increasing burnout and the poor outcomes associated with it.

During times of crisis, the Maslow hierarchy of needs takes precedence. Basic needs of food, drink, rest, and sleep take priority. Medical staff treating patients with COVID-19 in Hunan Province were interviewed and provided a psychosocial intervention package consisting of online courses, hotlines, and group interventions [47]. The staff was reluctant to take part in this [47]. Nurses, in particular, were anxious, irritable, unwilling to rest, and showing signs of distress, yet reported not needing psychological intervention [47]. In the acute crisis phase, staff concerned themselves with the anxiety of their families, uninterrupted breaks, adequate PPE, and more training [47]. As a result, the intervention efforts pivoted to provide more rest to their staff, supplies, videos to send to their families, and training [47]. Eventually, counselors could visit with the team and provide support [47]. This study shows that crises need to be managed initially by making sure nurses and healthcare staff can have their basic needs met.

The ability for nurses to maintain their ethical professionalism requires adequate staffing and resources in hospitals, but it also includes more social measures, such as availability of housing for patients on discharge, affordable medications, increased access to care, preventative care, care of other comorbidities, and the responsiveness of local, state, and federal governance. With these measures, the workloads can decrease, and patients can receive the empathy and attention they need and deserve.

A hospice agency reported on managing existing patients and the influx of patients during the COVID-19 pandemic [48]. COVID-19 interrupted the flow of patients into hospice settings. Workforce availability changed as the demand for nurses in acute care settings increased. The bereavement needs of patients and families grew, resulting in adverse patient outcomes because of negative psychosocial effects and inadequate symptom management [48]. Hospice and palliative care nurses and workers report stress related to managing patients, as well as their caretaking families, needing end-of-life care at increased and unprecedented rates [49]. Reframed as a public health issue [50], these nurses use advocacy, science-based solutions, and complex decision making to support those under their care. Laboratory testing for surveillance, detection of outbreaks, and containment for patients and staff continues to be a problem. Although these workers and families adapted to telehealth visits, this modality creates issues for families who must make decisions without in-person contact with their loved one.

Moral and Ethical Distress

The COVID-19 pandemic highlights some of the ethical dilemmas facing healthcare workers caring for patients on the front lines [51]. Nursing staff before COVID-19 were at high risk for burnout, compassion fatigue, and emotional exhaustion. In April 2020, a group of researchers at New York-Presbyterian/Columbia University Irving Medical Center screened clinicians for stress, anxiety, and depression symptoms [52]. Sixty-four percent of nurses reported acute stress, consisting of nightmares and inability to stop thinking about COVID-19, hypervigilance, numbness, or detachment from others and their environment [52].

For clinicians with preexisting workplace stress and fatigue, COVID-19 brought an increase in mental health strains, creating an acute-on-chronic condition.

Research demonstrates a preburnout prevalence rate of 35% among nurses prepandemic [53], likely secondary to staggering administrative tasks, mental stress, heavy workloads, etc. Burnout is a psychiatric condition originating from an extended destructive work environment. Its features include emotional and physical fatigue, feelings of ineffectiveness in the workplace, and depersonalization or detachment to feelings and thoughts [54]. In a 2010 study conducted on nurses, researchers identified a direct correlation between burnout and quality of care [55]. As burnout of nurses increases, the quality of care provided decreases [55]. Burnout also links to diminished empathy [56]. Empathy among clinicians toward their patients enhances their history-taking ability [57], medication compliance [58], and delivery and acceptance of bad news [59] and helps to reduce conflicts [60] and errors [61]. The pandemic's warlike, battlefield-like conditions created a vicious cycle, impeding the clinician's ability to reflect, think, analyze, emote, relate, and connect. This trajectory is worsening the prevalence of burnout among clinicians.

Utilitarianism has been a dominant ethical principle throughout the pandemic. It prioritizes the needs of many. The utilitarian concept depends on multiple variables, including the probability someone will record the duration of treatment and resources available [62]. An example of this would be allocating a ventilator to a patient with a greater chance of survival or a greater life expectancy and considering the duration of time the person would be on the ventilator, corresponding to saving the most significant number of lives. There may be some good reasons to depart from a sole utilitarianism approach, especially when human rights and equity are at stake [62].

The capacity of healthcare systems to advocate for clinicians with practice tools, such as appropriate education, specialist consultation, and PPE, has decreased. Ethical support is needed with a just allocation of resources and support for the frontline nurses and other clinicians experiencing moral and ethical adversity resulting from the pandemic.

Building Resilience

The term *resilience* should be used with caution when describing the impact of COVID-19 on nurses and other healthcare providers. There often has been an overemphasis on resilience amidst understaffing, death, extreme circumstances, and shortages of PPE – this can "let organization off the hook" [63]. Resilience should not be viewed as the individual's responsibility but the collective [64]. Team building and check-ins at the start and end of a shift can help build morale. Introductions and encouragement of new or temporary members to ask for help and support and pairing new team members with more experienced staff can help the team support each other [65, 66]. Optional end-of-the-shift or weekly team meetings to solve problems and share successes can help the decline in morale [65–67].

Managers and organizational leaders can make themselves accessible and approachable by inviting feedback and providing opportunities to do so, including anonymously [47, 65, 67, 68]. Regular emails communicating evolving guidelines or successes, even minor ones, can help staff feel acknowledged, valued, and informed [47, 65, 68]. Leaders should actively promote the recognition of psychological symptoms to reduce stigma and encourage them to seek help [69]. This recognition can be facilitated by appointing an organization lead for psychological health during the COVID pandemic and beyond [67]. Managers should be committed to addressing issues related to PPE, child care, staff illness, shortages, testing, etc. [47, 65, 68]. Nonurgent staff tasks (such as nonmandatory training and reviews) can be postponed to reduce the burden placed on personnel [67].

Addressing the long-term psychological impact on nurses remains critical to preventing burnout and combat fatigue for nurses and other healthcare workers. The creation of wellness activities that encourage self-care and peer support can alleviate that stress on the workforce [70]. Nurses should pay attention to their needs for safe working conditions, drinks, food, and regular breaks and make sure their peers do the same [47, 68]. The FACE COVID mnemonic developed by Dr. Russ Harris provides practical steps for remaining calm during stressful times. FACE stands for *focus* on what you can control; *acknowledge* thoughts and feelings; *come* back into your body; and *engage* in what you are doing [71]. Meditation and mindfulness strategies at work and home may also help support psychological and mental health [67].

Conclusion

Nursing is a profession with a longstanding reputation for trustworthiness. Nurses have been considered the most honest and ethical profession for nearly two decades [72]. 2020 was the year of the nurse. It was also the year that COVID-19 impacted our communities. Nurses became inventive problem-solvers creating compassionate solutions for patients. Although well deserved, this is not the attention that anyone had hoped for in the year of the nurse.

References

1 Iheduru-Anderson, K. (2021). Reflections on the lived experience of working with limited personal protective equipment during the COVID-19 crisis. *Nurs Inq.* 28 (1): e12382. https://doi.org/10.1111/nin.12382.

2 Rubinson, L., Nuzzo, J.B., Talmor, D.S. et al. (2005). Augmentation of hospital critical care capacity after bioterrorist attacks or epidemics: recommendations of the Working Group on Emergency Mass Critical Care. *Crit Care Med.* 33 (10): 2393–2403. https://doi.org/10.1097/01.ccm.0000173411.06574.d5.

3 Centers for Disease Control & Prevention. Optimizing supply of PPE and other equipment during shortages. CDC. http://www.cdc.gov/coronavirus/2019-ncov/hcp/ppe-strategy/general-optimization-strategies.html. Updated July 16, 2020. Accessed April 29, 2021.

4 Chang, E.F., Backer, H., Bey, T.A., and Koenig, K.L. (2008). Maximizing medical and health outcomes after a catastrophic disaster: defining a new "crisis standard of care" (abstract). *West J Emerg Med* 9 (3): S3. https://escholarship.org/uc/item/9j62f2b5.

5 Koenig, K.L., HCS, L., and Tsai, S.H. (2011). Crisis standard of care: refocusing care goals during catastrophic disasters and emergencies. *J Exp Clin Med* 3: 159–165. https://doi.org/10.1016/j.jecm.2011.06.003.

6 Powell, T., Christ, K.C., and Birkhead, G.S. (2008). Allocation of ventilators in a public health disaster. *Disaster Med Public Health Prep.* 2 (1): 20–26. https://doi.org/10.1097/DMP.0b013e3181620794.

7 Institute of Medicine (US) Forum on Medical and Public Health Preparedness for Catastrophic Events (2010). *Crisis Standards of Care: Summary of a Workshop Series.* Washington, DC: National Academies Press (US).

8 Centers for Disease Control & Prevention. Personal protective equipment (PPE) burn rate calculator. CDC. https://www.cdc.gov/coronavirus/2019-ncov/hcp-strategy/burn-calculator.html. Updated March 24, 2021. Accessed April 29, 2021.

9 Centers for Disease Control & Prevention. Strategies to mitigate healthcare personnel staffing shortages. CDC. https://www.cdc.gov/coronavirus/2019-ncov/hcp/mitigating-staff-shortages.html. Updated March 10, 2021. Accessed April 29, 2021.

10 Newby, J.C., Mabry, M.C., Carlisle, B.A. et al. (2020). Reflections on nursing ingenuity during the COVID-19 pandemic. *J Neurosci Nurs.* 52 (5): E13–E16. https://doi.org/10.1097/JNN.0000000000000525.

11 Zhang, X., Tai, D., Pforsich, H., and Lin, V.W. (2018). United States registered nurse workforce report card and shortage forecast: a revisit. *Am J Med Qual.* 33 (3): 229–236. https://doi.org/10.1177/1062860617738328.

12 Lasater, K.B., Aiken, L.H., Sloane, D.M. et al. (2021). Chronic hospital nurse understaffing meets COVID-19: an observational study. *BMJ Qual Saf.* 30: 639–647. https://doi.org/10.1136/bmjqs-2020-011512.

13 Dembosky A. California is overriding its limits on nurse workloads as COVID-19 surges. NPR. 2020. https://www.npr.org/sections/health-shots/2020/12/30/950177471/california-is-overriding-its-limits-on-nurse-workloads-as-covid-19-surges. Accessed April 27, 2021.

14 Holohan M. 'Silver lining' of 2020: Medical and nursing schools see an increase in applications. https://www.today.com/health/nursing-medical-schools-see-increase-applications-t204489. Published December 22, 2020. Accessed April 29, 2020.

15 Scaravilli, V., Grasselli, G., Castagna, L. et al. (2015). Prone positioning improves oxygenation in spontaneously breathing nonintubated patients with hypoxemic acute respiratory failure: a retrospective study. *J Crit Care* 30 (6): 1390–1394. https://doi.org/10.1016/j.jcrc.2015.07.008.

16 Wilcox, S.R. and Condella, A. (2021). Emergency department management of severe hypoxemic respiratory failure in adults with COVID-19. *J Emerg Med.* 60 (6): 729–742. https://doi.org/10.1016/j.jemermed.2020.12.014.

17 Taccone, P., Pesenti, A., Latini, R. et al. (2009). Prone positioning in patients with moderate and severe acute respiratory distress syndrome: a randomized controlled trial. *JAMA* 302 (18): 1977–1984. https://doi.org/10.1001/jama.2009.1614.

18 Raoof, S., Nava, S., Carpati, C., and Hill, N.S. (2020). High-flow, noninvasive ventilation and awake (nonintubation) proning in patients with coronavirus disease 2019 with respiratory failure. *Chest* 158 (5): 1992–2002. https://doi.org/10.1016/j.chest.2020.07.013.

19 Acute Respiratory Distress Syndrome Network, Brower, R.G., Matthay, M.A. et al. (2000). Ventilation with lower tidal volumes as compared with traditional tidal volumes for acute lung injury and the acute respiratory distress syndrome. *N Engl J Med.* 342 (18): 1301–1308. https://doi.org/10.1056/NEJM200005043421801.

20 Bellani, G., Laffey, J.G., Pham, T. et al. (2017). Noninvasive ventilation of patients with acute respiratory distress syndrome. Insights from the LUNG SAFE study. *Am J Respir. Crit Care Med.* 195 (1): 67–77. https://doi.org/10.1164/rccm.201606-1306OC.

21 Baroutjian, A., Sanchez, C., Boneva, D. et al. (2020). SARS-CoV-2 pharmacologic therapies and their safety/effectiveness according to level of evidence. *Am J Emerg Med.* 38 (11): 2405–2415. https://doi.org/10.1016/j.ajem.2020.08.091.

22 Beigel, J.H., Tomashek, K.M., Dodd, L.E. et al. (2020). Remdesivir for the treatment of Covid-19 – final report. *N Engl J Med.* 383 (19): 1813–1826. https://doi.org/10.1056/NEJMoa2007764.

23 Rosas, I.O., Bräu, N., Waters, M. et al. (2021). Tocilizumab in hospitalized patients with severe Covid-19 pneumonia. *N Engl J Med.* 384 (16): 1503–1516. https://doi.org/10.1056/NEJMoa2028700.

24 Centers for Disease Control & Prevention. Clinical care considerations for COVID-19 vaccination. CDC. https://www.cdc.gov/vaccines/covid-19/clinical-considerations/index.html. Updated March 11, 2021. Accessed May 7, 2021.

25 Centers for Disease Control & Prevention. V-safe after vaccination health checker. CDC. https://www.cdc.gov/coronavirus/2019-ncov/vaccines/safety/vsafe.html. Updated April 21, 2021. Accessed May 7, 2021.

26 Linn, D.D., Beckett, R.D., and Foellinger, K. (2015). Administration of enteral nutrition to adult patients in the prone position. *Intensive Crit Care Nurs.* 31 (1): 38–43. https://doi.org/10.1016/j.iccn.2014.07.002.

27 Elbaum, A. (2020). Black lives in a pandemic: implications of systemic injustice for end-of-life care. *Hastings Cent Rep* 50 (3): 58–60. http://doi.org/10.1002/hast.1135.

28 Centers for Disease Control & Prevention. Interim clinical guidance for management of patients with confirmed coronavirus disease (COVID-19). CDC. https://www.cdc.gov/coronavirus/2019-ncov/hcp/clinical-guidance-management-patients.html. Updated February 16, 2021. Accessed April 27, 2021.

29 Pannick, S., Davis, R., Ashrafian, H. et al. (2015). Effects of interdisciplinary team care interventions on general medical wards: a systematic review. *JAMA Intern Med.* 175 (8): 1288–1298. https://doi.org/10.1001/jamainternmed.2015.2421.

30 Waldman, G.J., Thakur, K.T., Der Nigoghossian, C. et al. (2020). Multidisciplinary guidance to manage comatose patients with severe COVID-19. *Ann Neurol.* 88 (4): 653–655. https://doi.org/10.1002/ana.25830.

31 Calligaro, K.D., Dougherty, M.J., Maloni, K. et al. (2020). Co-operative vascular intervention disease (COVID) team of greater Philadelphia. *J Vasc Surg.* 72 (4): 1178–1183.

32 Chun, T.T., Judelson, D.R., Rigberg, D. et al. (2020). Managing central venous access during a health care crisis. *J Vasc Surg.* 72 (4): 1184–95.e3. https://doi.org/10.1016/j.jvs.2020.06.112.

33 Centers for Medicare & Medicare Services (2019). Medicare and Medicaid Programs; Revisions to Requirements for Discharge Planning for Hospitals, Critical Access Hospitals, and Home Health Agencies, and Hospital and Critical Access Hospital Changes to Promote Innovation, Flexibility, and Improvement in Patient Care. *Federal Register* 84 (189): 51836–51884. https://www.federalregister.gov/documents/2019/09/30/2019-20732/medicare-and-medicaid-programs-revisions-to-requirements-for-discharge-planning-for-hospitals. Published September 30, 2019. Accessed May 30, 2021.

34 Gonçalves-Bradley, D.C., Lannin, N.A., Clemson, L.M. et al. (2016). Discharge planning from hospital. *Cochrane Database Syst Rev.* 2016 (1): CD000313. https://doi.org/10.1002/14651858.CD000313.pub5.

35 Brooks Carthon, J.M., Hedgeland, T., Brom, H. et al. (2019). "You only have time for so much in 12 hours" unmet social needs of hospitalised patients: a qualitative study of acute care nurses. *J Clin Nurs.* 28 (19–20): 3529–3537. https://doi.org/10.1111/jocn.14944.

36 Evans, M.K. (2020). Covid's color line – infectious disease, inequity, and racial justice. *N Engl J Med.* 383 (5): 408–410. https://doi.org/10.1056/NEJMp2019445.

37 Jiang, D.H. and McCoy, R.G. (2020). Planning for the post-COVID syndrome: how payers can mitigate long-term complications of the pandemic. *J Gen Intern Med.* 35 (10): 3036–3039. https://doi.org/10.1007/s11606-020-06042-3.

38 Lockwood, C. and Mabire, C. (2020). Hospital discharge planning: evidence, implementation and patient-centered care. *JBI Evid Synth.* 18 (2): 272–274. https://doi.org/10.11124/JBIES-20-00023.

39 Van Buren, N.R., Weber, E., Bliton, M.J., and Cunningham, T.V. (2021). In this together: navigating ethical challenges posed by family clustering during the Covid-19 pandemic. *Hastings Cent Rep.* 51 (2): 16–21. https://doi.org/10.1002/hast.1241.

40 Garg, S., Kim, L., Whitaker, M. et al. (2020). Hospitalization rates and characteristics of patients hospitalized with laboratory-confirmed coronavirus disease 2019 – COVID-NET, 14 States, March 1–30, 2020. *MMWR Morb Mortal Wkly Rep.* 60: 4580464. https://doi.org/10.15585/mmwr.mm6915e3.

41 Tenner-Hooban, S. (2021). Closing the loop of care, necessary changes during Covid. *DNA Reporter* 46 (1): 4.

42 Chopra, V., Flanders, S.A., O'Malley, M. et al. (2021). Sixty-day outcomes among patients hospitalized with COVID-19. *Ann Intern Med.* 174 (4): 576–578. https://doi.org/10.7326/M20-5661.

43 Atalla, E., Kalligeros, M., Giampaolo, G. et al. (2021). Readmissions among patients with COVID-19. *Int J Clin Pract.* 75 (3): e13700. https://doi.org/10.1111/ijcp.13700.

44 Stein, R.A. and Ometa, O. (2020). When public health crises collide: social disparities and COVID-19. *Int J Clin Pract.* 74 (9): e13524. https://doi.org/10.1111/ijcp.13524.

45 Kent, E.E., Ornstein, K.A., and Dionne-Odom, J.N. (2020). The family caregiving crisis meets an actual pandemic. *J Pain Symptom Manage.* 60 (1): e66–e69. https://doi.org/10.1016/j.jpainsymman.2020.04.006.

46 Smith, K. and Victor, C. (2019). Typologies of loneliness, living alone and social isolation, and their associations with physical and mental health. *Ageing Soc.* 39 (8): 1709–1730. https://doi.org/10.1017/S0144686X18000132.

47 Chen, Q., Liang, M., Li, Y. et al. (2020). Mental health care for medical staff in China during the COVID-19 outbreak. *Lancet Psychiatry* 7 (4): e15–e16. https://doi.org/10.1016/S2215-0366(20)30078-X.

48 Rogers, J.E.B., Constantine, L.A., Thompson, J.M. et al. (2021). COVID-19 pandemic impacts on U.S. hospice agencies: a national survey of hospice nurses and physicians. *Am J Hosp Palliat Care* 38 (5): 521–527. https://doi.org/10.1177/1049909121989987.

49 Kates, J., Gerolamo, A., and Pogorzelska-Maziarz, M. (2021). The impact of COVID-19 on the hospice and palliative care workforce. *Public Health Nurs.* 38 (3): 459–463. https://doi.org/10.1111/phn.12827.

50 Rosa, W.E., Gray, T.F., Chow, K. et al. (2020). Recommendations to leverage the palliative nursing role during COVID-19 and future public health crises. *J Hosp Palliat Nurs.* 22 (4): 260–269. https://doi.org/10.1097/NJH.0000000000000665.

51 Morley, G., Grady, C., McCarthy, J., and Ulrich, C.M. (2020). Covid-19: ethical challenges for nurses. *Hastings Cent. Rep.* 50 (3): 35–39. https://doi.org/10.1002/hast.1110.

52 New York Presbyterian. At height of COVID, nurses and doctors reported high levels of distress. https://www.nyp.org/news/levels-of-stress-during-covid. Published June 23, 2020. Accessed April 27, 2021.

53 Dyrbye, L.N., Shanafelt, T.D., Johnson, P.O. et al. (2019). A cross-sectional study exploring the relationship between burnout, absenteeism, and job performance among American nurses. *BMC Nurs.* 18: 57. https://doi.org/10.1186/s12912-019-0382-7.

54 Maslach, M. and Jackson, S.E. (1981). The measurement of experienced burnout. *J Occup Behav.* 2 (2): 99–113.

55 Poghosyan, L., Clarke, S.P., Finlayson, M., and Aiken, L.H. (2010). Nurse burnout and quality of care: cross-national investigation in six countries. *Res Nurs Health* 33 (4): 288–298. https://doi.org/10.1002/nur.20383.

56 Wilkinson, H., Whittington, R., Perry, L., and Eames, C. (2017). Examining the relationship between burnout and empathy in healthcare professionals: a systematic review. *Burn Res.* 6: 18–29. https://doi.org/10.1016/j.burn.2017.06.003.

57 Maguire, P., Faulkner, A., Booth, K. et al. (1996). Helping cancer patients disclose their concerns. *Eur J Cancer* 32A (1): 78–81. https://doi.org/10.1016/0959-8049(95)00527-7.

58 Kim, S.S., Kaplowitz, S., and Johnston, M.V. (2004). The effects of physician empathy on patient satisfaction and compliance. *Eval Health Prof.* 27 (3): 237–251. https://doi.org/10.1177/0163278704267037.

59 VandeKieft, G.K. (2001). Breaking bad news. *Am Fam Physician* 64 (12): 1975–1978.

60 Halpern, J. (2007). Empathy and patient-physician conflicts. *J Gen Intern Med.* 22 (5): 696–700. https://doi.org/10.1007/s11606-006-0102-3.

61 West, C.P., Huschka, M.M., Novotny, P.J. et al. (2006). Association of perceived medical errors with resident distress and empathy: a prospective longitudinal study. *JAMA* 296 (9): 1071–1078. https://doi.org/10.1001/jama.296.9.1071.

62 Savulescu, J., Persson, I., and Wilkinson, D. (2020). Utilitarianism and the pandemic. *Bioethics* 34 (6): 620–632. https://doi.org/10.1111/bioe.12771.

63 Traynor, M. (2018). Guest editorial: what's wrong with resilience. *J Res Nurs.* 23 (1): 5–8. https://doi.org/10.1177/1744987117751458.

64 Maben, J. and Bridges, J. (2020). Covid-19: supporting nurses' psychological and mental health. *J Clin Nurs.* 29 (15–16): 2742–2750. https://doi.org/10.1111/jocn.15307.

65 Billings J, Kember T, Greene T, et al. Guidance for planners of the psychological response to the stress experienced by hospital staff associated with COVID: early interventions. COVID trauma response working Ground rapid Guidance. 2020. www.aomrc.org.uk/wp-content/uploads/2020/03/Guidance-for-planners-of-the-psychological-response-to-stress-experienced-by-HCWs-COVID-trauma-response-working-group.pdf Accessed May 13, 2021.

66 Bridges, J., Nicholson, C., Maben, J. et al. (2013). Capacity for care: meta-ethnography of acute care nurses' experiences of the nurse-patient relationship. *J Adv Nurs.* 69 (4): 760–772. https://doi.org/10.1111/jan.12050.

67 Cole-King, A, Dykes, L. Wellbeing for HCWs during COVID-19. https://www.lindadykes.org/covid19. Updated May 19, 2020. Accessed May 13, 2021.

68 Adams, J.G. and Walls, R.M. (2020). Supporting the health care workforce during the COVID-19 global epidemic. *JAMA* 323 (15): 1439–1440. https://doi.org/10.1001/jama.2020.3972.

69 Greenberg, N., Docherty, M., Gnanapragasam, S., and Wessely, S. (2020). Managing mental health challenges faced by healthcare workers during covid-19 pandemic. *BMJ* 368: m1211. https://doi.org/10.1136/bmj.m1211.

70 Wallace, C.L., Wladkowski, S.P., Gibson, A., and White, P. (2020). Grief during the COVID-19 pandemic: considerations for palliative care providers. *J Pain Symptom Manage.* 60 (1): e70–e76. https://doi.org/10.1016/j.jpainsymman.2020.04.012.

71 Harris R. 'FACE COVID' – how to respond effectively to the corona crisis. 2020. https://www.actmindfully.com.au/wp-content/uploads/2020/03/FACE-COVID-eBook-by-Russ-Harris-March-2020.pdf. Accessed 13 May 2021.

72 Saad L. US ethics ratings rise for medical workers and teachers. *Gallup.* 22 December 2020. https://news.gallup.com/poll/328136/ethics-ratings-rise-medical-workers-teachers.aspx. Accessed 25 May 2021.

22

COVID-19 Vaccination

A Clinical Perspective

Anurag Singh[1], Simran P. Kaur[1], Mohd Fardeen Husain Shahanshah[1], Bhawna Sharma[1], Vijay K. Chaudhary[2], Sanjay Gupta[3], and Vandana Gupta[1]

[1] *Department of Microbiology, Ram Lal Anand College, University of Delhi, New Delhi, India*
[2] *Centre for Innovation in Infectious Disease Research, Education and Training, University of Delhi South Campus, New Delhi, India*
[3] *Independent Scholar (former Head, Centre for Emerging Diseases, Department of Biotechnology), Jaypee Institute of Information Technology, Noida, India*

Abbreviations

FDA	US Food and Drug Administration
IM	intramuscular
mAb	monoclonal antibody
SARS-CoV-2	severe acute respiratory syndrome coronavirus 2
WHO	World Health Organization

Severe acute respiratory syndrome coronavirus 2 (SARS-CoV-2), the causative agent of coronavirus disease 2019 (COVID-19), led to a pandemic claiming millions of lives across different age groups globally. The infected individuals primarily exhibit disease with varying severity and a wide variety of symptoms, including fever, dry cough, fatigue, shortness of breath, chills, weight loss, among others [1]. The secondary consequences of the disease include acute respiratory distress syndrome and an imbalance of liver and heart function, which may prompt multiple organ failure and death [2]. Viral shedding is prominent in the early phase of the infection, and contact tracing becomes a laborious task in the case of asymptomatic transmission [2]. Moreover, the effective use of masks, social distancing norms, and other nontherapeutic interventions are subject to the will and awareness of the user. The extreme variability of disease manifestation accentuates the need for a single perfect strategy that provides a sustained long-lasting immunity in everyone and mandates the hunt for both prophylactic and therapeutic measures. Possible off-target effects of approved therapeutics, heterologous protection from unrelated vaccines, and the use of monoclonal antibodies (mAbs) were initially explored to find an immediate cure [3, 4]. Interventions were channeled through clinical trials, with some of them gaining emergency use approval. Nevertheless, mass immunization with a safe and efficacious COVID-19 vaccine is essential to impede SARS-CoV-2 transmission and to restore social and economic activities. To combat the disease, accelerated efforts have been directed toward assessing various vaccine platforms, including protein subunit vaccines, viral vectored vaccines (replicating and nonreplicating), live attenuated vaccines, nucleic acid vaccines (DNA and RNA), and inactivated and virus-like particle vaccines (reviewed by Kaur and Gupta [5]).

In the initial section of this chapter, we describe a few terminologies related to the development and administration of vaccines and slowly shift toward the most clinical perspective of a few leading vaccine candidates. As of 1 January 2021, a total of 18 vaccine candidates were in phase 2 or higher trials [6], while 8 different vaccines gained regulatory approval in different countries [7]. Although the later-phase trials in a few thousand volunteers reflect on the most common adverse events that may be related to vaccines, larger public rollout might lead to several rare clinical symptoms and requires close regulatory monitoring. Therefore, symptom management holds

Coronavirus Disease 2019 (COVID-19): A Clinical Guide, First Edition. Edited by Ali Gholamrezanezhad and Michael P. Dube.
© 2023 John Wiley & Sons Ltd. Published 2023 by John Wiley & Sons Ltd.

important ground in the effective acceptance of prophylaxis and is dealt with in a dedicated section. Furthermore, the equitable and effective deployment of vaccines is equally significant to achieve the overall goal of immunization. Through a joint effort by the World Health Organization (WHO), the Coalition for Epidemic Preparedness Innovations, and Global Alliance for Vaccines and Immunization, the COVID-19 Vaccines Global Access Facility was created to accelerate the vaccine development process and to guarantee "fair and equitable" supply across the world [8]. Effective immunization drive is also dependent on the acceptability of vaccines among the general public, which in turn primarily depends on the vaccine's safety and efficacy. We close this chapter with insight on passive immunization and how it fares in this current pandemic. Convalescent plasma led to faster symptom resolution, but neither imparts mortality benefit nor hinders the disease progression [4]. However, several mAbs targeted against SARS-CoV-2 provided documented benefits, and three of them went on to gain approval for emergency use [9].

Terminologies

Storage and Handling

The availability of trained personnel and maintenance of cold chain are prerequisites for ensuring the safety and efficacy of the vaccination program. As per the worldwide WHO data, there is 50% wastage of the total vaccine stock, which is essentially attributed to the breach of cold chain and stock management issues [10]. To ensure the moderation of program cost by preventing high wastage, the vaccines (frozen or refrigerated)

should be stored as recommended by the manufacturer and must be safeguarded from exposure to temperature and light beyond the parameter range. The major elements for management of the cold-chain system are personnel (for vaccine management and administration), equipment (for storage and transportation of vaccine), and monitoring procedures (for ensuring the maintenance of appropriate temperature) [11].

Reactogenicity

The administration of vaccines with or without an adjuvant may induce a localized or systemic inflammatory response. A subset of symptoms, including injection-site pain, swelling and redness, development of fever, myalgia, headache, and rash, represent the reactogenicity of a vaccine. It is important to understand the reactogenicity profile of a vaccine by the healthcare professionals to ensure high vaccine coverage and acceptance in the population [12]. Factors that affect the reactogenicity of a vaccine are depicted in Figure 22.1, and an overview of the mechanism behind the progress of reactogenicity symptoms is depicted in Figure 22.2.

Efficacy and Immunogenicity

Vaccine efficacy is the proportionate reduction in disease incidence rate in the vaccinated and placebo group under optimal conditions [13]. The ratio of disease attack rates in vaccinated to the unvaccinated groups is the risk ratio, and one minus risk ratio, expressed in percentage, is called the *vaccine efficacy* [14]. However, immunogenicity accounts for the type and magnitude of the immune response mounted

Factors influencing reactogenicity

Vaccine factors	Vaccine administration factors	Individual factors
• Administration • Antigen dose • Type of adjuvant • Number of doses • Physicochemical characteristics	• Type and length of needle • Route of administration • Interval between doses	• Age • Body mass index (BMI) • Any underlying medical condition • Gender • Host genetics

Figure 22.1 Factors that influence the reactogenicity of a vaccine. The prevalence and severity of local and systemic adverse events are theoretically influenced by host factors, administration factors, and vaccine factors. *Source:* Hervé et al. [12].

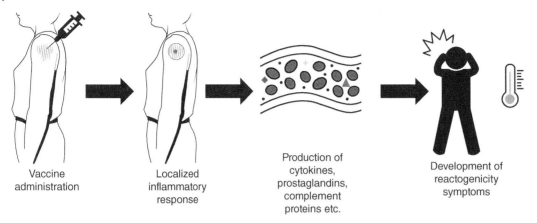

Figure 22.2 An overview of the mechanism of progression of reactogenicity symptoms after vaccination. The immune enhancers present in the vaccine formulation stimulate the resident immune cells, including macrophages, monocytes, and mast cells, and activate the innate immune arm. This results in the release of soluble factors, such as proinflammatory cytokines, vasodilators, and chemokines, which further allows the extravasation and recruitment of neutrophils and T lymphocytes to the site of injection. Prostaglandins, ATP, cytokines, and other soluble factors released by these immune cells are responsible for the development of typical cardinal signs of inflammation, while the paracrine activity of these cytokines stimulates the production of C-reactive proteins and some acute-phase proteins via liver, which later produce the systemic response.

by the vaccine. The evaluation of the immune response governs the dosage and immunization schedules of a vaccine candidate [15].

Contraindication

"A contraindication is a health condition in the recipient that increases the likelihood of a serious adverse reaction to a vaccine" [16]. Anaphylactic reaction to a vaccine component is a contraindication to all the vaccines that contain that particular component. Therefore, the administration of the vaccine must be avoided in the presence of contraindication. The individuals who previously exhibited an anaphylactic reaction to a preceding dose of the COVID-19 vaccine or any components of the vaccine, and immunocompromised individuals are contraindicated [16]. The list of contraindications varies from one vaccine to another and must be noted before administration of the COVID-19 vaccine.

Precaution

The condition that can enhance the severity of the risks of the postimmunization adverse reaction and can reduce the immune system's ability to generate an appropriate immune response against the antigen

leading to diagnostic confusion is referred to as *precaution*. Customarily, individuals with this condition should abstain from vaccine administration. Nevertheless, if the advantage of immunization exceeds the perils of the adverse reaction, then they may opt for immunization after expert consultation [16].

Authorized Candidate Vaccines

Eight vaccine candidates have gained Emergency Use Authorization in various parts of the world as of 1 January 2021 (Table 22.1) [7]. Notably, three prominent candidates—BNT162b2, mRNA-1273, and ChAdOX1 nCoV-19 vaccine—have *widely displayed* efficacy in phase 3 trials, whereas the rest have limited scientific evidence publicly available. The WHO in its "Draft Landscape of COVID-19 Candidate Vaccines" enlists 18 vaccine candidates in phase 2 or later trials [6]. Tables 22.1–22.6 provide information on these candidates classified under subgroups: nucleic acid vaccine (Table 22.2), inactivated vaccine (Table 22.3), viral vector vaccine (Table 22.4), protein subunit vaccine (Table 22.5), and virus-like particle (Table 22.6). According to the WHO [6], the EpiVacCorona vaccine is in phase 1/2 trial. However, it has gained regulatory approval in Russia [7].

Table 22.1 Vaccines candidates with regulatory approval in different countries on 1 January 2021.

Serial no.	Vaccine (developer)	Countries
1.	BNT162b2/Comirnaty (BioNTech/Pfizer/Fosun Pharma)	Bahrain, Canada, Chile, European Union, Kuwait, Mexico, Oman, Saudi Arabia, Singapore, United Kingdom, United States (World Health Organization has also provided emergency use validation)
2.	mRNA-1273 (Moderna)	Canada, European Union, Israel, United States
3.	ChAdOX1 nCoV-19 vaccine (AstraZeneca and Oxford University)	Argentina, Dominican Republic, El Salvador, Mexico, Morocco, United Kingdom
4.	Sputnik V (Gamaleya Research Institute of Epidemiology and Microbiology, Russia)	Russia
5.	CoronaVac (Sinovac Research and Development Co., Ltd)	China
6.	Unnamed (Sinopharm/Wuhan Institute of Biological Products Co., Ltd)	China
7.	BBIBP-CorV (Sinopharm/Beijing Institute of Biological Products)	Bahrain, China, Egypt, United Arab Emirates
8.	EpiVacCorona (State Research Center of Virology and Biotechnology VECTOR, Russia)	Russia

Source: Modified from Craven [7].

BNT162b2/Comirnaty (BioNTech/Pfizer/Fosun Pharma)

BNT162b2 contains a nucleoside-modified mRNA with two proline mutations, encoding a full-length prefusion stabilized conformation of SARS-CoV-2 spike protein. It is recommended to be administered intramuscularly (IM; in deltoid muscle) in two 30-µg doses (0.3 ml volume per dose), three weeks apart. It is formulated in preservative-free lipid nanoparticles and is supplied as a multidose vial stored between −80 and −60 °C, with each dose comprising lipids, sucrose, and salts: dibasic sodium phosphate dihydrate, monobasic potassium phosphate, potassium chloride, and sodium chloride (see Table 22.2). The vial once thawed is diluted with 1.8 ml 0.9% NaCl solution before administration. The diluted content can be stored between 2 and 25 °C for up to six hours. The thawed vial must never be refrozen [17, 18].

Data from a randomized, observer-blinded, 1:1 placebo-controlled, phase 2/3 study in 43 448 participants (21 720 in the intervention arm) aged 16 years and older reported BNT162b2 to have 95% efficacy in preventing symptomatic COVID-19 (assessed seven days after second dose), which was consistent among various subgroups such as sex, age, ethnicity, or individuals with comorbid conditions [18]. Two doses of BNT162b2 elicit a strong IgG antibody response, the 50% geometric mean titer of which is higher than those observed in convalescent plasma. It also elicits vigorous $CD8^+$ and T helper 1–$CD4^+$ T cell expansion [68].

Reactogenicity was observed in 8183 of 43 448 individuals and was more commonly reported in the intervention group than placebo recipient and in younger (16–55 years) than older (>55 years) participants [18]. Local events primarily were mild to moderate, including pain, redness, and swelling, while systemic ones included headache, fatigue, muscle and joint pain, fever, chills, and diarrhea. In this *subset*, 83% and 78% of the younger population and 71% and 66% among the older ones reported pain after the first and second doses, respectively. Redness was observed in 5% and 6% of younger participants after the first and second doses; it was 5% and 7% in older participants after the first and

Table 22.2 Nucleic acid vaccine undergoing phase 2/3 clinical trials.

Serial no.	Vaccine [developer]	Components	Reported data from trials (content can be written in a line or two)	References
1.	**BNT162b2/Comirnaty [BioNTech/ Pfizer/ Fosun Pharma] [mRNA]**	mRNA; **Lipids:** ((4-hydroxybutyl)azanediyl)bis(hexane-6,1-diyl)bis(2- hexyldecanoate), 2-[(polyethylene glycol)-2000]-N,N-ditetradecylacetamide, 1,2-distearoyl-snglycero-3-phosphocholine, and cholesterol; **sucrose;** and **salts:** dibasic sodium phosphate dihydrate, monobasic potassium phosphate, potassium chloride, and sodium chloride.	1) Dosage: Two IM dose (30 µg/0.3 ml) 3 wk apart 2) Reactogenicity: Mild-to-moderate local events including pain, redness and swelling. Systemic events include headache, fatigue, muscle and joint pain, fever, chills and diarrhea. 3) Efficacy: 95% 4) Storage: Stored between −80 °C and −60 °C	[17, 18]
2.	**mRNA-1273 [Moderna] [mRNA]**	mRNA; lipids (SM-102, 1,2-dimyristoyl-rac-glycero-3-methoxypolyethylene glycol-2000 [PEG2000-DMG], 1,2-distearoyl-sn-glycero-3-phosphocholine [DSPC], and cholesterol), acetic acid, sodium acetate, sucrose, tromethamine, and tromethamine hydrochloride	1) Dosage: Two IM dose (100 µg/0.5 ml) 4 weeks apart 2) Reactogenicity: Grade 1 and 2 local events including pain, swelling, redness, tenderness and induration. 3) Transient moderate-to-severe systemic events including fatigue, headache, myalgia, arthralgia, nausea, chills and fever. 4) Efficacy: 94.1% 5) Storage: Stored between −25 °C and −15 °C	[19, 20]
3.	**CVnCoV [CureVac] [mRNA]**	mRNA, lipid: 1,2-distearoyl-sn-glycero-3-phosphocholine (DSPC), a cationic lipid, PEG-ylated lipid and cholesterol.	1) Dosage: Two IM dose (0.5 ml) 4 weeks apart 2) Reactogenicity (Phase 1): Grade 1 and 2 pain at the injection site. Mild to moderate systemic events including fatigue, headache, chills and myalgia. Fever reported rarely. Transient lymphopenia was also reported. 3) Efficacy: Not known. Under Phase 2b/3, trial (36 500 participants) NCT04652102. 4) Storage: Stable for 3 mo at 5 °C and up to 24hr at room temperature.	[21, 22]

| 4. | **INO-4800 [Inovio Pharmaceuticals/ International Vaccine Institute]** [DNA] | It contains pGX9501 plasmid which express a synthetic optimized full length sequence of SARS-CoV-2S glycoprotein. | 1) Dosage: ID dose (0.1 ml) followed by electroporation using the CELLECTRAO 2000 device.
2) Reactogenicity (Phase 1): Pain and erythema at injection site. Grade 1 systemic event includes nausea. No increase in frequencies of adverse events after the second dose.
3) Efficacy: Not known.
4) Storage: Stable at 2–8 °C for more than 4.5 yr, at room temperature for 1 yr. | [23, 24] |

Efficacies of BNT162b2 and mRNA-1273 were assessed 7 and 14 days after the second dose, respectively.
ID, intradermal; IM, intramuscular.
Source: World Health Organization [6].

Table 22.3 Inactivated vaccines in phase 3 clinical trials.

Serial no.	Vaccine [developer]	Components	Reported data from trials (content can be written in a line or two)	References
1.	**CoronaVac [Sinovac Research and Development Co., Ltd]**	Alum absorbed inactivated SARS-CoV-2 (CN02 strain) diluted in a solution of sodium chloride, phosphate buffer saline, and water.	1) Dosage: Two IM doses (3 μg or 6 μg/0.5 ml), 3 or 4 wk apart. 2) Reactogenicity: Grade 1 (mild) adverse events and injection site pain, redness and swelling. One case of urticaria was also observed. 3) Efficacy: It showed 78% efficacy in a late-stage Brazilian trial. 4) Storage: Stored at 25 °C for 42 d, at 37 °C for 28 d, and at 2–8 °C for 5 mo.	[25–27]
2.	**Covaxin/BBV152 [Bharat Biotech International Limited]**	Inactivated SARS-CoV-2 whole-virion, adjuvanted with Algel (alum) and Algel-IMDG (TLR7/TLR8 agonist, an imidazoquinoline class molecule).	1) Dosage: Two IM doses (3 μg or 6 μg/0.5 ml), 3 or 4 wk apart. 2) Reactogenicity: Grade 1 (mild) adverse events, injection site pain, fatigue, headache, and fever. 3) Efficacy: Not known 4) Storage: Stored at 2–8 °C temperature	[28, 29]
3.	**Unnamed [Sinopharm/ Wuhan Institute of Biological Products Co., Ltd.]**	Inactivated WIV04 strain absorbed on 0.5-mg alum and diluted into 0.5 ml sterile phosphate buffer saline.	1) Dosage: Two IM doses (2.5, 5, or 10 μg/0.5 ml), at least 2 wk apart. 2) Reactogenicity: Grade 1 (mild) adverse events, including injection site pain followed by fever. 3) Efficacy: Not known 4) Storage: Data not available. 2–8 °C temperature is maintained while inactivating the virus.	[30]
4.	**BBIBP-CorV [Sinopharm/Beijing Institute of Biological Products (Beijing, China)]**	Liquid formulation of purified 19nCoV-CDC-Tan-HB02 (HB02) inactivated strain, adjuvanted to alum.	1) Dosage: Two IM doses (4 μg or 8 μg/0.5 ml), 3 or 4 wk apart. 2) Reactogenicity: local events such as injection site pain, swelling and itching. Systemic adverse events including fever, inappetence, constipation, mucocutaneous abnormalities, headache, vomiting, and itching at the non-injection site. 3) Efficacy: Sinopharm stated that the vaccine is 79.34% effective, without releasing any detailed efficacy data. 4) Storage: Data not available. 5) However, 2–8 °C temperature is maintained while inactivating the virus.	[31, 32]

IM, intramuscular; SARS-CoV-2, severe acute respiratory syndrome coronavirus 2; TLR, Toll-like receptor.
Data on a phase 2 inactivated vaccine, developed by Shenzhen Kangtai Biological Products Co., Ltd, are not available publically. Evaluation criteria for efficacy of CoronaVac and BBIBP-CorV are not available publically.
Source: World Health Organization [6].

Table 22.4 Viral vector vaccines undergoing phase 2/3 clinical trials.

Serial no.	Vaccine [developer]	Components	Reported data from trials	References
1.	**AZD1222/ChAdOx1/Covishield [University of Oxford & AstraZeneca]**	Replication-deficient Chimpanzee adenovirus (ChAd) encoding for S glycoprotein; Excipients: L-histidine, L-histidine hydrochloride monohydrate, magnesium chloride hexahydrate, polysorbate 80, ethanol, sodium chloride, sucrose, disodium edetate dihydrate, and water	1) Dosage: Two IM doses, at least 4 wk apart 2) Reactogenicity: 74% of participants depicted localized reactions and 75% of individuals depicted systemic reactions. 3) Efficacy: 70.4% 4) Storage: Shelf life 180 days; 2–8 °C	[33, 34]
2.	**Sputnik V [Gamaleya Research Institute of Epidemiology and Microbiology, Russia]**	Dual component recombinant adenoviral non-replicating vector (rAd26-S and rAd5-S) encoding for the spike protein	1) Dosage: Two IM doses of two-component vaccine administered 21 d apart. 2) Reactogenicity: mild local and systemic adverse events like localized pain, muscle and joint pain, headache, hyperthermia, asthenia, etc. 3) Efficacy: 92% 4) Storage: 2–8 °C	[35–37]
3.	**Ad5-nCoV/Convidecia [CanSino Biological Inc./ Beijing Institute of Biotechnology]**	It is constructed using the AdMax™ system which contains Adenovirus inactivated by gamma radiation.	1) Dosage: 5×10^{10} viral particles containing single IM dose. 2) Reactogenicity: Severe adverse reactions reported in 1% of the total volunteers in Phase 2 clinical trials. 3) Efficacy: Not known 4) Storage: 2–8 °C	[38, 39]
4.	**Ad26.CoV2.S [Janssen Pharmaceutical/Johnson & Johnson]**	It is prepared using the AdVac* technology which contains the non-replicating adenovirus vector	1) Dosage: Single-dose, IM administration 2) Reactogenicity: 43% volunteers depicted the localized adverse events while 50% individuals depicted the systemic adverse events with a few cases of grade 3 fever. 3) Efficacy: Not known 4) Storage: 2 yr at −20 °C; 2–8 °C for 3 mo	[6, 40]

Data on a phase 2 vaccine, DelNS1-2019-nCoV-RBD-OPT1 (Intranasal flu-based-RBD), developed by Jiangsu Provincial Centre for Disease Prevention, and control are not available publically. Efficacies of AZD1222/ChAdOx1 and Sputnik V were assessed 14 and 7 days after the second dose, respectively.
Source: World Health Organization [6].

Table 22.5 Protein/Peptide-based vaccines undergoing phase 2/5 clinical trials.

Serial no.	Vaccine [developer]	Components	Reported data from trials	References
1.	NVX-CoV2373 [Novavax Inc.]	Recombinant nanoparticle vaccine with mutations at the S1/S2 cleavage site along with certain substitutions in the full-length SARS-CoV-2 spike glycoprotein. Saponin based Matrix M comes as an adjuvant.	1) Dosage: Two IM doses of 10 µg/ml at an interval of 21 d. 2) Reactogenicity: It was either absent or mild which lasted for less than 2 d. Pain, erythema, tenderness and swelling at the site of injection was observed. One participant developed mild fever which lasted for a day. 3) Efficacy: Generates an effective and well tolerated immune response with an efficacy of 89.3% in UK phase 3 trials. However, it showed an efficacy of 60% in South African Phase 2b trials. All participants developed a strong anti-spike IgG neutralizing antibody reaction. 4) Storage: 2–8 °C.	[5, 41–46]
2.	Recombinant new coronavirus vaccine (CHO cell)/ZF2001 [Anhui Zhifei Longcom Biopharmaceutical, Institute of Microbiology Chinese Academy of Sciences]	RBD-dimer (aa residues 319–537 as tandem repeat) from the spike protein of SARS-CoV-2 with aluminum based adjuvant	1) Dosage: 0.5 ml of the vaccine is administered IM in two/three doses on Day 0, Day 14 (for two dose regimen), and Day 28 (for three dose regimen) 2) Reactogenicity: Mild pain at the site of the injection with redness and swelling. This wasn't common 3) Efficacy: No adverse side effects were reported. Sera of 93% of the participants showed significant titers of nAbs specific to the virus. 4) Storage: Data not available	[45, 47–53]
3.	Recombinant SARS-CoV-2 vaccine (Sf9 cell) [West China Hospital, Sichuan University]	The peptide between 319 and 545 aa residues of the receptor binding domain of the spike protein of SARS-CoV-2 is conjugated with a GP67 signal peptide sequence to produce a 34 kDa immunogen. Aluminum hydroxide is added as an adjuvant.	1) Dosage: It is administered intramuscularly in two doses at an interval of 28 d. 2) Reactogenicity: Data not available 3) Efficacy: The vaccine can mount an effective virus neutralizing immune response. The toxicology analysis confirms that it is safe to use. No obvious side effects have been reported. 4) Storage: Data not available	[54–58]
4.	EpiVacCorona [State Research Center of Virology and Biotechnology VECTOR, Russia]	The primary immunogenic component of this vaccine is the chemically synthesized peptide antigens of SARS-CoV-2 proteins. These peptide antigens are conjugated to a carrier protein and adsorbed on an aluminum-containing adjuvant such as aluminum hydroxide	1) Dosage: The vaccine is administered intramuscularly in two doses which are spaced 14–28 d apart. 2) Reactogenicity: Data not available 3) Efficacy: EpiVacCorona induces an effective immune response against the novel coronavirus without eliciting any side effects. From preclinical studies, the vaccine doesn't have any embryotoxic properties and does not affect the reproductive ability of the organisms even at higher doses. 4) Storage: 2–8 °C. Retain its viability for up to 2 yr.	[59–63]

According to the World Health Organization, EpiVacCorona is in phase 1/2 trial. However, it has gained regulatory approval in Russia. Evaluation criteria for efficacy of NVX-CoV2373 are not available publically.

aa, amino acid; IgG, immunoglobulin G; RBD, receptor-binding domain; nAb, neutralizing antibody; SARS-CoV-2, severe acute respiratory syndrome coronavirus 2.

Source: World Health Organization [6] and Craven [7].

Table 22.6 Virus-like particle vaccine undergoing phase 2/3 clinical trials.

Vaccine [developer]	Components	Reported data from trials	References
CoV-like particle (CoVLP) [Medicago]	CoVLP adjuvanted vaccine with AS03 adjuvant (squalene-based immunologic adjuvant/ GSK's pandemic adjuvant)	1) Dosage: 3.75 µg of CoVLP adjuvanted vaccine with AS03 adjuvant (squalene-based immunologic adjuvant/GSK's pandemic adjuvant) (0.5 ml) is administered intramuscularly to the deltoid region of the alternating arm in two doses which are spaced 21 d apart. 2) Reactogenicity: Both local and systemic reactogenicity events had similar frequency of occurrence. The severity and frequency of these adverse events increased after administration of the second dose. 3) Efficacy: Elicited a strong humoral and T cell response. nAb titers were 10 times higher than those observed in patients recovering from COVID-19. 4) Storage: CoVLP vaccine can be stored at 2–8 °C making cold chain management easier with the existing infrastructure.	[64–67]

CoVLP, coronavirus-like particle; GSK, GlaxoSmithKline; nAb, neutralizing antibody.
Source: World Health Organization [6].

second doses, respectively. Systemic reactogenicity was also frequent in younger recipients, with 47% and 59% reporting fatigue after the first and second doses, respectively, while it was conveyed by 34% and 51% of the older participants after the first and second doses. Similarly, headache was reported in 42%, 52%, 25%, and 39% in that order. Notably, placebo recipients also reported headache (24% and 14% after the second dose in younger and older recipients, respectively) and fatigue (23% and 17% after the second dose in younger and older recipients, respectively). Moreover, 16% of younger participants and 11% of older ones reported a body temperature greater than 38 °C. Overall, 0.2% and 0.8% of BNT162b2 recipients reported high fever after the first and second doses, respectively (38.9–40 °C), while two recipients reported body temperature greater than 40 °C. It was also found that the younger recipients tend to use antipyretics more often. Grade 4 reactogenicities, those requiring emergency hospitalization, were not reported in any participant.

Serious adverse responses (shoulder injury, lymphadenopathy, right leg paresthesia, and ventricular arrhythmia) were noted in four BNT162b2 recipients. The US Food and Drug Administration (FDA) considers shoulder injury and lymphadenopathy, to be related to vaccination. Furthermore, four cases of Bell's palsy were also noted in the vaccine group (no cases in the placebo group) [17]. Six deaths were also reported from this phase 2/3 study, which were unrelated to vaccine or placebo injection; two were in the intervention arm (one each from arteriosclerosis and cardiac arrest), and four from placebo group [17, 18].

Although phase 2/3 trial does not provide data to signify the efficacy and possible use of a single-dose regimen, the authors concluded that as early as 12 days after first jab, the vaccine efficacy to prevent COVID-19 was 52%, which increased to 91% within seven days after the second dose, and reached its peak at least seven days after the second jab. The UK government recently decided to delay the second dose by 12 weeks to inoculate as many people as possible with the first dose [69]. The study was not equipped to recommend vaccination to those younger than 16 years, pregnant or lactating women, those with immunocompromised conditions, or concomitant administration with other vaccines [18]. Nevertheless, this phase 2/3 study included participants with stable chronic illnesses, including HIV (human immunodeficiency virus), hepatitis B virus, and hepatitis C virus infections, but did not include those undergoing immunosuppressive therapy. With the vaccine being rolled out to the larger public, several reported side effects are now being investigated for their association with the jab. A Mexican doctor with a history of allergy was admitted to the intensive care unit with a possible encephalomyelitis, postvaccination, with regulators accessing the cause [70]. Norway also reported fatal outcomes in many elderly vaccine recipients. Causation could not be immediately ascertained; however, investigations into 13 deaths concluded that common adverse events from vaccination might have resulted in aggravating preexisting medical conditions [71].

mRNA-1273 (Moderna)

Jointly developed by Moderna and the National Institute of Allergy and Infectious Diseases, mRNA-1273 expresses SARS-CoV-2 spike protein stabilized in a prefusion conformation. The mRNA encapsulated in lipid nanoparticle comes frozen between −25 and −15 °C in a preservative-free multidose vial and is recommended to be administered undiluted IM (deltoid area of the same arm) in two doses of 100 µg (0.5 ml) each, four weeks apart. Other contents in a dose include lipids, acetic acid, sodium acetate, sucrose, tromethamine, and tromethamine hydrochloride. This preparation is stable for 30 days when stored between 2 and 8 °C before puncturing and can also be held for up to eight hours at room temperature before administration [19, 20]. Dry ice is not recommended for storing the vials; and once thawed, it must be used within six hours and must not be refrozen [20]. mRNA-1273 induces a high level of neutralizing antibodies, along with T helper 1–CD4$^+$ T cell response [72]. Data from phase 3 randomized COVE (coronavirus efficacy) trial in 30 420 volunteers of 18 years and older show mRNA-1273 to have 94.1% efficacy in preventing symptomatic COVID-19 (assessed 14 days after second dose), which was consistent across subgroups such as demography, age, sex, and so on. Clinical data from 28 207 participants (14 134 and 14 073 among vaccine and placebo groups, respectively) were used in primary efficacy analysis [19]. Reactogenicity was frequently observed in

the intervention group as compared with placebo and in participants aged between 18 and 65 years compared with those older than 65 years. Local events were more often observed after the second dose (88.6% and 18.8% in the vaccine and placebo groups, respectively) than the first dose (84.2% and 19.8% in the vaccine and placebo groups, respectively). Similar trends were observed for systemic reactogenicity, with 54.9% and 42.2% after the first dose and 79.4% and 36.5% after the second dose in the vaccine and placebo groups, respectively. Local adverse events (pain, swelling, redness, tenderness, and induration) were primarily of grade 1 and 2 severity and resolved after a mean of 2.6 days after the first and 3.2 days after the second dose. Notably, participants positive for SARS-CoV-2 at baseline experienced lesser adverse events. Treatment-related adverse events turned out to be higher among vaccine recipients (8.2% vs 4.5% in placebo), with fatigue in 1.5% and headache reported in 1.4%. Transient moderate-to-severe systemic events, such as myalgia, arthralgia, nausea, and chills, were reported in around 50% of mRNA-1273 recipients. About 0.8% and 15.6% of vaccine recipients reported fever after doses 1 and 2, respectively [19, 73]. Lymphadenopathy was also noted as an adverse event after any dose of vaccine administration in 21.4% of younger participants (<65 years) and in 12.4% of older participants (≥65 years). Hypersensitive reactions were found in 1.5% of vaccine recipients, and 13 fatal but treatment-unrelated serious adverse events were also described, 6 in the intervention group and 7 in the placebo group. However, investigators also reported seven vaccine-related serious adverse events in the intervention group (and five in placebo), including intractable nausea/vomiting, two cases of facial swelling, rheumatoid arthritis, dyspnea with exertion and peripheral edema, autonomic dysfunction, and B-cell lymphocytic lymphoma. The FDA considers the former three cases to be likely related to vaccination. Furthermore, cases of Bell's palsy were also noted in the mRNA-1273 group (n = 3) and placebo group (n = 1), which according to the FDA cannot be "definitively excluded" as unrelated to study vaccination [73].

Although limited preliminary data suggest prevention of asymptomatic infection after the first dose, additional studies are underway to better understand the impact of mRNA-1273 in cutting transmission chains [74]. Data from clinical trials were notably insufficient to provide evidence for use of mRNA-1273 vaccine as effective prophylaxis in various groups, such as individuals aged 17 years and younger, pregnant and lactating women, and immunocompromised individuals. These studies also do not reflect on the possible use of mRNA-1273 in single-dose regimens or concomitantly with other vaccines [73].

AZD1222/ChAdOx1/Covishield (University of Oxford and AstraZeneca)

The recombinant ChAdOx1 nCoV-19 vaccine, codeveloped by AstraZeneca and Oxford University, is capable of escalating the immunity against SARS-CoV-2 by stimulating the humoral and cell-mediated immune response. The replication-deficient chimpanzee adenovirus vector coding for the spike glycoprotein is produced in the genetically modified human embryonic kidney (HEK) 293 cells [75]. The vials contain a colorless (clear) to a slightly brown (opaque) solution at pH 6.6 and contain less than 1 mmol sodium. Other excipient molecules include L-histidine, L-histidine hydrochloride monohydrate, magnesium chloride hexahydrate, polysorbate 80, ethanol, sodium chloride, sucrose, disodium edetate dihydrate, and water. The vaccine-containing vials must be stored at 2–8 °C for six months (in the sealed state) and at 2–25 °C for six hours (during the use period). The product is light sensitive and should be maintained in the outer cartons to prevent photodegradation. Moreover, it is free of any preservatives; therefore, aseptic techniques must be used. The vaccine is to be administered IM (preferably in the deltoid muscle) in two doses (0.5 ml each), which must be 4 to 12 weeks apart, by a trained healthcare worker. Furthermore, the batch number and other details must be recorded clearly to ensure the traceability of the vaccine [33].

Sufficient clinical data on the impact of the vaccine on pregnant and lactating women are not available; however, the preclinical data do not specify any direct or indirect impact on the mother and fetus. There was no explicit impact on fertility after the administration of the vaccine in animal studies. Thrombocytopenic individuals must be vaccinated with caution, and individuals with a severe concurrent illness should get a shot at a later date [33]. However, ChAdOx1 has not been administered in children (<18 years old) and

immunocompromised individuals during the clinical studies, and it has limited data on people with comorbidities. The interim analysis report has documented that the vaccine is better tolerated by the older adults (age, ≥56 years) than the younger adults (age, 18–55 years). Local (induration, itching, pain, swelling, tenderness) and systemic (chills, fatigue, fever, headache, joint pain, malaise, muscle pain, nausea) reactions may be reported after the administration. In the clinical studies, a few individuals developed transverse myelitis (an unsolicited adverse event) that may be related to vaccine administration [34, 76, 77]. The adverse events can also include disorders of the circulatory system, nervous system, gastrointestinal system, skin or subcutaneous tissue, and connective tissues. These adverse events must be reported to the authorities as per the prescribed route [33].

Currently, there is no data on duration, the intensity of immune response, and interchangeability of vaccines; however, AstraZeneca will use the Ad26 vector-based component of the Sputnik V vaccine in the upcoming clinical trials to test the prospect of enhancing the efficacy of the vaccine [35]. The combined data from two dosing regimens of ChAdOx1 nCov-2019 vaccine have suggested an overall efficacy rate of 70.4% against the symptomatic disease, which was evaluated after 14 days of the administration of the second standard dose [77]. Furthermore, the vaccine was found to be 59% effective against the asymptomatic disease [78]. Persons with more than one comorbidity also exhibited an efficacy rate of 73.43%, which is equivalent to the average vaccine efficacy. The rate of seroconversion in individuals after securing the second dose of the vaccine is 99% [33]. However, the ultimate potential of the vaccine is to provide immunity against even asymptomatic infections.

Sputnik V (Gamaleya Research Institute of Epidemiology and Microbiology, Russia)

Sputnik V (earlier known as Gam-COVID-Vac) is a dual-component vaccine with recombinant adenoviral vectors (rAd26-S and rAd5-S) expressing a gene for spike glycoprotein [41]. IM administration twice at an interval of 21 days can prime the immune system against SARS-CoV-2, thus inducing the antigen-specific neutralizing IgG production and T cell responses [79]. The interim data analysis obtained 21 days postvaccination suggested an overall efficacy rate of 91.4%, thereby preventing the symptomatic infections and providing 100% protection against severe cases of COVID-19. The lyophilized form of the vaccine can be stored at refrigeration temperature (2–8 °C). The safety and tolerability of the vaccine among individuals between the ages of 18 and 60 years have been determined by phase 1/2 clinical trials. The studies and postapproval vaccination drives have reported mild local and systemic adverse events, such as localized pain, muscle and joint pain, headache, hyperthermia, asthenia, among others [36, 80]. Data on the efficacy of the vaccine in special conditions, such as pregnancy, immunocompromised conditions, and children, are currently unavailable [79].

CoronaVac (Sinovac Research and Development co., Ltd)

CoronaVac (previously known as PiCoVacc), developed by Sinovac Life Sciences (Beijing, China), is prepared by the absorption of inactivated SARS-CoV-2 (CN02 strain) on alum followed by dilution in the solution of sodium chloride, phosphate-buffered saline, and water [25]. It remains stable at 25 °C for 42 days, at 37 °C for 28 days, and at 2–8 °C for five months [26]. As per the reports, it showed 78% efficacy in the trials performed in Brazil [81]. Individuals with confirmed SARS-CoV-2 infection, adults who were at risk for contracting infection within 14 days before enrolment, participants having more than 37 °C axillary temperature, or those who were allergic to vaccine components were excluded from the clinical trials, thereby limiting the availability of data on these populations. Furthermore, the local events that manifested frequently were pain, redness, and swelling at the site of injection. Moreover, grade 1 (mild) adverse events with a single case of urticaria were observed. Notably, a high seroconversion rate was achieved by healthy adults 18–59 years old [25].

Unnamed (Sinopharm/Wuhan Institute of Biological Products co., Ltd.)

This unnamed it is prepared by the inactivation of SARS-CoV-2 WIV04 strain absorbed on 0.5-mg alum, followed by dilution in 0.5 ml sterile phosphate-buffered saline. The efficacy and long-term adverse events of the vaccine

are expected in the results of the phase 3 trials. The inactivated vaccine with a two-dose regimen must be stored at refrigeration temperatures. The exclusion of pregnant and lactating women, people with suspected or asymptomatic COVID-19, those allergic to vaccines, and those with more than 37 °C axillary temperature has resulted in the unavailability of data on the immunization of these special populations. Furthermore, grade 1 (mild) adverse events, including fever and injection-site pain, were more common in the healthy volunteers. Moreover, serious and special interest adverse events were not observed. Notably, 100% and 85.7% seroconversion rates were achieved in the 18- to 59 year-old participants in phase 1 and 2 trials, respectively [30].

BBIBP-CorV (Sinopharm/Beijing Institute of Biological Products)

BBIBP-CorV, co-developed by the Institute of Biological Products (Beijing, China) and the Sinopharm Group Co., Ltd., is prepared by the liquid formulation of purified 19nCoV-CDC-Tan-HB02 (HB02) inactivated strain, with aluminum hydroxide added as an adjuvant [30]. As per the reports, the provisional analysis of a phase 3 double-blinded randomized controlled trial has revealed an efficacy rate of nearly 79%, which was accompanied by the approval of this candidate in China and other nations [31]. The inactivated vaccine with a two-dose regimen must be stored at refrigeration temperatures. In addition, the exclusion of pregnant and lactating women and individuals with a history of COVID-19 from the clinical trials has resulted in the unavailability of data on the immunization of these special populations. Furthermore, the local events that manifested frequently were injection-site pain, swelling, and itching, although the observed systemic adverse events included fever, inappetence, constipation, mucocutaneous abnormalities, headache, vomiting, and itching at the noninjection site. Moreover, serious and special interest adverse events were not observed. Notably, a 100% seroconversion rate was achieved earlier by the 18- to 59-year-old age group [30].

EpiVacCorona (State Research Center of Virology and Biotechnology VECTOR, Russia)

EpiVacCorona is a peptide-based vaccine designed by the State Research Center of Virology and Biotechnology

VECTOR (Russia). The primary immunogenic component of this vaccine is the chemically synthesized peptide antigens of SARS-CoV-2 proteins. These peptide antigens are conjugated to a carrier protein and adsorbed on an adjuvant such as aluminum hydroxide [59]. The vaccine is administered IM in two doses, which are spaced 14–28 days apart [59, 60]. From the preliminary stage of human trials, it has been reported that EpiVacCorona induces an effective immune response against the novel coronavirus without eliciting any side effects [60]. The vaccine is yet to be approved by the FDA and is undergoing phase 3 clinical trials to evaluate and assess the reactogenicity, immunogenicity, and safety of the vaccine. The study will also look for any adverse reactions to vaccine administration. The clinical trial accepts participation from all healthy individuals between the ages of 18 and 60 years. However, this study excludes pregnant and lactating women, as well as children [60]. As per the report, approximately 30 000 healthy volunteers will be taking part in postregistration clinical trials of this vaccine [61, 62]. Notably, from the preclinical studies of EpiVacCorona conducted on rats, it was reported that this vaccine does not have any embryotoxic properties and does not affect the reproductive ability of the organisms even at higher doses [63]. Because it makes use of conserved epitopes of the virus, the expected advantage of this vaccine over other vaccine platforms is its effectiveness against antigenically evolving strains. Moreover, the vaccine can be stored and transported easily and safely at temperatures ranging between 2 and 8 °C. It also has been speculated that the vaccine shall retain its viability for up to two years [60, 82], although peptide-based subunit vaccines are poorly immunogenic and confer short-term immunity [82, 83].

Symptom Management

The anaphylactic response, a life-threatening event, which may include conditions such as angioedema, pulmonary edema, bronchospasm, or cardiovascular collapse, should be managed appropriately by the trained personnel at the vaccinating center [84]. The onset of symptoms often occurs within 15–30 minutes of vaccination; however, prognosis, severity, and clinical features are temperamental. As per the CDC guidelines, every individual must be monitored for at least 15 minutes, and those with a history of the immediate allergic response to any injectable must be monitored for 30 minutes postvaccination. Diagnosis of an anaphylactic event is established by the identification of clinical signs and symptoms (listed in Figure 22.3). The vaccination centers should have a prefilled syringe or autoinjector of epinephrine (with appropriate doses), H1 and H2 antihistamines, blood pressure cuff, stethoscope, pulse oximeter, oxygen

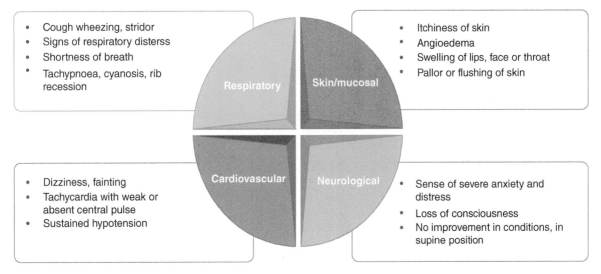

Figure 22.3   Early symptoms of postvaccination anaphylaxis. *Source:* Public Health England [85].

support, a bronchodilator, cardiopulmonary resuscitation mask, and so on. In case of an anaphylactic reaction, immediate action must be taken, as depicted in Figure 22.4. The aqueous solution of 1 mg/mL epinephrine (dilution 1:1000) is injected IM preferably at the "midpoint of the anterolateral aspect of the thigh" to manage these life-threatening symptoms. Multiple doses may be administered every few minutes (5–15 minutes) in case of persistence of the clinical signs and symptoms [85, 86].

Other less severe and more common symptoms, such as swelling and redness, do not usually lead to remarkable discomfort and can be locally managed by applying a cold compress. Systemic events, such as fever, headache, and body ache (commonly referred to as influenza-like symptoms), may however require administration of over-the-counter antipyretics or analgesics [12, 87].

Prioritization and Acceptance

Equitable distribution of vaccines is deemed important, especially with increasing economic disparity and the rich countries securing a majority of vaccine doses [88]. A descriptive study reports that around 68.4% of the world's population, amounting to around 3.7 billion people, is willing to be vaccinated [89]. Provided that most of the vaccines require a two-dose

regimen, the existing production capacity needs to be significantly ramped up to meet demand gaps. Moreover, lower- and middle-income countries have limited resources and expertise that could be dedicated to the immunization program. COVID-19 Vaccines Global Access Facility is an initiative in this prospect to ensure fair and equitable access to the COVID-19 vaccine [8] and has secured close to 2 billion vaccine doses that will be available by the end of 2021 [90].

Furthermore, prioritization of subgroups among a population is necessarily recommended to tackle the anticipated initial shortage of the vaccines. Three primary vaccination targets are: (i) ensuring core functioning of society (healthcare and frontline workers), (ii) decreasing fatal or serious outcomes (at-high-risk population, elderly, and those with comorbid conditions), and (iii) reducing community transmission (by targeting groups actively involved in economic and societal activities). Individuals with known SARS-CoV-2 infection may defer vaccination to a later time as current evidence disproves chances of reinfection so soon [91]. Similarly, patients who received passive immunotherapy may delay vaccination for 90 days to prevent unforeseen interaction of vaccine-induced immunity with antibody treatment [92]. An adequate degree of vaccine acceptance is required for achieving herd immunity in a population. Several factors contribute to this overall vaccine acceptance, including vaccine hesitance, availability of a

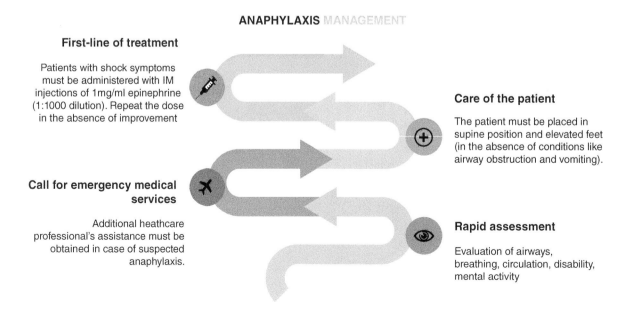

ANAPHYLAXIS MANAGEMENT

First-line of treatment

Patients with shock symptoms must be administered with IM injections of 1mg/ml epinephrine (1:1000 dilution). Repeat the dose in the absence of improvement

Care of the patient

The patient must be placed in supine position and elevated feet (in the absence of conditions like airway obstruction and vomiting).

Call for emergency medical services

Additional heathcare professional's assistance must be obtained in case of suspected anaphylaxis.

Rapid assessment

Evaluation of airways, breathing, circulation, disability, mental activity

Figure 22.4   Roadmap for the management of postvaccination anaphylactic events. *Source:* Public Health England [85].

safe and effective vaccine, reported adverse events, awareness level, among others [89]. Moreover, a better understanding of the reactogenicity profile of a vaccine candidate among healthcare workers could result in them being better aided to recommend the same. Publicly available safety data and compliance with standard scientific protocol during phase trials also mark an important component for public trust in vaccines. To this effect, nine leading pharmaceutical companies recently pledged to "stand with science" and vowed to thoroughly test the safety and efficacy profile of their vaccine candidate before putting it forward for public use [93].

Passive Immunotherapy

Convalescent Plasma

Convalescent plasma therapy has been authorized for emergency use by the FDA in patients with COVID-19 [94]. A high or low anti-SARS-CoV-2 antibody titer convalescent plasma is obtained from the patients who have recovered from COVID-19, and can be stored at temperatures less than −18 °C for up to one year, but it must be transfused within five days of thawing while storing at 2–8 °C in the registered blood establishments. The initial clinical dosage of COVID-19 convalescent plasma can comprise 200 ml, and further transfusion must be based on the clinical analysis and patient's response toward the treatment. A prolonged infusion or infusion of smaller volumes may be required in patients with comorbidities associated with cardiac functions. Furthermore, the advent of any side effects must be treated as per the medical protocol [94]. However, there is no statistically significant proof of reduced severity, swift recovery, or reduction in the number of deaths in patients with COVID-19 [4]. Therefore, the risk/benefit ratio must be evaluated before the administration of this immunotherapy.

Monoclonal Antibody

Thirteen mAb candidates are in phase 2/3 trials, and three of them—bamlanivimab, casirivimab, and imdevimab—have gained the FDA's emergency use approval in patients (age ≥ 12 years; weight ≥ 40 kg)

with mild to moderate COVID-19 and the possibility of severe disease progression in the due course of the time. They must be administered intravenously (over at least an hour) via gravity or pump. Casirivimab (REGN10933) and imdevimab (REGN10987) are administered as a diluted cocktail with a dosage of 1200 mg each. They are supplied in sealed vials and must be stored at refrigeration temperatures in their original cartons, while the diluted mixture of the two mAbs should not be stored for more than 36 hours at 2–8 °C [95]. Furthermore, bamlanivimab (LY-CoV555) is recommended in a 700 mg dose at the earliest after diagnosis of infection and within 10 days after symptoms manifest. It is supplied as a 20-ml concentrated solution that is required to be diluted in a 250 mL 0.9% NaCl injection. Postdilution, it can be stored between 2 and 8 °C for 24 hours and at room temperature for up to 7 hours, including the time required for infusion. Based on interim phase 2 results (BLAZE-1 trial), bamlanivimab was found to prevent hospitalization of patients with mild to moderate COVID-19 as compared with placebo [96]. The most common adverse events observed in the 700 mg dosing regimen (n = 101) were nausea, dizziness, headache, pruritus, diarrhea, and vomiting [97]. However, another randomized trial (ACTIV-3) found no clinical benefit of administering LY-CoV555 (along with remdesivir) in hospitalized patients with COVID-19 [98]. Notably, these mAbs should be administered only in clinical settings with immediate access to lifesaving medications to manage any potential severe infusion reactions. Postinfusion monitoring is mandatory for unapproved therapeutics because serious and unexpected adverse events may emerge as a result of the unavailability of substantial clinical trial data [95, 97]. Treatment of hospitalized patients or those requiring oxygen therapy because of SARS-CoV-2 infection is not recommended with any of these combinations.

Conclusion

We are currently amid the worst pandemic of the century, and it continues to surge. It has flabbergasted the health facilities in the majority of the most developed nations across the globe, and the world economy has been brought to an extraordinary collapse. This implausible pace of the pandemic is matched by the pace at which the scientific community has retorted to defy the situation. In the short span of a year, 8 vaccines acquired regulatory approval in different regions of the world, and 11 others are in phase 2 or later trials. Recognizing the urgency of the situation as posed by the pandemic and rising against all odds, the successful development of vaccines against COVID-19 was made possible only with the resolute and synchronized efforts of different governments, pharmaceutical companies, academia, and nonprofit organizations. The inspired and effective public–private cooperation and active involvement of regulatory and funding agencies made COVID-19 the first-ever disease in the history of vaccine development to have such an accelerated vaccine development [5]. This attests to what an effective and motivated collaboration among academia and industry can achieve and paves the way for new prospects in vaccine development for tackling not only future outbreaks but also current pathogens of concern, such as Dengue virus, HIV, and many more. The success of the COVID-19 vaccine initiative solely depends on the wide acceptance and willingness of the individuals to take all the recommended doses for a particular vaccine. Not just medical professionals but the onus also falls on government agencies, nongovernment organizations, the scientific community, and other community workers to sensitize people about the importance of vaccination and persuade them to get the vaccine. In addition to all of this, guaranteeing the safety and efficacy of vaccines is essential. This can be achieved through proper storage and handling, administration, monitoring the timing and spacing of vaccine doses, observation of precautions and contraindications, effective management of side effects, careful reporting of suspected side effects, and proper communication about vaccine benefits and risks [16].

Preferably, a vaccine should prompt long-term immunity; however, unfortunately, it does not seem to be the case for the SARS-CoV-2 vaccine. From previous experience, it has been confirmed that infections with other human coronaviruses result in a short-lived immunity. Callow et al. [99] demonstrated that just one year after inoculation with coronavirus 229E, most of the test subjects could be reinfected. The inoculated subjects elicited milder symptoms as compared with the noninoculated subjects, exhibiting a certain level of protection despite renewed infection. Notably, data from clinical trials of at least two vaccine candidates suggested against vaccine-mediated disease enhancement [18, 19]. For SARS-CoV-2, the longevity of the immune response due to the vaccine remains to be assessed in phase 4 analysis of the vaccine population. Vaccination is one of the most efficacious methods that aid in the successful eradication and restriction of infectious diseases. This assertion gains support from the disappearance of diseases such as smallpox and polio as a result of effective and widespread vaccination.

Acknowledgments

We acknowledge Dr. Rakesh Kumar Gupta, Principal, Ram Lal Anand College, University of Delhi for providing all the support required for the compilation of this chapter.

References

1 Sharma, Shahanshah, M.F., Gupta, S., and Gupta, V. (2021). Recent advances in the diagnosis of COVID-19: a bird's eye view. *Expert. Rev. Mol. Diagn.* 21: 475–491. https://doi.org/10.1080/14737159.2021.1874354.

2 Ortiz-Prado, E., Simbaña-Rivera, K., Gómez-Barreno, L. et al. (2020). Clinical, molecular, and epidemiological characterization of the SARS-CoV-2 virus and the coronavirus disease 2019 (COVID-19), a comprehensive literature review. *Diagn. Microbiol. Infect. Dis.* 98 (1): 115094.

3 Singh, A., Gupta, L., and Gupta, V. (2020). Heterologous protection to COVID-19 with BCG vaccine: deciphering the reality using meta-analysis approach. *J. Immunol. Sci.* 4 (4): 34–40.

4 Singh, A. and Gupta, V. (2021). SARS-CoV-2 therapeutics: how far do we stand from a remedy?

Pharmacol. Rep. 74: 750–768. https://doi.org/
10.1007/s43440-020-00204-0.

5 Kaur, S.P. and Gupta, V. (2020). COVID-19 vaccine: a comprehensive status report. *Virus Res.* 288: 198114. https://doi.org/10.1016/j.virusres.2020.198114.

6 WHO (2021). Draft landscape of COVID-19 candidate vaccines. https://www.who.int/publications/m/item/draft-landscape-of-covid-19-candidate-vaccines (accessed 1 January 2021).

7 Craven J. (2020). COVID-19 vaccine tracker. https://www.raps.org/news-and-articles/news-articles/2020/3/covid-19-vaccine-tracker (accessed 1 January 2021).

8 COVAX Facility (2021). COVAX. https://www.gavi.org/covax-facility (accessed 10 January 2021).

9 FDA (2020). Coronavirus (COVID-19) Update: FDA Authorizes Monoclonal Antibody for Treatment of COVID-19. November 9, 2020. https://www.fda.gov/news-events/press-announcements/coronavirus-covid-19-update-fda-authorizes-monoclonal-antibody-treatment-covid-19 (accessed 13 January 2021).

10 World Health Organization (2005). Monitoring Vaccine Wastage at Country Level : Guidelines for Programme Managers. WHO/V&B/03.18.Rev.1. World Health Organization. https://apps.who.int/iris/handle/10665/68463 (accessed 7 January 2021).

11 Lee, S., Lim, H.S., Kim, O. et al. (2012). Vaccine storage practices and the effects of education in some private medical institutions. *J. Prev. Med. Public Health* 45 (2): 78–89.

12 Hervé, C., Laupèze, B., Giudice, G.D. et al. (2019). The how's and what's of vaccine reactogenicity. *NPJ Vaccines* 4 (1): 1–11.

13 Hodgson, S.H., Mansatta, K., Mallett, G. et al. (2021). What defines an efficacious COVID-19 vaccine? A review of the challenges assessing the clinical efficacy of vaccines against SARS-CoV-2. *Lancet Infect. Dis.* 21: e26–e35. https://doi.org/10.1016/S1473-3099(20)30773-8.

14 Biswas A. (2021). A statistician explains: what does '90% efficacy' for a Covid-19 vaccine mean? Scroll.in. November 28, 2020. https://scroll.in/article/979627/a-statistician-explains-what-does-90-efficacy-for-a-covid-19-vaccine-mean (accessed 10 January 2021).

15 World Health Organization (2016). Guidelines on clinical evaluation of vaccines: regulatory expectations. https://www.who.int/biologicals/BS2287_Clinical_guidelines_final_LINE_NOs_20_July_2016.pdf (accessed 7 January 2021).

16 Pinkbook (2020). July 17, 2020. General recommendations on immunization. https://www.cdc.gov/vaccines/pubs/pinkbook/genrec.html#contraindications (accessed 9 January 2021).

17 FDA (2020). Vaccines and Related Biological Products Advisory Committee, December 10, 2020. Meeting Briefing Document – FDA. https://www.fda.gov/media/144245/download (accessed 4 January 2021).

18 Polack, F.P., Thomas, S.J., Kitchin, N. et al. (2020). Safety and efficacy of the BNT162b2 mRNA Covid-19 vaccine. *N. Engl. J. Med.* 383 (27): 2603–2615.

19 Baden, L.R., El Sahly, H.M., Essink, B. et al. (2021). Efficacy and safety of the mRNA-1273 SARS-CoV-2 vaccine. *N. Engl. J. Med.* 384: 403–416.

20 Centers for Disease Control and Prevention (2020). Moderna COVID-19 vaccine. https://www.cdc.gov/vaccines/covid-19/info-by-product/moderna/downloads/storage-summary.pdf (accessed 10 January 2021).

21 CureVac (2021). COVID-19 – CureVac. https://www.curevac.com/en/covid-19/ (accessed 9 January 2021).

22 Kremsner, P., Mann, P., Bosch, J. et al. (2020). Phase 1 assessment of the safety and immunogenicity of an mRNA- lipid nanoparticle vaccine candidate against SARS-CoV-2 in human volunteers. *medRxiv* doi:2020.11.09.20228551.

23 Smith, T.R.F., Patel, A., Ramos, S. et al. (2020). Immunogenicity of a DNA vaccine candidate for COVID-19. *Nat. Commun.* 11 (1): 1–13.

24 Tebas, P., Yang, S., Boyer, J.D. et al. (2020). Safety and immunogenicity of INO-4800 DNA vaccine against SARS-CoV-2: a preliminary report of an open-label, phase 1 clinical trial. *EClinicalMedicine* 31: 100689.

25 Zhang, Y., Zeng, G., Pan, H. et al. (2021). Safety, tolerability, and immunogenicity of an inactivated SARS-CoV-2 vaccine in healthy adults aged 18-59 years: a randomised, double-blind, placebo-controlled, phase 1/2 clinical trial. *Lancet Infect. Dis.* 21: 181–192. https://doi.org/10.1016/S1473-3099(20)30843-4.

26 Reuters (2020). China's Sinovac coronavirus vaccine candidate appears safe, slightly weaker in elderly. *Reuters*, September 7, 2020. https://www.reuters.com/article/us-health-coronavirus-vaccine-sinovac-idUSKBN25Y1QM (accessed 9 January 2021).

27 Simões E. (2021). Sinovac vaccine 78% effective in Brazil trial, experts call for more details. *Reuters*, January 7, 2021. https://www.reuters.com/article/health-coronavirus-brazil-sinovac-idINKBN29C1W5 (accessed 10 January 2021).

28 Ella, R., Mohan, K., Jogdand, H. et al. (2020). Safety and immunogenicity trial of an inactivated SARS-CoV-2 vaccine-BBV152: a phase 1, double-blind, randomised control trial. *medRxiv* https://doi.org/10.1101/2020.12.11.20210419.

29 Ella, R., Reddy, S., Jogdand, H. et al. (2020). Safety and immunogenicity clinical trial of an inactivated SARS-CoV-2 vaccine, BBV152 (a phase 2, double-blind, randomised controlled trial) and the persistence of immune responses from a phase 1 follow-up report. *medRxiv* https://doi.org/10.1101/2020.12.21.20248643.

30 Xia, S., Duan, K., Zhang, Y. et al. (2020). Effect of an inactivated vaccine against SARS-CoV-2 on safety and immunogenicity outcomes: interim analysis of 2 randomized clinical trials. *JAMA* 324 (10): 951–960. https://doi.org/10.1001/jama.2020.15543.

31 Gan N. (2020). China approves Sinopharm Covid-19 vaccine, promises free shots for all citizens – CNN. https://edition.cnn.com/2020/12/30/asia/china-sinopharm-vaccine-efficacy-intl-hnk/index.html (accessed 9 January 2021).

32 Xia, S., Zhang, Y., Wang, Y. et al. (2021). Safety and immunogenicity of an inactivated SARS-CoV-2 vaccine, BBIBP-CorV: a randomised, double-blind, placebo-controlled, phase 1/2 trial. *Lancet Infect. Dis.* 21 (1): 39–51. https://doi.org/10.1016/S1473-3099(20)30831-8.

33 MHRA (2021). Information for Healthcare Professionals on COVID-19 Vaccine AstraZeneca. https://www.gov.uk/government/publications/regulatory-approval-of-covid-19-vaccine-astrazeneca/information-for-healthcare-professionals-on-covid-19-vaccine-astrazeneca (accessed 7 January 2021).

34 Barrett, J.R., Belij-Rammerstorfer, S., Dold, C. et al. (2021). Phase 1/2 trial of SARS-CoV-2 vaccine ChAdOx1 nCoV-19 with a booster dose induces multifunctional antibody responses. *Nat. Med.* 27: 279–288.

35 SputnikV (2020). Vaccine. https://sputnikvaccine.com/about-vaccine/ (accessed 12 January 2021).

36 SputnikV (2020). The first registered COVID-19 vaccine. https://sputnikvaccine.com/ (accessed 12 January 2021).

37 Sputnik V (2020). AstraZeneca will test using component of Russia's Sputnik V in clinical trials of its own vaccine against coronavirus. December 11, 2020. http://sputnikvaccine.com/newsroom/pressreleases/astrazeneca-will-test-using-component-of-russia-s-sputnik-v-in-clinical-trials-of-its-own-vaccine-ag/ (accessed 12 January 2021).

38 Microbix (2020). Adenovirus, grade 2. August 2, 2020. https://microbix.com/product/adenovirus-grade-2/ (accessed 7 January 2021).

39 Zhu, F.C., Guan, X.H., Li, Y.H. et al. (2020). Immunogenicity and safety of a recombinant adenovirus type-5-vectored COVID-19 vaccine in healthy adults aged 18 years or older: a randomised, double-blind, placebo-controlled, phase 2 trial. *Lancet* 396 (10249): 479–488. https://doi.org/10.1016/S0140-6736(20)31605-6.

40 Sadoff, J., Gars, M.L., Shukarev, G. et al. (2020). Safety and immunogenicity of the Ad26.COV2.S COVID-19 vaccine candidate: interim results of a phase 1/2a, double-blind, randomized, placebo-controlled trial. *medRxiv* https://doi.org/10.1101/2020.09.23.20199604.

41 Kaur, S.P. and Gupta, V. (2020). SARS-CoV-2 vaccine: reconnoitering the prospects. *Vaccin. Res. Dev.* 1 (1): 1–5. https://doi.org/10.36959/669/745.

42 Keech, C. (2020). Phase 1–2 trial of a SARS-CoV-2 recombinant spike protein nanoparticle vaccine. *N. Engl. J. Med.* 383: 2320–2332.

43 ClinicalTrials.gov (2020). Clinical Trials Register. https://www.clinicaltrialsregister.eu/ctr-search/trial/2020-004123-16/GB (accessed 13 January 2021).

44 Novavax (2021). Novavax COVID-19 vaccine. January 28, 2021. https://ir.novavax.com/news-releases/news-release-details/novavax-covid-19-vaccine-demonstrates-893-efficacy-uk-phase-3 (accessed 30 January 2021).

45 Pollet, J., Chen, W.H., and Strych, U. (2021). Recombinant protein vaccines, a proven approach

against coronavirus pandemics. *Adv. Drug Deliv. Rev.* 170: 71–82.

46 TrackVaccines (2020). Novavax: NVX-CoV2373 – COVID19 Vaccine Tracker. https://covid19.trackvaccines.org/vaccines/25/ (accessed 13 January 2021).

47 Chictr (2020). "中国临床试验注册中心 - 世界卫生组织国际临床试验注册平台一级注册机构." www.chictr.org.cn/showproj.aspx?proj=58207 (accessed 7 January 2021).

48 ClinicalTrials.gov (2020). Phase I trial of a recombinant COVID-19 vaccine (CHO cell). https://clinicaltrials.gov/ct2/show/NCT04636333 (accessed 10 January 2021).

49 ClinicalTrials.gov (2020). Recombinant new coronavirus vaccine (CHO Cells) to prevent SARS-CoV-2 phase I clinical trial (≥60 years old). https://clinicaltrials.gov/ct2/show/NCT04550351 (accessed 11 January 2021).

50 Dai, L. and Gao, G.F. (2021). Viral targets for vaccines against COVID-19. *Nat. Rev. Immunol.* 21: 73–82.

51 Reuters Staff (2020). "China's CAS COVID-19 vaccine induces immune response in mid-stage tests. *Reuters*, December 23, 2020. https://www.reuters.com/article/us-health-coronavirus-china-vaccine-idUSKBN28X0RW (accessed 2 January 2021).

52 TrackVaccines (2020). Anhui Zhifei Longcom: RBD-dimer – COVID19 vaccine tracker. https://covid19.trackvaccines.org/vaccines/27/ (accessed January 11, 2021).

53 Yang, S., Li, Y., Dai, L. et al. (2020). Safety and immunogenicity of a recombinant tandem-repeat dimeric RBD protein vaccine against COVID-19 in adults: pooled analysis of two randomized, double-blind, placebo-controlled, phase 1 and 2 trials. *MedRxiv* https://doi.org/10.1101/2020.12.20.20248602.

54 Chictr (2020). 中国临床试验注册中心 - 世界卫生组织国际临床试验注册平台一级注册机构. www.chictr.org.cn/showproj.aspx?proj=60581 (accessed 11 January 2021).

55 ClinicalTrials.gov (2020). Safety and immunogenicity study of an inactivated SARS-CoV-2 vaccine for preventing against COVID-19 in people aged ≥60 years. https://clinicaltrials.gov/ct2/show/NCT04470609 (accessed 11 January 2021).

56 ETHealthworld (2020). West China Hospital's Covid-19 vaccine candidate enters mid-stage human trial. https://health.economictimes.indiatimes.com/news/pharma/west-china-hospitals-covid-19-vaccine-candidate-enters-mid-stage-human-trial/79260755 (accessed 13 January 2021).

57 Reuters Staff (2020). West China Hospital's COVID-19 vaccine candidate enters mid-stage human trial. *Reuters*, November 17, 2020. https://www.reuters.com/article/us-health-coronavirus-vaccine-china-idUSKBN27X0T1 (accessed 2 January 2021).

58 Yang, J., Wang, W., Chen, Z. et al. (2020). A vaccine targeting the RBD of the S protein of SARS-CoV-2 induces protective immunity. *Nature* 586 (7830): 572–577. https://doi.org/10.1038/s41586-020-2599-8.

59 ClinicalTrials.gov (2020). Study of the safety, reactogenicity and immunogenicity of 'EpiVacCorona' vaccine for the prevention of COVID-19. https://clinicaltrials.gov/ct2/show/record/NCT04527575 (accessed 13 January 2021).

60 PrecisionVaccinations (2021). EpiVacCorona Vaccine. https://www.precisionvaccinations.com/vaccines/epivaccorona-vaccine (accessed 9 January 2021).

61 Ray A. (2020). COVID-19 vaccine: WHO in talks with russia on its second vaccine EpiVacCorona. October 16, 2020. https://www.livemint.com/science/health/covid-19-vaccine-who-in-talks-with-russia-on-its-second-vaccine-epivaccorona-11602865577927.html (accessed 9 January 2021).

62 Reuters (2020). Russia begins mass trials of second coronavirus vaccine. *Reuters*, November 30, 2020. https://www.reuters.com/article/us-health-coronavirus-russia-cases-idUSKBN28A0P0 (accessed 9 January 2021).

63 Sputnik (2020). Russian EpiVacCorona vaccine has no negative effect on health of embryo, watchdog says. December 29, 2020. https://sputniknews.com/russia/202012291081595122-russian-epivaccorona-vaccine-has-no-negative-effect-on-health-of-embryo-watchdog-says/ (accessed 11 January 2021).

64 ClinicalTrials.gov (2020). Safety, tolerability and immunogenicity of a coronavirus-like particle COVID-19 vaccine in adults aged 18–55 years. https://clinicaltrials.gov/ct2/show/NCT04450004 (accessed 10 January 2021).

65 Medicago (2020). COVID-19 programs. https://www.medicago.com/en/covid-19-programs (accessed 10 January 2021).

66 Medicago (2020). Medicago announces positive phase 1 results for its COVID-19 vaccine candidate. https://www.medicago.com/en/newsroom/medicago-announces-positive-phase-1-results-for-its-covid-19-vaccine-candidate/#:~:text=About%20Phase%201%20results%20summary&text=Phase%201%20immunogenicity%20results%20demonstrate,to%20the%20non%2Dadjuvanted%20formulations (accessed 10 January 2021).

67 Ward, B.J., Gobeil, P., Séguin, A. et al. (2020). Phase 1 trial of a candidate recombinant virus-like particle vaccine for Covid-19 disease produced in plants. *medRxiv* https://doi.org/10.1101/2020.11.04.20226282.

68 Sahin, U., Muik, A., Vogler, I. et al. (2020). BNT162b2 induces SARS-CoV-2-Neutralising antibodies and T cells in humans. *medRxiv* https://doi.org/10.1101/2020.12.09.20245175.

69 Department of Health and Social Care (2020). Letter to the Profession from the UK Chief Medical Officers Regarding the UK COVID-19 Vaccination Programmes. GOV.UK. December 31, 2020. https://www.gov.uk/government/publications/letter-to-the-profession-from-the-uk-chief-medical-officers-on-the-uk-covid-19-vaccination-programmes/letter-to-the-profession-from-the-uk-chief-medical-officers-regarding-the-uk-covid-19-vaccination-programmes (accessed 7 January 2021).

70 Torres N. (2021). Mexican doctor hospitalized after receiving COVID-19 vaccine. *Reuters*, January 2, 2021. https://www.reuters.com/article/health-coronavirus-mexico-vaccines-idUSKBN2970H3. Accessed 7 January 2021.

71 Torjesen I (2021). Covid-19: Norway investigates 23 deaths in frail elderly patients after vaccination. *BMJ* 372: 149. https://doi.org/10.1136/bmj.n149.

72 Jackson, L.A., Anderson, E.J., Rouphael, N.G. et al. (2020). An mRNA vaccine against SARS-CoV-2 – preliminary report. *N. Engl. J. Med.* 383 (20): 1920–1931.

73 FDA (2020). Vaccines and Related Biological Products Advisory Committee, December 17, 2020: Meeting Briefing Document – FDA. https://www.fda.gov/media/144434/download (accessed 9 January 2021).

74 NIAID (2020). Peer-reviewed report on Moderna COVID-19 vaccine publishes. https://www.niaid.nih.gov/news-events/peer-reviewed-report-moderna-covid-19-vaccine-publishes (accessed 30 January 2021).

75 Doremalen, N., Lambe, T., Spencer, A. et al. (2020). ChAdOx1 nCoV-19 vaccination prevents SARS-CoV-2 pneumonia in rhesus macaques. *bioRxiv* https://doi.org/10.1101/2020.05.13.093195.

76 Ramasamy, M.N., Minassian, A.M., Ewer, K.J. et al. (2020). Safety and immunogenicity of ChAdOx1 nCoV-19 vaccine administered in a prime-boost regimen in young and old adults (COV002): a single-blind, randomised, controlled, phase 2/3 trial. *Lancet* 396 (10267): 1979–1993.

77 Voysey, M., Clemens, S., Madhi, S.A. et al. (2021). Safety and efficacy of the ChAdOx1 nCoV-19 vaccine (AZD1222) against SARS-CoV-2: an interim analysis of four randomised controlled trials in Brazil, South Africa, and the UK. *Lancet* 397 (10269): 99–111. https://doi.org/10.1016/S0140-6736(20)32661-1.

78 Mahase, E. (2020). Covid-19: Oxford vaccine could be 59% effective against asymptomatic infections, analysis shows. *BMJ* 371: m4777.

79 ClinicalTrials.gov (2020). Clinical trial of efficacy, safety, and immunogenicity of Gam-COVID-Vac vaccine against COVID-19. https://clinicaltrials.gov/ct2/show/NCT04530396 (accessed 7 January 2021).

80 ANI (2021). Arg reports adverse reaction to Sputnik V, doc gets side effects from Pfizer jab. Livemint. January 3, 2021. https://www.livemint.com/news/world/arg-reports-adverse-reaction-to-sputnik-v-doc-gets-side-effects-from-pfizer-jab-11609633103810.html (accessed 6 January 2021).

81 Asia N. (2021). China's Sinovac vaccine shows 78% efficacy in Brazilian trial." Nikkei Asia. January 8, 2021. https://asia.nikkei.com/Spotlight/Coronavirus/China-s-Sinovac-vaccine-shows-78-efficacy-in-Brazilian-trial (accessed 10 January 2021).

82 Sputnik (2020). Russia's EpiVacCorona vaccine helps create immunity 1 month after inoculation, developer says. November 27, 2020. https://sputniknews.com/russia/202011271081289686-russias-epivaccorona-vaccine-helps-create-immunity-1-month-after-inoculation-developer-says/ (accessed 11 January 2021).

83 Chung, Y.H., Beiss, V., Fiering, S.N., and Steinmetz, N.F. (2020). COVID-19 vaccine frontrunners and their nanotechnology design. *ACS Nano* 14 (10): 12522–12537.

84 Mali, S. and Jambure, R. (2012). Anaphylaxis management: current concepts. *Anesth. Essays Res.* 6 (2): 115–123.

85 Public Health England (2013). Vaccine safety and adverse events following immunisation: the Green Book, Chapter 8. GOV.UK. March 20, 2013. https:// www.gov.uk/government/publications/vaccine-safety-and-adverse-events-following-immunisation-the-green-book-chapter-8 (accessed 9 January 2021).

86 Centers for Disease Control and Prevention (2021). Management of anaphylaxis at COVID-19 vaccination sites. January 6, 2021. https://www.cdc.gov/vaccines/ covid-19/clinical-considerations/managing-anaphylaxis. html?CDC_AA_refVal=https%3A%2F%2Fwww.cdc. gov%2Fvaccines%2Fcovid-19%2Finfo-by-product%2Fpfizer%2Fanaphylaxis-management.html (accessed 10 January 2021).

87 Immunization Action Coalition (2019). Medical management of vaccine reactions in children and teens in a community setting. https://www.immunize. org/catg.d/p3082a.pdf (accessed 16 January 2021).

88 Rees V. (2020). Rich countries buy up majority of COVID-19 vaccine doses. December 10, 2020. https://www.europeanpharmaceuticalreview.com/ news/136170/rich-countries-buy-up-majority-of-covid-19-vaccine-doses-peoples-vaccine-alliance-says/ (accessed 8 January 2021).

89 Wang, W., Wu, Q., Yang, J. et al. (2020). Global, regional, and national estimates of target population sizes for covid-19 vaccination: descriptive study. *BMJ (Clin. Res. Ed.)* 371: m4704. https://doi.org/10.1136/ bmj.m4704.

90 World Health Organization (2020). Covax announces additional deals to access promising COVID-19 vaccine candidates; plans global rollout starting Q1 2021." https://www.who.int/news/item/18-12-2020-covax-announces-additional-deals-to-access-promising-covid-19-vaccine-candidates-plans-global-rollout-starting-q1-2021 (accessed 13 January 2021).

91 Centers for Disease Control and Prevention (2020). Duration of isolation and precautions for adults with COVID-19. December 1, 2020. https://www.cdc.gov/ coronavirus/2019-ncov/hcp/duration-isolation.html (accessed 10 January 2021).

92 Centers for Disease Control and Prevention (2021). Interim clinical considerations for use of Pfizer-BioNTech COVID-19 vaccine. January 6, 2021. https://www.cdc.gov/vaccines/covid-19/info-by-product/clinical-considerations.html (Accessed 9 January 2021).

93 Pfizer (2020). Biopharma leaders unite to stand with science. https://www.pfizer.com/news/press-release/ press-release-detail/biopharma-leaders-unite-stand-science (accessed 6 January 2021).

94 FDA (2020). Fact sheet for health care providers: Emergency Use Authorization (EUA) of COVID-19 convalescent plasma for treatment of COVID-19 in hospitalized patients. FDA. https://www.fda.gov/ media/141478/download (accessed 10 January 2021).

95 FDA (2020). Fact sheet for health care providers Emergency Use Authorization (eua) of casirivimab and imdevimab. https://www.fda.gov/media/143892/ download (accessed 13 January 2021).

96 National Institutes of Health (2020). The COVID-19 Treatment Guidelines Panel's Statement on the Emergency Use Authorization of Bamlanivimab for the Treatment of COVID-19. https://www.covid19treatmentguidelines.nih.gov/ statement-on-bamlanivimab-eua/ (accessed 28 January 2021).

97 FDA (2020). Fact sheet for health care providers Emergency Use Authorization (EUA) of bamlanivimab. http://pi.lilly.com/eua/ bamlanivimab-eua-factsheet-hcp.pdf (accessed 13 January 2021).

98 ACTIV-3/TICO LY-CoV555 Study Group (2020). A neutralizing monoclonal antibody for hospitalized patients with Covid-19. *N. Engl. J. Med.* 384: 905–941. https://doi.org/10.1056/nejmoa2033130.

99 Callow, K.A., Parry, H.F., Sergeant, M., and Tyrrell, D.A. (1990). The time course of the immune response to experimental coronavirus infection of man. *Epidemiol. Infect.* 105 (2): 435–446.

23

Post-COVID-19 Vaccine Imaging Findings

Shadi Asadollahi[1,2,], Liesl S. Eibschutz[1,*], Sanaz Katal[3], Vorada Sakulsaengprapha[4], Yasaswi Vengalasetti[5], Nikoo Saeedi[6], Sean K. Johnston[7], and Jennifer H. Johnston[8]*

[1] Department of Radiology, Keck School of Medicine, University of Southern California, Los Angeles, CA, USA
[2] Russell H. Morgan Department of Radiology and Radiological Science, Johns Hopkins University School of Medicine, Baltimore, MD, USA
[3] St Vincent's Hospital Medical Imaging Department, Melbourne, Victoria, Australia
[4] Johns Hopkins University School of Medicine, Baltimore, MD, USA
[5] Department of Epidemiology and Population Health, Stanford University School of Medicine, Stanford, CA, USA
[6] Medical School of Islamic Azad University of Mashhad, Mashhad, Iran
[7] Department of Radiology, Keck School of Medicine, University of Southern California, Los Angeles, CA, USA
[8] Department of Radiology, McGovern School of Medicine, UT Houston, Houston, TX, USA

Abbreviations

ADEM	acute disseminated encephalomyelitis
BI-RADS	Breast Imaging-Reporting and Data System
CTA	computed tomographic angiography
CVST	cerebral venous sinus thrombosis
FDA	US Food and Drug Administration
FDG	[^{18}F]-fluorodeoxyglucose
GBS	Guillain-Barré syndrome
LAP	lymphadenopathy
MRI	magnetic resonance imaging
mRNA	messenger RNA
PE	pulmonary embolism
PET/CT	positron emission tomography-computed tomography
PF4	platelet factor 4
SBI	Society of Breast Imaging
SIRVA	shoulder injury related to vaccine administration
T1W	T1-weighted
US	ultrasonography
VAERS	Vaccine Adverse Event Reporting System
VITT	vaccine-induced immune thrombotic thrombocytopenia

Throughout 2020 and 2021, coronavirus disease 2019 (COVID-19) spread rampantly across the globe, sparking an international research effort toward procuring a vaccine. Various companies worked tirelessly to rapidly design and deploy effective COVID-19 vaccination programs, in an attempt to impede the pandemic and facilitate a return to normalcy. Based on the platform used for preparing the vaccine, the commonly available COVID-19 vaccines are broadly classified into the following types: messenger RNA (mRNA), viral vector, inactivated virus, and protein subunits vaccines [1].

---

*Shadi Asadollahi and Liesl S. Eibschutz contributed equally to this work and should be considered as cofirst authors.

In the United States, the US Food and Drug Administration (FDA) granted Emergency Use Authorization to the two-dose mRNA-BNT162b2 (Pfizer-BioNTech) and mRNA-1273 (Moderna) vaccines and the single-dose Ad26.COV2·S (Johnson & Johnson/Janssen) viral vector vaccine [2–5]. In other countries, a variety of vaccines have been used, including the ChAdOx1 nCoV-19 (University of Oxford/ AstraZeneca) vaccine, Gam-COVID-Vac (Gamaleya Research Institute), Convidecia (CanSinoBIO-Beijing Institute of Biotechnology) Adenovirus-5-based vaccine, inactivated Covaxin (Bharat Biotech), and the more recently approved ZyCoV-D vaccine (Zydus Cadila), the world's first DNA vaccine against COVID-19 [6–8].

As with any immunization, side effects have been reported, ranging from self-limited, predictable responses to rare cases of severe or persistent complications. To identify both these expected and serious side effects associated with vaccination, various imaging modalities, such as ultrasonography (US), [18F]-fluorodeoxyglucose (FDG) positron emission tomography-computed tomography (PET/CT), and magnetic resonance imaging (MRI), have been used [5, 6, 9, 10].

Apart from the role of imaging in detecting these vaccine-induced side effects, it is imperative that radiologists are familiar with the expected imaging patterns of immune-mediated inflammatory changes, because they can mimic sinister pathologies such as malignancy/metastatic disease. For example, although vaccine-associated lymphadenopathy (LAP) can be anticipated post-COVID-19 vaccination, malignancies and diseases that predominantly involve the lymph nodes are prone to interpretive challenges on imaging. In cases where a thorough vaccination history is not appropriately recorded, unnecessary workups can occur and worsen patient anxiety. Thus, by elucidating typical post-COVID-19 vaccine imaging findings, highlighting potential imaging misinterpretation, and providing recommendations for optimal imaging timing, we can ensure effective clinical management and care of the patients. In this chapter, we will start by reviewing the postimmunization imaging challenges from past vaccines, then delve into the currently available COVID-19 vaccines, their potential side effects, and the challenges they might create for radiologists.

Vaccines and Imaging: Past Experience

What We Know from Previous Vaccines

For decades, vaccination has been proven and widely used as an effective strategy in preventing life-threatening infections, such as poliomyelitis, influenza, smallpox, measles, rabies, and tetanus. However, these vaccines are sometimes associated with adverse reactions that can be classified into two distinct categories: local and systemic reactions [11]. Local reactions are common and often caused by substandard injection or hypersensitivity to the adjuvant substances used in the vaccine. Systemic reactions, in contrast, are rare and attributed mainly to the vaccine itself.

Although vaccine-induced adverse effects are often mild and self-limited, severe or prolonged reactions may also occur, prompting further investigation with imaging of the affected region. Past reports describe the most common findings postvaccination, including local inflammation at the injection site, shoulder injuries, systemic immune response, and neurologic complications [12–14].

Local Reactions

A local inflammatory response is anticipated postvaccination and is often characterized on FDG PET/ CT imaging by hypermetabolism of the axillary lymph nodes draining the intramuscular injection site and ipsilateral deltoid muscle uptake. However, many authors have described several instances of more severe local inflammation after immunization, including vaccine-induced necrotizing granulomatous reactions, myositis, intramuscular sterile abscesses, and formation of fascial granulomas [5, 14–17]. These local reactions can mimic soft tissue neoplasms, resulting in further unnecessary workups. Yildirim et al. [17] reported a 14-year-old boy presenting with fascial granuloma formation in his deltoid muscle six months after tetanus vaccination. On ultrasound, the lesion was heterogeneously hypoechoic, with the upper pole containing subcentimetric anechoic foci. On color doppler study,

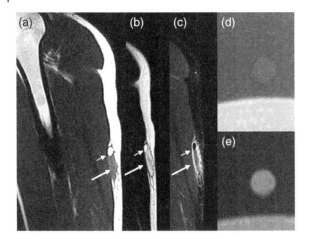

Figure 23.1 Granulomatous reaction after upper extremity fascial tetanus vaccination. Sagittal oblique MRIs of the left upper arm on precontrast T1W (a), T2W (b), and postcontrast T1W (c) sequences. The main lesion (*long arrows*) has a fusiform-shaped appearance with superficial and perifascial location to the deltoid muscle. The more cranial T1W hyperintense focus (*short arrows*) in the precontrast series appears hypointense on postcontrast fat-saturated image, which represents the lipoid admixture of the content. in vitro, the vaccine vial itself displays slightly hypointense signal characteristics on axial T1W and hyperintensity on T2W images (d, e), which are different from the patient lesion, warranting histopathologic evaluation. An excisional biopsy confirmed granulomatous inflammation. *Source:* Yildirim et al. [17].

moderately increased peripheral vascularity was noted. MRI examination was also performed, showing a space-occupying lesion in the deep subcutaneous fat layer, adjacent to the fascia. The lesion was mildly iso-hypointense on T1-weighted (T1W) imaging and apparently hyperintense on T2-weighted (T2W) imaging, with multiple subcentimeter hyperintense foci at its upper pole (Figure 23.1). On fat-saturated postcontrast T1W sequence, intense peripheral enhancement was demonstrated. Surgical excision of the left deltoid mass showed a local granulomatous reaction (associated with coagulation and liquefaction necrosis) in response to the vaccine material. Thus, it is imperative that clinicians consider both vaccination history and imaging findings when assessing such conditions to avoid misinterpretation of local inflammation as malignant neoplasms.

Lymphadenopathy

Vaccine-induced LAP has been widely debated in the previous literature because it varies based on the type of vaccine. In a study of 58 patients who received the H1N1 vaccine 1–14 days before PET-CT examination, 17 (29.3%) cases had FDG-positive lymph nodes with a mean standardized uptake value of 1.43 [18]. It was also reported that most of these cases also had increased FDG activity in their ipsilateral deltoid muscle. Thus, the authors concluded that the presence of ipsilateral deltoid uptake is a key finding for accurately labeling FDG-avid axillary nodes as being reactive/benign in nature. Other authors have reported similar findings with FDG accumulation in the axillary lymph nodes after vaccination [18]. Interestingly, the pattern of distribution, FDG intensity, and duration of nodal activation after immunization varies remarkably based on vaccine type. Although some authors suggest no abnormal activity seven days postvaccination, others report persistent tracer accumulation up to one month postvaccination. In addition, although most studies have found ipsilateral and less commonly contralateral axillary lymph node involvement, others have reported generalized nodal FDG uptake activity postvaccination [18]. Therefore, nodal activation postimmunization might pose a real challenge for clinicians and should be highly considered as a differential when dealing with unexplained nodal uptake.

Systemic Inflammation

In rare cases, a systemic inflammatory response postvaccination can occur [19]. A case report by Mingos et al. [19] described a 55-year-old man with a history of right lung cancer who demonstrated increased left axillary lymph node metabolic activity and intense splenic FDG uptake three days after influenza vaccine. Given the recent history of influenza vaccination, coupled with diffuse pattern and a relatively low level of FDG uptake in the spleen (as compared with primary neoplasm), underlying benign etiology was favored, most likely systemic immune-mediated inflammation [19]. Thus, it is imperative that clinicians take into account the vaccination history, pattern of FDG uptake, and time course on serial PET imaging to avoid making wrong a diagnosis of tumor progression and alteration of the therapy plan.

Neurologic Complications

Although rare, neurologic complications, such as encephalitis, myelitis, cerebellitis, and other neurologic syndromes, have been reported postvaccination. In these instances, neuroimaging modalities (especially MRI) offer valuable information for both detection and follow-up. For example, acute disseminated encephalomyelitis (ADEM) is an uncommon immune-mediated inflammatory demyelinating central nervous system disease, being reported after various vaccinations, such as poliomyelitis, influenza, smallpox, measles, rabies, and Japanese B encephalitis [20–23]. Postimmunization encephalomyelitis shares similar clinical and pathologic manifestations with postinfectious cases and often presents within three weeks of vaccination [24, 25]. For example, Ozawa et al. [20] reported a case of six-year-old girl with a history of high fever, headache, and gait disturbance after oral poliomyelitis vaccine administration. Neurologic examination revealing spastic palsy, sensory defects, urinary incontinence, and vision deterioration. On T2W MRI, multifocal high-intensity lesions were identified in the spinal cord. Combining the clinical picture, MRI findings, and increased myelin basic protein in the cerebrospinal fluid, the authors suggested ADEM associated with poliomyelitis vaccination. Similarly, Shoamanesh and Traboulsee [25] also described a patient with focal neurologic signs and significant brainstem involvement two days after seasonal influenza vaccination. MRI of neuraxis showed a long segment of T2 hyperintense extending from the caudal medulla down the entire length of the cervical cord, associated with cord expansion. Given her clinical presentation and neuroimaging pattern, a diagnosis of ADEM was made. Despite appropriate treatment, the patient's condition continued to deteriorate, and she passed away. Notably, most patients have a complete recovery, but brainstem dysfunction may serve as a poor prognostic indicator and may even cause death [25]. Ravaglia et al. [26] also reported a patient with previously diagnosed postinfectious ADEM who experienced a relapse after influenza vaccination. These findings may suggest a common pathogenic mechanism among postvaccine and postinfectious cases.

Other neurologic complications have also been reported after vaccination. Lessa et al. [27] reported four cases who had neurologic symptoms 4–15 days after H1N1 influenza vaccination. MRI detected abnormalities in all four patients, including high T2 signal in the cerebellum (acute cerebellitis), contrast enhancement within both internal auditory canals, gyriform hyperintensities on fluid-attenuated inversion recovery sequence with sulcal effacement in frontoparietal region, and thoracic myelitis. Ferraz-Filho et al. [28] presented a Brazilian infant who received the first dose of the oral polio vaccine and experienced vaccine-associated paralytic poliomyelitis 40 days later. MRIs of the cervical and thoracic spinal cord disclosed lesions involving the anterior horn, with increased signal intensity on T2W sequences. Consequently, these authors proposed that vaccine-associated paralytic poliomyelitis should be considered in patients with an MRI indicating spinal cord or medulla oblongata involvement and acute flaccid paralysis. Thus, vaccination history is essential in differentiating such an entity from other conditions. This is an important issue in countries such as India, where the oral polio vaccine is widely administrated as part of their nationwide immunization campaign [29].

In summary, combining imaging patterns, clinical presentation, and vaccination history can aid physicians in the early detection and prompt management of patients in such postimmunization scenarios. Although rare, the possibility that certain vaccines can provoke autoimmune disorders should also be considered in the appropriate context.

COVID-19 Vaccine: Types and Mechanisms

Before describing the expected imaging findings post-COVID-19 vaccination, it is imperative to quickly discuss the currently available vaccines against SARS-CoV-2. As of April 2021, 28 COVID-19 vaccines had entered phase III clinical trials, but only a few were granted emergency authorizations for use [30]. These include mRNA vaccines Pfizer-BioNTech and Moderna and the three adenoviral-vectored vaccines Oxford/AstraZeneca, Gam-COVID-Vac, and Johnson & Johnson/Janssen. Because the mechanisms behind the adenoviral-vectored and mRNA vaccines differ, both side effects and level of immunogenicity can vary. For example, most side effects related to Oxford/ AstraZeneca and Johnson & Johnson/Janssen involve hypercoagulability, while the most common side effects of mRNA-based vaccines involve myocarditis/ pericarditis. Also, certain studies indicate that mRNA biotechnology vaccines have greater immunogenicity and longer-lasting protection [31]. Although there is reasonable evidence that mRNA vaccines have an efficacy of ~95% after two doses, data from the viral-vectored vaccines are mixed. Although it is suggested that two doses of both mRNA and adenoviral-vectored vaccines elicit high levels of neutralizing antibodies (equivalent to or higher than those seen in the convalescence phase), the level of neutralizing antibodies with the mRNA vaccines is relatively higher.

Expected Findings Post-COVID-19 Vaccination

Lymphadenopathy

As vaccination rates in the general population have increased over time, the incidence of postvaccine regional LAP ipsilateral to the site of vaccination is also on the rise. The activation of the lymph node

post-COVID-19 vaccination can be attributed to local accumulation of viral antigen, because a sustained vaccination response requires localization of activated antigens at the injection site that subsequently move to the draining nodes. These findings can be detected on multiple imaging modalities and oftentimes reported as an incidental finding on imaging examinations during regular screening or oncologic surveillance assessments [32, 33].

Imaging in Vaccine-Related Lymphadenopathy

On US imaging, reactive LAP often manifests as diffuse or focal thickening of the cortex and preserved fatty hilum, indicating benign/reactive etiology. Findings on chest/breast MRI oftentimes show asymmetric axillary adenopathy with preserved fatty hilum or irregular or cortical thickening, which decreases in size and irregularity over time (Figure 23.2). Notably, lymph nodes can sometimes show abnormal size and loss of hilar fat shortly after vaccination, falsely indicating malignancy [35, 36]. For example, on CT, shortly after vaccine administration, lymph nodes may show abnormal morphology and appear completely rounded with loss of hilar fat. In such cases, short-term follow-up imaging can confirm the resolution of malignant features of LAP.

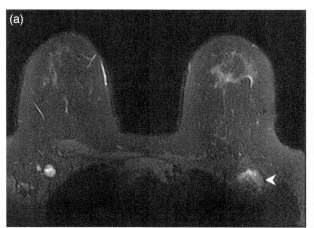
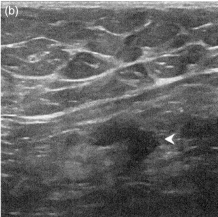

Figure 23.2 Images showing vaccine-related lymphadenopathy in a 41-year-old woman undergoing breast MRI for follow-up of a focal lesion. (a) T2W fat-saturated axial image through upper breasts and anterior chest five days after COVID-19 vaccination of the left shoulder, showing asymmetric left axillary adenopathy (3.0 × 1.7 cm at *arrowhead*) with preserved fatty hilum but irregular cortex. (b) Axillary sonography of same patient, performed at six-week follow-up, demonstrating decreased size (2.2 × 1.1 cm at *arrowhead*) and some residual cortical thickening of the lymph nodes, confirming benign/reactive nature. *Source:* Becker et al. [34].

On FDG-PET/CT imaging, lymph nodes in the axilla, supraclavicular region, and cervical region often exhibit substantial FDG uptake after intramuscular vaccination of the ipsilateral muscle, ranging from normal to considerably enlarged size. Generally, ipsilateral lymph nodes will show increased FDG uptake, although some of the contralateral lymph nodes may show uptake as well. Average reported maximum standardized uptake values of FDG-avid axillary and supraclavicular lymph nodes ipsilateral to the injection varied between 3.0 and 5.1 among different studies [37–39]. According to McIntosh et al. [40], the degree of FDG uptake depends on temporal proximity to the vaccination, ranging from intense uptake shortly after vaccination to hardly perceptible with a longer period postvaccination. In addition, vaccine-related FDG uptake typically occurs within seven days of vaccination and generally subsides by days 12–14. Clinically, benign axillary LAP develops within two to four days after the first or second dose of COVID-19 vaccination. Interestingly, Keshavarz et al. [41] reported that the median days of LAP after each dose of the vaccine was 12 (3–26 days) for the first dose and 5 (1–22 days) after the second dose. The LAP may persist for an average of 1–2 days (Moderna) and 10 days (Pfizer-BioNTech) with decreased lymph node size and residual cortical thickening over time [34]. Because vaccine-related LAP can be detected on PET/CT for roughly four to six weeks postvaccination, many authors suggest performing PET/CT at least two weeks after vaccine administration [40]. If imaging is not pertinent, four to six weeks should elapse after vaccination to avoid potential confounding findings.

In certain instances, a short period between vaccination and PET/CT imaging can lead to misinterpretation, misdiagnosis, or medical management dilemmas. Ozutemiz et al. [32] reported a case of a 32-year-old woman with a left-sided neck mass with biopsy showing a metastatic lymph node with BRAF-V600E mutant malignant melanoma. Staging PET/CT demonstrated hypermetabolic left intraparotid LAP and no other suspicious findings. After appropriate treatment, FDG-PET/CT showed complete resolution of the intraparotid LAP but indicated multiple slightly enlarged, hypermetabolic axillary lymph nodes with notable fat stranding (Figure 23.3). In addition, these authors noted an area of intramuscular FDG uptake in the left arm, which was initially reported as possible progression or pseudoprogression secondary to the patient's immunotherapy. Because the patient was assumed to be in remission, a biopsy was recommended. On further investigation, it was found that the patient had received their second Pfizer-BioNTech vaccine dose six days prior. Thus, these new imaging findings were attributed to the vaccine, and observation was elected over biopsy. Follow-up of the LAP was then included in the patient's three-month follow-up PET/CT for melanoma surveillance.

Many physicians also incidentally detected LAP during regular breast cancer screening and follow-up oncologic breast US imaging [42]. Shah et al. [43] reported a case of an 83-year-old woman who presented for a routine three-month follow-up for primary right-sided in situ breast cancer. On imaging, only the left supraclavicular and axillary lymph nodes contralateral to the breast cancer showed increased uptake. The rest of the lymph nodes were stable (as compared with the prior scan). It was then noted that she had received a COVID-19 vaccine injection on her left arm two weeks before FDG-PET/CT. The diagnosis of vaccine-related LAP was made based on the temporal connection between the history of immunization and morphologically normal but FDG-avid lymph nodes (Figure 23.4) [43].

In a study of COVID-19 vaccine–associated axillary LAP, Mortazavi [44] reported 23 women with axillary adenopathy on breast imaging after COVID-19 vaccination (with 74% receiving either the Pfizer-BioNTech or Moderna vaccine and 26% not specified/reported vaccine type). Of the 23 women, 13% were symptomatic with axillary lumps, 43% asymptomatic and undergoing imaging as part of a screening, and 43% asymptomatic and undergoing diagnostic imaging. Most underwent imaging between 2–6 (35%) and 7–13 days (35%) after their first vaccine dose. In addition, Mortazavi found that a majority (57%) had one abnormal lymph node, with maximal lymph node cortical thickness of 4 mm (43%) or 5–6 mm (43%) [44]. These patients (92%) were assigned a Breast Imaging-Reporting and Data System (BI-RADS) score of 3, indicating a probable benign finding, which follow-up in a short time frame suggested, ranging from 4 to 24 weeks.

LAP after COVID-19 vaccination detected on routine surveillance imaging can also be concerning in patients with a history of malignancy other than breast cancer. This is especially true in patients with a history

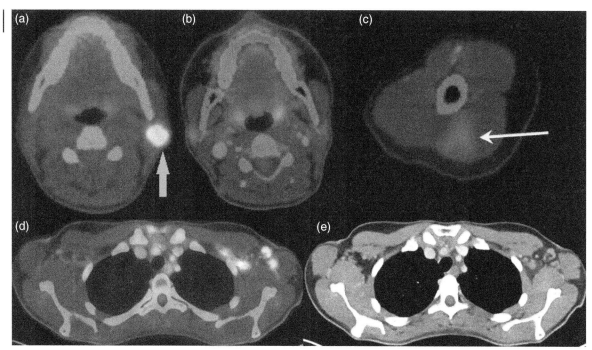

Figure 23.3 FDG-PET/CT images in a 32-year-old woman with metastatic malignant melanoma. (a) Axial fused FDG-PET/CT showing intensely hypermetabolic biopsy-proven metastatic left intraparotid lymph node (*green arrow*). (b) Axial fused FDG-PET/CT image at three-month follow-up showing complete resolution of nodal disease after chemotherapy. (c) Left arm with hypermetabolic triangular-shaped inflammation (*yellow arrow*) at the patient's COVID-19 vaccine injection site. (d) Axial fused images at the axilla level showing multiple new hypermetabolic lymph nodes. (e) Axial contrast-enhanced CT demonstrating mild fat stranding surrounding the ovoid lymph nodes with preserved fatty hilum, favoring vaccine-related lymphadenopathy. *Source:* Ozutemiz et al. [32].

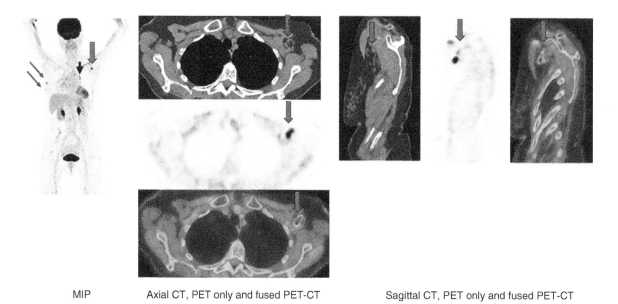

MIP   Axial CT, PET only and fused PET-CT   Sagittal CT, PET only and fused PET-CT

Figure 23.4 FDG-PET/CT (maximal intensity projection [MIP], axial PET only, fused PET/CT, CT only, sagittal PET only, fused PET/CT, and CT only) demonstrated intense uptake in two stable right breast nodules (*blue arrows*) and bilateral mediastinal and hilar lymph nodes (*black arrow*), unchanged from prior examination (not shown). Intense uptake in normal-size left axillary and subpectoral lymph nodes with normal fatty hilum (*red arrows*), typical appearance for vaccine-related lymphadenopathy. *Source:* Shah et al. [43].

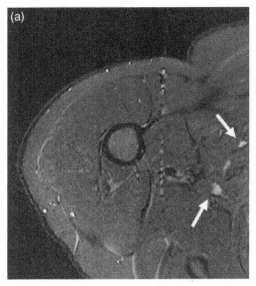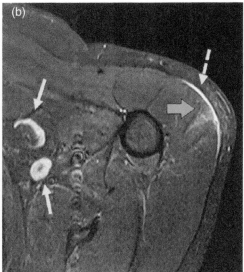

Figure 23.5 Left axillary lymphadenopathy in a patient with known malignancy. Axial T2 short-tau inversion-recovery (STIR) MRIs of the shoulders of a 41-year-old man with a history of oligometastatic myxoid liposarcoma. (a) Axial T2 STIR MRI of the right shoulder showing normal-appearing muscular and osseous structures and lymph nodes (*white arrows*). (b) Axial T2 STIR MRI of left shoulder at the same level as (a) showing new subcutaneous edema (*dashed yellow arrow*) overlying wedge-shaped intramuscular edema (*green arrow*) in the left deltoid muscle. In addition, new multiple prominent ovoid-shaped lymph nodes (*yellow arrows*) are seen, which, given the above imaging findings and recent history of ipsilateral COVID-19 vaccination, were favored to represent vaccine-related lymphadenopathy. *Source:* Ozutemiz et al. [32].

of known metastatic disease and, depending on the clinical context, may warrant further investigation. Ozutemiz et al. [32] reported a case of new clusters of left axillary lymph nodes, with one node measuring 20 mm in size and 7 mm in cortical thickness, as well as left deltoid intramuscular edema with subcutaneous edema around the muscle found on whole-body MRI surveillance in a 41-year-old man with a history of oligometastatic myxoid liposarcoma of the left thigh (Figure 23.5). Given that the patient received his second Pfizer-BioNTech vaccine four days prior to the MRI, the patient opted for clinical surveillance.

Vaccine-Related Imaging Misinterpretation

Recent studies indicate COVID-19 vaccine–induced LAP at the cervical, axillary, and supraclavicular lymph nodes. Conditions such as Castleman disease, lymphoma, head and neck malignancies, breast cancer, upper limb or trunk melanoma/sarcoma, lung cancer (particularly upper lobes), sarcoidosis, and advanced-stage cancers often also predominantly involve these lymph nodes, yielding interpretive challenges [40, 45]. Supraclavicular LAP is commonly seen in patients with gastric, esophageal, and pancreatic cancers and is usually considered as a distant metastasis and advanced-stage malignancy. In addition, the imaging presentation of mediastinal and axillary LAP after COVID-19 vaccination on FDG-PET/CT scan can resemble sarcoid-like granuloma or a concurrent hypermetabolic disease with high FDG-avid areas. Thus, it is imperative to take a thorough history regarding the type and time frame of COVID-19 vaccination to prevent imaging misinterpretation [46]. Ultimately, because postvaccination imaging findings can overlap with other diseases, notably malignancies, it is imperative that viral vaccination is considered as a possible cause of false-positive results. This in turn will help physicians avoid incorrect image interpretation and inadvertent staging of diseases showing similar PET/CT lymph node uptake.

Special Considerations for Oncologic Imaging with COVID-19 Vaccination

The presentation of a new-onset unilateral axillary LAP after vaccination can be challenging, especially in patients with current or prior history of malignancy. Ultimately, the management of this situation needs to analyze the probability of malignant spread versus benign immunologic reaction to recent vaccination. The primary points to consider when assessing the likelihood of malignancy recurrence include time of vaccination, site of primary malignancy, probable drainage pathways, patient prognosis, and general risk profile. With regard to risk assessment, a broad spectrum of therapeutic or diagnostic options may be considered, ranging from "no need for further imaging" (for the patients with the lowest risk for metastasis), "immediate further imaging tests," "short-interval clinical follow-up," and "excisional biopsy" (for the high risk for nodal metastasis).

Due to the absence of any established guidelines for the approach to LAP in patients with cancer, there are several recommendations suggested by the published literature. For instance, Lehman et al. [47, 48] stated that: (1) COVID-19 vaccine history should be documented for the time of subsequent imaging, (2) all the cancer care team members (especially the radiologists) should be educated and aware of the possible vaccine-induced LAP, and (3) patients should be reassured about this common side effect. However, concerns about vaccine-induced LAP are not a valid reason for vaccination delay because of the high rate of COVID-19-related deaths in cancer patient populations [49]. McIntosh et al. [40] noted that if the patient has a cancer with laterality, such as breast cancer, most melanomas, lung cancer, and head and neck cancers, the vaccine should be injected contralaterally to prevent the potential confounding LAP ipsilateral to the cancer. Moreover, patients with cancer are recommended to undergo PET/CT or CT scans at least two weeks after vaccination to avoid anticipated diagnostic challenges. However, if the PET/CT scan can be reasonably postponed, the best time for imaging after vaccination is four to six weeks to avoid probable confounding findings [47]. Furthermore, it is suggested that in the setting of screening breast imaging and

diagnostic imaging workup for breast-related symptoms in the patients who have a history of vaccination in the past six weeks, when the imaging findings do not show anything beyond unilateral axillary adenopathy ipsilateral to the vaccination site, it is reasonable to consider adenopathy as reactive in nature [47].

A recent article published in June 2021 [48] suggests that in cases with new unilateral LAP ipsilateral to the vaccine-administered arm and within six weeks after vaccination, clinical follow-up is sufficient and no further imaging is needed. In contrast, if the new unilateral LAP is at the contralateral site of vaccination or occurred later than six weeks, then imaging follow-up is highly recommended. Based on the type of primary malignancy, specific follow-up imaging may be indicated. For example, if the findings are localized, then ultrasound may be useful. In case of suspect abdominopelvic involvement, CT scan should be considered. PET/CT imaging can be reserved for the following scenarios: (1) evaluation of suspicious lymph node in the drainage pathway of the affected organ, (2) evaluation of a suspicious lymph node during remission, (3) evaluation of an undetermined lymph node in previously healthy individuals with a family history of malignancy, and (4) assessment of the extent of disease. If the LAP persists longer than two weeks or gets larger, then invasive diagnostic methods such as excisional biopsy may be helpful.

For breast cancer in particular, the Society of Breast Imaging (SBI), in their Fifth Edition of the *BI-RADS Atlas*, recommend that isolated unilateral axillary adenopathy on screening mammography should receive a BI-RADS category of 0 (meaning imaging was incomplete and additional imaging evaluation and/or comparison with prior mammograms is needed) in the absence of a known infectious or inflammatory cause [50]. This is to allow for further assessment of the ipsilateral breast and documentation of the patient's medical history, which may include COVID-19 vaccination. The SBI further recommends short-term follow-up within 4–12 weeks for women who were found to have unilateral axillary adenopathy and have received COVID-19 vaccination within the past four weeks. If axillary adenopathy persists after that time frame, lymph node sampling may be considered to exclude breast and nonbreast malignancy. Lastly, the SBI recommends that patients should schedule their screening examinations either before their first dose of vaccine or four to six weeks after the last required COVID-19 vaccine dose "when it does not unduly delay care" [50].

Other COVID-19 Vaccine–Induced Side Effects

Injection-Site Reaction

After COVID-19 vaccine administration, the most frequent side effect is a nonspecific inflammatory response characterized by local erythema, swelling, and tenderness. Different vaccine formulations induce different levels of inflammation, with exaggerated immune responses often occurring in inactivated vaccines because of the adjuvants used in their preparation (i.e. polyethylene glycol for the mRNA-based vaccines and polysorbates for the viral vector vaccines) [2, 51]. Although most COVID-19 vaccination side effects are mild and self-limited, severe inflammation may persist, involving deeper layers of the skin and soft tissues beyond the site of injection [4, 51]. US and MRI are often used to better characterize these findings because the former is a safe, available, and rapid diagnostic modality, while the latter offers a nonionizing method of imaging with high sensitivity to capture subtle soft tissue changes [7]. Ultimately, MRI is the optimal technique to assess soft tissue and quantify vaccine-induced tissue responses over time but is unfortunately resource limited [52–54].

Recently, rare cases of more severe local complications post-COVID-19 vaccination have been reported, including necrosis of the surrounding soft tissues, muscular fibrosis, and myositis [5, 16, 55]. In addition, both sterile and infectious intramuscular or subcutaneous abscesses can develop. Infectious abscesses occur because of bacterial inoculation at the site of injection via the vaccine needle. Sterile collections may result from a hypersensitivity reaction caused by the injected medication. These collections consist of liquefied fat and muscle tissue resulting from necrosis of the involved tissues [56]. With intramuscular vaccination and direct inoculation, the muscle is exposed to various contaminant agents triggering an immunologic response to the injected antigen. Many factors may contribute to induced muscle toxicity, such as inciting

substance and its components, and the host's immune system or inflammatory response. In myositis, nonenhanced fluid-sensitive sequences (proton density and T2W images) may indicate feathery edema infiltrating the affected muscle and adjoining perifascial fluid. On T1-enhanced sequence, the affected muscle may show intense enhancement reflecting inflammation [57, 58].

Musculoskeletal Complications

Although most postvaccination local reactions are typically mild and transient and limited to adjacent skin and underlying muscle, several studies reported bursitis and shoulder injury related to vaccine administration (SIRVA). Although an infrequent complication of COVID-19 immunization, the number of reported SIRVA cases is increasing. It is generally believed that SIRVA develops after improper administration of vaccine into the subdeltoid bursa, resulting in a long-lasting inflammation [59, 60]. SIRVA can have a significant impact on quality of life and job performance, because patients often suffer from severe pain and limited range of motion that may cause prolonged inability to use the shoulder. The hallmark of SIRVA is that the pain usually begins within 48 hours of vaccine administration and may persist for months [61].

Noninvasive imaging studies, such as MRI or US, can be helpful in differentiating this condition from other more common pathologies (e.g. arthritis, rotator cuff tears, calcific tendonitis) [62, 63]. Common imaging findings of SIRVA, including local subcortical edema of bone marrow without obvious cortical damage, periosseous soft tissue inflammatory changes, subacromial/subdeltoid bursal fluid, and intrasubstance edema-like signal in deltoid muscle, have all been reported post-COVID-19 vaccination [13].

Neurologic Complications

There is growing concern regarding neurologic consequences post-COVID-19 vaccination, after two individuals experienced transverse myelitis post-Oxford/AstraZeneca COVID-19 vaccine injection in the fall of 2020 [64]. On subsequent workup, one of the reported cases was found to have preexisting multiple sclerosis unrelated to the vaccine, while the other was found to be immune mediated and potentially linked to the vaccine [65, 66]. A 36-year-old man, with no prior comorbidities, presented to the emergency department eight days after Oxford/AstraZeneca vaccine with complaints of abnormal sensations in his lower limbs bilaterally. After the sensations began to ascend, MRI of the spine was ordered, showing a T2-hyperintense lesion dorsally at C6 and C7 (Figure 23.6). The patient was assumed to have vaccine-associated myelitis and responded well to intravenous methylprednisolone (1000 mg for five days). After a week-long hospital stay, the patient was discharged [67].

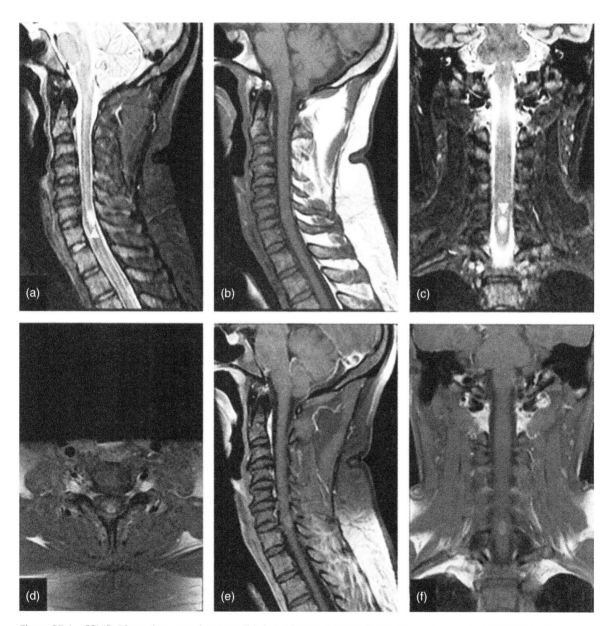

Figure 23.6 COVID-19 vaccine–associated myelitis in a 36-year-old man. Sagittal (a) and coronal (c) T2W MRIs of the cervical spine show a focal hyperintense lesion at C6-C7 level (*yellow arrowheads*). The lesion is isointense on precontrast sagittal T1W (b) image. Mild-to-moderate peripheral contrast enhancement (*red arrowheads*) was seen on corresponding postcontrast T1W axial (d), sagittal (e), and coronal (f) images. *Source:* Malhotra et al. [67].

Another neurologic complication that has been recently reported is Bell's palsy, particularly with mRNA-based vaccines. A clinical study based on both Moderna and the Pfizer-BioNTech COVID-19 vaccines showed that 7 cases out of 37 000 vaccination recipients experienced Bell's palsy. On further research, the FDA found that there was no significant increased risk for Bell's palsy in the vaccinated population [68]. However, Health Canada recently updated the label on the Pfizer-BioNTech vaccine to warn patients against the rare possibility of this condition [69]. Another recently reported neurologic condition is Guillain-Barré syndrome (GBS), particularly with the Johnson & Johnson/Janssen vaccine. In a clinical trial of the Johnson & Johnson/Janssen COVID-19 vaccine, one case of GBS was reported in the vaccinated group and one GBS case in the placebo group [70]. After 12.8 million administered doses of the Johnson & Johnson/Janssen COVID-19 vaccine, the Vaccine Adverse Event Reporting System (VAERS) reported 100 preliminary reports of GBS. Recently, a larger-scale study conducted by the VAERS received 9442 reports of postvaccination adverse effects linked to COVID-19 vaccines from Pfizer-BioNTech, Moderna, and Johnson & Johnson/Janssen. The reported results included 254 (2.69%) cases with neurologic adverse effects and 9 cases with transverse myelitis [65]. A number of transient neurologic symptoms were anticipated to develop within a short period after immunization, including dizziness and headaches, muscle pain and spasms, and paresthesia. In addition, the VAERS database contains instances of facial palsy, GBS, stroke, transverse myelitis, and ADEM [65].

Interestingly, a case report by Keir et al. [71] discussed a 57-year-old woman with phantosmia (olfactory hallucination) after she was given the second dose of the Pfizer-BioNTech vaccine. The patient described a strong reaction to the first dose of the vaccine, with symptoms such as fatigue, weakness, and random episodes of "smelling smoke." These intermittent phantosmia episodes progressed to being constant and became associated with hyposmia. The patient denied nasal congestion, rhinorrhea, and postnasal drip. Her COVID-19 polymerase chain reaction testing was negative, and physical examination showed normal cranial nerve function. CT angiography (CTA) of the head and neck was performed, indicating left (greater than right) olfactory tract enhancement (Figure 23.7). On MRI, T2 signal hyperintensity was reported in the left olfactory bulb and bilateral olfactory tracts, suggestive of edema (Figure 23.7). On further imaging, the olfactory nerve filia were also found to be thickened and clumped. Although the exact etiology of phantosmia is unknown, the radiographic findings may reflect an inflammatory response to the viral S antigen via the angiotensin-converting enzyme 2 coronavirus 2 (CoV-2) receptor protein and the S protein transmembrane protease serine 2 pathways [71]. Awareness of these findings, both clinically and radiographically, can help with understanding the pathophysiology and various manifestations of COVID-19, as well as the side effects of the vaccine.

Thrombotic Complications

Johnson & Johnson/Janssen Vaccine-Induced Immune Thrombotic Thrombocytopenia

Between March and April 2021, the VAERS received reports of headaches in six patients who received the Johnson & Johnson/Janssen COVID-19 vaccine, ranging from 6 to 13 days postvaccination [35]. One of these patients had abdominal pain, nausea, and vomiting. Four of the six had focal neurologic symptoms, such as focal weakness, aphasia, and visual disturbances, which prompted presentation to their local emergency departments. These patients were all eventually diagnosed with cerebral venous sinus thrombosis (CVST) by intracranial imaging, and two patients were also diagnosed with both portal vein and splanchnic thrombosis. All patients were found to have thrombotic thrombocytopenia, with the lowest platelet counts ranging from 10 000/ml to 127 000/ml during their hospitalizations. This vaccine-induced immune thrombotic thrombocytopenia (VITT) is a prothrombotic syndrome reported in some individuals who have received the Johnson & Johnson/Janssen vaccine. Although the exact incidence of VITT is still unknown, studies have shown that it appears to be a rare complication described in only a few cases per tens of millions of vaccinated individuals [72, 73]. The mechanism behind VITT involves antibodies targeting platelet factor 4 (PF4, or CXCL4), thus activating platelets through FcγIIa receptors and resulting in coagulation system activation and significant clinical

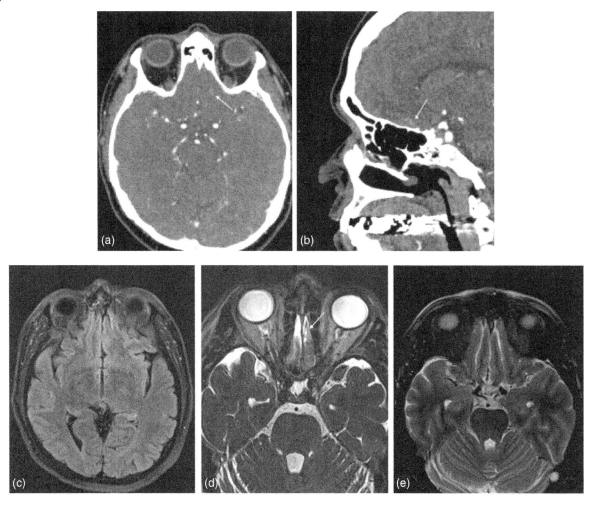

Figure 23.7 A 57-year-old woman with phantosmia after two doses of the Pfizer-BioNTech COVID-19 vaccine. (a, b) Axial (a) and sagittal (b) postcontrast CT angiogram images show faint enhancement of the left olfactory tract (*white arrows*). (c) Axial fluid-attenuated inversion recovery. (d) High-resolution thin-slice T2W imaging. (e) Axial T2 with fat saturation showing abnormal hyperintense signal in olfactory bulbs and tracts (*white arrow*) suggestive of edema. *Source:* Keir et al. [71].

thromboembolic complications. This syndrome begins 5–10 days postvaccination and usually presents as thrombocytopenia (with clinical presentation of petechial or mucosal bleeding), cerebral venous thrombosis, pulmonary embolism (PE), splanchnic vein thrombosis, adrenal vein thrombosis, ischemic stroke, limb ischemia, and coagulopathies, such as disseminated intravascular coagulation or bleeding.

Another case reported by Malik et al. [36] noted thrombocytopenia, PE, and transient ischemic attack 10 days after receiving the Johnson & Johnson/Janssen COVID-19 vaccine. The 43-year-old female patient presented to the hospital with an unbearable progressive headache and dyspnea. CTA of the head and neck showed a low-density filling defect in the venous sinus confluence, which was concerning for CVST. Further MRI of the head showed a focal filling defect in the region of the sinus confluence, as is typical for an arachnoid granulation with no evidence of dural venous sinus thrombosis. No intracranial hemorrhage or mass lesion was seen. Doppler images of the upper and lower extremities bilaterally were also performed to identify the cause of the patient's dyspnea and demonstrated no evidence of deep vein thrombosis.

However, her D-dimer was elevated, prompting a CT pulmonary angiogram to assess for PE. The patient was found to have right upper lobe, right lower lobe, and left lower lobe lobar and segmental pulmonary emboli. She was treated with intravenous immunoglobulin and daily subcutaneous fondaparinux (which was changed to apixaban on discharge), as well as supportive care for her headache. One day after discharge, she returned to the hospital with numbness and tingling of the face and right arm, with CTA of the head and neck showing a nonocclusive right internal carotid artery thrombus in the right carotid bulb/proximal right internal carotid artery. She was diagnosed with a transient ischemic attack, admitted for further management, and ultimately discharged.

Other case reports noted similar findings after vaccination with the Janssen vaccine. A healthy young woman with an unremarkable medical history experienced acute ischemic stroke eight days after vaccination with the Johnson & Johnson/Janssen vaccine. Laboratory findings were compatible with thrombocytopenia, and a positive anti-PF4 antibody was noted. After thrombectomy with recanalization, the patient showed a dramatic response to treatment [74]. To summarize, patients with new-onset symptoms of thrombosis after receiving the Johnson & Johnson/Janssen vaccine should undergo further workup for VITT and be treated appropriately.

Oxford/AstraZeneca Thrombotic Events

Similar to the Johnson & Johnson/Janssen vaccine, the Oxford/AstraZeneca (ChAdOx1 nCoV-19) vaccine is a viral vector vaccine that has also sparked controversy because of reports of thrombotic events. The most frequent side effects of the Oxford/AstraZeneca vaccine were pain, induration, itch, erythema, tenderness, swelling, and warmth at the injection site, as well as systemic side effects, such as general discomfort, fever, chills, malaise, fatigue, lethargy, headache, nausea, and arthralgia [75]. Most of these side effects commence between the first and second day after injection and subside at most within one week postvaccination [76, 77]. However, several studies have reported thrombosis and thrombocytopenia after the Oxford/AstraZeneca vaccine because of its ability to induce a hypercoagulable state. The mechanism behind this hypercoagulability relies on the fact that the Oxford/

AstraZeneca vaccine can trigger the expression of antiplatelet antibodies leading to thrombocytopenia and concomitant venous/arterial thromboses [78]. However, these side effects have proved to be rare because the German Society of Thrombosis and Hemostasis noted a total of 13 cases of sinus or cerebral vein thrombosis in 1.6 million Oxford/AstraZeneca COVID-19 vaccine injected doses. The thromboses occurred within 4–16 days after vaccination, and concomitant thrombocytopenia was noted in all patients, which was associated with a fatal clinical course in nine patients [79]. Consistent with this, Wolf et al. [78] reported the occurrence of CVST in three vaccinated individuals 4–17 days after vaccination with the Oxford/AstraZeneca vaccine.

Recent reports have also shown splanchnic vein thrombosis after Oxford/AstraZeneca COVID-19 vaccination. Three cases of thrombosis in the splanchnic veins were reported among young adults that initiated between 5 and 16 days after vaccination [68]. Another case report [80] described a 41-year-old man who presented to the emergency department with severe sudden-onset headache. He denied any other neurologic symptoms and had no relevant history except for the Oxford/AstraZeneca vaccine 11 days prior. Cranial CT was negative, but chest CT showed peripheral pulmonary emboli; four days later, the patient reported sudden abdominal pain. Abdominal CT scan showed massive thrombosis of the entire portal vein with no discernible enhancement in the portal, splenic, and superior mesenteric veins. Intraabdominal free fluid was detected with higher density around the spleen, along with splenomegaly with decreased spleen enhancement. Consistent with this, Umbrello et al. [81] described a case of concomitant thrombosis in portal vein, superior mesenteric vein, and splenic vein in a young female patient with no remarkable history, except for administration of ChAdOx1 nCoV-19 vaccine 17 days before. Garnier et al. [82] reported a case of a 26-year-old woman who initially presented with persistent nausea and headache shortly and was admitted for an acute stroke eight days after receiving the Oxford/AstraZeneca vaccine. She rapidly developed right hemiplegia and aphasia, resulting in a National Institutes of Health Stroke Scale score of 8 [82]. Left middle cerebral artery occlusion was diagnosed and treated angiographically (Figure 23.8a,b),

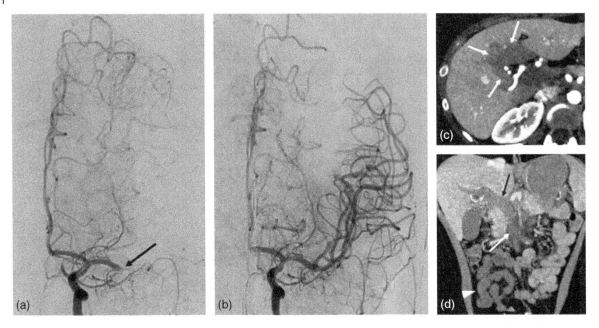

Figure 23.8 A 26-year-old woman admitted for acute stroke eight days after administration of the Oxford/AstraZeneca COVID-19 vaccine. (a) Anteroposterior projection digital subtracted angiography (DSA) of the left internal carotid artery showing occlusion of the M1 segment (*arrow*) of the left middle cerebral artery and absence of opacification of the Sylvian network. (b) Cerebral DSA after A Direct Aspiration, First Pass Technique (ADAPT) technique showing 2C recanalization of the left middle cerebral artery. (c) Arterial-phase CT image of the liver in axial plane showing global arterialization of the liver parenchyma with central and perihilar perfusion defects cause by portal trunk thrombosis (*arrows*). (d) Portal venous-phase CT image of the abdomen with portal (*black arrow*) and superior and inferior mesenteric vein (*white arrow*) thrombosis. Venous mesenteric ischemia, as shown by decreased ileal wall enhancement (*arrowhead*), was also present. *Source:* Garnier et al. [82].

and further CT imaging indicated segmental PE. The presence of anti-PF4 antibodies and thrombocytopenia raised suspicion for VITT. CT imaging of the liver further showed global arterialization of the liver parenchyma with central hypoattenuating areas that became iso-attenuating on portal venous phase, suggesting hepatic blood flow changes. In addition, portal venous and mesenteric vein thrombosis, as well as reduced ileal wall postcontrast enhancement and bowel wall edema, were also seen, suggesting mesenteric venous ischemia (Figure 23.8c,d). Subsequently, the patient was treated with corticosteroids, plasma exchange, and anticoagulants and was discharged 14 days later.

Myocarditis

Myocarditis refers to inflammation of the myocardium, leading to myocyte injury and necrosis. Although myocarditis is often idiopathic, there are some known etiologies, including infectious (especially viral), autoimmune, toxin induced, or even vaccination. A thorough analysis of VAERS data during 1990–2018 has reported myopericarditis as a rare complication after COVID-19 vaccines previously licensed for use in the United States [83]. Patients with vaccine-related myocarditis often present with non-specific symptoms, and diagnosis usually relies on the combination of clinical presentation, elevated cardiac enzymes, and cardiac imaging (mainly cardiac MRI) (Figure 23.9) [85].

Recently, an increasing number of myocarditis and pericarditis cases have been reported after mRNA COVID-19 immunization. In a review by Deb et al. [86], the authors identified 37 vaccine recipients who experienced myocarditis as an adverse event post-COVID-19 vaccination. They found that the median time of symptom onset was three days postvaccination, and that most cases occurred in male individuals. In addition, most cases ensued after the second vaccine dose, perhaps because of the heightened immune response. The majority (32/37) of the patients required

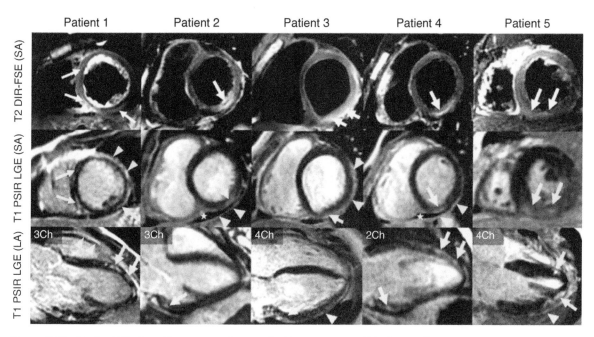

Figure 23.9 Cardiac MRIs from five patients diagnosed with acute myocarditis three to five days after a second dose of mRNA vaccine. Yellow arrows depict myocardial late gadolinium enhancement in a nonischemic pattern, white arrows depict corresponding T2 signal abnormalities, arrowheads depict pericardial enhancement, and stars depict pericardial effusion. *Source:* Starekova et al. [84].

hospitalization with an average hospital stay of three days, and one patient (1/37) died.

In a study from Israel, the authors noted 110 cases of myocarditis among the 5 million people who had received two doses of the Pfizer-BioNTech vaccine. Most cases occurred within a month postimmunization, and 90% of the cases were men [87]. Interestingly, the authors noted that among vaccinated young men, the probability of contracting myocarditis was 5–25 times higher than the background rate.

Rosner et al. [88] have also reported a case series of seven male patients hospitalized for acute myocarditis-like illness after COVID-19 vaccination. Six patients received an mRNA vaccine (Pfizer/BioNTech or Moderna), and one received the adenovirus vaccine (Johnson & Johnson/Janssen). They presented three to seven days after vaccination with acute-onset chest pain and biochemical evidence of myocardial injury by elevated cTnI (cardiac troponin I). A cardiac MRI was obtained for all patients between 3 and 37 days postvaccination (including multiplanar steady-state free precession sequences, short-axis T1 and T2 stacks, T1 mapping when available, and multiplanar myocardial late gadolinium enhancement). There was

multifocal subepicardial late gadolinium enhancement in all seven patients and additional midmyocardial late gadolinium enhancement in four of seven patients. Corresponding myocardial edema was also evident in three of seven patients. Two patients who underwent cardiac MRI (>7 days from presentation) had no edema. Endomyocardial biopsy was performed in one patient and showed no pathologic evidence of myocarditis. Although endomyocardial biopsy was negative in the single case in which it was performed, the authors stated that this might represent sampling bias, given the patchy nature of myocardial inflammation in myocarditis.

In another case report, Habib et al. [89] presented a young man who experienced acute myocarditis three days after the second dose of BNT162b2 (Pfizer) vaccine. The patient underwent cardiac MRI, which showed an early and late faint subepicardial enhancement of the basal lateral wall, suggestive of myocarditis. However, on T2W images, no clear evidence of myocardial edema was shown. Similarly, Singh et el. [90] reported a 24-year-old male patient who experienced chest pain after the second dose of the Pfizer-BioNTech COVID-19 vaccine and who was finally diagnosed with myocarditis on further workup. On cardiac MRI, there was linear subepicardial enhancement involving the lateral wall of the left ventricle, compatible with acute myocarditis.

Although these case studies may suggest a possible causal association between myocarditis and vaccination, given the temporal relationship, clinical presentations, and cardiac MRI findings, it is always difficult to distinguish causality from coincidence in vaccine-associated adverse events. More importantly, there is still a lack of evidence given the limited number of published cases. However, the temporal relationship of these conditions increases the likelihood that these complications are vaccination induced. Therefore, physicians should maintain a higher index of suspicion for postvaccination myocarditis, particularly in patients who have received mRNA-based vaccines. It cannot be overemphasized that the benefits of vaccination far outweigh the risk of SARS-CoV-2 infection, especially because the reported myocarditis is rare and most cases ultimately recover. Thus, vaccination is still an essential lifesaving measure to combat the ongoing COVID-19 global pandemic.

Summary of Recommendations and Conclusion

As previously stated, cancer-related imaging should occur before vaccination, unless urgent clinical indications occur, such as acute symptoms, short-term treatment monitoring, planning for urgent treatment, and screening for complications. For patients at low risk for supraclavicular or axillary nodal metastasis in whom the LAP is more likely to be due to vaccination rather than underlying malignancy (considering time frame, symptoms, location, and type of cancer), management strategies can exclude default follow-up imaging. In more ambiguous cases, a multidisciplinary discussion may be valuable. For other indications, including surveillance, screening, and staging, the postponement of imaging at least for six weeks after completion of vaccination should be considered [34]. Notably, some centers offer screening/surveillance examinations in concert with COVID-19 vaccination, to reduce patient burden and keep patient engagement in both domains. In addition, this patient population should receive the vaccine in the contralateral arm or thigh if possible.

As the global COVID-19 vaccine rollout continues, it is imperative that physicians are aware of the various vaccine-associated imaging findings, as well as the common misconceptions to prepare for potential imaging challenges in the vaccinated population. Vital information such as type of COVID-19 vaccine, date of injection, and the injection site should be easily accessible to radiologists and considered when interpreting potential vaccination-related abnormalities. Ultimately, by becoming familiar with the various signs, symptoms, and imaging findings associated with each vaccine, physicians will perform better at recognizing common vaccine-associated presentations and can initiate a directed workup sooner.

References

1 Mascellino, M.T., Di Timoteo, F., De Angelis, M., and Oliva, A. (2021). Overview of the main anti-SARS-CoV-2 vaccines: mechanism of action, efficacy and safety. *Infect Drug Resist.* 14: 3459–3476.

2 Pormohammad, A., Zarei, M., Ghorbani, S. et al. (2021). Efficacy and safety of COVID-19 vaccines: a systematic review and meta- analysis of randomized clinical trials. *Vaccine* 9 (5): 467.

3 Lin, Y. and He, Y. (2012). Ontology representation and analysis of vaccine formulation and administration and their effects on vaccine immune responses. *J Biomed Semantics* 3 (1): 17.

4 Siegrist, C.A. (2007). Mechanisms underlying adverse reactions to vaccines. *J Comp Pathol.* 137: S46–S50.

5 Polat, A.V., Bekci, T., Dabak, N. et al. (2015). Vaccine-induced myositis with intramuscular sterile abscess formation: MRI and ultrasound findings. *Skelet Radiol.* 44 (12): 1849–1852.

6 Lee, S., Choi, S., Kim, S.Y. et al. (2017). Potential utility of FDG PET-CT as a non-invasive tool for monitoring local immune responses. *J Gastric Cancer* 17 (4): 384–393.

7 Hung, E.H., Griffith, J.F., Yip, S.W. et al. (2020). Accuracy of ultrasound in the characterization of superficial soft tissue tumors: a prospective study. *Skelet Radiol.* 49 (6): 883–892.

8 India – COVID19 Vaccine Tracker. 2021. http://Covid19.trackvaccines.org. Accessed 12 Sep 2021.

9 Katal, S., Pouraryan, A., and Gholamrezanezhad, A. (2021). COVID-19 vaccine is here: practical considerations for clinical imaging applications. *Clin Imaging* 76: 38–41. https://doi.org/10.1016/j.clinimag.2021.01.023.

10 Hui H, Tang Y, Hu M, Zhao X. (2011). Stem cells: general features and characteristics. In: Gholamrezanezhad A, editors. Stem Cells in Clinic and Research. London: IntechOpen; 2011. doi:10.5772/23755. https://www.intechopen.com/chapters/18217.

11 Miliauskas, J.R., Mukherjee, T., and Dixon, B. (1993). Postimmunization (vaccination) injection-site reactions. A report of four cases and review of the literature. *Am J Surg Pathol.* 17 (5): 516–524.

12 Martín Arias, L.H., Sanz Fadrique, R., Sáinz Gil, M., and Salgueiro-Vazquez, M.E. (2017). Risk of bursitis and other injuries and dysfunctions of the shoulder following vaccinations. *Vaccine* 35 (37): 4870–4876.

13 Okur, G., Chaney, K.A., and Lomasney, L.M. (2014). Magnetic resonance imaging of abnormal shoulder pain following influenza vaccination. *Skelet Radiol.* 43 (9): 1325–1331. https://doi.org/10.1007/s00256-014-1875-9.

14 Frost, L., Johansen, P., Pedersen, S. et al. (1985). Persistent subcutaneous nodules in children hyposensitized with aluminum-containing allergen extracts. *Allergy* 40: 368–372.

15 Culora, G.A., Ramsay, A.D., and Theaker, J.M. (1996). Aluminium and injection site reactions. *J Clin Pathol.* 49: 844–847.

16 Katz, L.D. (2011). Vaccination-induced myositis with intramuscular sterile abscess formation. *Skelet Radiol.* 40 (8): 1099–1101. https://doi.org/10.1007/s00256-011-1158-7.

17 Yildirim, D., Gurses, B., Tamam, C. et al. (2011). Imaging findings after fascial injection of tetanus vaccine. *Med Ultrason.* 13 (2): 161–164.

18 Burger, I.A., Husmann, L., Hany, T.F. et al. (2011). Incidence and intensity of F-18 FDG uptake after vaccination with H1N1 vaccine. *Clin Nucl Med.* 36 (10): 848–853.

19 Mingos, M., Howard, S., Giacalone, N. et al. (2016). Systemic immune response to vaccination on FDG-PET/CT. *Nucl Med Mol Imaging* 50 (4): 358–361.

20 Ozawa, H., Noma, S., Yoshida, Y. et al. (2000). Acute disseminated encephalomyelitis associated with poliomyelitis vaccine. *Pediatr Neurol.* 23 (2): 177–179.

21 Arya, S.C. (2001). Acute disseminated encephalomyelitis associated with poliomyelitis vaccine. *Pediatr Neurol.* 24 (4): 325.

22 Ohya, T., Nagamitsu, S., Yamashita, Y., and Matsuishi, T. (2007). Serial magnetic resonance imaging and single photon emission computed tomography study of acute disseminated encephalomyelitis patient after Japanese encephalitis vaccination. *Kurume Med J.* 54 (3–4): 95–99.

23 Fukuda, H., Umehara, F., Kawahigashi, N. et al. (1997). Acute disseminated myelitis after Japanese B encephalitis vaccination. *J Neurol Sci.* 148 (1): 113–115.

24 Menge, T., Kieseier, B.C., Nessler, S. et al. (2007). Acute disseminated encephalomyelitis: an acute hit against the brain. *Curr Opin Neurol.* 20 (3): 247–254.

25 Shoamanesh, A. and Traboulsee, A. (2011). Acute disseminated encephalomyelitis following influenza vaccination. *Vaccine* 29 (46): 8182–8185.

26 Ravaglia, S., Ceroni, M., Moglia, A. et al. (2004). Post-infectious and post-vaccinal acute disseminated encephalomyelitis occurring in the same patients. *J Neurol.* 251 (9): 1147–1150.

27 Lessa, R., Castillo, M., Azevedo, R. et al. (2014). Neurological complications after H1N1 influenza vaccination: magnetic resonance imaging findings. *Arq Neuropsiquiatr.* 72 (7): 496–499. https://doi.org/10.1590/0004-282x20140064.

28 Ferraz-Filho, J.R., dos Santos, T.U., de Oliveira, E.P., and Souza, A.S. (2010). MRI findings in an infant with vaccine-associated paralytic poliomyelitis. *Pediatr Radiol.* 40 (Suppl 1): S138–S140.

29 Mathew, J.L. and Mittal, S.K. (2014). Vaccine associated paralytic poliomyelitis (VAPP) in India and its public health implications: a systematic review of literature. *Int J Infect Dis.* 21: 257.

30 Sadarangani, M., Marchant, A., and Kollmann, T.R. (2021). Immunological mechanisms of vaccine-induced protection against COVID-19 in humans. *Nat Rev Immunol.* 21: 475–484.

31 Cagigi, A. and Loré, K. (2021). Immune responses induced by mRNA vaccination in mice, monkeys and humans. *Vaccine* 9 (1): 61. https://doi.org/10.3390/vaccines9010061.

32 Ozutemiz, C., Krystosek, L.A., Church, A.L. et al. (2021). Lymphadenopathy in COVID-19 vaccine recipients: diagnostic dilemma in oncologic patients. *Radiology* 300: E296–E300.

33 Tu, W., Gierada, D.S., and Joe, B.N. (2021). COVID-19 vaccination-related lymphadenopathy: what to be aware of. *Radiol Imaging Cancer* 3: e210038.

34 Becker, A.S., Perez-Johnston, R., Chikarmane, S.A. et al. (2021). Multidisciplinary recommendations regarding post-vaccine adenopathy and radiologic imaging: radiology scientific expert panel. *Radiology* 300 (2): E323–E327.

35 CDC Health Alert Network. (2020). Cases of Cerebral Venous Sinus Thrombosis with Thrombocytopenia after Receipt of the Johnson & Johnson COVID-19 Vaccine. Centers for Disease Control and Prevention. 2020. https://emergency.cdc.gov/han/2021/han00442.asp. Accessed 8 Aug 2021.

36 Malik, B., Kalantary, A., Rikabi, K., and Kunadi, A. (2021). Pulmonary embolism, transient ischaemic attack and thrombocytopenia after the Johnson & Johnson COVID-19 vaccine. *BMJ Case Rep* 14 (7): e243975. https://doi.org/10.1136/bcr-2021-243975.

37 Eshet, Y., Tau, N., Alhoubani, Y. et al. (2021). Prevalence of increased FDG PET/CT axillary lymph node uptake beyond 6 weeks after mRNA COVID-19 vaccination. *Radiology* 300: E345–E347.

38 Skawran, S., Gennari, A.G., Dittli, M. et al. (2022). [18F] FDG uptake of axillary lymph nodes after COVID-19 vaccination in oncological PET/CT: frequency, intensity, and potential clinical impact. *Eur Radiol.* 32: 508–516.

39 Orevi, M., Chicheportiche, A., and Ben-Haim, S. (2021). Lessons learned from post-COVID-19 vaccination PET/CT studies. *J Nucl Med.* https://doi.org/10.2967/jnumed.121.262348.

40 McIntosh, L.J., Bankier, A.A., Vijayaraghavan, G.R. et al. (2021). COVID-19 vaccination-related uptake on FDG PET/CT: an emerging dilemma and suggestions for management. *AJR Am J Roentgenol.* 217 (4): 975–973.

41 Keshavarz, P., Yazdanpanah, F., Rafiee, F., and Mizandari, M. (2021). Lymphadenopathy following COVID-19 vaccination: imaging findings review. *Acad Radiol.* 28 (8): 1058–1071. https://doi.org/10.1016/j.acra.2021.04.007.

42 Mehta, N., Sales, R.M., Babagbemi, K. et al. (2021). Unilateral axillary adenopathy in the setting of COVID-19 vaccine. *Clin Imaging* 75: 12–15.

43 Shah, S., Wagner, T., Nathan, M., and Szyszko, T. (2021). COVID-19 vaccine-related lymph node activation–patterns of uptake on PET-CT. *BJR Case Rep* 7 (3): 20210040.

44 Mortazavi, S. (2021). COVID-19 vaccination-associated axillary adenopathy: imaging findings and follow-up recommendations in 23 women. *AJR Am J Roentgenol.* 217 (4): 857–858. https://doi.org/10.2214/AJR.21.25651.

45 Minamimoto, R. and Kiyomatsu, T. (2021). Effects of COVID-19 vaccination on FDG-PET/CT imaging: a literature review. *Glob. Health Med* 3 (3): 129–133.

46 Bauckneht, M., Aloè, T., Tagliabue, E. et al. (2021). Beyond Covid-19 vaccination-associated pitfalls on [18F] Fluorodeoxyglucose (FDG) PET: a case of a concomitant sarcoidosis. *Eur J Nucl Med Mol Imaging* 48 (8): 2661–2662.

47 Lehman, C.D., Lamb, L.R., and D'Alessandro, H.A. (2021). Mitigating the impact of coronavirus disease (COVID-19) vaccinations on patients undergoing breast imaging examinations: a pragmatic approach. *AJR Am J Roentgenol.* 217 (3): 584–586.

48 Lehman, C.D., D'Alessandro, H.A., Mendoza, D.P. et al. (2021). Unilateral lymphadenopathy after COVID-19 vaccination: a practical management plan for radiologists across specialties. *J Am Coll Radiol.* 18 (6): 843–852.

49 Saini, K.S., Tagliamento, M., Lambertini, M. et al. (2020). Mortality in patients with cancer and coronavirus disease 2019: a systematic review and pooled analysis of 52 studies. *Eur J Cancer* 139: 43–50.

50 Grimm L, Destounis S, Dogan B, et al. (2021). SBI recommendations for the management of axillary adenopathy in patients with recent COVID-19 vaccination. Society of Breast Imaging. 2021. https://

www.sbi-online.org/Portals/0/Position%20 Statements/2021/SBI-recommendations-for-managing-axillary-adenopathy-post-COVID-vaccination.pdf. Accessed 8 Aug 2021.

51 Rosenblatt, A.E. and Stein, S.L. (2015). Cutaneous reactions to vaccinations. *Clin Dermatol.* 33 (3): 327–332.

52 Fisher, M.R., Dooms, G.C., Hricak, H. et al. (1986). Magnetic resonance imaging of the normal and pathologic muscular system. *Magn Reson Imaging* 4 (6): 491–496.

53 Bernau, M., Kremer-Rücker, P.V., Kreuzer, L.S. et al. (2017). Magnetic resonance imaging to detect local tissue reactions after vaccination in sheep in vivo. *Vet Rec Open* 4 (1): e000200.

54 Bernau, M., Liesner, B.G., Schwanitz, S. et al. (2018). Vaccine safety testing using magnetic resonance imaging in suckling pigs. *Vaccine* 36 (13): 1789–1795.

55 Spouge, A.R., Thain, L.M., McMillan, C.S., and Hammerberg, O. (2000). Magnetic resonance imaging for differentiating delayed-onset sterile abscess complicating vaccination from soft-tissue neoplasm: case report. *Can Assoc Radiol J.* 51 (1): 28.

56 Peungjesada, S., Gupta, P., Rice, G.D. et al. (2010). Bilateral sterile gluteal abscesses following intramuscular injection of penicillin: CT appearance. *Int J Radiol.* 12 (1): https://doi.org/10.5580/22d9.

57 Theodorou, D.J., Theodorou, S.J., Axiotis, A. et al. (2021). COVID-19 vaccine-related myositis. *QJM.* 114 (6): 424–425.

58 Godoy, I.R., Rodrigues, T.C., and Skaf, A. (2021). Myositis ossificans following COVID-19 vaccination. *QJM.* 114 (9): 659–660.

59 Wiesel, B.B. and Keeling, L.E. (2021). Shoulder injury related to vaccine administration. *J Am Acad Orthop Surg.* 29: 732–739.

60 Szari, M.S., Belgard, C.A., Adams, L.C., and Freiler, C.J. (2019). Shoulder injury related to vaccine administration: a rare reaction. *Fed Pract.* 36 (8): 380.

61 Bancsi, A., Houle, S.K., and Grindrod, K.A. (2018). Getting it in the right spot: shoulder injury related to vaccine administration (SIRVA) and other injection site events. *Can Pharm J.* 151 (5): 295–299.

62 Cross, G.B., Moghaddas, J., Buttery, J. et al. (2016). Don't aim too high: avoiding shoulder injury related to vaccine administration. *Aust Fam Physician* 45 (5): 303–306.

63 Cantarelli Rodrigues, T., Hidalgo, P.F., Skaf, A.Y., and Serfaty, A. (2021). Subacromial-subdeltoid bursitis following COVID-19 vaccination: a case of shoulder injury related to vaccine administration (SIRVA). *Skeletal Radiol.* 50 (11): 2293–2297.

64 Allen A and Szabo L. 2020. Kaiser Health News. NIH "Very Concerned" about Serious Side Effect in Coronavirus Vaccine Trial. Scientific American. https://www.scientificamerican.com/article/ nih-very-concerned-about-serious-side-effect-in-coronavirus-vaccine-trial/. Accessed 27 Feb 2021.

65 Goss, A.L., Samudralwar, R.D., Das, R.R., and Nath, A. (2021). ANA investigates: neurological complications of COVID-19 vaccines. *Ann Neurol.* 89 (5): 856.

66 Voysey, M., Clemens, S.A., Madhi, S.A. et al. (2021). Safety and efficacy of the ChAdOx1 nCoV-19 vaccine (AZD1222) against SARS-CoV-2: an interim analysis of four randomized controlled trials in Brazil, South Africa, and the UK. *Lancet* 397 (10269): 99–111.

67 Malhotra, H., Gupta, P., Prabhu, V. et al. (2021). COVID-19 vaccination-associated myelitis. *QJM.* 114 (8): 591–593. https://doi.org/10.1093/qjmed/hcab069.

68 Ledford, H. (2020). US authorization of first COVID vaccine marks new phase in safety monitoring. *Nature* 588 (7838): 377–378.

69 Health Canada. 2021. Health Canada updates Pfizer-BioNTech COVID-19 vaccine label to reflect very rare reports of Bell's palsy – recalls and safety alerts. https://healthycanadians.gc.ca/recall-alert-rappel-avis/hc-sc/2021/76203a-eng.php.

70 Centers for Disease Control and Prevention. 2021. COVID-19 vaccination considerations for persons with underlying medical conditions. Centers for Disease Control and Prevention 2021. https://www. cdc.gov/coronavirus/2019-ncov/vaccines/ recommendations/underlying-conditions.html. Accessed 11 Mar 2021.

71 Keir, G., Maria, N.I., and Kirsch, C.F.E. (2021). Unique imaging findings of neurologic Phantosmia following Pfizer-BioNtech COVID-19 vaccination: a case report. *Top Magn Reson Imaging* 30 (3): 133–137. https://doi.org/10.1097/RMR.0000000000000287.

72 Greinacher, A., Thiele, T., Warkentin, T.E. et al. (2021). Thrombotic thrombocytopenia after ChAdOx1 nCov-19 vaccination. *N Engl J Med.* 384 (22): 2092–2101.

73 Scully, M., Singh, D., Lown, R. et al. (2021). Pathologic antibodies to platelet factor 4 after ChAdOx1 nCoV-19 vaccination. *N Engl J Med.* 384 (23): 2202–2211.

74 Costentin, G., Ozkul-Wermester, O., Triquenot, A. et al. (2021). Acute ischemic stroke revealing ChAdOx1 nCov-19 vaccine-induced immune thrombotic thrombocytopenia: impact on recanalization strategy. *J Stroke Cerebrovasc Dis.* 30 (9): 105942.

75 Sah, R., Shrestha, S., Mehta, R. et al. (2021). AZD1222 (Covishield) vaccination for COVID-19: experiences, challenges, and solutions in Nepal. *Travel Med Infect Dis.* 40: 101989.

76 Folegatti, P.M., Ewer, K.J., Aley, P.K. et al. (2020). Safety and immunogenicity of the ChAdOx1 nCoV-19 vaccine against SARS-CoV-2: a preliminary report of a phase 1/2, single-blind, randomised controlled trial. *Lancet* 396 (10249): 467–478.

77 Abu-Hammad, O., Alduraidi, H., Abu-Hammad, S. et al. (2021). Side effects reported by Jordanian healthcare workers who received COVID-19 vaccines. *Vaccine.* 9 (6): 577.

78 Wolf, M.E., Luz, B., Niehaus, L. et al. (2021). Thrombocytopenia and intracranial venous sinus thrombosis after "COVID-19 vaccine AstraZeneca" exposure. *J Clin Med.* 10 (8): 1599.

79 Oldenburg, J., Klamroth, R., Langer, F. et al. (2021). Diagnosis and management of vaccine-related thrombosis following AstraZeneca COVID-19 vaccination: guidance statement from the GTH. *Hamostaseologie.* 41 (3): 184–189.

80 Öcal, O., Stecher, S.-S., and Wildgruber, M. (2021). Portal vein thrombosis associated with ChAdOx1 nCov-19 vaccination. *Lancet Gastroenterol Hepatol.* 6 (8): 676.

81 Umbrello, M., Brena, N., Vercelli, R. et al. (2021). Successful treatment of acute spleno-Porto-mesenteric vein thrombosis after ChAdOx1 nCoV-19 vaccine. A case report. *J Crit Care* 65: 72–75.

82 Garnier, M., Curado, A., Billoir, P. et al. (2021). Imaging of Oxford/AstraZeneca® COVID-19 vaccine-induced immune thrombotic thrombocytopenia. *Diagn Interv Imaging* 102 (10): 649–650. https://doi.org/10.1016/j.diii.2021.04.005.

83 Su, J.R., McNeil, M.M., Welsh, K.J. et al. (2021). Myopericarditis after vaccination, vaccine adverse event reporting system (VAERS), 1990-2018. *Vaccine* 39 (5): 839–835. https://doi.org/10.1016/j.vaccine.2020.12.046.

84 Starekova, J., Bluemke, D.A., Bradham, W.S. et al. (2021). Myocarditis associated with mRNA COVID-19 vaccination. *Radiology.* 301: 211430.

85 Sagar, S., Liu, P.P., and Cooper, L.T. Jr. (2012). Myocarditis. *Lancet* 379 (9817): 738–747.

86 Deb, A., Abdelmalek, J., Iwuji, K., and Nugent, K. (2021). Acute myocardial injury following COVID-19 vaccination: a case report and review of current evidence from vaccine adverse events reporting system database. *J Prim Care Community Health* 12: 21501327211029230.

87 Vogel, G. and Couzin-Frankel, J. (2021). Israel reports link between rare cases of heart inflammation and COVID-19 vaccination in young men. *Science* https://doi.org/10.1126/science.abj7796.

88 Rosner, C.M., Genovese, L., Tehrani, B.N. et al. (2021). Myocarditis temporally associated with COVID-19 vaccination. *Circulation* 144 (6): 502–505.

89 Habib, M.B., Hamamyh, T., Elyas, A. et al. (2021). Acute myocarditis following administration of BNT162b2 vaccine. *IDCases* 25: e01197.

90 Singh, B., Kaur, P., Cedeno, L. et al. (2021). COVID-19 mRNA vaccine and myocarditis. *Eur J Case Rep Intern Med.* 8 (7): 002681.

24

COVID-19: Long-Term Pulmonary Consequences

Liesl S. Eibschutz[1], Tianyuan Fu[2], Boniface Yarabe[1], Narges Jokar[3], Sanaz Katal[4], Charlotte Sackett[5], Michael Repajic[1], and Ching-Fei Chang[6]

[1] Department of Radiology, Keck School of Medicine, University of Southern California, Los Angeles, CA, USA
[2] Department of Radiology, University Hospitals Cleveland Medical Center, Cleveland, OH, USA
[3] Department of Molecular Imaging and Radionuclide Therapy, The Persian Gulf Nuclear Medicine Research Center, Bushehr Medical University Hospital, Bushehr, Iran
[4] St Vincent's Hospital Medical Imaging Department, Melbourne, Victoria, Australia
[5] USC Master of Public Health Program, University of Southern California, Los Angeles, CA, USA
[6] Division of Pulmonary and Critical Care, Department of Medicine, Keck School of Medicine, University of Southern California, Los Angeles, CA, USA

Abbreviations

ARDS	acute respiratory distress syndrome
BTS	British Thoracic Society
CO-RADS	COVID-19 Reporting and Data System
CPET	cardiopulmonary exercise testing
CT	computed tomography
CT-LSIM	lung subtraction iodine mapping computed tomography
CXR	chest x-ray
DECT	dual-energy computed tomography
DLCO	diffusing capacity for carbon monoxide
ECHO	echocardiogram
FVC	forced vital capacity
GGO	ground-glass opacity
HRCT	high-resolution computed tomography
ICU	intensive care unit
ILD	interstitial lung disease
LDCT	low-dose computed tomography
MERS	Middle East respiratory syndrome
MERS-CoV	Middle East respiratory syndrome coronavirus
MRI	magnetic resonance imaging
OP	organizing pneumonia
PCR	polymerase chain reaction
PE	pulmonary embolism
PET	positron emission tomography
PFT	pulmonary function test
SARS	severe acute respiratory syndrome
SOB	shortness of breath
SPECT	single-photon emission computed tomography
V/Q	ventilation-perfusion

Previous coronavirus diseases, such as severe acute respiratory syndrome (SARS) and Middle East respiratory syndrome (MERS), have demonstrated that even after recovery, patients can suffer from irreversible pulmonary dysfunction and demonstrate residual imaging or functional abnormalities. Similar radiographic findings and clinical syndromes of prolonged fatigue and disability have also been described in recovered coronavirus disease 2019 (COVID-19) patients. Thus, valuable insights and parallels can be drawn between these three viruses to extrapolate preexisting knowledge toward managing the current crisis.

Although the first phase of the pandemic was spent on intense efforts toward containment, resource allocation, and acute treatment of this novel virus, the second phase will now need to include a focus on the management of long-term pulmonary complications, such as persistent shortness of breath (SOB) and exercise limitation of unclear etiology. In that regard, it is imperative to establish the expected baseline and long-term imaging findings when tracking this disease. A summary of the most common early, mid, and late-stage radiographic findings in COVID-19 will be presented in this chapter, as well as helpful advice regarding which imaging modalities should be ordered at the time of diagnosis, before discharge, and during serial follow-up visits as an outpatient.

More importantly, physicians who inherit the care of these post-COVID patients need to understand that refractory dyspnea may not be related to the lung at all. Up to 70% of all chronically debilitated post-COVID patients have grossly normal chest computed tomography (CT) scans and pulmonary function tests (PFTs), suggesting that pulmonary fibrosis is not the primary culprit. Indeed, with the use of cardiopulmonary exercise testing (CPET), researchers now realize that the chronic dyspnea seen in the so-called long hauler's syndrome may be neuromuscular weakness in origin, likely from deconditioning and myopathies induced by prolonged mechanical ventilation and use of steroids and paralytic agents. Other potential non-lung etiologies include pulmonary microangiopathy, occult thromboembolic disease, cardiac dysfunction, and a new entity called *hyperventilation syndrome* from viral-induced dysautonomic regulation of breathing. Throughout this chapter, we will discuss the pathophysiology behind the top five etiologies responsible for post-COVID SOB, explain which tests should be ordered to differentiate between them, and provide appropriate disease-specific management recommendations once an accurate diagnosis has been made.

Only by keeping an open mind and learning to integrate the radiographic, physiologic, and clinical findings will clinicians be able to meet the future challenge of caring for an incredibly large number of chronically symptomatic COVID-19 survivors.

Long-Term Pulmonary Complications from Past Viral Pandemics

Historically, long-term pulmonary disability is not uncommon in patients who have recovered from severe viral pneumonia. These survivors are not only at risk for physical and psychological damage but also lingering complications resulting from aggressive treatment, such as adverse medication effects and prolonged mechanical ventilation. Given that there are many similarities between past coronavirus crises and the current one (e.g. presenting symptoms, radiographic findings, and clinical sequelae), a review of SARS and MERS may provide insight and guidance into the management of COVID-19.

Severe Acute Respiratory Syndrome

From 2002 to 2003, thousands of individuals in China were diagnosed with SARS, a viral infection caused by SARS-CoV-1 [1]. Similar to COVID-19, it is postulated that this zoonotic virus originated from the live-animal markets in China. Over the course of the outbreak, SARS mortality rate was roughly 15% and reached 45% in patients older than 60 years [2].

Clinically, SARS presents very similarly to COVID-19 with influenza-like symptoms, such as upper respiratory complaints, cough, fever, chills, and myalgias. The illness progresses to a respiratory phase that may require intubation. Diarrhea has been reported in roughly 25% of patients. Although this viral illness is fatal primarily in the older population, deaths in young people without comorbidities have also been reported [2].

A comprehensive study conducted by Zhang et al. [3] followed 71 healthcare workers who survived nosocomial SARS infections in 2003 for 15 years. In 27 of these patients (38%), ground-glass opacities (GGOs) or cordlike consolidations were observed on CT during their 15-year follow-up period. The incidence of pulmonary lesions gradually decreased each year, and most of the evolution and healing of the pulmonary disease occurred within the first year postinfection and then remained stable [3].

In a study conducted by Dundamadappa et al. [4], high-resolution CT (HRCT) scans of 65 patients who had imaging postdischarge were analyzed at six weeks, three months, six months, and one year. They found that SARS can cause scarring and fibrosis, both parenchymal and interstitial. Of the 65 patients, 28 had a normal first scan and were not followed up any further. Among the rest, abnormalities noted were parenchymal scarring (25/37), GGOs (22/37), consolidation

(3/37), traction bronchiectasis (9/37), interstitial thickening (15/37), pleural abnormalities (effusion and thickening) (4/37), air trapping (12/37), mediastinal adenopathy (1/37), and a lung cyst (1/37). Although seven of these patients showed no changes in their abnormalities, the rest of them had various degrees of improvement over time.

In another study conducted by Wu et al. [5], the authors performed HRCT of 11 patients with SARS at 3, 6, and 84 months postdischarge. They found that the number of damaged lung segments decreased over time, with 10 segments per patient at three months, 9.6 segments per patient at six months, and ultimately 6.7 segments per patient at 84 months. At three months, the most common CT feature of residual lung abnormality was the presence of GGOs, with or without consolidation. At six months, GGOs were still the predominant imaging finding, but approximately 25% of patients demonstrated reticulation and interlobular thickening. At 84 months, only 1 of the 11 patients had no lung abnormalities, and the rest had primarily reticulation and interlobular thickening. Three of these patients still had GGOs or traction bronchiectasis. Overall, the authors noted a decrease of GGOs with an increase in reticulation over time [5].

Zhang et al. [3] also monitored pulmonary function in patients with SARS over a 15-year time span. They reported that the forced expiratory flow 25–75% value and the ratio of forced expiratory volume in one second to forced vital capacity (FVC) were significantly reduced in patients with residual chest CT abnormalities compared with those with complete radiologic recovery. Even in those whose initial postrecovery CT scans looked normal, there was still evidence of incremental improvement in pulmonary function from 2006 to 2018. These findings indicate that, even in patients with early complete resolution of chest CT abnormalities, pulmonary function can take several years to return to normal [3].

Middle East Respiratory Syndrome

Middle East respiratory syndrome coronavirus (MERS-CoV) is another zoonotic, enveloped, single-stranded RNA virus from the Coronaviridae family that is known for causing viral pneumonias [6].

MERS-CoV is the sixth coronavirus to cause infection in humans, bearing more similarities to strains isolated from bats, as compared with SARS [7]. From 2012, at its discovery, to 2015, MERS-CoV spread to more than 200 countries with a mortality rate that approached 35% [8].

Clinically, MERS presents as an influenza-like illness with symptoms including fever and a dry cough. Between one fourth and one third of patients experienced gastrointestinal symptoms [7]. In addition, patients often developed acute kidney injury during their hospital visit. Unlike SARS and COVID-19, which usually progress into severe disease after one week of presenting symptoms, MERS increased in severity after hours to days of symptom onset [9].

Long-term clinical findings in these patients include lung function abnormalities in a restrictive pattern and reduced exercise capacity [10]. A MERS outbreak at a Korean hospital in 2015 indicated that FVC and diffusing capacity for carbon monoxide (DLCO) were reduced in severe MERS pneumonia infection compared with patients with MERS with no or mild pneumonia at one year of follow-up [11]. The average FVC in this study was 93% of the expected volume, and the DLCO was 77% of expected diffusion capacity [11]. In this study, severity or presence of pneumonia did not have any statistically significant effect on exercise capacity, as measured by six-minute walking test, where the mean six-minute walking distance was 540 m.

Just as in SARS-CoV, there are several known radiologic long-term sequelae. However, because of the higher mortality rate of MERS, fewer survivors are available to conduct long-term outcomes research. In the few studies that do exist, some of the common radiologic findings documented include GGOs, pleural thickening, and lung fibrosis. The latter finding was shown to be significantly more common in patients with a greater number of intensive care unit (ICU) admission days, older age, higher chest radiographic scores, chest radiographic deterioration patterns, and peak lactate dehydrogenase levels [12]. Although pleural effusion is not often seen in viral pneumonia, it can be seen in MERS and in late acute COVID-19 infection. The presence of pleural effusion in MERS had adverse prognostic correlations [13].

Monitoring for Long-Term Pulmonary Consequences of COVID-19 Infection

Imaging Modalities for the Diagnosis and Follow-Up of COVID-19

Long-term chest imaging findings after COVID-19 infection are often variable and do not necessarily correlate with clinical symptomatology. Visible lung injury may develop even after clinical symptoms have subsided and can persist for months to years. In some cases, radiographic findings of lung injury may be persistent. Thus, a chest CT obtained during the acute phase of infection will provide a "new baseline" comparison for future follow-up, as well as for research in the radiographic evolution of COVID-19. Ideally, this should be obtained prior to discharge if not already done on admission [14].

For acute infection, the most common radiographic scans used are chest x-ray (CXR) and HRCT, mostly because of cost and widespread availability in emergency departments. Although often mentioned in the literature, magnetic resonance imaging (MRI) and positron emission tomography-CT (PET-CT) are useful only in select situations of initial diagnosis of COVID-19. A "radiographic signature" of COVID-19 on CXR or chest CT is usually the presence of bilateral GGOs distributed in a peripheral and lower lobe fashion. This radiographic pattern is said to evolve through four stages – early, progressive, peak, and absorption – before resolving or becoming fibrotic (Figure 24.1) [15–17]. Certain patients may have a mixed pattern of pulmonary parenchymal opacities consisting of ground-glass and consolidation, and less commonly, consolidative opacities only [18, 19]. Subsequent chest radiographs in patients with active COVID-19 infection may demonstrate progression of GGOs to predominantly consolidative opacities, as well as a greater distribution or diffuse involvement of both lungs. Additional findings may include pulmonary nodules and reticulonodular opacities [19]. Some nonspecific findings that may be observed include perihilar vascular congestion, cardiomegaly, pleural effusion, and

Time course of CT changes in COVID-19

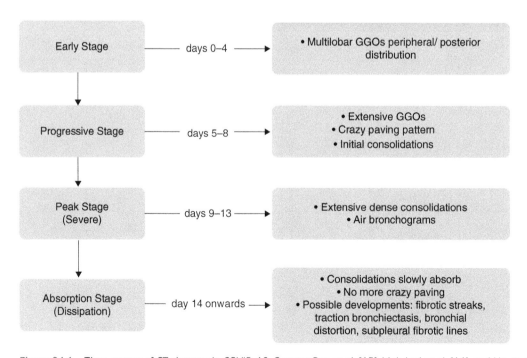

Figure 24.1   Time course of CT changes in COVID-19. *Sources:* Pan et al. [15], Mahdavi et al. [16], and Hu et al. [17].

pneumothorax [19]. These findings may peak in severity around 10–12 days from symptom onset [20]. It is important to note, however, that some patients with only mild COVID-19 infection may present with a normal initial CXR or chest CT scan.

For long-term follow-up, stable patients may undergo serial CXR or low-dose CT (LDCT) imaging to document resolution of findings with minimal radiation exposure. However, in patients with significant lingering respiratory symptoms and minimal findings on chest CT, other types of imaging modalities may be helpful. This includes selective use of PET-CT and various types of lung perfusion scan (ventilation-perfusion [V/Q], dual-energy CT [DECT], lung subtraction iodine mapping CT (CT-LSIM)), which may help elucidate other causes of ongoing dyspnea that are not readily explained by a relatively normal chest CT.

Chest Radiograph

CXRs are often the first-line imaging modality for patients with suspected acute COVID-19 because they are easy to obtain and low cost in most healthcare settings. They also give significantly less radiation to the patient compared with a chest CT scan. CXRs may also be used for long-term follow-up of noncomplicated patients who are recovering well from COVID-19 infection. However, compared with chest CT, CXRs have limited sensitivity in detecting subtle parenchymal changes because of lower tissue resolution and overlapping soft tissues obscuring underlying pulmonary abnormalities [18]. As a result, more complex COVID-19 patients with clinical or functional lung impairment should obtain an HRCT for further characterization of underlying pulmonary parenchymal abnormalities (ground-glass, fibrosis, bronchiectasis, etc.), which can be tracked over time.

Chest CT

Since the onset of the COVID-19 pandemic, chest CT has frequently been used to both diagnose the infection (more sensitive than nasal swab reverse transcription-polymerase chain reaction [PCR]) and quantitate the extent of initial lung damage. This has been accomplished using the COVID-19 Reporting and Data System (CO-RADS). CO-RADS combines chest CT findings, clinical presentation, and laboratory test results to determine the likelihood of

COVID-19 infection [21]. The scoring scale ranges from 0 to 5, with 0 representing absence of infection and 5 representing a high degree of suspicion for acute COVID-19. Patients receive a 6 if reverse transcription-PCR is positive for COVID-19 infection. Thus, this scoring system has a high level of diagnostic utility in addition to risk stratification.

In most healthcare settings, HRCT is the preferred modality given its availability and relatively low cost, but with higher detailed anatomic resolution of the lung parenchyma than regular CT scans. Although it would be logical to continue tracking the long-term follow-up of complex COVID-19 patients with HRCT, certain authors advocate for the use of LDCT instead given the reduced radiation exposure and adequate visibility of features such as consolidation, nodular infiltrates, and crazy paving [22].

Notably, the severity of CT findings does not always correlate with the severity of clinical presentation, and the findings of lung abnormalities will often lag behind clinical improvement. Thus, although scoring systems such as the CT severity scoring system are useful to identify the level of GGOs, crazy paving, and consolidation in the lung, oftentimes there is a distinct discordance between radiographic imaging and symptomatology [21]. For example, postacute patients may present with normalized chest CT scans and yet still have significant SOB on exertion. Further research is needed in not only the tracking of COVID-19 radiographic changes over time, but also whether it has prognostic significance, and whether it can detect the level of contagiousness in patients.

Pulmonary MRI

The utility of MRI in COVID-19 infection is limited, both in the acute setting and for long-term follow-up. In general, MRI is not considered routine in the evaluation of suspected lower respiratory tract infections. First, MRI is costly to obtain and not readily available in all healthcare settings. In addition, characterization of pulmonary lesions with MRI is limited because of cardiac and respiratory motion artifact. Because the acquisition time for obtaining an MRI is also significantly longer than that of CXR or chest CT, its use is limited in acute COVID-19 infections because of increased risk for exposure to imaging staff.

In select instances of patients with high suspicion of or confirmed COVID-19 infection that cannot undergo regular CT scanning (e.g. pregnant patients, children), pulmonary MRI may be of benefit for the assessment of the extent of lung damage. A more common scenario is when the patient undergoes an MRI of a different part of the body and incidentally captures evidence in the lungs that is suspicious for COVID-19 infection and thus prompts confirmatory testing.

When pulmonary abnormalities are present, MRI has been shown to correlate well with CT findings of GGOs, consolidation, and mixed ground-glass/consolidative lesions [23, 24]. On pulmonary MRI, GGOs and consolidation are hyperintense relative to the surrounding tissues secondary to exudative fluid accumulation and increased proton density. If the patient happens to receive an MRI for other reasons during long-term follow-up, findings of residual GGOs may be seen suggestive of persistent pulmonary parenchymal damage. However, unless there are continued contraindications to radiation exposure, the use of MRI for routine follow-up of COVID-19 lung damage is not supported given the disadvantages previously listed.

PET-CT

^{18}F-FDG-PET is a nuclear imaging modality that uses ^{18}F-fluorodeoxyglucose, a glucose analog and positron-emitting radiotracer, to identify and localize functional malignancies. The level of FDG uptake is proportional to the cellular metabolic rate and the density of glucose transporters; thus, FDG often accumulates at sites of infection and inflammation [25]. When the functional aspects of PET are combined with the structural underlays of CT fusion, PET-CT allows for correlation of functional processes to anatomic components [25].

Because PET-CT is so nonspecific, lighting up indiscriminately in any area of increased metabolism, it has a limited role in the diagnosis and management of most infections. Indeed, it is more expensive and delivers more radiation to the patient without much additional benefit compared with regular chest CT, and in the setting of COVID-19, the prolonged acquisition time may pose an additional risk of exposure to the technologists and staff. However, there are select situations in which PET-CT might be of benefit in the diagnosis and management of COVID-19, both in the acute phase of infection and in long-term follow-up when symptoms are still persistent.

For subclinical acute infections, PET-CT may be able to pick up radiographic evidence of COVID-19 when regular chest CT scans are grossly normal. Studies show that cases of active COVID-19 infection demonstrate pulmonary parenchymal uptake in regions corresponding to GGOs or consolidative opacities, as well as the regional lymph nodes [26]. Thus, when patients present with nonspecific mild symptoms and a clear CXR or CT scan, PET-CT findings of occult nodal uptake in the axillary and mediastinal stations, as well as mild early lung parenchymal damage in the peripheral and basilar regions of the lung, will raise suspicion for COVID-19 and prompt laboratory testing to preemptively diagnose COVID-19 infection and curb asymptomatic spread [25]. Other authors have noted persistent FDG-positive pulmonary parenchymal GGOs/consolidative opacities and FDG-avid lymph nodes even in patients who have recovered from COVID-19 and been discharged from the hospital [27]. Asymptomatic oncologic patients who undergo routine PET-CT scanning for malignancy monitoring may be found to have unexpected subtle GGOs or consolidations, along with increased regional nodal uptake. This pattern is not typical of metastatic disease and may trigger a workup for COVID-19, thus potentially saving their lives [25].

Due to cost, radiation burden, and lengthy scan times, PET-CT scans should not be used for routine outpatient follow-ups of patients with COVID-19. Indeed, studies have shown that pathologic evidence of residual abnormalities in the lungs may persist long after discharge from the hospital without clinical significance. Autopsy studies of patients with COVID-19 who were discharged and then later died have shown viral inclusion bodies still present in their lungs. Other studies confirm persistent FDG-positive pulmonary parenchymal GGOs/consolidative opacities and FDG-avid lymph nodes in patients who have fully recovered clinically from the acute infection [27]. However, if the patient is experiencing unexplained lingering symptoms, a PET-CT may be warranted in follow-up because it can potentially identify and quantify areas of residual inflammation that may not be visible on traditional anatomic imaging techniques and allow targeted workup [28].

Importantly, PET-CT can also detect areas of decreased metabolic activity that suggest post-COVID damage, especially in extrapulmonary sites. For example, some authors report evidence of decreased metabolic activity in the orbitofrontal cortex associated with COVID-19-induced anosmia [25, 29]. Patients with COVID-19-induced facial nerve palsy may demonstrate reduced metabolic activity of the facial nerve. Also, during acute COVID-19 infection through six months after recovery and potentially beyond, there may be evidence of reduced radiotracer uptake in multiple areas of the brain, including the prefrontal cortex, which may explain the "brain fog" found in many long hauler patients [25].

Notably, the effects of COVID-19 vaccination should be recognized in the context of PET-CT scans in oncologic patients. Specifically, a review published by Eibschutz et al. [25] discusses how PET-CT scans may demonstrate reactive hypermetabolic lymphadenopathy several weeks after vaccination, which may trigger unnecessary biopsies and restaging unless the physician is aware of this phenomenon.

Timeline of Chest CT Findings During Different Phases of COVID-19 Infection

Acute Infection (0–2 Weeks)

Acute COVID-19 infection commonly presents on chest CT as scattered bilateral GGOs or mixed GGOs and consolidative opacities, often with a peripheral and lower lung–predominant distribution [28]. During the acute infection, these will progress as diffuse worsening GGOs and increasing consolidations, possibly with subsequent development of crazy-paving pattern, interlobular septal thickening, fibrotic bands, and findings of organizing pneumonia (OP) [28]. Less common findings include pulmonary nodules, bronchial wall thickening, strandlike opacities, pleural effusions, and enlarged mediastinal lymph nodes [28].

Several authors have organized the evolution of chest CT findings in cases of mild COVID-19 infection into four stages: stage 1 (early: 0–4 days), predominantly multilobar GGOs; stage 2 (progressive: 5–8 days), extensive GGO in a crazy-paving pattern, with the early development of consolidation; stage 3 (peak: 9–13 days), with spread and worsening of the consolidation; and stage 4 (absorption: 14 days

onward), disappearance of crazy-paving pattern and gradual resolution of consolidations [15–17]. Findings suggestive of improvement include shrinking pulmonary opacities and the melted sugar sign. Pleural effusions are not common; if present, they may start to manifest after two weeks, coincident with lack of improvement. Notably, in the patients with more severe COVID-19, such progression from stage 1 to 4 may not be seen because of the rapid deterioration of the patient's clinical course.

In both SARS-CoV-1 and MERS literature, the trajectory of radiographic recovery over time can manifest in four different ways [17]:

- Type I: Scans will deteriorate and then improve and recover to baseline.
- Type II: Scans will have a static, unchanging course.
- Type III: Scans will have a fluctuating course of worsening and improvement.
- Type IV: Scans will have a progressive deterioration without improvement.

Given that it shares many similarities with the other two coronaviruses, it would not be unreasonable to assume that these four patterns may also apply in the case of COVID-19 [30]. These findings are visually represented in Figure 24.2.

Within the first one to three weeks postinfection, certain authors have reported a shift in lesions from predominantly GGOs to a mixed pattern of basilar consolidation and reticular pattern [31]. In a series of 81 patients with COVID-19, serial CT monitoring also showed the persistence of GGOs, bronchiolectasis, reticular patterns, pleural thickening, and effusions. At three weeks, the primary radiologic abnormalities were GGOs, fibrous stripe, and thickening of the adjacent pleura [32].

Short-Term Follow-up (1–3 Months)

At the four-week mark, most patients will continue to demonstrate CT evidence of lung abnormality, even after they have clinically recovered and been discharged from the hospital [33]. Findings are variable and may present as subtle GGOs, residual parenchymal consolidation, interstitial pulmonary fibrosis, and subpleural fibrotic bands. These tend to be peripheral and may gradually present more centrally over time. Additional findings may include persistent crazy

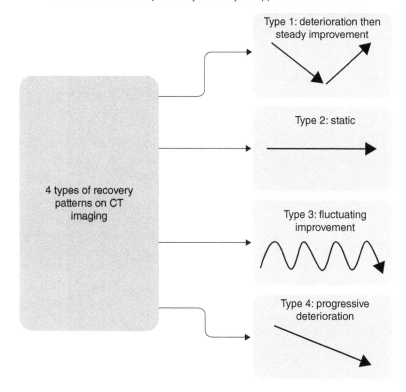

Four Types of Recovery Trajectories

Seen in SARS/MERS previously and may be applicable to COVID-19

4 types of recovery patterns on CT imaging

Type 1: deterioration then steady improvement

Type 2: static

Type 3: fluctuating improvement

Type 4: progressive deterioration

Figure 24.2   Trajectory of radiographic recovery over time in SARS and MERS that may be applicable to COVID-19.

paving, traction bronchiectasis, honeycombing, mosaic attenuation, scattered linear/curvilinear opacities, and pneumatoceles [33].

Several case reports exist of patients with COVID-19 with an OP pattern on chest CT while still hospitalized for their acute infection. Pogatchnik et al. [34] reported a case of a woman with OP on CT scan after three weeks of cough, fevers, and dyspnea. Because her PCR was negative for COVID-19, she underwent bronchoscopic lung biopsy that histologically proved OP; the bronchoalveolar lavage PCR was positive for COVID-19. Although this patient had only mild to moderate disease and recovered without requiring any high-dose steroids (just remdesivir), her case illustrates the potential presence of OP during her acute illness [34]. Similarly, a Brazilian case series of three ventilated patients with OP on their CT scans illustrates the utility of using high-dose steroids to expedite a dramatic recovery [35].

Notably, although rare, some patients present an OP pattern well beyond four weeks postdischarge. Out of a population of 837 patients, Myall et al. [36] reported that 4.8% of patients with continued symptoms after discharge had an interstitial lung disease (ILD) pattern, mostly OP. After presentation to a multidisciplinary ILD board, the decision was made to treat these patients with high-dose prednisolone with excellent response. Thus, despite receiving steroids as part of their initial inpatient care, select patients will still benefit from more steroids as an outpatient if their follow-up CT scans show OP [36].

At six weeks, follow-up chest CT findings for patients with COVID-19 demonstrated extensive diffuse bilateral pulmonary GGOs, air-space disease with architectural distortion bronchiectasis, residual parenchymal consolidations suggesting fibrotic damage, peribronchial thickening, traction bronchiectasis, and bronchiolectasis [37]. A post-COVID-19 autopsy case with no prior history of pulmonary disease demonstrated various regions with severe and organizing alveolar damage and fibrosis with honeycomb-like remodeling and bronchial metaplasia 39 days after infection [38].

In another study, three-month follow-up HRCT demonstrated that 17% of patients had HRCT abnormalities affecting more than 5% of their lung parenchyma, while signs of fibrosis were found in 21%. CT imaging at this time point notes that common features such as pure GGOs, interstitial thickening, and crazy paving were nearly resolved, but manifestations of fibrosis, such as interstitial thickening, were still present [39]. Ultimately, patients with severe radiologic findings on acute infection may be more likely to demonstrate fibrotic changes and architectural distortion on follow-up scans. Although an exact correlation has yet to be identified, a multiple linear regression model also indicated a correlation between ICU hospitalization and the extent of persisting lesions on HRCT, with intubation associated with signs of fibrosis at follow-up [40].

Mid-Term Follow-up (3–6 Months)

Studies have shown that three to six months postinfection, around 70% of recovered patients will still demonstrate radiologic abnormalities, such as GGOs, interstitial thickening, and crazy-paving pattern [39]. In addition, there may be reticular opacities, architectural distortion, and bronchiectasis with lung volume loss suggestive of fibrotic changes [41].

At four months postdischarge of patients hospitalized for COVID-19, fibrotic-like patterns were reported as the most frequent CT finding for those who underwent mechanical ventilation [42]. Similarly, a case study by the COMEBAC (Consultation Multi-Expertise de Bicêtre Après COVID-19) group reported that findings on chest CT of intubated and nonintubated individuals four months after hospitalization showcased predominantly subtle GGOs and fibrotic lesions [43]. Guler et al. [44] also investigated pulmonary sequelae of COVID-19 survivors at four-month follow-up. In agreement with previous studies, unilobular or multilobular hypoattenuated areas without or with bulging of the lobular margins, GGOs with a mosaic attenuation pattern, reticulations, linear/curvilinear densities, honeycombing, traction bronchiectasis with architectural distortion, as well as pneumatoceles

were the typical radiologic follow-up sequelae of COVID-19. However, in this study, considerable pulmonary fibrosis was rarely observed [44].

A prospective study by Han et al. [45] explored the probability risk factors for fibrotic-like changes in the lung during a six-month follow-up of 114 survivors recovering from acute COVID-19 pneumonia. They observed some evidence of fibrotic-like changes in almost one third of the participants, whereas the remaining patients showed either complete radiologic resolution or residual GGOs or interstitial thickening (Figure 24.3). In multivariate analysis, important prognostic factors included heart rate greater than 100 beats/min at admission, noninvasive mechanical ventilation, age older than 50 years, duration of hospitalization ≥17 days, acute respiratory distress syndrome (ARDS), and total CT score of ≥18 at initial CT as independent predictors for fibrotic-like changes in the lung [45]. They also found that bronchiectasis was evident in 24% of the patients at follow-up, compared with only 7% in the acute stage of the infection. These findings suggest that bronchiectasis can occur in up to a quarter of patients who suffered from severe COVID-19 pneumonia (at least from a radiologic point of view) [46], although the long-term prevalence of bronchiectasis in patients postdischarge is yet to be determined. Although the exact etiology of bronchiectasis is still unknown, certain authors suggest that it may stem from traction (secondary to pulmonary fibrosis) rather than prolonged inflammation [47].

In addition, a cohort study by Huang et al. [48] evaluated the long-term pulmonary consequences of COVID-19 in 353 survivors six months after hospital discharge. They noted that patients who were more acutely ill during hospitalization had more strictly impaired pulmonary diffusion capacities and abnormal chest imaging appearances. In addition, these patients demonstrated a significant proportion of pulmonary interstitial change (GGOs and irregular lines) [48].

Long-Term Follow-up (One Year and Beyond)

Wu et al. [49] assessed 83 patients hospitalized for severe COVID-19 at 3-month intervals, up to 12 months after hospital discharge. The authors stated that although most patients improved over time, radiologic abnormalities remained in 24% of patients even 12 months after discharge [49].

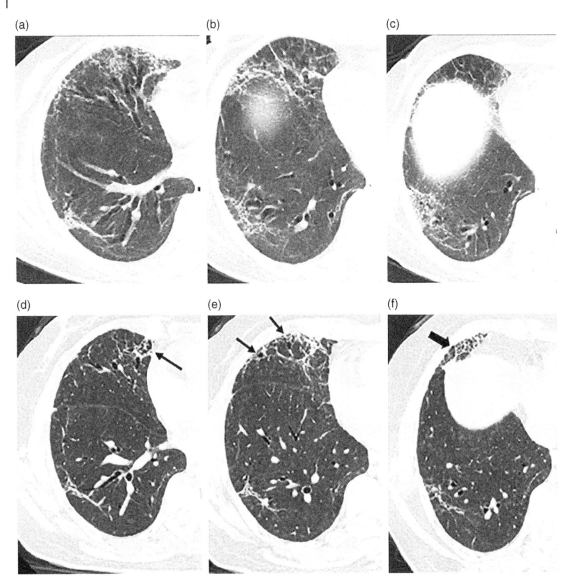

Figure 24.3 Serial CT scans in a 46-year-old woman with severe COVID-2019 pneumonia. (a–c) Scans obtained on day 32 after symptom onset show multiple GGOs and interstitial thickening with mild cylindrical traction bronchiectasis involving the middle lobe and lower lobe of the right lung. (d–f) Scans obtained on day 198 show partial absorption of the abnormalities, reduced extension, traction bronchiectasis (*arrows* in d and e), and localized "honeycombing" (*arrow* in f) in the subpleural region of the right middle lobe. *Source:* Han et al. [45].

These radiographic abnormalities correlated with peak HRCT pneumonia scores at the time of hospitalization. At three months, the most common CT features found in 78% of patients were residual GGOs, reticular opacities, interlobular septal thickening, and subpleural curvilinear opacities at three-month follow-up. At six months, 48% of patients still had abnormal chest radiographs with GGOs, inter-lobular septal thickening, reticular opacities, subpleural curvilinear opacities, mosaic attenuation, and bronchiectasis. At nine months, features such as interlobular septal thickening, reticular opacities, and subpleural curvilinear opacities had resolved, while GGOs were still present in 27% of patients. Notably, there was no significant improvement between 9 and 12 months [49].

Ultimately, long-term follow-up with either LDCT or HRCT can help physicians understand the natural evolution of radiographic changes after COVID-19 infection and thus identify patients who may need additional treatment (such as steroids for persistent OP). In addition, establishing a "new radiographic baseline" is important for future comparisons when patients present with recurrent pulmonary symptoms, and clinicians need to know what changes are new or old.

Pathologic Findings After Discharge

In patients who have recovered from COVID-19 and have been discharged from the hospital, pathologic evidence of residual abnormalities in the lungs may persist. These include persistent FDG-positive pulmonary parenchymal GGOs/consolidative opacities and FDG-avid lymph nodes [27].

In patients who had recovered from COVID-19 and died of a different cause at or immediately after discharge, autopsy findings have demonstrated viral particles within pulmonary epithelial cells. Other postmortem pathologic findings may include evidence of persistent lung injury, such as diffuse alveolar damage, desquamation of type II alveolar epithelial cells, interstitial inflammatory infiltrate, and hyaline membrane formation [50].

Long-Term Clinical Sequelae of COVID-19

Pathophysiology

The most challenging aspect of managing post-COVID respiratory symptoms is the wide heterogeneity of etiologies. In patients who had severe COVID-19 infection that required prolonged mechanical ventilation for ARDS, complaints of persistent dyspnea and follow-up CT findings of architectural distortion and pulmonary fibrosis are unsurprising. However, the clinical conundrum lies in patients who describe pulmonary symptoms but lack PFT abnormalities.

Based on a recent prospective study by Wu et al. [49] of long-term respiratory symptoms after COVID-19 infection, only 24% of patients developed permanent lung fibrosis, and the remaining 76% had no abnor-

malities on their 1-year follow-up CT scan. Most of these patients also showed normalization of their PFTs (except for a reduction in DLCO), so the residual pulmonary symptoms are difficult to explain. Arnold et al. [51] noted similar findings and reported that only 10% of COVID-19 survivors with residual symptoms at three months had PFT abnormalities. Thus, the persistence of pulmonary symptoms can often not be explained by impairment of lung function alone.

In the three to four weeks following acute COVID-19 infection, the two most persistent symptoms are dyspnea and fatigue. In a meta-analysis that detailed respiratory symptoms postdischarge, either dyspnea or fatigue was present in up to 87% of patients at 60 days postdischarge [52, 53]. Often known as "post-COVID-19 syndrome" or "long hauler's syndrome," lingering dyspnea and fatigue may be accompanied by additional pulmonary symptoms, such as persistent cough (16%), chest pain (14%), sore throat (4%), and rhinorrhea (4.1%) [54].

Although the mechanisms behind these symptoms have not been clearly established, understanding the pathophysiology of COVID-19 infection may be the key to differentiating between the various potential causes of the most common and debilitating symptom: SOB [54]. Besides overt pulmonary fibrosis, several other possibilities of why patients are dyspneic on long-term follow-up include muscular deconditioning and weakness, occult myocardial damage, pulmonary vascular disease (including chronic microemboli and pulmonary hypertension), and autonomic dysfunction leading to an inappropriate hyperventilation syndrome. In the following sections, we will explore the theoretical basis of each and suggest different management strategies based on the specific etiology.

Post-COVID Pulmonary Fibrosis

The British Thoracic Society (BTS) defines "severe" COVID-19 infection by the following risk factors: (1) severe pneumonia, (2) requirement of ICU care, or (3) elderly or with multiple comorbidities [55]. Recent studies have noted that severe infection by COVID-19 can trigger lung epithelial cell destruction, thrombosis, hypercoagulation, vascular leak leading to sepsis, and ultimately ARDS and pulmonary fibrosis. Studies estimate that about 20–30% of these patients often progress to ARDS and subsequent pulmonary fibrosis [56]. In addition to direct viral invasion and damage of alveolar and interstitial cells, pulmonary fibrosis can also result from the side effects of prolonged mechanical ventilation with high oxygen requirement, as well as the constant inflammatory milieu of the cytokine storm.

Virus-specific pathophysiologic changes refer to the invasion of nasal and bronchial epithelial cells, as well as pneumocytes, by SARS-CoV-2. This occurs through interactions with the angiotensinogen-converting enzyme 2 receptor, which binds the structural spike (S) protein, as well as the type 2 transmembrane serine protease, which promotes viral uptake by activating the SARS-COV-2 S protein, mediating viral entry into cells [52].

Historically, a high fraction of inspired oxygen (FiO_2) environment has been shown to promote oxidative stress and free radical production, which leads to a higher risk for pulmonary fibrosis. During later stages of infection, the epithelial–endothelial barrier in the lungs is compromised, leading to an increased inflammatory response and influx of monocytes and neutrophils [57]. In addition, it has been hypothesized that COVID-19 can cause an inflammatory response that impairs lymphopoiesis and increases lymphocyte apoptosis. Thus, the long-term pulmonary sequelae of COVID-19 are believed to be due to the microvascular ischemia and injury, immobility, and metabolic alterations that promote the development of fibrosis [52].

Muscular Deconditioning and Weakness

Similar to SARS, recent reports suggest that patients with COVID-19 have reduced levels of physical function and fitness postinfection compared with healthy control subjects, with physical impairment lasting one to two years postinfection [58]. In an Italian study, the authors found that about half of patients with COVID-19 postdischarge had severe impairment in physical functioning and activities of daily living at discharge [59].

Ong et al. [60] showed that many SARS survivors had reduced exercise capacity three months postdischarge. Interestingly, when these authors compared exercise capacity and resting PFT results, many cases of discordance occurred (e.g. normal PFTs with abnormal CPETs). Such discordance supports the complementary role of CPET in the exercise impairment evaluation, especially when symptoms are inconsist-

ent with the degree of impairment on PFT. CPET provides a more global assessment of dyspnea as compared with PFT because it examines the integrated influence of multiple factors (e.g. pulmonary mechanics, cardiac, peripheral muscle, and psychosocial factors) and thus is ideal for post-COVID evaluation of dyspnea. Based on the guidelines established by the American Thoracic Society/American College of Chest Physicians, the most appropriate protocol for this setting is a symptom-limited CPET (stage II type of exercise testing). Most centers use a modern ramping protocol with a cycle ergometer interfaced with MedGraphics software [61–64].

Ultimately, in Ong et al.'s study [60], exercise limitation in recovered SARS patients was primarily caused by extrapulmonary entities rather than lung damage. The authors found that impaired muscle function was the most important contributor to the reduced functional outcomes of these patients. Thus, many clinicians should consider an exercise rehabilitation program to reduce dyspnea and improve exercise capacity in post-COVID patients [60].

In a study of 24 patients with COVID-19 who had been mechanically ventilated in the ICU, Blokland et al. [65] also found that 23 of the 24 patients could perform a maximal exercise test, but that their cardiorespiratory fitness was poor with a median peak oxygen uptake of 15.0 mL/kg/min (57% of the predicted value). Only 7 of these 23 patients were primarily limited by ventilatory function, while the rest were restricted by the decreased peripheral muscle mass from their ICU stay [65]. Several other authors also found similar results on CPET, with physical deconditioning and loss of muscle mass being the primary determinants of dyspnea and exercise limitation post-COVID [66].

Occult Myocardial Damage

Although myocardial infarction, myocarditis, and arrhythmias have all been described in the course of acute COVID-19 infection, they can also occur after discharge as well. Three types of COVID-19-induced cardiac injury have been described [67]:

1) Myocardial infarction (type I: due to plaque rupture and thrombosis, type II: nonobstructive, due to generalized ischemia)

2) Left ventricular dysfunction from ischemia or myocarditis
3) Right-heart failure (from pulmonary embolism [PE] or pulmonary hypertension)

To further elucidate these findings, Puntmann et al. [68] performed cardiac MRI scans on 100 post-COVID patients and found occult heart disease in 78% and ongoing cardiac inflammation in 60% at two months after discharge (Figure 24.4). Rajpal et al. [69] noted similar findings after subjecting 26 college athletes to cardiac MRI after asymptomatic infection with COVID-19. Surprisingly, these authors found 46% of them had evidence of occult myocarditis and cardiac damage, even with just a mild disease course. Therefore, in the workup of unexplained dyspnea post-COVID, echocardiography and cardiac MRI testing should be considered, even if the patient does not present with classic signs and symptoms of heart disease. CPET can also uncover occult cardiovascular complications.

Pulmonary Vascular Disease and Decreased Lung Perfusion

One of the hallmarks of COVID-19 infection is hypercoagulability with thromboembolic complications. Pulmonary emboli, strokes, and myocardial infarctions are just some of the catastrophic consequences of COVID-19 in addition to fulminant respiratory failure from diffuse pneumonitis and ARDS. In fact, patients with severe COVID-19 are at such high risk for PE that therapeutic dosages of anticoagulation are often started at the time of admission. However, once discharged, patients can still be at risk for pulmonary vascular microangiopathy and chronic microemboli.

Autopsy reports have demonstrated not only the presence of diffuse alveolar damage in the lungs of deceased COVID-19 patients, but also small microthrombi in pulmonary capillaries, intravascular fibrin aggregates in the lumen of larger vessels, and intussusceptive angiogenesis, which is a phenomenon also seen in chronic thromboembolic pulmonary hypertension [70].

In addition, a discordantly decreased DLCO in the setting of normal spirometric and lung volume measures often suggests a pulmonary vascular problem. Some authors report that the mechanism behind this pathology relies on the concept of inadequate "pulmonary perfusion" caused by obstruction of small vessels at the periphery of the lungs [71]. This phenomenon of small vessel angiopathy is not quite the same as acute pulmonary emboli, which usually involves the larger, more central pulmonary artery branches, nor does it produce the same degree of appreciable pulmonary hypertension as chronic thromboembolic disease. However, poor pulmonary perfusion could result in a sensation of discomfort and dyspnea.

To diagnose this unusual entity, however, clinicians should consider a V/Q single-photon emission computed tomography-CT (SPECT-CT) scan. Previously, this modality of imaging was restricted mostly for the workup of chronic thromboembolic pulmonary hypertension or PE in patients who cannot tolerate exposure to radiation. Based on limited data thus far, COVID-19 has a distinct V/Q pattern of enhancement that is quite different from a normal PE. Unlike larger clots that obstruct the lumens of large vessels, the "small vessel footprint" of COVID-19 looks like bilateral subpleural nongeometric enhancement at the very periphery of the lungs (Figure 24.5). This pattern can also be seen in entities such as scleroderma, connective tissue disorders, veno-occlusive disease, and sickle cell anemia; but in the context of a post-COVID patient, this pattern is pathognomonic for a lung perfusion problem. Newer imaging modalities, such as DECT and CT-LSIM, may provide one-stop shopping regarding three pieces of critical information: (1) lung perfusion mapping, (2) ruling out luminal clot burden, and (3) detecting parenchymal lung damage. However, they are still experimental in nature and need further validation studies [71].

Autonomic Dysfunction with Resultant Hyperventilation Syndrome

One of the most intriguing concepts of why post-COVID patients may feel dyspneic in the absence of appreciable chest CT changes or PFT defects is the syndrome of inappropriate hyperventilation [72]. This is often diagnosed by CPET findings of exercise ventilatory inefficiency – i.e. an elevated minute ventilation/carbon dioxide production, hypocapnia, and reduction in end-tidal carbon dioxide.

In the pre-COVID era, this pattern was often seen in patients with high anxiety levels, liver disease, and chronic ILD with architectural distortion of the lungs

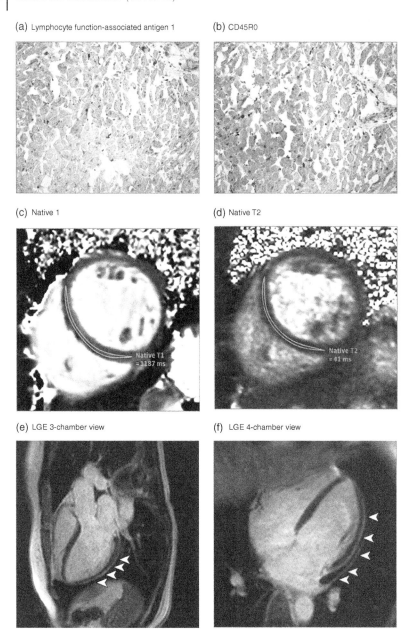

Figure 24.4 (a and b) Histologic findings in an adult man with severe cardiac MRI abnormalities 67 days after COVID-19 diagnosis. High-sensitivity troponin T level on the day of cardiac MRI was 16.7 pg/ml. The patient recovered at home from COVID-19 illness with minimal symptoms, which included loss of smell and taste and only mildly increased temperature lasting two days. There were no known previous conditions or regular medication use. Histology showed intracellular edema as enlarged cardiomyocytes with no evidence of interstitial or replacement fibrosis. Immunohistochemical staining shows acute lymphocytic infiltration (lymphocyte function–associated antigen 1 and activated lymphocyte T antigen CD45R0), as well as activated intercellular adhesion molecule 1. (c–f) Representative cardiac MRIs of an adult woman with COVID-19-related perimyocarditis. (c and d) Significantly raised native T1 and native T2 in myocardial mapping acquisitions. (e and f) Pericardial effusion and enhancement (*yellow arrowheads*) and epicardial and intramyocardial enhancement (*white arrowheads*) in late gadolinium enhancement (LGE) acquisition. *Source:* Puntmann et al. [68].

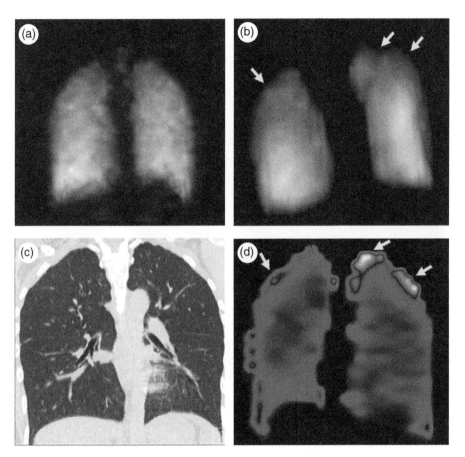

Figure 24.5 V/Q SPECT-CT in a 22-year-old woman 6 weeks after acute COVID-19 illness who did not receive anticoagulation for thromboembolic prophylaxis during acute hospitalization. (b) ^{99m}Tc macroaggregated albumin (MAA) perfusion coronal maximum intensity projection (MIP) showing subtle, tiny peripheral subpleural perfusion deficits (*green arrows*) in the upper zones with relatively preserved ^{99m}Tc diethylenetriamine pentaacetic acid (DTPA) aerosol ventilation (a). (c) Coronal lung CT (from V/Q SPECT-CT template) showing no abnormal lung morphology. (d) V/Q parametric images showing V/Q quotient abnormalities highlighted in pink-orange tones (*green arrows*) at sites of V/Q discordance, representing V/Q mismatch. This pattern of tiny subpleural upper zone V/Q mismatches is atypical for classical pulmonary thromboembolism and taken in the COVID-19 context to represent residual small vessel insult. *Source:* Dhawan et al. [71].

triggering various intrathoracic receptors that stimulate breathing [72]. Inappropriate hyperventilation can also be seen in acute PE or pneumonia, in which the hypoxia-induced activation of peripheral chemoreceptors causes the respiratory control center to increase the output of signals to breathe. This dysregulation of breathing in turn causes an alkalosis, which lowers the threshold membrane potential and allows hyperexcitability and excessive muscular contraction. Arterial vasoconstriction in response to the alkalosis may then result in subsequent hypoperfusion of various organ systems.

In patients with COVID-19, occult ischemia occurs in various organ systems because the endothelium contains a high concentration of angiotensinogen-converting enzyme 2 receptors, so widespread vascular damage is a hallmark of this disease. In addition, hyperinflammation and cytokine storm also contribute to endothelial dysfunction and damage [73]. Some authors postulate that endothelial injury and microangiopathy in the brainstem and spinal cord may lead to autonomic dysfunction in select post-COVID patients [72]. This dysregulation could explain many features of long hauler's syndrome, including fatigue, palpitations, chest pain, orthostatic hypotension, postural orthostatic tachycardia, and unexplained dyspnea.

In the case of hyperventilation, damage to the respiratory control center can result in either: (1) stimulation of activator systems (automatic and cortical ventilatory control, peripheral afferents, and sensory cortex), or (2) suppression of inhibitory systems [72]. Treatment is primarily educational: a combination of respiratory physiotherapy and various retraining techniques to control breathing (e.g. Papworth and Buteyko). In the Papworth method, patients are trained to focus on diaphragmatic breathing and controlled slow nasal breathing. In the Buteyko method, nasal breathing is intermixed with controlled pauses to reduce the habit of hyperventilation [67, 70, 72]. Fortunately, this problem usually self-resolves with time.

Clinical Management

In the first waves of COVID-19, hospitals across the globe struggled to contain the virus and offer effective, acute treatment. Now that these waves are subsiding in parts of the world, clinicians everywhere need to focus on the aftermath – i.e. how best can we treat the patients who survived but have residual debilitating SOB and other symptoms. By outlining the currently available treatment options, physicians can further investigate and understand COVID-19-induced long-term sequelae. Ultimately, it is imperative to identify the long-term pulmonary consequences of COVID-19 and create standardized guidelines for follow-up.

Clinical management strategies from previous viral epidemics can offer important insight into COVID-19 long-term pulmonary management. Given the pathologic similarities seen in both SARS and MERS, treatment strategies and rehabilitation techniques for improved exercise tolerance may apply. Several different factors may play a role in the likelihood and severity of persistent imaging and functional abnormalities. For example, patient age, previous pulmonary and extrapulmonary comorbidities, severity and progression of the infection, hospital course, and whether certain medications such as antiviral agents or anti-inflammatories were given will clearly make

an impact. A correlation between ICU hospitalization and the extent of persisting lesions on HRCT has been recognized, as well as a link between intubation and fibrosis at follow-up [40]. Ultimately, the development of ARDS portends long-term COVID-19 pulmonary complications, especially if it evolves into pulmonary fibrosis with impaired alveolar oxygenation and chronic respiratory acidosis [51].

Depending on the severity of the disease, initial management may include airway clearance techniques, physical and breathing exercises, activity guidance, and patient education [74]. Because muscle weakness is an important cause of persistent dyspnea in many COVID-19 survivors, clinicians should focus on initiating pulmonary and physical rehabilitation immediately after discharge. Those who are older, who have significant comorbidities, and who have a severe course of infection will benefit from follow-up evaluation by their primary care provider or a pulmonologist.

For long-term follow-up, stable patients may undergo serial CXR or LDCT imaging to document resolution of findings with minimal radiation exposure. The BTS guideline recommends follow-up CXR at 12 weeks postdischarge for patients with COVID-19 pneumonia to assess for abnormalities [55, 75]. If there are persistent CXR changes on the second CXR and/or ongoing respiratory symptoms, further investigations are indicated, such as full PFTs (i.e. spirometry, lung volume tests, lung diffusion capacity, pulse oximetry, arterial blood gas tests, and fractional exhaled nitrous oxide tests), echocardiogram, desaturation walk test, and sputum sampling for other respiratory pathogens, as well as precontrast HRCT and a CT pulmonary angiogram to detect both ILD and PE. In the event of ILD, pulmonary hypertension, or PE, patients should be considered for further referral to a regional specialist. Other complications or residual symptoms should be managed on a case-by-case basis depending on the clinical setting [55, 75].

Unexplained cardiopulmonary symptoms, such as dyspnea, despite a normal CXR or chest CT should be evaluated for other potential causes, such as cardiac dysfunction, muscular weakness, viral-induced dysautonomic regulation of breathing, or pulmonary thromboembolic disease [75]. In this patient population, other types of imaging modalities may be indicated, such as PET-CT to differentiate between active and resolved inflammation, suggesting further diagnostic evaluation (e.g. bronchoscopy, CT-guided biopsy) [28]. Various types of lung perfusion scan (SPECT V/Q, DECT, CT-LSIM) may also be useful in elucidating other causes of ongoing dyspnea that are not readily explained by a relatively normal chest CT. CPET should also be considered in the monitoring and assessment of COVID-19 survivors, especially when the symptoms are inconsistent with the degree of impairment on PFTs.

Ultimately, in patients with significant lingering respiratory symptoms and minimal findings on chest CT, it is imperative to look beyond standard chest imaging and consider nonpulmonary causes. Figure 24.6 demonstrates a potential workup plan for management of nonresolving dyspnea after COVID-19 recovery.

In post-COVID patients who have pulmonary fibrosis, persistent dyspnea and hypoxemia are expected outcomes. Much like for idiopathic pulmonary fibrosis, interventions include: (1) supplemental oxygen, (2) pulmonary rehabilitation, (3) trial of antifibrotic agents, and (4) consideration for lung transplantation [76–78]. As Maher and colleagues [79] have highlighted in a recent *Lancet* editorial, the evolving need to manage post-COVID pulmonary fibrosis may be a call to arms regarding the use of preexisting antifibrotic agents for experimental trials. These include drugs for idiopathic pulmonary fibrosis (pirfenidone, nintedanib), mineralocorticoid receptor antagonists (spironolactone), and traditional Chinese herbal medicine. Hyperbaric

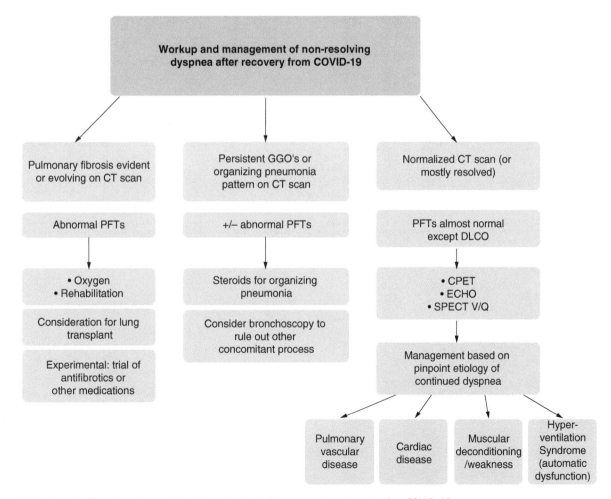

Figure 24.6 Suggested workup and management of nonresolving dyspnea after COVID-19 recovery.

oxygen and human amniotic fluid have also been considered but are clearly controversial. Ultimately, the best way of preventing pulmonary fibrosis in established disease is to intervene early in the course of severe infection with timely administration of antiviral agents (remdesivir), glucocorticoids (dexamethasone), anti–IL-6 monoclonal antibodies (tocilizumab, sarilumab), or JAK inhibitors (baricitinib, tofacitinib) [76] (Figure 24.7).

Patients who still have persistent GGOs or OP on CT more than a month after discharge should be considered for a trial of high-dose steroids, even if they already received steroids during acute hospitalization [36]. Bronchoscopy can be requested to rule out concomitant processes but is not mandatory in the right clinical setting.

When pulmonary parenchymal damage is not the cause of persistent dyspnea, the ultimate management plan will differ based on the specific etiology. Following are suggested treatment algorithms for the four major nonlung etiologies of post-COVID dyspnea.

1) **Pulmonary vascular disease** (e.g. pulmonary embolic disease, small vessel angiopathy, reduced peripheral lung perfusion)
   a) Evaluate for pulmonary hypertension with echocardiography and consideration of right-heart catheterization
   b) Trial of select pulmonary vasodilators
   c) Long-term anticoagulation
   d) Referral for lung transplantation
2) **Cardiac disease** (e.g. coronary occlusion, heart failure, arrhythmias, myocarditis)
   a) Cardiac catheterization to rule out and treat significant coronary artery disease
   b) Heart failure medications, such as diuretics, beta-blockers, angiotensin-converting enzyme inhibitors, afterload reducing agents; mechanical support devices as needed
   c) Anticoagulation and antiarrhythmics as needed

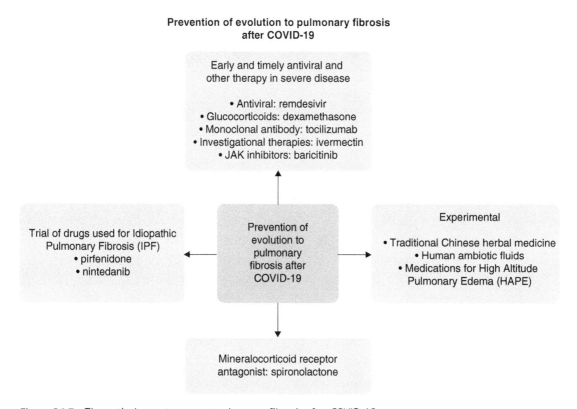

Prevention of evolution to pulmonary fibrosis after COVID-19

Early and timely antiviral and other therapy in severe disease
- Antiviral: remdesivir
- Glucocorticoids: dexamethasone
- Monoclonal antibody: tocilizumab
- Investigational therapies: ivermectin
- JAK inhibitors: baricitinib

Trial of drugs used for Idiopathic Pulmonary Fibrosis (IPF)
- pirfenidone
- nintedanib

Prevention of evolution to pulmonary fibrosis after COVID-19

Experimental
- Traditional Chinese herbal medicine
- Human ambiotic fluids
- Medications for High Altitude Pulmonary Edema (HAPE)

Mineralocorticoid receptor antagonist: spironolactone

Figure 24.7   Theoretical ways to prevent pulmonary fibrosis after COVID-19.

d) Consideration of nonsteroidal anti-inflammatory drugs or steroids to resolve ongoing cardiac inflammation
e) Cardiac rehabilitation
3) **Neuromuscular weakness** (e.g. loss of muscle mass, deconditioning, neuropathies)
a) Refer to an acute rehabilitation program
b) Correct electrolyte imbalances
c) Improve nutritional status
d) Avoid any other insult that could worsen muscular strength (such as steroids and statins)
4) **Hyperventilation syndrome** (dysfunctional breathing caused by autonomic nervous system damage)
a) Respiratory physiotherapy
b) Retraining of breathing (Papworth and Buteyko methods)
c) Meditation

In summary, for both the acute and long-term management of COVID-19 pneumonia, it is imperative that clinicians serially monitor and document radiographic and functional data over time. Although many patients will recover from COVID-19 over time, complaints of persistent SOB should prompt a timely workup of potential causes beyond just overt pulmonary fibrosis. Potential conditions such as muscular deconditioning and weakness, occult myocardial damage, pulmonary vascular disease, and inappropriate hyperventilation syndrome should be identified rapidly using a robust algorithm and managed appropriately.

Summary Points

- Based on our prior experiences with past coronavirus infections, such as SARS and MERS, long-term pulmonary consequences should be expected in post-COVID-19 patients. Residual symptoms of SOB and fatigue may persist for months to years and, in certain cases, become permanent.
- Whereas many chest CT scans may normalize after one year, radiographic pulmonary abnormalities can linger indefinitely in some patients. The most common findings include persistent GGOs, residual parenchymal consolidation, interstitial fibrosis, and subpleural fibrotic bands.
- Baseline imaging should be considered at the time of hospital discharge for patients with severe lung damage or who are at higher risk for development of future viral infections, including reinfection with COVID-19. Those with preexisting lung disease and significant medical comorbidities may also benefit from serial imaging and follow-up with a pulmonologist.
- Baseline imaging and subsequent follow-up are best accomplished by chest CT, although initially, CXR may be the only practical option in symptomatic unstable patients. PET-CT may serve as a useful ancillary tool, specifically in the case of identifying residual pulmonary or nodal inflammation or screening for other sites of involvement.
- The BTS guidelines recommend that PFTs be considered at three months postdischarge, especially for the follow-up of patients with possible residual interstitial disease. Serial testing will be based on patient and physician preference. Over time, most patients will have normalization of their PFTs, except for the DLCO, which may be an important clue toward a nonparenchymal etiology of continued dyspnea.
- Because of its global and integrated assessment, CPET should also be considered in the evaluation of post-COVID survivors, especially when their respiratory symptoms are inconsistent with the degree of impairment on PFTs.
- Because muscle weakness is an important cause of lingering SOB in the majority of COVID-19 survivors, clinicians should initiate pulmonary and physical rehabilitation as soon as possible after hospital discharge.
- In many patients with post-COVID long hauler's syndrome, persistent respiratory symptoms do not always correlate with chest imaging and PFTs. Keeping an open mind and pinpointing the correct etiology (or etiologies) using a variety of testing modalities is vital to ensure accurate and effective treatment planning.
- Immunization against SARS-CoV-2 and influenza according to established guidelines is critical for preventing future infections and further loss of lung and physical functioning.

References

1 Poon, L.L., Guan, Y., Nicholls, J.M. et al. (2004). The aetiology, origins, and diagnosis of severe acute respiratory syndrome. *Lancet Infect Dis.* 4: 663–671.

2 Sampathkumar, P., Temesgen, Z., Smith, T.F., and Thompson, R.L. (2003). SARS: epidemiology, clinical presentation, management, and infection control measures. *Mayo Clin Proc* 78 (7): 882–890. https://doi.org/10.4065/78.7.882.

3 Zhang, P., Li, J., Liu, H. et al. (2020). Long-term bone and lung consequences associated with hospital-acquired severe acute respiratory syndrome: a 15-year follow-up from a prospective cohort study. *Bone Res.* 8: 34.

4 Dundamadappa S, Kaw G, Koteyar S, Goh J, Chee T. High-resolution CT (HRCT) in severe acute respiratory syndrome (sars) patients post hospital discharge: a long-term follow-up study. Radiological Society of North America. Presented at the RSNA Annual Scientific Assembly and Meeting, 28 November 2004. https://archive.rsna.org/2004/4411116.html.

5 Wu, X., Dong, D., and Ma, D. (2016). Thin-section computed tomography manifestations during convalescence and long-term followup of patients with severe acute respiratory syndrome (SARS). *Med Sci Monit Int Med J Exp Clin Res.* 22: 2793–2799.

6 Zumla, A., Hui, D.S., and Perlman, S. (2015). Middle East respiratory syndrome. *Lancet* 386 (9997): 995–1007.

7 Gao, H., Yao, H., Yang, S., and Li, L. (2016). From SARS to MERS: evidence and speculation. *Front Med.* 10 (4): 377–382. https://doi.org/10.1007/s11684-016-0466-7.

8 Das, K.M., Lee, E.Y., Langer, R.D., and Larsson, S.G. (2016). Middle East respiratory syndrome coronavirus: what does a radiologist need to know? *AJR Am J Roentgenol.* 206 (6): 1193–1201. https://doi.org/10.2214/AJR.15.15363.

9 Liya, G., Yuguang, W., Jian, L. et al. (2020). Studies on viral pneumonia related to novel coronavirus SARS-CoV-2, SARS-CoV, and MERS-CoV: a literature review. *APMIS* 128 (6): 423–432. https://doi.org/10.1111/apm.13047.

10 Ahmed, H., Patel, K., Greenwood, D.C. et al. (2020). Long-term clinical outcomes in survivors of severe acute respiratory syndrome and Middle East respiratory syndrome coronavirus outbreaks after hospitalisation or ICU admission: a systematic review and meta-analysis. *J Rehabil Med.* 52 (5): jrm00063. https://doi.org/10.2340/16501977-2694.

11 Park, W.B., Jun, K.I., Kim, G. et al. (2018). Correlation between pneumonia severity and pulmonary complications in Middle East respiratory syndrome. *J. Korean Med. Sci.* 33 (24): e169. https://doi.org/10.3346/jkms.2018.33.e169.

12 Das, K.M., Lee, E.Y., Singh, R. et al. (2017). Follow-up chest radiographic findings in patients with MERS-CoV after recovery. *Indian J Radiol Imaging* 27 (3): 342–349. https://doi.org/10.4103/ijri.IJRI_469_16.

13 Wong, K.T., Antonio Gregory, E., Hui, D.S. et al. (2003). Severe acute respiratory syndrome: radiographic appearances and pattern of progression in 138 patients. *Radiology* 228: 401–406.

14 Katal, S., Myers, L., and Gholamrezanezhad, A. (2021). SARS-CoV-2 reinfection: "New baseline" imaging concept in the era of COVID-19. *Clin Imaging* 78: 142–145. https://doi.org/10.1016/j.clinimag.2021.03.021.

15 Pan, Y., Guan, H., Zhou, S. et al. (2020). Initial CT findings and temporal changes in patients with the novel coronavirus pneumonia (2019-nCoV): a study of 63 patients in Wuhan, China. *Eur. Radiol.* 30: 3306–3309. https://doi.org/10.1007/s00330-020-06731-x.

16 Mahdavi, A., Haseli, S., Mahdavi, A. et al. (2020). The role of repeat chest CT scan in the COVID-19 pandemic. *Acad. Radiol.* 27 (7): 1049–1050. https://doi.org/10.1016/j.acra.2020.04.031.

17 Hu, T., Liu, Y., Zhao, M. et al. (2020). A comparison of COVID-19, SARS and MERS. *PeerJ* 8: e9725. https://doi.org/10.7717/peerj.9725.

18 Jin, Y.-H., Cai, L., Cheng, Z.-S. et al. (2020). A rapid advice guideline for the diagnosis and treatment of 2019 novel coronavirus (2019-nCoV) infected pneumonia (standard version). *Mil Med Res.* 7 (1): 4.

19 Cozzi, D., Albanesi, M., Cavigli, E. et al. (2020). Chest X-ray in new coronavirus disease 2019 (COVID-19) infection: findings and correlation with clinical outcome. *Radiol Med.* 125: 730–737.

20 Wong, H.Y.F., Lam, H.Y.S., Fong, A.H.-T. et al. (2020). Frequency and distribution of chest radiographic findings in patients positive for COVID-19. *Radiology* 296 (2): E72–E78.

21 Zayed, N.E., Bessar, M.A., and Lutfy, S. (2021). CO-RADS versus CT-SS scores in predicting severe COVID-19 patients: retrospective comparative study. *Egypt J Bronchol.* 15: 13. https://doi.org/10.1186/s43168-021-00060-3.

22 Shiri, I., Akhavanallaf, A., Sanaat, A. et al. (2021). Ultra-low-dose chest CT imaging of COVID-19 patients using a deep residual neural network. *Eur Radiol.* 31 (3): 1420–1431.

23 Yang, S., Zhang, Y., Shen, J. et al. (2020). Clinical potential of UTE-MRI for assessing COVID-19: patient-and lesion-based comparative analysis. *J Magn Reson Imaging* 52 (2): 397–406.

24 Ates, O.F., Taydas, O., and Dheir, H. (2020). Thorax magnetic resonance imaging findings in patients with coronavirus disease (COVID-19). *Acad Radiol.* 27 (10): 1373–1378.

25 Eibschutz, L.S., Rabiee, B., Asadollahi, S. et al. (2022). FDG-PET/CT of COVID-19 and other lung infections. *Semin Nucl Med.* 52 (1): 61–70. https://doi.org/10.1053/j.semnuclmed.2021.06.017.

26 Kamani, C.H., Jreige, M., Pappon, M. et al. (2020). Added value of 18F-FDG PET/CT in a SARS-CoV-2-infected complex case with persistent fever. *Eur J Nucl Med Mol Imaging* 47 (8): 2036–2037. https://doi.org/10.1007/s00259-020-04860-5.

27 Fu, C., Zhang, W., Li, H. et al. (2020). FDG PET/CT evaluation of a patient recovering from COVID-19. *Eur J Nucl Med Mol Imaging.* 47 (11): 2703–2705.

28 Salehi, S., Reddy, S., and Gholamrezanezhad, A. (2020). Long-term pulmonary consequences of coronavirus disease 2019 (COVID-19): what we know and what to expect. *J Thorac Imaging* 35 (4): W87–W89.

29 Alavi, A., Werner, T.J., and Gholamrezanezhad, A. (2021). The critical role of FDG-PET/CT imaging in assessing systemic manifestations of COVID-19 infection. *Eur J Nucl Med Mol Imaging* 48 (4): 956–962. https://doi.org/10.1007/s00259-020-05148-4.

30 Liya, G., Yuguang, W., Jian, L. et al. (2020). Studies on viral pneumonia related to novel coronavirus SARS-CoV-2, SARS-CoV, and MERS-CoV: a literature review. *APMIS* 128 (6): 423–432. https://doi.org/10.1111/apm.13047.

31 Shi, H., Han, X., Jiang, N. et al. (2020). Radiological findings from 81 patients with COVID-19 pneumonia in Wuhan, China: a descriptive study. *Lancet Infect Dis.* 20 (4): 425–434. https://doi.org/10.1016/S1473-3099(20)30086-4.

32 Liu, D., Zhang, W., Pan, F. et al. (2020). The pulmonary sequalae in discharged patients with COVID-19: a short-term observational study. *Respir Res.* 21: 125. https://doi.org/10.1186/s12931-020-01385-1.

33 Ding, X., Xu, J., Zhou, J. et al. (2020). Chest CT findings of COVID-19 pneumonia by duration of symptoms. *Eur J Radiol.* 127: 109009.

34 Pogatchnik, B.P., Swenson, K.E., Sharifi, H. et al. (2020). Radiology-pathology correlation in recovered COVID-19, demonstrating organizing pneumonia. *Am J Respir Crit Care Med.* 202 (4): 598–599.

35 de Oliveira Filho, C.M., Vieceli, T., de Fraga, B.C. et al. (2021). Organizing pneumonia: a late phase complication of COVID-19 responding dramatically to corticosteroids. *Braz J Infect Dis.* 25 (1): 101541. https://doi.org/10.1016/j.bjid.2021.101541.

36 Myall, K.J., Mukherjee, B., Castanheira, A.M. et al. (2021). Persistent post-COVID-19 interstitial lung disease. An observational study of corticosteroid treatment. *Ann Am Thorac Soc.* 18 (5): 799–806. https://doi.org/10.1513/AnnalsATS.202008-1002OC.

37 Malik, B., Abdelazeem, B., and Ghatol, A. (2021). Pulmonary fibrosis after COVID-19 pneumonia. *Cureus* 13 (3): e13923. https://doi.org/10.7759/cureus.13923.

38 Schwensen, H.F., Borreschmidt, L.K., Storgaard, M. et al. (2021). Fatal pulmonary fibrosis: a post-COVID-19 autopsy case. *J Clin Pathol.* 74: 400–402. https://doi.org/10.1136/jclinpath-2020-206879.

39 Zhao, Y.M., Shang, Y.M., Song, W.B. et al. (2020). Follow-up study of the pulmonary function and related physiological characteristics of COVID-19 survivors three months after recovery. *EClinicalMedicine* 25: 100463. https://doi.org/10.1016/j.eclinm.2020.100463.

40 Froidure, A., Mahsouli, A., Liistro, G. et al. (2021). Integrative respiratory follow-up of severe COVID-19 reveals common functional and lung imaging sequelae. *Respir. Med.* 181: 106383. https://doi.org/10.1016/j.rmed.2021.106383.

41 Zha, L., Shen, Y., Pan, L. et al. (2021). Follow-up study on pulmonary function and radiological changes in critically ill patients with COVID-19. *J Infect.* 82 (1): 159–198. https://doi.org/10.1016/j.jinf.2020.05.040.

42 McGroder, C.F., Zhang, D., Choudhury, M.A. et al. (2021). Pulmonary fibrosis 4 months after COVID-19 is associated with severity of illness and blood leucocyte telomere length. *Thorax* 76 (12): 1242–1245. https://doi.org/10.1136/thoraxjnl-2021-217031.

43 Writing Committee for the COMEBAC Study Group, Morin, L., Savale, L. et al. (2021). Four-month clinical status of a cohort of patients after hospitalization for COVID-19. *JAMA* 325 (15): 1525–1534. https://doi.org/10.1001/jama.2021.3331.

44 Guler, S.A., Ebner, L., Aubry-Beigelman, C. et al. (2021). Pulmonary function and radiological features 4 months after COVID-19: first results from the national prospective observational Swiss COVID-19 lung study. *Eur Respir J.* 57 (4): 2003690. https://doi.org/10.1183/13993003.03690-2020.

45 Han, X., Fan, Y., Alwalid, O. et al. (2021). Six-month follow-up chest CT findings after severe COVID-19 pneumonia. *Radiology* 299 (1): E177–E186.

46 Ambrosetti, M.C., Battocchio, G., Zamboni, G.A. et al. (2020). Rapid onset of bronchiectasis in COVID-19 pneumonia: two cases studied with CT. *Radiol Case Rep.* 15 (11): 2098–2103. https://doi.org/10.1016/j.radcr.2020.08.008.

47 Martinez-Garcia, M.A., Aksamit, T.R., and Aliberti, S. (2021). Bronchiectasis as a long-term consequence of SARS-COVID-19 pneumonia: future studies are needed. *Arch. Bronconeumol. (Engl Ed)* (12): 739–740. https://doi.org/10.1016/j.arbres.2021.04.021.

48 Huang, C., Huang, L., Wang, Y. et al. (2021). 6-month consequences of COVID-19 in patients discharged from hospital: a cohort study. *Lancet* 397 (10270): 220–232. https://doi.org/10.1016/S0140-6736(20)32656-8.

49 Wu, X., Liu, X., Zhou, Y. et al. (2021). 3-Month, 6-month, 9-month, and 12-month respiratory outcomes in patients following COVID-19-related hospitalisation: a prospective study. *Lancet Respir Med.* 9 (7): 747–754. https://doi.org/10.1016/S2213-2600(21)00174-0.

50 Grillo, F., Barisione, E., Ball, L. et al. (2021). Lung fibrosis: an undervalued finding in COVID-19 pathological series. *Lancet Infect Dis.* 21 (4): e72.

51 Arnold, D.T., Hamilton, F.W., Milne, A. et al. (2021). Patient outcomes after hospitalisation with COVID-19 and implications for follow-up: results from a prospective UK cohort. *Thorax* 76: 399–401.

52 Nalbandian, A., Sehgal, K., Gupta, A. et al. (2021). Post-acute COVID-19 syndrome. *Nat Med.* 27: 601–615. https://doi.org/10.1038/s41591-021-01283-z.

53 Carfì, A., Bernabei, R., and Landi, F.; Gemelli against COVID-19 post-acute care study group(2020). Persistent symptoms in patients after acute COVID-19. *JAMA* 324 (6): 603–605. https://doi.org/10.1001/jama.2020.12603.

54 Cares-Marambio, K., Montenegro-Jiménez, Y., Torres-Castro, R. et al. (2021). Prevalence of potential respiratory symptoms in survivors of hospital admission after coronavirus disease 2019 (COVID-19): a systematic review and meta-analysis. *Chron. Respir. Dis.* 18: 14799731211002240. https://doi.org/10.1177/14799731211002240.

55 British Thoracic Society. British Thoracic Society guidance on respiratory follow up of patients with a clinico-radiological diagnosis of COVID-19 pneumonia. 2020. https://www.brit-thoracic.org.uk/document-library/quality-improvement/covid-19/resp-follow-up-guidance-post-covid-pneumonia.

56 Tsatsakis, A., Calina, D., Falzone, L. et al. (2020). SARS-CoV-2 pathophysiology and its clinical implications: an integrative overview of the pharmacotherapeutic management of COVID-19. *Food Chem. Toxicol.* 146: 111769. https://doi.org/10.1016/j.fct.2020.111769.

57 Wiersinga, W.J., Rhodes, A., Cheng, A.C. et al. (2020). Pathophysiology, transmission, diagnosis, and treatment of coronavirus disease 2019 (COVID-19): a review. *JAMA* 324 (8): 782–793. https://doi.org/10.1001/jama.2020.12839.

58 Rooney, S., Webster, A., and Paul, L. (2020). Systematic review of changes and recovery in physical function and fitness after severe acute respiratory syndrome-related coronavirus infection: implications for COVID-19 rehabilitation. *Phys. Ther.* 100 (10): 1717–1729. https://doi.org/10.1093/ptj/pzaa129.

59 Belli, S., Balbi, B., Prince, I. et al. (2020). Low physical functioning and impaired performance of activities of daily life in COVID-19 patients who survived hospitalisation. *Eur Respir J.* 56 (4): 2002096. https://doi.org/10.1183/13993003. 02096-2020.

60 Ong, K.C., Ng, A.W., Lee, L.S. et al. (2004). Pulmonary function and exercise capacity in survivors of severe acute respiratory syndrome. *Eur Respir J.* 24 (3): 436–442. https://doi.org/10.1183/090 31936.04.00007104.

61 Davis, R., Dixon, C., Millar, A.B. et al. (2021). A role for cardiopulmonary exercise testing in detecting physiological changes underlying health status in idiopathic pulmonary fibrosis: a feasibility study. *BMC Pulm Med.* 21: 147. https://doi.org/10.1186/ s12890-021-01520-8.

62 Clavario, P., De Marzo, V., Lotti, R. et al. (2021). Cardiopulmonary exercise testing in COVID-19 patients at 3 months follow-up. *Int J Cardiol.* 340: 113–118. https://doi.org/10.1016/j.ijcard.2021.07.033.

63 Rinaldo, R., Mondoni, M., Parazzini, E. et al. (2021). Deconditioning as main mechanism of impaired exercise response in COVID-19 survivors. *Eur Respir J.* 58 (2): 2100870. https://doi.org/10.1183/13993003. 00870-2021.

64 American Thoracic Society; American College of Chest Physicians (2003). ATS/ACCP statement on cardiopulmonary exercise testing. *Am J Respir Crit Care Med.* 167 (2): 211–277.

65 Blokland, I.J., Ilbrink, S., Houdijk, H. et al. (2020). Inspanningscapaciteit na beademing vanwege covid-19 [Exercise capacity after mechanical ventilation because of COVID-19: Cardiopulmonary exercise tests in clinical rehabilitation]. *Ned Tijdschr Geneeskd.* 164: D5253.

66 Gao, Y., Chen, R., Geng, Q. et al. (2021). Cardiopulmonary exercise testing might be helpful for interpretation of impaired pulmonary function in recovered COVID-19 patients. *Eur Respir J.* 57 (1): 2004265. https://doi.org/10.1183/13993003. 04265-2020.

67 Motiejunaite, J., Balagny, P., Arnoult, F. et al. (2021). Hyperventilation: a possible explanation for long-lasting exercise intolerance in mild COVID-19 survivors? *Front Physiol* 11: 614590. https://doi. org/10.3389/fphys.2020.614590.

68 Puntmann, V.O., Carerj, M.L., Wieters, I. et al. (2020). Outcomes of cardiovascular magnetic resonance imaging in patients recently recovered from coronavirus disease 2019 (COVID-19). *JAMA Cardiol.* 5 (11): 1265–1273. https://doi.org/10.1001/ jamacardio.2020.3557.

69 Rajpal, S., Tong, M.S., Borchers, J. et al. (2021). Cardiovascular magnetic resonance findings in competitive athletes recovering from COVID-19 infection. *JAMA Cardiol.* 6 (1): 116–118. https://doi.org/10.1001/jamacardio. 2020.4916.

70 Aparisi, Á., Ybarra-Falcón, C., García-Gómez, M. et al. (2021). Exercise ventilatory inefficiency in post-COVID-19 syndrome: insights from a prospective evaluation. *J Clin Med.* 10 (12): 2591. https://doi.org/10.3390/jcm10122591.

71 Dhawan, R.T., Gopalan, D., Howard, L. et al. (2021). Beyond the clot: perfusion imaging of the pulmonary vasculature after COVID-19. *Lancet Respir Med.* 9 (1): 107–116. https://doi.org/10.1016/ S2213-2600(20)30407-0.

72 Becker, R.C. (2021). Autonomic dysfunction in SARS-COV-2 infection acute and long-term implications COVID-19 editor's page series. *J Thromb Thrombolysis* 52: 692–707. https://doi. org/10.1007/s11239-021-02549-6.

73 Nägele, M.P., Haubner, B., Tanner, F.C. et al. (2020). Endothelial dysfunction in COVID-19: current findings and therapeutic implications. *Atherosclerosis* 314: 58–62. https://doi.org/10.1016/ j.atherosclerosis.2020.10.014.

74 Wang, T.J., Chau, B., Lui, M. et al. (2020). Physical medicine and rehabilitation and pulmonary rehabilitation for COVID-19. *Am J Phys Med Rehabil.* 99 (9): 769–774. https://doi.org/10.1097/ PHM.0000000000001505.

75 George, P.M., Barratt, S.L., Condliffe, R. et al. (2020). Respiratory follow-up of patients with COVID-19 pneumonia. *Thorax* 75: 1009–1016.

76 Lechowicz, K., Drożdżal, S., Machaj, F. et al. (2020). COVID-19: the potential treatment of pulmonary fibrosis associated with SARS-CoV-2 infection. *J Clin Med.* 9 (6): 1917. https://doi.org/10.3390/ jcm9061917.

77 Gentile, F., Aimo, A., Forfori, F. et al. (2020). COVID-19 and risk of pulmonary fibrosis: the importance of planning ahead. *Eur J Prev Cardiol.* 27 (13): 1442–1446. https://doi.org/10.1177/2047487320932695.

78 George, P.M., Wells, A.U., and Jenkins, R.G. (2020). Pulmonary fibrosis and COVID-19: the potential role for antifibrotic therapy. *Lancet Respir Med.* 8 (8): 807–815. https://doi.org/10.1016/S2213-2600(20)30225-3.

79 Spagnolo, P., Balestro, E., Aliberti, S. et al. (2020). Pulmonary fibrosis secondary to COVID-19: a call to arms? *Lancet Respir Med.* 8 (8): 750–752. https://doi.org/10.1016/S2213-2600(20)30222-8.

25

Psychological Effects and Neuropsychiatric Sequelae in COVID-19 Patients

Elpitha Sakka[1], Arturas Kalniunas[2], Elzbieta Vitkauskaite[2], Wala Salman[2], Subhana Chaudhri[3], and Sofia Pappa[2,4]

[1] School of Pharmacy and Biomolecular Sciences, University of Brighton, Brighton, United Kingdom
[2] West London NHS Trust, London, United Kingdom
[3] Greater Manchester Mental Health NHS Foundation Trust, Manchester, United Kingdom
[4] Faculty of Medicine, Department of Brain Sciences, Imperial College London, London, United Kingdom

Abbreviations

CBT	cognitive behavioral therapy
HCW	healthcare worker
ICU	intensive care unit
MERS	Middle East respiratory syndrome
PTSD	posttraumatic stress disorder
SARS-CoV-2	severe acute respiratory syndrome coronavirus 2

The emergence of the novel severe acute respiratory syndrome coronavirus 2 (SARS-CoV-2) has caused an ongoing global health crisis, which has significantly impacted all aspects of day-to-day life. SARS-CoV-2 is homologous with previous coronaviruses that were transmissible in humans, such as SARS-CoV-1 and Middle East respiratory syndrome (MERS)-CoV, which were responsible for causing two notable infectious disease outbreaks in the twenty-first century.

Evidence from previous outbreaks shows that infected patients are at an increased risk for experiencing symptoms of psychological distress and developing mental health disorders, including depression, anxiety, posttraumatic stress disorder (PTSD), and sleep-related disorders [1]. However, it is thought that the psychological implications of the COVID-19 pandemic may exceed that of previous outbreaks because of its massive scale and significant implications, including the spread of misinformation through social media [2].

Indeed, a large proportion of early research following COVID-19 focused on the physiological effects of the virus; however, a substantial body of subsequent studies have shown that the psychological burden of the infection is considerable [3]. Alongside a number of other psychosocial factors, a COVID-19 diagnosis is more likely to increase susceptibility in developing mood, cognitive, and sleep disturbances because infected patients often require hospitalization in the intensive care unit (ICU) and mechanical ventilation, both of which are considered risk factors for the acquisition of acute psychiatric disorders; direct bioimmunologic effects have also been implicated [4].

These disorders should be diagnosed adequately and in a timely manner to improve prognosis, reduce the duration of hospital stay and admission to ICU, and prevent the development of long-term mental health issues in patients suffering from COVID-19. Therefore, it is imperative to continue recording prevalence rates in different populations, identify predictive and mitigating factors, and evaluate effective interventions. In this chapter, we will summarize the evidence to date and discuss relevant management strategies.

Depression and Anxiety

The COVID-19 crisis has had a significant impact on the physical and mental well-being of the global population, accompanied by a marked increase in anxious and depressive symptoms, especially during the early stages of the pandemic. Still, the prevalence of these symptoms diminished over time among the general population [5]. However, symptoms persisted in individuals diagnosed with COVID-19, showing higher rates of anxiety (47%) and depression (34%) compared with the general population (rates of 34% and 32%, respectively) [1]. Prevalence rates were found to be highest during the first week of hospitalization and persisted 6 months postinfection [6, 7]. It is important to note that despite the significant impact of COVID-19 on Black and Asian minority groups, these groups are largely underrepresented in studies [8]. This may be because of cultural differences in articulating or associating symptoms with mental health and/or relevant behaviors being considered culturally unacceptable [9].

Individuals with a mental health diagnosis in the year prior to contracting COVID-19 were at higher risk (65%) for development of depression and/or anxiety [10]. Likewise, patients with no history of mental illness and COVID-19 infection were also more likely to receive a diagnosis of anxiety and/or depression for the first time compared with those without a COVID-19 infection [11]. As reported by Taquet et al. [10], the development of symptoms of depression and anxiety may be directly associated with SARS-CoV-2 because patients with COVID-19 presented with considerably higher levels depression and anxiety in comparison with hospitalized patients with other respiratory illnesses (Figure 25.1).

Cause or Consequence

Further exploring whether COVID-19 causes anxiety and depression or vice versa can help our understanding of the direction and nature of this relationship. Mazza et al. [3] proposed that anxiety and depression may be caused by an immune response to SARS-CoV-2 because the same biomarkers have been implicated in both major depressive disorder and COVID-19 [12]. Prolonged high concentrations of these biomarkers were associated with greater COVID-19 severity and, in turn, higher levels of depression [6, 13]. Thus, it is postulated that those with long COVID are at a higher risk of developing depressive and/or anxious symptoms and may partly explain why anxiety improves but depression persists in patients with COVID-19 postinfection [14]. However, oxygen saturation levels at baseline and at one-month follow-up were not associated with anxiety and depression levels [3].

However, not all patients with COVID-19 develop anxiety and/or depression, nor does the severity of COVID-19 contribute equally to the likelihood of experiencing mood symptoms [15–17], indicating that a variety of psychosocial factors may play a role in the development of anxiety and depression in patients with COVID-19 [10].

Worry about the future, uncertainty of new infections, and self-blame when contracting COVID-19 were all associated with anxiety [18]. Individuals who tested positive for COVID-19 and were required to self-isolate reported increased feelings of loneliness, frustration, and boredom because of not being able to physically see loved ones and a loss of usual routine, resulting in increased levels of depression [18]. In addition, once returning from self-isolation, they reported a sense of stigma toward them by neighbors – being treated differently, being avoided, and comments being made about them, which also increased levels of anxiety and depression [19].

Mitigating Factors and Management Strategies

Social support has been identified to be a predominant buffer against the development of anxiety and depression in individuals with COVID-19 because it compensates for low resilience, which is typically observed in patients [20, 21]. Specifically, social support from family, in comparison with that of friends or partners, has been found to be most influential because of its perceived stability and material support [22]. This includes face-to-face person support and online and telephone communication that patients can use when self-isolating or in hospital because it reduces feelings of loneliness and a sense of missing out on socializing and, in turn, depression [5, 18]. In addition, within hospitals, having support from healthcare workers (HCWs) and engaging in a range of activities further promotes personal resilience because it encourages patients to adapt to the hospital environment in a positive manner [23].

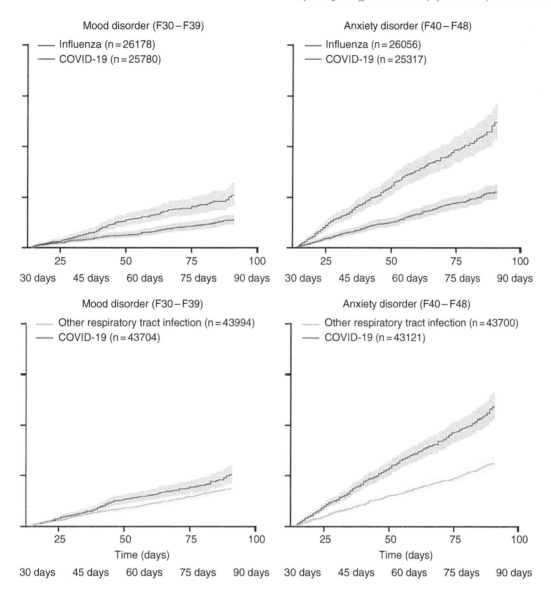

Figure 25.1 Depression and anxiety levels of COVID-19 patients versus hospitalized patients with other respiratory illnesses. *Source:* Taquet et al. [10].

Psychological support has been found to be effective for patients with COVID-19 and anxiety/depression. A randomized control trial by Li et al. [24] compared patients receiving cognitive behavioral therapy (CBT) with those with only routine treatment for physical symptoms of COVID-19. Results found CBT to be more effective, especially for those with longer hospital stays who generally displayed higher levels of anxiety. The cognitive aspects of CBT increase tolerance to uncertainty, ability to reappraise the situation, and enhance self-efficacy; all of which

increase resilience and ultimately reduce feelings of anxiety and depression [25]. The behavioral aspects of CBT, such as self-protective behaviors (e.g. washing hands), behavioral activation, relaxation, and grounding techniques, improve self-confidence and stimulate the parasympathetic nervous system, which is related to improved mental health [26]. Changes in cognitions and behavior, and the increased availability of CBT online has led CBT to be a favorable intervention for patients of COVID-19 with anxiety and/or depression [27].

Due to the large number of patients with COVID-19 and anxiety and/or depression, there is a need for assertive mental health support. The provision of mental health screening tests during hospital admission would be beneficial to monitor levels of anxiety and/or depression and to prevent them from exacerbating. Training HCWs who support patients with COVID-19 to identify signs of poor mental health and an increase in available mental health professionals/services may further prevent affective disturbances in patients with COVID-19. Furthermore, using CBT, maintaining strong support networks, and following a daily routine can promote resilience and mitigate mood problems.

Posttraumatic Stress Disorder

PTSD, according to the International Classification of Disease, Tenth Revision, is a mental health illness that develops after exposure to a traumatic and stressful life event that is sufficient to result in pervasive distress [28]. Core manifestations include flashbacks of the traumatic event, sleep problems, avoidance of situations or places reminiscent of the trauma, low mood, hyperarousal, and anxiety. Such symptoms can develop shortly after the traumatic event, but in some, the development of PTSD symptoms can have a latency period of a few months [28]. Several different scales are used in the screening of PTSD, including the Impact of Event Trauma scale, Davidson Trauma Scale, and Posttraumatic Diagnostic Scale [29].

Previous evidence has demonstrated that large-scale pandemics significantly influence a population's mental health, increasing the prevalence of different psychiatric illnesses, including PTSD [30]. Moreover, pandemics caused by infectious diseases, like COVID-19, appear to be more traumatic when compared with other stressful life events, increasing the risk for PTSD following exposure. A systematic review found the risk of developing PTSD after an infectious disease outbreak to be higher than the risk after major traumatic events and natural disasters such as floods [30].

Furthermore, COVID-19 infection can have a profound impact on the mental health of those who survived the disease, with findings suggesting that the psychological trauma brought about by the symptoms of the disease may lead to an increased risk for PTSD. Hence a number of studies demonstrated an increased prevalence of PTSD among those who had recovered from COVID-19 infection. However, there was significant heterogeneity as the numbers reported by different studies varied considerably [30–33]. These variations can be a result of different methods adopted by individual studies, as well as factors related to the outbreak and/or the study population [30]. A meta-analysis reported that approximately 3 in every 10 COVID-19 survivors and 1 in every 10 individuals of the general public experienced PTSD-type symptoms.

Specifically, the severity of the disease was shown to play a role in modifying the risk for development of PTSD symptoms postinfection. A study examining 13 000 patients in the United Kingdom with confirmed or suspected COVID-19 infection found 35% of those who had a severe infection requiring respiratory support (assisted ventilation) had symptoms of PTSD compared with only 18% of those who did not require ventilatory support [32].

The prevalence of PTSD may differ depending on whether the population infected with COVID-19 is hospitalized or in the community. One study found as much as 96.2% of hospitalized patients with COVID-19 in China in 2020 experienced symptoms of PTSD [31]. This sharply contrasts with the prevalence rate of 12.4% found by another study conducted in China in the same year among patients who have recovered from COVID-19 and were discharged from the hospital. However, Liu et al. [33] postulated that the significantly higher prevalence of PTSD rates among hospitalized populations with the infection may be a result of an overlap between the physical symptoms of the disease, mental health effects of COVID-19, and circumstances of hospital admission (i.e. poor sleep, hospital environment).

However, social, and economic factors can also explain part of the link between COVID-19 infection and the development of PTSD symptoms. Fear of death from the infection, seeing others suffer and die of the disease, social isolation, fear of exclusion, uncertainty, and economic costs were previously identified as contributing factors to a high level of stress after infectious disease outbreaks [33–35]. Moreover, the immune response to SARS-CoV-2 is possibly implicated in the development of psychiatric conditions (including PTSD) after the infection [3].

Table 25.1 Factors associated with posttraumatic stress disorder after infectious disease outbreaks, including COVID-19.

Personal	Familial and societal	Infection related	Subgroup specific
• Age – Older (5)[a] – Younger (10) Gender – Male (4) – Female (25) • Low annual income • Occupation – Business units – HCWs • Education – Lower level of education – Being a final-year student • Living in a city • Smoking • Physiologic and psychological comorbidity or history • Comorbidity: anxiety, depression, poor sleep quality, higher stress level, and having physical comorbidity • History: psychiatric or neurologic disorder history, neurotic and psychopathic personality, low distress tolerance, trauma, or adverse experience • Family member having higher PTSD score • Inappropriate coping strategy • High internet addiction • Anxiolytic substances use • Negative or passive coping strategy	• Poor support network • Have/live with children • Limited living space • Marital status – Married (4) – Unmarried (4)	• Decreased support status – Quarantine – Economic loss – Poorer social life – Impact on livelihood (change in routine, less activity, work life) • Perceived high risk for infection – Being infected or having infection-associated symptoms – Knowing of/exposure to someone infected – Perception of poor hygiene in the workplace – Negative information exposure • Psychological response toward infection – Having anxious or depressive affect – Having uncertainty of the possibility of contracting infection – Perceived negative feeling toward the infection – Elevated stress level – Feel horrified, apprehensive, and helpless/loneliness because of infection – Regarding oneself as having been the target of discrimination, stigma	• Factors specific to patients – Higher disease severity – Lower levels of SaO_2 during hospitalization – Feeling discriminated against – Death of family members from infection • Factors specific to HCWs – Work in high-risk units/communities – Nurses (3) – Frontline (6) – Working in a hospital or high-risk community (1) – Technician (inadequate protection) (1) – General practitioner (1) – Nonlocal aid worker (1) • Work experience – Fewer working experiences (with exception in one study) – Lower degree of job satisfaction – Longer work shifts • Psychological response – Insecurity (fear of potential harm, death, and life out of control) followed by instability (work environment changes and assignment to high-risk units) and infection – Having colleagues infected/hospitalized/in quarantine/deceased – Concerned that people they live with may be infected

[a] Numbers in parentheses refer to the number of studies that support the identified risk factors of PTSD.
HCW, healthcare worker; PTSD, posttraumatic stress disorder.
Source: Yuan et al. [30].

In fact, the risk is not uniform, and some patients are at more risk for development of PTSD than others [32]. A number of studies focused on understanding the different predictors for the development of PTSD symptoms in patients who have recovered from COVID-19 infection. A systemic review and meta-analysis by Yuan et al. [30] examining the prevalence of PTSD after infectious disease pandemics (including COVID-19) identified a number of risk factors across 70 studies. Table 25.1 summarizes these findings.

The findings underscore the importance of looking beyond treating the physical symptoms of infectious diseases and dedicating efforts to early detection and treatment of PTSD. In fact, there are significant individual and societal gains from early detection and management of PTSD, while if left untreated it can adversely impact people's personal, family, and social life [31, 36, 37]. Available treatment for PTSD includes psychological therapy, such as group or individual trauma-focused CBT, eye movement desensitization or reprocessing therapy, as well as pharmaceutical intervention, usually in the form of antidepressants, or a combination of the two [38].

Sleep Dysfunction

Sleep-related disorders prevent an individual from getting an appropriate amount of sleep or result in poor sleep quality long term. Sleep plays a crucial role in the maintenance of normal bodily functions, and sleep deficiency gives way to a plethora of chronic physical and mental health problems [39]. Previous studies have demonstrated the significant impact of infectious disease outbreaks on the well-being of the general population, and especially HCWs and infected individuals, as observed during the MERS and SARS epidemics [1].

The Bidirectional Relationship of SARS-CoV-2 Infection and Sleep Dysfunction

Existing studies have shown a great variability in the prevalence of sleep problems in patients with COVID-19, yet a general trend of poor sleep persists in patients. This heterogeneity in rates of sleep dysfunction across studies is speculated to be partly because of the use of different psychometric scales (such as the Insomnia Severity Index, Pittsburgh Sleep Quality Index, and Athens Insomnia Scale) and researcher-designed questionnaires to quantify sleep problems [40]. Richter et al. [41] found symptoms of insomnia persisted in 36–88% of the patient cohort; this range is significantly inflated in comparison with the rate of insomnia recorded before the COVID-19 outbreak, estimated to affect anywhere between 10% and 40% of the general population [42, 43].

In addition, a recent systematic review and meta-analysis by Alimoradi et al. [44] comprising 345 270 participants from 39 countries found the estimated prevalence of sleep problems to be highest in COVID-19 sufferers, with 57% of them presenting with symptoms of sleep dysfunction. Lower rates were reported in HCWs at 31%, while only 18% of the general population reported problems in sleep throughout the first year of the pandemic. Moreover, poor sleep quality was positively correlated with symptoms of psychological distress and higher levels of both anxiety and depression in all subgroups [44].

Similarly, a systematic review by Jahrami et al. [45] found the global pooled prevalence rate of poor sleep quality was 35.7% among all populations. Of these populations, patients with COVID-19 appeared to be the most affected, with a prevalence rate of 74.8%, which was higher than the incidence rates reported in both HCWs and the general population, who had comparative rates of 36% and 32.3%, respectively. This is not wholly unexpected given that COVID-19 is characterized by respiratory distress, and core symptoms include difficulty breathing, coughing, and fever, all of which are associated with worsened sleep quality [46, 47].

Reports are also starting to emerge detailing the residual effects of SARS-CoV-2 infection on the physical and mental health of survivors [48]. In a prospective cohort study by Huang et al. [6] in Wuhan, China, sleep abnormalities and fatigue were some of the most common causes for concern in discharged patients six months after disease onset, affecting 26% and 63% of the total cohort of 1733 survivors. Similar findings were reported in studies from the United Kingdom and France. Sleep difficulties, dyspnea, cough, and fatigue were reported in approximately a third (ranging from 24% to 30.8%) of the survivors three to four months postinfection [15, 49].

Moreover, impaired sleep appears to predict a greater susceptibility to COVID-19 and is generally associated with a worse clinical course and outcome in affected individuals [50, 51]. Huang et al. [50] compared adults with symptomatic COVID-19 and uninfected adults in China; they found that individuals who experienced poorer sleep quality and reduced sleep hours in the week leading up to a COVID-19 diagnosis had a 6- to 8-fold increased risk for severe infection.

Factors Associated with Sleep Dysfunction

Various studies have attempted to map predictive factors for the acquisition of sleep-related disorders in patients with COVID-19. Current evidence suggests that a history of poor mental health and psychological vulnerability characterized by symptoms of depression and anxiety, as well as hospital and ICU admission, longer hospital stays, mechanical ventilation, and patient stressors, to be associated with sleep dysfunction in patients [45, 52].

Studies to date are at discourse whether there is a significant correlation between sleep dysfunction and sex or mean age of those infected [1]. Subgroup analysis conducted by Jahrami et al. [45] found that the male gender and advancing age are factors associated with a higher prevalence rate of sleep difficulties. However, analysis by Alimoradi et al. [44] found female-only studies demonstrated a higher prevalence of sleep problems in comparison with both gender studies: 82% in female-only studies and a significantly lower prevalence of 54% in both gender studies. Notably, being male and advancing age are risk factors associated with more severe obstructive sleep apnea and COVID-19 infections, while sleep deprivation is believed to contribute to the pathogenesis of both [50, 53].

Understandably, patients with severe symptoms of COVID-19 reported a considerably higher rate of insomnia and troubled sleep than patients who presented with moderate or mild symptoms [41]. Severe symptoms of COVID-19 are typically accompanied by increased rates of hospitalization, longer duration of stay at medical facilities, as well as a greater risk for requiring oxygen support, mechanical ventilation, and ICU care [51, 54–56]. Such factors, typically not seen in asymptomatic or mild cases of COVID-19, may contribute to poor sleep parameters [1].

Another study of 572 patients noted a much lower prevalence of sleep disturbances in individuals hospitalized for COVID-19 (11%), but this cohort also suffered from other neuropsychiatric conditions, including obstructive sleep apnea, restless leg syndrome, and periodic limb movements, which may play a role in determining the severity of sleep dysfunction [57]. Furthermore, Zhang et al. [51] found that poor sleep in hospitalized COVID-19 patients was associated with lymphopenia, presenting as a lower absolute number of lymphocytes, which was not reported in individuals who were good sleepers. Lymphopenia in these patients was linked to a slower recovery rate, as well as an increased neutrophil/lymphocyte ratio. As such, it has been established that poor sleep dampens the immune response elicited to fight off infection in patients with COVID-19, resulting in worsened symptomatology and prognosis [51]. However, the causal relationship remains undefined because it is unclear as to what degree poor sleep results from a specific virus itself [58].

Nevertheless, studies regarding sleep dysfunction in patients with COVID-19 remain limited and for the most part do not sufficiently address important aspects, such as whether patients are symptomatic or asymptomatic, hospitalized or in the community. Moreover, among hospitalized individuals, whether patients were admitted to ICU or admitted to the respiratory unit with COVID-19 as the primary cause are largely overlooked in the current literature. As such, most studies to date report the overall impact of SARS-CoV-2 infection on the sleep quality of patients. This provides general insight into the relationship between sleep and infection status, but we cannot draw robust conclusions concerning predictive factors or the long-term effects of COVID-19 on sleep [59].

Management of Sleep-Associated Disorders

Appropriate management strategies and interventions are necessary to tackle the pandemic-related sleep dysfunction observed throughout the different societal populations. Data clearly demonstrate that symptoms of sleep dysfunction persist in a great portion of the patients diagnosed with COVID-19, exceeding the portion of the general population who are affected by sleep-related disorders. This highlights the need to improve sleep quality, because it may be a decisive factor in recovery progression and disease outcome for individuals suffering from COVID-19.

Tailored and appropriate management strategies are required to reduce environmental and iatrogenic stressors, ensuring patients are offered suitable psychological and pharmacologic support as needed. Sleeping conditions can be improved by reducing exposure to light and noise during the duration of hospitalization, as well as by ensuring patients are given privacy during sleeping hours [41]. Accompanying these preventative measures, CBT is recommended as a first-line treatment option for patients with insomnia, as outlined by the European Sleep Research Society and American Academy of Sleep Medicine [60, 61]. Alternative nonpharmacologic interventions to tackle pandemic-related sleep problems could potentially include progressive muscular relaxation or yoga [60]. Medication strategies can be explored in cases of chronic insomnia where CBT has failed and in the presence of psychiatric comorbidities, such as depression or anxiety, because they are believed to have a reciprocal relationship with insomnia [62, 63].

In terms of pharmacologic means, adjuvant treatment with melatonin or melatonin receptor agonists has been suggested to improve sleep quality in patients with COVID-19 [64, 65] and delirium in hospitalized patients with COVID-19 [66]. The antiviral action of melatonin is indirect, as summarized by Reiter et al. [67], acting through its anti-inflammatory, antioxidant, and immune-enhancing properties, making it suitable as an adjuvant treatment for COVID-19 [65, 67, 68]. In addition, fluvoxamine, a selective serotonin reuptake inhibitor, has shown promising results in limiting disease progression in COVID-19 outpatients with symptoms ranging from mild to moderate [69]. Fluvoxamine may have a beneficial effect on the sleep–wake cycle of patients with COVID-19 through its well-characterized effect on the plasma concentration of melatonin in the body, increasing levels by 2- to 3-fold at nighttime [70]. A multidisciplinary approach can help improve sleep quality in patients with COVID-19 and, in turn, improve the chances of a faster recovery and a better clinical outcome. Table 25.2 summarizes these management strategies.

Neuropsychiatric Sequelae

A plethora of existing evidence suggests that a significant proportion of patients with COVID-19 are at risk for developing various psychiatric and neuropsychiatric complications, which are one of the fundamental constituents of long COVID syndrome. Neuropsychiatric sequelae associated with COVID-19 comprise neurologic, psychiatric, and cognitive problems because of direct or indirect effects on the brain caused by the SARS-CoV-2 virus [72].

Table 25.2 Management strategies for sleep dysfunction.

Prevention	• Early and accurate detection of sleep dysfunction and associated psychological distress • Personalized treatment
Improvement of sleep hygiene	• Adopt measures to reduce noise and lighting • Chronotherapy • Ensure privacy of patients during hospital stay • Provision of psychological and emotional support • Provision of sedation and analgesia when necessary
Medication strategies	• Melatonin and melatonin receptor agonists
Insomnia	• CBT, possible even via telemedicine • Progressive muscular relaxation • Medication, administered for chronic insomnia where CBT is not possible/has failed or in the presence of other psychiatric comorbidities
Obstructive sleep apnea	• Sleep laboratories should adapt according to local COVID-19 prevalence • Home testing in uncomplicated patients • Home positive airway pressure could be employed using telemonitoring in uncomplicated patients • Telemedicine may be used for evaluation and follow-up appointments

CBT, cognitive behavioral therapy.
Source: Pataka et al. [71].

The evidence thus far has shown a significant variability in the prevalence of neuropsychiatric sequelae. A systematic review by Kumar et al. [73] suggests that 20–40% of patients may be at risk for development of neuropsychiatric complications during or shortly after COVID-19 infection, such as cerebrovascular events, headache, dizziness, encephalopathies, anosmia, ageusia, and mood problems. In addition, a retrospective study by Delorme et al. [74] selected 245 patients, who were hospitalized with COVID-19 and who developed de novo neuropsychiatric complications, which included motor weakness (41%), cognitive disturbances (35%), impaired consciousness

(26%), psychiatric disturbance (24%), headache (20%), and behavioral disturbance (18%). Interestingly, nearly half of the patients were admitted to ICU, which could have contributed to such a high number of neurologic complications.

Generally, the existing studies indicate the pattern of improvement in neuropsychiatric symptoms over time. Similarly, the severity of COVID-19 infection seems to be of relevance, although patients with mild or asymptomatic COVID-19 and especially those who do not require hospital admission remain underrepresented in current research, which makes it difficult to generalize the data and draw firm conclusions around the predictive factors [75]. The impact of ethnicity and the course and frequency of neuropsychiatric symptoms in the long run also remain unclear [75].

Pathophysiology of Neuropsychiatric Complications Associated with COVID-19

The underlying pathophysiologic mechanisms of neuropsychiatric sequelae associated with COVID-19 are not fully understood; however, different routes of entry and mechanisms of potential viral damage have been proposed. Based on previous experience with SARS-CoV-1 and MERS-CoV, four such mechanisms leading to neuropsychiatric complications have been most commonly described [76, 77]:

1) Neurotropism and neuroinvasion via blood–brain barrier and/or axonal migration across olfactory neurons
2) Damage caused to cerebral vessels and coagulopathies leading to ischemic or hemorrhagic strokes
3) Extreme systemic inflammatory responses ("cytokine storm") leading to immune cell infiltration and subsequent brain damage
4) Peripheral organ dysfunctions leading to global ischemia secondary to, for example, respiratory insufficiency and acute respiratory distress syndrome; complex multisystem failures, including electrolyte imbalances, renal and liver impairments, that may lead to delirium

Some authors reported that 34% of patients with COVID-19 showed several brain abnormalities, such as white matter hyperintensities and hypodensities, microhemorrhages, hemorrhages, and infarcts [78,

79]. Furthermore, Delorme et al. [74] found that acute cerebrovascular disorders consisted mostly of ischemic strokes, and the authors cautioned that delirium without a focal deficit could be an unusual first stroke presentation in patients with COVID-19. Both magnetic resonance imaging and electroencephalographic abnormalities associated with COVID-19 have been widely described, although screening of the cerebrospinal fluid showed no evidence of SARS-CoV-2.

Cognitive Impairment Associated with COVID-19

Cognitive deficits have been reported during both acute illness and as a persisting symptom after recovery from COVID-19. The World Health Organization has recognized acute confusion as one of the core symptoms of COVID-19 illness at presentation. A rapid review of 229 studies by Hawkins et al. [80] found that more than 50% of patients admitted to ICU experienced delirium. Even though the included studies had limited data on the clinical outcomes and their results were also largely dependent on the population and the setting, delirium was found to be linked with poorer outcomes, including longer duration of hospital and ICU stay, increased mortality, worse physical function, and prolonged cognitive impairment.

A recent comprehensive review by Schou et al. [81] identified 27 studies reporting a wide range of cognitive deficits in patients who were followed up between one day and seven months after disease onset. Highlighted risk factors were disease severity, duration of symptoms, and female sex. The cognitive deficits included concentration problems; short-term memory deficits; general memory loss; a specific decline in attention, memory, language, and praxis abilities; encoding and verbal fluency; and an International Classification of Disease, Tenth Revision diagnosis of dementia.

Another systematic review of 12 studies by Daroische et al. [76] concluded that patients with COVID-19 are at a higher risk for development of a global cognitive impairment compared with healthy control subjects. It is also worth noting that attention and executive function were reportedly the most frequently affected cognitive domains. In addition, a large electronic health records study by Taquet et al. [10] found new-onset dementia to be two to three times higher in patients after hospitalization for COVID-19 compared with other medical events [74].

Long COVID Syndrome

Long COVID is a patient-coined term that has been widely used to describe the long-lasting symptoms of COVID-19 that persist beyond acute infection. However, a clear consensus surrounding the universally agreed definition is yet to be reached. The National Institute for Health and Care Excellence [82] suggests that long COVID comprises ongoing symptomatic COVID-19, sometimes called post-acute COVID (symptoms linger for 4–12 weeks after acute disease) and post-COVID-19 syndrome (symptoms last longer than 12 weeks and when an alternative diagnosis is not plausible).

The gradually emerging evidence indicates that long COVID can manifest in a wide range of physical and neuropsychiatric symptoms. Aiyegbusi et al. [83] have attempted to rank the top 10 most prevalent symptoms associated with long COVID; the list included fatigue (pooled prevalence of 47%), shortness of breath (32%), muscle pain (25%), joint pain (20%), headache (18%), cough (18%), chest pain (15%), altered smell (14%), altered taste (7%), and diarrhea (6%).

Meanwhile, d'Ettorre et al. [84] found that headaches (up to 38%), muscle weakness, dizziness, and cognitive blunting (self-reported "brain fog"), which often present along with fatigue and breathlessness, were the most common long-term neuropsychiatric sequelae, particularly in hospitalized patients. In addition, they found that both the number and the severity of acute COVID-19 symptoms, along with high levels of D-dimer, were associated with the increased risk for development of long COVID syndrome.

In contrast, a prospective study about persistent subjective neurocognitive symptoms six months postinfection, conducted by Dressing et al. [85], found only minor levels of cognitive impairment and no distinct pathologic changes in functional brain imaging (cerebral ^{18}F-FDG PET). However, fatigue was found to be highly prevalent, which is in keeping with other studies. Huang et al. [6] assessed 1733 patients and found that the most common complaints after recovery were fatigue (63%) and disturbed sleep (26%). Schou et al. [81] noted that fatigue can be reported in both more severe COVID-19 cases (requiring hospitalization) and in milder cases. Ursini et al. [86] found that a total of 189 individuals (30.7%) were diagnosed with fibromyalgia after three to nine months from COVID-19 infection. The male gender and obesity were associated with significantly increased risk for post-COVID fibromyalgia.

Management of Delirium and Long COVID Syndrome

Current literature around management of delirium is limited by the lack of use of validated screening tools and published randomized controlled trials. Nonetheless, expert consensus articles suggest that prevention of delirium and identification of the underlying and precipitating factors should be the primary management strategy. Nonpharmacologic management remains the mainstay of delirium treatment. There does not appear to be a consensus on pharmacologic management of delirium because many of the studies showed differing opinions, and further research is required before evidence-based recommendations can be made [80].

Because long COVID affects many systems in the body, rehabilitation with a multidisciplinary approach should be used. It has been suggested that this service should include mental health input, nutrition, breathing exercises, and resistance training alongside pharmaceutical treatment. A systematic review on the topic suggested that more investment needs to be targeted toward psychological and social support to aid recovery, including peer support groups and face-to-face contact with healthcare professionals [87].

Conclusions

Ultimately, the ongoing pandemic has had a profound effect on the physiologic and mental well-being of patients with COVID-19, as well as HCWs and the general population. Stressors such as government lockdowns, social isolation, financial instability, fear of viral transmission, and death affected the entirety of the global population. Moreover, evidence suggests a significant impact on both the physical and the mental health of patients with COVID-19, as they continue to be disproportionately affected by the pandemic. This results in a variety of neurologic, psychiatric, and cognitive problems caused by the direct and indirect effects of the SARS-CoV-2 virus. However, the impact of both acute and chronic phases of the illness remains largely elusive, and long-term implications for these patients are yet to be determined with the continuity of the current health crisis. Because patients with COVID-19 remain a vulnerable group who are highly susceptible to developing symptoms of psychological distress, it is important that tailored and appropriate management strategies are used in a timely manner to support their physical and mental health well-being. Study of the prolonged neuropsychiatric sequelae after recovery from COVID-19 is also imperative in establishing a multidisciplinary approach to caring for patients during both active infection and recovery.

References

1 Deng, J., Zhou, F., Hou, W. et al. (2021). The prevalence of depression, anxiety, and sleep disturbances in COVID-19 patients: a meta-analysis. *Ann. N. Y. Acad. Sci.* 1486 (1): 90–111. https://doi.org/10.1111/nyas.14506.

2 Zarocostas, J. (2020). How to fight an infodemic. *Lancet* 395 (10225): 676. https://doi.org/10.1016/S0140-6736(20)30461-X.

3 Mazza, M.G., De Lorenzo, R., Conte, C. et al. (2020). Anxiety and depression in COVID-19 survivors: role of inflammatory and clinical predictors. *Brain Behav. Immun.* 89: 594–600. https://doi.org/10.1016/j.bbi.2020.07.037.

4 Hatch, R., Young, D., Barber, V. et al. (2018). Anxiety, depression and post traumatic stress disorder after critical illness: a UK-wide prospective cohort study. *Crit. Care* 22 (1): 310. https://doi.org/10.1186/s13054-018-2223-6.

5 Fancourt, D., Steptoe, A., and Bu, F. (2021). Trajectories of anxiety and depressive symptoms during enforced isolation due to COVID-19 in England: a longitudinal observational study. *Lancet Psychiatry* 8 (2): 141–149. https://doi.org/10.1016/S2215-0366(20)30482-X.

6 Huang, C., Huang, L., Wang, Y. et al. (2021). 6-month consequences of COVID-19 in patients discharged from hospital: a cohort study. *Lancet* 397 (10270): 220–232. https://doi.org/10.1016/S0140-6736(20)32656-8.

7 Matalon, N., Dorman-Ilan, S., Hasson-Ohayon, I. et al. (2021). Trajectories of post-traumatic stress symptoms, anxiety, and depression in hospitalized COVID-19 patients: a one-month follow-up. *J. Psychosom. Res.* 143: 110399. https://doi.org/10.1016/j.jpsychores.2021.110399.

8 Phiri, P., Delanerolle, G., Al-Sudani, A., and Rathod, S. (2021). COVID-19 and black, Asian, and minority ethnic communities: a complex relationship without just cause. *JMIR Public Health Surveill.* 7 (2): e22581. https://doi.org/10.2196/22581.

9 Memon, A., Taylor, K., Mohebati, L.M. et al. (2016). Perceived barriers to accessing mental health services among black and minority ethnic (BME) communities: a qualitative study in Southeast England. *BMJ Open* 6 (11): e012337. https://doi.org/10.1136/bmjopen-2016-012337.

10 Taquet, M., Geddes, J.R., Husain, M. et al. (2021). 6-month neurological and psychiatric outcomes in 236 379 survivors of COVID-19: a retrospective cohort study using electronic health records. *Lancet Psychiatry* 8 (5): 416–427. https://doi.org/10.1016/S2215-0366(21)00084-5.

11 Writing Committee for the COMEBAC Study Group, Morin, L., Savale, L. et al. (2021). Four-month clinical status of a cohort of patients after hospitalization for COVID-19. *JAMA* 325 (15): 1525–1534. https://doi.org/10.1001/jama.2021.3331.

12 Lorkiewicz, P. and Waszkiewicz, N. (2021). Biomarkers of post-COVID depression. *J. Clin. Med.* 10 (18): 4142. https://doi.org/10.3390/jcm10184142.

13 Huang, C., Wang, Y., Li, X. et al. (2020). Clinical features of patients infected with 2019 novel coronavirus in Wuhan, China. *Lancet* 395 (10223): 497–506. https://doi.org/10.1016/S0140-6736(20)30183-5.

14 Parker, C., Shalev, D., Hsu, I. et al. (2021). Depression, anxiety, and acute stress disorder among patients hospitalized with COVID-19: a prospective cohort study. *J. Acad. Consult. Liaison Psychiatry*

62 (2): 211–219. https://doi.org/10.1016/j.psym.2020.10.001.

15 Arnold, D.T., Hamilton, F.W., Milne, A. et al. (2021). Patient outcomes after hospitalisation with COVID-19 and implications for follow-up: results from a prospective UK cohort. *Thorax* 76 (4): 399–401. https://doi.org/10.1136/thoraxjnl-2020-216086.

16 de Graaf, M.A., Antoni, M.L., Ter Kuile, M.M. et al. (2021). Short-term outpatient follow-up of COVID-19 patients: a multidisciplinary approach. *EClinicalMedicine* 32: 100731. https://doi.org/10.1016/j.eclinm.2021.100731.

17 Scarr, E., Millan, M.J., Bahn, S. et al. (2015). Biomarkers for psychiatry: the journey from fantasy to fact, a report of the 2013 CINP think tank. *Int. J. Neuropsychopharmacol.* 18 (10): pyv042. https://doi.org/10.1093/ijnp/pyv042.

18 Serafini, G., Parmigiani, B., Amerio, A. et al. (2020). The psychological impact of COVID-19 on the mental health in the general population. *QJM* 113 (8): 531–537. https://doi.org/10.1093/qjmed/hcaa201.

19 Brooks, S.K., Webster, R.K., Smith, L.E. et al. (2020). The psychological impact of quarantine and how to reduce it: rapid review of the evidence. *Lancet* 395 (10227): 912–920. https://doi.org/10.1016/S0140-6736(20)30460-8.

20 Hajure, M., Tariku, M., Mohammedhussein, M., and Dule, A. (2020). Depression, anxiety and associated factors among chronic medical patients amid COVID-19 pandemic in Mettu Karl referral hospital, Mettu, Ethiopia, 2020. *Neuropsychiatr. Dis. Treat.* 16: 2511–2518. https://doi.org/10.2147/NDT.S281995.

21 Li, F., Luo, S., Mu, W. et al. (2021). Effects of sources of social support and resilience on the mental health of different age groups during the COVID-19 pandemic. *BMC Psychiatry* 21 (1): 16. https://doi.org/10.1186/s12888-020-03012-1.

22 Liu, C.H., Zhang, E., Wong, G. et al. (2020). Factors associated with depression, anxiety, and PTSD symptomatology during the COVID-19 pandemic: clinical implications for U.S. young adult mental health. *Psychiatry Res.* 290: 113172. https://doi.org/10.1016/j.psychres.2020.113172.

23 Qian, Y., Xu, H., Diao, J. et al. (2021). Influence of life intervention on anxiety, depression, and quality of life of COVID-19 patients: a protocol for systematic review and meta-analysis. *Medicine* 100 (18): e25391. https://doi.org/10.1097/MD.0000000000025391.

24 Li, J., Li, X., Jiang, J. et al. (2020). The effect of cognitive behavioral therapy on depression, anxiety, and stress in patients with COVID-19: a randomized controlled trial. *Front. Psychiatry* 11: 580827. https://doi.org/10.3389/fpsyt.2020.580827.

25 Hofmann, S.G., Asmundson, G.J., and Beck, A.T. (2013). The science of cognitive therapy. *Behav. Ther.* 44 (2): 199–212. https://doi.org/10.1016/j.beth.2009.01.007.

26 Jerath, R., Edry, J.W., Barnes, V.A., and Jerath, V. (2006). Physiology of long pranayamic breathing: neural respiratory elements may provide a mechanism that explains how slow deep breathing shifts the autonomic nervous system. *Med. Hypotheses* 67 (3): 566–571. https://doi.org/10.1016/j.mehy.2006.02.042.

27 Liu, Z., Qiao, D., Xu, Y. et al. (2021). The efficacy of computerized cognitive behavioral therapy for depressive and anxiety symptoms in patients with COVID-19: randomized controlled trial. *J. Med. Internet Res.* 23 (5): e26883. https://doi.org/10.2196/26883.

28 ICD-10 Version (2010). Available at: https://icd.who.int/browse10/2010/en#!F43.0 (accessed: 15 November 2021)

29 Forman-Hoffman, V., Middleton, J.C., Feltner C, et al. (2018). Psychological and pharmacological treatments for adults with posttraumatic stress disorder: a systematic review update [Comparative Effectiveness Review, No. 207, Table B-1]. Rockville, MD: Agency for Healthcare Research and Quality; https://www.ncbi.nlm.nih.gov/books/NBK525129/table/appb.tab1 (accessed 15 Nov 2021).

30 Yuan, K., Gong, Y.M., Liu, L. et al. (2021). Prevalence of posttraumatic stress disorder after infectious disease pandemics in the twenty-first century, including COVID-19: a meta-analysis and systematic review. *Mol. Psychiatry* 26 (9): 4982–4998. https://doi.org/10.1038/s41380-021-01036-x.

31 Bo, H.X., Li, W., Yang, Y. et al. (2021). Posttraumatic stress symptoms and attitude toward crisis mental health services among clinically stable patients with COVID-19 in China. *Psychol. Med.* 51 (6): 1052–1053. https://doi.org/10.1017/S0033291720000999.

32 Chamberlain, S.R., Grant, J.E., Trender, W. et al. (2021). Post-traumatic stress disorder symptoms in COVID-19 survivors: online population survey. *BJPsych Open* 7 (2): e47. https://doi.org/10.1192/bjo.2021.3.

33 Liu, D., Baumeister, R.F., Veilleux, J.C. et al. (2020). Risk factors associated with mental illness in hospital discharged patients infected with COVID-19 in Wuhan, China. *Psychiatry Res.* 292: 113297. https://doi.org/10.1016/j.psychres.2020.113297.

34 Jeong, H., Yim, H.W., Song, Y.J. et al. (2016). Mental health status of people isolated due to Middle East respiratory syndrome. *Epidemiol. Health* 38: e2016048. https://doi.org/10.4178/epih.e2016048.

35 Viseu, J., Leal, R., de Jesus, S.N. et al. (2018). Relationship between economic stress factors and stress, anxiety, and depression: moderating role of social support. *Psychiatry Res.* 268: 102–107. https://doi.org/10.1016/j.psychres.2018.07.008.

36 Kirkpatrick, H.A. and Heller, G.M. (2014). Post-traumatic stress disorder: theory and treatment update. *Int. J. Psychiatry Med.* 47 (4): 337–346. https://doi.org/10.2190/PM.47.4.h.

37 Liu, N., Zhang, F., Wei, C. et al. (2020). Prevalence and predictors of PTSS during COVID-19 outbreak in China hardest-hit areas: gender differences matter. *Psychiatry Res.* 287: 112921. https://doi.org/10.1016/j.psychres.2020.112921.

38 (2018). National Institute for Health Excellence (NICE). In: *Recommendations: post-traumatic stress disorder*. NICE https://www.nice.org.uk/guidance/ng116/chapter/Recommendations#recognition-of-post-traumatic-stress-disorder. Accessed 19 Apr 2022.

39 Alvarez, G. and Ayas, N. (2004). The impact of daily sleep duration on health: a review of the literature. *Prog. Cardiovasc. Nurs.* 19 (2): 56–59. https://doi.org/10.1111/j.0889-7204.2004.02422.x.

40 Pappa, S., Sakkas, N., and Sakka, E. (2021). A year in review: sleep dysfunction and psychological distress in healthcare workers during the COVID-19 pandemic. *Sleep Med.* https://doi.org/10.1016/j.sleep.2021.07.009.

41 Richter, K., Kellner, S., Hillemacher, T., and Golubnitschaja, O. (2021). Sleep quality and COVID-19 outcomes: the evidence-based lessons in the framework of predictive, preventive and personalised (3P) medicine. *EPMA J.* 12 (2): 221–241. https://doi.org/10.1007/s13167-021-00245-2.

42 Bhaskar, S., Hemavathy, D., and Prasad, S. (2016). Prevalence of chronic insomnia in adult patients and its correlation with medical comorbidities. *J. Fam. Med. Prim. Care* 5 (4): 780–784. https://doi.org/10.4103/2249-4863.201153.

43 Patel, D., Steinberg, J., and Patel, P. (2018). Insomnia in the elderly: a review. *J. Clin. Sleep Med.* 14 (6): 1017–1024. https://doi.org/10.5664/jcsm.7172.

44 Alimoradi, Z., Broström, A., Tsang, H. et al. (2021). Sleep problems during COVID-19 pandemic and its' association to psychological distress: a systematic review and meta-analysis. *EClinicalMedicine* 36: 100916. https://doi.org/10.1016/j.eclinm.2021.100916.

45 Jahrami, H., BaHammam, A.S., Bragazzi, N.L. et al. (2021). Sleep problems during the COVID-19 pandemic by population: a systematic review and meta-analysis. *J. Clin. Sleep Med.* 17 (2): 299–313. https://doi.org/10.5664/jcsm.8930.

46 Ferrando, C., Suarez-Sipmann, F., Mellado-Artigas, R. et al. COVID-19 Spanish ICU Network(2020). Clinical features, ventilatory management, and outcome of ARDS caused by COVID-19 are similar to other causes of ARDS. *Intensive Care Med.* 46 (12): 2200–2211. https://doi.org/10.1007/s00134-020-06192-2.

47 Singh, K., Chaubey, G., Chen, J., and Suravajhala, P. (2020). Decoding SARS-CoV-2 hijacking of host mitochondria in COVID-19 pathogenesis. *Am. J. Physiol. Cell Physiol.* 319 (2): C258–C267. https://doi.org/10.1152/ajpcell.00224.2020.

48 Nalbandian, A., Sehgal, K., Gupta, A. et al. (2021). Post-acute COVID-19 syndrome. *Nat. Med.* 27 (4): 601–615. https://doi.org/10.1038/s41591-021-01283-z.

49 Garrigues, E., Janvier, P., Kherabi, Y. et al. (2020). Post-discharge persistent symptoms and health-related quality of life after hospitalization for COVID-19. *J. Infect.* 81 (6): e4–e6. https://doi.org/10.1016/j.jinf.2020.08.029.

50 Huang, B., Niu, Y., Zhao, W. et al. (2020). Reduced sleep in the week prior to diagnosis of COVID-19 is associated with the severity of COVID-19. *Nat. Sci. Sleep* 12: 999–1007. https://doi.org/10.2147/NSS.S263488.

51 Zhang, J., Xu, D., Xie, B. et al. (2020). Poor-sleep is associated with slow recovery from lymphopenia and an increased need for ICU care in hospitalized patients with COVID-19: a retrospective cohort study. *Brain Behav. Immun.* 88: 50–58. https://doi.org/10.1016/j.bbi.2020.05.075.

52 LeBlanc, M., Mérette, C., Savard, J. et al. (2009). Incidence and risk factors of insomnia in a population-based sample. *Sleep* 32 (8): 1027–1037. https://doi.org/10.1093/sleep/32.8.1027.

53 Salles, C. and Mascarenhas Barbosa, H. (2020). COVID-19 and obstructive sleep apnea. *J. Clin. Sleep Med.* 16 (9): 1647. https://doi.org/10.5664/jcsm.8606.

54 Ahmed, G.K., Khedr, E.M., Hamad, D.A. et al. (2021). Long term impact of Covid-19 infection on sleep and mental health: a cross-sectional study. *Psychiatry Res.* 305: 114243. https://doi.org/10.1016/j.psychres.2021.114243.

55 Hu, Y., Chen, Y., Zheng, Y. et al. (2020). Factors related to mental health of inpatients with COVID-19 in Wuhan, China. *Brain Behav. Immun.* 89: 587–593. https://doi.org/10.1016/j.bbi.2020.07.016.

56 Vitale, J.A., Perazzo, P., Silingardi, M. et al. (2020). Is disruption of sleep quality a consequence of severe Covid-19 infection? A case-series examination. *Chronobiol. Int.* 37 (7): 1110–1114. https://doi.org/10.1080/07420528.2020.1775241.

57 Goldstein, C.A., Rizvydeen, M., Conroy, D.A. et al. (2021). The prevalence and impact of pre-existing sleep disorder diagnoses and objective sleep parameters in patients hospitalized for COVID-19. *J. Clin. Sleep Med.* 17 (5): 1039–1050. https://doi.org/10.5664/jcsm.9132.

58 Wesselius, H.M., van den Ende, E.S., Alsma, J. et al. (2018). Quality and quantity of sleep and factors associated with sleep disturbance in hospitalized patients. *JAMA Intern. Med.* 178 (9): 1201–1208. https://doi.org/10.1001/jamainternmed.2018.2669.

59 Bhat, S. and Chokroverty, S. (2021). Sleep disorders and COVID-19. *Sleep Med.* https://doi.org/10.1016/j.sleep.2021.07.021.

60 Altena, E., Baglioni, C., Espie, C.A. et al. (2020). Dealing with sleep problems during home confinement due to the COVID-19 outbreak: practical recommendations from a task force of the European CBT-I academy. *J. Sleep Res.* 29 (4): e13052. https://doi.org/10.1111/jsr.13052.

61 Shamim-Uzzaman, Q., Bae, C., Ehsan, Z. et al. (2021). The use of telemedicine for the diagnosis and treatment of sleep disorders: an American Academy of Sleep Medicine update. *J. Clin. Sleep Med.* 17 (5): 1103–1107. https://doi.org/10.5664/jcsm.9194.

62 Edinger, J., Arnedt, J., Bertisch, S. et al. (2021). Behavioral and psychological treatments for chronic insomnia disorder in adults: an American Academy of Sleep Medicine clinical practice guideline. *J. Clin. Sleep Med.* 17 (2): 255–262. https://doi.org/10.5664/jcsm.8986.

63 Oh, C.M., Kim, H.Y., Na, H.K. et al. (2019). The effect of anxiety and depression on sleep quality of individuals with high risk for insomnia: a population-based study. *Front. Neurol.* 10: 849. https://doi.org/10.3389/fneur.2019.00849.

64 Zhang, Q., Gao, F., Zhang, S. et al. (2019). Prophylactic use of exogenous melatonin and melatonin receptor agonists to improve sleep and delirium in the intensive care units: a systematic review and meta-analysis of randomized controlled trials. *Sleep Breath.* 23 (4): 1059–1070. https://doi.org/10.1007/s11325-019-01831-5.

65 Zhang, R., Wang, X., Ni, L. et al. (2020). COVID-19: melatonin as a potential adjuvant treatment. *Life Sci.* 250: 117583. https://doi.org/10.1016/j.lfs.2020.117583.

66 Zambrelli, E., Canevini, M., Gambini, O., and D'Agostino, A. (2020). Delirium and sleep disturbances in COVID-19: a possible role for melatonin in hospitalized patients? *Sleep Med.* 70: 111. https://doi.org/10.1016/j.sleep.2020.04.006.

67 Reiter, R., Ma, Q., and Sharma, R. (2020). Treatment of ebola and other infectious diseases: melatonin "goes viral". *Melatonin Res.* 3 (1): 43–57.

68 Boga, J.A., Coto-Montes, A., Rosales-Corral, S.A. et al. (2012). Beneficial actions of melatonin in the management of viral infections: a new use for this "molecular handyman"? *Rev. Med. Virol.* 22 (5): 323–338. https://doi.org/10.1002/rmv.1714.

69 Lenze, E.J., Mattar, C., Zorumski, C.F. et al. (2020). Fluvoxamine vs placebo and clinical deterioration in outpatients with symptomatic COVID-19: a randomized clinical trial. *JAMA* 324 (22): 2292–2300. https://doi.org/10.1001/jama.2020.22760.

70 Anderson, G. (2021). Fluvoxamine, melatonin and COVID-19. *Psychopharmacology (Berl)* 238 (2): 611. https://doi.org/10.1007/s00213-020-05753-z.

71 Pataka, A., Kotoulas, S., Sakka, E. et al. (2021). Sleep dysfunction in COVID-19 patients: prevalence, risk factors, mechanisms, and management. *J. Pers. Med.* 11 (11): 1203. https://doi.org/10.3390/jpm11111203.

72 Rogers, J.P., Chesney, E., Oliver, D. et al. (2020). Psychiatric and neuropsychiatric presentations associated with severe coronavirus infections: a systematic review and meta-analysis with comparison to the COVID-19 pandemic. *Lancet Psychiatry* 7 (7): 611–627. https://doi.org/10.1016/S2215-0366(20)30203-0.

73 Kumar, S., Veldhuis, A., and Malhotra, T. (2021). Neuropsychiatric and cognitive sequelae of COVID-19. *Front. Psychol.* 12: 577529. https://doi.org/10.3389/fpsyg.2021.577529.

74 Delorme, C., Houot, M., Rosso, C. et al. (2021). The wide spectrum of COVID-19 neuropsychiatric complications within a multidisciplinary Centre. *Brain Commun.* 3 (3): fcab135. https://doi.org/10.1093/braincomms/fcab135.

75 Badenoch, J.B., Rengasamy, E.R., Watson, C.J. et al. (2022). Persistent neuropsychiatric symptoms after COVID-19: a systematic review and meta-analysis. *Brain Commun* 4: fcab297.

76 Daroische, R., Hemminghyth, M.S., Eilertsen, T.H. et al. (2021). Cognitive impairment after COVID-19-a review on objective test data. *Front. Neurol.* 12: 699582. https://doi.org/10.3389/fneur.2021.699582.

77 Nakamura, Z.M., Nash, R.P., Laughon, S.L., and Rosenstein, D.L. (2021). Neuropsychiatric complications of COVID-19. *Curr. Psychiatry Rep.* 23 (5): 25. https://doi.org/10.1007/s11920-021-01237-9.

78 Egbert, A.R., Cankurtaran, S., and Karpiak, S. (2020). Brain abnormalities in COVID-19 acute/subacute phase: a rapid systematic review. *Brain Behav. Immun.* 89: 543–554. https://doi.org/10.1016/j.bbi.2020.07.014.

79 Helms, J., Kremer, S., Merdji, H. et al. (2020). Neurologic features in severe SARS-CoV-2 infection. *N. Engl. J. Med.* 382 (23): 2268–2270. https://doi.org/10.1056/NEJMc2008597.

80 Hawkins, M., Sockalingam, S., Bonato, S. et al. (2021). A rapid review of the pathoetiology, presentation, and management of delirium in adults with COVID-19. *J. Psychosom. Res.* 141: 110350. https://doi.org/10.1016/j.jpsychores.2020.110350.

81 Schou, T.M., Joca, S., Wegener, G., and Bay-Richter, C. (2021). Psychiatric and neuropsychiatric sequelae of COVID-19 – a systematic review. *Brain Behav. Immun.* 97: 328–348. https://doi.org/10.1016/j.bbi.2021.07.018.

82 National Institution for Health Excellence (NICE). (2020). NICE, SIGN and RCGP set out further details about the UK guideline on management of the long-term effects of COVID-19. www.nice.org.uk/news/article/nice-sign-and-rcgp-set-out-further-details-about-the-uk-guideline-on-management-of-the-long-term-effects-of-covid-19 (accessed 15 Nov 2021)

83 Aiyegbusi, O.L., Hughes, S.E., Turner, G. et al. (2021). Symptoms, complications and management of long COVID: a review. *J. R. Soc. Med.* 114 (9): 428–442. https://doi.org/10.1177/01410768211032850.

84 d'Ettorre, G., Gentilini Cacciola, E., Santinelli, L. et al. (2021). Covid-19 sequelae in working age patients: a systematic review. *J. Med. Virol.* https://doi.org/10.1002/jmv.27399.

85 Dressing, A., Bormann, T., Blazhenets, G. et al. (2021). Neuropsychological profiles and cerebral glucose metabolism in neurocognitive long COVID-syndrome. *J. Nucl. Med.* https://doi.org/10.2967/jnumed.121.262677.

86 Ursini, F., Ciaffi, J., Mancarella, L. et al. (2021). Fibromyalgia: a new facet of the post-COVID-19 syndrome spectrum? Results from a web-based survey. *RMD Open* 7 (3): e001735. https://doi.org/10.1136/rmdopen-2021-001735.

87 Akbarialiabad, H., Taghrir, M.H., Abdollahi, A. et al. (2021). Long COVID, a comprehensive systematic scoping review. *Infection* 49 (6): 1163–1186. https://doi.org/10.1007/s15010-021-01666-x.

26

Mental Health Effects of the COVID-19 Pandemic on Healthcare Professionals

Liesl S. Eibschutz[1], Charlotte Sackett[2], Vorada Sakulsaengprapha[3], Masoomeh Faghankhani[4], Glenn Baumann[1], and Sofia Pappa[5,6]

[1] *Keck School of Medicine, University of Southern California, Los Angeles, CA, USA*
[2] *USC Master of Public Health Program, University of Southern California, Los Angeles, CA, USA*
[3] *Johns Hopkins University School of Medicine, Baltimore, MD, USA*
[4] *Tehran University of Medical Sciences, Tehran, Iran*
[5] *Faculty of Medicine, Department of Brain Sciences, Imperial College London, London, United Kingdom*
[6] *West London NHS Trust, London, United Kingdom*

Abbreviations

CDC	US Centers for Disease Control and Prevention
GAD	generalized anxiety disorder
GHQ-12	12-item General Health Questionnaire
HCW	healthcare worker
ICU	intensive care unit
MDD	major depressive disorder
PPE	personal protective equipment
PSS	perceived stress score
PTSD	posttraumatic stress disorder
SARS	severe acute respiratory syndrome
WHO	World Health Organization

The emergence of the novel coronavirus disease 2019 (COVID-19) in Wuhan, China, quickly threatened the normalcy of everyday life for millions of people as it rapidly spread across the world. In an effort to slow its transmission, many national and local governing bodies implemented policies such as social distancing, self-isolation, quarantine, mask wearing, lockdowns, and curfews. Although these mandates aimed to protect physical health by decreasing the transmission rates of COVID-19, they simultaneously jeopardized many aspects of mental well-being.

Previous disease outbreaks have demonstrated their potential to inflict grave consequences on mental health, and COVID-19 was perhaps the most harmful in this regard [1–3]. In addition to social isolation, the fear of infection from a highly contagious and potentially fatal virus, shortages of personal protective equipment (PPE), ongoing media coverage, and copious amounts of misinformation contributed to unprecedented feelings of anxiety [4]. The closure of schools and businesses disrupted daily routines, threatened employment, and engendered financial instability. Considering these upheavals, it is unsurprising that many people experienced adverse psychological symptoms during the pandemic, which was particularly true for high-risk and vulnerable groups such as healthcare workers (HCWs), who had the additional strain of working at the forefront of the fight against COVID-19. HCWs at the frontline confronted high risks for infection, unprecedented exposure to death and dying, inadequate emotional support, isolation from their families because of fear of transmitting the virus, shortages of necessary drugs and medical supplies, and an unremitting workload.

Although the prevalence of adverse psychological symptoms increased among the general population compared with prepandemic times, HCWs appear to have endured an overall greater psychological burden [5–8]. Thus, identifying both the initial impact and long-term effects of the COVID-19 pandemic on the well-being of HCWs remains of critical importance, alongside effective interventions that offer support, mitigate vulnerability, and enhance resilience.

Overview of Psychological Impact on Healthcare Professionals

Since the start of the pandemic, a fast-growing body of evidence confirmed the worsening mental health effects of the pandemic on HCWs around the world, including high prevalence rates of depressive symptoms, anxiety, insomnia, traumatic stress, and post-traumatic stress disorder (PTSD). Reports of substance abuse, burnout, and suicidal ideation and behavior in this population have also increased.

In fact, a plethora of studies confirmed the presence of high levels of affective symptoms such as depression and anxiety in HCWs around the world. In the first meta-analysis identifying the pooled prevalence of adverse mental health effects in HCWs globally, rates of depression and anxiety in HCWs ranged from 10% to 34% and 15% to 48%, respectively, depending on the questionnaire used, while pooled prevalence was estimated at around 23% for both depression and anxiety [9]. Other studies note rates of depression and anxiety as high as 78% and 60%, respectively [10].

Traumatic stress and PTSD were also frequently reported, with certain studies noting one third of participants describing moderate to severe stress and 45% of HCWs reporting symptoms in line with possible PTSD [11]. In this capacity, many HCWs indicated struggling with traumatic flashbacks, nightmares, and low social support.

Sleep dysfunction in HCWs during the COVID-19 pandemic was also a common finding; in four different systematic reviews with meta-analysis, pooled prevalence rates for sleep problems in HCWs ranged from 36% to 45%, with some studies describing up to 68% of physicians reporting poor or disturbed sleep [12]. These sleep disturbances can be characterized by decreased sleep quality/quantity and a variety of sleep-related issues (need to use sedative medications, difficulty falling or staying asleep). Recent studies also demonstrated a direct correlation between risk for contracting COVID-19 and likelihood of experiencing sleep disturbances [12]. Reduced quantity of sleep can adversely affect the immune system, thus increasing the risk for COVID-19 infection. Ultimately, sleep dysfunction or deprivation can affect cognitive functioning and increase the risk for errors, long-term psychological consequences, and HCW burnout.

In fact, a cross-sectional survey of residents, fellows, and attending physicians in New York between late April and mid-May of 2020 found that 19.6% reported burnout [13]. Even more concerning, another survey of US physicians during the pandemic revealed that 58% of physicians reported they "often have feelings of burnout," with 30% feeling hopeless or purposeless "because of [COVID-19's] effects on their practice/employment" [14]. In a UK study, the authors noted a high prevalence of burnout, with rates of emotional exhaustion and low/moderate personal accomplishment exceeding 50% [15]. Furthermore, high rates of burnout among physicians have been shown to be associated with increased suicide rates [16] and may even almost double the odds of suicidal ideation [17].

Even before the COVID-19 pandemic, a 2019 systematic review analyzing 25 studies across the world reported that the physicians are 44% more likely to attempt suicide than the general population [18]. These authors also noted that 17% of physicians showed suicidal ideation and 1% attempt suicide [18]. However, there was a considerable statistical heterogeneity in this study. In addition to these findings, the authors reported that the risk for suicide was higher among female physicians, as well as some specialties such as anesthesiology, psychiatry, general practitioner, and general surgery [18], which may correlate to greater access to lethal medications [19].

However, during the pandemic, HCWs were at an even greater risk for suicide [20–23]. In the same study that examined mental wellness in US physicians during the pandemic, the authors noted that 26% of survey respondents stated that they knew a physician who had considered suicide, while 18% reported that they knew a physician who had committed suicide [14]. Early research in this area used retrospective media reports to estimate actual COVID-19-related suicides among HCWs and identified 26 cases as of 5 August 2020, 11 of whom were physicians [24].

The press cited work-related stress, depression, suicidal tendencies, mental detachment from witnessing deaths, fear of COVID-19 infection, and confirmed infection by COVID-19 as possible suicide reasons in this sample of physicians [24].

The unprecedented toll on HCWs' mental health has also led to increased alcohol and substance misuse both among the general population and HCWs [25]. A survey administered to the US public in June 2020 noted that 13.3% of respondents had started or increased substance use as a mechanism to cope with the pandemic [26]. In addition, in a survey of intensive care HCWs, including physicians, nurses, and care assistants, 15.0% of respondents reported an increase in tobacco consumption, while 22.2% of respondents reported an increase in alcohol consumption as a coping mechanism [27].

Across most psychological outcomes, there has been a significant variability in reported figures. Confounding factors include differences in viral activity in different areas, as well as discrepancies in quarantine measures, healthcare system preparedness, HCW workload, and social support across various countries. In addition, outcome measure selection can also partly explain the heterogeneity in prevalence rates across different studies [28]. Most studies quantified mental health symptoms with the use of self-administered validated psychometric scales, while some used researcher-designed questionnaires. Different assessment tools and case definitions may compromise generalizability.

In the following section, we attempt to summarize the evidence regarding the presence of mental health symptoms in HCWs by country, occupation, and setting, while highlighting individual, environmental, and organizational predictors of poor outcomes. Furthermore, we emphasize the role of resilience and tailored interventions at different levels to enhance staff well-being and ultimately strengthen the healthcare systems.

Impact on Healthcare Workers by Country

The countries in the following subsections were selected as representative examples on the basis that they were either a COVID-19 hotspot and/or have produced a substantial amount of data on this topic.

China

One of the first studies study conducted between February and March 2020 revealed the prevalence of depression, anxiety, and insomnia among Chinese frontline HCWs to be between 23% and 30%, 17% and 20%, and 7% and 14%, respectively [5]. Conversely, in the general public, rates of depression, anxiety, and insomnia were 18–23%, 9–13%, and 7–11%, respectively [5]; Figure 26.1 graphically shows these findings. In addition to their close proximity to patients with coronavirus, frontline HCWs were also reported to endure social stigma, burnout, dwindling medical supplies, and a lack of support [7]. Hao et al. [7] summarized the findings of 20 Chinese and Singaporean

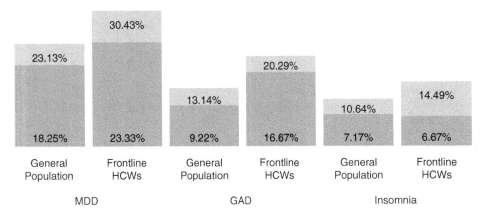

Figure 26.1 Ranges in prevalence of depression, anxiety, and insomnia in the general population versus frontline HCWs in China (2020).

studies conducted from late January through March 2020 and described a comparable 24% pooled prevalence of depression and notably higher pooled prevalence of 29% and 44% for anxiety and insomnia, respectively. This meta-analysis also reported a high prevalence of other mental health conditions among Chinese medical staff, including PTSD (26%), obsessive-compulsive disorder (16%), somatization symptoms (11%), and phobia (35%) [7].

Although it is unsurprising that a greater proportion of Chinese frontline HCWs experienced higher rates of mental health effects compared with the Chinese public, certain cultural and environmental factors may conflate these numbers. For example, Chinese culture historically stigmatizes mental illness; thus, the overall reported prevalence rates may be falsely low [29]. In contrast, due to Southeast Asia's prior history of coronavirus epidemics, such as severe acute respiratory syndrome (SARS) between 2002 and 2004, those living in the region may have had heightened responses to the COVID-19 outbreak [1, 30]. Thus, the fear of reliving the same or worse devastation that was experienced nearly two decades ago could potentially elevate the prevalence of adverse mental health effects [1, 30].

Interestingly, the 2002–2004 SARS pandemic shed light on a "typhoon eye effect," where hospitals closer to the epicenter of a crisis correlate with worse mental health outcomes [31]. This relationship has also proved to be true with the COVID-19 pandemic as HCWs in epicenters have reported serious adverse psychological symptoms [32]. This was observed in the Hubei province of China, where HCWs in Wuhan experienced higher incidences of depression, anxiety, posttraumatic stress syndrome, stress, and insomnia compared with those in the rest of the country [33–35]. Taking anxiety as an example, the prevalence among HCWs in Hubei province was 38%, which was more than 7% higher than the prevalence among HCWS working in other regions of China [34]. In addition, Wuhan HCWs were more likely to report feeling isolated, lonely, and fearful of backlash from others because of working with patients with COVID-19 [35, 36].

Another study conducted in China compared poor mental well-being between frontline HCWs and the general population, and further stratified each comparison group by those in Hubei versus those outside of Hubei [5]. This study found that those within the epicenter had a higher prevalence of depression, anxiety, and insomnia when compared with those outside of the epicenter (Figure 26.2). Specifically, the rates of depression, anxiety, and insomnia were 30%, 20%, and 14%, respectively, among frontline HCWs in Hubei, all of which were higher than the rates among frontline HCWs outside of Hubei at 23%, 17%, and 7%, respectively [5]. Similarly, the prevalence of depression, anxiety, and insomnia among the general population living in Hubei (23%, 13%, and 11%, respectively) was again higher than the prevalence among those outside of Hubei [5]. These findings demonstrate that the epicenter effect can impact both HCWs and the general population alike.

United States of America

Although COVID-19 originated in China, the United States has endured one of the most severe impacts in the world and has surpassed China in crude morbidity and mortality counts with more than 47 million confirmed cases and 775 000 deaths as of November 2021 [37]. The gravity of the COVID-19 situation in the United States may have, in part, contributed to the overall higher psychological burden observed in HCWs in New York and other hard-hit areas in the United States compared with those in China.

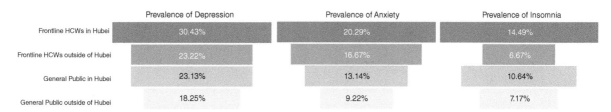

Figure 26.2 Prevalence of depression, anxiety, and insomnia in Hubei province and outside of Hubei province, demonstrating the epicenter effect among HCWs and the general public.

For example, in April 2020, a study found that 48%, 33%, and 57% of HCWs in New York City (NYC) screened positive for symptoms of depression, anxiety, and traumatic stress, respectively, which was substantially higher than the prevalence recorded in Chinese HCWs surveyed in early 2020 [8]. Around the same time, approximately one month after the United States declared a state of emergency due to COVID-19, an online survey of US adults indicated that 43%, 45%, 32%, and 62% screened positive for high levels of depression, anxiety, PTSD, and loneliness, respectively [38]. Thus, although the prevalence of depression was similar between NYC HCWs and the general US population, the latter appeared to have substantially higher rates of anxiety than HCWs in NYC. This finding, albeit counterintuitive, may be attributed to social isolation, shutdowns of businesses and schools, excessive media coverage surrounding the pandemic, and the United States' recent classification of the pandemic as a state of emergency – all of which likely fueled concern and public fear.

The epicenter effect was also shown to be present in the United States. NYC, an early epicenter of the epidemic in America, was reported to have HCWs with a higher mental health burden than those in the Midwest (Midwest HCWs served as the reference population) [33]. In fact, HCWs in the Northeast had 19%, 50%, 50%, and 34% higher odds of probable depression, anxiety, traumatic stress/PTSD, and alcohol use disorder, respectively, when compared with HCWs in the Midwest [33]. Hence these data demonstrate that HCWs in the Northeast – the region surrounding one of the most prominent early epicenters of the pandemic in the United States – had higher odds of experiencing negative mental health symptoms compared with those in the Midwest, further substantiating the epicenter effect.

United Kingdom

The United Kingdom has had fewer confirmed cases of and deaths from COVID-19 than both the United States and India since it spread to their islands in January 2020 [37, 39]. Nonetheless, England, Scotland, Wales, and Northern Ireland have similarly seen a high prevalence of poor mental health outcomes within their National Health Service (NHS), particularly during the peak of the pandemic [40, 41]. In a multicenter survey of NHS staff during the first wave of the pandemic from April to June 2020, Gilleen et al. [40] reported that 67% of respondents screened positive for mild depression. Debski et al. [41] administered a similar questionnaire to all UK HCWs between April and May 2020 and found that 28% were actually above the cutoff for moderate to severe depression. The rates of moderate, moderately severe, and severe depression in this study were 15%, 8%, and 5%, respectfully. Both Gilleen et al. [40] and Debski et al. [41] reported comparable prevalence of anxiety among NHS workers, at roughly 31%. As far as COVID-19-related stress and PTSD, both author groups indicated that 27% of those surveyed were in the top quartile for stress, 15% screened positive for at least partial PTSD, and 61% had experienced a stressful or traumatic event related to COVID-19. Other studies revealed equally harrowing findings; in a cross-sectional study of 387 U.K. mental HCWs, more than half of respondents reported moderate or severe emotional exhaustion and low/moderate personal accomplishment, thus highlighting the burnout prevalent in this population [15]. In addition, 52% of respondents noted sleep dysfunction. This study also described an increase in potentially harmful coping strategies, such as overeating, increased alcohol consumption, and smoking.

Interestingly, the epicenter effect was not evident in the United Kingdom, because working outside of London – the epicenter of COVID-19 in the United Kingdom – was significantly associated with higher depression and anxiety compared with working in London [40]. For depression, anxiety, PTSD, and severe stress, the mean and median scores of those living in London were all slightly lower than those for HCWs outside of London [40]. When examining depressive symptoms by severity, HCWs in London had a slightly higher prevalence of mild depression than those outside of London (30% vs. 29.5%), but the reverse was true for moderate, moderately severe, and severe depression (15% vs. 13%, 9% vs. 7%, and 6% vs. 3%, respectively). Logistic regression also confirmed that those outside of London had a 31.8% higher chance of depression than those working in London [40].

Similar results were seen for anxiety with HCWs in London experiencing higher levels of mild anxiety (29% vs. 24%) and those working outside of London higher levels of both moderate and severe anxiety (20% vs. 17% and 15% vs. 10%, respectively) [40]. Furthermore, those working outside of London had 56% higher odds of experiencing anxiety than those in London.

It is unclear why the epicenter effect is not consistent across countries. Specifically, London workers were significantly less likely to be female, which has been associated with increased odds of poor mental well-being in numerous studies [7, 33, 35, 40]; this may suggest that gender is a stronger risk factor for adverse mental health outcomes than working in an epicenter. In addition, clinical staff in London were less likely to be pressured to reuse PPE, which may have contributed to decreased stress levels [40] and may have worked in a better-resourced healthcare setting, while those outside of London may have been subjected to greater deficits of critical medical supplies at least in the early stages of the outbreak. Lastly, HCWs in London may simply be more accustomed to city-related stressors, which could have translated to increased levels of resilience compared with those living in the countryside [40].

India

India has also faced incredibly high morbidity and mortality at the hands of COVID-19. Second to the United States in crude morbidity, there have been more than 34 million confirmed cases and 461 000 deaths in India as of November 2021 [37]. Two separate surveys have described a high prevalence of depression, anxiety, stress, and PTSD. In a questionnaire sent to HCWs in Karnataka between July and September 2020, 20% of those with clinical responsibilities (physicians, nurses, and hospital assistants) experienced symptoms of depression, compared with only 14% of those in supportive roles (Figure 26.2) [42]. Among those with clinical responsibilities, 24% suffered from anxiety, which declined to 15% among those in supportive roles (Figure 26.3) [42]. Another Indian study that focused specifically on the mental health of attending physicians reported that 41% of survey respondents suffered from symptoms of depression [43]. In the same sample of physicians, 38% and 32% screened positive for anxiety and stress, respectively.

The impact of COVID-19 in India was likely aggravated by shortages in both human resources and medical supplies/PPE. Although the World Health Organization (WHO) advocates for 44.5 physicians, nurses, and midwives per 10 000 population, India is far below this threshold, with roughly 5–6 physicians, nurses, and midwives per 10 000 people [44]. This deficit is likely to have contributed to the increased adverse mental health effects among HCWs. In addition, like many other countries, the impact of COVID-19 was exacerbated by deficits in lifesaving resources such as oxygen tanks [44].

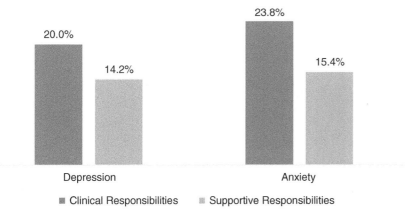

Figure 26.3 Prevalence of depression and anxiety among those with clinical versus supportive responsibilities in India. *Source:* Based on Sahoo [43].

Iran

Despite Iran's case-fatality rate of 2.2%, which was higher than that of the United States, India, and the United Kingdom as of November 2021, Iran has reported fewer confirmed cases and deaths than each of those aforementioned countries [37]. Nevertheless, the introduction of the virus into the country has caused a surge in the rates of stress and mental health issues in both HCWs and the general population.

In March 2020, a mixed-methods study conducted among the general population in all 31 provinces used the 10-item Cohen perceived stress scale (PSS-10) [45]. A total of 2204 HCWs had a median perceived stress score (PSS) of 19, which is much higher than many other groups of the general population (PSS-10 scores range from 0 to 40 with scores ≤ 13 considered as a mild level of stress and scores ≥ 27 considered as a severe level of stress) [45]. Interestingly, no significant difference in PSS was observed among different groups of HCWs. The healthcare professionals mentioned that the most common stressors were fear of disease transmission to others, competency in the management of the disease because of minimal knowledge about COVID-19 natural prognosis, a higher rate of delivering bad news to patients, and fear of death as a result of COVID-19. In this study, the second most common stressor was shortage of PPE, medical supplies and equipment, and professional human resources, while financial and job instability in private sectors ranked as the third most common stressor [45]. They also mentioned self-isolation, social stigma, difficulty in taking care of their kids, familial dispute on quitting their job, and insufficient policies against the COVID-19 pandemic at the societal level. In another survey, 487 HCWs completed a web-based Hospital Anxiety and Depression Scale in April 2020 [46]. Of 127 physicians, 25% of physicians met depression criteria and 33% met absolute anxiety criteria. Of 105 nurses, 26% reported depression symptoms and 41% symptoms of anxiety. Figure 26.4 highlights the rates of both possible depression and anxiety and absolute depression and anxiety in these HCWs.

Interestingly, the prevalence of anxiety in specialist physicians was significantly higher than in general physicians; however, the prevalence of depression did not follow the same pattern [46]. Another study conducted in Tehran recruited 296 HCWs from an inpatient setting and 532 matched control subjects from the general population to evaluate and compare the levels of stress, anxiety, and depression using Depression, Anxiety, and Stress Scale short-form (DASS-21) questionnaire from February to March 2020 [47]. Both HCWs and the community population reported clinically severe stress, extremely severe anxiety, and severe depression [47]. Although the mean scores for anxiety and depression were slightly higher for HCWs than those for the general population, there was no clinically significant difference between HCWs and the community population. Another

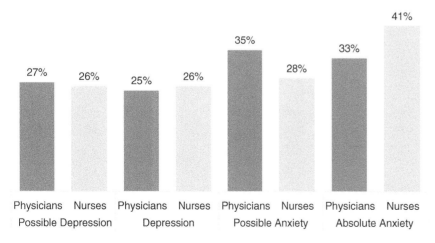

Figure 26.4 Prevalence of possible depression, depression, possible anxiety, and absolute anxiety among physicians and nurses in Iran.

hospital-based study in Tehran screened HCWs' mental health status using Impact of Event Scale–Revised and 12-item General Health Questionnaire (GHQ-12) [48]. Of 222 HCWs, 27% reported severe impact of posttraumatic distress, and 31.5% showed moderate levels of posttraumatic distress [48]. These authors also noted that nurses were most affected by the impact of COVID-19 pandemic, with 43% and 27% of them showing a severe and moderate level of posttraumatic distress, respectively. Furthermore, 62% of the participants who completed the GHQ-12 showed probable risk for nonpsychotic psychiatric morbidity. Caring for COVID-19 inpatients was associated with a higher GHQ-12 score and poorer psychological well-being.

Country-specific factors that may contribute to Iran's increased susceptibility to virus-related mental health problems include the economic fallout as a result of US-enacted sanctions, inefficient national policies to prevent the COVID-19 pandemic, and dissatisfaction with the government in addressing financial and social concerns.

Southeast Asia

Few studies describe the mental health effects of COVID-19 on HCWs in Southeast Asia. A recent systemic review by Pappa et al. [49] noted that the reported rates of depression, anxiety, and insomnia in Southeast Asian HCWs were 16%, 22%, and 19%, respectively. These rates were lower than that of other countries, but also lower than the previously reported mental health effects of HCWs in this region after Middle East respiratory syndrome and SARS. These findings may be because of the initial swift and effective COVID-19 response in Southeast Asian countries and the experience with previous outbreaks that was lacking from other countries and areas. Another potential explanation is the lower infection rates among HCWs within this region, thus decreasing the adverse mental health effects in this population. However, it is still unclear whether the lower infection rates are due to the effective COVID-19 response, lower workforce density in this region, or lack of testing availability [50]. Both HCWs and the general population reported clinically significant adverse psychological outcomes, and rates of anxiety were higher in the general population than in HCWs [49].

COVID-19 Impact by Occupation and Healthcare Setting

Frontline Healthcare Workers

As indicated earlier, healthcare professionals at all levels faced stressors such as increased workload, canceled leave of absences, unsafe working environments, as well as disruption to education, certifications, and licensing exams, all of which contributed to adverse mental health effects during the COVID-19 pandemic. However, because of the nature of their jobs, frontline medical staff experienced the highest exposure to the virus itself and to the gravity of the epidemic situation. Therefore, it is not surprising that these HCWs reported both greater prevalence and severity of most mental health symptoms.

Frontline HCWs tend to experience a higher prevalence of anxiety symptoms and generalized anxiety disorder (GAD) when compared with non-frontline workers [7, 42]. Overall, the prevalence of anxiety was 33.5% and 25%, respectively, for frontline versus second-line HCWs in China and Singapore (Figure 26.5) [7]. Furthermore, the prevalence of moderate to severe anxiety was nearly three times that among frontline workers compared with second-line HCWs, reported at 12% and 4.5%, respectively (Figure 26.5) [7].

Other authors reported similar findings regarding anxiety symptoms and prevalence of GAD, with HCWs having 54% higher odds of GAD compared with non-frontline workers [40]. An Indian study reported that HCWs with frontline responsibilities had a higher prevalence of anxiety (27%) than those with only general clinical duties (21%) [40]. In addition, frontline work was also associated with 119% and 43.5% higher odds of PTSD and severe stress, respectively, compared with non-frontline staff. Many authors have noted that the increased responsibility of taking care of patients with COVID-19 was associated with poorer psychological well-being, with one study noting "working on the frontline" as a risk factor for both PTSD and insomnia [7, 51, 52].

Studies were less congruent regarding the comparative prevalence of depressive symptoms. In frontline HCWs in China and Singapore, the overall prevalence of depressive symptoms among frontline HCWs was

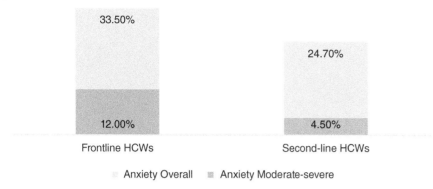

Figure 26.5 Prevalence of moderate to severe and overall anxiety in frontline versus non-frontline HCWs in China. *Source:* Based on Hao et al. [7].

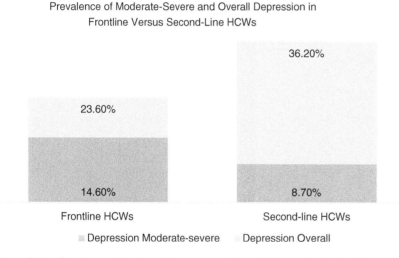

Figure 26.6 Prevalence of moderate to severe and overall depression in frontline versus non-frontline HCWs in China.

24%, while 36% of second-line staff reported depression overall (Figure 26.6) [7]. However, the proportion of moderate to severe depression was greater among frontline HCWs, with rates of 15% compared with 9% of second-line staff (Figure 26.6) [7]. Parthasarathy et al. [42] reported similar findings and stated that Indian workers with frontline responsibilities had a higher prevalence of depression at 24%, compared with the 18% prevalence among those with only general clinical duties.

The association between adverse mental health outcomes as a result of COVID-19 can be further broken down based on job title and setting. For instance, senior/attending physicians, advanced practice providers, resident physicians, medical students, nurses, allied health professionals, and administrative and management staff all faced common and distinct challenges during the pandemic and may have been impacted differently, as detailed in the following section.

Different Medical Professionals

In a survey distributed to attending physicians of the American Society for Apheresis between 26 August 2020 and 16 September 2020, the authors evaluated mental health at four time points – pre-COVID-19, during COVID-19, reopening, and the present day – and found that pre-COVID-19 well-being scores were significantly higher than any other time point [53]. Interestingly, the largest change in well-being among

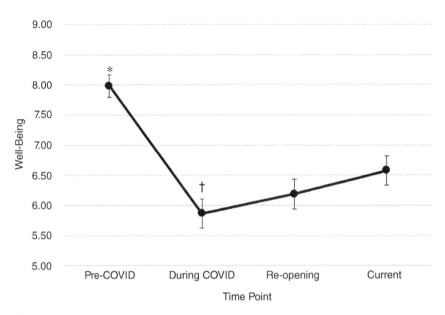

Figure 26.7 Change in mental health among attending physicians in United States during four time points. The asterisk denotes *P < 0.01 compared with "during COVID," "reopening," and "current." *Source:* Tanhehco et al. [53].

these attending physicians occurred between the pre-COVID-19 and during COVID-19 scores, indicating that this transition had the greatest impact on negative health outcomes [53]. Figure 26.7 graphically represents these findings.

True figures of the mental health effects on physicians may be even higher because of underreporting. Some authors, for example, argued that falsely low numbers may be attributed to physicians potentially experiencing self-stigmatization or fear of judgment from their colleagues [54]. A 2016 UK study indicated that although 82% of the physicians surveyed were aware of other physicians with mental health conditions, the overwhelming majority (84%) of respondents stated that they would be unlikely to seek mental health help for themselves because of fear of discrimination or stigma from their colleagues [55].

Trainees and resident physicians comprise another group of frontline HCWs who faced additional stressors related to COVID-19, aggravating traditional pressures that already put them at risk for mental illness, such as work–life imbalance, lack of control, sleep deprivation, and financial concerns. In addition to the stressors other frontline HCWs face, medical residents have also had to exercise flexibility and

resiliency by commonly enduring increased caseloads and redeployments to high-need areas at short notice and without the guarantee of adequate training or support [56].

Medical students have also experienced disruptions to their education and training, retraction from clinical experiences, modified curricula, virtual instruction, and a lack of enriching on-campus interactions and in-person activities and lack of social and peer support [26, 38, 55, 57, 58].

A global meta-analysis conducted before the pandemic reported that 34% of medical students experience anxiety [54]. Although this statistic already exceeds that among the general population, research in Australia, India, Morocco, and the United States all highlight the fact that the prevalence of anxiety, among other adverse psychological symptoms in medical students, has increased dramatically during the COVID-19 pandemic [26, 38, 55, 57].

A cross-sectional survey found that nearly two thirds of respondents self-reported a deterioration of overall mental health since the onset of COVID-19 [38] (Figure 26.8).

Rates of depression in medical students followed a similar trend. In a longitudinal study conducted on undergraduate medical students in India, 44.7% of those surveyed scored higher in depression in the follow-up survey compared with their pre-COVID-19 responses [26]. Medical students in Morocco in early April 2020 had a 75% prevalence of depression among survey respondents (Figure 26.9), while US medical students reported that 50% felt depressed since the pandemic's onset [55, 57]. Notably, those who reported at least one depressive episode during this time were also 60% more likely to experience high levels of anxiety than those who had not had a depressive episode, demonstrating the link between depression and anxiety during COVID-19 [55].

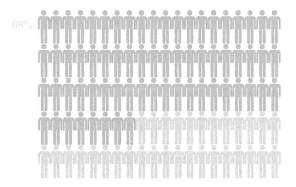

Figure 26.8 Proportion of Australian medical students who reported poorer mental health since the onset of COVID-19. *Source:* Based on Liu et al. [38].

Nursing Staff

There is overwhelming evidence that nurses were the most severely affected among all HCWs, experiencing a plethora of adverse mental health effects, including depression, anxiety, traumatic stress, and PTSD [7, 33–35, 40]. In a cross-sectional study conducted in frontline HCWs in Greece, being a nurse was a risk factor for depression, anxiety, emotional exhaustion, and depersonalization [11]. These findings may be a result of the nature of their jobs, because nurses provide the most bedside care and support to their patients. Nurses reported a larger workload, assessed by NASA-Task Load Index, compared with the other HCWs in Iran during the pandemic [52]. These nurses described more pressure in the following domains of NASA-Task Load Index than other HCWs: mental pressure, physical pressure, time pressure (temporal), and frustration.

Most study findings concur that both prevalence and odds of depression were greater among nurses compared with other medical staff. In an influential study conducted by Hao et al. [7], 25% of nurses experienced depression, but that number declined to 23.6% among the combined medical and nursing workforce. Dong et al. [34] reported similar findings, with the prevalence of depression estimated at 34% among nurses and 29% among other HCWs. Two further

Prevalence of Overall Depression and Breakdown of Depression by Severity

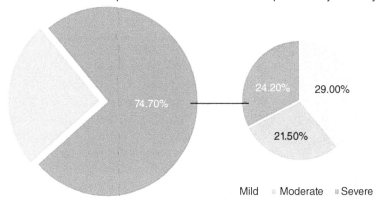

Figure 26.9 Prevalence of overall depression and breakdown of overall depression by mild, moderate, and severe levels among Moroccan medical students. *Source:* Rimmer [55].

studies showed that nurses had 132% and 56%, respectively, higher odds of probable depression compared with physicians.

Nursing staff have also experienced increased rates of anxiety symptoms compared with physicians and other HCWs [7, 34, 40]. The prevalence of anxiety among nurses (37%) was notably higher than that reported among mixed staff (23.5%) [7]. Another study provided further evidence of this discrepancy, because the prevalence of anxiety was estimated to be 44% among nurses and 29% among other HCWs [34]. Moreover, the odds of GAD were found to be 63% higher among nurses than physicians, further substantiating these findings [40].

Finally, the proportion of those experiencing stress was also greater among nurses than physicians [35, 40]. Specifically, nurses had 121% and 78% higher odds of PTSD and severe stress, respectively, compared with physicians [40]. These results were upheld in a second study that found that the odds of psychological stress were 124% higher among nurses than physicians [35].

Taken together, these studies indicate that nurses may have faced the greatest mental health burden as a result of COVID-19 compared with other HCWs.

Non-frontline Healthcare Workers

Non-frontline HCWs also appeared to experience worsening rates of mental health symptoms and in some studies even worse than those observed in physicians [5–8, 33, 35, 37, 40].

Allied health personnel constitute a large cluster of non-frontline professionals who are, nonetheless, involved in patient care and health promotion; examples include laboratory and radiologic personnel; physical, respiratory, and occupational therapists; audiologists and speech-language pathologists, and Emergency Medical Technicians [59]. One study comparing the rates of major depressive disorder (MDD), GAD, PTSD, and stress between allied health personnel and physicians [40] showed that they had 83%, 89%, 97%, and 41% higher odds of the respective mental health conditions than attending physicians [40]. The same study also reported that ambulance and healthcare assistants, specifically, had 102%, 126%, 173%, and 114% higher odds of MDD, GAD, PTSD, and stress, respectively, compared with physicians.

Two further studies reported that medical technicians had 57% higher odds of psychological stress and 334% higher odds of anxiety compared with physicians [33, 35].

The elevated levels of adverse mental health symptoms among non-frontline HCWs are possibly due to decreased clinical understanding regarding the virus' behavior and manifestations, associated protocols and management resulting in increased fear and stress.

Nonclinical Healthcare Personnel

The rapid transmission and severity of COVID-19 resulted in crippling rates of hospital and ICU admissions in many highly populated regions, forcing hospital managers to encounter medical staff, hospital bed, and equipment deficiencies.

Perhaps counterintuitively, several studies described higher odds of severe mental health symptoms among those working in nonclinical roles compared with physicians, findings similar to non-frontline staff [33, 40]. One study demonstrated that those holding nonclinical roles had 148% and 106% higher odds of probable GAD and PTSD, respectively, than attending physicians [33], while a second study noted 142%, 181%, 424%, and 226% higher odds of depression, GAD, PTSD, and stress, respectively, among healthcare management compared with physicians [40]. Similarly, in the United Kingdom, managers had a 5.2 times greater likelihood of reporting PTSD-like symptoms when compared with physicians [40].

It is evident that the pandemic has put a substantial burden on healthcare providers, creating major logistic and financial challenges for those in managerial and administrative roles.

Identifying Risk/Predisposing Factors

Risk factors for adverse mental health outcomes in HCWs during COVID-19 have been suggested. We have stratified these into three socioecological levels, as summarized in Table 26.1. Several studies suggest subpopulations who may require special attention to address and mitigate adverse mental outcomes as a result of COVID-19.

Table 26.1 Risk factors for targeted mental health intervention stratified by socioecological level.

Sociodemographic factors	Occupational factors	Circumstantial factors
Female sex	Nursing > physician	Isolation
Younger age	Medical > nonmedical HCWs	Underlying physical illness
Living close to epicenter	Longer work hours	Underlying psychiatric illness
Living in rural areas	Sleep deprivation	Viewing self as higher risk
	Shortage of PPE	Uncertainty about infection in family
		Uncertainty about infection in coworkers

HCW, healthcare worker; PPE, personal protective equipment.

Gender

A number of studies from China, Singapore, the United States, the United Kingdom, and elsewhere have provided evidence that both the prevalence and odds of several mental health conditions are greater among female than male individuals [7, 33, 35, 40].

A meta-analysis examining Asian HCWs demonstrated the prevalence of depression among female HCWs as 39%, which decreased to 30% among male HCWs [7]. Separate studies in China and the United Kingdom reported that the odds of depression were 75% and 53% higher, respectively, among women than men [35, 40]. The rates and odds of anxiety followed parallel trends to those of depression, as shown in Figure 26.10. The same meta-analysis found that 27% of female HCWs, compared with only 14% of male HCWs, experienced anxiety symptoms [7]. Similarly, the odds of anxiety were found to be 33% and 61% higher among female than male HCWs in China and the United Kingdom, respectively [35, 40].

Finally, being female was a risk factor for traumatic stress and PTSD-type symptoms. Although one study in China showed that women had only 31% higher odds of psychological stress than men, research in the United States and the United Kingdom reported that the odds of probable PTSD and severe stress were 105% and 149% higher, respectively, in female compared with male individuals [7, 33, 35, 40].

Ample evidence supports potentially important gender differences with female staff. This may be partially reflecting the already established gender gap for mood symptoms, as well as the composition of the nursing workforce. Female nurses constitute the vast majority of nurses in each major region of the world [60], and nurses have been found to experience higher rates and more severe symptoms of mental illness during this pandemic [7, 33, 35, 40].

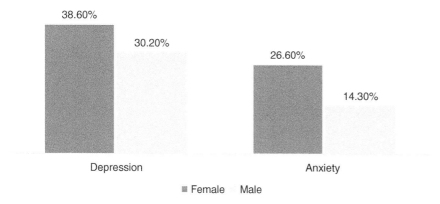

Figure 26.10 Prevalence of depression and anxiety between female and male Asian HCWs.

Age

Interestingly, several studies demonstrated that older age was associated with lower odds of mood symptoms, stress, and alcohol misuse [33, 40]. Specifically, a one-year increase in age was associated with 3% and 2% lower odds of probable GAD and AUD, respectively, among US HCWs [33]. Studies in the United Kingdom found that all age groups of HCWs older than 25 years had a decreased prevalence of severe stress compared with those younger than 25 years. For example, the oldest age group (composed of those ≥64 years old) had 63.8% lower odds of severe stress compared with those younger than 25 years [40].

Although the previous studies demonstrated older age may be a protective factor, HCWs of different age groups still reported a variety of concerns and stressors during the pandemic. A study of Chinese HCWs found that the subject matter of worry may vary greatly by age group [61]. For example, staff aged 31–40 years were more worried about infecting their family members, whereas those older than 50 years were more likely to be stressed about patient deaths. In older staff, there was also increased stress because of lack of PPE and exhaustion caused by prolonged work hours. Regardless of age, the safety of colleagues and lack of treatment for COVID-19 were universally perceived as factors that induced stress [61].

Underlying Medical Conditions

In studies conducted in China, Singapore, the United States, and the United Kingdom, underlying medical conditions were a risk factor for symptoms of depression, anxiety, PTSD/stress, insomnia, and somatization [7, 33, 35, 40].

A study from China and Singapore identified poor physical health status as a risk factor for depression [7]. Similarly, Chinese HCWs with a chronic noncommunicable disease and those with a history of mental disorders had 35% and 578% higher odds, respectively, of depression compared with those in good health [35]. Similarly, an American study found that those who were diagnosed with a prepandemic mental health condition had 149% higher odds of probable MDD than those who were not [33].

Finally, HCWs in the United Kingdom who were diagnosed with a mental health illness had 114% higher odds of depression compared with those who were not [40].

The presence of poor physical health status also provides a risk factor for anxiety and stress [7]. Chinese HCWs with a chronic noncommunicable disease or a history of mental disorders had 38% and 403% higher odds, respectively, of anxiety, and 51% and 227% higher odds of psychological stress compared with those in good health [35]. Results were similar in the United States, with one study reporting that a prepandemic mental health diagnosis was associated with 130% higher odds of probable GAD and 88% higher odds of probable PTSD among US HCWs [33]. UK HCWs with a mental health diagnosis had 61.5% higher odds of GAD compared with those who had not been diagnosed with a mental health illness [40]. Finally, previous psychiatric history was also found to be associated with more severe psychiatric symptoms in HCWs.

Alcohol use in Chinese HCWs correlated with 63% higher odds of experiencing depressive symptoms compared with nondrinkers [35]. In addition, eating disorders and changes in eating habits among HCWs were also associated with poor mental health outcomes during the COVID-19 pandemic [27]. More specifically, a significant portion of ICU HCW respondents (32%) in the aforementioned survey reported eating more than usual, while 13.4% reported eating less. In the same survey using multiple psychiatric scales, eating less was consistently identified as a risk factor for high psychiatric scores and low well-being scales in both ICU and non-ICU HCWs.

Risk for Infection and Level of Precaution at Home

A national survey of 2145 practicing internists in 2020 from the American College of Physicians assessed the prevalence of mental health diagnoses, as well as the associations between self-rated risk for COVID-19 and mental health outcomes [62]. Based on 810 respondents, the prevalence of positive screening for depression, generalized anxiety, and PTSD were 12%, 15%, and 13%, respectively, all of which were lower than previously estimated in other studies, suggesting possible resilience in this population. Of those surveyed, 13% had previously been infected with COVID-19 and reported a higher level of depression, but not anxiety or PTSD. Among those who had not been infected with COVID-19, 28% rated themselves as high risk for becoming infected and 8% rated themselves as high risk for death if infected. For those who rated their risk for death as high or very high, high levels of depression and PTSD, but not anxiety, were reported in the former population, while there were significantly higher odds of screening positive for all three adverse outcomes in the latter population.

In another survey of 3083 individuals, including but not limited to physicians, nurses, technicians, Emergency Medical Service professionals, and nondirect patient care HCWs, factors such as isolation, living alone, and taking precautions at home while continuing to live with cohabitants were associated with higher anxiety symptoms [63]. Those who reported not taking precautions at home reported lower levels of depressive, anxiety, and burnout symptoms. Thus, it seems that individuals who took more precautions in their daily life from the onset of the pandemic onset had higher levels of anxiety. However, there may be other factors that increase these individuals' anxiety, such as lack of a strong support system, work burnout, and high-risk family members.

Living Circumstances

Reports regarding the effect of living circumstances on mental health among HCWs complicates the findings reported earlier [35]. Although the survey conducted in the United States found that those living alone had higher anxiety symptoms, a Chinese study reported that HCWs with two or more children (n = 668) had 56% higher odds of psychological stress than those without children [35, 63]. This finding may be partly because of the fact that, as of July 2021, the WHO had not yet recommended the COVID-19 vaccine for younger age groups, making children more susceptible to the virus [64]. Although those who lived entirely alone may have suffered from greater anxiety because of contributing factors such as social isolation, increased vulnerability in children may have contributed to higher levels of stress among parents.

Infection Rate Among Peers

Infection among respondents, their family members, and coworkers was also related to psychological well-being. Being unsure whether a family member has contracted COVID-19 correlated with greater anxiety levels. Similarly, having a coworker contract, or be admitted to the hospital for, COVID-19 was associated with worse psychological outcomes [63]. This effect was amplified in HCWs who spent more time working with patients with COVID-19, highlighting their heightened vulnerability possibly as a result of the stress of caring for the sick and trying to protect loved ones, and the knowledge of their own increased exposure risk.

Time Spent Focusing on COVID-19

Several other risk factors have been shown to increase the risk for negative mental health symptoms. Among the Chinese general population, greater time spent focusing on COVID-19 was associated with increased odds of experiencing anxiety symptoms and poor sleep quality. Those who spent at least three hours per day focusing on the pandemic had a 91% chance of experiencing mood symptoms and poor sleep, while those who focused on the pandemic less than one hour per day had an 18% chance [36]. This is visually represented in Figure 26.11.

Similarly, exposure to COVID-19-related media coverage was also associated with adverse psychological symptoms among HCWs. Although widespread reporting played a crucial role in disseminating real-time factual information, it also increased the level of distress [5, 7, 33]. One study found that for each one-hour increase in daily media consumption, the odds of probable GAD and PTSD among American HCWs increased by 37% and 22%, respectively [33].

Demand for Personal Protective Equipment

One of the challenges that COVID-19 posed to healthcare systems was the immediate and universal demand for PPE [65, 66]. For COVID-19 specifically, PPE consists of head, face, and shoe covers, as well as impervious gown, gloves, eye protection, and respirator with a rating of N95 or higher [66, 67].

Chance of experiencing GAD symptoms and poor sleep

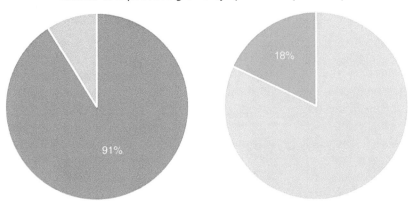

■ 3+ hours/day focusing on the pandemic   ■ <1 hour/day focusing on the pandemic

Figure 26.11 Chance of experiencing anxiety symptoms and poor sleep quality for those who spent three or more hours per day focusing on the pandemic compared with those who spent less than one hour per day focusing on the pandemic. *Source:* Yang et al. [36].

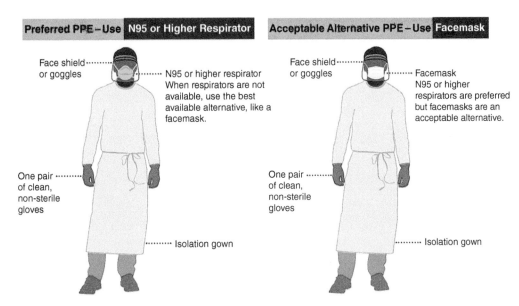

Figure 26.12 CDC guidelines regarding the proper use of PPE. *Source:* Figure reproduced with permission from COVID-19 personal protective equipment (PPE) for healthcare personnel. Infographic: Centers for Disease Control and Prevention. https://stacks.cdc.gov/view/cdc/86559.

The US Centers for Disease Control and Prevention (CDC) also attempted to aid the shortages by releasing a contingency guideline that approved the extended use, reuse, and reprocessing of N95 respirators, even though they are designed for single use [66]. If a N95 was unavailable, the CDC noted the use of a face mask as an acceptable alternative form of PPE (Figure 26.12) [68].

It became evident that these practices were not ideal. In a survey distributed to US nurses in May 2020, 87% reported having to reuse a single-use disposable mask or N95 respirator, potentially increasing the likelihood of COVID-19 exposure [69]. In addition, 28% of respondents stated that they were forced to reuse a decontaminated respirator with confirmed

COVID-19 patients, despite a lack of evidence at the time that decontamination is effective or safe. More disturbing is the finding that 27% of these nurses also described being exposed to confirmed COVID-19 patients without wearing appropriate PPE [69]. This is of particular concern given the results of a Chinese study that found that inadequate or improper use of PPE resulted in 182% greater risk for contracting COVID-19 among HCWs in Wuhan [70].

The PPE shortage also contributed to disease transmission among US HCWs, as well as increased morbidity and mortality [71, 72]. As of 2 August 2021, there have been more than 519 000 cases of COVID-19 and more than 1600 COVID-related deaths among US healthcare personnel [72]. COVID-19 exposure or infection in HCWs is extremely consequential, because it reduces the quantity of available staff to treat patients with COVID-19.

Healthcare facilities' PPE reuse directives further exacerbated the stress placed on clinical staff, who were familiar with the practice of donning and doffing traditionally single-use items such as N95 masks [73]. A meta-analysis that included studies conducted in China and Singapore noted that depletion of PPE acted as a risk factor for poor mental health among HCWs [7]. Additional studies have demonstrated that feelings of inadequate safety because of insufficient PPE resulted in symptoms of depression, anxiety, and PTSD, specifically [40, 65].

With these findings, there are opportunities for identifying individuals at higher risk for targeted interventions, as well as ways to proactively protect HCWs. Preventing mental harm and promoting well-being are essential, because future pandemics and epidemics are bound to reoccur, and preparation can help mitigate negative mental health outcomes. In addition, familiarity with protective factors should also be prioritized to prevent the progression of mental health effects.

Mental Health Interventions and Strategies for HCWs

Various models have been proposed for supporting HCWs during the COVID-19 pandemic. The National Academy of Medicine describes a tiered public health approach, using universal resources and information, targeted logistical and psychological interventions, and intensive mental health services [74]. This model enables triaging based on needs to appropriately allocate specific interventions, services, and resources. The National Child Trauma Stress Network and the National Center for PTSD have also proposed a model called "psychological first aid," which includes information gathering to identify needs, addressing immediate needs and concerns, and connecting and linking individuals in need of social support and other services [75]. These key themes may be useful when creating interventions and strategies to address specific mental health needs of HCWs [76]. Ultimately, it is imperative that mental health interventions and strategies exist at various levels, spanning from international to individual, and are used simultaneously for optimal outcomes to respond proactively and reactively to needs in the HCW population.

Interventions and Strategies at the International, National, and Regional Levels

Given the chaos surrounding the pandemic, particularly in the first few months of 2020, there were several instances of harassment against HCWs. There were reports of vandalism of public and private hospital property, particularly in hospitals that did not accept patients. Stigmatization against HCWs and lack of medical infrastructure also resulted in both physical and verbal assaults. The combination of pandemic uncertainty coupled with this increase in HCW harassment, engendered an increase in psychological distress internationally [77].

At the regional level and beyond, various campaigns have been executed to combat stigma and misinformation, which ultimately played a role in supporting HCWs. For example, international organizations, governments, and regulatory bodies began labeling HCWs as "heroes of the pandemic." Slogans such as "Not all heroes wear capes, some wear scrubs" were also circulated. In addition, measures were taken to stop misinformation through visual, print, and social media sources (Figure 26.13). The International Committee of the Red Cross and the WHO also published a checklist for HCWs to address the issue of violence against this population. This checklist included risk assessment

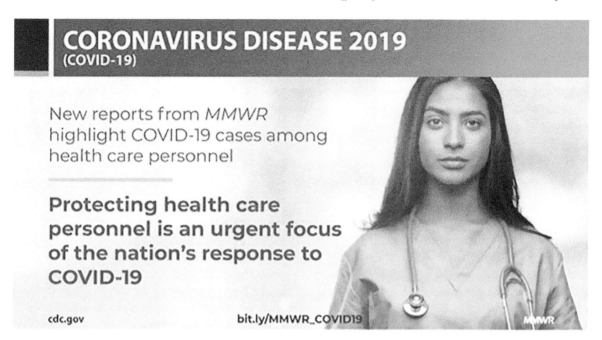

Figure 26.13 Example of a message circulated by the Centers for Disease Control regarding protecting and supporting HCWs during the COVID-19 pandemic. *Source:* Sharif and Amin [77].

procedures, as well as guidelines on response and accountability toward those receiving care.

In addition, ensuring public health information systems were accurate, up to date, and easily accessible also helped reduce the psychological impact of misinformation and uncertainty in HCWs. Many international and national agencies have created web-based resources that give HCWs current COVID-19 information and help them develop skills for addressing their mental health needs. Local governments should be encouraged to regulate how news and broadcast agencies report COVID-19-related news, ensuring that the reporting is responsible and fact based. The airing of motivational and morale-boosting programs may also allay the psychological distress experienced by HCWs, as well as the public to some degree [78].

Interventions and Strategies at the Institutional Level

Barriers to the success of mental health interventions include themes of uncertainty, inaccessibility, stigma surrounding mental health, as well as a lack of time for and access to resources. There is also evidence that HCWs tend to seek help reactively, only after the onset of distress or burnout [79]. Given these obstacles, targeted interventions addressing these specific needs are vital.

Methods that have been used in previous pandemics, such as the 2002–2004 SARS outbreak, include multidisciplinary mental health teams (composed of psychiatrists, psychiatric nurses, clinical psychologists, and other mental health workers) that were established by health authorities at national and regional levels to provide support for HCWs [80]. These specialized teams can provide treatments and services, especially for those with preexisting psychiatric disorders [80]. Medications may also be used while ensuring minimal harmful interactions with COVID-19 treatment. Counseling should also be available on digital platforms (online or phone based). Being able to share stress and having ethical support for treatment decisions has been shown to be significantly associated with fewer adverse psychiatric symptoms [40]. Both individual and group counseling would likely be beneficial, because each may cater to HCWs' unique needs. Although psychoeducation and mindfulness have been proved to be beneficial, cognitive-behavioral therapy can also be quite useful.

Studies have found that mental health programs for HCWs, in the setting of COVID-19, were implemented quickly, with little preparation, and at times overlooked safety issues such as PPE availability and training [81], which must also be addressed. Clear communication about the pandemic can provide HCWs with information that may help assuage uncertainty or fear.

Involving HCWs in planning and strategizing for the pandemic may also boost self-esteem and trust, allowing HCWs to feel that they are essential to the healthcare team. Involving HCWs has been shown to have beneficial results, including decreased job-related stress, uncertainties, fear, depression, and anxiety [82]. Papoutsi et al. [50] reported similar findings and noted that putting more experienced HCWs in organizational positions could protect against adverse mental health effects.

For those directly caring for patients with COVID-19, additional protective measures include redesigning procedures that pose a high risk for infectious spread, reducing patient density on each ward, providing better ventilation systems or safer isolation rooms, avoiding compulsory care, and allowing more flexible work scheduling [82].

Institutions have also found success in creating tiered, multifold systems whereby different HCWs are matched with designated mental health clinicians to provide emotional support and mental health support systems [76]. These clinicians were also provided the opportunity to join regular, recurring staff huddles to introduce themselves, listen to concerns, and normalize fear and stress associated with the new and uncertain realities of the pandemic. In addition, concerns can be escalated to leadership, which would allow for further tailored institutional response and support. One concrete example of this paradigm was seen at an emergency department in a hospital in Los Angeles, California. Mental health clinicians discovered that HCWs in the unit were experiencing insomnia and sleep disturbances, which prompted the work group to coordinate an educational and supportive session to address sleep and insomnia [76]. In addition, when these clinicians learned that supervisors were struggling to inspire and manage their nonclinical HCW teams given the prolonged uncertainty and ever-changing protocols, the group developed a series of department-specific leadership development courses. These sessions educated supervisors on the tenets of stress and psychological first aid, and provided them with opportunities for peer support and self-reflection so that they could use these experiences with their own teams. An additional positive outcome of this feedback system is the formation of community pods that enable HCWs' families and loved ones to connect with each other for shared child care, educational opportunities, and to share experiences with each other [76]. Parenting forums with information and communication channels to help with child development and parent strategies, especially in the setting of disasters, pandemics, and crises, were also implemented.

Proactive, prophylactic mental health support may also be beneficial. For example, at the Princess Margaret Cancer Centre in Canada, the CREATE (Compassion, REsilience And TEam-building) team-based intervention was established during the 2002–2004 SARS outbreak to provide psychological first aid and adaptive coping interventions in the frontline and oncology clinic workflow for HCWs [79]. Its goals were to enhance team cohesion and social support, facilitate emotional validation, normalize traumatic reactions, and provide mutual instruction on effective coping [79]. This intervention was designed to be delivered at the point of care, either remotely or in-person, by psychosocial coaches, which include psychiatrists, psychologists, occupational therapists, spiritual care, and music therapy.

Because CREATE uses existing psychosocial staff, it is cost-effective and can be rapidly mobilized. As such, the program was subsequently implemented during the COVID-19 pandemic. HCWs' needs, addressed by psychosocial coaches, were largely characterized by four main themes: physical (15%), social (28%), psychological (46%), and spiritual (11%) [79]. Overall, the emotional tone expressed within teams trended positively over the study period, indicating reduced team-level distress and an increase in team resilience. This model may serve as a framework for other institutions to emulate. However, limitations to this program may include difficulty in implementation if such a team did not previously exist, highlighting the importance of establishing these systems before a pandemic to allow for adequate training and preparation.

Another model used to address mental health concerns in HCWs has been the Psychological Resilience Intervention, which was founded on a peer support model ("Battle Buddies"), developed by the US Army [83]. The intervention incorporates evidence-informed "stress inoculation" methods to help manage psychological stress exposure in providers deployed to disasters. More specifically, it includes a peer support "Battle Buddy" and a designated mental health consultant who can facilitate training in stress inoculation methods, provide any necessary additional support, as well as coordinate referrals to external resources, such as external professional consultations [83].

In the "Battle Buddy" system, daily stressors and suffering are shared between many people. Buddies were assigned based on common factors such as areas of practice, clinical responsibilities, experience, seniority, and life circumstances. Pairings were made between individuals who did not have established friendships to ensure that difficult conversations could occur without the fear of jeopardizing the preexisting relationship. An example of a pocket card with information on the rationale behind the intervention is shown in Figure 26.14.

The second prong of this intervention consisted of stress inoculation in small groups, to help HCW participants recognize the importance of cognitively and emotionally anticipating and preparing for specific stressors they may face. Then, a personal resilience plan is drafted for various situations, including unique coping skills and resources. Participants are also encouraged to self-monitor for stress and ask for additional help as needed.

Interventions such as these are highly scalable, virtually costless, and require very few resources aside from the endorsement and support from institutional leaders. Although there are no numerical data yet, early anecdotal evidence suggests that this program is beneficial and easy to implement in the setting of large-scale emergencies, such as the COVID-19 pandemic [83].

In addition to direct mental health interventions, other factors related to an institution's response to the pandemic have also been found to be protective. For example, confidence in infection-control measures and intensive training on personal protective measures have been found to be associated with psychological resilience during the COVID-19 pandemic [84]. Occupational adjustments such as scheduled rest periods, shorter work hours, and flexible staffing resources may also be beneficial [35]. Rotating employees between higher- and lower-stress functions, partnering workers and creating a "buddy system" to monitor stress and reinforce safety procedures, and implementing flexible schedules for workers who have been impacted directly or have a family member affected by COVID-19 are additional strategies [85].

The WHO's Mental Health Gap Action Program Humanitarian Intervention Guide provides recommendations for first-line management of mental health conditions in humanitarian emergencies in cases where access to specialists and treatment options is limited [86]. It serves as a tool for facilities and institutions affected by emergencies such as the pandemic to assess and manage acute stress, grief, depression, PTSD, suicide risk, and other poor mental health outcomes. In low-resource settings, these guidelines may be useful as a reference for appropriate and expeditious training by institutions [86]. These guidelines are available in multiple languages, including Arabic, Bengali, English, French, Portuguese, Russian, Spanish, and Ukrainian.

Interventions and Strategies at the Individual Level

At the individual level, it is imperative that HCWs recognize signs of burnout, secondary traumatic stress, and changes in their own mental health [85]. Signs of burnout include sadness, depression, apathy, isolation, or disconnection from others and feelings of indifference or hopelessness [86]. Signs of secondary traumatic stress may include excess worry or fear about something bad happening, being easily startled, recurring thoughts, feeling ownership of others' trauma, as well as physiological signs of stress, such as an increased heart rate [85].

On recognizing these signals, it is important to take breaks and be reminded that maintaining one's own health is an important aspect of fulfilling a role in health care. Some strategies include talking to family, friends, other loved ones, supervisors, and colleagues about one's experiences. An additional benefit of seeking out social support is the production of positive psychological states, including having a sense of purpose,

COVID 19 Battle Buddy Support Program

Background: COVID-19 is a pandemic that threatens not only our patients but ourselves and our sense of safety and control. Like soldiers on a battlefield, our front line staff are coping with ongoing uncertainty about the scope of the threat, concerns about adequate PPE, and worry about the complex decisions that will be required of them. Many of us are experiencing unusual levels of professional anxiety and stress under these "battlefield conditions." This places all of us at increased risk for burnout and psychological trauma reactions. In order to mitigate these risks, we must develop cognitive and emotional resilience in ourselves and our colleagues. Our goal is to provide you with tools based on the *Anticipate, Plan, and Deter* model fostering resilience in healthcare workers who are deployed in hazardous situations.[1] The first tool is the Battle Buddy system.

What Are Battle Buddies?
The US Army uses the Battle Buddy for peer mentoring and emotional support. Having a Battle Buddy helps you to: 1) Validate your experiences; 2) Identify and address stressors early; 3) Keep work at work; 3) Develop and maintain resilience.

Who Is the Ideal Battle Buddy?
Battle Buddies (BBs) are usually chosen by a third party but in some instances pair up spontaneously. BBs are matched based on a common working environment, clinical responsibilities, level of seniority, and stage in life, but without being close friends. BBs need to be able to be supportive <u>and</u> objective when assessing stress behavior and providing feedback.

What Does a Battle Buddy Do?
The BB is a listener. BBs do a brief check-in as they share their reactions to stressors and anxieties and validate each other's experiences (e.g. "I'm afraid I'm going to bring the virus home", "I keep doing chart checks on my patients late into the evening"). BBs understand the daily challenges of a particular unit, provide each other an additional perspective, support resilience and encourage additional help if stresses and anxieties escalate. Listening and validating is not debating or arguing. If this is occurring, it is best to reach out to a mental health professional or to your employee assistance program.

How Do Battle Buddies Help to Find Solutions?
BB's support resilience: figuring out adaptive ways to cope with challenges so we can all perform successfully in a less-than-perfect environment. Daily BB conversations can also help identify specific issues that need to be addressed locally (within their unit) or that need to be escalated to leadership.

BATTLE BUDDY CHECK-IN
1-10 MINUTES

- Aim to contact your Battle Buddy 2-3 times per week or more (daily if needed)
- Contact can be a quick text to check in; a short call to debrief; a zoom meeting to hash something out
- Listen, validate, and provide feedback; identify any issues that need more support or attention
- Identify any operational issues that need escalation

Sample questions for your check-in:
- What is hardest right now?
- What worried you today?
- What went well today?
- How are things at home?
- What challenges are you facing with sleep/rest, exercise, healthy nutrition?

If you or your Battle Buddy are ready to support one another in anticipating and planning for specific stressors you may encounter, please see the back of the card.

What is The End State for the Battle Buddy Program?
1. A working environment where everyone feels supported and validated. No one is left out.
2. Work stays at work. Home is a place for relaxation and recovery.
3. A cognitively and emotionally resilient team culture.

---

[1] Schreiber et al. Maximizing the Resilience of HealthCare Workers in Multi Hazard Events: Lessons from the 2014-2015 Ebola Response in Africa. *Military Medicine* 184,:114. 2019

Figure 26.14 Part of the Battle Buddy pocket card. *Source:* Albott et al. [83].

belongingness, security, and self-worth [36]. If social distancing is a concern, journaling and participating in online communities are also potential strategies [87]. Additional coping methods include having family support, positive thinking, as well as worship according to faith, ensuring adequate sleep and food intake, exercise and physical activity, reading, and participating in hobbies and non-work-related activities [87]. Mindfulness activities and meditation have also been proven to be safe and beneficial [88]. Active mind-body therapies, such as meditation, yoga, Tai Chi, and Qigong, are considered helpful practices for improving HCWs' mental and physical health. It has been shown that active mind-body therapies had therapeutic effects for those suffering from PTSD [34]. These interventions can effectively help HCWs take their attention off stressors and are simple and low cost.

Conclusion

SARS-coronavirus 2 and the pandemic have simultaneously jeopardized both physical and mental health for billions of people across the world. Many of those who contracted COVID-19 or were psychologically impacted by the pandemic were members of the general public, who faced stressors such as social isolation, shutdowns, financial instability, misinformation or lack of information, and fear of transmission and death. However, these effects were more pronounced in HCWs who reported feelings of burnout and fear of infection and transmission, exacerbated by shortages of PPE; unparalleled exposures to death; deficits in lifesaving equipment; lack of support; social stigmatization; misinformation-fueled violence, unsafe working environments as a result of insufficient infection control and incompetence in hospital management; and familial problems, including childcare arrangements. It is unsurprising that HCWs have suffered poor mental health outcomes as a result of COVID-19. Because HCWs constitute a particularly vulnerable population, it is imperative that timely and targeted interventions are put in place at the international, national, regional, community, and institutional levels to support the well-being of HCWs and prevent long-term consequences.

References

1 De Brier, N., Stroobants, S., Vandekerckhove, P. et al. (2020). Factors affecting mental health of health care workers during coronavirus disease outbreaks (SARS, MERS & COVID-19): a rapid systematic review. *PLoS One* 15 (12): e0244052.

2 Ren, F.F. and Guo, R.J. (2020). Public mental health in post-COVID-19 era. *Psychiatr. Danub.* 32 (2): 251–255.

3 Park, J.S., Lee, E.H., Park, N.R. et al. (2018). Mental health of nurses working at a government-designated hospital during a MERS-CoV outbreak: a cross-sectional study. *Arch. Psychiatr. Nurs.* 32 (1): 2–6.

4 Islam, M.S., Sarkar, T., Khan, S.H. et al. (2020). COVID-19-related infodemic and its impact on public health: a global social media analysis. *Am. J. Trop. Med. Hyg.* 103 (4): 1621–1629.

5 Liang, Y., Wu, K., Zhou, Y. et al. (2020). Mental health in frontline medical workers during the 2019 novel coronavirus disease epidemic in China: a comparison with the general population. *Int. J. Environ. Res. Public Health* 17 (18): 6550.

6 Wang, C., Pan, R., Wan, X. et al. (2020). Immediate psychological responses and associated factors during the initial stage of the 2019 coronavirus disease (COVID-19) epidemic among the general population in China. *Int. J. Environ. Res. Public Health* 17 (5): 1729.

7 Hao, Q., Wang, D., Xie, M. et al. (2021). Prevalence and risk factors of mental health problems among healthcare workers during the COVID-19 pandemic: a systematic review and meta-analysis. *Front. Psychiatry* 12: 567381.

8 Shechter, A., Diaz, F., Moise, N. et al. (2020). Psychological distress, coping behaviors, and preferences for support among New York healthcare workers during the COVID-19 pandemic. *Gen. Hosp. Psychiatry* 66: 1–8.

9 Pappa, S., Ntella, V., Giannakas, T. et al. (2020). Prevalence of depression, anxiety, and insomnia among healthcare workers during the COVID-19 pandemic: a systematic review and meta-analysis. *Brain Behav. Immun.* 88: 901–907.

10 Sahebi, A., Nejati-Zarnaqi, B., Moayedi, S. et al. (2021). The prevalence of anxiety and depression among healthcare workers during the COVID-19 pandemic: an umbrella review of meta-analyses. *Prog. Neuro-Psychopharmacol. Biol. Psychiatry* 107: 110247.

11 Pappa, S., Athanasiou, N., Sakkas, N. et al. (2021). From recession to depression? Prevalence and correlates of depression, anxiety, traumatic stress and burnout in healthcare workers during the COVID-19 pandemic in Greece: a multi-center, cross-sectional study. *Int. J. Environ. Res. Public Health* 18 (5): 2390.

12 Pappa, S., Sakkas, N., and Sakka, E. (2021). A year in review: sleep dysfunction and psychological distress in healthcare workers during the COVID-19 pandemic. *Sleep Med.* https://doi.org/10.1016/j.sleep.2021.07.009.

13 Al-Humadi, S., Bronson, B., Muhlrad, S. et al. (2021). Depression, suicidal thoughts, and burnout among physicians during the COVID-19 pandemic: a survey-based cross-sectional study. *Acad. Psychiatry* 45 (5): 557–565.

14 Berlin, J. (2021). No escape: COVID-19 continues to exacerbate physician burnout. *Tex. Med.* 117 (2): 16–21.

15 Pappa, S., Barnett, J., Berges, I. et al. (2021). Tired, worried and burned out, but still resilient: a cross-sectional study of mental health workers in the UK during the COVID-19 pandemic. *Int. J. Environ. Res. Public Health* 18 (9): 4457.

16 Dyrbye, L.N., West, C.P., Satele, D. et al. (2014). Burnout among US medical students, residents, and early career physicians relative to the general US population. *Acad. Med.* 89 (3): 443–451.

17 Shanafelt, T.D., Balch, C.M., Dyrbye, L. et al. (2011). Special report: suicidal ideation among American surgeons. *Arch. Surg.* 146 (1): 54–62.

18 Dutheil, F., Aubert, C., Pereira, B. et al. (2019). Suicide among physicians and health-care workers: a systematic review and meta-analysis. *PLoS One* 14 (12): e0226361.

19 Gulati, G. and Kelly, B.D. (2020). Physician suicide and the COVID-19 pandemic. *Occup. Med. (Lond.)* https://doi.org/10.1093/occmed/kqaa104.

20 Hawton, K., Agerbo, E., Simkin, S. et al. (2011). Risk of suicide in medical and related occupational groups: a national study based on Danish case population-based registers. *J. Affect. Disord.* 134 (1): 320–326.

21 Schernhammer, E.S. and Colditz, G.A. (2004). Suicide rates among physicians: a quantitative and gender assessment (meta-analysis). *Am. J. Psychiatry* 161 (12): 2295–2302.

22 Hawton, K., Simkin, S., Rue, J. et al. (2002). Suicide in female nurses in England and Wales. *Psychol. Med.* 32 (2): 239–250.

23 Katz, R.M. (1983). Causes of death among registered nurses. *J. Occup. Med.* 25 (10): 760–762.

24 Jahan, I., Ullah, I., Griffiths, M.D. et al. (2021). COVID-19 suicide and its causative factors among the healthcare professionals: case study evidence from press reports. *Perspect. Psychiatr. Care* 57 (4): 1707–1711.

25 Greenberg, N. (2020). Mental health of health-care workers in the COVID-19 era. *Nat. Rev. Nephrol.* 16 (8): 425–426.

26 Czeisler, M., Wiley, J.F., Facer-Childs, E.R. et al. (2021). Mental health, substance use, and suicidal ideation during a prolonged COVID-19-related lockdown in a region with low SARS-CoV-2 prevalence. *J. Psychiatr. Res.* 140: 533–544.

27 Wozniak, H., Benzakour, L., Moullec, G. et al. (2021). Mental health outcomes of ICU and non-ICU healthcare workers during the COVID-19 outbreak: a cross-sectional study. *Ann. Intensive Care* 11 (1): 106.

28 Pappa, S., Giannakoulis, V.G., Papoutsi, E. et al. (2021). Author reply – letter to the editor "the challenges of quantifying the psychological burden of COVID-19 on heathcare workers". *Brain Behav. Immun.* 92: 209–210.

29 Yu, S., Kowitt, S.D., Fisher, E.B. et al. (2018). Mental health in China: stigma, family obligations, and the potential of peer support. *Community Ment. Health J.* 54 (6): 757–764.

30 Centers for Disease Control and Prevention (2013). CDC SARS Response Timeline. https://www.cdc.gov/about/history/sars/timeline.htm.

31 Xie, X.-F., Stone, E., Zheng, R. et al. (2011). The 'typhoon eye effect': determinants of distress during the SARS epidemic. *J. Risk Res.* 14 (9): 1091–1107.

32 Yáñez, J.A., Afshar Jahanshahi, A., Alvarez-Risco, A. et al. (2020). Anxiety, distress, and turnover intention of healthcare workers in Peru by their distance to the epicenter during the COVID-19 crisis. *Am. J. Trop. Med. Hyg.* 103 (4): 1614–1620.

33 Hennein, R., Mew, E.J., and Lowe, S.R. (2021). Socio-ecological predictors of mental health outcomes among healthcare workers during the COVID-19 pandemic in the United States. *PLoS One* 16 (2): e0246602.

34 Dong, F., Liu, H.L., Yang, M. et al. (2021). Immediate psychosocial impact on healthcare workers during COVID-19 pandemic in China: a systematic review and meta-analysis. *Front. Psychol.* 12: 645460.

35 Zhu, Z., Xu, S., Wang, H. et al. (2020). COVID-19 in Wuhan: sociodemographic characteristics and hospital support measures associated with the immediate psychological impact on healthcare workers. *EClinicalMedicine* 24: 100443.

36 Yang, Y., Lu, L., Chen, T. et al. (2021). Healthcare worker's mental health and their associated predictors during the epidemic peak of COVID-19. *Psychol. Res. Behav. Manag.* 14: 221–231.

37 Johns Hopkins University & Medicine. Mortality analyses. (2021). https://coronavirus.jhu.edu/data/mortality.

38 Liu, C.H., Zhang, E., Wong, G.T.F. et al. (2020). Factors associated with depression, anxiety, and PTSD symptomatology during the COVID-19 pandemic: clinical implications for US young adult mental health. *Psychiatry Res.* 290: 113172.

39 Public Health England. Coronavirus (COVID-19) in the UK. (2021). https://coronavirus.data.gov.uk/details/cases.

40 Gilleen, J., Santaolalla, A., Valdearenas, L. et al. (2021). Impact of the COVID-19 pandemic on the mental health and well-being of UK healthcare workers. *BJPsych Open* 7 (3): e88.

41 Debski, M., Abdelaziz, H.K., Sanderson, J. et al. (2021). Mental health outcomes among British healthcare workers – lessons from the first wave of the Covid-19 pandemic. *J. Occup. Environ. Med.* 63 (8): e549–e555.

42 Parthasarathy, R., Jaisoorya, T.S., Thennarasu, K. et al. (2021). Mental health issues among health care workers during the COVID-19 pandemic – a study from India. *Asian J. Psychiatr.* 58: 102626.

43 Sahoo, A.,.,B.S. (2020). Impact of Covid-19 pandemic on mental health of healthcare workers in India: a questionnaire based study. *Integr. J. Med. Sci.* 7: 1–4. https://doi.org/10.15342/ijms.7.205.

44 Karan, A., Negandhi, H., Hussain, S. et al. (2021). Size, composition and distribution of health workforce in India: why, and where to invest? *Hum. Resour. Health* 19 (1): 39.

45 Faghankhani, M., Sodagari, F., Shokrani, M. et al. (2021). Perceived stress among Iranians during COVID-19 pandemic; stressors and coping mechanisms: a mixed-methods approach: stress percu chez les Iraniens Durant la pandemie de la COVID-19; stresseurs et mecanismes d'adaptation: Une approche de methodes mixtes. *Can. J. Psychiatr.* https://doi.org/10.1177/07067437211004881.

46 Hassannia, L., Taghizadeh, F., Moosazadeh, M. et al. (2021). Anxiety and depression in health workers and general population during COVID-19 in IRAN: a cross-sectional study. *Neuropsychopharmacol. Rep.* 41 (1): 40–49.

47 Saffari, M., Raei, M., Pourhoseingholi, M.A. et al. (2021). Psychological aspects of COVID-19 in Iran: how the disease may affect mental health of medical staff and general population? *Int. J. Travel Med. Glob. Health* 9 (2): 94–99.

48 Kheradmand, A., Mahjani, M., Pirsalehi, A. et al. (2021). Mental health status among healthcare workers during COVID-19 pandemic. *Iran. J. Psychiatry* 16 (3): 250–259.

49 Pappa, S., Chen, J., Barnet, J. et al. (2022). A systematic review and meta-analysis of the mental health symptoms during the Covid-19 pandemic in Southeast Asia. *Psychiatry Clin. Neurosci* 76 (2): 41–50.

50 Papoutsi, E., Giannakoulis, V.G., Ntella, V. et al. (2020). Global burden of COVID-19 pandemic on healthcare workers. *ERJ Open Res.* 6 (2): 00195–02020.

51 Ahmadi, Z.H., Mousavizadeh, M., Nikpajouh, A. et al. (2021). COVID-19: a perspective from Iran. *J. Card. Surg.* 36 (5): 1672–1676.

52 Shoja, E., Aghamohammadi, V., Bazyar, H. et al. (2020). Covid-19 effects on the workload of Iranian healthcare workers. *BMC Public Health* 20 (1): 1636.

53 Tanhehco, Y.C., Li, Y., Zantek, N.D. et al. (2021). Apheresis physician well-being during the COVID-19 pandemic: results of a survey. *Transfusion* 61 (5): 1542–1550.

54 Henderson, M., Brooks, S.K., del Busso, L. et al. (2012). Shame! Self-stigmatisation as an obstacle to sick doctors returning to work: a qualitative study. *BMJ Open* 2 (5): e001776.

55 Rimmer, A. (2016). Over 80% of doctors know a colleague with mental health issues, survey finds. *BMJ* 352: i1677.

56 Gregory, E. (2020). Resident physicians' mental health during COVID-19: advocating for supports during and post pandemic. *Can. Med. Educ. J.* 11 (6): e188–e190.

57 Essangri, H., Sabir, M., Benkabbou, A. et al. (2021). Predictive factors for impaired mental health among medical students during the early stage of the COVID-19 pandemic in Morocco. *Am. J. Trop. Med. Hyg.* 104 (1): 95–102.

58 Frank, V., Doshi, A., Demirjian, N.L. et al. (2022). Educational, psychosocial, and clinical impact of SARS-CoV-2 (COVID-19) pandemic on medical students in the United States. *World J Virol* 11: 150–169.

59 Institute of Medicine (US) Committee to Study the Role of Allied Health Personnel (1989). What does "Allied Health" mean? In: *Allied Health Services: Avoiding Crises*. Washington, DC: National Academies Press.

60 Boniol, M., McIsaac, M., Xu, L. et al. (2019). *Gender equity in the health workforce: analysis of 104 countries*. Geneva: World Health Organization.

61 Cai, H., Tu, B., Ma, J. et al. (2020). Psychological impact and coping strategies of frontline medical staff in Hunan between January and march 2020 during the outbreak of coronavirus disease 2019 (COVID-19) in Hubei, China. *Med. Sci. Monit.* 26: e924171.

62 Sonis, J., Pathman, D.E., Read, S. et al. (2021). Generalized anxiety, depression and posttraumatic stress disorder in a national sample of US internal medicine physicians during the COVID-19 pandemic. *Gen. Hosp. Psychiatry* 71: 142–144.

63 Firew, T., Sano, E.D., Lee, J.W. et al. (2020). Protecting the front line: a cross-sectional survey analysis of the occupational factors contributing to healthcare workers' infection and psychological distress during the COVID-19 pandemic in the USA. *BMJ Open* 10 (10): e042752.

64 Centers for Disease Control and Prevention (2021). COVID-19 children & teens. https://www.cdc.gov/coronavirus/2019ncov/vaccines/recommendations/adolescents.html.

65 Muller, A.E., Hafstad, E.V., Himmels, J.P.W. et al. (2020). The mental health impact of the covid-19 pandemic on healthcare workers, and interventions to help them: a rapid systematic review. *Psychiatry Res.* 293: 113441.

66 Jain, U. (2020). Risk of COVID-19 due to shortage of personal protective equipment. *Cureus* 12 (6): e8837.

67 Ortega, R., Gonzalez, M., Nozari, A. et al. (2020). Personal protective equipment and Covid-19. *N. Engl. J. Med.* 382 (26): e105.

68 Centers for Disease Control and Prevention (2020). Using personal protective equipment (PPE). CDC. https://www.cdc.gov/coronavirus/2019-ncov/hcp/using-ppe.html.

69 National Nurses United. New survey of nurses provides frontline proof of widespread employer, government disregard for nurse and patient safety, mainly through lack of optimal PPE. https://www.nationalnursesunited.org/press/new-survey-results.

70 Zhan, M., Anders, R.L., Lin, B. et al. (2020). Lesson learned from China regarding use of personal protective equipment. *Am. J. Infect. Control* 48 (12): 1462–1465.

71 Chou, R., Dana, T., Buckley, D.I. et al. (2020). Epidemiology of and risk factors for coronavirus infection in health care workers: a living rapid review. *Ann. Intern. Med.* 173 (2): 120–136.

72 Ha, J.F. (2020). The COVID-19 pandemic, personal protective equipment and respirator: a narrative review. *Int. J. Clin. Pract.* 74 (10): e13578.

73 De Kock, J.H., Latham, H.A., Leslie, S.J. et al. (2021). A rapid review of the impact of COVID-19 on the mental health of healthcare workers: implications for supporting psychological well-being. *BMC Public Health* 21 (1): 104.

74 Anderson, G.F., Dahlberg, M., and Whicher, D. (ed.) (2017). *Effective Care for High-need Patients: Opportunities for Improving Outcomes, Value, and Health Executive Summary*. Washington, DC: National Academy of Sciences.

75 The National Child Traumatic Stress Network, National Center for PTSD (2005). *Psychological First*

Aid: Field Operations Guide. Los Angeles, CA: The National Child Traumatic Stress Network.

76 Sanford, J., Agrawal, A., and Miotto, K. (2021). Psychological distress among women healthcare workers: a health system's experience developing emotional support services during the COVID-19 pandemic. *Front. Glob. Womens Health* 2: 614723.

77 Sharif, S. and Amin, F. (2021). COVID-19 pandemic; anxiety and depression among frontline healthcare workers: rising from the ashes. *IntechOpen* https://doi.org/10.5772/intechopen.98274.

78 Gupta, S. and Sahoo, S. (2020). Pandemic and mental health of the front-line healthcare workers: a review and implications in the Indian context amidst COVID-19. *Gen. Psychiatr.* 33 (5): e100284.

79 Shapiro, G., Schulz-Quach, C., Mosher, P. et al. (2021). An institutional model for health care workers' mental health during Covid-19. *NEJM Catalyst* https://catalyst.nejm.org/doi/full/10.1056/CAT.20.0684.

80 Xiang, Y.T., Yang, Y., Li, W. et al. (2020). Timely mental health care for the 2019 novel coronavirus outbreak is urgently needed. *Lancet Psychiatry* 7 (3): 228–229.

81 Priede, A., López-Álvarez, I., Carracedo-Sanchidrián, D. et al. (2021). Mental health interventions for healthcare workers during the first wave of COVID-19 pandemic in Spain. *Rev. Psiquiatr. Salud Ment. (Engl. Ed.)* 14 (2): 83–89.

82 Thatrimontrichai, A., Weber, D.J., and Apisarnthanarak, A. (2021). Mental health among healthcare personnel during COVID-19 in Asia: a systematic review. *J. Formos. Med. Assoc.* 120 (6): 1296–1304.

83 Albott, C.S., Wozniak, J.R., McGlinch, B.P. et al. (2020). Battle buddies: rapid deployment of a psychological resilience intervention for health care workers during the COVID-19 pandemic. *Anesth. Analg.* 131 (1): 43–54.

84 Heath, C., Sommerfield, A., and von Ungern-Sternberg, B.S. (2020). Resilience strategies to manage psychological distress among healthcare workers during the COVID-19 pandemic: a narrative review. *Anaesthesia* 75 (10): 1364–1371.

85 Nguyen, J., Swartz, K., MacKrell, K. et al. (2020). Managing stress and coping with COVID-19. In: *Johns Hopkins Psychiatry Guide*. https://www.hopkinsguides.com/hopkins/view/Johns_Hopkins_Psychiatry_Guide/787387/all/Managing_Stress_and_Coping_with_COVID_19.

86 World Health Organization and United Nations High Commissioner for Refugees. mhGAP Humanitarian Intervention Guide (mhGAP-HIG): Clinical management of mental, neurological and substance use conditions in humanitarian emergencies. (2021). Geneva: WHO

87 Htay, M.N.N., Marzo, R.R., Bahari, R. et al. (2021). How healthcare workers are coping with mental health challenges during COVID-19 pandemic? A cross-sectional multi-countries study. *Clin. Epidemiol. Glob. Health* 11: 100759.

88 Rodriguez-Vega, B., Palao, Á., Muñoz-Sanjose, A. et al. (2020). Implementation of a mindfulness-based crisis intervention for frontline healthcare workers during the COVID-19 outbreak in a public general Hospital in Madrid, Spain. *Front. Psychiatry* 11: 562578.

27

COVID-19: Ethical Considerations in Clinical Practice

Kiarash Aramesh

The James F. Drane Bioethics Institute, Edinboro University of Pennsylvania, Edinboro, PA, USA

Abbreviations

ICU   intensive care unit

In March 2020, Italy was experiencing the first reported major outbreak of coronavirus disease 2019 (COVID-19) outside of China. Then, for the first time, the burdensome decision of allocating a limited number of lifesaving ventilators among too many patients who needed them emerged in the hospitals and found its way to the headlines. Soon afterward, the pandemic struck New York City on a record scale and raised the same ethical questions [1].

The pandemic had started to bring up challenging ethical questions; none of them was new or unique, but the scale was so unprecedented that they needed new approaches and new answers. The COVID-19 pandemic is a new example of operating under the crisis standard of care and all its challenging implications and consequences.

This chapter provides a brief review of some of the most challenging ethical issues raised by the pandemic in clinical settings, including resource allocation, professional duties of healthcare providers, off-label use of medications, dealing with medical pseudoscience, and contact tracing. Other issues related to research ethics or public health ethics, although important and impactful, are beyond the scope of this chapter.

The nature of a pandemic entails the involvement of many countries with various cultures, economies, and systems of beliefs. The specific and detailed guidelines should be tailored based on the cultural and socioeconomic variations and subtleties. This chapter, however, focuses on the most general ethical issues that have been common among almost all the involved countries and adopts an ethical perspective based on universally consensual values and principles of bioethics. These values and principles do not belong to any specific country, nation, or religion, but they can be considered a part of the common intellectual heritage of humankind [2].

Crisis Standard of Care

In the event of a public health crisis, to which the COVID-19 pandemic is a typical example, abidance to the usual and normal standards of care falls beyond the realm of possibilities, not only because of the overwhelming demands and scarce supplies but also because of the new ethical priorities that require new approaches and practices. Under these new standards, a balance is required between the norms of clinical ethics under normal conditions (i.e. the patient-centered standard of care) and the need to consider all the affected people and their rights and interests (i.e. public-focused duties) [3].

Crisis standard of care entails a significant change in usual healthcare operations and the level of care [4]. Healthcare institutions need to foresee the possible need to adopt crisis standards of care in the event of a public health crisis and be prepared for that. This preparedness included preparing the relevant guidelines and providing the appropriate training for their healthcare providers. Hospital ethics committees and ethics consultation services should be involved in the process.

Clinicians usually have a patient-centered mindset, and the usual standard of care has the same approach. However, the crisis standard of care centers around paying attention to the needs of the community and vulnerable groups. Fairness in distributing scarce resources, in some cases, demands some degree of deviation from the usual patient-centered care. For instance, a physician may consider releasing her patient from the intensive care unit (ICU) to make a bed available for other patients while she believes her patient's best interest is staying in the ICU for a few more days.

In addition, the leadership of healthcare institutions has a duty to safeguard their personnel and professionals. The frameworks and guidelines need to consider the importance of safeguarding the frontline healthcare providers, not only by providing safety measures but also by foreseeing and preventing their possible exhaustion and burnout.

Resource Allocation and the Pandemic

Even in the most developed countries, the overwhelming number of patients caught healthcare institutions unprepared. From the direst questions in the ICUs on the allocation of lifesaving instruments to other questions about the distribution of tests, medications, and lastly, vaccines, the health system wrestled with the challenge of applying the principle of justice into various aspects of its fight with the pandemic. Even at the global level, the observed unfairness in the distribution of vaccines has raised serious ethical debates. This chapter, however, focuses on the clinical implications of the principles of justice and fairness.

One of the most important aspects of resource allocation in the realm of clinical ethics is the allocation of scarce ICU resources. The shortage of ICU resources, including beds, oxygen, ventilators, and even skilled

personnel, has been a constant headline of the news coming from the most affected areas. For most seriously affected patients, ICU admission is a matter of life and death.

Admission to the ICU should be reserved for the patients who would benefit from it. If the demand is more than supply, the principle of distributive justice demands it to be reserved for the patients who are most likely to benefit and would benefit most from it. In other words, priority should be given to the patients who are not going to die anyway, are in critical need of ICU care, and are expected to recover after receiving it. This principle guides the decisions on preferential admission or early release of patients to and from the ICU [5]. Also, empirical studies show that the healthcare providers believe that the allocation of scarce ICU resources should be based on the expected clinical outcomes [6]. Having this guiding principle in mind, the hospitals who are or expected to be in the frontline of fighting against the pandemic should prepare or adopt guidelines for the triage of patients with COVID-19 in case of overwhelming demand. They also need to establish triage committees in anticipation of future surges of the disease. The triage committee takes part in preparing the guidelines for resource allocation under crisis standards of care. Clinical Ethics Committees should be involved in the process. The guidance created by the US Department of Health and Human Services provides an example and resource for that purpose [7].

In the case of an overwhelming number of patients, it may become impossible to involve the triage committee in decision making for each and every case. In such situations, the clinicians make the decisions at the bedside. Healthcare institutions should educate the potential bedside clinicians for such challenging decision making. Although, as mentioned earlier, the priority should be given to the patients who are in direst need and are expected to benefit most from the treatment, the egalitarian principles, including nondiscrimination and equal respect for all the patients, should be part of the ethical framework, the guidelines, and the ethical education [8, 9]. These principles (including the need-based utilitarian principles and egalitarian principles) can be relied on in allocation of any type of scarce resource, including ICU beds, ventilators, medications, oxygen supply, and even vaccines.

The Duty of Healthcare Providers

In the spring of 2020, some photos of nurses of New York City hospitals were published and stunned the nation. They wore plastic trash bags instead of proper protective garb. The problem was simply a shortage in supply because the pandemic had caught the city unprepared [10]. The underlying ethical question was unavoidable. Do the healthcare workers have a duty to provide critical care even in the face of higher-than-normal risk and shortage of personal protective equipment? The answer of the American Medical Association was affirmative. But that answer predated the pandemic [11]. In addition, it does not specify the limits of the acceptable risk.

The essence of medical professionalism is giving priority to the patients' needs over one's welfare [12]. Therefore, medical professionalism requires the members of the profession, healthcare providers, to accept degrees of risk to save patients' lives. Here, one can see an implication of virtue ethics, when virtues such as courage, care, and compassion lead the healthcare professionals to sacrifice their own welfare to help people in desperate need. These virtues are the merging points of the traditional Aristotelian virtue ethics and the feminist ethics of care. In the absence of such virtues, mere reliance on utilitarianism or duty-based ethics fail to justify such big sacrifices that are needed at the time of a health crisis, such as COVID-19 [13, 14]. It has been argued that virtue ethics is not only needed for the professionals to fulfill their duties but also is relevant to the duties of the public to keep abidance to the public health measures to prevent the spread of the infection [15].

A more recent related question is about the responsibility of healthcare providers to get vaccinated. Although they have given the highest priority in receiving the shots, some of them might be hesitant to receive them because of a variety of reasons, including religious, ideological, or health concerns. However, the physicians have a duty not to harm their patients, their colleagues, and other people to whom they are in contact. In the presence of scientifically approved vaccines, avoiding vaccination equals harming others. Therefore, physicians have a duty to both get vaccinated and encourage and educate their patients to do so when they are eligible [16].

A conflict may arise between the physicians' personal beliefs (including the ones that embrace antivaccination ideas) and their ethical duty to get vaccinated. Are physicians allowed to adopt antiscientific and health-related superstitious beliefs? It seems that following scientific standards and methods is part of medical professionalism. In other words, deviation from scientific measures of efficacy and safety is a violation of professional values and duties. A healthcare provider is free to adopt any type of idea and personal belief. However, if those personal ideas come in conflict with their professional duties, the only acceptable choice is either disregarding those ideas or forsaking the profession.

The Problem of Pseudoscience

The COVID-19 pandemic has been accompanied by a surge of antiscientific and pseudoscientific claims, sometimes made or supported by popular political, religious, or ideological leaders. False claims about the nature of the disease (such as denying its existence), its treatments (such as promoting risky and futile treatments), and its vaccine (such as bizarre conspiracy theories) can be very harmful to the people who believe and follow them or are in contact with those people. When such claims are supported by political role-players, it becomes an example of biopolitics. The health sector should follow its genuine ethical standards and safeguard its independence from the influence of biopolitics [17].

Because of the magnitude of pseudoscientific claims, the risks and costs they inflict, and their popularity, healthcare professionals need to take them seriously [18]. They need to ask their patients about any possible use of so-called alternative medicine, and then educate patients about the possible harms of pseudoscientific treatments. Healthcare professionals also have a duty to educate society about the risks of pseudoscientific approaches in preventing or treating COVID-19.

Off-Label Use of Medications

In the absence of evidence-based curative treatment, many physicians tried to use other medications in the hope of their effectiveness against COVID-19. In some cases, such as using hydroxychloroquine for treating patients with COVID-19, the debate found its way to political conversations [19].

Off-label use of drugs is potentially harmful. Relying on the clinical judgment of expert physicians, in the absence of more reliable evidence, is not in contract with evidence-based practice. As a matter of fact, expert opinion is a type of evidence, although at a level much lower than clinical trials. In some cases, the severity of the condition and the urgency of treatment justify some sorts of off-label use of medications based on the clinicians' judgment.

However, the associated risk or even the potential of abuse implies that such a practice should be limited and well regulated. Healthcare institutions need to have guidelines for off-label use of medications, so that this practice would be allowed when needed and justified, but banned when too risky and burdensome [20].

Contact Tracing

Contact tracing is an integral part of the public health response to infectious disease outbreaks and epidemics. Effective, rapid contact tracing has been called the cornerstone of effective public health response against infectious outbreaks, including pandemics. Because contact tracing needs to be practiced at the individual level by clinicians, it is also related to clinical ethics.

This practice has always raised concerns about people's right to confidentiality and privacy. The high presymptomatic transmission rate of COVID-19 was a challenge for the standard measures of contact tracing. Using high-tech instruments such as mobile apps for controlling and ensuring social distancing, contact tracing has been practiced in China and other countries; however, their use in democratic countries encounters considerable resistance and concerns about the rights of citizens [21]. An alternative to using force for such purposes is relying on virtues such as compassion and solidarity. Without a sense of solidarity and cooperation in fighting against the pandemic, it is impossible to convince people to impose limitations on themselves and follow the burdensome requirements for a long period [22].

Solidarity is very important, partly because virtues such as solidarity do not belong to certain cultures; rather, they are part of the common intellectual and ethical heritage of humanity [23].

In short, it is necessary that clinicians encourage people with positive COVID-19 tests to inform all the people they have been in contact with and to practice self-quarantine. However, adopting public health measures that include degrees of control over their private life is ethically challenging and, in most cases, inapplicable.

Conclusions

The COVID-19 pandemic brought up a set of ethical challenges. Not one of those challenges was unique or new. However, amid the chaos created by the pandemic, they demanded new answers and new approaches.

Theoretically speaking, no single moral theory can provide all the normative fundaments to create frameworks to address the various ethical issues of the pandemic. Utilitarianism (e.g. in allocating scarce ICU resources), duty-based ethics (e.g. in safeguarding the human dignity of the patients), principlism (e.g. in avoiding harm to patients by untested treatments), virtue ethics (e.g. in cultivating courage and compassion in frontline healthcare workers), and other theories are to be appealed to develop comprehensive and practical frameworks and guidelines.

The key point is to be prepared for the next waves of the current or any future unpredicted infectious outbreak, not only by having the needed supply, knowledge, and technology but also by preparing the relevant ethical frameworks and guidelines and providing the appropriate training for the actual and potential frontline healthcare providers. This necessity of preparedness, or "the duty to plan," is the most important lesson learned from this costly pandemic.

References

1 Fins, J.J. and Prager, K.M. (2020). The COVID-19 crisis and clinical ethics in New York City. *J Clin Ethics* 31 (3): 228–232.

2 UNESCO (2005). The UNESCO universal declaration on bioethics and human rights. UNESCO. http://portal.unesco.org/en/ev.php-URL_ID=31058&URL_

DO=DO_TOPIC&URL_SECTION=201.html (accessed 4 May 2021).

3 Berlinger, N., Wynia, M., Powell, T., Hester, M., Milliken, A., Fabi, R. et al. (2020).Ethical framework for health care institutions responding to novel coronavirus SARS-CoV-2 (COVID-19) guidelines for institutional ethics services responding to COVID-19: managing uncertainty, safeguarding communities, guiding practice. https://www.thehastingscenter.org/wp-content/uploads/HastingsCenterCovidFramework2020.pdf (accessed 10 August 2021).

4 American Nurses Association (2020). Crisis standard of care: COVID-19 pandemic. https://www.nursingworld.org/~496044/globalassets/practiceandpolicy/work-environment/health--safety/coronavirus/crisis-standards-of-care.pdf (accessed 10 August 2021).

5 Vincent, J.L. and Creteur, J. (2020). Ethical aspects of the COVID-19 crisis: how to deal with an overwhelming shortage of acute beds. *Eur Heart J Acute Cardiovasc Care* 9 (3): 248–252. doi: 10.1177/2048872620922788.

6 Biddson, E.L.D., Gwo, H.S., Schoch-Spana, M. et al. (2018). Scarce resource allocation during disasters: a mixed-method community engagement study. *Chest* 153: 187–195.

7 US Department of Health & Human Services (2021). Interim guidance on critical care resources allocation for direct-service IHS hospitals. https://www.hhs.gov/civil-rights/for-providers/civil-rights-covid19/ihs-interim-guidance/index.html (accessed 28 May 2021).

8 Laventhal, N., Basak, R., Dell, M.L. et al. (2020). The ethics of creating a resource allocation strategy during the COVID-19 pandemic. *Pediatrics* 146 (1): e20201243. https://doi.org/10.1542/peds.2020-1243.

9 Supady, A., Curtis, J.R., Abrams, D. et al. (2021). Allocating scarce intensive care resources during the COVID-19 pandemic: practical challenges to theoretical frameworks. *Lancet Respir Med.* 9 (4): 430–434. https://doi.org/10.1016/s2213-2600(20)30580-4.

10 Bowden, E., Campanile, C., Golding, B. (25 March 2020). Worker at NYC hospital where nurses wear trash bags as protection dies from coronavirus. *New York Post.* https://www.healthleadersmedia. com/nursing/worker-nyc-hospital-where-nurses-wear-trash-bags-protection-dies-coronavirus.

11 Smith, T.M. (2020). Doctors obliged to provide pandemic care. It wasn't always that way. AMA. https://www.ama-assn.org/delivering-care/public-health/doctors-obliged-provide-pandemic-care-it-wasn-t-always-way (accessed 20 April 2020).

12 Jecker, N.S. (2004). The theory and practice of professionalism. *Am J Bioethics* 4 (2): 47–48. https://doi.org/10.1162/152651604323097790.

13 Gelhaus, P. (2012). The desired moral attitude of the physician: (II) compassion. *Med Health Care Philos.* 15 (4): 397–410. https://doi.org/10.1007/s11019-011-9368-2.

14 ter Meulen, R. (2011). Ethics of care. In: *The SAGE handbook of health care ethics: core and emerging issues* (eds. R. Chadwick, H. ten Have and E.M. Meslin), 39–49. Sage.

15 Bellazzi, F. and Boyneburgk, K.V. (2020). COVID-19 calls for virtue ethics. *J Law Biosci.* 7 (1): lsaa056. https://doi.org/10.1093/jlb/lsaa056.

16 American Medical Association (n.d.). Do physicians have a responsibility to be vaccinated? https://www.ama-assn.org/delivering-care/ethics/do-physicians-have-responsibility-be-vaccinated (accessed 10 August 2021).

17 Aramesh, K. (2019). Biopolitics, pseudoscience, and alternative-facts medicine. Impact Ethics. https://impactethics.ca/2019/07/29/biopolitics-pseudoscience-and-alternative-facts-medicine/#respond (accessed 10 August 2021).

18 Aramesh, K. (2020). The COVID-19 pandemic and the problem of pseudoscience. Bioethics.net. http://www.bioethics.net/2020/06/the-covid-19-pandemic-and-the-problem-of-pseudoscience (accessed 10 August 2021).

19 Lewis, S. (2021). Hydroxychloroquine, once touted by Trump, should not be used to prevent COVID-19, WHO experts say. CBS News. https://www.cbsnews.com/news/hydroxychloroquine-not-effective-prevention-covid-19-world-health-organization-donald-trump (accessed 3 May 202).

20 Shojaei, A. and Salari, P. (2020). COVID-19 and off label use of drugs: an ethical viewpoint. *Daru* 28 (2): 789–793. https://doi.org/10.1007/s40199-020-00351-y.

21 Parker, M.J., Fraser, C., Abeler-Dörner, L., and Bonsall, D. (2020). Ethics of instantaneous contact tracing using mobile phone apps in the control of the COVID-19 pandemic. *J Med Ethics* 46 (7): 427–431. https://doi.org/10.1136/ medethics-2020-106314.

22 Galang, J.R.F., Gopez, J.M.W., Capulong, H.G.M., and Gozum, I.E.A. (2021). Solidarity as a companion virtue in response to the COVID-19 pandemic. *J* *Public Health* 43 (2): e315–6. https://doi.org/10.1093/ pubmed/fdab024.

23 Elungu, A. (2009). Solidarity and cooperation. In: *The UNESCO universal declaration on bioethics and human rights: background, principles, and application* (eds. H. ten Have and M.S. Jean), 211–218. UNESCO.

28

Racial, Ethnic, and Other Disparities in the Epidemiology and Care of COVID-19

Liesl S. Eibschutz[1], Charlotte Sackett[2], Kalpana Dave[2], Sarah Cherukury[2], Christian Vega[3], Mauricio Bueno[4], and Hector Flores[4]

[1] Department of Radiology, Keck School of Medicine, University of Southern California, Los Angeles, CA, USA
[2] USC Master of Public Health Program, University of Southern California, Los Angeles, CA, USA
[3] University of Southern California, Los Angeles, CA, USA
[4] Department of Family Medicine, Adventist Health White Memorial, Los Angeles, CA, USA

Abbreviations

AI	American Indian
AN	Alaska Native
CDC	Centers for Disease Control and Prevention
CI	confidence interval
HCW	healthcare worker
ICU	intensive care unit
PPE	personal protective equipment
RR	relative risk
SARS-CoV-2	severe acute respiratory syndrome coronavirus 2
SES	socioeconomic status
WHO	World Health Organization

For well over a year, the novel coronavirus, severe acute respiratory syndrome coronavirus 2 (SARS-CoV-2), pushed many healthcare systems beyond their limits. The coronavirus disease 2019 (COVID-19) pandemic overwhelmed global healthcare infrastructure and resulted in many countries facing the greatest healthcare crisis in recent history. Because the clinical presentation of COVID-19 varied in many patients, and clinicians were unclear how preexisting comorbidities would play a role in patient outcomes, healthcare workers (HCWs) and hospital systems navigated this emerging virus unprepared and underequipped [1].

By the time government officials began to enact a serious public health response to the COVID-19 pandemic, infection had spread far beyond the margin of containment. Unfortunately, COVID-19, like many other illnesses, disproportionately affected minorities and people of color. Discrepancies in the impact of the pandemic included risk for exposure to the virus, geographic distribution, diagnostic disparities, and issues in COVID-19 management once diagnosed. This pandemic also exposed the preexisting incongruities present in neighborhoods and physical environments, health and health care, occupation and job conditions, income and wealth, and education. Throughout this chapter, we will discuss global disparities in exposure risk and identify disparities in COVID-19 diagnosis, patient outcome, hospitalization rates, and vaccination inherent within our healthcare systems.

Disparities in Risk for Exposure in the United States

In March 2020, Jason Hargrove was working as a bus driver in the city of Detroit. He became rightfully concerned when he noticed a passenger coughing without covering her mouth. He vocalized his fear and asked for better personal protective equipment (PPE) to continue working. Two weeks later, he contracted the virus. He was a Black essential worker who experienced the firsthand risk of COVID-19, asked for his life and health to matter, and ultimately died in part because of his occupation. His story cannot be ignored.

Unfortunately, Jason's story is not an outlier. During the COVID-19 pandemic of 2020, many racial, ethnic, environment-based social, and economic inequities increased the risk for exposure to COVID-19. Many Americans felt obligated to continue working during the pandemic to provide for their families, even if it meant increasing their risk for acquiring COVID-19. Many of these jobs had high exposure to vulnerable populations with little protection, such as driving a public transit bus or working in the American prison system. In addition, many families lived in overcrowded conditions, putting their vulnerable elderly relatives at risk. Simultaneously facing the global COVID-19 pandemic, the US healthcare system also had to combat its own public health crises: racism and a lack of health equity [2].

Racial and Ethnic Disparities

According to the US Centers for Disease Control and Prevention (CDC), racial and ethnic minority groups were at significantly greater risk for exposure to COVID-19 because of the social determinants of health [3]. To identify the root cause of these disparities, the COVID Racial Data Tracker was created to collect and share the most up-to-date data regarding COVID-19 in the United States and its relationship with race and ethnicity. Although not comprehensive, the database examines state-level statistics and county-level data to track inequity [4]. Ultimately, they found that the 20 counties with the highest level of infections per capita were in areas where more than 60% of the population was Black or Latino [4]. Furthermore, in Minnesota, Black people represent 6% of the state population, yet disproportionately comprised 29% of COVID-19 cases (Figure 28.1) [4].

This information is unsurprising because there is overwhelming evidence that Black people experience worse outcomes in the US healthcare system. Many studies note that this population experiences higher prevalence of chronic disease and lower-quality health care for certain conditions, and Black women have higher maternal mortality than women of other racial and ethnic backgrounds [2]. In addition, many members of the Black community continue to distrust the US medical system because of the historical mistreatment of Black patients, as seen in the Tuskegee experiments conducted on Black men by the US Public Health Service [5]. Although the Affordable Care Act increased access to the healthcare market to purchase insurance and pushed for Medicaid expansion in many states, people of color still experience a disproportionate lack of health insurance [6]. This coverage gap impacts uninsured Black populations even more significantly because they are more likely to reside in Southern states that have not enacted this Medicaid expansion (Figure 28.2) [7]. This increases the

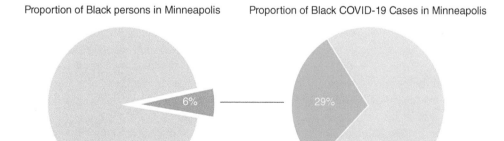

Proportion of Black persons in Minneapolis   Proportion of Black COVID-19 Cases in Minneapolis

6%   29%

Figure 28.1   Proportions of Black population versus Black COVID-19 cases in Minneapolis.

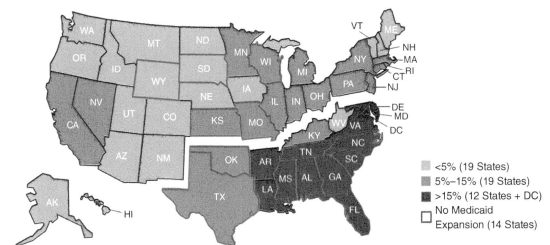

Note: Includes nonelderly individuals 0–64 years of age and non-Hispanic Blacks.
Source: KFF analysis of 2018 American Community Survey, 1-Year Estimates and KFF, Status of State Action on the Medicaid Expansion Decision, as of April 2020, https://www.kff.org/health-reform/state-indicator/state-activity-around-expanding-medicaid-under-the-affordable-care-act/.

Figure 28.2 Share of total nonelderly population that is Black by state and Medicaid expansion status as of April 2020. *Source:* Artiga et al. [7].

prevalence of chronic disease in these populations and hinders reliable access to health care, often leaving these individuals few options, if any, to seek care with safety net providers [6]. Thus, people of color are already more likely to experience comorbidities that leave them vulnerable to being exposed to COVID-19 and developing complications.

Neighborhood and Environment

Communities in largely Black counties experienced both higher morbidity and mortality rates of COVID-19 [8]. These outcomes may be, in part, because of the fact that these regions already had a higher prevalence of comorbidities and air pollution than other areas with different racial and ethnic composition [8]. However, studies indicate that counties with higher proportions of Black residents had a 24% higher rate of COVID-19 diagnoses and an 18% higher rate of death even after adjusting for age, poverty, comorbidities, and pandemic duration [8].

In Western states, such as Utah, the COVID-19 pandemic devastated economically deprived communities that were largely Hispanic and non-White in population [9]. Deprivation burden, which is defined as a geographic region's social and economic inequity, is highest in Utah's communities of color [9]. These communities were more likely to live in overcrowded housing, as well as experience food and healthcare insecurity. As an example of the intersection between social determinants of health, health inequalities, and the pandemic, the incidence of COVID-19 infections was three times higher in Utah's communities of color compared with regions of very low deprivation between 3 March and 9 July 2020 [9].

The impact of COVID-19 has also been magnified in sustained hot spot areas such as Los Angeles County, where longstanding health inequities also disproportionately impact vulnerable and underserved populations. Not surprisingly, the region's Latinx residents and other racial/ethnic minorities have borne the brunt of COVID-19-related illness and death. As of 23 August 2021, Hispanics/Latinx accounted for more than half of all Los Angeles County's COVID-19 laboratory-confirmed cases [10]. Interestingly, a report published that same week revealed that more than 11 000 pregnant women in Los Angeles county tested positive for COVID-19, and 77% of them were Latina/Latinx [11].

In addition, the mortality rate caused by the virus among Latinx increased to staggeringly high levels during the peak of the pandemic. After the virus's major surge in fall 2020, the COVID-19 mortality rate for Latinx residents in Los Angeles county increased more than 1000%, with 3.5 daily deaths per 100 000 in November 2020 to 40 daily deaths per 100 000 in January 2021 [12]. The average COVID-19 death rate among Latinx in Los Angeles County peaked in mid-January at a daily rate of 48 deaths per 100 000 Latinx residents, three times greater than the rate for White residents.

Tribal and Rural Communities

In the United States, 1.7% of the total population identify as American Indian (AI) and Alaska Native (AN) alone or in combination with other races [13]. Most of these individuals reside in rural areas of the nation and face similar issues that increase the risk for exposure to COVID-19 infection, such as poverty, lack of access to transportation, and overcrowded housing [13]. A commentary emphasized the particular social vulnerabilities experienced by the Navajo Nation, with an average poverty rate of 40.2% and per capita income of $12 117, approximately 17.4% of the population is forced to live in overcrowded, multigenerational housing environments [13].

Ultimately, CDC surveillance data noted that 2.7% of COVID-19 cases occurred in AI/AN persons, more than double the percentage of non-Hispanic AI/AN cases (1.3%) [14]. Although the exact association behind this elevated prevalence has yet to be elucidated, it could be because of the higher levels of shared transportation, smaller average housing size, and limited access to running water [14]. Unfortunately, most data on comorbidities within this population are lacking, and thus the role of race/ethnicity may be falsely elevated. Conversely, the CDC surveillance data were obtained through a passive reporting system, which may underestimate the actual burden of cases.

Unemployment and Occupational Risk

While the unemployment rate increased for Asian, Black, and White workers at the pandemic's onset, it plateaued for White workers in April 2020 but continued to increase for Asians and Blacks through May 2020 [15]. Hispanic workers continued to experience high unemployment rates through May 2021 [15]. Black and Hispanic workers were thus at greater risk for living in overcrowded housing situations, experiencing the threat of eviction, and ultimately suffering from homelessness, all factors that make social distancing and quarantining nearly impossible [16].

For those fortunate to remain employed and in their current housing despite the pandemic, Black people were more likely to be employed in occupationally segregated low-wage essential worker positions that increased the risk for exposure to COVID-19 [17]. Similarly, Hispanic and non-White workers were likely to be employed in manual, essential, or public-facing occupations that increased the risk for exposure to COVID-19 [9]. Particularly, women of color across all education levels were segregated into lower-wage jobs in comparison with White women in similar roles [18]. In these jobs, people of color faced increased exposure to infected persons as well as crowding and limited access to PPE [17]. As essential workers unable to work from home, these individuals were also more likely to use public transportation, where adequate social distancing is often difficult to accomplish [2].

The American Prison and Correctional System

The US criminal justice system has also been responsible for the disparate mass incarceration of many racial and ethnic minorities (Figure 28.3). Currently, almost 2.3 million people of the total American population are imprisoned, disproportionately Black men and women [20]. From 1980 to 2016, incarceration of women has increased by 742% [21]. In US correctional and detention facilities, there have been 531 280 COVID-19 cases among residents and 109 846 cases among staff to date from 31 March 2020 to 27 August 2021 [22]. Furthermore, much of the population is elderly, burdened with preexisting chronic disease and comorbidities, and poorly educated. At baseline, prisoners are a vulnerable population who are more likely to develop severe complications and require hospitalization.

In April 2020, the COVID-19 infection rate at Rikers Island jail in New York City was 5.1%, almost five times the overall rate in the state of New York [21].

Blacks, Hispanics make up larger shares of prisoners than of U.S. population

U.S. adult population and U.S. prison population by race and Hispanic origin, 2018

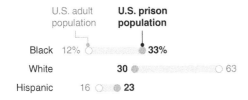

Notes: Blacks and whites iclude those who report being only one race and are non-Hispanic. Hispanics are of any race. Prison population is defined as inmates sentenced to more than a year in state or federal prison.
Source: U.S. Census Bureau, Bureau of Justice Statistics.

PEW RESEARCH CENTER

Figure 28.3 Racial and ethnic disparities in US correctional facilities in 2018. *Source:* Gramlich et al. [19].

Overcrowding, transfer between facilities, circulating correctional staff, inadequate ventilation, and limited access to personal hygiene items were just some of the factors contributing to increased risk for exposure [21]. Furthermore, the incapacitating environment debilitates an individual's access to accurate and trustworthy information [21]. Distrust, fear, and misinformation about COVID-19, health care, and vaccination spread rampantly in the prison system.

Although the CDC released guidance for management of COVID-19 in correctional and detention facilities, such as detailed protocols for prevention, public health information-sharing communications, and management, limited resources and capacity often make it difficult to adhere to these recommendations [23]. In collaboration with Harvard Law School and the National Commission on Correctional Health Care, a two-month survey examined COVID-19 effects in jails, prisons, and juvenile detention facilities [24]. Incidence rates of cases and suspected cases were two to four times higher each week among Black compared with White inmates [24]. Ultimately, the US prison system is an environment where multiple social determinants of health converge to increase the risk for exposure to COVID-19, and further research is necessary to identify how best we can combat these disparities.

Access to Education and the American School System

Education is a social determinant that is associated with better health and longevity of life. Several risk factors, such as having a disability, experiencing social discrimination, and arising from a low-income family, expose children to a decreased likelihood of graduating from high school and experiencing math/reading difficulties [25]. In addition, these students are more likely to be employed in unsafe and low-wage jobs [25] disproportionately held by people of color.

Certain authors report that a general lack of COVID-19 knowledge is more likely in Hispanic and non-Hispanic Black individuals [3]. In addition, less education often leads to employment in conditions that increase the risk for exposure to COVID-19 infection.

Furthermore, the COVID-19 pandemic led to unprecedented school closures across the country and the world. Early in the pandemic, this containment strategy likely helped to mitigate the risk for COVID-19 exposure in children and staff [26]. However, the rate of infection in children could increase as schools reopen, especially for those from low-income families, because of crowded living situations and less access to resources such as masks and hand sanitizer.

According to the CDC, the risk for exposure in schools depends on several coinciding factors, including the nature of the variants that are circulating, the rates of community transmission and vaccine uptake, as well as the public health prevention strategies that are in effect [26]. A series of studies suggest that taking a strong "layered prevention strategy" approach through the implementation of measures such as social distancing, enforcement of mask wearing, and frequent disinfection can help to greatly reduce COVID-19 transmission in educational settings [26]. The recent US Food and Drug Administration approval for the use of COVID-19 vaccines in children aged 12 years and older might help to further mitigate viral transmission. However, there are disparities in vaccine uptake for different racial/ethnic and income groups, which will be discussed in detail later in this chapter.

Despite the effectiveness of school closures in reducing COVID-19 transmission among children, this measure had negative consequences. In addition to significant social isolation from peers, this disrupted the primary point of access for food, health care, and mental health services for many children in the United States. A recent study at Northwestern University investigated the effect of the closure of in-school learning on children's mental health during the pandemic [27]. The researchers surveyed 32 217 caregivers of children in kindergarten through grade 12 in the Chicago public school system [27]. Black or Latino respondents had greater exposure than White respondents for almost all stressors and faced significant uncertainties (Figure 28.4). With the loss of in-person education, children lost a sense of security and

community connection, and resultantly experienced deep stress during the pandemic.

Although the loss of in-school learning posed many challenges, the transition to a hybrid or online learning environment that still allows students to connect with one another could help to reduce feelings of social isolation, as well as to ensure that education is continued during the pandemic. However, students from low-income families may have living conditions that make learning difficult, such as reduced access to the Internet and unstable housing [28]. In addition, many low-income students lacked high-speed Internet

COVID–19 family exposure	No. (%)			
		Race/ethnicity		
	All participants	Black	Hispanic/Latinx	White
Stopped working temporarily	6074 (18.9)	1205 (19.5)	2115 (25.4)	1487 (13.7)
Permanently lost job	2688 (8.3)	570 (9.2)	803 (9.7)	742 (6.9)
Kept working outside of home	14208 (44.1)	2886 (46.8)	4606 (55.4)	3785 (35.0)
Health care practitioner	4052 (12.6)	896 (14.5)	835 (10.0)	1264 (11.7)
Cut basic hours	7313 (22.7)	1114 (18.1)	2222 (26.7)	2389 (22.1)
Moved out of home	184 (0.6)	48 (0.8)	60 (0.7)	30 (0.3)
Lost health insurance	634 (2.0)	133 (2.2)	200 (2.4)	145 (1.3)
Family income decreased	10577 (32.8)	1647 (26.7)	3257 (39.1)	3360 (31.0)
Difficulty				
Getting other essentials	4308 (13.4)	1296 (21.0)	1475 (17.7)	628 (5.8)
Getting medicine	1102 (3.4)	369 (6.0)	335 (4.0)	128 (1.2)
Getting health care	1728 (5.4)	450 (7.3)	497 (6.0)	326 (3.0)
Getting food	1881 (5.8)	571 (9.3)	661 (7.9)	239 (2.2)
Getting face masks, sanitizer, or other products	9461 (29.4)	2197 (35.6)	3268 (39.3)	2079 (19.2)
Could not pay				
Rent	1840 (5.7)	433 (7.0)	800 (9.6)	256 (2.4)
Bills	2496 (7.7)	694 (11.3)	988 (11.9)	325 (3.0)
Children took on job outside of home	275 (0.9)	57 (0.9)	101 (1.2)	44 (0.4)
Children assumed childcare responsibilities	1983 (6.2)	422 (6.8)	605 (7.3)	487 (4.5)
Someone in family				
Was exposed to COVID–19	4746 (14.7)	949 (15.4)	1469 (17.7)	1378 (12.7)
Had COVID–19 symptoms or was diagnosed	3407 (10.6)	829 (13.4)	1268 (15.2)	715 (6.6)
Died of COVID–19	1403 (4.4)	521 (8.4)	481 (5.8)	175 (1.6)
Overall CEFIS score, mean (SD)[a]	2.5 (2.2)	2.8 (2.4)	3.1 (2.3)	1.8 (1.8)

Figure 28.4 COVID-19 exposure and family impacts for all participants and by race/ethnicity. CEFIS, COVID-19 Exposure and Family Impact Scale. [a]Range 0–20, with higher scores indicating more exposure. *Source:* Raviv et al. [27].

connections, causing lags and outages that cut into learning hours. Other students reported lack of consistent access to devices or broken devices but lacked the funds to contact IT (Information Technology) support or replace them [29]. Ultimately, these issues further increase the many disparities in access to education that these children face during the COVID-19 pandemic.

International Risk for Exposure to COVID-19

These disparities in exposure risk are not limited to the United States. In this section, we will discuss the international risk for exposure to COVID-19 for citizens residing in China, Italy, India, Brazil, and Iran, respectively.

China

Let us begin in China, where the first case of COVID-19 was identified in the city of Wuhan and allegedly linked to the Huanan Seafood Wholesale Market in December 2019 [30]. Although the wet markets allow access to fresh and affordable food, they also create a favorable environment for viral mutation and zoonotic spillover, which leads to a heightened risk for viral acquisition and ensuing human-to-human transmission [31, 32].

China's large population size and density further increases the risk for exposure to COVID-19 [33]. This nation has the largest population in the world of approximately 1.4 billion, with an estimated density of 154/km^2 [34, 35]. Approximately 60% live in urban areas, while 40% live in rural areas [35]. According to the World Health Organization (WHO), China's population is aging rapidly, and 176 million Chinese residents are 65 years or older, as of 2019 [36]. Moreover, there is a larger ratio of men to women at 120 : 100 [34]. The risk for severe infection or mortality substantially increases after age 65 years [37]. Although rates of infection with COVID-19 are similar between men and women, men are more likely to have severe manifestations of disease, regardless of age [38]. Furthermore, individuals living in rural areas have lower socioeconomic status (SES) and educational

levels, as well as less access to health care, healthcare resources, and sanitation [39]. All these social determinants of health disproportionately increase the susceptibility to infections such as COVID-19, as well as the potential for adverse outcomes in certain vulnerable Chinese populations [39].

Chinese hospitals were initially overwhelmed by COVID-19 patients and soon became short on essential resources such as beds, ventilators, and medication, as well as PPE [40]. Without an effective vaccine at this early stage of the pandemic, HCWs had high risk for acquiring COVID-19 [40]. In addition, the scarcity of resources made it difficult for all COVID-19-infected patients to be isolated in the hospital, which further increased the risk for exposure to their families at home [40]. However, China was soon able to contain the virus through swift implementation of several innovative strategies. For instance, "Fangcang hospitals" were quickly assembled in public venues, where patients without severe COVID-19 illness could be isolated, monitored, and treated [40, 41]. In addition, the use of Internet hospitals and 5G robots helped alleviate the healthcare burden and further reduced risk for HCW exposure and transmission [40]. Lastly, the implementation of large-scale lockdowns and an increase in testing also helped to mitigate the number of new COVID-19 cases [42]. These are all key examples of how strong public health infrastructures and containment measures can play a major role in mitigating COVID-19 risk.

Italy

Italy was one of the first countries to encounter COVID-19, and it was hit especially hard by the virus. Although Italy only makes up 0.78% of the world's total population, Italy has a large population size (60 367 477) relative to its geographical region area of 294 140 km^2, which creates a high population density of 205/km^2 [43]. The most densely populated Italian cities are Rome, Naples, and Milan, which are also among some of the most popular cities for tourism [43–45].

The elderly adults comprise approximately 23% of the Italian population as of 2019 [43]. In addition, a larger portion of the elderly in Italy live with their children and grandchildren [46]. Italy also has a relatively large homeless population of approximately 49 000–52 000 individuals, particularly in larger cities such as Rome and Milan with crowded living situations and disproportionately low access to health care and basic sanitation [47]. These factors significantly heighten the risk for infection and subsequent transmission, especially for elderly homeless [43, 46, 47].

Occupation is another major factor in risk of COVID-19 exposure. Iavicoli et al. [48] assessed the occupational risk for exposure in Italy, which is depicted in Figure 28.5. The individuals at highest risk for COVID-19 exposure are those who work in human health and social work activities (Figure 28.5). Individuals at medium-high risk have occupations in public administration and defense; compulsory social security; activities of households; and undifferentiated goods and service producing activities of households for own use as employers. Lastly, workers at medium-low risk are employed in education, arts, entertainment, and recreation, as well as other services

Risk class and working population by employment sector.

Description of employment sectors (ATECO classification)		Risk class	No. of workers (per 1,000)
A	Agriculture, forestry and fishing	Low	908.8
B	Mining and quarrying	Low	24.7
C	Manufacturing	Low	4,321.4
D	Electricity, gas, steam and air conditioning supply	Low	114.1
E	Water supply; sewerage, waste management and remediation activities	Low	242.8
F	Construction	Low	1,339.4
G	Wholesale and retail trade; repair of motor vehicles and motorcycles	Low	3,286.5
H	Transportation and storage	Low	1,142.7
I	Accommodation and food services activities	Low	1,480.2
J	Information and communication	Low	618.1
K	Financial and insurance activities	Low	635.6
L	Real estate activities	Low	164.0
M	Professional, scientific and technical activities	Low	1,516.4
N	Administrative and support services activities	Low	1,027.9
O	Public administration and defense; compulsory social security	Medium-High	1,242.6
P	Education	Medium-Low	1,589.4
Q	Human health and social work activities	High	1,922.3
R	Arts, entertainment and recreation	Medium-Low	318.2
S	Other services activities	Medium-Low	711.6
T	Activities of households as employers; undifferentiated goods and services producing activities of households for own use	Medium-High	738.9
U	Activities of extraterritorial organization and bodies	Low	14.1

Figure 28.5 Occupational risk assessment according to the Italian Classification of Economic Activities (ATECO). Risk class and working population by employment sector. *Source:* Iavicoli et al. [48].

sectors [48]. Unsurprisingly, the occupations with highest exposure risk are those that involve necessary direct contact between individuals. For instance, at the time of this study, data from the Italian National Institute of Health indicated that 12.2% of all COVID-19 infections occurred in HCWs, which fall into the highest risk sector of human health and social work activities [48]. However, the implementation of policies that allow citizens to work from home whenever possible, in combination with other safety measures, greatly reduced the risk for COVID-19 exposure and transmission [48].

Several studies regarding the observed COVID-19 pandemic trends in Italy suggest that the risk for exposure may be greater in the northern regions because of demographic and environmental aspects, although additional evidence is needed to support this hypothesis [46, 49, 50]. For instance, Northern Italy has high concentrations of atmospheric pollution, which might be an important environmental factor in the context of COVID-19 risk for exposure [50]. In addition, Northern Italy has a large business district, so many individuals work and travel here from other parts of Italy and across the world [49]. Furthermore, the north has a large portion of elderly residents [50]. These may help to explain the higher rates of COVID-19 incidence and mortality that were observed early in the pandemic for Northern Italy compared with Southern Italy [49, 50].

India

India is the second most populous nation in the world after China, with a 2021 population of 1.39 billion and population density of 460 people/km^2 [51]. Unfortunately, the country's large population lends itself to heavily concentrated areas, which can increase susceptibility to viral infections such as COVID-19. In one study that used a vulnerability assessment model to determine COVID-19 exposure risk in the most affected nations, India was considered the highest-risk group [52]. Of the hundreds of countries included in the study, India had the highest potential damage, calculated as exposure risk times population normalized, because it had the highest speed of cases, moderately high incidence, and one of the largest potentially exposed populations [52]. Several factors were identified as contributors to India's heightened vulnerabil-

ity, including sociodemographic (life expectancy at birth and population median age), health care (mortalities, water supply, and hospital beds), political-domestic (public services and governance), and public health (immunization). Thus, although cases initially remained more concentrated in urban areas such as New Delhi, Mumbai, Ahmedabad, and Chennai, the virus steadily spread to all states [53]. A serologic survey found that, by May 2021, more than two thirds of the population aged six years and older had been exposed to the virus [54].

The COVID-19 pandemic brought focus to the long-standing social class hierarchies and segregational practices that continue to plague Indian culture and health care [55]. When Indian Prime Minister Narendra Modi announced the national lockdown, poor and migrant workers in the cities were left suddenly unemployed and were initially unable to access transportation to return to their homes in rural regions of the country. As fears of infection and lack of adequate food and housing grew, masses of men, women, and children risked the dangerous journey home by foot. Many of those undertaking the brutal, yet unavoidable trek home were already part of a disadvantaged, vulnerable population because of occupational characteristics [56]. A report from the Stranded Workers Action Network found that of those workers who attempted the long walk home, 9 of 10 had been dismissed by their employers and about 75% left with food supplies sufficient for only two days [56]. Eventually, local governments arranged buses to shuttle migrant workers back to their homes, yet the capacity was inadequate [56]. Some migrants risked physical injury by grasping onto the buses' footboards and rooftops just to get home, and all were in crowded conditions in which COVID-19 is easily transmitted [56]. Hundreds of migrant workers died on the road home from fatigue, starvation, and injury [55]. Millions of workers and their families traveled from cities with high incidence rates to rural villages with limited healthcare resources, providing opportunities for nationwide spread (Figure 28.6).

In April 2020, United Nations-Habitat released a COVID-19 Response Plan that discussed the urban-centric nature of COVID-19 [57]. Because more than 95% of all COVID-19 cases occurred in urban areas at the time of the publication, the guide predicted that

Proportion of Black COVID-19 cases in Louisiana

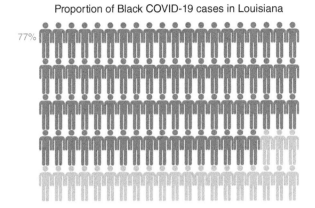

Figure 28.6 Proportion of Black COVID-19 cases in Louisiana.

the ramifications of COVID-19 would be the most catastrophic in poor and densely populated urban regions, particularly in slums and areas with high concentrations of migrants or refugees [57]. United Nations-Habitat specifically noted the susceptibility of the Asia-Pacific region, given the substantial proportions of urban dwellers in slums or slum-like conditions [57]. Social distancing and self-quarantine are unfeasible [58]. The Indian Council of Medical Research reported that the risk for COVID-19 was 1.09 and 1.89 times higher in urban and urban slum-like areas, respectively, compared with rural regions [59]. Presence in an urban population significantly affected the total number of COVID-19-positive patients more so than other demographic variables [60].

Brazil

Brazil is the largest South American country and has an ethnically diverse and complex population size of 214 million, where more than half of the population is Black or Brown [61]. The Brazilian Institute of Geography and Statistics racially classifies this diverse population into five categories through self-identification: Branco (White), Preto (Black), Amarelo (East Asian), Indígeno (Indigenous), or Pardo (mixed ethnic ancestry), yet many Blacks often self-identify as Pardo [62]. Brazil's average population density is 26/km^2, and approximately 87% of citizens reside in urban areas; notably, most (62%) are younger than 29 years and have many preexisting comorbidities,

such as diabetes, hypertension, HIV, tuberculosis, and obesity [61, 63, 64]. Although the first case of COVID-19 was confirmed in São Paulo on 25 February 2020, data monitoring infection spread in the subsequent months is limited because of a weak epidemiologic infrastructure in the country [65]. The Brazilian Ministry of Health had already declared a national public health emergency on 10 January 2020, an action that mobilizes emergency response protocols, but prioritized SARS-CoV-2 testing in only patients with severe clinical symptoms, such as those requiring intensive care unit (ICU)-level care [64, 65]. Thus, data regarding population-level prevalence early on in the pandemic, where significant asymptomatic transmission likely occurred in dense urban areas such as São Paulo and Rio de Janeiro, has been limited and underreported [65].

The Brazilian healthcare system is well-known to be weak, fragmented, and inequitable in quality of care. This region of Latin America already carries significant infectious disease burden, and crises in neighboring nations, such as Venezuela, have led to massive migrations into the northern regions of the country [66]. The nation is plagued by socioeconomic determinants of health that cause disparities, such as lower income, overcrowded housing, and lack of access to education, all hardships disproportionately affecting people of color and northern regions [67]. A population-based study of COVID-19 deaths among São Paulo residents from March to September 2020 found higher mortality rates in Blacks (relative risk [RR] = 1.77, 95% confidence interval [CI]: 1.67–1.88) and mixed residents (RR = 1.42, 95% CI: 1.37–1.47) in comparison with Whites; lower mortality was found in Asian residents (RR = 0.63, 95% CI: 0.58–0.68) [67]. Furthermore, Blacks and mixed individuals were more likely to die in public institutions (75.5% and 76.5%, respectively) in comparison with Whites (49.4%) and Asians (72.2%), who would receive care in private or nonprofit health facilities [67].

Previous studies have concluded that serious structural racial and ethnic disparities are present within the Brazilian healthcare system – one that is divided into public and private healthcare sectors. A cross-sectional study examined COVID-19 hospital mortality in 11 321 patients from the SIVEP-Gripe (Sistema de Informação de Vigilância Epidemiológica da Gripe) dataset [62]. Pardo and Black Brazilians had higher risk for mortality (hazard ratio, 1.45 and 1.32, respectively; 95% CI: 1.33–1.58 and 1.15–1.52, respectively) [62]. Most striking, being of Pardo ethnicity was the second most important risk factor for death, after age [62]. These deaths are likely attributable to the social inequities that continue to limit equitable healthcare access to people of color, such as admission to ICU-level care in private hospital settings [62]. In addition, Black Brazilian women with COVID-19 were more likely to receive hospitalized care only in more severe conditions, in comparison with White women. In addition, they experienced maternal mortality caused by COVID-19 that was two times higher than that of White women [68].

The transmission of the highly infectious gamma (P.1) COVID-19 variant, first identified in Brazil, has been observed to have a high reinfection rate among individuals who previously contracted the virus [69, 70]. It is also suspected that the gamma variant is able to infect and produce severe outcomes in younger patients more easily compared with other variants [69, 71]. In contrast with global trends of COVID-19 in which higher incidence and mortality rates have been observed in older individuals, many Brazilians aged 40 years and younger have succumbed to the virus [69]. This is especially concerning given the prevalence of young citizens in Brazil. Oliveira et al. [71] found increased rates of mortality among pediatric patients aged 2 years and younger, as well as those aged 12–19 years. This study also suggests that risk for mortality is greater for pediatric patients who are Indigenous, live in poverty, and have underlying medical conditions. Children of Black and Brown ethnicity had worse outcomes compared with children of White ethnicity [71]. Here again, these factors are closely intertwined and lead to health disparities.

An essential factor throughout the pandemic has been the Brazilian government's weak approach to public health containment strategies. An inadequate nonpharmacologic public health strategy has led to varying policies across the nation, so there has been limited standardized enforcement of mask wearing and social distancing [65, 66, 72]. In addition, a small percentage of the population is fully vaccinated [72, 73]. These conditions may have coalesced, aiding the spread of the virulent gamma variant [73].

Iran

Iran is one of the largest countries in the Middle East, with a population size of 85 million and an average population density of 52/km^2 [74]. Approximately 75% of the population resides in urban areas, and the median age of citizens is 30.3 years [75]. The cities with the largest densities are located in the north, such as Iran's capital of Tehran, as well as the holy city of Qom, which is a notable pilgrimage site [76]. As with other major industrious or frequently visited cities, the risk for exposure to COVID-19 may be higher in these areas. There were higher COVID-19 incidence rates in cities that had closer proximity to Qom and large elderly populations [76]. However, regions with smaller population densities compared with Tehran had higher incidence rates of COVID-19 infection [76]. These results suggest that population density is just one of many factors that must be accounted for in determining exposure risk [76].

The occupational risk for COVID-19 exposure in Iran appears to mirror global trends, with a higher risk in occupations that involve exposure to other individuals such as patients or customers [77]. The risk for exposure to COVID-19 may be greater in small Iranian industries compared with larger industries, because the latter may have better screening measures and administrative controls to prevent infection and protect workers [78]. In addition, Poustchi et al. [77] assessed SARS-CoV-2 antibody seroprevalence throughout Iran and found that rates of infection may in fact be higher than what was previously thought according to data on confirmed cases. There was no statistically significant difference between seropositivity in high-risk occupational groups compared with that of the general population, perhaps because of a lack of general preventative measures [77]. Furthermore, there have been reports of reinfection in Iran [79], highlighting the importance of public health strategies to combat viral transmission for all individuals, but especially those in high-risk groups.

The delta variant, as of August 2021, is responsible for most of the COVID-19 cases in Iran [80]. The COVID-19 level in Iran is currently characterized as "Level 4: Very High" by the CDC [81]. As the gravity of the situation has been understated, minimal and delayed action was taken to mitigate viral transmission. This, along with scientific misinformation, has led to mistrust by citizens, which in turn may have resulted in low compliance with public health strategies [80]. There is also a low vaccination rate and a scarcity of protective equipment [80]. As the delta variant continues to spread, it is essential to continue enactment of effective public health mitigation strategies. These include the implementation of health policy and an adequate supply of resources, plus strong public health education and motivation to engage in preventive behavior [80].

An interesting study by Jahangiry et al. [82] suggests that risk perception plays a vital role in COVID-19 containment among different groups. These authors report that Iranians who are older, female, single, and of higher SES, as well as those who reside in rural areas, are likely to have greater self-efficacy in response to the current pandemic. In contrast, older married men with higher education levels tend to have greater perceptions of COVID-19 susceptibility [82]. This study highlights that risk for exposure may be higher in groups with less self-efficacy. The current pandemic situation in Iran is yet another example of how there are many aspects to consider while determining risk for COVID-19 exposure, which are crucial to understand before creating targeted interventions to decrease the rate of viral transmission.

The remainder of this chapter will primarily focus on disparities within the United States, interspersed with some global trends.

Diagnostic Disparities

Diagnostic Disparity in COVID-19 Testing

The Infectious Diseases Society of America has defined practice guidelines for COVID-19 testing in the forms of molecular, serology, and antigen testing. However, in certain geographic areas, limited resources and capacity continues to prevent equity in access to testing for suspected cases [83].

In the United States, a significant factor contributing to diagnostic disparities throughout the pandemic has been access to SARS-CoV-2 testing sites [84]. A recent study by the *Wall Street Journal* noted that in Wayne County, Michigan, which includes Detroit, roughly 77% of rapid testing sites are in ZIP codes with a median

income above that of the county [85]. Similarly, in both Harris County, TX (which includes Houston), and Los Angeles, CA, 60% and 64% of rapid testing sites were in more affluent areas, respectively [85].

The Indian Health Service also faced critical shortages in COVID-19 tests, testing materials, and PPE for HCWs, while others faced a lack of funding and clinical site distribution issues [86]. Certain proprietary testing centers used online registration almost exclusively, leaving out communities experiencing the digital divide [87]. In addition, a study analyzing two national datasets reported a significant disparity in the distribution of healthcare resources needed for COVID-19 testing [84]. Unfortunately, this distribution disparity particularly impacts minority, uninsured, and rural population areas [84].

Interestingly, travel time is surprisingly short for uninsured minority populations in urban areas, but testing rates continue to remain low for unexplained reasons [84]. Certain authors hypothesize that these clinics may only be accessible by car, refuse to test children, or charge for tests, thus creating barriers for many low-income families [85]. In addition, many low-income families may be fearful of the COVID-19 test result they may receive. If they test positive, who will pay the bills, take care of their families, and put food on the table? Thus, the lack of flexibility inherent in staying home from work may push many people to avoid getting tested altogether.

The CDC cites limited transportation, lack of health insurance, cost, inability to take time off from work or paid time off during clinic testing hours, inequitable access for those with disabilities, and a fundamental lack of trust in the government as additional disparities impeding fair access to testing [3]. In addition, financial, cultural, and language barriers may impede clinic visits [85]. Even though mobile testing and clinic access expanded over the course of the pandemic year and more testing locations and options became available, people of color and low SES still faced a variety of barriers.

The Kaiser Family Foundation reported that at community health centers, people of color consist of 57% of patients tested, as well as 56% of confirmed cases. Of those confirmed cases, most patients identified as Hispanic [88]. More so, Black and Hispanic neighborhoods experienced a greater demand for testing than White areas [88, 89]. This is due in large part to lower median household income in minority communities, fewer testing site locations, a lack of funding for testing resources, limited clinic hours, and the testing sites that are accessible usually being last-line safety net providers [89].

Diagnostic Workup of COVID-19 and the Role of Imaging Utilization

The role of imaging utilization and whether a disparity arose during the pandemic has been debated. Certain authors note a significant increase in imaging utilization consistent with the known health disparities observed in patients with COVID-19, i.e. higher imaging utilization in male ($P < 0.0001$), non-White (Black, Asian, other, unknown; $P < 0.05$) patients 60–79 years old ($P = 0.0025$) who are covered by Medicaid or uninsured ($P < 0.05$) and have income <$80 000 ($P < 0.05$) [90]. Conversely, a significant decrease in imaging utilization was reported among patients who are younger (<18 years old; $P < 0.0001$), female ($P < 0.0001$), White ($P = 0.0003$), commercially insured ($P < 0.0001$), and have income ≥$80 000 ($P < 0.05$) [90].

Yet, another study that examined 4110 patients who underwent COVID-19 testing from 3 March to 4 April 2020 reported no significant difference in imaging utilization or outcomes in racial/ethnic minorities or low-socioeconomic groups [91]. Larsen et al. [92] reported no statistically significant difference in imaging utilization and clinical outcomes for COVID-19 in Hispanic and non-Hispanic patients. However, these findings do not entirely exclude the possibility of diagnostic disparity affecting management of COVID-19 in racial and ethnic minority groups. Further studies that describe the associations with social injustices, such as overall lack of access to health care or health insurance, are warranted.

Clinical Disparities

Hospitalizations and Inpatient Admissions

There have been notable discrepancies in the populations who are most severely affected. In a retrospective cohort study in Louisiana, residence in a low-income area, public insurance (Medicare or Medicaid), increasing age, higher Charlson Comorbidity Index scores (measure of burden of illness), and obesity were associated with increased odds of hospital admission [93]. In addition, Black people had an increased prevalence of hospital admission. Of the 39.7% of patients who were hospitalized, nearly 77% were Black (Figure 28.6) [93].

Other ethnic groups may have even more profound differences in COVID-19-related hospitalizations. As of 16 July 2021, while Black and Hispanic persons both had 2.8 times the odds of hospitalization compared with White people, AI/AN non-Hispanic persons had 3.4 times the odds of hospitalization, making them the highest-risk ethnic group (Figure 28.7) [94].

In the United Kingdom, several studies reported that being non-White was associated with increased odds of hospitalization for COVID-19 compared with their White counterparts [95, 96]. In data from the UK Biobank, Black participants had 2.4 times the odds of hospitalization compared with White participants, after adjusting for Townsend Deprivation Index (measure of SES), household income, various comorbidities, smoking status, statin use, and body mass index (95% CI: 1.5, 3.7) [95]. Asian participants also had 80% higher odds of hospitalization compared with White participants, after adjusting for the aforementioned confounders [95]. A second study using the UK Biobank reported that being from a Black ethnic background had 4.32 times the odds of hospitalization for

	American Indian/Alaska Native (AI/AN) non-Hispanic individuals	Hispanic/Latinx individuals	Black non-Hispanic individuals	Asian non-Hispanic individuals
Cases	1.7	1.9	1.1	0.7
Hospitalizations	3.4	2.8	2.8	1.0
Deaths	2.4	2.3	2.0	1.0
Reference group: White non-Hispanic individuals				

Figure 28.7   Rates of cases, hospitalizations, and deaths based on race/ethnicity. *Source:* Centers for Disease Control and Prevention [94].

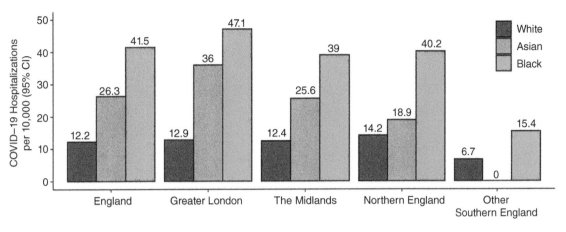

Figure 28.8 COVID-19 hospitalizations in the United Kingdom, stratified by region and ethnicity. *Source:* Patel et al. [95].

COVID-19 compared with White subjects, after adjusting for age and sex (95% CI: 3.00–6.23) [96]. Asian ethnic background was associated with 112% higher odds of COVID-19-related hospitalization compared with White participants, after adjusting for age and sex [96]. Taken together, these findings demonstrate that racial background clearly played a role in COVID-19-related hospitalization rates (Figure 28.8).

In addition to racial disparities, SES may impact the risk for hospitalization for COVID-19 in the United Kingdom. Specifically, subjects with lower SES were at substantially higher risk for COVID-19 hospitalization [95]. The researchers also noted a similar pattern based on self-reported household income [95]. Likewise, another UK-based study noted that hospitalized patients more commonly lived in deprived neighborhoods with higher prevalence of physical inactivity and cigarette smoking [96].

ICU Admission

ICU admission rates followed a parallel trend to hospitalizations and inpatient admissions. In CDC data, after adjusting for sex, age, and comorbidities, non-Hispanic Whites had a decreased risk for requiring ICU admission [97]. Hispanic Whites, Hispanic Blacks, and Hispanic Multiracial/Other individuals had 11%, 106%, and 84%, respectively, higher risk for ICU admission compared with the baseline group of non-Hispanic Whites (95% CI: 1.03–1.21, 1.76–2.42, and 1.73–1.96, respectively) [97].

Complicating the association between race and risk for ICU admission, the disparities in ICU admission between Blacks and Whites increased with progressing age such that as age increased, the gap in risk for ICU admission between Black and White individuals widened [97]. These findings are shown in Figure 28.9.

SES also affected the relationship between race and risk for ICU admission. Although a study conducted in a large midwestern academic health system in the United States reported no statistically significant difference in ICU admissions between African American patients and patients from other racial groups, the race and SES interaction term was statistically significant [98]. In other words, the effect of poverty on ICU admissions was accentuated by racial group. Specifically, poverty increased the odds of ICU admission by 50% among African Americans and 300% among other racial groups [98].

SES was also shown to be independently associated with ICU admission rates, because poverty increased the odds of ICU admission 3.58-fold (95% CI: 1.08–11.80) [98]. This finding may be because of characteristics of lower SES populations. For example, those with low SES may be more likely to work in service industries that do not offer flexible telework policies and present the potential for greater exposure to SARS-CoV-2 [98]. In addition, these individuals may have comorbidities or underlying physical or immunologic conditions that increase their susceptibility to COVID-19 [98]. Finally, those with low SES may also be more likely to lack health insurance and therefore

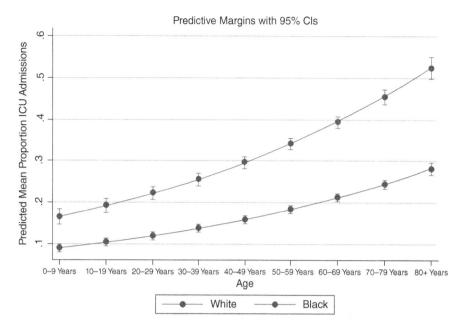

Figure 28.9 Risk for ICU admission for COVID-19 by age, stratified by race. *Source:* Poulson et al. [97].

may delay seeking care, resulting in advanced illness when they present for care [98].

Treatment Disparities

In addition to drastic increases in inpatient admissions compared with a prepandemic era, the proportion of severe COVID-19 cases resulted in a scarcity of ICU beds. In fact, one Chinese study conducted in early 2020 reported that 44.1% of hospitalized COVID-19 patients required admission to the ICU because of disease progression [99].

Many healthcare facilities exceeded their regular ICU capacity during the outbreak. In Madrid, Spain, the COVID-19 outbreak resulted in reaching ICU capacity within a matter of days [100]. Four new ICUs were established, generating a 340% surge capacity of ICU beds [100]. Other areas in Spain were even more impacted. By early March 2020, the ICU capacity in Madrid was 89%, compared to 216% in Vitoria (Figure 28.10) [101]. Optimizing oxygenation and clinical criteria-based intubation may have helped alleviate the burden in the ICU [101].

Other countries in the Mediterranean faced similar ICU demands as a result of COVID-19. In Lombardy,

Italy, the prepandemic ICU capacity was approximately 720 beds, which constituted less than 3% of all hospital beds [102]. Hospitals in Lombardy were forced to increase their surge capacity by adding 482 ICU beds [102]. ICU capacity in South Korea was exceeded by approximately 60 beds across all Daegu hospitals before 9 March 2020 [103]. This surge resulted in Daegu hospitals remaining at maximum capacity for just under four weeks [103].

Rural India maintains only 3.2 government hospital beds per 10 000 persons, while urban India boasts 11.9 per 10 000 [104]. Many individual states have substantially fewer rural beds than the rural average [105]. There is also a dearth of medical specialists working at Community Health Centers [106]. Adding to this dilemma, the systemic inequity has sustained a culture of deep mistrust toward healthcare and medical providers, which hinders many from seeking care. Thus, although those living in cities may be at greater risk for exposure to COVID-19, those in rural environments because of limited resources, are particularly susceptible to serious illness if infected [107].

In addition to the expansion of surge capacities, hospitals established principles of critical care triage, which emphasize the allocation of scarce resources to those

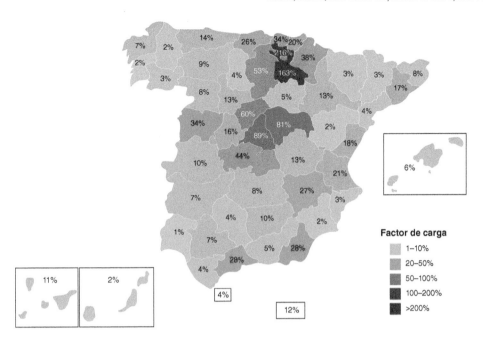

Figure 28.10 Percentages of Spanish ICU beds occupied on 18 March 2020, by region. *Source:* Barrasa et al. [101].

who are most likely to benefit from them [103, 108]. The triaging system prioritizes lifesaving equipment, such as ICU beds and mechanical ventilators, for patients with signs of clinical deterioration [103]. However, this also necessitates that patients who recover from serious illness are either promptly relocated to noncritical care units or are discharged from the hospital entirely [103]. Similarly, some nations chose to cohort patients in first-responder hub hospitals before recommending a patient for ICU admission [102]. In other instances, critically ill patients were transferred to hospitals that were not at maximum capacity [103].

In some cases, a lack of resources was not the defining issue. A review of ICU capacity in the WHO's Eastern Mediterranean Region found that biomedical equipment was ample but remained unused because of a lack of knowledge about their function [109]. Unfortunately, many countries suffered from inadequate staffing for lifesaving equipment. Initiatives were implemented to provide online and on-site training that covered the fundamentals of critical care management and the skills necessary for operating life support equipment [109]. These programs immediately filled gaps in ICU care when the issue was an inadequate workforce [109].

The surge in ICU bed demand offered lessons on how to better prepare for hospital capacity issues in the future. Researchers have recommended a long-term capacity building program in critical care and ICU management so that healthcare systems are equipped for other emergency situations [109]. This proposed program incorporates long-term clinical specialty training and mentorship, as well as the development of operations and management capabilities of ministries of health, host health facilities for ICUs, and local institutions [109].

Disparities in Patient Outcome

Certain demographic characteristics, such as obesity and older age, are associated with hospitalizations and deaths related to COVID-19 [93], contributing to disparate outcomes between rural and urban communities. Specifically, rural communities are more likely to have a high proportion of older, overweight/obese, and tobacco-using residents, increasing the risk for COVID-19 [110]. In addition, rural communities may have limited availability of ICU facilities and lifesaving

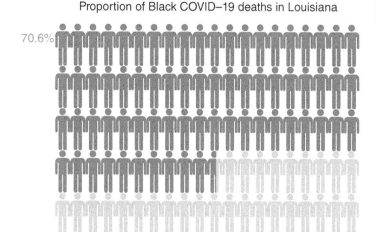

Proportion of Black COVID–19 deaths in Louisiana

70.6%

Figure 28.11 Proportion of Black COVID-19 deaths in Louisiana.

equipment. Although ICU beds were being added to US hospitals, these beds were concentrated in large, urban hospitals, whereas smaller hospitals experienced decreased ICU capacity [111]. Rural communities may also lack an adequate physician workforce, which can lead to delays and decreased quality of care [112].

Racial disparities were not only seen in hospital admission rates but also in patient outcomes. Discrepancies in mortality between Black and non-Black patients were particularly prominent in Louisiana. Even though Louisiana's population is only 32% Black, 70.6% of the patients who died as a result of COVID-19 in this state were Black (Figure 28.11) [93].

Another US study found that mortality rates for Black or African American non-Hispanic persons were two times that of their non-Hispanic White counterparts [94]. Hispanic and AI/AN non-Hispanic persons had 2.3 and 2.4 times the rate of mortality, respectively, than that of White non-Hispanic individuals [94]. A cross-sectional study on COVID-19 deaths in 28 US states and New York City reported substantial variation in the association between Black race and mortality across states [113]. However, in most states (22 states) and New York City, Blacks had significantly higher risk for COVID-19-associated death than Whites. In aggregated data from all locations, the risk ratio of death for Black versus White populations was 3.57 (95% CI: 2.84–4.48), with the magnitude of risk as

high as 18-fold in Wisconsin [113]. Overall, the Latino population experienced 88% higher risk for death as a result of COVID-19 than Whites (95% CI: 1.61–2.19) [113]. Data from the CDC also adjusted for sex, age, and comorbidities [94, 97]. The risk for mortality increased by 36%, 72%, and 68% for Hispanic Whites, Hispanic Blacks, and Hispanic Multiracial/Other individuals, respectively, compared with non-Hispanic Whites [94, 97]. The disparities in mortality between Black and White individuals increased with progressing age (Figure 28.12).

Other factors have been shown to be related to in-hospital mortality. In Louisiana, older age and clinical findings, such as elevated respiratory rate, elevated levels of venous lactate, creatinine, or procalcitonin, and low platelet or lymphocyte counts, were all associated with COVID-19-related deaths [93]. An ecologic study conducted in the United States assessed COVID-19 mortality rates from the seven most affected states as of April 2020 (Michigan, New York, New Jersey, Pennsylvania, California, Louisiana, and Massachusetts) and found that counties with a higher proportion of disability, poverty, and people on Medicaid were each independently classified as risk factors [113]. Higher percentages of Asians, women, individuals with higher education levels (bachelor's degree or higher), people insured, and larger total population were each independently found to be protective factors against COVID-19-related mortality [113].

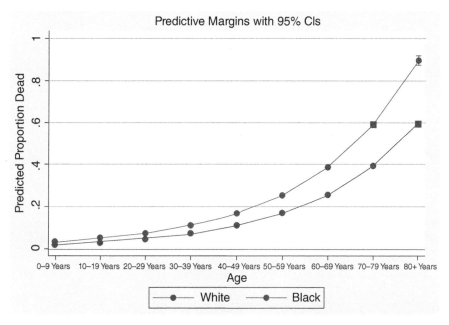

Figure 28.12 Risk for COVID-19-related mortality by age, stratified by race. *Source:* Poulson et al. [97].

Disparities in Vaccination

In a questionnaire distributed to US adults in May 2020, before COVID-19 vaccines were available, several characteristics were associated with increased likelihood of accepting immunization [114]. Specifically, males, adults 55 years or older, Asians, and individuals with college and/or graduate degrees were more likely to accept the vaccine [114]. Groups with lower vaccine acceptance included those who were unemployed and Black Americans [114]. Many of these same findings were corroborated by a survey administered to the US public several weeks later in late May to early June (Figure 28.13) [115]. Nearly 18% of individuals who did not intend to pursue the vaccine felt that it was unsafe, while 15.55% questioned its efficacy [115]. Interestingly, women and Black individuals were more likely than men and White individuals, respectively, to believe that the vaccine is unsafe or ineffective [115]. The largest effect was reported for women, however, who were 71% more likely not to pursue vaccination [115]. Similarly, but to a lesser degree, Black individuals were 41% more likely not to pursue immunization against SARS-CoV-2 [115]. In addition, they found that conservatives, those who intended to vote for President Donald Trump in 2020, and highly religious individuals had higher odds of COVID-19 vaccine refusal [115]. Other justifications for not pursuing the vaccine included a lack of insurance (6.22%), lack of financial resources to be vaccinated (6.17%), and belief that an individual had already contracted COVID-19 (3.31%) [115].

After the COVID-19 vaccine rollout, the CDC analyzed county-level vaccine administration data in all 50 US jurisdictions, examining Americans who received either the first dose of a Pfizer-BioNTech or Moderna immunization, or a single dose of the Johnson & Johnson vaccine [116]. At the time, adult COVID-19 vaccination coverage was lower in rural counties compared with urban counties both overall (38.9% versus 45.7%, respectively), and among several groups [116]. This trend was also seen for adults aged 65 years and older; rural counties reported that 67.6% of their older population was vaccinated, while this statistic increased to 76.1% in urban counties [116]. In addition, rural counties reported smaller percentages of vaccinated men and women than urban counties. These findings are demonstrated graphically in Figure 28.14.

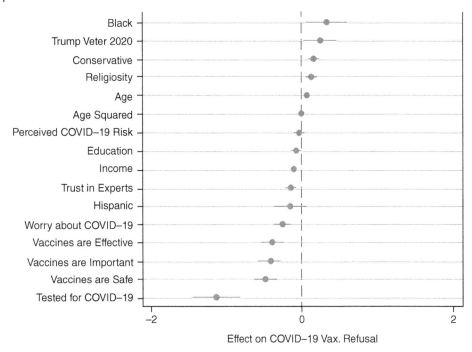

Figure 28.13 Factors associated with increased odds of vaccine refusal in US adults, before vaccine rollout. *Source:* Callaghan et al. [115].

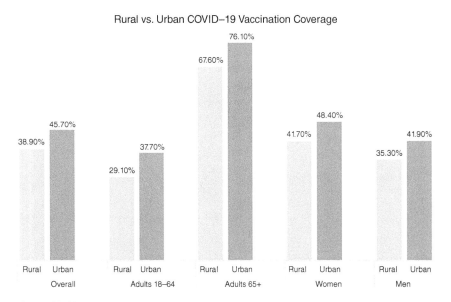

Figure 28.14 Proportion of COVID-19-vaccinated individuals in rural and urban communities in the United States in April 2021. *Source:* Based on Murthy et al. [116].

Several factors may have contributed to the disparity in vaccination rates between rural and urban counties. First, individuals in rural counties may be more likely to be conservative and may have been more likely to vote for President Trump in 2020 – two variables that were previously shown to be associated with vaccine hesitancy [115]. In addition, those residing in rural areas may be less likely to have a higher educational degree or may be more likely to be unemployed than their urban counterparts – both of which were, again, more likely to be associated with vaccine reluctance [114].

The vaccine rollout also lacked equity – big pharmacy chains had direct access to vaccine procurement on a national scale, favoring sites in more affluent communities. In certain states like California, multi-county health systems received vaccines directly from the state, whereas safety net providers and small private practices relied heavily on the local public health authorities [117].

Other countries experienced similar discrepancies in vaccination coverage. An ecologic study that was conducted using Israel's Ministry of Health database among older adults ($\geq$60 years) found that the proportion of vaccinated individuals was strongly correlated with municipal SES ($r = 0.83$; 95% CI: 0.79–0.87) such that lower COVID-19 immunization percentage was associated with lower SES (Figure 28.15) [118].

India has also been plagued by intranational disparities with logistical delays in distributing vaccines to infection hot spots throughout the rural regions of the country [119]. In addition, a recent study found a gender gap, with for every 100 men vaccinated, only 90 women have received the vaccine [120]. In earlier vaccine distribution phases, women constituted greater proportions of HCWs, and so this disparity was not immediately evident. Much of this has been attributed to widespread fear of the vaccine, misinformation, and lack of equal access to information because of gender and racial disparities.

There are also substantial discrepancies on an international scale. For instance, the United Arab Emirates have reported 166 vaccine doses per 100 population, while most African countries have administered fewer than 10 doses per 100 population [121]. Highlighting this imbalance further, only four countries in Africa have administered more than 10 doses per 100 population [121]. Interestingly, immunization rates in Africa do not appear to be dependent on how quickly a country received the vaccine. As an example, South Africa was one of the first African countries to receive the vaccine, but only 5.7 and 2.8 persons per 100 population were partially and fully vaccinated, respectively, at the time of the study [121]. In contrast, 58.0 and 49.2 individuals per 100 population had been partially and fully vaccinated, respectively, in the US as of July 2021 [121]. As Figure 28.16 shows, there are stark contrasts in vaccination rates by country.

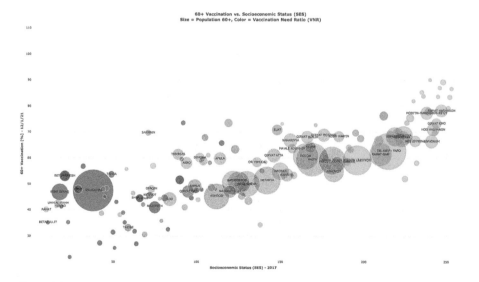

Figure 28.15 Correlation between proportion of vaccinated older adults by municipality and municipality SES in Israel. *Source:* Caspi et al. [118].

(a)

(b)

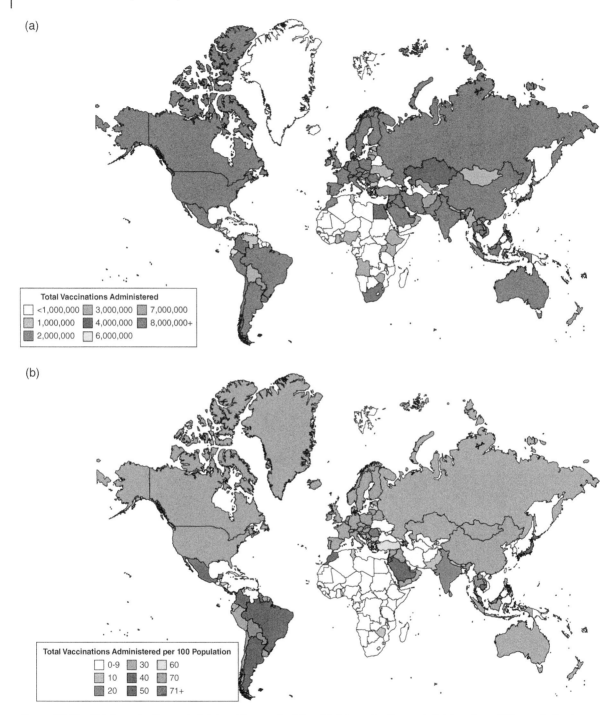

Figure 28.16 Total vaccinations administered by country (a) and total vaccinations administered per 100 population by country (b). *Source:* Sen-Crowe et al. [121].

Combating These Disparities

Overall, combating these disparities begins with identifying their presence and understanding their cascading effects. The COVID-19 pandemic revealed gaping differences between geographic regions and highlighted the racial and economic inequalities that are structurally ingrained in the public health infrastructure within and between many countries. With these limited-resource areas identified, efforts should focus on addressing economic and social deprivation. Specifically, COVID testing, contact tracing, quarantine and isolation options, preventative care, disease management, and prevention guidance should all be improved so that these services are equally accessible to all people [3]. In addition, diagnostic disparities can be addressed through the establishment of available testing sites with adequate healthcare resources. Legislative efforts must be made to provide financial support to local communities, focusing particularly on funding healthcare facilities in less affluent areas to ensure the ongoing availability of medical services and care in vulnerable communities [122].

Public health officials should target rural areas with campaigns promoting physical activity and discouraging tobacco use to help mitigate the effects of COVID-19 infection. In addition, local and state governing bodies should allocate substantial financial resources to increase accessibility of healthcare institutions, as well as ample medical supplies and equipment. Finally, there needs to be incentives for doctors and other healthcare professionals to serve rural areas.

Because vaccination rates vary quite markedly between different groups of Americans, such as by race, sex, and political view, it is imperative to attenuate misinformation that contributes to vaccine hesitancy. Specifically, news media outlets should present accurate, current, and practical advice, and visible community leaders should be enlisted to promote vaccination [110, 122]. Barriers to vaccine access must be relieved. Local organizations can partner with the CDC and state health departments to improve access to vaccines by identifying and eradicating obstacles such as language barriers. For example, the CDC has used multiple channels to distribute vaccines, including federal partners such as the Indian Health Service, the Health Resources and Services Administration, and the Federal Retail Pharmacy Program [116]. Finally, efforts should be made to engage underserved populations both directly and through community partners to better understand their needs [116].

On a global scale, nations should be encouraged to join in a collective effort to both decrease risk for exposure and ensure the equitable allocation of COVID-19 vaccines. International public health organizations may implement targeted vaccine distribution strategies to increase vaccination rates in high-need areas, preserve healthcare systems' resources, and avoid preventable deaths [121]. Countries with a high proportion of their overall population vaccinated should consider redistributing their vaccines to countries with small percentages of their nation vaccinated. For instance, despite the growing number of COVID-19 cases in the United States, America has elected to increase vaccine exports to countries in dire need [121]. Some researchers have also recommended prioritizing partially immunizing a larger proportion of people over fully immunizing half that number [121]. As an example, the WHO Regional Director for Africa suggested administering a single vaccine dose to the greatest proportion of high-risk individuals, as opposed to fully vaccinating half of their high-risk population [121]. This may be an effective strategy, particularly in nations that have a limited supply of vaccines.

Conclusion

Certain individuals are disproportionately predisposed to COVID-19 infection and/or mortality, based on a myriad of factors such as race/ethnicity, age, sex, and the social determinants of health. These factors may also increase susceptibility to chronic disease in these populations, which further exacerbates the crisis. Strong public health mitigation approaches, such as social distancing, mask wearing, vaccination, health education, access to information, and the enforcement of effective health policy, remain some of the most vital strategies in eradicating COVID-19. However, we have seen repeatedly that the inequitable distribution of resources, underrepresentation of racial and ethnic minority groups in medicine, economic deprivation, limited access to health care and trustworthy information sources, and uncontrollable living situations make these public health approaches obsolete in a plethora of the most vulnerable communities. In fact, they lead to further distrust in healthcare providers, novel treatments that emerge, and the fundamental health system [123, 124]. Although some of these contributing factors are inevitable, many are also attributable to social factors that demand to be addressed, such as racial injustice and systemic poverty. The

implementation of proper containment strategies, enforcement of health policy, and provision of key information through health education are all crucial to not only protect our citizens but also to help them make informed and autonomous decisions regarding their health and safety. The people of this world demand equity in access to safety and health care as a right, not a privilege.

References

1 Koley, T.K. and Dhole, M. (2020). *COVID-19 Pandemic: The Deadly Coronavirus Outbreak in the 21st century*. New Delhi, India: Routledge India.

2 Carroll, A.E. (2020). Health disparities among black persons in the US and addressing racism in the health care system. *JAMA Health Forum* 1 (6): e200769. https://doi.org/10.1001/jamahealthforum.2020.0769.

3 Centers for Disease Control and Prevention (2020). *COVID-19 Racial and Ethnic Disparities*. CDC https://www.cdc.gov/coronavirus/2019-ncov/community/health-equity/racial-ethnic-disparities/index.html.

4 The Covid Racial Data Tracker. The COVID Tracking Project. 2021. https://covidtracking.com/race.

5 Centers for Disease Control and Prevention (2021). *The U.S. Public Health Service Syphilis Study at Tuskegee: The Tuskegee Study*. CDC https://www.cdc.gov/tuskegee/timeline.htm.

6 Blumenthal, D., Fowler, E.J., Abrams, M., and Collins, S.R. (2020). Covid-19 – implications for the health care system. *N. Engl. J. Med.* 383 (15): 1483–1488. https://doi.org/10.1056/NEJMsb2021088.

7 Artiga, S., Garfield, R., and Orgerg, K. (2020). *Communities of color at higher risk for health and economic challenges due to COVID-19*. KFF https://www.kff.org/coronavirus-covid-19/issue-brief/communities-of-color-at-higher-risk-for-health-and-economic-challenges-due-to-covid-19.

8 Millett, G.A., Jones, A.T., Benkeser, D. et al. (2020). Assessing differential impacts of COVID-19 on black communities. *Ann. Epidemiol.* 47: 37–44.

9 Lewis, N.M., Friedrichs, M., Wagstaff, S. et al. (2020). Disparities in COVID-19 incidence, hospitalizations, and testing, by area-level deprivation – Utah, march 3–July 9, 2020. *MMWR Morb. Mortal. Wkly Rep.* 69: 1369–1373.

10 LA County Department of Public Health. COVID-19 Locations & Demographics. 2021. http://publichealth.lacounty.gov/media/coronavirus/locations.htm. Accessed 20 Oct 2021.

11 County of Los Angeles Public Health (2021). As COVID-19 cases among pregnant women increase, public health encourages expecting and new moms to get vaccinated - 5 new deaths and 2,426 new confirmed cases of COVID-19 in Los Angeles County. Listing of Department of Public Health press releases. http://publichealth.lacounty.gov/phcommon/public/media/mediapubhpdetail.cfm?prid=3317. Accessed 20 Oct 2021.

12 Lin, R.-G. II and Money, L. (2021). Latino COVID-19 deaths hit "horrifying" levels, up 1,000% since November in L.A. County. *Los Angeles Times* https://www.latimes.com/california/story/2021-01-29/la-latino-covid-19-deaths-up-1000-percent-since-november. Accessed 20 Oct 2021.

13 Hathaway, E.D. (2021). American Indian and Alaska native people: social vulnerability and COVID-19. *J. Rural. Health* 37 (1): 256–259.

14 Hatcher, S.M., Agnew-Brune, C., Anderson, M. et al. (2020). COVID-19 among American Indian and Alaska native persons – 23 states, January 31–July 3, 2020. *MMWR Morb. Mortal. Wkly Rep.* 69: 1166–1169.

15 Congressional Research Service. (2021). Unemployment rates during the COVID-19 pandemic. https://fas.org/sgp/crs/misc/R46554.pdf.

16 Galea, S. and Abdalla, S.M. (2020). COVID-19 pandemic, unemployment, and civil unrest: underlying deep racial and socioeconomic divides. *JAMA* 324 (3): 227–228. https://doi.org/10.1001/jama.2020.11132.

17 Hawkins, D. (2020). Differential occupational risk for COVID-19 and other infection exposure according to race and ethnicity. *Am. J. Ind. Med.* 63 (9): 817–820. https://doi.org/10.1002/ajim.23145.

18 Equitable Growth. Fact sheet: Occupational segregation in the United States. Washington Center for Equitable Growth. 2019. https://equitablegrowth.org/fact-sheet-occupational-segregation-in-the-united-states.

19 Gramlich, J. (2020). *Black Imprisonment Rate in the U.S. has Fallen by a Third Since 2006*. Washington, DC: Pew Research Center https://www.pewresearch.org/fact-tank/2020/05/06/share-of-black-white-hispanic-americans-in-prison-2018-vs-2006.

20 Sawyer W, Wagner P (n.d.). Mass incarceration: The whole pie 2020. Prison Policy Initiative. 2020. https://www.prisonpolicy.org/reports/pie2020.html.

21 Montoya-Barthelemy, A.G., Lee, C.D., Cundiff, D.R., and Smith, E.B. (2020). COVID-19 and the correctional environment: the American prison as a focal point for public health. *Am. J. Prev. Med.* 58 (6): 888–891. https://doi.org/10.1016/j.amepre.2020.04.001.

22 Centers for Disease Control and Prevention. CDC COVID Data Tracker. CDC. https://covid.cdc.gov/covid-data-tracker/#datatracker-home.

23 Centers for Disease Control and Prevention. (2022). Interim guidance on management of Coronavirus DISEASE 2019 (COVID-19) in correctional and detention facilities. CDC. https://www.cdc.gov/coronavirus/2019-ncov/community/correction-detention/guidance-correctional-detention.html#Overview.

24 Nelson, B. and Kaminsky, D.B. (2020). A COVID-19 crisis in US jails and prisons. *Cancer Cytopathol.* 128 (8): 513–514.

25 Office of Disease Prevention and Health Promotion. Education access and quality. Healthy People 2030. https://health.gov/healthypeople/objectives-and-data/browse-objectives/education-access-and-quality.

26 Centers for Disease Control and Prevention (2021). Science brief: Transmission of SARS-CoV-2 in k-12 schools and early care and education programs – updated. CDC. https://www.cdc.gov/coronavirus/2019-ncov/science/science-briefs/transmission_k_12_schools.html.

27 Raviv, T., Warren, C.M., Washburn, J.J. et al. (2021). Caregiver perceptions of children's psychological well-being during the COVID-19 pandemic. *JAMA Netw. Open* 4 (4): e2111103. https://doi.org/10.1001/jamanetworkopen.2021.11103.

28 Van Lancker, W. and Parolin, Z. (2020). COVID-19, school closures, and child poverty: a social crisis in the making. *Lancet Public Health* 5 (5): e243–e244. https://doi.org/10.1016/S2468-2667(20)30084-0.

29 Richards, E., Aspegren, E., and Mansfield, E. (2021). A year into the pandemic, thousands of students still can't get reliable WIFI for school. the digital divide remains worse than ever. *USA Today*. https://www.usatoday.com/story/news/education/2021/02/04/covid-online-school-broadband-internet-laptops/3930744001 accessed 20 Oct 2021.

30 Zhu, N., Zhang, D., Wang, W. et al. (2020). A novel CORONAVIRUS from patients with pneumonia in CHINA, 2019. *N. Engl. J. Med.* 382 (8): 727–733. https://doi.org/10.1056/nejmoa2001017.

31 Woo, P.C., Lau, S.K., and Yuen, K.Y. (2006). Infectious diseases emerging from Chinese wet-markets: zoonotic origins of severe respiratory viral infections. *Curr. Opin. Infect. Dis.* 19 (5): 401–407. https://doi.org/10.1097/01.qco.0000244043.08264.fc.

32 Plowright, R.K., Parrish, C.R., McCallum, H. et al. (2017). Pathways to zoonotic spillover. *Nat. Rev. Microbiol.* 15 (8): 502–510. https://doi.org/10.1038/nrmicro.2017.45.

33 Khan, I.M., Haque, U., Zhang, W. et al. (2021). COVID-19 in China: risk factors AND R0 REVISITED. *Acta Trop.* 213 (105731): 1–8. https://doi.org/10.1016/j.actatropica.2020.105731.

34 World Population Review. (2021). China population 2021 (Live). China Population 2021 (Demographics, Maps, Graphs). https://worldpopulationreview.com/countries/china-population.

35 Worldometers.info. (2020). China demographics. Worldometer. https://www.worldometers.info/demographics/china-demographics/#median-age.

36 World Health Organization. (2021). Ageing and health – China. WHO. https://www.who.int/china/health-topics/ageing.

37 Centers for Disease Control and Prevention. (2021). Certain medical conditions and risk for severe COVID-19 illness. CDC. https://www.cdc.gov/coronavirus/2019-ncov/need-extra-precautions/

people-with-medical-conditions.html?CDC_AA_refVal=https%3A%2F%2Fwww.cdc.gov%2Fcoronavirus%2F2019-ncov%2Fneed-extra-precautions%2Fgroups-at-higher-risk.html.

38 Jin, J.M., Bai, P., He, W. et al. (2020). Gender differences in patients with COVID-19: focus on severity and mortality. *Front. Public Health* 8: 152. https://doi.org/10.3389/fpubh.2020.00152.

39 Wang, Q. and Jiao, J. (2016). Health disparity and cancer health disparity in China. *Asia Pac. J. Oncol. Nurs.* 3 (4): 335–343. https://doi.org/10.4103/2347-5625.195899.

40 Sun, S., Xie, Z., Yu, K. et al. (2021). COVID-19 and healthcare system in China: challenges and progression for a sustainable future. *Glob. Health* 17 (1): 14. https://doi.org/10.1186/s12992-021-00665-9.

41 Fang, D., Pan, S., Li, Z. et al. (2020). Large-scale public venues as medical emergency sites in disasters: lessons from COVID-19 and the use of Fangcang shelter hospitals in Wuhan, China. *BMJ Glob. Health* 5 (6): e002815. https://doi.org/10.1136/bmjgh-2020-002815.

42 Lee, Y. N. (2021). From Beijing to Wuhan, China orders mass testing and restrictions as Covid cases rise. *China Economy*. https://www.cnbc.com/2021/08/04/china-orders-wuhan-mass-testing-beijing-restrictions-as-covid-delta-spreads.html.

43 World Population Review. (2021). Italy population 2021 (Live). Italy Population 2021 (Demographics, Maps, Graphs). https://worldpopulationreview.com/countries/italy-population.

44 Worldometer. (2021). Italy population (live). Worldometer. https://www.worldometers.info/world-population/italy-population.

45 Statista. (2021). Topic: Tourism in Italian cities. Statista. https://www.statista.com/topics/5972/tourism-in-italian-cities.

46 Di Lorenzo, G. and Di Trolio, R. (2020). Coronavirus disease (COVID-19) in Italy: analysis of risk factors and proposed remedial measures. *Front. Med.* 7: 140. https://doi.org/10.3389/fmed.2020.00140.

47 Barbieri, A. (2020). CoViD-19 in Italy: homeless population needs protection. *Recenti Prog. Med.* 111: 295–296. https://doi.org/10.1701/3366.33409.

48 Iavicoli, S., Boccuni, F., Buresti, G. et al. (2021). Risk assessment at work and prevention strategies on COVID-19 in Italy. *PLoS One* 16 (3): e0248874. https://doi.org/10.1371/journal.pone.0248874.

49 Rudan, I. (2020). A cascade of causes that led to the COVID-19 tragedy in Italy and in other European Union countries. *J. Glob. Health* 10 (1): 010335. https://doi.org/10.7189/jogh-10-010335.

50 Fattorini, D. and Regoli, F. (2020). Role of the CHRONIC air pollution levels in the COVID-19 outbreak risk in Italy. *Environ. Pollut.* 264: 114732. https://doi.org/10.1016/j.envpol.2020.114732.

51 Worldometer (2020). *India Demographics*. Worldometer https://www.worldometers.info/demographics/india-demographics.

52 Cartaxo, A.N.S., Barbosa, F.I.C., de Souza Bermejo, P.H. et al. (2021). The exposure risk to COVID-19 in most affected countries: a vulnerability assessment model. *PLoS One* 16 (3): e0248075. https://doi.org/10.1371/journal.pone.0248075.

53 Ram, V.S., Babu, G.R., and Prabhakaran, D. (2020). COVID-19 pandemic in India. *Eur. Heart J.* 41 (40): 3874–3876. https://doi.org/10.1093/eurheartj/ehaa493.

54 Bajpai, N., Wadhwa, M. (2021). COVID-19 in India: Disease Burden, managing the second wave and innovations. Columbia University Libraries. https://academiccommons.columbia.edu/doi/10.7916/d8-xgtr-jj83.

55 Breman, J. (2020). The pandemic in India and its impact on footloose labour. *Indian J. Labour Econ.* 63: 901–919. https://doi.org/10.1007/s41027-020-00285-8.

56 Iyengar, K.P. and Jain, V.J. (2021). COVID-19 and the plight of migrants in India. *Postgrad. Med. J.* 97: 471–472.

57 UN Habitat. *UN-Habitat COVID-19 response plan*. United Nations Human Settlements Program. 2020. https://unhabitat.org/sites/default/files/2020/04/final_un-habitat_covid-19_response_plan.pdf

58 Wasdani, K.P. and Prasad, A. (2020). The impossibility of social distancing among the urban poor: the case of an Indian slum in the times of COVID-19. *Local Environ.* 5: 414–418.

59 Swarajya Staff. ICMR serosurvey: Just 0.73 per cent of population had evidence of past exposure to coronavirus. 2020. https://swarajyamag.com/insta/icmr-serosurvey-just-073-per-cent-of-population-had-evidence-of-past-exposure-to-coronavirus

60 Pandey, A. and Sazena, N.K. (2022). Effectiveness of government policies in controlling COVID-19 in

India. *Int. J. Health Serv.* 52: 30–37. https://doi.org/10.1177/0020731420983749.

61 Worldometer. (2021). *Brazil demographics.* Worldometer. https://www.worldometers.info/demographics/brazil-demographics.

62 Baqui, P., Bica, I., Marra, V. et al. (2020). Ethnic and regional variations in hospital mortality from COVID-19 in Brazil: a cross-sectional observational study. *Lancet Glob. Health* 8 (8): e1018–e1026. https://doi.org/10.1016/S2214-109X(20)30285-0.

63 World Population Review. (2021). Brazil population 2021 (Live). Brazil Population 2021 (Demographics, Maps, Graphs). https://worldpopulationreview.com/countries/brazil-population.

64 Croda, J. et al. (2020). COVID-19 in Brazil: advantages of a socialized unified health system and preparation to contain cases. *Rev. Soc. Bras. Med. Trop.* 53: e20200167.

65 Marson, F.A.L. (2020). COVID-19 – 6 million cases worldwide and an overview of the diagnosis in Brazil: a tragedy to be announced. *Diagn. Microbiol. Infect. Dis.* 98 (2): 115113. https://doi.org/10.1016/j.diagmicrobio.2020.115113.

66 Rodriguez-Morales, A.J., Gallego, V., Escalera-Antezana, J.P. et al. (2020). COVID-19 in Latin America: the implications of the first confirmed case in Brazil. *Travel Med. Infect. Dis.* 35: 101613. https://doi.org/10.1016/j.tmaid.2020.101613.

67 Ribeiro, K.B., Ribeiro, A.F., Sousa Mascena Veras, M.A., and de Castro, M.C. (2021). Social inequalities and COVID-19 mortality in the city of São Paulo, Brazil. *Int. J. Epidemiol.* 50 (3): 732–742. https://doi.org/10.1093/ije/dyab022.

68 de Souza, S.D., de Oliveira, M.M., Andreucci, C.B. et al. (2021). Disproportionate impact of coronavirus disease 2019 (COVID-19) among pregnant and postpartum black women in Brazil through structural racism lens. *Clin. Infect. Dis.* 72 (11): 2068–2069. https://doi.org/10.1093/cid/ciaa1066.

69 Trevisani, P., Pearson, S., & Magalhaes, L. (2021, March 27). Covid-19 variant rages in BRAZIL, Posing global risk. *The Wall Street Journal.* https://www.wsj.com/articles/covid-19-variant-rages-in-brazil-posing-global-risk-11616845889.

70 Taylor, L. (2021). Covid-19: researchers find higher than expected reinfections with P.1 variant among the Brazilian Amazon. *BMJ* 373: n1353. https://doi.org/10.1136/bmj.n1353.

71 Oliveira, E.A., Colosimo, E.A., Simões e Silva, A.C. et al. (2021). Clinical characteristics and risk factors for death among hospitalised children and adolescents with COVID-19 in Brazil: an analysis of a nationwide database. *Lancet Child Adolesc. Health* 5 (8): 559–568. https://doi.org/10.1016/s2352-4642(21)00134-6.

72 Guerra, S., & Filho, P. G. (2021, May 24). Risk regulation and Brazil's battle Against COVID-19. *The Regulatory Review.* https://www.theregreview.org/2021/05/24/guerra-filho-risk-regulation-brazil-battle-against-covid-19.

73 Taylor, L. (2021). Covid-19: how the Brazil variant took hold of South America. *BMJ* 373: n1227. https://doi.org/10.1136/bmj.n1227.

74 World Population Review. (2021). *Iran population 2021 (Live).* Iran Population 2021 (Demographics, Maps, Graphs). https://worldpopulationreview.com/countries/iran-population.

75 Worldometer. (2021). *Iran demographics.* Worldometer. https://www.worldometers.info/demographics/iran-demographics.

76 Dadar, M., Fakhri, Y., Bjørklund, G., and Shahali, Y. (2020). The association between the incidence of COVID-19 and the distance from the virus epicenter in Iran. *Arch. Virol.* 165 (11): 2555–2560. https://doi.org/10.1007/s00705-020-04774-5.

77 Poustchi, H., Darvishian, M., Mohammadi, Z. et al. (2021). SARS-CoV-2 antibody seroprevalence in the general population and high-risk occupational groups across 18 cities in Iran: a population-based cross-sectional study. *Lancet Infect. Dis.* 21 (4): 473–481. https://doi.org/10.1016/S1473-3099(20)30858-6.

78 Malekpour, F., Ebrahimi, H., Yarahmadi, R. et al. (2021). Prevention measures and risk factors FOR COVID-19 in Iranian workplaces. *Work* 69 (2): 327–330. https://doi.org/10.3233/wor-205045.

79 Zare, F., Teimouri, M., Khosravi, A. et al. (2021). COVID-19 re-infection in Shahroud, Iran: a follow-up study. *Epidemiol. Infect.* 149: e159. https://doi.org/10.1017/S095026882100087X.

80 Calabrese, J. (2021, August 17). Iran's COVID-19 PANDEMIC RESPONSE: Mission critical. MEI@75. Middle East Institute. https://www.mei.edu/

publications/irans-covid-19-pandemic-response-mission-critical.

81 Centers for Disease Control and Prevention. (2021). COVID-19 in Iran – COVID-19 very high – Level 4: COVID-19 very high – travel Health Notices. CDC. https://wwwnc.cdc.gov/travel/notices/covid-4/covid-19-iran.

82 Jahangiry, L., Bakhtari, F., Sohrabi, Z. et al. (2020). Risk perception related to COVID-19 among the Iranian general population: an application of the extended parallel process model. *BMC Public Health* 20: 1571. https://doi.org/10.1186/s12889-020-09681-7.

83 Caliendo, A., & Hanson, K. COVID-19: diagnosis. Uptodate. https://www.uptodate.com/contents/covid-19-diagnosis?search=covid+diagnosis&source=search_result&selectedTitle=1~150&usage_type=default&display_rank=1. Accessed 1 Aug 2021.

84 Rader, B., Astley, C.M., Sy, K.T.L. et al. (2020, 2020). Geographic access to United States SARS-CoV-2 testing sites highlights healthcare disparities and may bias transmission estimates. *J. Travel Med.* 27 (7): taaa076. https://academic.oup.com/jtm/article/27/7/taaa076/5837479.

85 Krouse, S, Abbott B, Hernandez D. COVID-19 tests are still hard to get in many communities. *Wall Street Journal.* 2021. https://www.wsj.com/articles/covid-19-testing-challenges-remain-for-many-urban-rural-communities-11611320400.

86 Heisler, E.J. (2020). COVID-19 and the Indian Health Service [IN11333, version 3, updated]. Washington, DC: Congressional Research Service.

87 The Digital Divide Is Deepening Vaccine Frustrations. (2022). Retrieved 26 June 2022, from https://www.govtech.com/health/the-digital-divide-is-deepening-vaccine-frustrations.html.

88 Artiga S. Racial disparities in COVID-19: key findings from available data and analysis. Kaiser Family Foundation. https://www.kff.org/racial-equity-and-health-policy/issue-brief/racial-disparities-covid-19-key-findings-available-data-analysis.

89 Kim, S. R., Vann, M., Bronner, L., & Manthey, G. (2020). Which cities have the biggest racial gaps in COVID-19 testing access? FiveThirtyEight. https://fivethirtyeight.com/features/white-neighborhoods-have-more-access-to-covid-19-testing-sites.

90 Naidich, J.J., Boltyenkov, A., Wang, J.J. et al. (2021). Imaging utilization during the COVID-19 pandemic highlights socioeconomic health disparities. *J. Am. Coll. Radiol.* 18 (4): 554–565. https://doi.org/10.1016/j.jacr.2020.10.016.

91 Toy, D., Mahmood, S.S., Rotman, J. et al. (2020). Imaging utilization and outcomes in vulnerable populations during COVID-19 in New York City. *Radiol. Cardiothoracic Imaging* 2 (6): –e200464. https://doi.org/10.1148/ryct.2020200464.

92 Larsen, L.H., Desai, B., Cen, S.Y. et al. (2021). Addressing ethnic disparities in imaging utilization and clinical outcomes for COVID-19. *Clin. Imaging* 77: 276–282. https://doi.org/10.1016/j.clinimag.2021.06.018.

93 Price-Haywood, E.G., Burton, J., Fort, D., and Seoane, L. (2020). Hospitalization and mortality among black patients and white patients with Covid-19. *N. Engl. J. Med.* 382: 2534–2543.

94 Centers for Disease Control and Preventions. Hospitalization and death by race/ethnicity. CDC. https://www.cdc.gov/coronavirus/2019-ncov/covid-data/investigations-discovery/hospitalization-death-by-race-ethnicity.html

95 Patel, A.P., Paranjpe, M.D., Kathiresan, N.P. et al. (2020). Race, socioeconomic deprivation, and hospitalization for COVID-19 in English participants of a national biobank. *Int. J. Equity Health* 19: 114.

96 Lassale, C., Gaye, B., Hamer, M. et al. (2020). Ethnic disparities in hospitlisation for COVID-19 in England: the role of socioeconomic factors, mental health, and inflammatory and pro-inflammatory factors in a community-based cohort study. *Brain Behav. Immun.* 88: 44–49.

97 Poulson, M., Neufeld, M., Geary, A. et al. (2021). Intersectional disparities among Hispanic groups in COVID-19 outcomes. *J. Immigr. Minor. Health* (23): 4–10.

98 Muñoz-Price, L.S., Nattinger, A.B., Rivera, F. et al. (2020). Racial disparities in incidence and outcomes among patients with COVID-19. *JAMA Netw. Open* 3: e2021892.

99 Lei, S., Jiang, F., Su, W. et al. (2020). Clinical characteristics and outcomes of patients undergoing surgeries during the incubation period of COVID-19 infection. *EClinicalMedicine* 21: 100331.

100 Bardi, T., Gómez-Rojo, M., Candela-Toha, A.M. et al. (2021). Rapid response to COVID-19, escalation and de-escalation strategies to match surge capacity of intensive care beds to a large scale epidemic. *Rev. Esp. Anestesiol. Reanim.* 68: 21–27.

101 Barrasa, H., Rello, J., Tejada, S. et al. (2020). SARS-CoV-2 in Spanish intensive care units: early experience with 15-day survival in Vitoria. *Anaesth. Crit. Care Pain Med.* 39: 553–561.

102 Grasselli, G., Pesenti, A., and Cecconi, M. (2020). Critical care utilization for the COVID-19 outbreak in Lombardy, Italy. *JAMA* 323: 1545–1546.

103 Lee, S.H., Park, S.Y., Seon, J.Y. et al. (2020). Intensive care unit capacity and its associated risk factors during the COVID-19 surge in the Republic of Korea: analysis using Nationwide health claims data. *Risk Manag. Healthc. Policy* 13: 2571–2581.

104 Kumar, A., Nayar, K.R., and Koya, S.F. (2020). COVID-19: challenges and its consequences for rural health care in India. *Public Health Pract. (Oxf).* 1: 100009. http://doi.org/10.1016/j.puhip.2020.100009.

105 Mampatta, S.P (2020). Rural India vs. Covid-19: Train curbs a relief but challenges remain. *Business Standard.* https://www.business-standard.com/article/economy-policy/rural-india-vs-covid-19-train-curbs-a-relief-but-challenges-remain-120032300007_1.html

106 Kumar, A., Rajasekharan Nayar, K., and Koya, S.F. (2020). COVID-19: challenges and its consequences for rural health care in India. *Public Health Pract (Oxf)* 1: 100009. https://doi.org/10.1016/j.puhip.2020.100009.

107 Venkata-Subramani, M. and Roman, J. (2020). The coronavirus response in India – World's largest lockdown. *Am. J. Med. Sci.* 360 (6): 742–748. https://doi.org/10.1016/j.amjms.2020.08.002.

108 Maves, R.C., Dwonar, J., Dichter, J.R. et al. (2020). Triage of scarce critical care resources in COVID-19 an implementation guide for regional allocation: an expert panel report of the task force for mass critical care and the American College of Chest Physicians. *Chest* 158: 212–225.

109 Kodama, C., Kuniyoshi, G., and Abbubakar, A. (2021). Lessons learned during COVID-19: building critical care/ICU capacity for resource limited countries with complex emergencies in the World Health Organization Eastern Mediterranean region. *J. Glob. Health* 11: 03088.

110 Lakhani, H.V., Pillai, S.S., Zehra, M. et al. (2020). Systematic review of clinical insights into novel coronavirus (CoVID-19) pandemic: persisting challenges in U.S. rural population. *Int. J. Environ. Res. Public Health* 17: 4279.

111 Wallace, D.J., Seymour, C.W., and Kahn, J.M. (2017). Hospital-level changes in adult ICU bed supply in the United States. *Crit. Care Med.* 45: e67–e76.

112 Ricketts, T.C. (2000). Health care in rural communities. *West. J. Med.* 173: 294–295.

113 Gross, C.P., Essien, U.R., Pasha, S. et al. (2020). Racial and ethnic disparities in population-level Covid-19 mortality. *J. Gen. Intern. Med.* 35: 3097–3099.

114 Malik, A.A., McFadden, S.M., Elharake, J., and Omer, S.B. (2020). Determinants of COVID-19 vaccine acceptance in the US. *EClinicalMedicine* 26: 100495.

115 Callaghan, T., Moghtaderi, A., Lueck, J.A. et al. (2021). Correlates and disparities of intention to vaccinate against COVID-19. *Soc. Sci. Med.* 272: 113638.

116 Murthy, B.P., Sterrett, N., Weller, D. et al. (2021). Disparities in COVID-19 vaccination coverage between urban and rural counties – United States, December 14, 2020-April 10, 2021. *MMWR Morb. Mortal. Wkly Rep.* 70: 759–764.

117 Snow, J. (2022). California's "Equity" Algorithm Could Leave 2 Million Struggling Californians Without Additional Vaccine Supply | ACLU of Northern CA. Retrieved 29 June 2022, from https://www.aclunc.org/blog/californias-equity-algorithm-could-leave-2-million-struggling-californians-without-additional.

118 Caspi, G., Dayan, A., Eshal, Y. et al. (2021). Socioeconomic disparities and COVID-19 vaccination acceptance: a nationwide ecologic study. *Clin. Microbiol. Infect.* 27: 1502–1506.

119 Padma, T.V. (2021). India's COVID-vaccine woes – by the numbers. *Nature (London)* 592 (7855): 500–501. https://doi.org/10.1038/d41586-021-00996-y.

120 Centre for Economic Data & Analysis. Picture this: COVID vaccination leaving women behind (2021). CEDA, Ashoka University. https://ceda.ashoka.edu.in/picture-this-covid-vaccination-leaving-women-behind.

121 Sen-Crowe, B., McKenney, M., and Elkbuli, A. (2021). Disparities in global COVID-19 vaccination rates & allocation of resources to countries in need. *Ann. Med. Surg. (Lond.)* 68: 102620.

122 Carethers, J.M. (2021). Rectifying COVID-19 disparities with treatment and vaccination. *JCI Insight* 6: e147800.

123 Shan, A., Baumann, G., and Gholamrezanezhad, A. (2021). Patient race/ethnicity and diagnostic imaging utilization in the emergency department: a systematic review. *J. Am. Coll. Radiol.* 18 (6): 795–808. https://doi.org/10.1016/j.jacr.2020.12.016.

124 Shin, H., Abdelhalim, A., Chau, S. et al. (2020). Responding to coronavirus disease 2019: LA County hospital experience. *Emerg. Radiol.* 27 (6): 785–790. https://doi.org/10.1007/s10140-020-01818-w.

29

Global Impact of COVID-19 on Healthcare Systems

Liesl S. Eibschutz[1]*, Alexander A. Bruckhaus[2]*, Alexis Bennett[2], Dominique Duncan[2], Charlotte Sackett[3], Kalpana Dave[3], Sarah Cherukury[3], Victoria Uram[4], and Calvin M. Smith[5]

[1] Department of Radiology, Keck School of Medicine, University of Southern California, Los Angeles, CA, USA

[2] Laboratory of Neuro Imaging, USC Stevens Neuroimaging and Informatics Institute, Keck School of Medicine, University of Southern California, Los Angeles, CA, USA

[3] USC Master of Public Health Program, University of Southern California, Los Angeles, CA, USA

[4] Department of Clinical Research, University Hospitals, Cleveland, OH, USA

[5] Department of Internal Medicine, Nashville General Hospital at Meharry, Nashville, TN, USA

*Liesl S. Eibschutz and Alexander A. Bruckhaus contributed equally to this work and should be considered as cofirst authors.

Abbreviations

COVAX	COVID-19 Vaccines Global Access
EBV	Ebola virus disease
GDP	gross domestic product
HCW	healthcare worker
MENA	Middle East/North Africa
MERS	Middle East respiratory syndrome
PPE	personal protective equipment
SARS	severe acute respiratory syndrome
SARS-CoV-2	severe acute respiratory syndrome coronavirus 2
WHO	World Health Organization

Over the course of the coronavirus disease 2019 (COVID-19) pandemic, severe acute respiratory syndrome coronavirus 2 (SARS-CoV-2) has been cited as "the great equalizer," because it has disregarded wealth, age, location, and prestige when spreading across the globe [1]. In addition to the devastating impact COVID-19 had on the general population, this novel virus exacerbated struggling healthcare systems and revealed stark weaknesses in others. Hospitals around the world consumed vital medical supplies and human resources quicker than they were replenished, while simultaneously suffering enormous human and financial losses. Thus, the COVID-19 pandemic engendered a paradigm shift as an increasing number of healthcare facilities were forced to adapt or risk closing their doors altogether. Ultimately, countries around the world have tirelessly fought the COVID-19 pandemic by enacting their own unique healthcare responses while also collaborating with other countries to curb the spread of disease. Throughout this chapter, we will identify the varying impacts of COVID-19 on different healthcare systems around the world and discuss the unprecedented public health strategies used to mitigate the significant effects of this novel virus.

Healthcare Systems Before COVID-19

While the modern world has never experienced a disease as widespread and devastating as the SARS-CoV-2- induced COVID-19, previous viral outbreaks also had an impact on global healthcare systems and provided valuable lessons that can be adapted to combat COVID-19.

As the first pandemic of the twenty-first century, severe acute respiratory syndrome (SARS) spread to more than two dozen countries while infecting more than 8000 people and causing nearly 1000 deaths [2]. This outbreak demonstrated the importance of enacting quarantine measures, real-time information gathering, and collaboration among scientists and laboratories across the world [3]. The detriments of the 2003 SARS pandemic led to revisions of the International Health Regulations, which outline the duties of countries and leadership responsibilities of the World Health Organization (WHO) [4].

These revised guidelines helped lead the fight against the 2009 influenza A (H1N1 or swine flu), which resulted in an estimated 151 700–575 400 deaths worldwide during the first year [5]. Although the world gained invaluable knowledge and experience from this pandemic, public health officials were nonetheless provided with the grim reminder that "the world is ill-prepared to respond to a severe influenza pandemic or to any similar global, sustained and threatening public health emergency" [6].

In 2012, yet another public health crisis struck with the first few cases of Middle East respiratory syndrome (MERS) detected in the Middle East, Africa, and Asia [7]. With a 35% mortality rate, its spread to 27 countries led to 886 confirmed deaths worldwide [7]. This outbreak highlighted the necessity of infection control, as transmission within healthcare facilities and between patients and healthcare workers (HCWs) was observed, inevitably worsening the impact of MERS [7].

Just two years later, the 2014 Ebola virus disease (EVD) originated in southeastern Guinea and rapidly spread throughout parts of West Africa [8]. This epidemic demonstrated how weak and inadequate public health infrastructure and surveillance systems can fail to contain a deadly virus, as it was rapidly transmitted within densely populated areas and to neighboring countries. The fear of international spread became a reality when EVD was transmitted to the United States, United Kingdom, Italy, Spain, Mali, Senegal, and Nigeria, resulting in approximately 11 300 deaths [8]. However, this outbreak also showcased how international efforts can translate into effective action; the EVD outbreak ended in 2016 after partnerships between national bodies, such as ministries of health, and international public health organizations collaborated to slow its transmission and aid the most heavily affected countries. Figure 29.1 details the timeline and impact of past viral outbreaks.

After the Ebola outbreak, certain authors, such as Kruk et al. [9], detailed specific prerequisites that encompass a resilient healthcare system, including the following: (1) recognition of the global potential of severe health crises and establishment of clear roles at all levels of the global health system, (2) legal and policy framework to direct the public health response and establish accountability, and (3) the need for a strong and committed healthcare workforce. Furthermore, they characterized resilient health systems as possessing the following five traits: (1) awareness, particularly in the current health trends across the world; (2) diversity, or being able to address a multitude of health

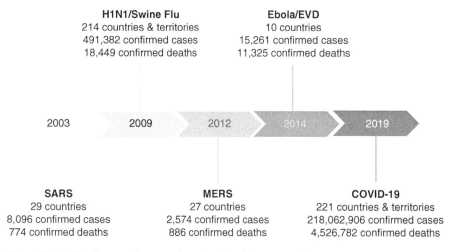

Figure 29.1 Timeline and impact of pandemics of the twenty-first century.

challenges; (3) self-regulation, or the ability to manage current health crises while also tending to other health services; (4) integration of all aspects of care, from HCWs to public health officials to the public; and (5) adaptability, or the ability to react quickly to changing conditions and meet the needs of the volatile state of health in the world [9]. Although neither official nor comprehensive, these traits can undoubtedly guide healthcare systems across the world and prepare them for future emergencies.

Unfortunately, during the current COVID-19 pandemic, several of these traits are absent from many healthcare systems, and the virus is still devastating global healthcare systems at an unprecedented pace. As of September 2021, COVID-19 has infected more than 200 million individuals and led to more than four million deaths globally [10] (Figure 29.2). Ultimately, although these public health crises improved our pandemic response knowledge and highlighted the resilience of modern healthcare systems, they did not sufficiently fortify healthcare systems in preparation for the COVID-19 pandemic.

International Trends and Collaboration

Fortunately, the increase in international collaboration helped mitigate the destructive consequences of SARS-CoV-2. Many countries throughout the world faced severe shortages of medical equipment and supplies, and thus relied on high-income countries for support. As early as December 2019, the WHO released a document discussing the rationing of personal protective equipment (PPE) [11]. This was one of the initial impacts that COVID-19 had on global healthcare systems, because medical supply chains were severely disrupted, yielding massive PPE shortages [12]. In addition to the lack of PPE, the surge of patients with COVID-19 created widespread shortages of intensive care unit (ICU) beds and ventilators [12]. Many hospitals were also at risk for financial collapse because many facilities decided to either cancel or postpone nonemergency appointments, eliminating a significant source of income for healthcare facilities [12]. This decision not only impacted these

Global cummulative cases of COVID-19 reported

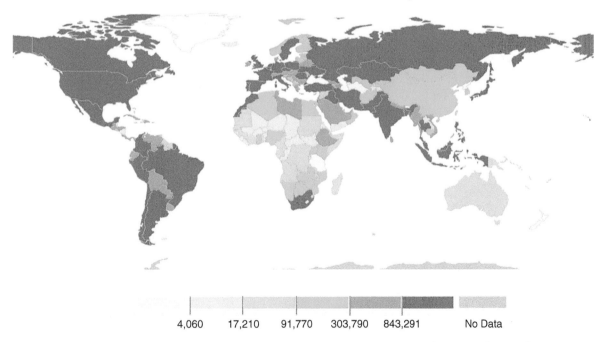

| 4,060 | 17,210 | 91,770 | 303,790 | 843,291 | No Data |

Figure 29.2 Cumulative cases of COVID-19 worldwide. *Source:* Data are provided by the Centers for Disease Control and Prevention's COVID Data Tracker (https://covid.cdc.gov/covid-data-tracker/#datatracker-home).

facilities but also had harrowing ramifications for patients with noncommunicable diseases who were unable to receive adequate levels of treatment [12]. In low- and middle-income countries, these consequences were exacerbated, and it was estimated that the COVID-19 pandemic cost around US$52 billion every four weeks to provide effective healthcare responses [12]. Thus, in May 2020, the World Bank announced its emergency operations to fight COVID-19, including US$160 billion in grants and financial support to help strengthen developing countries' health systems and their ability to respond to the pandemic's impacts. For example, the Philippines received US$100 million to procure medical supplies such as PPE, medicines, and test kits, and Iraq received US$33.6 million to help finance its need for medical supplies and strengthen its hospital ICU capacity [13].

Aside from financial assistance, healthcare systems benefited by learning from the novel public health strategies and innovative medical technology adapted in other countries. Many vital lessons were provided by Singapore, one of the first countries to be affected by COVID-19. The combination of swift government action, stringent contact tracing, and implementation of infectious disease centers all helped aid healthcare systems in their battle against COVID-19. Throughout the country, more than 800 public health preparedness clinics were created to enhance detection of the virus [14]. Singapore also proactively built a 330-bed facility with integrated clinical, laboratory, and epidemiologic functions [14, 15]. In terms of the financial burden of COVID-19, the government of Singapore financed treatment costs incurred by patients with COVID-19 in public hospitals, allowing for higher quality and quantity of health care [16]. Furthermore, private insurers also extended coverage for hospitalizations as a result of COVID-19 [14]. Although cases surged months later in April 2020, Singapore provided valuable lessons to the rest of the world, including the importance of (1) consistency and transparency in information communicated, (2) clear legal framework to reduce possibilities of misinformation and enhance clearer communication, (3) increased testing and contact tracing to identify and isolate cases, and (4) emphasis on dense or at-risk populations to mitigate community transmission [14]. Although it is by no

means a comprehensive guide for a COVID-19 response, Singapore serves as an example of how a healthcare system quickly adapted to the evolving situation, while undergoing trial and error to identify both effective and ineffective strategies. Although Singapore's measures played an integral role in gaining invaluable knowledge of the dynamics of the virus early in the pandemic, it should be noted that regions across the world were impacted differently and possessed varying levels of resources and funding that shaped their ability to fight the COVID-19 pandemic. We will discuss Singapore's response in more detail later in the "Southeast Asia" section.

In some developing countries, lack of preparedness proved to be a major contributor to pandemic-induced struggles. For many people, social distancing was a nearly impossible feat due to overcrowding in households, limited access to basic necessities such as fresh water and sanitation, and reliance on public transportation. Shortages of PPE, healthcare personnel, and medical equipment, as well as the lack of adequate database technologies, largely contributed to the negative outcomes that occurred. A worldwide survey of HCWs indicated that 52% of respondents reported at least one piece of standard PPE was unavailable, 44% reported an additional need for PPE, and only 44% of HCWs were confident in the adequacy of PPE they received, while 14% were not confident at all (Figure 29.3) [17]. Yet, even in prodigiously developed countries like the United States, 80% of HCWs reported having to repeatedly reuse PPE [12].

In some cases, a lack of resources was not the defining issue. A review by the WHO of the ICU capacity in the Eastern Mediterranean indicated no shortage of medical equipment, but it all remained unused because of a lack of knowledge about their function [18]. For example, ventilators and oxygen delivery devices, which were highly valuable due to their lifesaving capacity in patients with COVID-19, required operation by specially trained medical staff [18]. Unfortunately, an adequate supply of HCWs was deficient in many areas of the world, with even fewer experienced HCWs available to operate these lifesaving machines.

Many countries, developing countries in particular, also did not have sophisticated database and surveillance technologies, which are vital to help gather and

Results from a Worldwide Survey of Healthcare Workers Assessing PPE Shortage

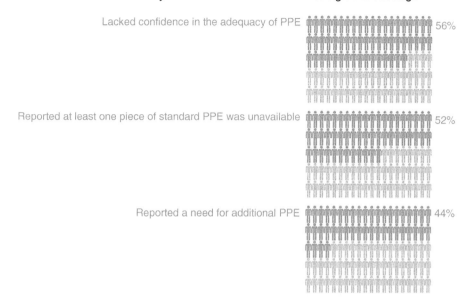

Figure 29.3 Results from a worldwide survey assessing PPE adequacy among HCWs.

disseminate information in real time to inform healthcare responses. Ideally, these health information technology systems, which include civil registration and vital statistics, would be able to track birth, death, and cause of death data. However, because many countries lacked this infrastructure, they instead evaluated COVID-19 death data through the use of "excess mortality," a statistical measure defined as "the difference between the total observed deaths for the year and those expected in the absence of COVID-19" [19]. However, this model is based only on available data from 50 European countries and 15 countries from the Americas, with no adjustments included for underreporting. As a result, data gaps exist in the African, Eastern Mediterranean, Southeast Asian, and Western Pacific regions [19]. These serious flaws in the estimation and reporting process continue to prevent accurate global measurements of COVID-19 deaths that would guide future public policy and health emergency preparedness plans.

In short, the COVID-19 pandemic gravely impacted healthcare systems around the world and posed massive challenges of varying effects on different regions. We will now discuss the impact of COVID-19 on healthcare systems according to region, including Africa, Asia Pacific, Europe, the Middle East/North Africa (MENA), and the Americas.

Africa

As SARS-CoV-2 spread across the globe, Africa felt the effects of COVID-19 relatively late as the first case on the continent was reported nearly two months (in Egypt on 14 February 2020) after the first case in Wuhan, China. However, by March, the speed of transmission across the continent increased, and by early April, almost every country in Africa reported COVID-19 cases [20]. Yet, the COVID-19 case numbers in Africa were much lower compared with the rest of the world. To put this in perspective, as of 13 April 2020, there were about 14 000 COVID-19 cases in Africa, whereas Italy and the United States had 160 000 and 560 000 confirmed cases, respectively [21, 22]. Although the WHO asserted in May 2020 that the COVID-19 case numbers in Africa remained low because of its strong leadership and unique population demographics, the low case count may instead

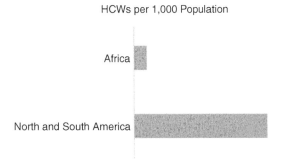

Figure 29.4 HCWs per 1000 population in Africa and North and South America.

be because of the lack of testing availability [23]. In addition, reverse transcription polymerase chain reaction diagnostic capacity was extremely limited because of the presence of only one to three qualified testing labs throughout 40 African countries [24].

Across all African regions, COVID-19 deleteriously impacted the already fragile healthcare systems in place. Africa contains 22 of the 25 most vulnerable countries to infectious diseases [25] and has been historically plagued by fatal diseases, where 26 million people are estimated to be infected with HIV, 2.5 million with tuberculosis, 71 million with hepatitis B or C, and approximately 200 million with malaria [26]. To make matters worse, Africa currently suffers an HCW shortage, with about 2.3 HCWs per 1000 population, while both North and South America have approximately 24.8 HCWs per 1000 population (Figure 29.4) [27].

Poverty is also widespread throughout Africa, where approximately 85% of Africans make less than US$6 per day [28]. Thus, the combination of these factors made African health systems particularly vulnerable to the COVID-19 pandemic, which will be explored by region in the upcoming section.

West Africa

Although COVID-19 was late to reach West Africa, this region was particularly vulnerable to the outbreak due to its lack of resources, widespread poverty, and meager investments into health care, including HCWs, medical supplies, and infrastructure [29]. In the early stages of the pandemic, Nigeria's head of Centers for Disease Control and Prevention stated, "Our health system is not as strong as we'd like it to be. It is because we are a bit worried about our capacity to deal with a large outbreak that we are focused so intensively on prevention and early detection" [30]. This disconcerting truth was highlighted by the fact that, in 13 of 16 West African countries, there exists less than two medical doctors for every 10 000 people [29, 31, 32]. According to the World Bank, West Africa is home to 9 of the 25 poorest countries in the world, with little room to fund health care [32]. Furthermore, in the West African region, healthcare spending per capita is extremely low, with 8 of the 16 West African countries spending less than $50 per capita on healthcare expenses [29, 33]. In contrast, the per capita spending on healthcare in the United States is around $11 582 per person [34]. These country-based differences in healthcare spending are highlighted in Figure 29.5.

Due to learned experiences from the 2014 Ebola outbreak and the subsequent creation of strong regional partnerships, the ministers of health of all 15 Economic Community of West African States met and swiftly decided on a unified regional approach to the crisis. This included strengthening national diagnosing and managing capacities, infrastructure for adequate quarantine, ICU facilities, and availability of medical supplies and PPE [35].

Thus, although West African countries received generous donations from the World Bank to help strengthen immediate healthcare capacity and combat the virus long term, many shortcomings within their healthcare systems hindered their outbreak response [36]. For example, West Africa has only a handful of ventilators to accommodate millions of people – an amount far too small to sustain the COVID-19-stricken healthcare systems of these countries [37]. Liberia has only five ventilators for 4.94 million residents, and Nigeria has less than 100 ventilators for 200 million residents [38]. Moreover, most countries in West Africa possess fewer than five hospital beds per 10 000 of the population [32]. COVID-19 also exacerbated the widespread PPE shortages in the region, with many West African countries unable to adequately supply HCWs, let alone the general population [38].

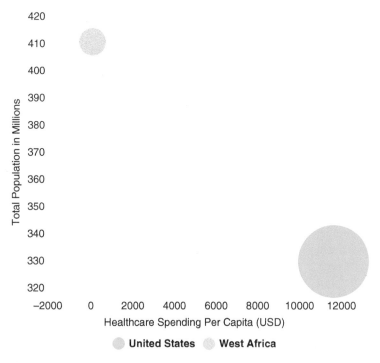

Figure 29.5 Difference in total population and comparative healthcare spending per capita between West Africa and the United States.

The rapid influx of patients with COVID-19 also forced West African countries to expand their current healthcare facilities or build new ones. In Niger, Médecins Sans Frontières, a medical humanitarian group, helped construct a new treatment center that houses up to 100 beds [36]. In Liberia, the Incident Management System created treatment units and precautionary observation centers by means of renovating public buildings and 14 military hospitals [36]. Public health officials also created self-quarantine shelters to host displaced persons with contact history and ensure self-isolation [33].

To further fund testing and PPE, the West African Health Organization provided 50000 specimen transport kits, more than 30000 diagnostic test kits, and 10000 PPE supplies [38]. Through a combination of new health service delivery approaches, public health actions, and a wealth of donations, West Africa's healthcare systems have further strengthened their resilience. Yet, further steps, such as investing in research and developing health technologies, need to occur to decrease the gap between an adequate and successful response [39].

East Africa

East Africa consists of 20 countries in the eastern region of Africa, including some of the poorest nations in the world [40]. To understand COVID-19's impact on East Africa, it is vital to first recognize that the region has been plagued by civil unrest and disease before the arrival of the novel coronavirus. East African countries have a bleak infectious disease history, most notably AIDS, tuberculosis, and malaria. Malawi has one of the highest prevalences of HIV/AIDS in the world, with 9.2% of the adult population suffering from the disease [41]. COVID-19 further worsened these public health crises in rural Uganda, where COVID-19 restrictions prevented residents from accessing HIV testing services [42]. East African residents also suffer exorbitant healthcare costs, with residents in Comoros and Uganda paying up to 70% of healthcare expenses out of pocket [43–45]. Thus, most East Africans were unable to afford healthcare treatment, with COVID-19-induced lockdowns exacerbating this issue by making it increasingly difficult to find income [46]. East Africa's underfunded healthcare systems, along with its disease and poverty-stricken population, makes the region a disconcerting area of concern for the COVID-19 pandemic.

As East Africa continues to be one of the poorest regions across the globe, COVID-19 truly tested the resilience of their healthcare systems as they battled extensive resource scarcities in addition to the virus. In Kenya, COVID-19 yielded substantial shortages of ICU beds and ventilators, with reports that only 200 ICU beds existed for a population of 50 million [37]. Somalia also experienced a resource shortage, with only 46 ICU beds and 15 ventilators available for the whole country [23].

Many strategies were adopted to try and combat these shortages at both the national and international level. For example, many East African countries postponed or canceled elective medical procedures to shift medical focus to COVID-19-related matters [36]. Other countries blocked the exportation of certain PPE such as face masks [47]. As far as international measures, the WHO gave East African countries more than US$250 000 worth of medical equipment [36].

HCW shortages also debilitated East African countries because countries like Uganda have only one third of the minimum WHO-recommended number of HCWs [48]. To address these HCW shortages, additional HCWs were contracted to East African countries for the first six months of COVID-19, to support the mass influx of cases [36]. In Mozambique, staff at the National Institute of Health, medical residents, and students from the Field Epidemiology and Laboratory Training program helped carry out contact tracing tasks in an effort to better understand and contain the spread of the virus in East Africa [36]. In addition, these workers increased national testing capacity, set out rationing guidelines for PPE, and helped refurbish and construct health facilities to accommodate cases [36]. Ultimately, East African healthcare systems were forced to adapt in an unprecedented fashion, and only time will tell how COVID-19 will affect the region's healthcare systems over the long term.

Southern Africa

Southern Africa, which consists of Botswana, Eswatini, Lesotho, Namibia, and South Africa, fared better than other African regions (aside from the North African region) because of the previous infectious disease outbreaks and higher average income of its countries, particularly South Africa [49, 50]. Because of Southern Africa's historical experiences with Ebola, tuberculosis, malaria, and HIV, the region was able to quickly activate preexisting community engagement programs and emergency public health interventions, as well as redirect trained emergency medical staff toward COVID-19 [50]. Thus, these established programs likely guided public health officials when designing interventions specific to COVID-19.

Early efforts against COVID-19 emphasized preventive measures, rapid case identification, and contact tracing to mitigate transmission [51]. For example, Namibia enacted several policies and practices aimed at preventing the spread of COVID-19, including stay-at-home orders apart from essential activities, limiting capacity and hours of operation for public transportation, physical distancing mandates, and daily media updates to the public [52]. Similarly, both South Africa and Botswana initiated early testing of suspected COVID-19 cases and established specific facilities for COVID-19 testing and care [53, 54]. More specifically, by mid-March 2020, both South Africa and Botswana had prohibited mass gatherings and nonessential travel within the country, encouraged remote work for private and government institutions, and closed schools [55, 56]. Just a few days later, these countries increased these measures by initiating border closures for noncitizens and nonessential workers, implementing border screening at ports of entry, and recommending 14-day self-quarantines for all incoming travelers [57, 58]. Finally, by the end of the month, both countries established widespread lockdowns and strict enforcement of social distancing guidelines [59, 60]. A visual representation of the enactment timeline of these COVID-19 measures in South Africa and Botswana is shown in Figure 29.6.

Despite these efforts, COVID-19 still infiltrated Southern Africa and overwhelmed certain regions more than others. Interestingly, while Botswana suffered nearly 160 000 confirmed cases and slightly less than 2300 COVID-19 deaths as of September 2021, South Africa has tallied almost three million confirmed cases and approximately 83 000 deaths [61]. However, this stark discrepancy may be attributed to

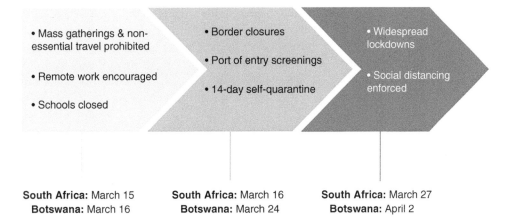

• Mass gatherings & non-essential travel prohibited

• Remote work encouraged

• Schools closed

• Border closures

• Port of entry screenings

• 14-day self-quarantine

• Widespread lockdowns

• Social distancing enforced

South Africa: March 15
Botswana: March 16

South Africa: March 16
Botswana: March 24

South Africa: March 27
Botswana: April 2

Figure 29.6   Timeline of COVID-19 measures in South Africa and Botswana.

the lack of accurate data collection and testing occurring in Botswana. This may also be true of Lesotho, a country surrounded entirely by South Africa, as the first COVID-19 case was not reported until May 2020, yet many authors also attribute this to the successful implementation of lockdown measures [62].

Although South Africa has a higher per capita income than many Southern African countries, this region still had severe health outcomes, because of the long history of income polarization and racial/gender-based discrimination present within this country [63]. South Africa is considered one of the globe's most inequitable countries, with 30.3 million South Africans living in poverty [64]. Despite South Africa having one of the best healthcare systems in the Southern African region, the nation struggled with a lack of healthcare facilities, workers, and equipment. Not only were ventilators in short supply, but there were also less than 1000 ICU beds for a population of more than 56 million people [65]. To try to mitigate the effects of lost resources from COVID-19 surges in healthcare facilities, South Africa brought in doctors from Cuba and adopted digital health technologies at an unprecedented rate, which is less common in other parts of Africa [66, 67].

Ultimately, throughout Southern Africa, the COVID-19 pandemic has spurred the adaptation of preexisting public health strategies and the diversion of emergency health workforce staff, while also necessitating atypical responses to adapt to the unprecedented damage to its healthcare systems. For example,

some countries within Southern Africa created a 24-hour hotline and used social media platforms to disseminate real-time information [68, 69]. In general, this part of Africa coped with COVID-19 relatively well because Southern Africa's prior experiences fighting infectious disease outbreaks have indisputably fortified their healthcare systems, which likely contributed to the region's success against COVID-19.

Central Africa

Like many other African regions, Central Africa was not spared in terms of historical epidemics and public health crises. Although some authors note that Central Africa's previous experience with infectious disease may better equip them with knowledge to fend off COVID-19, this has not proven to be true because of the lack of available healthcare funding. Due to the high prevalence of measles, polio, cholera, yellow fever, tetanus, and meningitis still present in this region, many central African countries were unable to fund further health expenses and pay their employees [63, 70]. Thus, many HCWs emigrated from Central African countries to other parts of Africa in search of better pay. Overall, it is no surprise that Central Africa's already weak healthcare systems were greatly exacerbated by the monumental surge of COVID-19 cases.

Aside from healthcare resource shortages, Central Africa is notoriously known for its wars and conflicts, which oftentimes have devastating consequences on healthcare systems [70]. The Central African region is also poverty ridden, with reports that this jurisdiction has one of the lowest human development indices in the world, with 73% of the Democratic Republic of Congo living on less than $2 per day in 2018 [70]. Together, Central Africa's history of diseases, already weak healthcare systems, conflicts, and poverty created an uphill battle against COVID-19.

Future Directions for Africa

Despite Africa's hefty resilience to the pandemic, their already derelict healthcare systems compounded with the high prevalence of comorbidities, poverty, and an underinsured population have left them continuing to struggle under COVID-19's grasp (Figure 29.7). Nonetheless, from adapting and creating healthcare delivery services, to unprecedented public health actions, to receiving generous aid, African health systems have indeed battled back

fiercely against this pandemic. Many authors push for the emergence of telemedicine and digital health in Africa [71], which can reduce overcrowded health facilities, decrease the risk for disease transmission, and eliminate travel costs [72]. However, these ideas are naive and unrealistic in many African regions due to the lack of reliable Wi-Fi, electricity, and adequate technology.

Regarding vaccination against COVID-19, most African countries have administered fewer than 10 doses per 100 population [73]. Although this delayed distribution of COVID-19 vaccines may be attributed to high demand, high costs, and low supply, Sen-Crowe et al. [73] note that immunization rates in Africa do not seem to be dependent on how quickly a country received the vaccine. For example, South Africa was one of the first African countries to receive the vaccine, but only 5.7 and 2.8 persons per 100 population were partially and fully vaccinated, respectively, at the time of the study [73]. However, the COVID-19

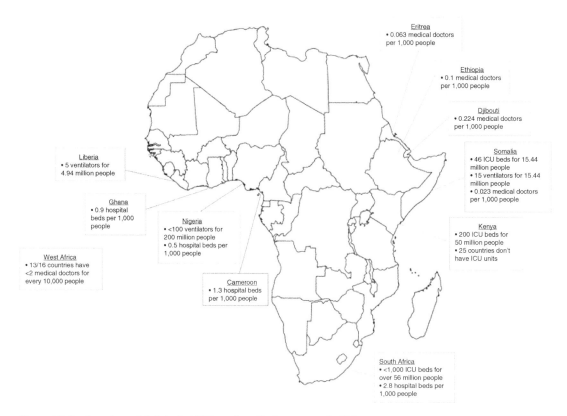

Figure 29.7 Overview of deficits in HCWs and medical resources in Africa.

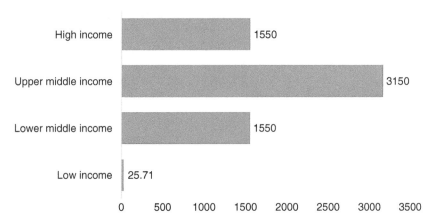

Figure 29.8 Disparities in COVID-19 vaccine availability based on the income group of countries worldwide. *Source:* Data are extrapolated with permission from Our World in Data: https://ourworldindata.org/grapher/cumulative-covid-vaccinations?country=High+income~Upper+middle+income~Lower+middle+income~Low+income.

Vaccines Global Access (COVAX) facility, a cofinancing vaccine acquisition program, continues to help African countries cover at least 20% of their population, which will drastically decrease the burden faced by African healthcare systems (Figure 29.8) [74, 75].

Asia Pacific

Although the five subregions of Asia-Pacific – East Asia, Central Asia, South Asia, Southeast Asia, and Oceania – are politically, culturally, economically, and geographically diverse, the high rates of infection disabled healthcare systems throughout the entire continent. However, some regions of Asia were more vulnerable to the effects of the pandemic due to lack of resources, insufficient intervention policies, and impoverished populations (Figure 29.9).

East Asia

As the COVID-19 pandemic first struck East Asia, healthcare systems in this region were forced to adapt in an unprecedented amount of time. However, compared with the other Asian regions, East Asia had greater success in managing the spread of COVID-19, because of the rapid governmental intervention and the general population's willingness to comply with guidelines [76]. In addition, this region was no stranger

to public health crises due to prior experience with SARS and MERS outbreaks [77].

Overall, the East Asian region was more equipped to handle COVID-19 infection because of higher income, government structure, and production capabilities. In addition, healthcare systems in these developed countries were better prepared to manage stark increases in patient load, thus further contributing to the containment of COVID-19. For example, China's well-resourced health system features 41 HCWs and 42 hospital beds per 10 000 people [77]. In terms of medical equipment and supplies, East Asian countries have an advantage because it is home to some of the world's largest economies and production sites of many supplies. Thus, when faced with medical equipment shortages, many countries such as Taiwan had the ability to increase production of supplies like masks and halt the exportation of medical supplies [78]. A majority of the East Asian population also have more access to health care. China's strong health system provides more than 95% of citizens with healthcare coverage [77]. Moreover, Taiwan has a single-payer system, in which the government covers comprehensive benefits for a majority of citizens [78].

Despite those facts, these countries were still overwhelmed with initial increases in COVID-19 cases. In China, more than 80 000 cases were reported in less than two months, making it the original epicenter of the pandemic (Figure 29.10) [76]. To manage the

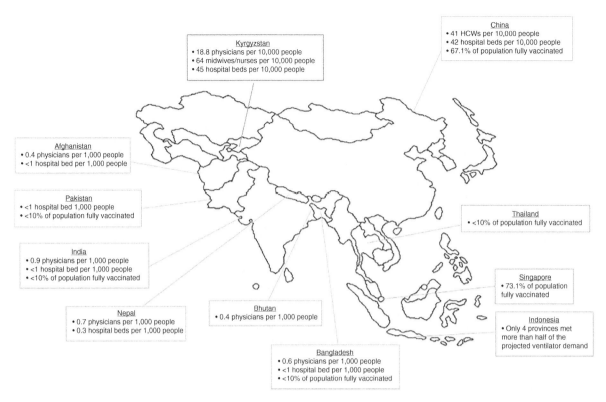

Figure 29.9 Overview of vaccination rates, as well as deficits in HCWs and medical resources, in Asia.

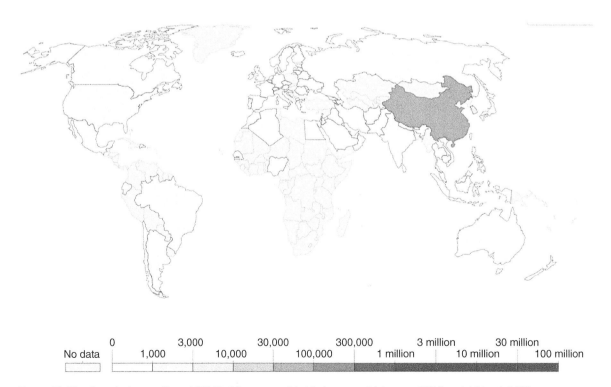

No data   0   3,000   30,000   300,000   3 million   30 million
           1,000   10,000   100,000   1 million   10 million   100 million

Figure 29.10 Cumulative confirmed COVID-19 cases worldwide between 11 January 2020 and 1 March 2020.
Source: Ritchie et al. [79].

initial exponential patient increase, China constructed specialty hospitals, such as Leishenshan Hospital and Huoshenshan Hospital, to deliver treatment for severe respiratory illness [36]. In addition, shelter hospitals were created from large public facilities to provide more space to admit patients [80]. Governmental policies and other healthcare strategies were also adopted to reduce transmission.

Other countries in East Asia enacted similar policies, such as increased contact tracing, strict testing policies, free treatment for patients with COVID-19, and mobilization of resources [12, 76]. Taiwan, although expected to have a catastrophically high rate of COVID-19 cases because of its proximity to China, was able to quickly mobilize public health efforts to manage the pandemic. This targeted approach was supported by proactive testing and contact tracing. For example, patients on the National Health Insurance database with severe respiratory symptoms who previously tested negative for influenza were retested for COVID-19 [81]. In addition, national datasets were analyzed to ensure PPE was successfully distributed to the most vulnerable populations [82]. New technologies, including quick response code scanning and online travel history reporting, were also used to classify infection risk of travelers. Those with high infection risks were mandated to quarantine at home and were tracked through mobile phones to ensure compliance with quarantine guidelines [81]. Contact tracing methods in South Korea were also elevated by digital technologies, because HCWs were able to identify exposed members of the population using electronic medical records, credit card transactions, Global Position System data, and closed-circuit television [83]. Ultimately, although the introduction of digital methods, extensive testing, and tracing tactics have proved successful in combating COVID-19 in certain East Asian countries, it is unlikely that more democratic countries will adopt these strategies because of privacy and equity concerns.

Central Asia

The five countries of Central Asia – Kazakhstan, Uzbekistan, Tajikistan, Kyrgyzstan, and Turkmenistan – are geographically and culturally remote [84]. Interestingly, this region did not report a positive COVID-19 case until two months after the first case in Wuhan. Shortly thereafter, the virus spread to every country in the region except Turkmenistan, who has yet to report a single COVID-19 case [85, 86]. However, a lack of comprehensive testing is a great concern in this country [87].

Compared with the rest of Central Asia, Kyrgyzstan's healthcare system was best equipped to handle a pandemic because of recent reform and support from many international organizations [88]. This resulted in 45 hospital beds, 18.8 physicians, and 64 nurses and midwives per 10000 people [89]. Yet, even with Kyrgyzstan's moderately strong healthcare system and the enactment of strict lockdowns, none of the countries of Central Asia had an adequate infrastructure to accommodate the vast number of cases [88]. Therefore, when lockdown mandates were lifted and infections began to rise, medical facilities were forced to turn patients away [88]. In addition, half of the country's ventilators were dysfunctional, one in four COVID-19 cases occurred in HCWs, and patients suffering from other diseases had limited access to treatment because all focus shifted to battling the effects of COVID-19 [88, 89].

Parts of Central Asia worked tirelessly to mitigate this outbreak, with countries such as Kyrgyzstan creating COVID-19 departments and outpatient facilities [88]. Uzbekistan also committed to increasing medical equipment, constructing new treatment facilities, and encouraging international cooperation in response to COVID-19 [84]. Conversely, other countries, such as Tajikistan and Turkmenistan, have been criticized for denying the seriousness of the pandemic and potentially reporting false information regarding cases and deaths [85]. Thus, the COVID-19 pandemic not only shed light on faults in Central Asian healthcare systems but also emphasized the corruption occurring in parts of this region.

South Asia

South Asia, which includes India, Pakistan, Bangladesh, Nepal, Sri Lanka, Afghanistan, Maldives, and Bhutan, is one of the most densely populated and poorest regions in the world [90]. Therefore, when infection rates inevitably surged in this region, healthcare systems were unprepared and unequipped to mount an effective response. The first confirmed case in South Asia was discovered in Nepal on 14 January 2020 [82, 91]. Cases quickly spread to other countries, with Sri Lanka and India having confirmed cases on 17 January and 30 January 2020, respectively. By 18 June 2020, India became the fourth most affected country in the world and the most impacted country in South Asia with more than 354 000 cases [91, 92], devastating the weak healthcare system in place.

The underdeveloped state of the healthcare systems in South Asia can be attributed to lack of funding, resources, and HCWs. While the United States spends 17.06% of its gross domestic product (GDP) on health care, India and Bangladesh spend only 3.53 and 2.27% of their GDPs, respectively [93]. This directly translates to the large gap in the availability of necessary hospital resources. For example, Nepal has only 0.3 hospital bed per 1000 people, one of the lowest rates in the world. Other countries, such as Afghanistan, India, Pakistan, and Bangladesh, also have less than one hospital bed available per 1000 people [94]. This region also faces a HCW shortage as well, with Afghanistan and Bhutan having only 0.4 physician per 1000 people. Bangladesh, Nepal, and India do not have much higher rates, with only 0.6, 0.7, and 0.9 physician per 1000 people, respectively [95]. In addition, the available frontline workers were faced with a high risk for COVID-19 infection because of a shortage of PPE. In Pakistan, only 37.4% of HCWs had access to N95 respirators, 34.5% to gloves, 13.8% to face shields or goggles, and only 12.9% had access to full suits and gowns [12]. These characteristics reflect the weak state of healthcare systems in South Asia, which ultimately resulted in overburdened hospitals and high morbidity and mortality.

Southeast Asia

Although COVID-19 spread to every nation in Southeast Asia, each country undertook vastly different strategies to manage the pandemic. As mentioned previously, Singapore took a stringent approach to suppressive strategies, as well as widespread testing and contact tracing. In addition, Singapore took the unprecedented step of closing international borders [96]. Conversely, Indonesia's initial relaxed governmental response burdened its already inadequate healthcare system. Although COVID-19 spread rapidly throughout neighboring countries, it was not until 2 March 2020 that the first cases were reported in Indonesia. The decentralized healthcare system in Indonesia was characterized by a scarcity of resources and insufficient testing and tracing, thus making it unequipped to handle the large influx of cases. Sadly, Indonesia quickly had one of the largest fatality rates in the world [97]. In addition, only four provinces in Indonesia were deemed "safe," meaning they met more than half of the projected ventilator demand [98]. With insufficient resources, widespread poverty, overworked HCWs, and unabated infection rates, Indonesia continues to experience a dire healthcare crisis and has already surpassed 100 000 COVID-19 deaths [99].

Other countries in Southeast Asia, such as Thailand, Vietnam, and Malaysia, initially had relative success managing the pandemic. However, in 2021, cases began to soar in these countries. As seen in other regions of Asia, the combination of the new delta variant and low vaccination rates engendered a devastating outcome [99]. Many Southeast Asian countries have less than 10% of the population fully vaccinated [100]. In fact, in Vietnam, only 3.40% of the population was fully vaccinated as of September 2021 [100]. Thus, it is imperative that these countries quickly increase inoculation rates and consider reinstating strict lockdown procedures to better combat COVID-19.

Oceania/Pacific

Overall, the impacts of the COVID-19 pandemic in the Oceania/Pacific region were much milder than what occurred throughout the rest of the developed world [101]. This can be attributed to geographic isolation, widespread testing and containment measures, and strict border closures [101]. Australia and New Zealand in particular demonstrated rapid and effective COVID-19 responses, resulting in relatively low case and death numbers. New Zealand also ensured equitable access to diagnostic and treatment strategies, with a particular focus on Māori and Pacific islander populations [36]. As of August 2021, New Zealand has reported only 2936 cumulative COVID-19 cases and 26 COVID-19-related deaths [102]. Similar to Singapore, New Zealand and Australia quickly enacted strict international border closures to reduce imported transmission of the virus [101]. Further, returning Australians were subjected to a mandatory 14-day hotel quarantine [103]. Despite low case numbers in Australia, the healthcare systems were still indirectly impacted. In New South Wales, the most populous state in Australia, the stable healthcare system is publicly funded and features more than 110 000 HCWs [103]. Efforts to increase healthcare capacities for COVID-19 outbreaks resulted in the postponement of unrelated medical procedures, and a study in New South Wales notes that the number of elective surgeries has decreased by 32.6% compared with 2019, creating a significant financial burden [103].

Although many of the Pacific Islands have avoided disastrous consequences of COVID-19 through border closures, the region has still faced challenges throughout the pandemic because of limited access to quality health care. Unlike Australia and New Zealand, the healthcare systems in the smaller Pacific Island countries lack infrastructure, resources, and qualified workers [104]. Further, a shortage of laboratory equipment needed to analyze test samples made identifying COVID-19 cases in these countries a difficult task [104]. Health delivery in the Pacific Island countries also presents a unique challenge, because a significant portion of the population is widely dispersed throughout remote areas even though hospital-based care is localized in densely populated areas [105]. To combat this, the WHO created a Pacific Action COVID-19 Preparedness and Response Plan, which outlines methods to minimize virus transmission and optimize treatment capabilities for this region. Countries were advised to close international borders, enforce quarantines, and send medical resources to Pacific Island countries in greater need [106]. Fortunately, these vulnerable Pacific Island countries have been only mildly impacted by the pandemic. Only five countries worldwide have yet to report any COVID-19 cases, of which three are Pacific Island countries: Tonga, Tuvalu, and Nauru [107, 108]. It is unclear whether this is due to insufficient testing [106].

Future Directions for the Asia-Pacific Region

Ultimately, the Asia-Pacific region is vastly diverse, and the impacts of COVID-19 on healthcare systems vary. In wealthier, developed areas such as East Asia,

containment of the virus was relatively successful due to strong healthcare infrastructure, access to resources, and availability of care to the population. However, countries such as India and Indonesia with weaker healthcare systems, impoverished populations, and social inequality quickly became epicenters of COVID-19, with devastating surges of cases and deaths. Thus, countries such as India and Indonesia should consider enacting digital tracing technology to identify and isolate potential new cases. In addition, strict international border closures and supervised quarantines after travel can help lessen the burden on healthcare systems in some regions.

Recent outbreaks of the delta variant throughout Asia present new challenges for healthcare systems, especially in countries with low vaccination rates. As of August 2021, wealthier countries such as Singapore and China have 73.1 and 67.1% of their populations fully vaccinated [100, 109]. In comparison, developing countries in Asia, such as India, Pakistan, Thailand, and Bangladesh, all have less than 10% of their populations fully vaccinated [100]. Low vaccination rates ultimately result in a greater amount of severe disease cases, hospitalizations, and deaths [110]. Therefore, it is imperative to close the gap between vaccine supply and distribution in low-income countries.

Europe

Although most European countries are high income and predominantly based on socialized health care, there are unique political, social, and financial nuances that affect quality of care, healthcare delivery, and how each healthcare system managed its response to the COVID-19 pandemic. Thus, when the COVID-19 pandemic arrived in Europe, it was an unprecedented crisis that affected each healthcare system to varying degrees.

On 21 February 2020, Italy became one of the first European countries to identify a COVID-19-positive individual [111]. The virus quickly spread throughout the country, resulting in lockdown measures that were implemented around Lombardy – the area of the initial outbreak in Italy – only one day later [111]. However, Italy's management of COVID-19 was marked by uncertainty, perhaps because of the country's decentralization [112]. Throughout the pandemic, there were power struggles between the central and regional governments, a lack of policy coordination, and unclear communication to the public [113]. Nevertheless, by 9 March 2020, the entire nation underwent lockdown and more severe prevention measures were established, including travel restrictions [112]. However, these travel constraints triggered an economic crisis that increased nationwide tension [113]. To make matters worse, Italy had only a modest number of hospital beds, with a mere 8.4 beds per 100 000 population, that were not appropriately rationed [112]. Initially, patients with moderate symptoms were admitted, resulting in limited bed availability for severe cases [113]. Hospitals were also rapidly left short-staffed; by late March, nearly 9000 HCWs were infected with COVID-19, resulting in insufficient workforce capacity in many areas of the country [112]. Ultimately, the healthcare system has been devastated with more than 4.5 million COVID-19 cases and approximately 129 290 deaths as of 1 September 2021 [114, 115].

In Spain, political unrest also delayed a time-sensitive government response, which resulted in increased COVID-19 cases and deaths [116]. In fact, Spain has been one of the hardest-hit countries in terms of morbidity and mortality rates. Although the first diagnosed case of COVID-19 occurred in Spain on 31 January 2020, when a German tourist tested positive in the Spanish Canary Islands, several weeks passed before transmission was observed [117]. As a result, it was not until March 2020 that the Spanish Government established a series of preventive strategies, including educational class cancelations, flight cancelations, localized quarantines, prohibition of large-scale gatherings and nonessential travel, and encouragement of remote work [117]. Figure 29.11 demonstrates the timeline of the COVID-19 measures implemented in Spain.

Despite these efforts, initial transmission rates of COVID-19 were not favorable. By the end of March 2020, approximately 6000 ICU beds were being used by patients with COVID-19, and within eight weeks, about 250 000 cases and 25 000 deaths had occurred – constituting the highest mortality rate per million population at the time [118]. However, these statistics likely underestimate the true burden of COVID-19 in Spain, because there was a severe shortage of diagnostic tests [118]. Unfortunately, deficits in essential medical resources were not just limited to tests; Spain also experienced a paucity of PPE and healthcare providers, the latter of which was partially attributable to the high infection rate among HCWs [118]. Overall, Spain has been highly impacted by COVID-19, with more than 4.87 million confirmed cases and nearly 85 000 deaths in the country [61].

France was also heavily burdened by COVID-19. As of 3 September 2021, France has tallied approximately 6.9 million cases and 115 thousand deaths [61]. The high morbidity and mortality rates are likely due in part to wariness in leadership after previous overresponses and overspending during the 2008 H1N1 crisis [116, 119]. Due to this flawed perception, France was ill-prepared with an inadequate supply of PPE, COVID tests, and ICU beds [116]. In March 2020, a model-based study anticipated that approximately half of the regions in France would be at full capacity before mid-April 2020 [120]. Research published in January of 2021 confirmed these predictions; by the end of March 2020, France was forced to increase short-term ICU capacity by 3000 [121]. In addition to supplementing medical equipment, other preventive strategies were established. From 24 March to 11 May 2020, the President of the Republic declared a State of Sanitary Emergency, placing the country in a full lockdown [121]. However, despite France's executive centralism, which allowed top-down management of the COVID-19 crisis, the nation has fared poorly compared with other European countries, perhaps because of lack of confidence in national leadership and insufficient reserves of medical resources [121].

In contrast, Germany, with its decentralized system, initially used a bottom-up strategy in managing COVID-19 [121]. Germany approached preventative measures through containment from January to March 2020, and then transitioned to stringent rules thereafter with a national lockdown, stay-at-home orders, and legally binding social distancing rules [121, 122]. Expecting an onslaught of cases, as was seen in other parts of the world, Germany established approximately 12 000 additional ICU beds by the end of March 2020 [121]. Unlike the trends seen in other countries, Germany's containment policies were

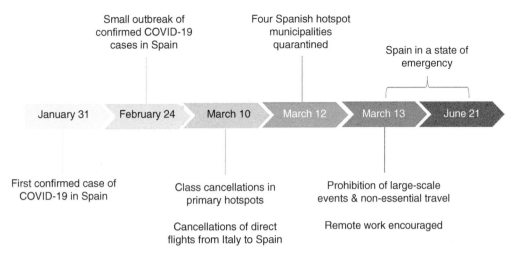

Figure 29.11 Timeline of COVID-19 measures implemented in Spain.

successful, and the surplus of ICU beds proved unnecessary as many remained unused [121]. However, even with these precautions in place, the nation has experienced 4.0 million cases and 92 849 deaths as of September 2021 [123].

In general, the UK Government initially delayed implementing policies that could have contributed to viral containment because of hesitancy in placing residents in lockdown for prolonged periods and the hope that herd immunity by natural infection would occur before COVID-19 overwhelmed the country [124]. However, not all regions hesitated in enacting public health strategies during the COVID-19 crisis. The Irish government established immediate restrictions with a nationwide lockdown on 12 March 2020, while England initially wavered before experiencing an increase in COVID-19 cases and later initiated a lockdown on 20 March 2020 [116]. In addition to these regulations, other strategies were also mandated, such as the use of face masks when using public transportation [124]. Moreover, one of the UK healthcare system's primary components, the National Health Service, which provides free health care to all permanent residents, helped to mitigate the consequences of COVID-19. Despite these systems in place, the United Kingdom still suffered at the hands of COVID-19, with nearly 7 million cases and more than 133 000 deaths as of September 2021 [61].

Future Directions for Europe

Although Europe addressed the COVID-19 pandemic from a place of higher income and strong healthcare infrastructure compared with many other regions discussed in this chapter, COVID-19 still greatly impacted this region. Although Europe's socialized healthcare systems and predominantly universal healthcare access allowed for more structure and efficiency as COVID-19 cases began to increase, domestic miscommunication and lack of clarity in policy implementation led to a disconnect between national and local government leadership. In some countries, such as Italy, a lack of a standardized national pandemic response caused regional division in pandemic response. Future healthcare crisis response in this region would largely benefit from national and continental coordination, communication in public health prevention, and outbreak mitigation strategies.

Interestingly, the European Union initially struggled with vaccine rollout because of purchasing delays and high rates of vaccine hesitancy [125]. The latter finding is especially surprising because this contradicts the results of numerous surveys that found that socioeconomic status was positively associated with vaccine acceptance [126]. In fact, both Italy and France were initially among those nations with the lowest COVID-19 vaccination acceptance rates (53.7 and 58.9%, respectively) in a study that assessed vaccine adoption in 33 different countries [127]. Individuals in Spain have echoed similar uncertainty, which was exacerbated by rare adverse side effects related to the AstraZeneca and Johnson and Johnson vaccines [128]. Yet, informational campaigns, vaccine mandates, and stringent guidelines have greatly increased the rate of vaccination. In fact, a recent article noted that Europe has vaccinated its public at four times the American pace [127]. Despite the initial reluctance, many European nations still urged, and in some cases even mandated, that their residents get inoculated. For example, Italy required COVID-19 vaccination among HCWs [129]. In other countries such as France, residents must show a "health pass" to enter indoor spaces [125]. As of 3 September 2021, well more than 541 million doses have been administered in the European Union, with 76.8 and 69.1% of the adult population having received at least one dose and full vaccination, respectively, constituting some of the highest vaccination rates in the world [130]. Specific to Italy, France, Spain, and Germany, each country respectively boasts full vaccination rates of 71.4, 76.5, 78.1, and 72.7% (Figure 29.12) [130]. Thus, many countries that initially struggled with vaccine rollout should learn from Europe's progress.

Middle East and North Africa

The MENA region has a complex interrelational political and social dynamic that spans from nations at civil war, such as in Syria, Iraq, Libya, and Yemen, to massive refugee crises of almost 15 million people fleeing to Jordan, Lebanon, Djibouti, and Tunisia [131]. With so much ongoing turmoil, prioritization of the healthcare system has not been a major focus for many MENA nations; thus, each healthcare system varies extensively (Figure 29.13) [132]. For example, Gulf countries have prospering economies and strong healthcare infrastructure, whereas developing economies in North Africa have weak health systems and fragile governments at war, leaving much of their healthcare facilities and resources already destroyed from conflict [132]. In strained regions such as Iran, Syria, Iraq, the Palestinian territories, Yemen, and Libya, accessing even water, sanitation, and hygiene services can be a challenge.

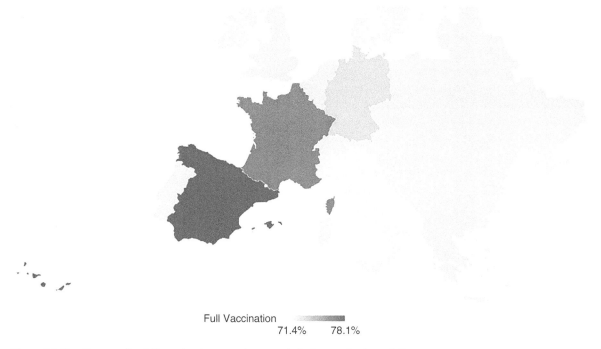

Full Vaccination
71.4%   78.1%

Figure 29.12 Comparative full vaccination rates between Italy, France, Spain, and Germany.

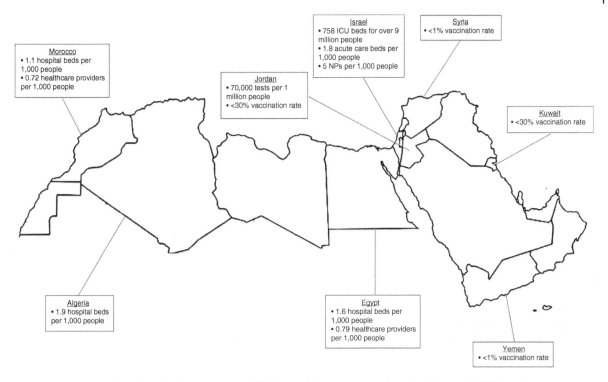

Figure 29.13 Overview of vaccination rates and deficit in healthcare personnel and equipment in MENA nations.

With more than 2.2 million confirmed COVID-19 cases in this area, the general initial government response to the COVID-19 pandemic was to declare a national state of emergency and implement strict containment policies in all nations. However, the capacity in which each healthcare system responded to the government varied greatly. For example, in Jordan, Saudi Arabia, and the United Arab Emirates, the containment policies were enforced by their respective governments through penalties, such as substantial fines and imprisonment [132]. In addition, these wealthy countries were able to quickly adapt to the influx of patients by increasing both funding and healthcare providers to improve efficiency and quality of care.

Although Israel, a country with a flourishing economy, provides universal healthcare service to all residents, including primary and secondary care, hospital services, pharmaceuticals, and diagnostic examinations, it lacked essential resources necessary to combat COVID-19 [133]. With a population of more than 9 million, Israel has only 758 ICU beds, along with only 1.8 acute care hospital beds per 1000 people [134]. In addition, Israel has only 5 practicing nurses per 1000 people [134]. The COVID-19 pandemic intensified these shortages, especially among the minority populations of the ultra-Orthodox Jewish community and the Arab population. However, Israel quickly rose to the occasion and implemented aggressive containment strategies, medical staff training, and ICU preparation strategies for suspected patient isolation. In addition, the Ministry of Health focused on building isolated COVID-19 units and diverting patients who needed mechanical ventilation to avoid overwhelming hospital capacity [134].

In contrast with Israel's robust response, the Palestinian territories' poor socioeconomic and living conditions hindered their ability to fend off the effects of the COVID-19 pandemic [135]. Moreover, the ongoing Israeli–Palestinian conflict further stressed their already fragile healthcare system. That said, the Palestinian Authority's health system response was reported to be satisfactory earlier on in the pandemic [135].

Other developing MENA nations also suffered from limited healthcare capacities and a dearth of physicians. For instance, in Morocco and Egypt, the number of healthcare providers per 1000 population is merely 0.72 and 0.79, respectively [132]. Similarly, according to the WHO, only 30% of HCWs remain in Syria, while the rest have either migrated or sought refuge elsewhere [132]. Therefore, these poorer countries were left particularly vulnerable and unequipped to deal with the COVID-19 crisis at hand.

In Lebanon, the COVID-19 pandemic caused an overwhelming crisis. Once containment measures were enacted, even political activists halted mass public gatherings. However, Lebanon's fragile healthcare system, particularly public hospitals and their providers, was devastated during the first wave of the pandemic [132]. In contrast, Jordan and Morocco were again better prepared and resourced to withstand the arrival of the virus. Jordan quickly expanded its testing capacity to 70 000 tests per 1 million individuals, implemented telemedicine visits to physicians, and introduced robotics for sanitation [132]. Similarly, in Morocco, the resilient healthcare system sprang into action with mask and COVID-19 test production and vaccine research [132]. Figure 29.14 describes the healthcare system responses in these countries and other MENA nations in more detail. The figure provides several examples of how a nation's health system capacity directly influences its ability to implement quick and effective containment measures to mitigate the impact of the COVID-19 crisis. Notable is the stark contrast between the responses of the aforementioned wealthier nations compared with the responses of poorer nations such as Syria and Yemen. This highlights the dire need of strong healthcare infrastructures to combat the COVID-19 virus in both wealthy and impoverished MENA nations alike.

Further Directions for MENA Countries

The aftermath of the COVID-19 pandemic has left the MENA region both in devastation and striving to reform its healthcare infrastructure. According to the United Nations Economic and Social Commission for West Asia, an estimated 8.3 million people will fall into poverty after this healthcare crisis [132]. Although many healthcare systems in the region have responded to this with expanded safety net care and welfare support, inequalities will continue to disproportionately affect the vulnerable – women, youth, elderly, informal workers, and refugees [132]. With ongoing political instability, economic crisis, and fallout from the pandemic, future government reform demands more healthcare funding, resources, and humanitarian assistance to the region.

In terms of vaccination, vaccine hesitancy and misinformation in parts of the MENA region also compromise vaccine rollout programs [136]. For example, Jordan and Kuwait were found to have some of the lowest rates of vaccine acceptance globally, with values less than 30% [127]. These issues compounded with variants spreading rampant throughout the MENA region have further distressed healthcare systems. For future relief, procurement of additional doses and a strong vaccination distribution campaign is necessary.

Systemic issues apparent in the MENA region also contributed to the lagging vaccination rate in some countries. Although wealthier countries, such as the United Arab Emirates, Qatar, Israel, and Bahrain, are leaders in vaccination rates worldwide [136], other countries plagued by poverty and conflict have had greater troubles securing doses and planning effective distribution methods. This is reflected in vaccination rates less than 1% in countries such as Syria and Yemen [136]. In contrast, Israel has led the world in the COVID-19 vaccination rollout because of its strong infrastructure and well-coordinated planning [137]. Some of the strengths noted in their vaccine rollout include a separate trained workforce to deliver the vaccines, as well as a comprehensive data tracking system for minorities to ensure they would not fall through the cracks [137]. Ultimately, countries around the world should use Israel as a model for effective vaccine rollout.

Americas

The Americas, comprising North America, Central America, South America, and the Caribbean are composed of vastly differing healthcare systems among their heterogeneous populations. From fragile to robust healthcare systems, COVID-19 has impacted

	Curfews / Lockdowns / Movement restrictions	Social distancing measures	Barrier gestures	Health screening / Tracking / Quarantine
Algeria	Full lockdown in Blida wilaya (March-April) Partial lockdown (curfew) in all other wilayas	Prohibition of all public gatherings	Masks mandatory in all public venues and outdoor public spaces	
Bahrain	Night-time curfew (March-May)	Prohibition of gatherings of more than 5 people in public spaces	Masks mandatory in all public venues and public transportation	Screening of all incoming passengers Mandatory quarantine for positive patients
Egypt	Night-time curfew (March-June) Restrictions on opening hours of public venues		Masks mandatory in all public venues and public and private transportation	Mandatory Covid-19 test for incoming passengers Mandatory quarantine for positive patients
Iran	Partial lockdown (March-April) Localised, short-term full lockdowns in certain areas Restrictions on travel in and out of certain provinces/cities		Masks mandatory in all enclosed public spaces	Screening of all incoming passengers
Iraq	Night-time curfew		Masks mandatory in all public venues and public transportation	Mandatory Covid-19 test for incoming passengers Mandatory quarantine for positive patients
Jordan	Full lockdown (March) Night-time curfew Restrictions on opening hours of public venues	Public gatherings restricted to 20 people	Masks and gloves mandatory in all public venues and public transportation	Mandatory Covid-19 test for incoming passengers Health tracking app mandatory Mandatory quarantine for all incoming passengers
Kuwait	Partial lockdown (March-May) Full lockdown (May) Night-time curfew		Masks mandatory in all public venues and public transportation	Random testing of population Mandatory Covid-19 test for incoming passengers Mandatory quarantine for all incoming passengers
Libya	Partial lockdown (curfew on weekdays, full lockdown on weekends) Restrictions on re-opening of certain public venues		Masks mandatory in all public venues	Mandatory Covid-19 test for incoming passengers Mandatory quarantine for all incoming passengers
Lebanon	Full lockdown (March, May) Night-time curfew		Masks mandatory in all public venues and public transportation	Mandatory Covid-19 test for incoming passengers
Morocco	Night-time curfew Restrictions on opening hours of public venue Movement restrictions on certain cities/areas	Public gatherings restricted to 50 people	Masks mandatory in all public venues, public transportation and in the workplace	Mandatory Covid-19 test (PCR and serology) for incoming passengers
Oman	Night-time curfew (ended August 15)	Prohibition of all public gatherings	Masks mandatory in all public venues and public transportation	Screening of all incoming passengers Mandatory quarantine for incoming passengers

Figure 29.14 Overview of the health system responses and extent of containment measures in MENA countries. *Source:* Organisation for Economic Co-operation and Development [132].

Palestinian Authority	Localised night-time curfew Restrictions on re-opening of certain public venues	Prohibition of all public gatherings	Masks and gloves mandatory in public transportation	
Qatar		Gatherings limited to 15 people indoors / 30 people outdoors	Masks mandatory in all public venues and public transportation	Health tracking app mandatory Thermal screening in all public venues
Saudi Arabia	Full lockdown or night-time curfew depending on areas (ended end of June)	Umrah pilgrimage suspended Public gatherings limited to 50 people	Masks mandatory in all public venues and public transportation	Mandatory Covid-19 test for incoming passengers Mandatory quarantine (2 days) for incoming passengers Health tracking app available
Syria	Partial curfew Restrictions on re-opening of certain public venues	Prohibition of large public gatherings		
Tunisia	Full lockdown (March-May) Night-time curfew (May-June)		Masks mandatory in all public venues Thermal cameras for fever screening in airports and at border crossings with neighboring countries	Mandatory Covid-19 test for incoming passengers Strict quarantine programme for 18.000 repatriated Tunisians Mandatory self-quarantine for incoming passengers from medium- to high-risk countries
United Arab Emirates	Night-time curfew (March-July) 2-week full lockdown (April) Travel restrictions in and out of Abu Dhabi	Social gatherings limited to 10 people	Masks mandatory in all public venues and public transportation	Health tracking app mandatory Mandatory Covid-19 test for incoming passengers Mandatory self-quarantine & mandatory GPS tracking bracelet for incoming travellers to Abu Dhabi
Yemen	Night-time curfew (April-July) Localised, short-term full lockdowns in certain areas Travel restrictions between provinces			

Sources & notes: This table has been prepared based on official sources, the OECD's Country Policy Tracker, and media reporting. Given the rapid developments of events and measures, the information in the table may not be comprehensive or fully up to date. It will be updated periodically.

Figure 29.14   (Continued)

them all (Figure 29.15). North America, containing some of the stronger healthcare networks in the region, still suffered under COVID-19's grasp, because their healthcare systems were overwhelmed and many times forced to turn away patients because of overflowing hospital beds and ventilators. In Central America, South America, and the Caribbean, similar impacts ensued, but healthcare systems in these regions were already vastly underresourced and underlabored. In this section, the impact of COVID-19 on the Americas' healthcare systems will be explored in further depth.

North America

This section will focus on the United States, Canada, and Mexico. Other North American countries, such as Caribbean countries, are covered in subsequent sections. The United States, Canada, and Mexico are all considered at least upper-middle income [142], with

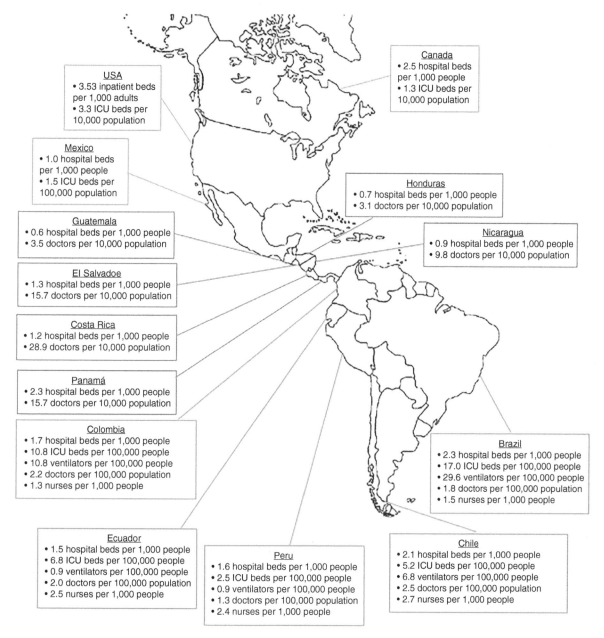

Figure 29.15 Overview of the supply of medical professionals and equipment in the Americas. *Source:* McKee and Rajan [137] and Refs. [138–141].

healthcare systems that tend to be more resilient than other regions of the world. Yet, since 2018, Mexico has spent only 5.37% of its GDP on healthcare systems [143], which is less than the 6% recommended value by the WHO, making it vulnerable to stressors [144].

Despite the strength of health care in these three North American countries, COVID-19 did not spare them, because the infrastructure in place was insufficient to address the virus's catastrophic impacts. All three countries endured massive surges to their healthcare organizations, which were shorthanded and underresourced. Nonetheless, each country adapted to the COVID-19 pandemic in unprecedented ways in efforts to sustain and mitigate the impact of COVID-19.

To accommodate for massive surges in patients with COVID-19, hospitals in the United States were forced to institute significant changes. Among the plethora of consequences faced by US healthcare systems, the most drastic ones included a shortage of HCWs, PPE, and other equipment/supplies such as hospital beds and ventilators. Thus, in response to this need, the president of the United States directed private companies to manufacture medical supplies, such as ventilators, under the Defense Production Act [36]. In hotspots across America, an increased amount of healthcare staff were hired, with many states also allowing recent medical graduates and health workers to work across states that endured surges [36]. In addition, a plethora of volunteers and workers were hired to assist with contact tracing throughout the pandemic [36]. To combat the excess number of cases, certain states built field hospitals with respiratory units and ICU capability [36].

In terms of economic impact, the US healthcare sector was devastated. Healthcare employment declined by 1.58 million jobs between February and April 2020 (healthcare workforce was 4.2% smaller than it was pre-COVID-19 in September 2020). Other consequences included a decrease in physician and clinical services by 34.4% from April 2019 to April 2020, and hospital spending was decreased by 34.5% from April 2019 to April 2020 [145]. Moreover, hospitals and healthcare providers lost vast amounts of income because of the lack of demand for non-COVID-19-related health issues [146]. Furthermore, drug prices, per adjusted discharge, increased 36% from 2020 to 2021 [147]. Insurance was also a big area of concern, because many millions of US workers lost their employer-sponsored insurance during the pandemic, which heightened the existing lack of insurance coverage among US residents [146]. These stark numbers provide only a snapshot of the severe impact COVID-19 had on US healthcare systems.

The decentralized universal healthcare system in neighboring Canada quickly instituted plans to cancel or delay elective surgeries; implement early, safe discharges; and adapt recovery and operating rooms to accommodate for increases in COVID-19 cases [148]. Canada also shifted the paradigm of their healthcare network, with mass migration to digital healthcare systems [72]. Digitizing the healthcare process minimized the risk of exposure for HCWs, as well as others in the hospital, while also reducing public transportation use, in which the spread of the virus may also occur [149]. Digital healthcare also reduced the use of physical medical supplies, which helped Canada preserve its resources [150].

Unfortunately, COVID-19 had a huge impact on Mexico's population because it was among the countries with the highest mortality rates in 2020 [151]. This could be primarily because of the fact that Mexico has the highest prevalence of diabetes and obesity in the world, which are dangerous comorbidities that can increase the severity of COVID-19 infection [66, 152]. In addition, adequate testing and reporting of COVID-19 cases were greatly lacking in Mexico, because the federal government focused testing primarily on the most severe hospital cases. Moreover, Mexico was unable to utilize digital health care and surveillance because it lacked system-wide health information management systems [152].

Lack of adequate resources also played a role as Mexican healthcare facilities quickly became overwhelmed and underresourced by COVID-19's high transmissibility and widespread prevalence. In densely populated Mexico City, Mexico, a report indicated that 22 hospitals designated as COVID-19 treatment sites had run out of hospital beds [153]. To combat this shortage, the General Health Council of Mexico worked to convert 143 certified private hospitals to COVID-19 hospitals when government facilities surpassed capacity limits [154]. This action added more than 1700 hospital beds to Mexico [154]. To deal with the increased demand for HCWs, Mexico hired 6500 physicians and 12 600 nurses on a temporary basis [66, 151]. Despite these efforts, the pandemic greatly strained healthcare resources and massively impacted both Mexican people and healthcare systems alike.

Central America

Central America, consisting of Costa Rica, El Salvador, Guatemala, Honduras, Nicaragua, and Panama, possesses healthcare systems of differing qualities. On one hand, Costa Rica and Panama, the wealthier countries in the region, have stronger, more resilient healthcare systems with a higher disposition to fight off the pandemic [155]. Costa Rica has one of the best healthcare networks in Central America that provides universal health care to all residents and contains a high-functioning primary care system [138]. Conversely, the remaining, poorer countries possess fragile healthcare systems that are less prepared to handle pandemics [155]. These realities are evidenced by the fact that Costa Rica and Panama have an average of 22.3 physicians per 10 000 people, whereas Guatemala, El Salvador, Honduras, and Nicaragua have an average of only about 8 physicians for every 10 000 people (as of 2018) [155]. To further demonstrate the impact of COVID-19 on scarce healthcare resources, in the beginning months of the pandemic, about 80% of Nicaragua's 160 ventilators were already in use [139]. In terms of resources throughout the region, Costa Rica and Panama, on average, have a considerably higher health expenditure per capita (US$1528.5 as of 2017) than the remaining countries (US$489.875), along with more hospital beds per 1000 people (1.75 versus 0.875, respectively, as of 2015) [155]. Fortunately, Costa Rica built a field hospital at its border to expand its healthcare capacity to assist neighboring Nicaraguans [140]. Certain authors also report that poorer countries such as Nicaragua may be reporting unreliable numbers because of the lack of infrastructure and resources necessary to have an accurate testing system [155]. For example, a physician from Honduras stated, "For those of us doctors who are attending cases day-after-day, we can see that official figures of COVID-19 cases should be double or triple what is reported" [155]. These falsehoods could be costly, because they are not conducive to proper preparation for the pandemic.

In Honduras, health systems were largely disrupted, as many hospitals reached or were close to reaching capacity limits because of the influx of COVID-19 cases [141]. Although Honduras further tried to help patients with COVID-19 by opening health sites that were open 24 hours a day, 7 days a week, they lacked HCWs because of the burden of COVID-19 [141]. El Salvador also faced a shortage of hospital beds and worked tirelessly to build more than 100 ICU beds per month [156]. These beds helped prevent El Salvadorian

healthcare systems from overflowing. Guatemala's healthcare systems also faced deleterious effects because COVID-19 severely disrupted other healthcare services, with HIV testing decreasing by 54.7% and fatalities increasing by 10.7% because of opportunistic infections during the pandemic [157].

South America

Compared with countries in the Eastern Hemisphere, the arrival of COVID-19 in South America was delayed, thus allowing these countries more time to institute pandemic preparedness. Several countries, such as Chile, Colombia, Ecuador, and Peru, quickly implemented movement restrictions and attempted to improve health system capacities [158]. However, these efforts were unsuccessful due to prepandemic factors, such as social and economic inequalities, disease burden, and weak testing and contact tracing systems [159, 160].

As healthcare systems across South America were already overburdened with diseases such as dengue, chikungunya, yellow fever, and tuberculosis, most countries lacked adequate resources or capacity to handle the added burden of COVID-19 [159]. Brazil, the most populous country in South America, was among the hardest-hit countries in the world. Political issues translated into the public health sector and contributed to the continually climbing case and death toll. The Brazilian Administration initially dismissed the severity of the pandemic and failed to implement an effective national public health response [159]. Without lockdown mandates, comprehensive testing, or tracing and isolation methods, Brazil health systems were left overloaded with infected patients [159]. Despite having a universal healthcare system [154], the Brazilian health system boasts only 1.8 physicians, 17 ICU beds, and 29.6 ventilators per 100 000 people. Further, there are only 1.5 nurses and 2.3 hospital beds per 1000 people [141]. These values are below the WHO benchmark, highlighting the uphill battle Brazil faced when presented with a stark increase in cases [158]. Unfortunately, many South American countries faced the same issue with workforce and capacity values below the WHO benchmark as well [152].

Other factors have contributed to the health crisis in South America, including widespread poverty, high incidences of comorbidities, economic informalities, and corruption relating to the use of resources leading to inequitable access to health care [161]. For example, 231 million people are estimated to be living below the poverty line in Latin America [161]. Diseases that are prominent in South America, namely, diabetes, obesity, and dengue, among others, disproportionately affect those living in poverty [160]. Compounding this with unequal access to health care, the spread of COVID-19 in this environment became rampant, and Latin America soon had one of the highest COVID-19 mortality rates globally [161]. This reality is exacerbated by the informal labor market, with informal workers (individuals with casual work arrangements or no fixed salary) representing about 54% of the regional population [161]. Informal workers have less access to health care and minimal ability to social distance or isolate, which results in an unequal threat of COVID-19 for this at-risk population [161]. Other vulnerable populations throughout South America also have an increased risk for endangerment. Indigenous populations, such as Amazonian Iquitos in Peru, are underresourced and have little access to health care, medical equipment, and oxygen, leaving them unprotected from the fatal effects of the virus [154]. Ultimately, COVID-19 not only engendered a health crisis but also highlighted the humanitarian crisis in South America.

Caribbean

The Caribbean region, defined by a chain of islands consisting of 16 countries, reported its first COVID-19 case in the Dominican Republic on 1 March 2020 [162]. The delayed emergence of the virus in this region may be attributed to the Caribbean countries quickly restricting international travel [163]. Border closures and interstate movement were maintained for several months and successfully helped flatten the curve in the Caribbean. However, the region depends heavily on tourism for economic stimulation. In 2019 only, tourists brought US$59 billion to the region [163]. Therefore, in June 2020, several Caribbean nations began reopening their borders despite the looming threat of COVID-19 [163]. Ultimately, cases remain high in this region as the emphasis has shifted from public health concerns to

appeasing partisan leadership by strengthening the economy.

Because the majority of Caribbean healthcare systems have limited ICU capacity, they are able to treat only those with severe symptoms [164]. In addition, the health systems have limited financial support, with only an average of 3.7% of GDP in the region being spent on health care [165]. Consequently, these countries depend on imports for medical equipment, which were ultimately blocked by the US Customs and Border Protection [164]. In addition, developing countries in this region had only a fraction of the workforce present in developed countries and lacked the proper equipment needed for virus testing [164, 165]. Overall, most Caribbean health systems were generally unequipped to handle increases in infections.

Due to the finite resources, limited capacities, weak infrastructure, health inequities, and poor health information systems present in the Caribbean, the durability of these healthcare systems was greatly tested [166]. Interestingly, Trinidad and Tobago, a developing island state, rose to the occasion and adapted their healthcare system. Their effective response included increasing testing and tracing, enforcing isolation, implementing a separate health system to diagnose and treat patients with COVID-19, and providing free COVID-19-related health services [166]. As a result, Trinidad and Tobago's pandemic response was ranked first by the Oxford COVID-19 Government Response Tracker [166]. Although the impact of COVID-19 in most developing nations has been catastrophic, countries that face similar social and economic struggles should learn from the efforts of Trinidad and Tobago.

Further Directions for the Americas

Ultimately, the COVID-19 pandemic introduced unparalleled challenges to both strong and weak healthcare systems in the Americas. In Central American countries with weaker healthcare system infrastructures, themes of financial and human power constraints were highly prevalent. Yet, although lower-income countries throughout the Western Hemisphere faced a greater healthcare burden, as of September 2021, the United States has the highest cumulative case (39 198 072) and death

(640 108) numbers worldwide [167]. The severe toll COVID-19 has taken on the United States is primarily attributed to a disjointed political response rather than a failure in healthcare mobilization. For example, each state responded differently to the outbreak in terms of mask and vaccine mandates and public restrictions. Further work is necessary to combat the political divide within both the United States and Central America and help unify the COVID-19 response.

As far as vaccine rollout, differences also exist between the American regions. Countries in North America, which benefit from stronger healthcare and economic stability, have greater access to vaccines. As of September 2021, Canada and the United States have fully vaccinated 67.74 and 52.53% of their populations, respectively [100]. Conversely, lower-income countries throughout Latin America have had greater difficulty in acquiring doses of approved vaccines. Fortunately, vaccine rollout began to expand because of donations from other countries, as well as arrivals of COVAX-procured vaccines. In March, Colombia was the first country in the region to receive vaccines through COVAX [164]. Shortly after, 2.3 million COVAX doses were set to arrive in Bolivia, El Salvador, Guatemala, Honduras, Jamaica, Nicaragua, and Peru [168]. Overall, 36 countries in the Americas have received aid through COVAX, which has helped to bridge the gap between vaccination rates in low-income and wealthier countries [168].

Conclusion

Since early 2020, COVID-19 has impacted nearly every region of the world to varying extents, pushing healthcare facilities to their breaking points. Limited resources, inadequate capacities, poor infrastructure, healthcare disparities, and weak information systems caused a plethora of previously unforeseen issues throughout the globe and exacerbated the detrimental impact of this virus. To mitigate enormous surges in patients with COVID-19, hospitals were forced to create and implement substantial changes [79, 169–174]. Although some regions folded under the pressure, many countries worked tirelessly to evolve and adapt to this unprecedented public health crisis. From building makeshift hospitals and ICU beds, to instituting stringent quarantine procedures, to recruiting and training thousands of healthcare volunteers, to the introduction of digital methods and extensive testing/tracing tactics, it goes without saying that many countries miraculously rose to this immense challenge despite political, financial, and social impediments. By identifying the extensive strategies used to combat COVID-19 throughout Africa, Asia, Europe, the Middle East, and the Americas, we were able to identify effective tools and strengths in some countries, while simultaneously revealing gaps in technical ability and infrastructure in others. Although the future of the COVID-19 pandemic remains unknown, it is imperative that we learn from our weaknesses and further develop our healthcare systems to improve healthcare outcomes around the world [175–179].

References

1 Mein, S.A. (2020). COVID-19 and health disparities: the reality of "the great equalizer.". *J. Gen. Intern. Med.* 35 (8): 2439–2440. https://doi.org/10.1007/S11606-020-05880-5.

2 Centers for Disease Control and Prevention. CDC SARS Response Timeline. CDC. (2013). https://www.cdc.gov/about/history/sars/timeline.htm. Accessed 30 Aug 2021.

3 Chew, S.K. (2007). SARS: how a global epidemic was stopped. *Bull. World Health Organ.* 85 (4): 324. https://doi.org/10.2471/BLT.07.032763.

4 Fineberg, H.V. (2014). Pandemic preparedness and response – lessons from the H1N1 influenza of 2009.

N. Engl. J. Med 370 (14): 1335–1342. https://doi.org/10.1056/NEJMRA1208802.

5 Centers for Disease Control and Prevention. 2009 H1N1 Pandemic (H1N1pdm09 virus). CDC. 2019. https://www.cdc.gov/flu/pandemic-resources/2009-h1n1-pandemic.html. Accessed 30 Aug 2021.

6 Ross, A.G.P., Crowe, S.M., Tyndall, M.W., and Petersen, E. (2015). Planning for the next global pandemic. *Int. J. Infect. Dis.* 38: 89–94. https://doi.org/10.1016/J.IJID.2015.07.016.

7 World Health Organization. (n.d.). Middle East respiratory syndrome coronavirus (MERS-CoV). WHO. https://www.who.int/health-topics/middle-east-respiratory-syndrome-coronavirus-mers#tab=tab_1. Accessed 30 Aug 2021.

8 Centers for Disease Control and Prevention. CDC Releases Detailed History of the 2014-2016 Ebola Response in MMWR. CDC. 2016. https://www.cdc.gov/media/releases/2016/p0707-history-ebola-response.html. Accessed 30 Aug 2021.

9 Kruk, M.E., Myers, M., Varpilah, S.T., and Dahn, B.T. (2015). What is a resilient health system? Lessons from Ebola. *Lancet* 385 (9980): 1910–1912. https://doi.org/10.1016/S0140-6736(15)60755-3.

10 World Health Organization *WHO Coronavirus (COVID-19) Dashboard*. WHO https://covid19.who.int. Accessed 20 Aug 2021.

11 World Health Organization. (2020). Rational use of personal protective equipment for coronavirus disease (COVID-19) and considerations during severe shortages. WHO. https://www.who.int/publications/i/item/rational-use-of-personal-protective-equipment-for-coronavirus-disease-(covid-19)-and-considerations-during-severe-shortages. Accessed 30 Aug 2021.

12 Kaye, A.D., Okeagu, C.N., Professor, A. et al. (2021). Economic impact of COVID-19 pandemic on healthcare facilities and systems: international perspectives. *Best. Pract. Res. Clin. Anaesthesiol.* 35 (3): 293–306. https://doi.org/10.1016/j.bpa.2020.11.009.

13 World Bank. World Bank Group: 100 countries get support in response to COVID-19 (coronavirus). 2020. https://www.worldbank.org/en/news/press-release/2020/05/19/world-bank-group-100-countries-get-support-in-response-to-covid-19-coronavirus. Accessed 30 Aug 2021.

14 Qijia Chua, A., Mei Jin Tan, M., Verma, M. et al. (2020). Health system resilience in managing the COVID-19 pandemic: lessons from Singapore practice handling editor Seye Abimbola. *BMJ Glob. Health* 5: 3317. https://doi.org/10.1136/bmjgh-2020-003317.

15 Lee, V.J., Chiew, C.J., and Khong, W.X. (2020). Interrupting transmission of COVID-19: lessons from containment efforts in Singapore. *J. Travel Med.* 27 (3): taaa039. https://doi.org/10.1093/JTM/TAAA039.

16 Ting Chung, Y. (2020). Coronavirus: Singapore Government to foot bills of infected patients at public hospitals, except outpatient expenses. *The Straits Times.* https://www.straitstimes.com/singapore/health/coronavirus-government-to-foot-bills-of-infected-patients-at-public-hospitals

17 Tabah, A., Ramanan, M., Laupland, K. et al. (2020). Personal protective equipment and intensive care unit healthcare worker safety in the COVID-19 era (PPE-SAFE): an international survey. *J. Crit. Care* 59: 70–75. https://doi.org/10.1016/J.JCRC.2020.06.005.

18 Guerra, S., & Filho, P. G. (2021). Risk regulation and Brazil's battle against COVID-19. The Regulatory Review. https://www.theregreview.org/2021/05/24/guerra-filho-risk-regulation-brazil-battle-against-covid-19.

19 World Health Organization. The true death toll of COVID-19: estimating global excess mortality. WHO. 2021. https://www.who.int/data/stories/the-true-death-toll-of-covid-19-estimating-global-excess-mortality

20 Rosenthal, P.J., Breman, J.G., Djimde, A.A. et al. (2020). COVID-19: shining the light on Africa. *Am. J. Trop. Med. Hyg.* 102 (6): 1148.

21 Johns Hopkins University & Medicine. COVID-19 dashboard by the center for systems science and engineering (CSSE) at Johns Hopkins University (JHU): Italy. 2020. https://coronavirus.jhu.edu/map.html.

22 African Union, African Centres for Disease Control and Prevention. Coronavirus Disease 2019 (COVID-19). https://africacdc.org/covid-19. Accessed 30 Aug 2021.

23 Mohamed, A.A., Adan, M.A., and Mohamoud, S.A. (2020, 2020). *COVID-19 Outbreak and The Horn of Africa: An Analysis of How Less-Developed Healthcare Systems are Tackling Coronavirus Pandemic,* 163–169. Health and Society.

24 Kobia, F. and Gitaka, J. (2020). COVID-19: are Africa's diagnostic challenges blunting response effectiveness? *AAS Open Res.* 3: 4. https://doi.org/10.12688/AASOPENRES.13061.1.

25 World Health Organization. COVID-19 cases top 10 000 in Africa. WHO, Regional Office for Africa. 2020. https://www.afro.who.int/news/covid-19-cases-top-10-000-africa

26 World Health Organization. Malaria. WHO, Regional Office for Africa. https://www.afro.who.int/ health-topics/malaria. Accessed 30 Aug 2021.

27 Quadri, N.S., Sultan, A., Ali, S.I. et al. (2021). COVID-19 in Africa: survey analysis of impact on health-care workers. *Am. J. Trop. Med. Hyg.* 104 (6): 2169–2175. https://doi.org/10.4269/AJTMH.20-1478.

28 World Bank Blogs. 85% of Africans live on less than $5.50 per day. https://blogs.worldbank.org/ opendata/85-africans-live-less-550-day. Accessed 31 Aug 2021.

29 Taboe, H.B., Salako, K.V., Tison, J.M. et al. (2020). Predicting COVID-19 spread in the face of control measures in West Africa. *Math. Biosci.* 328: 108431. https://doi.org/10.1016/J.MBS.2020.108431.

30 Abba, A. (2020) COVID-19: Nigeria lacks sufficient hospital beds in face of viral pandemic – data. International Center for Investigative Reporting. https://www.icirnigeria.org/covid-19-nigeria-lacks-sufficient-hospital-beds-in-face-of-viral-pandemic-data. Accessed 30 Aug 2021.

31 World Health Organization. Global Health Observatory data repository. WHO. 2016. https://apps.who.int/gho/data/node.main. HWFGRP_0020%3Flang%3Den. Accessed 2 Sep 2021.

32 Martinez-Alvarez, M., Jarde, A., Usuf, E. et al. (2020). COVID-19 pandemic in West Africa. *Lancet Glob. Health* 8 (5): e631–e632. https://doi.org/10.1016/S2214-109X(20)30123-6.

33 Hernández-Peña, P. (2019). *Global Spending on Health: A World in Transition* [Global Report 2019]. Geneva: World Health Organization https://www.who.int/publications/i/item/WHO-HIS-HGF-HFWorkingPaper-19.4.

34 Martin, A.B., Hartman, M., Lassman, D., and Catlin, A. (2021). National health care spending in 2019: steady growth for the fourth consecutive year. *Health Aff.* 40 (1): 14–24. https://doi.org/10.1377/HLTHAFF.2020.02022.

35 Ahanhanzo, C., Johnson, E.A.K., Eboreime, E.A. et al. (2021). COVID-19 in West Africa: regional resource mobilisation and allocation in the first year of the pandemic. *BMJ Glob. Health* 6 (5): e004762. https://doi.org/10.1136/BMJGH-2020-004762.

36 Haldane, V., De Foo, C., Abdalla, S.M. et al. (2021). Health systems resilience in managing the COVID-19 pandemic: lessons from 28 countries. *Nat. Med.* 27 (6): 964–980. https://doi.org/10.1038/s41591-021-01381-y.

37 El-Sadr, W.M. and Justman, J. (2020). Africa in the path of Covid-19. *N. Engl. J. Med.* 383 (3): e11. https://doi.org/10.1056/NEJMP2008193.

38 Bouraima, M. B., & Zonon, I. (2020). COVID-19 pandemic and socio-economic and elections implications in the Economic Community of West African States (ECOWAS). SSRN. https://ssrn.com/abstract=3683816

39 Ahanhanzo, C., Ameswue Kpogbe Johnson, E., Amaize Eboreime, E. et al. (2021). COVID-19 in West Africa: regional resource mobilisation and allocation in the first year of the pandemic handling editor Seye Abimbola. *BMJ Glob. Health* 6: 4762. https://doi.org/10.1136/bmjgh-2020-004762.

40 University of Pittsburgh Library System. *African Studies and African Country Resources @ Pitt: East African Countries.* https://pitt.libguides.com/c.php?g=12378&p=65814. Accessed 30 Aug 2021.

41 UNAIDS. Malawi. https://www.unaids.org/en/regionscountries/countries/malawi. Accessed 31 Aug 2021.

42 Ponticiello, M., Mwanga-Amumpaire, J., Tushemereirwe, P. et al. (2020). "Everything is a mess": how COVID-19 is impacting engagement with HIV testing Services in Rural Southwestern Uganda. *AIDS Behav.* 24: 3006–3009. https://doi.org/10.1007/s10461-020-02935-w.

43 Ataguba, J.E. (2020). COVID-19 pandemic, a war to be won: understanding its economic implications for Africa. *Appl. Health Econ. Health Policy* 18 (3): 325–328. https://doi.org/10.1007/S40258-020-00580-X.

44 Mills, A. Constraints to Scaling Up and Costs: Working Group 1 Report. https://www.who.int/pmnch/media/membernews/2009/htltf_wg1_report_EN.pdf. Accessed 5 Sep 2021.

45 Mills, A. (2014). Health care systems in low- and middle-income countries. *N. Engl. J. Med.* 370 (6): 552–557. doi: 10.1056/NEJMRA1110897.

46 Social Science in Humanitarian Action Platform. COVID-19: supporting forcibly displaced people in the Middle East and East Africa. SSHAP. https://opendocs.ids.ac.uk/opendocs/bitstream/handle/20.500.12413/15503/SSHAP_Infographic_

forcibly_displaced_v3.pdf?sequence=5. Accessed 31 Aug 2021.

47 Zhou, Y.R. (2020). The global effort to tackle the coronavirus face mask shortage. The Conversation. https://theconversation.com/the-global-effort-to-tackle-the-coronavirus-face-mask-shortage-133656

48 World Health Organization. (2012). World Health Statistics 2012. https://www.who.int/gho/publications/world_health_statistics/EN_WHS2012_Full.pdf

49 The World Bank. Where we work. https://www.worldbank.org/en/where-we-work. Accessed 31 Aug 2021.

50 Africa Renewal. WHO: How the lessons from Ebola are helping Africa's COVID-19 response. 2020. https://www.un.org/africarenewal/magazine/who-how-lessons-ebola-are-helping-africa%E2%80%99s-covid-19-response. Accessed 3 Sep 2021.

51 Umviligihoza, G., Mupfumi, L., Sonela, N., Naicker, D., Obuku, E.A., Koofhethile, C., et al. (2020). Sub-Saharan Africa preparedness and response to the COVID-19 pandemic: A perspective of early African scientists. Wellcome Open Res. 5: 163.

52 Lane, J., Means, A., Bardosh, K. et al. (2021). *A comparative Analysis of COVID-19 Physical Distancing Policies in Botswana, India, Jamaica, Mozambique, Namibia, Ukraine, and the United States*, vol. 17, 124. Globalization and Health.

53 Health Department Republic of South Africa. Government is identifying accommodation facilities. COVID-19 South African Online Portal. 2020. https://sacoronavirus.co.za/2020/03/07/government-is-identifying-accommodation-facilities. Accessed 3 Sep 2021.

54 Republic of Botswana Task Force. About COVID-19 COVID-19: what are we doing in Botswana. 2020. https://covid19portal.gov.bw/about-covid-19. Accessed 3 Sep 2021.

55 Health Department Republic of South Africa. Social distancing guidelines. COVID-19 South African Online Portal. 2020. https://sacoronavirus.co.za/2020/03/16/social-distancing-guidelines. Accessed 3 Sep 2021.

56 Republic of Botswana. Public Notice COVID-19 press release. 2020. https://www.gov.bw/sites/default/files/2020-03/Covid19.pdf. Accessed 3 Sep 2021.

57 Health Department Republic of South Africa. South African closures due to COVID-19. 2020. https://sacoronavirus.co.za/2020/03/16/south-african-closures-due-to-covid-19. Accessed 3 Sep 2021.

58 Republic of Botswana. Government Gazette Extraordinary no. 26 on 24 March 2020. Public Health (Prevention of Introduction of Covid-19 into Botswana) Order, 2020. Statutory Instrument 36 of 2020. 2020. https://gazettes.africa/archive/bw/2020/bw-government-gazette-dated-2020-03-24-no-26.pdf. Accessed 3 Sep 2021.

59 Health Department Republic of South Africa. National lockdown regulations. COVID-19 South African Online Portal. 2020. https://sacoronavirus.co.za/2020/03/26/national-lockdown-regulations. Accessed 3 Sep 2021.

60 Republic of Botswana. (2020). Government Gazette Extraordinary Gaborone, Vol. LVIII, No 32. https://covid19portal.gov.bw/sites/default/files/2020-05/ExtraordinaryGazette02-04-2020.pdf. Accessed 3 Sep 2021.

61 Johns Hopkins University & Medicine. COVID-19 Dashboard. https://coronavirus.jhu.edu/map.html. Accessed 3 Sep 2021.

62 Makateng, D. (2020). Implications of social adaptation in the Kingdom of Lesotho during 2019-nCoV pandemic. *Electron. Res. J. Soc. Sci. Humanities* 2 (3): 165–183.

63 Coovadia, H., Jewkes, R., Barron, P. et al. (2009). The health and health system of South Africa: historical roots of current public health challenges. *Lancet* 374 (9692): 817–834. https://doi.org/10.1016/S0140-6736(09)60951-X.

64 World Bank Group. Poverty & Equity Brief: Sub-Saharan Africa: South Africa. 2020. https://databank.worldbank.org/data/download/poverty/33EF03BB-9722-4AE2-ABC7-AA2972D68AFE/Global_POVEQ_ZAF.pdf

65 Dzinamarira, T., Dzobo, M., and Chitungo, I. (2020). COVID-19: a perspective on Africa's capacity and response. *J. Med. Virol.* 92 (11): 2465–2472. https://doi.org/10.1002/JMV.26159.

66 Shuchman, M. (2020). Low- and middle-income countries face up to COVID-19. *Nat. Med.* 26 (7): 986–988. https://doi.org/10.1038/D41591-020-00020-2.

67 Webster, P. (2020). Virtual health care in the era of COVID-19. *Lancet* 395 (10231): 1180–1181. https://doi.org/10.1016/S0140-6736(20)30818-7.

68 Government of Botswana. COVID-19 contacts. 2020. https://www.gov.bw/covid-19-contacts. Accessed 3 Sep 2021.

69 Health Department Republic of South Africa. Coronavirus: tool kits. 2020. https://sacoronavirus.co.za/category/tool-kits. Accessed 3 Sep 2021.

70 Ditekemena, J., Doumbia, S., and Ebrahim, S.H. (2020). COVID-19's final frontier: the Central Africa region. *Travel Med. Infect. Dis.* 37: 101694. https://doi.org/10.1016/J.TMAID.2020.101694.

71 Akintunde, T.Y., Akintunde, O.D., Musa, T.H. et al. (2021). Expanding telemedicine to reduce the burden on the healthcare systems and poverty in Africa for a post-coronavirus disease 2019 (COVID-19) pandemic reformation. *Glob. Health J.* 5: 128–134. https://doi.org/10.1016/J.GLOHJ.2021.07.006.

72 Monaghesh, E. and Hajizadeh, A. (2020). The role of telehealth during COVID-19 outbreak: a systematic review based on current evidence. *BMC Public Health* 20 (1): 1193. https://doi.org/10.1186/S12889-020-09301-4.

73 Sen-Crowe, B., McKenney, M., and Elkbuli, A. (2021). Disparities in global COVID-19 vaccination rates & allocation of resources to countries in need. *Ann. Med. Surg. (Lond.)* 68: 102620.

74 Aborode, A.T., Olofinsao, O.A., Osmond, E. et al. (2021). Equal access of COVID-19 vaccine distribution in Africa: challenges and way forward. *J. Med. Virol.* 93 (9): 5212–5215. https://doi.org/10.1002/JMV.27095.

75 World Health Organization. COVAX. https://www.who.int/initiatives/act-accelerator/covax. WHO. Accessed 31 Aug 2021.

76 Ma, M., Wang, S., & Wu, F. (2021). COVID-19 prevalence and well-being: lessons from East Asia. World Happiness Report. New York: Sustainable Development Solutions Network. https://worldhappiness.report/ed/2021/covid-19-prevalence-and-well-being-lessons-from-east-asia

77 Renzaho, A.M.N. (2021). Challenges associated with the response to the coronavirus disease (COVID-19) pandemic in Africa – an African diaspora perspective. *Risk Anal.* 41 (5): 831–836. https://doi.org/10.1111/risa.13596.

78 Maizland, L., & Felter, C. Comparing six health-care systems in a pandemic. Council on Foreign Relations. 2020. https://www.cfr.org/backgrounder/comparing-six-health-care-systems-pandemic

79 Ritchie, H., Mathieu, E., Rodés-Guirao, L., Appel, C., Giattino, C., Ortiz-Ospina, E., Hasell, J., Macdonald, B., Beltekian, D., Roser, M. Coronavirus pandemic (COVID-19). 2020. https://ourworldindata.org/coronavirus

80 Shang, L., Xu, J., and Cao, B. (2020). Fangcang shelter hospitals in COVID-19 pandemic: the practice and its significance. *Clin. Microbiol. Infect.* 26 (8): 976–978. https://doi.org/10.1016/J.CMI.2020.04.038.

81 Wang, C.J., Ng, C.Y., and Brook, R.H. (2020). Response to COVID-19 in Taiwan: big data analytics, new technology, and proactive testing. *JAMA* 323 (14): 1341–1342. https://doi.org/10.1001/JAMA.2020.3151.

82 Johns Hopkins University & Medicine. Johns Hopkins Coronavirus Resource Center. https://coronavirus.jhu.edu. Accessed 31 Aug 2021.

83 COVID-19 National Emergency Response Center, Epidemiology & Case Management Team, Korea Centers for Disease Control & Prevention (2020). Contact transmission of COVID-19 in South Korea: novel investigation techniques for tracing contacts. *Osong Public Health Res. Perspect.* 11 (1): 60–63. https://doi.org/10.24171/J.PHRP.2020.11.1.09.

84 Shadmanov, A., Boklage, E., Storozhenko, O., and Jansen, A. (2021). COVID-19 in Central Asia: Uzbekistan's new approach to international cooperation. *Lancet Reg. Health Eur* 1: 100007. https://doi.org/10.1016/J.LANEPE.2020.100007.

85 Lemon, E. and Antonov, O. (2021). Responses to COVID-19 and the strengthening of authoritarian governance in Central Asia. In: *COVID-19 pandemic and Central Asia* (ed. M. Laruelle), 51–59. Washington, DC: Central Asia Program, The George Washington University https://www.researchgate.net/publication/350965127.

86 World Health Organization. Turkmenistan: WHO coronavirus disease (COVID-19) dashboard with vaccination data. https://covid19.who.int/region/euro/country/tm. Accessed 31 Aug 2021.

87 Ibbotson, S. (2020). COVID-19: approaches, outlooks, and power dynamics in Central Asia

COVID-19: approaches, outlooks, and power dynamics in Central Asia Sophie Ibbotson. *Asian Aff.* 51 (3): 528–541. https://doi.org/10.1080/03068374.2020.1805891.

88 Dzushupov, K., Lucero-Prisno, D.E. III, Vishnyakov, D. et al. (2021). COVID-19 in Kyrgyzstan: navigating a way out. *J. Glob. Health* 11: 03020. https://doi.org/10.7189/JOGH.11.03020.

89 United Nations Office for the Coordination of Humanitarian Affairs. Kyrgyzstan. Humanitarian Response. https://www.humanitarianresponse.info/en/operations/Kyrgyzstan. Accessed 31 Aug 2021.

90 Hom Nath, C. (2020). South Asia is more vulnerable to COVID-19 pandemic. *Arch. Psychiatry Men. Health* 4 (1): 046–047. https://doi.org/10.29328/JOURNAL.APMH.1001018.

91 Jain, M., Sharma, G.D., Goyal, M. et al. (2021). Econometric analysis of COVID-19 cases, deaths, and meteorological factors in South Asia. *Environ. Sci. Pollut. Res.* 28 (22): 28518–28534. https://doi.org/10.1007/S11356-021-12613-6.

92 Worldometer. COVID live update: 218,540,994 cases and 4,533,609 deaths from the coronavirus. https://www.worldometers.info/coronavirus/?utm_campaign=homeAdUOA?Si. Accessed 31 Aug 2021.

93 Stone, R. (2020). COVID-19 in South Asia: mirror and catalyst COVID-19 in South Asia: mirror and catalyst Rupert Stone. *Asian Aff.* 51 (3): 542–568. https://doi.org/10.1080/03068374.2020.1814078.

94 World Bank. Hospital beds (per 1,000 people). https://data.worldbank.org/indicator/SH.MED.BEDS.ZS?most_recent_value_desc=false. Accessed 31 Aug 2021.

95 World Bank. Physicians (per 1,000 people). https://data.worldbank.org/indicator/SH.MED.PHYS.ZS?most_recent_value_desc=false. Accessed 31 Aug 2021.

96 Djalante, R., Nurhidayah, L., Van Minh, H. et al. (2020). COVID-19 and ASEAN responses: comparative policy analysis. *Prog. Disaster Sci.* 8: 100129. https://doi.org/10.1016/J.PDISAS.2020.100129.

97 Fauzi, M.A. and Paiman, N. (2020). COVID-19 pandemic in Southeast Asia: intervention and mitigation efforts. *Asian Educ. Dev. Stud.* 10 (2): 176–184. https://doi.org/10.1108/AEDS-04-2020-0064.

98 Olivia, S., Gibson, J., and Nasrudin, R.'a. (2020). Indonesia in the time of Covid-19. *Bull. Indones. Econ. Stud.* 56 (2): 143–174. https://doi.org/10.1080/00074918.2020.1798581.

99 Regan, H. Covid-19 Delta variant is pushing Southeast Asia to breaking point. CNN. 2021. https://www.cnn.com/2021/08/04/asia/southeast-asia-delta-covid-explainer-intl-hnk/index.html. Accessed 31 Aug 2021.

100 Ritchie, H., Mathieu, E., Rodés-Guirao, L., Appel, C., Giattino, C., Ortiz-Ospina, E., Hasell, J., Macdonald, B., Beltekian, D., & Roser, M. Coronavirus (COVID-19) Vaccinations. Our World in Data. 2020. https://ourworldindata.org/covid-vaccinations. Accessed 31 Aug 2021.

101 Fitzgerald, D.A. and Wong, G.W.K. (2020). COVID-19: a tale of two pandemics across the Asia Pacific region. *Paediatr. Respir. Rev.* 35: 75–80. https://doi.org/10.1016/J.PRRV.2020.06.018.

102 Our World in Data. New Zealand: coronavirus pandemic country profile. Our World in Data. 2021. https://ourworldindata.org/coronavirus/country/new-zealand

103 Sutherland, K., Chessman, J., Zhao, J. et al. (2020). Impact of COVID-19 on healthcare activity in NSW, Australia article history key points. *Public Health Res. Pract.* 30 (4): 3042030. https://doi.org/10.17061/phrp3042030.

104 COVID-19: Pacific Community Updates. The Pacific Community. 2021. https://www.spc.int/updates/blog/2021/08/covid-19-pacific-community-updates. Accessed 31 Aug 2021.

105 World Health Organization. Strengthening Pacific Health Systems. WHO. https://www.who.int/westernpacific/activities/strengthening-pacific-health-systems. Accessed 31 Aug 2021.

106 Filho, W.L., Lütz, J.M., Sattler, D.N., and Nunn, P.D. (2020). Coronavirus: COVID-19 transmission in Pacific Small Island developing states. *Int. J. Environ. Res. Public Health* 17: 5409. https://doi.org/10.3390/IJERPH17155409.

107 World Health Organization. Tonga: WHO coronavirus disease (COVID-19) dashboard with vaccination data. https://covid19.who.int/region/wpro/country/to. Accessed 31 Aug 2021.

108 Koryo Tours. List of countries without coronavirus. 2021. https://koryogroup.com/blog/are-there-countries-without-coronavirus

109 Mainland China: the latest coronavirus counts, charts and maps. https://graphics.reuters.com/world-coronavirus-tracker-and-maps/countries-and-territories/china. Accessed 31 Aug 2021.

110 Centers for Disease Control and Prevention. (2021). COVID-19 breakthrough case investigations and reporting. CDC. https://www.cdc.gov/vaccines/covid-19/health-departments/breakthrough-cases.html. Accessed 31 Aug 2021.

111 Giordano, G., Blanchini, F., Bruno, R. et al. (2020). Modelling the COVID-19 epidemic and implementation of population-wide interventions in Italy. *Nat. Med.* 26: 855–860.

112 Boccia, S., Ricciardi, W., and Ioannidis, J.P.A. (2020). What other countries can learn from Italy during the COVID-19 pandemic. *JAMA Intern. Med.* 180: 927–928.

113 Malandrino, A. and Demichelis, E. (2020). Conflict in decision making and variation in public administration outcomes in Italy during the COVID-19 crisis. *Eur. Policy Anal.* 6 (2): 138–146. https://doi.org/10.1002/EPA2.1093.

114 Italy Population. Worldometer. 2021. https://www.worldometers.info/world-population/italy-population. Accessed 1 Sep 2021.

115 Italy COVID: 4,546,487 cases and 129,290 deaths. Worldometer. (2021). https://www.worldometers.info/coronavirus/country/italy. Accessed 1 Sep 2021.

116 Colfer, B. (2020). Public policy responses to COVID-19 in Europe. *Eur. Policy Anal.* 6 (2): 126–137. https://doi.org/10.1002/EPA2.1097.

117 Oliver, N., Barber, X., Roomp, K., and Roomp, K. (2020). Assessing the impact of the COVID-19 pandemic in Spain: Large-scale, online, self-reported population survey. *J. Med. Internet Res* 22: e21319.

118 Soriano, V. and Barreiro, P. (2020). Why such excess of mortality for COVID-19 in Spain? *Ther. Adv. Infect. Dis.* 7: 2049936120932755.

119 France population (2021). Worldometer. https://www.worldometers.info/world-population/france-population. Accessed 1 Sep 2021.

120 Massonnaud, C., Roux, J., Crépey, P. (2020). *COVID-19: Forecasting short term hospital needs in France.* medRxiv. https://www.medrxiv.org/content/10.1101/2020.03.16.20036939v1.article-info

121 Kuhlmann, S., Hellström, M., Ramberg, U., and Reiter, R. (2021). Tracking divergence in crisis governance: responses to the COVID-19 pandemic in France, Germany and Sweden compared. *Int. Rev. Admin. Sci.* 87: 556–575.

122 Naumann, E., Möhring, K., Reifenscheid, M. et al. (2020). COVID-19 policies in Germany and their social, political, and psychological consequences. *Eur. Policy Anal.* 6 (2): 191–202. https://doi.org/10.1002/EPA2.1091.

123 Germany COVID: 3,970,033 cases and 92,757 deaths. Worldometer. https://www.worldometers.info/coronavirus/country/germany. Accessed 1 Sep 2021.

124 Anderson, R.M., Hollingsworth, T.D., Baggaley, R.F. et al. (2020). COVID-19 spread in the UK: the end of the beginning? *Lancet* 396: 587–590.

125 Peltier, E. and Holder, J. (2021). How Europe, after a fumbling start, overtook the U.S. in vaccination. *The New York Times.* https://www.nytimes.com/interactive/2021/07/29/world/europe/europe-us-vaccination.html

126 Caspi, G., Dayan, A., Eshal, Y. et al. (2021). Socioeconomic disparities and COVID-19 vaccination acceptance: a nationwide ecologic study. *Clin. Microbiol. Infect.* 27: 1502–1506.

127 Sallam, M. (2021). COVID-19 vaccine hesitancy worldwide: a concise systematic review of vaccine acceptance rates. *Vaccines* 9: 160.

128 Lazarus, J.V., Bassat, Q., Crespo, J. et al. (2021). Vaccinate fast but leave no one behind: a call to action for COVID-19 vaccination in Spain. *Commun. Med.* 1: 12.

129 Paterlini, M. (2021). Covid-19: Italy makes vaccination mandatory for healthcare workers. *BMJ* 373: n905.

130 European Centre for Disease Prevention and Control. COVID-19 vaccine tracker. ECDC. 2021. https://vaccinetracker.ecdc.europa.eu/public/extensions/COVID-19/vaccine-tracker.html#uptake-tab. Accessed 4 Sep 2021.

131 The World Bank. Middle East and North Africa overview. (2021). https://www.worldbank.org/en/region/mena/overview

132 Organisation for Economic Co-operation and Development. (2020).COVID-19 crisis response in MENA countries. Paris: OECD. https://read.oecd-ilibrary.org/view/?ref=129_129919-4li7bq8asv&

title=COVID-19-Crisis-Response-in-MENA-Countries&_ga=2.94027549.1655410805.1630430766-719051120.1630430766

133 Waitzberg, R., Davidovitch, N., Leibner, G. et al. (2020). Israel's response to the COVID-19 pandemic: tailoring measures for vulnerable cultural minority populations. *Int. J. Equity Health* 19 (1): 71. https://doi.org/10.1186/S12939-020-01191-7.

134 Leshem, E., Afek, A., and Kreiss, Y. (2020). Buying time with COVID-19 outbreak response, Israel. *Emerg. Infect. Dis.* 26 (9): 2253. https://doi.org/10.3201/EID2609.201476.

135 AlKhaldi, M., Kaloti, R., Shella, D. et al. (2020). Health system's response to the COVID-19 pandemic in conflict settings: Policy reflections from Palestine. *Global Public Health* 15 (8): 1244–1256. https://doi.org/10.1080/17441692.2020.1781914.

136 Dyer, P., Schaider, I., and Letzkus, A. (2021). *Infographic: COVID-19 vaccination efforts in the Middle East and North Africa*. Brookings https://www.brookings.edu/interactives/covid-19-vaccination-efforts-in-the-middle-east-and-north-africa.

137 McKee, M. and Rajan, S. (2021). What can we learn from Israel's rapid roll out of COVID 19 vaccination? *Isr. J. Health Policy Res.* 10 (1): 5. https://doi.org/10.1186/S13584-021-00441-5.

138 Garcia, P.J., Alarcón, A., Bayer, A. et al. (2020). COVID-19 response in Latin America. *Am. J. Trop. Med. Hyg.* 103 (5): 1765–1772. https://doi.org/10.4269/AJTMH.20-0765.

139 Aburto, M. W. *Hospitales de Nicaragua sin ventiladores para pacientes de coronavirus. Confidencial*. 2020. https://www.confidencial.com.ni/nacion/hospitales-sin-ventiladores-suficientes-pacientes-criticos-por-covid-19

140 Pearson, A.A., Prado, A.M., and Colburn, F.D. (2020). Nicaragua's surprising response to COVID-19. *J. Glob. Health* 10 (1): 010371. https://doi.org/10.7189/JOGH.10.010371.

141 Fuentes-Barahona, C.I., Henriquez-Márquez, I.K., Muñoz-Lara, F. et al. (2021). COVID-19 situation in Honduras: lessons learned. *Gaceta Medica de Caracas* 128: S242–S250.

142 The World Bank. World Bank country and lending groups. https://datahelpdesk.worldbank.org/

knowledgebase/articles/906519. Accessed 31 Aug 2021.

143 The World Bank. Current health expenditure (% of GDP) – Mexico. https://data.worldbank.org/indicator/SH.XPD.CHEX.GD.ZS?locations=MX. Accessed 1 Sep 2021.

144 Kanavos, P., Parkin, G.C., Kamphuis, B., and Gill, J. (2019). *Latin America Healthcare System Overview: a Comparative Analysis of Fiscal Space in Healthcare*. London: The London School of Economics and Political Science.

145 Rhyan, C., Turner, A., and Miller, G. (2020). Tracking the U.S. health sector: the impact of the COVID-19 pandemic. *Bus. Econ.* 55 (4): 267–278. https://doi.org/10.1057/S11369-020-00195-Z.

146 Blumenthal, D., Fowler, E.J., Abrams, M., and Collins, S.R. (2020). Covid-19 – implications for the health care system. *N. Engl. J. Med.* 383 (15): 1483–1488. https://doi.org/10.1056/NEJMSB2021088.

147 American Hospital Association. Hospitals face continued financial challenges one year into the COVID-19 pandemic. 2021. https://www.aha.org/system/files/media/file/2021/03/hospitals-face-continued-financial-challenges-one-year-into-covid-19-pandemic-fact-sheet.pdf

148 Government of Canaa (2020). COVID-19 pandemic guidance for the health care sector. Public Health Agency of Canada. https://www.canada.ca/en/public-health/services/diseases/2019-novel-coronavirus-infection/health-professionals/covid-19-pandemic-guidance-health-care-sector.html

149 Nicol, G.E., Piccirillo, J.F., Mulsant, B.H., and Lenze, E.J. (2020). Action at a distance: geriatric research during a pandemic. *J. Am. Geriatr. Soc.* 68 (5): 922–925. https://doi.org/10.1111/JGS.16443.

150 Shaker, M.S., Oppenheimer, J., Grayson, M. et al. (2020). COVID-19: pandemic contingency planning for the allergy and immunology clinic. *J. Allergy Clin. Immunol. Pract.* 8 (5): 1477–1488.e5. https://doi.org/10.1016/J.JAIP.2020.03.012.

151 Block, M.Á.G., Reyes, H., Lucero, M. et al. (2020). Mexico: Health system review. In: *Health Systems in Transition*, vol. 22(2), i–222. https://apps.who.int/iris/bitstream/handle/10665/334334/HiT-22-2-2020-eng.pdf.

152 Ejaz, H., Alsrhani, A., Zafar, A. et al. (2020). COVID-19 and comorbidities: deleterious impact on infected patients. *J. Infect. Public Health* 13 (12): 1839. https://doi.org/10.1016/J.JIPH.2020.07.014.

153 McDonnell, J. P. and Sanchez, C. (2020). Mexico's fragile health system running out of room for coronavirus patients. *Los Angeles Times*. https://www.latimes.com/world-nation/story/2020-05-04/mexican-hospitals-brace-for-coronavirus-crunch. Accessed 1 Sep 2021.

154 Andrus, J.K., Evans-Gilbert, T., Santos, J.I. et al. (2020). Perspectives on battling COVID-19 in countries of Latin America and the Caribbean. *Am. J. Trop. Med. Hyg.* 103 (2): 593–596. https://doi.org/10.4269/AJTMH.20-0571.

155 Pearson, A.A., Prado, A.M., and Colburn, F.D. (2021). The puzzle of COVID-19 in Central America and Panama. *J. Glob. Health* 11: 03077.

156 Bello, M., Segura, V., Camputaro, L. et al. (2021). Hospital El Salvador: a novel paradigm of intensive care in response to COVID-19 in Central America. *Lancet Glob. Health* 9 (3): e241–e242. https://doi.org/10.1016/S2214-109X(20)30513-1.

157 Medina, N., Alastruey-Izquierdo, A., Bonilla, O. et al. (2021). Impact of the COVID-19 pandemic on HIV care in Guatemala. *Int. J. Infect. Dis.* 108: 422–427. https://doi.org/10.1016/J.IJID.2021.06.011.

158 Cometto, G. and Witter, S. (2013). Tackling health workforce challenges to universal health coverage: setting targets and measuring progress. *Bull. World Health Organ.* 91 (11): 881–885. https://doi.org/10.2471/BLT.13.118810.

159 Benítez, M.A., Velasco, C., Sequeira, A.R. et al. (2020). Responses to COVID-19 in five Latin American countries. *Health Policy Technol.* 9 (4): 525–559. https://doi.org/10.1016/J.HLPT.2020.08.014.

160 Litewka, S.G. and Heitman, E. (2020). Latin American healthcare systems in times of pandemic. *Dev. World Bioeth.* 20 (2): 69–73. https://doi.org/10.1111/DEWB.12262.

161 The Lancet (2020). COVID-19 in Latin America: a humanitarian crisis. *Lancet* 396 (10261): 1463. https://doi.org/10.1016/S0140-6736(20)32328-X.

162 Escobedo, A.A., Rodríguez-Morales, A.J., Almirall, P. et al. (2020). SARS-CoV-2/COVID-19: evolution in the Caribbean islands. *Travel Med. Infect. Dis.* 37: 101854. https://doi.org/10.1016/J.TMAID.2020.101854.

163 Burki, T.K. (2021). COVID-19 in the Caribbean. *Lancet Respir. Med.* 9 (4): e46. https://doi.org/10.1016/S2213-2600(21)00090-4.

164 Knight, W.A. and Reddy, K.S. (2020). Caribbean response to COVID-19: a regional approach to pandemic preparedness and resilience. *Commonw. J. Int. Affairs* 109 (4): 464–465. https://doi.org/10.1080/00358533.2020.1790759.

165 Economic Commission for Latin America and the Caribbean (ECLAC) and the Pan American Health Organization (PAHO). COVID-19 report: health and the economy: a convergence needed to address COVID-19 and retake the path of sustainable development in Latin America and the Caribbean. PAHO and United Nations. 2020. https://repositorio.cepal.org/bitstream/handle/11362/45841/S2000461_en.pdf?sequence=4&isAllowed=y

166 Hunte, S.-A., Pierre, K., Rose, R.S., and Simeon, D.T. (2020). Health systems' resilience: COVID-19 response in Trinidad and Tobago. *Am. J. Trop. Med. Hyg.* 103 (2): 590–592. https://doi.org/10.4269/AJTMH.20-0561.

167 Johns Hopkins Univerisity & Medicine. Mortality analyses. Johns Hopkins Coronavirus Resource Center. https://coronavirus.jhu.edu/data/mortality. Accessed 1 Sep 2021.

168 Pan American Health Organization. COVID-19 vaccine rollout expanded in the Americas, PAHO Director reports. PAHO/WHO. 2021. https://www.paho.org/en/news/10-3-2021-covid-19-vaccine-rollout-expanded-americas-paho-director-reports

169 Kooraki, S., Hosseiny, M., Velez, E.M. et al. (2021). COVID-19 pandemic revisited: lessons the radiology community has learned a year later. *Emerg. Radiol.* 28 (6): 1083–1086.

170 Larsen, L.H., Desai, B., Cen, S.Y. et al. (2021). Addressing ethnic disparities in imaging utilization and clinical outcomes for COVID-19. *Clin. Imaging* 77: 276–282.

171 Assadi, M., Gholamrezanezhad, A., Jokar, N. et al. (2020). Key elements of preparedness for pandemic coronavirus disease 2019 (COVID-19) in nuclear

medicine units. *Eur. J. Nucl. Med. Mol. Imaging* 47 (8): 1779–1786.

172 Azam, S.A., Myers, L., Fields, B.K.K. et al. (2020). Coronavirus disease 2019 (COVID-19) pandemic: review of guidelines for resuming non-urgent imaging and procedures in radiology during Phase II. *Clin. Imaging* 67: 30–36.

173 Katal, S., Azam, S., Bombardieri, E. et al. (2020). Reopening the country: recommendations for nuclear medicine departments. *World J. Nucl. Med.* 20 (1): 1–6.

174 Fields, B.K.K., Demirjian, N.L., and Gholamrezanezhad, A. (2020). Coronavirus disease 2019 (COVID-19) diagnostic technologies: a country-based retrospective analysis of screening and containment procedures during the first wave of the pandemic. *Clin. Imaging* 67: 219–225.

175 Pan, J., St Pierre, J.M., Pickering, T.A. et al. (2020). Coronavirus disease 2019 (COVID-19): a modeling study of factors driving variation in case fatality rate by country. *Int. J. Environ. Res. Public Health* 17 (21): 8189.

176 Demirjian, N.L., Fields, B.K.K., Song, C. et al. (2020). Impacts of the coronavirus disease 2019 (COVID-19) pandemic on healthcare workers: a nationwide survey of United States radiologists. *Clin. Imaging* 68: 218–225.

177 Radmard, A.R., Gholamrezanezhad, A., Montazeri, S.A. et al. (2020). A multicenter survey on the trend of chest CT scan utilization: tracing the first footsteps of COVID-19 in Iran. *Arch. Iran Med.* 23 (11): 787–793.

178 Shin, H., Abdelhalim, A., Chau, S. et al. (2020). Responding to coronavirus disease 2019: LA County hospital experience. *Emerg. Radiol.* 27 (6): 785–790.

179 Abbasi, F., Gholamrezanezhad, A., Jokar, N., and Assadi, M. (2021). A path to new normal of nuclear medicine facilities: considerations for reopening. *Asia Ocean J. Nucl. Med. Biol.* 9 (1): 80–85.

30

COVID-19: Mass Casualty Planning

Lee Myers

Keck School of Medicine, University of Southern California, Los Angeles, CA, USA

Abbreviations

ECMO	extracorporeal membrane oxygenation
ED	emergency department
EMS	Emergency Medical Service
ICU	intensive care unit
MCI	mass casualty incident
PPE	personal protective equipment

A mass casualty incident (MCI) can be defined as an event that overwhelms hospital resources. Triage is necessary to help the greatest number of patients with the least amount of compromise in patient care. The majority of these events occur at a discrete moment with variability in the length of the MCI. An example would be a major earthquake with the mainshock and aftershocks inflicting serious injuries from falling debris, landslides, and liquefaction, as well as hazards of fire and flood leading to additional casualties. After the immediate aftermath of an MCI, search and rescue efforts will be instituted. In this scenario, the majority of the injuries will occur within the first 24 hours. Soon after a major earthquake, injured people will seek care at the closest hospital (walking wounded), while others will be transported via ambulance. Hospital resources will be overwhelmed quickly, which will start with emergency departments (EDs) and then lead to other parts of the hospital, including the operating rooms, intensive care units (ICUs), and then finally other inpatient units. After a major incident occurs and search and rescue efforts have ceased, the burden on hospital resources will continue until these patients are discharged from the hospital. A viral disease, such as coronavirus disease 2019 (COVID-19), can have many of the same effects on a hospital system but with a few additional ramifications.

Viral Pandemic

A viral pandemic can simulate other MCIs in that hospital system resources can become overwhelmed quickly during a surge; however, there are differences as well. Many factors will shape a viral pandemic, some of which are the type of organism, route of spread, incubation period, virulence, duration of illness and infectiousness, and mortality rate. The incubation period is the time between being exposed and the start of symptoms. In COVID-19, the incubation period can be up to 2 weeks. During the end of the incubation period, patients may be infectious 2–3 days before the symptoms start [1]. This poses the biggest obstacle for limiting the transmission of COVID-19 – spreading the disease without having signs or symptoms of being ill. Although initial infections will start slowly, they may accelerate at an exponential rate.

MCI plans will generally categorize an MCI into one of five levels, based on the number of victims or the number of resources needed to treat the wounded. These levels do not apply to the worst-case scenario in the COVID-19 pandemic, because COVID-19 cases can be orders of magnitude higher than the highest MCI levels as a result of multiple hospital systems being affected. In addition, international assistance may be stifled by the global threat [2].

A viral pandemic can occur and spread contemporaneously in different cities, states, and countries. This puts tremendous stress on the supply chain for personal protective equipment (PPE) and other equipment that hospitals and hospital providers need to treat patients with or without COVID-19. Shortages of PPE can place healthcare workers at risk for exposure to COVID-19.

The Surge

The surge phase is generally considered the rapid increase in victims immediately after an event, during which the hospital systems may become overwhelmed with victims. In COVID-19, the surge phase is protracted over days or weeks and may be occurring in numerous health systems across the world. The surge phase has the most potential to lack the appropriate resources to treat both COVID-19 and non-COVID-19 patients. The surge may contribute to long wait times in the ED and triage tents, lack of proper boarding of patients, and inability to receive patients from ambulances.

The goal of social distancing and mask wearing is to "flatten the curve," which simply means to curtail the exponential infectious rates to keep the number of hospitalized patients at less than the maximum limit of the hospital system. See Figure 30.1 for a graphical representation of the effects of flattening the curve during a surge.

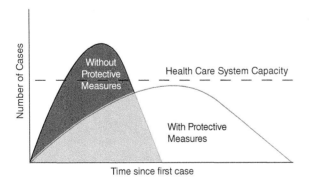

Figure 30.1 Graphical representation of "flattening of the curve" of infections in the population.

Prehospital Planning

Mitigation

In a viral outbreak, such as a COVID-19, community education is extremely important. The major challenge of community education of a novel virus is the constantly evolving and sometimes contradictory recommendations, which can lead to confusion or distrust. Keeping communities informed with the most current information in clear and concise language will help mitigate fear and transmission. Key components of the message should include route of transmission, symptoms, morbidity, and mortality associated with the virus; comorbidities that have the greatest risk for severe disease or complications; and when to seek medical attention.

Additional restrictions can be placed on the population to decrease the spread of the disease. Mask wearing, social distancing, stay-at-home orders, business closure, and restricting travel are some of the ways that local, state, or federal governments can decrease the burden on the hospital systems. In the medical field, we have seen the rescheduling of elective or nonurgent procedures, nonurgent healthcare inquiries, and nonurgent imaging.

Incorporating telemedicine early in a viral pandemic can help ensure people are able to receive health care from outside the hospital or clinic setting. Telemedicine visits are helpful for both patients with symptoms of COVID-19 and for patients with other pressing medical conditions.

Emergency Medical Service Preparedness

Emergency Medical Service (EMS) providers play a critical role in prehospital health care during a pandemic because they are often the first to see patients who may have infections. It is important to minimize exposure of COVID-19 by having an adequate supply of PPE and clear protocols to mitigate patient-to-provider and provider-to-patient transmission. Inadequate PPE supply leads to personal safety concerns for our first responders [3]. EMS call centers should be prepared for an increased number of calls. In Tehran, Iran, EMS calls increased by 347% in the first 28 days after the country's first confirmed case [4]. Other EMS call centers experienced a decrease in phone call volume. A strategy to handle an increased volume of calls is to have a dedicated COVID-19 support track [5]. It is also crucial that EMS providers and emergency medicine providers should work closely together to set up protocols or changes in standard practice to mitigate exposure to both EMS and emergency medicine personnel. One example to decrease transmission is discontinuation of nebulizer treatments that are actively aerosolizing particles because these treatments can generate copious amounts of small particles [6]. Once ED resources become overwhelmed, there may be prolonged EMS transfers that can cause a delay in definite care.

Field Hospitals

Field hospitals can be used to quarantine and treat confirmed infections, easing the demand on hospital resources and hospital bed shortages. China was the first to establish two field hospitals, Huoshenshan Hospital and Leishenshan Hospital, with 1000- and 1600-bed capacities, respectively. Both hospitals were operational in less than 2 weeks [7].

Hospital Planning

Strategies for planning for a viral pandemic at the hospital level will differ based on hospital system size and community size. Important factors involved in hospital planning are to create triage areas, increase capacity, limit transmission, and create specific plans for a surge and recovery phase. Creating an interdepartmental task force can promote cooperation between departments, with members having logistical insights into another member's respective department.

Triage and Emergency Department Capacity

The ED is on the frontline of the pandemic for the hospital system. Emergency medicine providers triage patients daily, which makes the ED the perfect place to plan, set up, and execute COVID-19 triaging protocols. During a viral pandemic, EDs may be flooded with patients and may be overwhelmed quickly. The priority

in a viral epidemic is managing the increased volume of patients both in the triaging and in adding capacity [6]. Algorithm-based processes for testing patients can assist in limiting rapid testing of patients who can otherwise self-monitor at home, especially if rapid tests are in short supply. This can be accomplished by adding on-site triaging areas, such as triaging tents. The patients who are deemed low risk for complications of the infection can self-monitor at home, while high-risk patients can be seen in the "COVID-19 unit." Conversion of a portion of the ED to a COVID-19 unit and grouping patients with COVID-19 can help streamline management and decrease transmission of the disease.

Priority should also be afforded to the highest risk populations, including patients older than 65 years, patients with chronic medical conditions (e.g. hypertension and diabetes), and close contacts with a patient with known COVID-19 in the past 14 days.

Infection Control

Mitigating the spread of COVID-19 in the hospital setting is of utmost importance. Severe acute respiratory syndrome coronavirus 2 predominately spreads from person to person through contact and droplet transmission under normal circumstances. The potential for airborne transmission can be enhanced during medical procedures that generate aerosolized particles that can remain suspended in the air. Policies should be instituted to protect healthcare providers, including identifying specific criteria to increase the level of PPE.

Proper PPE, including an N95 mask, gown, gloves, and eye protection, should be used during interactions with patients with known or suspected infection (https://www.cdc.gov/coronavirus/2019-ncov/hcp/infection-control-recommendations.html). It is essential to have adequate PPE to protect both patients and healthcare workers. Of the 72 314 people who were originally infected in China, 3.8% of them were healthcare providers, and 14.8% of the healthcare providers were classified as severe or critical [8]. Another study found healthcare workers were seven times more likely to have severe COVID-19 compared with other workers [9].

Recommendations for the proper PPE use from the Centers for Disease Control and Prevention and the

World Health Organization may differ from hospitals and professional societies, causing confusion. This may lead to additional shortages in PPE, especially N95 masks [10]. The Centers for Disease Control and Prevention has provided guidance for optimizing N95 availability during supply shortages [11]. The infection control department can help guide the clinical departments in the most up-to-date information and help develop policies to ensure patient and healthcare provider safety.

Identification and appropriate management of transmission hot spots within the hospital can also reduce transmission. Transmission hot spots will have a high throughput and mixing of COVID-19 and non-COVID-19 patients. Triaging areas are the first transmission hot spots that a patient may pass through; another potential transmission hot spot is the radiology department. Although the American College of Radiology does not recommend computed tomography imaging for the diagnosis of COVID-19, patients with COVID-19 may have underlying or superimposed disease that warrants urgent imaging (e.g. acute appendicitis, stroke, pulmonary embolism). A dedicated computed tomographic scanner for patients with confirmed COVID-19 may limit the spread of the virus. Portable sonographic and radiographic imaging is recommended to limit transport of patients with COVID-19 within the hospital and the time to clean radiology rooms. Cleaning protocols for radiologic equipment should be created with collaboration between the infection control and radiology departments. Requesting air exchange rates from environmental services for imaging rooms can determine droplet settle time per room [12].

Conversion of Inpatient Units

Converting portions of inpatient units to dedicated COVID-19 units will be required as patient volumes increase. Planning for bed allocation before a surge will streamline admission from the ED. In worst-case scenarios, the capacity of hospital beds will be reached, with additional patients arriving in the ED who need hospital resources. Conversations and decisions for alternative boarding of patients in unique areas of the hospital should be considered before the surge. The hospital may not be equipped for additional patient volume, which may be related to equipment or staffing. Having the ability to increase staff volume in the time of a surge may help the burden on the already-weary staff.

Staff and Equipment Shortages

As more patients become critically ill, the need for a higher level of care in an ICU increases. In turn, as the burden on ICUs increase, ICU staff will be overextended, leading to burnout. A strategy that has been used is to have subspecialties, such as anesthesia and surgical teams, aid in ICUs as elective surgeries were canceled [13]. This takes advantage of personnel who may be less busy during a viral pandemic but have specialized skills that can assist the most burdened areas.

Staffing coverage also will be affected by healthcare workers with infection or employees who are unable to work because of school and daycare closures. Hospital-based childcare plans may be used to maintain staff who would otherwise not be able to work.

Critical equipment shortages, including PPE for healthcare workers, should be anticipated during a viral pandemic. Shortages may be because of a large portion of the population acquiring PPE, leading to diminished supply, disrupted global supply chain, and increased use. A few solutions to the problem have been instituted or proposed. One of the first helpful solutions was medical supply donations of face masks, N95 masks, face shields, and disposable gowns and gloves. Many of these programs were instituted in cities around the world. Another solution is for the government to step in and require private companies to produce equipment needed for a national emergency, such as under the US Defense Production Act. One major obstacle is to ensure the hospitals with a COVID-19 surge have the appropriate PPE. A proposed program would include a collaboration between government and private technology companies to track and distribute PPE to hospitals undergoing a surge to fill in the gaps during equipment shortages [14].

Mechanical ventilators, extracorporeal membrane oxygenation (ECMO) machines, and other specialized equipment can also undergo critical shortages in a viral pandemic. Respiratory illness such as COVID-19 can cause severe acute respiratory failure, which may necessitate the use of a ventilator or ECMO. A study of

80 409 diagnosed cases from China revealed 3.2% of patients required intubation and ventilation at some point during the disease course [15]. From a survey of acute care hospitals in the United States, there were an estimated 62 188 full-feature mechanical ventilators [16]. Although the number of ventilators exceeded other developed countries by population, a surge can overwhelm ventilator inventory in a city or region. During a time of resource crisis, there are three major efforts that can be instituted, including reducing the demand for mechanical ventilation, maximizing existing supply, and increasing supply during peak supply demands. Using noninvasive oxygenation with continuous positive airway pressure or recommending self-proning can help reduce demand. Use of local or regional unused supply in ambulatory surgical suites or use of the Strategic National Stockpile can maximize existing supplies. Lastly, conversion of bilevel positive airway pressure or continuous positive airway pressure to invasive ventilation or using alternative ventilator devices can increase supply [17].

ECMO machines are typically used as a last option in patients whose condition has progressed to acute respiratory distress syndrome. ECMO machines are relatively scarce in the United States when compared with ventilators and are currently not a Strategic National Stockpile product.

Outpatient Planning

Not all patients need to be hospitalized for COVID-19 or other diseases but continue to need healthcare support. As local or national governments place restrictions on nonurgent procedures, imaging studies, or routine visits to the primary care providers, the care that will be offered to patients will diminish, especially in the outpatient setting.

Telemedicine

The use of technology has been a sufficient stopgap in the need to evaluate and engage with patients without being seen in person [18]. Although videoconferencing technologies have been around for decades, the use of this technology skyrocketed in the medical field during the COVID-19 pandemic. It helps engage patients and providers in routine clinic visits and follow-up. The use of telemedicine also helps isolate at-risk patients and providers. Videoconferencing has also evolved in other applications, such as triaging patients.

There are barriers in the telemedicine landscape, including patients generally revert to what they are used to, that is, seeing physicians in person; patients preferring to see their own provider; or patients being unable to connect through telemedicine for various reasons [19]. The Telehealth Impact survey offers insight into physician barriers to continue telemedicine after COVID-19. The top three responses in this survey included low or no reimbursement, technology challenges for patients, and liability [20].

Radiology is unique in that other than procedural interventions, the radiologist does not need to see patients. The advent of the picture archiving and communication system (PACS) and high-speed Internet connections have increased teleradiology over the last few decades. During COVID-19, private practice groups and academic groups have at least temporarily transitioned to teleradiology [21].

Recovery Phase

The recovery phase should start as soon as the COVID-19 infections subside and government regulations are lifted. This is a critical time for the recovery of providers who have undergone enormous stress and burnout in the preceding days or weeks. Extended hours, financial burden on practices during COVID-19 shutdowns, and psychosocial impact have taken a toll on healthcare workers. The financial impact has been estimated to be $202.6 billion in lost revenue from the American Hospital Association [22].

A comprehensive plan for rescheduling nonurgent procedures, surgeries, and imaging eases the financial impact that many of our practices have and continue to face during COVID-19 shutdowns. As systems improve in efficiency of scheduling around surges, the financial impact will diminish. It is unknown how many surges each hospital system will encounter in the coming months or years, but taking advantage of the recovery phase will be of paramount importance.

References

1 Wei, W.E., Li, Z., Chiew, C.J. et al. (2020). Presymptomatic transmission of SARS-CoV-2 - Singapore, January 23 march 16, 2020. *MMWR Morb. Mortal. Wkly Rep.* 69 (14): 411–415. https://doi.org/10.15585/mmwr.mm6914e1.

2 Coccolini, F., Sartelli, M., Kluger, Y. et al. (2020). COVID-19 the showdown for mass casualty preparedness and management: the Cassandra syndrome. *World J. Emerg. Surg.* 15 (1): 26. https://doi.org/10.1186/s13017-020-00304-5.

3 Ehrlich, H., McKenney, M., and Elkbuli, A. (2021). Defending the front lines during the COVID-19 pandemic: protecting our first responders and emergency medical service personnel. *Am. J. Emerg. Med.* 40: 213–214. https://doi.org/10.1016/j.ajem.2020.05.068.

4 Saberian, P., Conovaloff, J.L., Vahidi, E. et al. (2020). How the COVID-19 epidemic affected prehospital emergency medical services in Tehran, Iran. *West. J. Emerg. Med.* 21 (6): 110–116. https://doi.org/10.5811/westjem.2020.8.48679.

5 Jensen, T., Holgersen, M.G., Jespersen, M.S. et al. (2021). Strategies to handle increased demand in the COVID-19 crisis: a coronavirus EMS support track and a web-based self-triage system. *Prehosp. Emerg. Care* 25 (1): 28–38. https://doi.org/10.1080/10903127.2020.1817212.

6 Whiteside, T., Kane, E., Aljohani, B. et al. (2020). Redesigning emergency department operations amidst a viral pandemic. *Am. J. Emerg. Med.* 38 (7): 1448–1453. https://doi.org/10.1016/j.ajem.2020.04.032.

7 Luo, H., Liu, J., Li, C. et al. (2020). Ultra-rapid delivery of specialty field hospitals to combat COVID-19: lessons learned from the Leishenshan hospital project in Wuhan. *Autom. Constr.* 119: 103345. https://doi.org/10.1016/j.autcon.2020.103345.

8 Wu, Z. and McGoogan, J.M. (2020). Characteristics of and important lessons from the coronavirus disease 2019 (COVID-19) outbreak in China: summary of a report of 72 314 cases from the Chinese Center for Disease Control and Prevention. *JAMA* 323 (13): 1239–1242. https://doi.org/10.1001/jama.2020.2648.

9 Mutambudzi, M., Niedwiedz, C., Macdonald, E.B. et al. (2020). Occupation and risk of severe COVID-19: prospective cohort study of 120 075 UK biobank participants. *Occup. Environ. Med.* 78 (5): 307–314. https://doi.org/10.1136/oemed-2020-106731.

10 Rhee, C., Baker, M.A., and Klompas, M. (2020). The COVID-19 infection control arms race. *Infect. Control Hosp. Epidemiol.* 41 (11): 1323–1325. https://doi.org/10.1017/ice.2020.211.

11 Centers for Disease Control and Prevention (2021). Summary for healthcare facilities: strategies for optimizing the supply of N95 respirators during shortages. CDC. https://www.cdc.gov/coronavirus/2019-ncov/hcp/checklist-n95-strategy.html (accessed 31 August 2021).

12 Myers, L., Balakrishnan, S., Reddy, S., and Gholamrezanezhad, A. (2020). Coronavirus outbreak: is radiology ready? Mass casualty incident planning. *J. Am. Coll. Radiol.* 17 (6): 724–729. https://doi.org/10.1016/j.jacr.2020.03.025.

13 Hasan, Z. and Narasimhan, M. (2020). Preparing for the COVID-19 pandemic: our experience in New York. *Chest* 157 (6): 1420–1422. https://doi.org/10.1016/j.chest.2020.03.027.

14 Ranney, M.L., Griffeth, V., and Jha, A.K. (2020). Critical supply shortages – the need for ventilators and personal protective equipment during the Covid-19 pandemic. *N. Engl. J. Med.* 382 (18): e41. https://doi.org/10.1056/NEJMp2006141.

15 Meng, L., Qiu, H., Wan, L. et al. (2020). Intubation and ventilation amid the COVID-19 outbreak: Wuhan's experience. *Anesthesiology* 132 (6): 1317–1332. https://doi.org/10.1097/aln.0000000000003296.

16 Rubinson, L., Vaughn, F., Nelson, S. et al. (2010). Mechanical ventilators in US acute care hospitals. *Disaster Med. Public Health Prep.* 4 (3): 199–206. https://doi.org/10.1001/dmp.2010.18.

17 Dar, M., Swamy, L., Gavin, D., and Theodore, A. (2021). Mechanical-ventilation supply and options for the COVID-19 pandemic. Leveraging all available

resources for a limited resource in a crisis. *Ann. Am. Thorac. Soc.* 18 (3): 408–416. https://doi.org/10.1513/AnnalsATS.202004-317CME.

18 Monaghesh, E. and Hajizadeh, A. (2020). The role of telehealth during COVID-19 outbreak: a systematic review based on current evidence. *BMC Public Health* 20 (1): 1193. https://doi.org/10.1186/s12889-020-09301-4.

19 Portnoy, J., Waller, M., and Elliott, T. (2020). Telemedicine in the era of COVID-19. *J Allergy Clin Immunol Pract* 8 (5): 1489–1491. https://doi.org/10.1016/j.jaip.2020.03.008.

20 Telehealth impact: physician survey analysis. The MITRE Corporation (2021). https://c19hcc.org/telehealth/physician-survey-analysis (accessed 19 July 2021).

21 ACR Statement on Teleradiology During the COVID-19 Pandemic. American College of Radiology (2021). https://www.acr.org/Advocacy-and-Economics/ACR-Position-Statements/Teleradiology-during-the-COVID-19-Pandemic (accessed 31 August 2021).

22 Kaye, Okeagu, A.D., C.N., Pham, A.D. et al. (2021). Economic impact of COVID-19 pandemic on healthcare facilities and systems: international perspectives. *Best Pract. Res. Clin. Anaesthesiol.* 35: 293–306. https://doi.org/10.1016/j.bpa.2020.11.009.

Index

Coronavirus Disease 2019 (COVID-19): A Clinical Guide, First Edition. Edited by Ali Gholamrezanezhad and Michael P. Dube.
© 2023 John Wiley & Sons Ltd. Published 2023 by John Wiley & Sons Ltd.